Pulmonary
Rehabilitation
Guidelines to Success

Pulmonary Rehabilitation
Guidelines to Success

John E. Hodgkin, MD

Medical Director, Pulmonary Rehabilitation Program
Redbud Community Hospital
Clearlake, California
Medical Director, Smoke-Free Life Program
St. Helena Center for Health
St. Helena, California

Bartolome R. Celli, MD

Chief, Pulmonary and Critical Care Medicine
St. Elizabeth's Medical Center
Professor of Medicine
Tufts University
Boston, Massachusetts

Gerilynn L. Connors, BS, RRT, RCP

Clinical Manager
Pulmonary Rehabilitation
Inova Fairfax Hospital
Falls Church, Virginia

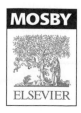

MOSBY

ELSEVIER

11830 Westline Industrial Drive
St. Louis, Missouri 63146

PULMONARY REHABILITATION: GUIDELINES TO
SUCCESS, FOURTH EDITION

ISBN: 978-0-323-04549-0

Notice

Knowledge and best practice in this field are constantly changing. As new research and experience broaden our knowledge, changes in practice, treatment and drug therapy may become
necessary or appropriate. Readers are advised to check the most current information provided
(i) on procedures featured or (ii) by the manufacturer of each product to be administered, to
verify the recommended dose or formula, the method and duration of administration, and
contraindications. It is the responsibility of the practitioner, relying on their own experience and
knowledge of the patient, to make diagnoses, to determine dosages and the best treatment for
each individual patient, and to take all appropriate safety precautions. To the fullest extent of the
law, neither the Publisher nor the Editors assume any liability for any injury and/or damage to
persons or property arising out of or related to any use of the material contained in this book.

The Publisher

Library of Congress Cataloging-in-Publication Data

Pulmonary rehabilitation : guidelines to success/[edited by] John E. Hodgkin,
Bartolome R. Celli, Gerilynn L. Connors. - 4th ed.
     p. ; cm.
   Includes bibliographical references and index.
   ISBN 978-0-323-04549-0 (hardcover : alk. paper)   1. Lungs–Diseases, Obstructive–
Patients–Rehabilitation. 2. Lungs–Diseases–Patients–Rehabilitation. I. Hodgkin, John E.
(John Elliott), 1939- II. Celli, Bartolome R. III. Connors, Gerilynn Long.
   [DNLM: 1. Lung Diseases, Obstructive-rehabilitation. WF 600 P9866 2009]
   RC776.O3P85 2009
   616.2'406-dc22

                                                                          2008017578

Managing Editor: Billi Sharp
Senior Developmental Editor: Mindy Hutchinson
Publishing Services Manager: Patricia Tannian
Project Manager: Claire Kramer
Design Direction: Teresa McBryan

Printed in United States of America

Last digit is the print number: 9   8   7   6   5   4   3   2   1

With much love to my wife, Jeanie; children, Steve, Kathryn, Carolyn, Jon, and Jamie; and 10 grandchildren, Savannah, Sophie, Alex, Summer, Kaia, Kaelyn, Lynae, Hollyn, Joel, and Annie.

JEH

To my wife, Doris, family, and peers who have made my profession possible.

BRC

To my loving husband, Frank: I am only able to pursue my passion for pulmonary rehabilitation because of you. You are the reason I am. You are all my reasons. Thank you! To my daughter, Shannon Mae: You are my greatest love, my Irish Princess, whose laughter and smile inspire me. To my parents, my pulmonary rehabilitation teams, medical directors, colleagues, and patients: Thank you for your perseverance, strength, and dedication.

GLC

Contributors

Àlvar Agusti, MD, FRCP
Certified in Respiratory Medicine
Professor
Health Sciences
Universitat de les Illes Balears
Head of Pulmonary Department
Hospital Unieversitari Son Dureta
Executive Director
International Centre for Advanced Respiratory Medicine
Scientific Director
CIBER Enfermedades Respiratorias
Instituto de Salud Carlos III
Palma Mallorca, Balearic Islands, Spain

James J. Barnett, RRT, RCP
Pulmonary Rehabilitation Coordinator
Community Benefit
Mission Hospital Regional Medical Center
Mission Viejo, California

Joshua O. Benditt, MD
Professor of Medicine
University of Washington
Director of Respiratory Care Services Medicine
University of Washington Medical Center
Seattle, Washington

Louis J. Boitano, MSC, RRT
Respiratory Care
University of Washington Medical Center
Seattle, Washington

Mary Burns, BS, RN
Executive Vice President
Pulmonary Education and Research Foundation
Lomita, California

Andrea K. Busby, BA
Doctoral Teaching Assistant
Psychology
The Ohio State University
Columbus, Ohio

Brian W. Carlin, MD
Assistant Professor of Medicine
Department of Internal Medicine
Drexel University School of Medicine
Philadelphia, Pennsylvania
Division of Pulmonary and Critical Care Medicine
Allegheny General Hospital
Pittsburgh, Pennsylvania

Virginia Carrieri-Kohlman DNSC, RN, FAAN
UCSF School of Nursing Professor
Physiological Nursing
University of California, San Francisco
San Francisco, California

Christopher L. Carroll, MD
Assistant Professor
Pediatrics
University of Connecticut School of Medicine
Farmington, Connecticut
Attending Physician
Pediatric Critical Care
Connecticut Children's Medical Center
Hartford, Connecticut

Rick Carter, PhD, MBA
Professor and Chair
Health, Exercise and Sports Sciences and Physiology
Texas Tech University and Texas Tech Health Sciences
Lubbock, Texas

Bartolome R. Celli, MD
Chief, Pulmonary and Critical Care Medicine
St. Elizabeth's Medical Center
Professor of Medicine
Tufts University
Boston, Massachusetts

Gerilynn L. Connors, BS, RRT, RCP, FAAACVP
Clinical Manager
Pulmonary Rehabilitation
Inova Fairfax Hospital
Falls Church, Virginia

Susan Coppola, MS, OTR/L, BCG
Clinical Associate Professor
Division of Occupational Science
University of North Carolina at Chapel Hill
Chapel Hill, North Carolina

Rebecca Crouch, MS, PT, FAACVPR
Clinical Associate
Doctoral Program of Physical Therapy
Duke University
Coordinator of Pulmonary Rehabilitation–Physical
  Therapy
Duke University Medical Center
Durham, North Carolina

J. Randall Curtis, MD, MPH
Professor of Medicine
University of Washington
Harborview Medical Center
Seattle, Washington

DorAnne Donesky-Cuenco, PhD, RN
Assistant Adjunct Professor
Department of Physiological Nursing
University of California
San Francisco, California

Charles F. Emery, PhD
Professor of Psychology
The Ohio State University
Director, Cardiopulmonary Behavioral Medicine Clinic
Center for Wellness and Prevention
Columbus, Ohio

Steven E. Gay, MD, MS
Clinical Assistant Professor of Internal Medicine
Director, Critical Care Support Services
Director, Bronchoscopy Service
Associate Director, Lung Transplantation Program
University of Michigan Medical Center
Ann Arbor, Michigan

MeiLan K. Han, MD
Critical Care Practitioner, Pulmonologist
University of Michigan Medical Center
Ann Arbor, Michigan

R. Scott Harris, MD
Assistant Professor of Medicine
Harvard Medical School
Boston, Massachusetts
Assistant in Medicine
Pulmonary and Critical Care Unit
Massachusetts General Hospital
Boston, Massachusetts

John E. Heffner, MD
Garnjobst Chair of Graduate Medical Education
Department of Medical Education
Providence Portland Medical Center
Portland, Oregon

Lana R. Hilling, RCP, FAACVPR
Coordinator, Lung Health Care
John Muir Health
Concord, California

Phillip D. Hoberty, EdD, RRT
Associate Professor and Director of Clinical Education
Respiratory Therapy Division, School of Allied Medical
    Professions
The Ohio State University
Columbus, Ohio

Rebecca J. Hoberty, BS, RRT, RCP
Pulmonary Rehabilitation Therapist
Central Ohio Pulmonary Disease, Inc—Meridian
    Healthcare Clinic
Columbus, Ohio

John E. Hodgkin, MD
Medical Director, Pulmonary Rehabilitation Program
Redbud Community Hospital
Clearlake, California
Medical Director, Smoke-Free Life Program
St. Helena Center for Health
St. Helena, California

Michelle J. Huffman, MA
Doctoral Trainee, Cardiopulmonary Behavioral Medicine
    Laboratory
Psychology
The Ohio State University
Columbus, Ohio

Robert M. Kacmarek, PhD RRT
Professor of Anesthesiology
Department of Anesthesiology and Critical Care
Director, Respiratory Care
Respiratory Care Services
Massachusetts General Hospital
Boston, Massachusetts

Robert M. Kaplan, PhD
Professor and Chair
Health Services
University of California, Los Angeles
Los Angeles, California

Bruce P. Krieger, MD
Professor of Medicine
Pulmonary and Critical Care
University of Miami
Miami, Florida
Associate Medical Director
Critical Care Center
Memorial Hospital
Jacksonville, Florida

James P. Lamberti, MD
Assistant Clinical Professor
Medicine
Georgetown University
Washington, District of Columbia
Medical Director
Respiratory Care Services
Inova Fairfax Hospital
Falls Church, Virginia

Donald A. Mahler, MD
Professor of Medicine
Department of Medicine
Dartmouth Medical School
Hanover, New Hampshire
Director of Pulmonary Function and Cardiopulmonary
    Exercise Laboratories
Section of Pulmonary and Critical Care Medicine
Dartmouth Hitchcock Medical Center
Lebanon, New Hampshire

Thomas P. Malinowski, RRT, FAARC
Director of Respiratory Care Services
Inova Fairfax Hospital
Falls Church, Virginia

Fernando J. Martinez, MD, MS
Professor of Internal Medicine
Division of Pulmonary and Critical Care Medicine
University of Michigan
Ann Arbor, Michigan

Susan L. McInturff, RRT, RCP
Continuous Positive Airway Pressure Coordinator
Sleep Disorder Center
Harrison Medical Center
Bremerton, Washington

James A. Murray, DO
Instructor of Medicine
Department of Medicine
Dartmouth Medical School
Senior Pulmonary and Critical Care Fellow
Section of Pulmonary and Critical Care Medicine
Dartmouth Hitchcock Medical Center
Lebanon, New Hampshire

Steven D. Nathan, MD
Medical Director
Lung Transplant Program
Inova Fairfax Hospital
Falls Church, Virginia

Linda Nici, MD
Clinical Associate Professor of Medicine
Director, Pulmonary Rehabilitation Program
Pulmonary and Critical Care Medicine
Providence VAMC and Brown University
Providence, Rhode Island

James A. Peters, MD, DrPH, MPH, RD, RRT, LDN, FACPM
Nutrition & Lifestyle Medical Clinic
St. Helena, California

Andrew L. Ries, MD, MPH
Associate Dean for Academic Affairs
Professor of Medicine and Family and Preventive
    Medicine
University of California, San Diego
Medical Director
Pulmonary Rehabilitation Program
San Diego Medical Center
San Diego, California

Carolyn L. Rochester, MD
Associate Professor of Medicine
Section of Pulmonary and Critical Care
Yale University School of Medicine
New Haven, Connecticut
Medical Director, Pulmonary Rehabilitation
Section of Pulmonary and Critical Care
VA Connecticut Healthcare System
West Haven, Connecticut

Daniel O. Rodenstein, MD
Head, Pneumology
Cliniques Universitaires Saint-Luc
Université Catholique de Louvain
Brussels, Belguim

David P.L. Sachs, MD
Director
Palo Alto Center for Pulmonary Disease Prevention
Palo Alto, California
Clinical Associate Professor
Division of Pulmonary Medicine and Critical Care
    Medicine
Stanford Hospital and Clinics
Stanford, California

Ernest Sala, MD
Hospital Universitario Son Dureta
Palma Mallorca, Balearic Islands, Spain

Annemie Schols, MWJ, PhD
Professor
Respiratory Diseases, University Hospital Maastricht
NUTRIM School for Nutrition, Toxicology, and
    Metabolism
Maastricht, The Netherlands

Paul A. Selecky, MD, FACP, FCCP
Clinical Professor of Medicine
University of California, Los Angeles
Los Angeles, California
Medical Director
Pulmonary Department
Hoag Hospital
Newport Beach, California

Georgianna G. Sergakis, MS, RRT
Assistant Professor of Clinical Allied Medicine
School of Allied Medical Professions
The Ohio State University
Columbus, Ohio

Shelley Shapiro, MD, PhD, FACC, FCCP
Clinical Professor of Medicine
Cardiology and Pulmonary Critical Care Division
David Geffen UCLA School of Medicine
Los Angeles, California
Director of Pulmonary Hypertension
VA Greater Los Angeles Healthcare System
Clinical Professor of Medicine
Pulmonary Critical Care
UCLA Medical Center
Los Angeles, California

Oksana A. Shlobin, MD
Transplant Pulmonologist
Advanced Lung Disease and Transplant Program
Inova Fairfax Hospital
Falls Church, Virginia

Vijay Subramaniam, MD
Division of Pulmonary and Critical Care Medicine
Allegheny General Hospital
Pittsburgh, Pennsylvania

Cheryl D. Thomas-Peters, BS, RD, LDN
Nutrition & Lifestyle Medical Clinic
St. Helena, California

Brian L. Tiep, MD
Medical Director and Program Designer
Respiratory Disease Management Institute
Pomona, California
Director of Pulmonary Rehabilitation
City of Hope National Medical Center
Duarte, California
Associate Professor of Family Medicine
Western University of Health Sciences
Pomona, California

Glenna L. Traiger, MSN, RN
Cardiovascular Clinical Nurse Specialist
Pulmonary Arterial Hypertension Program
Greater Los Angeles VA Healthcare System/UCLA
Los Angeles, California

Wendy Wood, PhD, OTR/L FAOTA
Professor and Department Head
Department of Occupational Therapy
Colorado State University
Fort Collins, Colorado

Richard ZuWallack, MD
Professor of Medicine
University of Connecticut School of Medicine
Farmington, Connecticut
Associate Chief, Pulmonary and Critical Care
St. Francis Hospital and Medical Center
Hartford, Connecticut

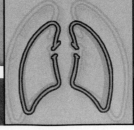

Reviewers

Shane Keene, MBA, MS, RRT-NPS, CPPT
Director of Clinical Education
East Tennessee State University
Consultant, Board of Respiratory Care
Nashville, Tennessee

Trina Limberg, BS, RRT
Pulmonary Rehabilitation Department Director
University of California San Diego
San Diego, California

June Schulz, RRT, FAACVPR
Pulmonary Rehabilitation Coordinator
Sioux Valley Hospital
Sioux Falls, South Dakota

Ken Wyka, MS, RRT, FAARC
Respiratory Clinical Specialist
Home Therapy Equipment
Clifton, New York

Foreword

Pulmonary rehabilitation has now become the standard of care for patients with chronic obstructive pulmonary disease (COPD) or related disorders with physiologic impairment and impaired quality of life. Advances in pulmonary rehabilitation have improved dramatically during the last 40 years. Forty years has elapsed since the realization that a comprehensive program of education, physical reconditioning, breathing retraining, behavioral and social adjustments, and ambulatory oxygen in selected patients can improve both the length and quality of life. New pharmacologic agents improve airflow, reduce exacerbations, and may slow the rate of decline of lung function. Many of these advances have been led by the pioneering work of the authors of this book.

COPD is now recognized as a systemic disease with multiple manifestations and an often insidious course. Early identification should be the goal, and this is advocated by the nationwide movement known as the National Lung Health Education Program. Office spirometry should become widespread so that occult disease can be detected and smoking cessation encouraged. The discovery of such disease and a patient's discontinuance of smoking are fundamental steps in stemming the progress of a disease that covers two or more decades before becoming disabling.

Pulmonary rehabilitation was the standard by which lung volume reduction surgery was evaluated, assessed, and found equivalent in measured outcomes in all but a subset of patients with poor exercise tolerance and hyperinflation in the upper lungs. The remaining challenge is appropriate reimbursement and promotion of the concepts and principles that have been championed by John Hodgkin and his colleagues over many years. The future appears bright for millions of Americans—both those who have received a diagnosis and those who have not—with progressive respiratory impairment because we can find COPD by means of simple spirometry and treat it effectively in all stages of disease.

Thomas L. Petty, MD
Professor of Medicine
University of Colorado Health Science Center
President, Snowdrift Pulmonary Conference

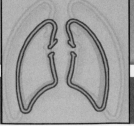

The act of breathing is synonymous to life itself. The first cry of a newborn is associated with health, whereas at the other end, death is characterized by the inability to breathe spontaneously. It is not surprising that the specialty dedicated to the physiology, pathology, and treatment of respiratory disease has achieved ever-increasing importance in the curriculum of different health care practitioners. The progressive elimination of many acute problems as major causes of death and the cornering of tuberculosis and other infectious diseases, at least in the developed world, have led to the emergence of several chronic diseases as the most important causes of morbidity and mortality today and in the near future.

Many patients affected by acute injury will have substantial deconditioning after recovery, and with many chronic diseases, most patients have important limitations in their capacity to perform activities of daily living. By their nature, diseases such as chronic obstructive pulmonary disease (COPD), cystic fibrosis, uncontrolled asthma, deformities of the rib cage, neuromuscular degenerative maladies, and respiratory insufficiency of many types affect the act of breathing and as such lead to dyspnea and limitations to perform physical activities. Frequently, patients with such diseases limit their activities to avoid the perception of dyspnea and adopt a more sedentary lifestyle; the result is worse deconditioning. It is in this context that primary and secondary rehabilitation plays a crucial role. The recognition that this branch of our therapeutic armamentarium has importance in patients with chronic respiratory illnesses led to the development of the first edition of this book in 1984, which was entirely devoted to dissecting the nature of pulmonary rehabilitation and its scope. Indeed, the recent publications of evidence-based guidelines on pulmonary rehabilitation reaffirm the value of the concepts discussed in the first and subsequent editions of the book.

Pulmonary Rehabilitation: Guidelines to Success is the only book entirely devoted to pulmonary rehabilitation that has evolved as the field has expanded. Whereas the field was originally based primarily on anecdotal experience, it is now grounded on evidence, a fact that is reflected in each of the rewritten chapters to present such evidence. Each edition has reflected the changes in the field at the moment of its publication. The recent expansion of sleep-related disorders, the reality of changes in the pharmacotherapeutic treatment of COPD, and the application of the concepts of rehabilitation to diseases different from the obstructive diseases are now given prominence in this edition. This book is not just a repository of information for the academician but, rather, a handbook that should prove useful for the multidisciplinary members of the teams that define the nature of rehabilitation. In its pages, all professionals interested in the field should find information that is useful to them and for the patients for whom they care.

We are grateful that, over the more than two decades since the first edition of this book appeared, pulmonary rehabilitation has moved from being a controversial therapeutic intervention to becoming the standard of care for patients with COPD, as well as being recommended for individuals with many other chronic respiratory conditions.

We express our appreciation to Mindy Hutchinson, Senior Developmental Editor, and Claire Kramer, Project Manager, for their assistance with the production of the book.

John E. Hodgkin, MD
Bartolome R. Celli, MD
Gerilynn L. Connors, BS, RRT, RCP

Contents

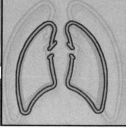

I Historical Perspective of Pulmonary Rehabilitation, 1

1 Pulmonary Rehabilitation: History and Definition, 1
   JOHN E. HODGKIN

II Basic Concepts of Pulmonary Rehabilitation, 9

2 Selection and Assessment of the Patient with Chronic Respiratory Disease for Pulmonary Rehabilitation, 9
   LINDA NICI

3 Pathophysiology of Chronic Obstructive Pulmonary Disease, 18
   BARTOLOME R. CELLI

4 Systemic Effects of Chronic Obstructive Pulmonary Disease, 30
   ERNEST SALA, ÀLVAR AGUSTI

5 Dyspnea: Assessment and Management, 39
   VIRGINIA CARRIERI-KOHLMAN, DORANNE DONESKY-CUENCO

6 Education in Pulmonary Rehabilitation, 74
   PHILLIP D. HOBERTY, GEORGIANNA G. SERGAKIS, REBECCA J. HOBERTY

III Therapeutic Intervention in Pulmonary Rehabilitation, 83

7 Pharmacologic Therapy for Chronic Obstructive Pulmonary Disease, 83
   BARTOLOME R. CELLI

8 Aerosol Therapy, 95
   ROBERT M. KACMAREK, R. SCOTT HARRIS

9 Therapeutic Oxygen, 115
   BRIAN L. TIEP, RICK CARTER

10 Exercise in the Rehabilitation of Patients with Respiratory Disease, 129
   BARTOLOME R. CELLI

11 Inspiratory Muscle Training, 143
   JAMES A. MURRAY, DONALD A. MAHLER

12 Physical and Respiratory Therapy for the Medical and Surgical Patient, 154
   REBECCA CROUCH

13 Occupational Therapy to Promote Function and Health-Related Quality of Life, 180
   SUSAN COPPOLA, WENDY WOOD

14 Nutritional Assessment and Support, 209
   ANNEMIE SCHOLS

15 Complementary Alternative Medicine for Patients with Chronic Lung Disease, 220
   JAMES A. PETERS, CHERYL D. THOMAS-PETERS

16 Medical Management of Tobacco Dependence: Concepts and Treatment Objectives, 234
   DAVID P.L. SACHS

17 Behavioral Medicine in Pulmonary Rehabilitation: Psychological, Cognitive, and Social Factors, 269
   CHARLES F. EMERY, MICHELLE J. HUFFMAN, ANDREA K. BUSBY

18   *Sexuality in the Patient with Pulmonary Disease*, 285
PAUL A. SELECKY

19   *Preventive Strategies for the Patient with Chronic Lung Disease*, 303
BRIAN W. CARLIN, VIJAY SUBRAMANIAM

IV   Special Considerations in Pulmonary Rehabilitation, 316

20   *Adherence in the Patient with Pulmonary Disease*, 316
ROBERT M. KAPLAN, ANDREW L. RIES

21   *Outcome Assessment*, 330
RICHARD ZuWALLACK

22   *Home Mechanical Ventilation*, 351
JOSHUA O. BENDITT, LOUIS J. BOITANO

23   *Pulmonary Rehabilitation and Lung Transplantation*, 361
STEVEN D. NATHAN, OKSANA A. SHLOBIN

24   *Pulmonary Rehabilitation and Lung Volume Reduction Surgery*, 385
MeiLan K. HAN, STEVEN E. GAY, FERNANDO J. MARTINEZ

25   *Ethical and End-of-Life Issues for the Care of Patients with Advanced Lung Disease*, 393
JOHN E. HEFFNER, J. RANDALL CURTIS

26   *Social and Recreational Support of the Patient with Pulmonary Disease*, 406
JAMES J. BARNETT, MARY BURNS

27   *Sleep Disorders in Patients with Pulmonary Disease*, 417
DANIEL O. RODENSTEIN

28   *Role of Respiratory Home Care*, 432
SUSAN L. MCINTURFF

29   *Travel for the Patient with Respiratory Disease*, 454
BRUCE P. KRIEGER

30   *Management of and Reimbursement for Pulmonary Rehabilitation*, 467
GERILYNN L. CONNORS, THOMAS P. MALINOWSKI, LANA R. HILLING, JAMES P. LAMBERTI

V   Pulmonary Rehabilitation for Miscellaneous Disorders, 497

31   *Pulmonary Rehabilitation for Patients with Disorders Other Than Chronic Obstructive Pulmonary Disease*, 497
CAROLYN L. ROCHESTER

32   *Exercise and Pulmonary Hypertension*, 518
SHELLEY SHAPIRO, GLENNA L. TRAIGER

33   *Rehabilitation for the Pediatric Patient with Pulmonary Disease*, 529
CHRISTOPHER L. CARROLL

VI   Benefits and the Future of Pulmonary Rehabilitation, 543

34   *Benefits and the Future of Pulmonary Rehabilitation*, 543
JOHN E. HODGKIN

Index, 562

Chapter 1

Pulmonary Rehabilitation: History and Definition

John E. Hodgkin

CHAPTER OUTLINE

Impact of Chronic Pulmonary Disease
Definition of Pulmonary Rehabilitation

Candidates for Pulmonary Rehabilitation
Conclusion

PROFESSIONAL SKILLS

On completion of this chapter, the reader will be able to do
the following:
* Review the development of pulmonary rehabilitation
* State the prevalence of asthma and chronic obstructive pulmonary disease (COPD)
* Discuss morbidity and mortality information for asthma and COPD
* Discuss the economic consequences of chronic lung disease
* Define pulmonary rehabilitation
* List disease states that should be considered as appropriate for pulmonary rehabilitation

Although rehabilitation has been practiced for several decades, its application to patients with pulmonary disorders is relatively recent. In 1942, the American Medical Association Council on Rehabilitation defined *rehabilitation* as the restoration of the individual to the fullest medical, mental, emotional, social, and vocational potential of which he or she is capable.

Lavoisier, a French scientist, discussed the concept of oxygen and carbon dioxide, in association with lung function, back in 1775 to 1794. As a result of this enlightenment, Thomas Beddoes established the Pneumatic Institute at Bristol for the treatment of patients with heart disease and asthma.[1,2] Laënnec described the concept of rehabilitation in 1821 in "Treatise on the Diseases of the Chest and Mediate Auscultation." Charles L. Denison, who had pulmonary tuberculosis, was an early advocate for exercise. In 1880, Dr. Denison authored a book entitled *Rocky Mountain Health Resorts*, an analytic study of chronic pulmonary disease, in which he recommended exercise for those with tuberculosis.[1] He also authored a monograph, in 1895, entitled Exercise for Pulmonary Invalids.

The pioneer for treatment of chronic pulmonary disease in the 20th century was Alvan L. Barach. In 1922, he wrote a landmark article on the

1

therapeutic use of oxygen.[3] Barach subsequently authored many other articles and monographs promoting inhalation therapy and therapeutic techniques based on physiologic principles.[4-7] Of interest is the fact that Dr. Barach was a cigarette smoker, as were many physicians in the early 1940s and 1950s. It was not until after the Surgeon General's report in 1964 that antismoking programs became accepted.

In the 1950s, William F. Miller studied and reported on techniques that became part of pulmonary rehabilitation programs.[8,9] By the 1960s, the term *rehabilitation* was beginning to be used to describe comprehensive care programs for individuals with chronic obstructive pulmonary disease (COPD).[10,11] Other proponents for pulmonary rehabilitation in the 1960s included Thomas L. Petty and Louise M. Nett,[12,13] Al Haas,[14] and Oscar J. Balchum.[15]

By the 1970s, numerous reports began to appear regarding the effectiveness of pulmonary rehabilitation modalities from a wide variety of investigators: H. Bass,[16] Phil Kimbel,[17] D. P. Agle,[18] George Burton,[19] John E. Hodgkin,[20] Ken Moser and Carol Archibald,[21] Reuben Cherniack and M. M. Lertzman,[22] and Irving Kass.[23,24]

In the mid-1970s, a study by the Human Interaction Research Institute in Los Angeles, California, showed that many physicians in the United States either were not aware of or were not using various facets of care for patients with pulmonary disease that had been shown previously to be useful.[25] As part of this Human Interaction Research Institute project, which was funded by the National Science Foundation, a state-of-the-art paper on the diagnosis and treatment of COPD was developed and published in the *Journal of the American Medical Association* in 1975.[20] Hundreds of physicians and allied health personnel around the country were invited to critique this paper, after which the article was modified, expanded, and published in 1979 as a book by the American College of Chest Physicians.[26] It was the goal of those involved in this project to disseminate widely to physicians and allied health professionals those principles of care that had been demonstrated to produce both subjective and objective benefits in respiratory patients. Although this goal, in large part, has been realized, many primary care physicians still seem unaware of the benefits of pulmonary rehabilitation.

Since the 1980s, pulmonary rehabilitation programs have rapidly gained in acceptance and number. The decade began with the report of a 10-year follow-up study of a comprehensive program, that is, pulmonary rehabilitation for patients with COPD.[27] Dudley and colleagues[28] reported on the importance of assessing and dealing with psychological issues as part of a rehabilitation program. In 1981, the American Thoracic Society (ATS) issued an official position statement supporting pulmonary rehabilitation for patients with chronic lung disease.[29] The committee, chaired by Dr. John Hodgkin, developed a statement that not only defined pulmonary rehabilitation, but also described the essential components of such a program. In 1984, the first edition of *Pulmonary Rehabilitation: Guidelines to Success* was published,[30] and the structure for pulmonary rehabilitation programs was created.[2] Multiple professional organizations, worldwide, have contributed to the promotion and acceptance of pulmonary rehabilitation, including the American Association for Respiratory Care, American Association of Cardiovascular and Pulmonary Rehabilitation, American College of Chest Physicians, American Thoracic Society, European Respiratory Society, and National Association for Medical Direction of Respiratory Care.

IMPACT OF CHRONIC PULMONARY DISEASE

The term *chronic obstructive pulmonary disease* (COPD) is best reserved for those individuals with chronic bronchitis or emphysema who have obstruction to airflow on a spirogram. It should be recognized that those with COPD may also have a component of bronchial asthma.

It is estimated that bronchial asthma has been diagnosed in 24.3 million individuals in the United States, chronic bronchitis in 9.4 million, and emphysema in 4.1 million.[31] Most individuals with emphysema also have chronic bronchitis, whereas most people with chronic bronchitis do not have concomitant emphysema. Although COPD has been diagnosed in approximately 12 million people in the United States, it is estimated that there are an additional 12 million who also have COPD but remain undiagnosed.[32,33] This compares with an estimated 51.5 million with hypertension, 14 million with coronary heart disease, 5.6 million with stroke,[31] and 5.2 million with congestive heart failure.[32] Whereas emphysema is

TABLE 1-1 Prevalence Data for Obstructive Airway Disease in the United States

Disease	NUMBER (IN MILLIONS)	
	Males	Females
Bronchial asthma	10.1	14.2
Chronic bronchitis	2.9	6.5
Emphysema	2.5	1.6

From Pleis JR, Lethbridge-Çejku M: Summary health statistics for U.S. adults: National Health Interview Survey, 2006. National Center for Health Statistics, Vital Health Stat 10(235), 2007. Available at http://www.cdc.gov/nchs/data/series/sr_10/ sr10_233.pdf. Retrieved February 14, 2008.

TABLE 1-2 Leading Chronic Conditions Causing Limitations of Activity, U.S., 2005

Chronic Condition	Persons (in millions)
Arthritis	6.5
Back/neck conditions	6.1
Heart condition	4.5
Diabetes	3.2
Mental condition	3.2
Hypertension	3.2
Musculoskeletal condition	2.9
Lung condition	2.7
Bone or joint injury	2.7
Nervous condition	2.6
Vision condition	2.1
Stroke	1.6
Cancer	1.4

From National Heart, Lung, and Blood Institute, National Institutes of Health, Public Health Service, U.S. Department of Health and Human Services: Morbidity & mortality: 2007 chart book on cardiovascular, lung, and blood diseases. June 2007. Available at http://www.nhlbi.nih.gov/resources/docs/07-chtbk.pdf. Retrieved February 2008.

more common in males, chronic bronchitis and asthma are more common in females (Table 1-1). Bronchial asthma, chronic bronchitis, and emphysema are among the leading chronic conditions in the United States (Table 1-2).

In 2004, COPD was the first-listed discharge diagnosis for 636,000 hospitalizations and in 2003 for 15,401,000 physician office visits.[32] This compares with asthma as the first-listed discharge diagnosis for 497,000 hospitalizations and 12,855,000 physician office visits.[32]

The death rate from coronary heart disease increased 10% from 1950 to its peak in 1968; by 2004, it was 66% lower than it was in 1950. Stroke mortality, on the other hand, declined for most of those years and by 2004 was 72% lower than it was in 1950. Death rates for lung cancer and COPD increased during the same period (Figure 1-1).[32] Asthma mortality declined between 1950 and 1978 but then increased until the mid-1990s and subsequently declined again.[32] COPD and allied conditions constitute the fourth leading cause of death in the United States (Table 1-3).[32]

Although cardiovascular disease is the leading contributor to the economic burden of health care in the United States, chronic lung disease also is a significant factor (Table 1-4).[32] Approximately 85% of patients with COPD have this problem as a direct result of smoking cigarettes, with the remainder due to such factors as previous serious lung infections, environmental and occupational exposures, or genetic abnormalities such as α_1-antitrypsin deficiency.[34] Although progress has been made in reducing the number of persons who smoke in the United States, efforts to help individuals avoid or cease smoking must be intensified. In 1965, 40% of individuals (52% of men and 34% of women) aged 18 years and older in the United States smoked cigarettes

compared with approximately 21% (23% of men and 18% of women) in 2006.[31] The decline began in the late 1960s for men and a decade later for women, whose rate of decrease has been much more gradual. Between 2003 and 2005, the percentage of high school students who reported smoking cigarettes remained stable at 23%, after declining from 36% in 1997.[35] Despite this decline in smoking in the United States, it is estimated that approximately 440,000 individuals in the United States die each year as a result of smoking cigarettes.[31]

DEFINITION OF PULMONARY REHABILITATION

Attempts have been made to define pulmonary rehabilitation. In 1974, a committee of the American College of Chest Physicians developed the following definition[36]:

> Pulmonary rehabilitation may be defined as an art of medical practice wherein an individually tailored, multi-disciplinary program is formulated which through accurate diagnosis, therapy, emotional support, and education, stabilizes or reverses both the physio- and psychopathology of pulmonary disease and attempts to return the patient to the highest possible functional capacity allowed by his pulmonary handicap and overall life situation.

In the late 1970s, pulmonary rehabilitation programs began to spring up around the country.

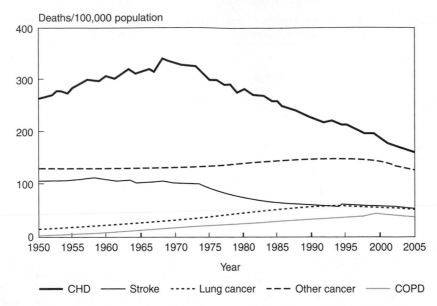

FIGURE 1-1 Crude death rates for selected causes, United States, 1950-2005. CHD, coronary heart disease; COPD, chronic obstructive pulmonary disease.

TABLE 1-3 Leading Causes of Death, U.S., 2004	
Cause of Death	**Number**
Total deaths	2,397,615
Heart disease*	652,486
Cancer	553,888
Cerebrovascular disease (stroke)	150,074
COPD and allied conditions†	121,987
Accidents	112,012
Diabetes	73,138
Alzheimer's disease	65,965
Influenza and pneumonia	59,664
Nephritis	42,480
Septicemia	33,373
All other causes of death	532,648

*Includes 451,326 deaths from coronary heart disease.
†Chronic lower respiratory diseases (includes asthma).
COPD, Chronic obstructive pulmonary disease.
From National Heart, Lung, and Blood Institute, National Institutes of Health, Public Health Service, U.S. Department of Health and Human Services: Morbidity & mortality: 2007 chart book on cardiovascular, lung, and blood diseases. June 2007. Available at http://www.nhlbi.nih.gov/resources/docs/07-chtbk.pdf. Retrieved February 14, 2008.

Because of a growing recognition that the term *pulmonary rehabilitation* was defined differently by many pulmonary specialists, in 1979 an ad hoc committee of the ATS Assembly on Clinical Problems was delegated the responsibility of defining pulmonary rehabilitation.

The ATS statement[29] listed the two principal objectives of pulmonary rehabilitation as (1) to control and alleviate as much as possible the symptoms and pathophysiologic complications of respiratory impairment and (2) to teach the patient how to achieve optimal capability for carrying out his or her activities of daily living. This 1981 statement also stated that:

> In the broadest sense, pulmonary rehabilitation means providing good, comprehensive respiratory care for patients with pulmonary disease.

A logical sequence for an individual participating in a pulmonary rehabilitation program is as follows[23]: (1) select the individual, (2) evaluate the individual to determine his or her needs, (3) develop goals, (4) determine components of care, (5) assess the individual's progress, and (6) arrange for long-term follow-up.

Two principles from the 1981 ATS statement[29] are worth repeating:

1. A physician knowledgeable about respiratory disease should perform the initial complete examination and assist in outlining a proper regimen of treatment.
2. The specific provider for the program's services may vary from program to program. A large, multidisciplinary team is appropriate for settings where large numbers of patients are referred and for teaching or research purposes. However, in other settings, it may be possible to provide similar services with fewer individuals if they are highly qualified and specially trained in evaluation and management of the patient.

In 1987, the ATS published a statement dealing with the standards for the diagnosis and care

TABLE 1-4 Economic Cost of Cardiovascular, Lung, and Blood Diseases, U.S., 2007

Disease	Dollars (Billions)			
	Total	Direct	Morbidity	Mortality
Total CVD	431.8	283.2	36.3	112.3
Heart disease	277.1	164.9	22.3	89.9
Coronary	151.6	83.6	9.8	58.2
Congestive heart failure	33.2	30.2	*	3.0
Stroke	62.7	41.6	6.5	14.6
Hypertensive disease	66.4	49.3	7.8	9.3
Selected lung diseases	153.6	94.8	27.9	30.9
COPD	42.6	26.7	8.0	7.9
Asthma	19.7	14.7	3.1	1.9
Selected blood diseases	13.8	10.2	0.7	2.9
Anemias	8.5	6.9	0.6	1

*No estimate available.
COPD, *Chronic obstructive pulmonary disease*, CVD, *cardiovascular disease*.
From National Heart, Lung, and Blood Institute, National Institutes of Health, Public Health Service, U.S. Department of Health and Human Services: *Morbidity & mortality: 2007 chart book on cardiovascular, lung, and blood diseases.* June 2007. Available at http://www.nhlbi.nih.gov/resources/docs/07-chtbk.pdf. Retrieved February 2008.

of patients with COPD and asthma.[37] Many of the components of care used in pulmonary rehabilitation programs are discussed in this statement.

In 1994, the National Heart, Lung, and Blood Institute published the results of a consensus conference on pulmonary rehabilitation.[38] The individuals participating in this conference developed the following definition of pulmonary rehabilitation:

> A multidimensional continuum of services directed to persons with pulmonary disease and their families, usually by an interdisciplinary team of specialists, with a goal of achieving and maintaining the individual's maximum level of independence and functioning in the community.

In 1995, an update on the diagnosis and care of patients with COPD was published by the ATS.[39] This new statement included pulmonary rehabilitation in the algorithm of care for patients with COPD.

The ATS published a new official statement on pulmonary rehabilitation in 1999.[40] The following definition was developed and included in this statement:

> Pulmonary rehabilitation is a multidisciplinary program of care for patients with chronic respiratory impairment that is individually tailored and designed to optimize physical and social performance and autonomy.

In 2006, the ATS and European Respiratory Society published a joint statement on pulmonary rehabilitation.[41] The document states that "The impressive rise in interest in pulmonary rehabilitation is likely related to both a substantial increase in the number of patients being referred as well as the establishment of its scientific basis by the use of well-designed clinical trials that use valid, reproducible, and interpretable outcome measures." The statement, based on "our understanding of the science and process of pulmonary rehabilitation," offers the following definition:

> Pulmonary rehabilitation is an evidence-based, multidisciplinary, and comprehensive intervention for patients with chronic respiratory diseases who are symptomatic and often have decreased daily life activities. Integrated into the individualized treatment of the patient, pulmonary rehabilitation is designed to reduce symptoms, optimize functional status, increase participation, and reduce health care costs through stabilizing or reversing systemic manifestations of the disease.

CANDIDATES FOR PULMONARY REHABILITATION

Pulmonary rehabilitation is most commonly used for individuals with COPD; however, patients with other diseases leading to chronic respiratory impairment can also benefit from this process. The following quotations comment on when pulmonary rehabilitation should be considered:

> *Any patient whose breathlessness from COPD has resulted in functional limitations that affect his or her quality of life should be considered a candidate for pulmonary rehabilitation.*[42]

Historically, pulmonary rehabilitation has been used primarily for patients with COPD. However, it has also been applied successfully to patients with other chronic lung conditions such as interstitial diseases, cystic fibrosis, bronchiectasis, thoracic cage abnormalities, and neuromuscular disorders as well as part of the evaluation, preparation for, and recovery from surgical interventions such as lung transplantation and lung volume reduction surgery. Pulmonary rehabilitation is appropriate for any patient with stable disease of the respiratory system and disabling symptoms.[43]

Pulmonary rehabilitation is indicated for patients with chronic respiratory impairment who, despite optimal medical management, are dyspneic, have reduced exercise tolerance, or experience a restriction in activities. It should be emphasized that symptoms, disability, and handicap, not the severity of physiologic impairment of the lungs, dictate the need for pulmonary rehabilitation. Thus, no specific pulmonary function criteria exist to indicate the need for pulmonary rehabilitation.[40]

The timing of pulmonary rehabilitation depends on the clinical status of the individual patient and should no longer be viewed as a "last ditch" effort for patients with severe respiratory impairment. Rather, it should be an integral part of the clinical management of all patients with chronic respiratory disease, addressing their functional and/or psychologic deficits.[41]

Pulmonary rehabilitation should be considered for COPD patients with an FEV_1/FVC less than 0.7 and FEV_1 less than 80% of predicted.[44]

It should be noted that there are inconsistencies among the statements quoted, representing the diversity of opinions regarding this issue. In the United States, Medicare Fiscal Intermediaries (to be replaced by Medicare Administrative Contractors) for the various states have various pulmonary function criteria for admission to a pulmonary rehabilitation program, which is confusing and frustrating.

CONCLUSION

Pulmonary rehabilitation programs may vary in size and configuration. All allied health professions may not be represented on every team in every hospital; however, all the services needed must be available and provided by someone from the appropriate discipline. Although every patient with chronic lung disease does not need all these services, many patients need them all.

Although most patients participating in pulmonary rehabilitation programs have COPD, these programs may also be helpful for patients with other types of pulmonary dysfunction. Fortunately, pulmonary rehabilitation is more widely accepted now than in 1984, when the first edition of this book was published.[30] The remainder of this book is devoted to describing the components of pulmonary rehabilitation and providing guidelines that can lead to the successful rehabilitation of patients with pulmonary impairment.

References

1. Berra K: Cardiac and pulmonary rehabilitation: historical perspectives and future needs, J Cardiopulm Rehabil 11:8-15, 1991.
2. Wilson PK, Williams MA, Humphrey R, Hodgkin JE, Lui K et al: Contemporary cardiovascular & pulmonary rehabilitation: AACVPR—the first 20 years, American Association of Cardiovascular and Pulmonary Rehabilitation, 2005, Tampa, Faircount.
3. Barach AL: The therapeutic use of oxygen, JAMA 79:693-698, 1922.
4. Barach AL: Physiological methods in diagnosis and treatment of asthma and emphysema, Ann Intern Med 12:454-481, 1938.
5. Barach AL: Principles and practice of inhalation therapy, Philadelphia, 1944, JB Lippincott.
6. Barach AL: Physiological therapy in respiratory diseases, Philadelphia, 1948, JB Lippincott.
7. Barach AL: Breathing exercises in pulmonary emphysema and allied chronic respiratory diseases, Arch Phys Med Rehabil 36:379-390, 1955.
8. Miller WF: A physiologic evaluation of the effects of diaphragmatic breathing training in patients with chronic pulmonary emphysema, Am J Med 17:471-477, 1954.
9. Miller WF: Physical therapeutic measures in the treatment of chronic bronchopulmonary disorders: methods for breathing training, Am J Med 24:929-940, 1958.
10. Miller WF, Taylor HD, Jasper L: Exercise training in the rehabilitation of patients with obstructive lung disease: the role of oxygen breathing, South Med J 55:1216, 1962.
11. Miller WF, Taylor HD, Pierce AK: Rehabilitation of the disabled patient with chronic bronchitis and pulmonary emphysema, Am J Public Health 53:18-24, 1963.
12. U.S. Public Health Service: Principles of management of chronic obstructive lung diseases. In Petty TL, editor: Proceedings of the Eighth Aspen Emphysema Conference, Washington, DC, 1966 (USPHS publication No. 1457), Rockville, Md, 1966, U.S. Department of Health, Education, and Welfare.
13. Petty TL, Nett LM, Finigan MM et al: A comprehensive care program for chronic airway obstruction: methods and preliminary evaluation of symptomatic and functional improvement, Ann Intern Med 70:1109-1120, 1969.
14. Haas A, Cardon H: Rehabilitation in chronic obstructive pulmonary disease: a five-year study of 252 male patients, Med Clin North Am 53:593-606, 1969.
15. Balchum OJ: Rehabilitation in chronic obstructive pulmonary disease, Arch Environ Health 16:614, 1968.
16. Bass H, Whitcomb JF, Forman R: Exercise training: therapy for patients with chronic obstructive pulmonary disease, Chest 57:116-121, 1970.

17. Kimbel P, Kaplan AS, Alkalay I, Lester D: An in-hospital program for rehabilitation of patients with chronic obstructive pulmonary disease, Chest 60(suppl):6S-10S, 1971.

18. Agle DP, Baum GL, Chester EH et al: Multidiscipline treatment of chronic pulmonary insufficiency. I. psychologic aspects of rehabilitation, Psychosom Med 35:41-49, 1973.

19. Burton GG, Gee G, Hodgkin JE et al: Respiratory care warrants studies for cost-effectiveness, Hospitals 49:61-71, 1975.

20. Hodgkin JE, Balchum OJ, Kass I, Glaser EM et al: Chronic obstructive airway diseases: current concepts in diagnosis and comprehensive care, JAMA 232:1243-1260, 1975.

21. Modrak M, Moser KM, Archibald C et al: Better living and breathing: a manual for patients, St. Louis, CV Mosby, 1975.

22. Lertzman MM, Cherniak RM: Rehabilitation of patients with chronic obstructive pulmonary disease, Am Rev Respir Dis 114:1145-1165, 1976.

23. Kass I, Dyksterhuis JE: A program to identify the factors involved in the rehabilitation of patients with chronic obstructive pulmonary diseases: a multidisciplinary study of 140 patients [Nebraska COPD Rehabilitation Project]. Final report, Social and Rehabilitation Service, U.S. Department of Health, Education, and Welfare, Project RD-2517-M, Washington, DC, December 1971.

24. Daughton DM, Fix AJ, Kass I et al: Psychological intellectual components of rehabilitation success in patients with chronic obstructive pulmonary disease, J Chronic Dis 32:405-409, 1979.

25. Glaser EM: Strategies for facilitating knowledge utilization in the biomedical field: final report to the National Science Foundation, grant No. DAR73-07767 A06. Washington DC, 1975, National Science Foundation.

26. In Hodgkin JE, editor: Chronic obstructive pulmonary disease: current concepts in diagnosis and comprehensive care, Park Ridge, Ill, 1979, American College of Chest Physicians.

27. Sahn SA, Nett LM, Petty TL: Ten year follow-up of a comprehensive rehabilitation program for severe COPD, Chest 77:311-314, 1980.

28. Dudley DL, Glaser EM, Jorgenson BL et al: Psychological concomitants to rehabilitation in chronic obstructive pulmonary disease, Chest 77:413-420, 544-551, 677-684, 1980.

29. American Thoracic Society: Position statement on pulmonary rehabilitation, Am Rev Respir Dis 124:663-666, 1981.

30. In Hodgkin JE, Zorn EG, Connors GL, editors: Pulmonary rehabilitation: guidelines to success, Boston, 1984, Butterworth.

31. Pleis JR, Lethbridge-Çejku M: Summary health statistics for U.S. adults: National Health Interview Survey, 2005. National Center for Health Statistics, Vital Health Stat 10(235), 2007. Available at http://www.cdc.gov/nchs/data/series/sr_10/sr10_232.pdf. Retrieved February 2008.

32. National Heart, Lung, and Blood Institute, National Institutes of Health, Public Health Service, U.S. Department of Health and Human Services: Morbidity & mortality: 2007 chart book on cardiovascular, lung, and blood diseases. Available at http://www.nhlbi.nih.gov/resources/docs/07-chtbk.pdf. Retrieved February 14, 2008.

33. National Heart, Lung, and Blood Institute. Available at http://www.nhlbi.nih.gov/health/public/lung/copd. Retrieved February 2008.

34. American Thoracic Society/European Respiratory Society Task Force: Standards for the diagnosis and management of patients with COPD [Internet], version 1.2. New York, American Thoracic Society, 2004 (updated September 8, 2005). Available at http://www.thoracic.org/go/copd. Retrieved February 2008.

35. Centers for Disease Control and Prevention. Cigarette use among high school students-United States, 1991-2005. Morbidity and Mortality Weekly Report (serial online) 2006: 55(26): 724-726. Available at http://www.cdc.gov/mmwr/preview/mmwrhtml/mm5526a2.htm. Retrieved February 2008.

36. Petty TL: Pulmonary rehabilitation. In Basics of RD, vol 4, New York, 1975, American Thoracic Society.

37. American Thoracic Society: Standards for the diagnosis and care of patients with chronic obstructive pulmonary disease (COPD) and asthma, Am Rev Respir Dis 136:225-244, 1987.

38. Fishman AP: Pulmonary rehabilitation research: NIH workshop summary, Am J Respir Crit Care Med 149:825-833, 1994.

39. American Thoracic Society: Standards for the diagnosis and care of patients with chronic obstructive pulmonary disease, Am J Respir Crit Care Med 152(5 pt 2):S77-S121, 1995.

40. American Thoracic Society: Pulmonary rehabilitation—1999: official statement of the American Thoracic Society, Am J Respir Crit Care Med 159:1666-1682, 1999.

41. American Thoracic Society/European Respiratory Society: Statement on pulmonary rehabilitation, Am J Respir Crit Care Med 173:1390-1413, 2006. Available at http://www.thoracic.org/sections/publications/statements/pages/respiratory-disease-adults/atserspr0606.html. Retrieved February 2008.

42. Staats BA, Simon PM: Comprehensive pulmonary rehabilitation in chronic obstructive pulmonary disease. In Fishman AP, editor: Pulmonary rehabilitation, New York, 1996, Marcel Dekker, pp 651-681.

43. ACCP/AACVPR Pulmonary Rehabilitation Guidelines Panel: Pulmonary rehabilitation: Joint ACCP/AACVPR evidence-based guidelines, J Cardiopulm Rehabil 17:371-405, 1997.

44. Pauwels RA, Buist AS, Calverly PM, Jenkins CR, et al.; GOLD Scientific Committee: Global strategy for the diagnosis, management, and prevention of chronic obstructive pulmonary disease. NHLBI/WHO Global Initiative for Chronic Obstructive Lung Disease (GOLD) workshop summary, Am J Respir Crit Care Med 163:1256-1276, 2001. Available at http://www.goldcopd.com (last major revision, November 2006). Retrieved February 2008.

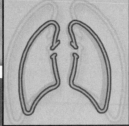

Chapter 2

Selection and Assessment of the Patient with Chronic Respiratory Disease for Pulmonary Rehabilitation

LINDA NICI

CHAPTER OUTLINE

Patient Selection
  Exclusions
  Program Logistics
Patient Assessment
  Medical History and Physical
    Examination
  Diagnostic Tests
  Symptom Assessment
  Exercise Assessment

Pain Assessment
Activities of Daily Living Assessment
Nutritional Assessment
Educational Assessment
Psychosocial Assessment
Goal Development and Rehabilitation
  Potential
Conclusion

PROFESSIONAL SKILLS

On completion of this chapter, the reader will be able to do
the following:
* Understand the patient selection criteria for entrance into pulmonary rehabilitation
* Explain the difference between physiologic impairment and functional impairment
* List the chronic lung diseases appropriate for pulmonary rehabilitation
* Know the components of the initial patient assessment
* State why functional goal development is critical for successful pulmonary rehabilitation

*P*ulmonary rehabilitation should be considered for any patient with chronic respiratory disease who continues to have symptoms, reduced performance, or decreased health-related quality of life despite otherwise optimal medical management.[1,2]

Although individuals with chronic obstructive pulmonary disease (COPD) still comprise the largest proportion of those referred for pulmonary rehabilitation, it has become clear that patients with many types of respiratory disease experience common comorbidities including peripheral muscle disease, cardiac dysfunction, nutritional abnormalities, and psychosocial maladaptation. Because pulmonary rehabilitation interventions address these secondary impairments, it is likely to show substantial benefit in all patients whose respiratory disease is associated with functional impairment or decreased health-related quality of life.

The timing of pulmonary rehabilitation depends on the clinical status of the individual patient and should not be reserved only for those patients with severe respiratory impairment. Rather, it should be an integral part of the clinical management of all patients with chronic respiratory disease, tailored to the individual's specific needs. Reserving pulmonary rehabilitation for patients with end-stage respiratory disease results in many individuals being denied the opportunity to benefit from pulmonary rehabilitation. Although patients with severe disease derive considerable benefit from the rehabilitation process, patients with moderate disease may benefit from additional prevention strategies such as smoking cessation, nutritional therapy, and higher intensity exercise training.

Evidence-based support for pulmonary rehabilitation in the management of patients with chronic respiratory disease has grown tremendously in the last decade, and this comprehensive intervention has been clearly demonstrated to reduce dyspnea, increase exercise performance, and improve health-related quality of life.[3,4] Less than 50% of individuals with COPD based on airflow limitation have a doctor's diagnosis of COPD. Prevalence and morbidity data greatly underestimate the total burden of COPD because the disease is usually not diagnosed until it is clinically apparent and moderately advanced.[1] Therefore as pulmonary rehabilitation specialists we need to educate the public, the medical community, and governmental agencies about the importance of prevention, early detection, and rehabilitation of patients with chronic respiratory disease.

The initial component of a pulmonary rehabilitation program is the interdisciplinary team assessment. It is the foundation for all services provided during pulmonary rehabilitation, directing the patient's individualized plan of care. The components of exercise training, patient education, and nutritional and psychosocial interventions alone or together do not constitute pulmonary rehabilitation unless an initial and ongoing individualized assessment is included.

PATIENT SELECTION

Pulmonary rehabilitation should be considered for all patients with chronic respiratory disease who have persistent symptoms, reduced exercise ability, limited activity, or suboptimal adjustment to their illness despite standard medical management.[5] The literature to date has focused on patients with COPD, with limited studies describing rehabilitation in other chronic respiratory diseases.[6] However, the benefits are likely to extend to these patients because their secondary impairments, which are addressed by the process of pulmonary rehabilitation, are similar. Gains can be achieved from pulmonary rehabilitation regardless of age, sex, lung function, or smoking status. A list of conditions considered appropriate for pulmonary rehabilitation is shown in Box 2-1.

Nutritional status and peripheral muscle weakness may influence the outcome of rehabilitation. Peripheral muscle weakness is a positive predictor of successful outcome, whereas severe nutritional depletion and low-fat free mass may be associated with an unsatisfactory response to rehabilitation.[7-9]

Traditionally, abnormal results of pulmonary function testing (done within 1 year of initiating pulmonary rehabilitation for stable patients) have been used as the primary selection criterion in judging patient eligibility for pulmonary rehabilitation. Although helpful in assessing the degree of physiologic impairment, pulmonary function test data alone are not sufficient selection criteria. Symptoms, disability, and handicap despite standard medical therapy dictate the need for pulmonary rehabilitation, not the degree of physiologic impairment such as the FEV_1 (forced expiratory volume in 1 second) or the diffusing capacity. Symptoms, especially dyspnea, correlate better with functional ability than FEV_1 or other measures of pulmonary function.[10] A simple dyspnea rating such as the modified Medical Research Council (MMRC) Dyspnea Scale may be a general

BOX 2-1	Conditions Appropriate for Pulmonary Rehabilitation

OBSTRUCTIVE DISEASES
- COPD (including α_1-antitrypsin deficiency)
- Persistent asthma
- Bronchiectasis
- Cystic fibrosis
- Bronchiolitis obliterans

RESTRICTIVE DISEASES
- Interstitial diseases
  - Interstitial fibrosis
  - Occupational or environmental lung disease
  - Sarcoidosis
- Chest wall diseases
  - Kyphoscoliosis
  - Ankylosing spondylitis
- Neuromuscular diseases
  - Parkinson's disease
  - Postpolio syndrome
  - Amyotrophic lateral sclerosis
  - Diaphragmatic dysfunction
  - Multiple sclerosis
  - Posttuberculosis syndrome

OTHER CONDITIONS
- Lung cancer
- Primary pulmonary hypertension
- Before and after thoracic and abdominal surgery
- Before and after lung transplantation
- Before and after lung volume reduction surgery
- Ventilator dependency
- Pediatric patients with respiratory disease
- Obesity-related respiratory disease

indicator for when pulmonary rehabilitation may be of benefit (grades 0-4).[11]

In addition to symptoms, reductions in physical activity, occupational performance, activities of daily living, and increases in medical resource consumption should be evaluated and used in the selection process.[12]

In general, symptoms and functional limitations from chronic respiratory disease become clinically apparent with one or more of the following objective abnormalities[1,6]:

- FEV_1 less than 80% of predicted
- FEV_1/FVC (forced vital capacity) less than 70% of predicted
- Diffusing capacity for carbon monoxide adjusted for hemoglobin less than or equal to 65% of predicted
- Resting hypoxemia: Sao_2/Spo_2 (arterial oxygen saturation/pulse oximetry–based oxygen saturation) less than or equal to 90%
- Exercise testing demonstrating hypoxemia (Sao_2/Spo_2 less than or equal to 90%),

ventilatory limitation (expired volume per unit time/maximal voluntary ventilation [V_E/MVV] equal to or more than 0.8), or a rising ratio of dead space volume to tidal volume (V_D/V_T)

However, as described earlier, there are exceptions to these criteria. Clinical issues that commonly lead to referral to pulmonary rehabilitation include dyspnea/fatigue, impaired health-related quality of life, decreased functional status, decreased occupational performance, difficulty in performing activities of daily living, difficulty with the medical regimen, psychosocial problems attendant to the underlying respiratory illness, nutritional depletion, increased use of medical resources (e.g., hospitalizations, emergency department visits, physician visits), and gas exchange abnormalities including hypoxemia. There may also be some specific indications for rehabilitation before transplantation or lung volume reduction surgery.[13]

Enrolling active smokers in pulmonary rehabilitation is a controversial issue. Some programs exclude these patients from participating in pulmonary rehabilitation because some are thought to be less motivated and may adversely affect group dynamics. There is no research to substantiate this belief, and cigarette smokers may, in fact, significantly benefit from rehabilitation with a focus on smoking cessation.

Patient motivation is also a necessary consideration in patient selection, although difficult to assess. Patients obviously must agree to participate in the program, with a commitment to attend most, if not all, sessions. However, patients who initially appear resistant to rehabilitation often show dramatic improvement and become highly motivated attendees. Therefore patient motivation should not be considered too strongly in the initial assessment.

Exclusions

Concurrent diseases or conditions that may interfere with the rehabilitation process or place the patient at substantial risk during exercise should be corrected or stabilized before the patient enters the program. Permanent or temporary conditions that may be considered contraindications to pulmonary rehabilitation include, but are not limited to, significant orthopedic, neurologic, or psychiatric problems that prohibit ability or cooperation with physical training; unstable cardiac disease; and severe pulmonary hypertension. Stable cardiac disease with a practitioner's clearance is not a contraindication to pulmonary rehabilitation. The clinical judgment of the medical director and rehabilitation team during the initial assessment is necessary to determine whether any comorbidity would preclude participation in pulmonary rehabilitation.

Program Logistics

Patients must be informed of the anticipated expenses of pulmonary rehabilitation, including verbal and written information regarding program fees and coverage before admission. Transportation to and from the program must also be considered. This can be provided by family, friends, institutional support services, or public transit. Patients too ill to regularly attend outpatient pulmonary rehabilitation may be more appropriate candidates for admission to an inpatient rehabilitation facility or home care.

PATIENT ASSESSMENT

The pulmonary rehabilitation assessment is performed by the medical director/program coordinator or trained health care designee and appropriate team members. This assessment is the basis on which the patient's individualized plan of care is developed. The initial assessment begins with an interview that serves not only to obtain information about the patient, but also to describe the pulmonary rehabilitation process and discuss the patient's concerns and goals. The importance of the initial interview cannot be overstated. Not only is information gathered and goals formulated, but also the foundations of trust and credibility are generated at this time. The interview allows the patient to interact on a personal level with the rehabilitation staff, see the program, and possibly meet current participants or recent graduates.

After the interview, the patient should undergo a medical history and physical examination, diagnostic tests, symptoms assessment, musculoskeletal and exercise assessment, activities of daily living assessment, nutritional assessment, educational assessment, psychosocial assessment, and goal development.

Medical History and Physical Examination

A thorough review of the patient's medical history is essential during the initial assessment. This information can be obtained from the patient, family members, primary health provider office records, or hospital records. This information is important in identifying comorbid conditions that may directly influence the patient's participation and progress in the pulmonary rehabilitation program. It is often very useful for the pulmonary rehabilitation staff to directly communicate with the referring physician to determine which factors are contributing to the patient's limitations. Important components of the medical history include the type and degree of chronic respiratory disease, other comorbid illnesses, smoking history, number of exacerbations and hospitalizations, and medications including the use of systemic steroids and oxygen.

The physical examination, although primarily focused on the respiratory system, must also assess other systems that will have direct bearing on the pulmonary rehabilitation prescription. In addition to chest examination and evaluation for use of accessory muscles, clubbing, and signs of cor pulmonale, the physical assessment should include measurement of vital signs, signs of left heart failure, musculoskeletal examination, neurologic examination, and evaluation of nutritional state. Measurement of arterial oxygen saturation with pulse oximetry at rest and with activity is frequently performed during the initial physical assessment.

Diagnostic Tests

Diagnostic tests aid in identifying the patient's respiratory disease and establishing a clinical baseline. Some tests, such as a field test of exercise capacity or cardiopulmonary exercise testing, are extremely useful not only during the initial assessment, but also as outcomes to evaluate response to the intervention. Diagnostic tests that are useful during the initial patient assessment include but are not limited to spirometry, arterial oxygen saturation at rest and with exercise, chest radiograph, electrocardiogram, and complete blood count. Additional laboratory tests may also be helpful for selected patients such as complete pulmonary function testing, bronchial challenge, and cardiovascular testing such as Holter monitor, echocardiogram, and thallium stress test.

Symptom Assessment

The two major symptoms that lead to referral for pulmonary rehabilitation are dyspnea and fatigue[14-17] (see Chapter 5). These symptoms are complex, with multiple mechanisms of action.[10]

By nature, dyspnea and fatigue are subjective and require self-reporting. In the pulmonary rehabilitation setting, dyspnea or fatigue can be assessed either in "real time" or through recall.[18] Real-time evaluation of symptoms will only determine how short of breath or fatigued the patient is at the moment of testing. The Borg Scale[19] and the Visual Analog Scale[20] are most commonly used for this purpose, with either being useful in assessing dyspnea or fatigue during exercise testing or training. Recall of symptoms such as dyspnea or fatigue is usually accomplished through the use of questionnaires. Some questionnaires require patients to rate overall dyspnea, whereas others ask about dyspnea related to activities. The impact of dyspnea on physical function can be measured with the Baseline Dyspnea Index, (BDI), the modified Medical Research Council (MMRC), Dyspnea Scale, the Oxygen Cost Diagram, (OCD), the UCSD Shortness of Breath Questionnaire, (SOBQ), or the dyspnea domain of the Chronic Respiratory Disease Questionnaire (CRQ or CRDQ).[21] When a questionnaire is selected, certain technical issues should be taken into account including the length of time to complete/administer the questionnaire, mode of administration (self-administered or given by another), complexity of scoring, purchase cost, and whether written permission is required to use the questionnaire.

Other important symptoms in patients referred for pulmonary rehabilitation include cough, sputum production, wheeze, chest pain, postnasal drainage, reflux, edema, extremity pain and weakness, loss of appetite, anxiety, depression, patient's perception of abilities, and sleep disturbances.

Exercise Assessment

Before exercise training, clinicians must establish optimal medical treatment, including bronchodilator therapy, long-term oxygen therapy, and treatment of comorbidities. The safety and appropriateness of exercise training, as well as the exercise prescription, are determined during the initial exercise assessment. This assessment includes evaluation of the patient's physical limitations including orthopedic limitations, limitations in the ability to perform activities of daily living, gait and balance evaluation, and the need for supplemental oxygen. The exercise assessment should establish a baseline of exercise capacity, endurance, strength, range of motion, and functional abilities. The evaluation should also highlight any restrictions to activity that require exercise modification (see Chapter 10).

Measurement of exercise capacity can be accomplished in several ways, including field tests, activity monitors, and cardiopulmonary exercise testing. Field tests are simple to perform, require little additional equipment, are conducted in a nonlaboratory setting, and have been shown to be responsive to the rehabilitation intervention. They include the 6-minute walk test (6MWT),[22-24] which is self-paced, and externally paced tests such as the incremental and endurance shuttle walk tests.[25,26] Both types of test measure distance walked. The 6MWT has been shown to have the most variability in its administration,[27-30] which can be minimized by using published guidelines that standardize the performance of this test.[31] Although these tests are effective objective measures for programs, it is unclear how they translate into improvement in day-to-day activities.

A thorough patient assessment may also include a maximal cardiopulmonary exercise test to assess the safety of exercise, the factors contributing to exercise limitation, and the exercise prescription. Cardiopulmonary exercise testing can be of considerable help in the initial assessment of exercise limitation and formulating the exercise prescription. Physiologic measurements also provide valuable insight into mechanisms of exercise intolerance. Cardiopulmonary exercise testing can be performed incrementally to maximal symptom limitation or at a constant work rate.[32]

Pain Assessment

It is also worthwhile to assess pain during the initial assessment and during the exercise program. Pain may directly affect the ability of the patient to complete the program and may also lead to suboptimal benefits. Special attention should be paid to location, character, intensity, and duration and to factors that aggravate or ameliorate the pain. Pain can be assessed with a numeric rating system or a facial descriptor.

Activities of Daily Living Assessment

Chronic respiratory disease and its resultant dyspnea may negatively affect on the patient's ability and willingness to perform activities of daily living (ADL). This often leads to dependence on family and friends. Frustration with this loss of independence can present in the form of irritability, pessimism, a hostile attitude toward others, and depression. Therefore it is important that the patient's ability to function independently in ADL and leisure activities be part of the initial assessment (see Chapter 13).

The ADL assessment should include breathing and pacing techniques, energy conservation techniques, extremity strength and range of motion, need for adaptive equipment, and impairment in leisure activities. Sexual dysfunction resulting from chronic respiratory disease is another important area to be assessed.[33] Understanding the patient's (and significant other's) concerns and previous patterns of sexual activity will help in the plan for counseling, if necessary. If appropriate, functional task performance (such as food procurement and preparation) and a vocational evaluation should be included before goal development and treatment planning. Including a significant other during the ADL assessment will add complementary information to the patient's own report.

Most pulmonary rehabilitation programs rely on patient self-reports to assess activity levels, using both the intensity of dyspnea with activities and the degree to which a patient may perform activities in a real-life situation[34]; however, patients may overestimate their activity levels when assessed with questionnaires as compared with direct assessment. An emerging method of evaluating activities in the nonlaboratory setting is the use of activity monitors or motion detectors.[35] Activity monitors, which provide an objective measure of patients' daily activity,[36] can be simple (such as a pedometer, which evaluates the number of steps a patient takes) or more complex devices that measure movement in three planes (such as a triaxial accelerometer).[37] These devices are generally less sensitive to arm activities than to activities requiring lower extremity movement. The role of activity monitors in clinical pulmonary rehabilitation assessment requires further study.

Nutritional Assessment

The rationale for addressing and treating body composition abnormalities in patients with chronic respiratory disease is based on the high prevalence of abnormalities and their impact on morbidity, mortality, and success of structured exercise training (see Chapter 14).

Individuals with moderate-to-severe COPD are frequently underweight, including up to one third of outpatients[38-40] and two thirds of those referred for pulmonary rehabilitation or participating in clinical trials.[41-44] Muscle wasting associated with COPD is more common in, but by no means limited to, underweight patients. Chronic respiratory disease causes increased energy expenditure during breathing, which results in increased caloric needs,[45] and difficulty in maintaining adequate nutrition is seen in 40% to 60% of patients with COPD.[46] Underweight patients with COPD have significantly greater impairment in health-related quality of life than those of normal weight.[47] Poor nutritional status is also a significant predictor of mortality,[48-51] independent of the degree of airflow obstruction.[52] Perhaps more important, weight gain in those with a body mass index below 25 kg/m^2 is associated with decreased mortality.[48]

At a minimum, simple screening should be a component of the initial patient assessment. This can be most easily accomplished by calculating the body mass index (BMI), which is defined as the weight (in kilograms) divided by the height (in meters squared). On the basis of the BMI, patients can be categorized as underweight (less than 21 kg/m^2), normal weight (21-25 kg/m^2), overweight (25-30 kg/m^2), and obese (more than 30 kg/m^2). Recent weight loss (more than 10% in the past 6 months or more than 5% in the past month) is also an important independent predictor of morbidity and mortality in chronic respiratory disease. Other assessments should be based on the needs of the patient and may include laboratory tests of nutritional status (serum albumin and prealbumin) and determination of drug-nutrient interactions, fat-free mass (FFM) determination, need for nutritional supplements, use of nutritional/herbal supplements, and dentition/mastication.

Educational Assessment

Patient education is a core component of pulmonary rehabilitation and permeates all aspects of the program. The style of teaching used in pulmonary rehabilitation is changing from traditional, didactic lectures to self-management education.[53] Whereas the former provides information related to the disease and its therapy, the latter teaches self-management skills that emphasize illness control through health behavior modification, thus increasing self-efficacy, with the goal of improving clinical outcomes including adherence.[54-56] Self-management interventions emphasize how to integrate the demands of the disease into daily routine (see Chapter 6).

The curriculum of an individualized educational program is based on addressing knowledge deficits of the patients and their significant others. These specific educational requirements and the goals of patients are determined at the time of their initial evaluation and are reevaluated during the program. There is limited information in COPD regarding the relationship between self-management, self-efficacy, and specific behavior modification. Self-efficacy can be assessed with the COPD Self-Efficacy Scale (CSES) developed by Wigal, Creer, and Kotses,[57] a 34-item self-administered questionnaire, divided into five domains: negative affect, emotional arousal, physical exertion, weather or environment, and behavioral risk factors. The CSES can be used to measure patients' confidence in transforming their knowledge into effective action and may be useful in measuring increases in self-efficacy subsequent to a pulmonary rehabilitation program. However, it has not been externally validated as an outcome measure in pulmonary rehabilitation research and there is no known minimal, clinically important difference. The Pulmonary Rehabilitation Knowledge Test[58] is the only published validated questionnaire that assesses a COPD patient's knowledge. This questionnaire is a self-administered multiple-choice test consisting of 40 questions that cover the component areas identified as relevant to rehabilitation programs. It may provide additional useful information as an evaluative tool for individual programs; however, knowledge change may not translate into behavior change.

A number of areas in addition to patients' knowledge of their disease should also be evaluated, including the ability to read or write, hearing or vision impairment, cognitive impairment, language barriers, and cultural diversity (ethnicity, cultural beliefs, and customs). This information can be ascertained during the initial interview session.

The degree of adherence to healthy behaviors is enhanced when the relationship between the patient, family, and health care providers is a partnership. Pulmonary rehabilitation is a venue that supports the strengthening of this partnership.

Psychosocial Assessment

The initial patient assessment should include a psychosocial evaluation. The interview should allow adequate time for patients to openly express concerns about the psychosocial adjustment to their disease. Questions should cover perception of quality of life, ability to adjust to the disease, self-efficacy, motivation, emotional distress, substance abuse, interpersonal conflict, coping, adherence, and neuropsychological impairment (e.g., memory, attention/concentration, problem-solving abilities). Common feelings and concerns that are expressed in this component of the evaluation include guilt, anger, resentment, fear of abandonment anxieties, helplessness, isolation, grief, pity, sadness, stress, poor sleep, and poor marital relations.[59] If possible, interviewing the significant other (with the patient's consent) may help to explore issues related to dependency, interpersonal conflict, and intimacy. Screening questionnaires such as the Hospital Anxiety and Depression Questionnaire or Beck Depression Inventory may aid in the recognition of significant anxiety and depression[60,61] (see Chapter 17).

Patients identified with significant psychosocial problems should be referred to appropriate professionals for further evaluation and treatment, if indicated. Failure to detect the presence of significant psychosocial abnormalities may result in poor progress with rehabilitation.

The findings from the psychosocial assessment are most useful if they lead to specific and individually tailored treatment goals and are integrated into the overall interdisciplinary treatment plan.

GOAL DEVELOPMENT AND REHABILITATION POTENTIAL

The mutually agreed on treatment plan is a direct reflection of the success and thoroughness of the initial patient assessment. Measurable, patient-specific goals, both short-term and long-term, are formulated during this assessment. The treatment plan must incorporate and reflect these goals. In addition, these goals must be realistic and compatible with the patient's underlying disease, the patient's needs and expectations, and the program's objectives. Examples include the ability to return to work, care for family, walk to the mailbox, bowl, play golf, perform proper breathing techniques, and better understand the disease and its therapy.

The patient must have a clear understanding of the goals and should agree to work toward their attainment. Reviewing progress toward goals throughout the program facilitates their attainment. Involving family in the goal-setting process at the beginning of the program helps to ensure that everyone understands what can and cannot be expected as a result of the program.

CONCLUSION

Assessment of the pulmonary rehabilitation patient by an interdisciplinary team sets the foundation for an individualized and comprehensive pulmonary rehabilitation program. Assessment is one of the most critical components of a program, a precursor to all pulmonary rehabilitation interventions and strategies that follow.

References

1. Global Initiative for Chronic Obstructive Pulmonary Disease: Global strategy for diagnosis, management, and prevention of COPD [GOLD report, 2006 revision]. Available at http://www.goldcopd.com. Retrieved May 2007.
2. American Thoracic Society/European Respiratory Society: Standards for the diagnosis and management of patients with COPD. Available at http://www.thoracic.org/sections/copd. Retrieved May 2007.
3. Nici L, Donner C, Wouters E et al: American Thoracic Society/European Respiratory Society statement on pulmonary rehabilitation, Am J Respir Crit Care Med 173:1390-1413, 2006.
4. Troosters T, Casaburi R, Gosselink R et al: Pulmonary rehabilitation in chronic obstructive pulmonary disease, Am J Respir Crit Care Med 172:19-38, 2005.
5. Donner CF, Muir JF: Rehabilitation and Chronic Care Scientific Group of the European Respiratory Society: Selection criteria and programmes for pulmonary rehabilitation in COPD patients, Eur Respir J 10:744-757, 1997.
6. Crouch RH, ZuWallack R, Connors G et al: American Association of Cardiovascular and Pulmonary Rehabilitation: Guidelines for pulmonary rehabilitation programs, ed 3, Champaign, Ill, 2004, Human Kinetics.
7. Gosselink R, Troosters T, Decramer M: Distribution of muscle weakness in patients with stable chronic obstructive pulmonary disease, J Cardiopulm Rehabil 20:353-360, 2000.
8. Steiner MC, Barton RL, Singh SJ et al: Nutritional enhancement of exercise performance in chronic obstructive pulmonary disease: a randomised controlled trial, Thorax 58:745-751, 2003.
9. Troosters T, Gosselink R, Decramer M: Exercise training in COPD: how to distinguish responders from nonresponders, J Cardiopulm Rehabil 21:10-17, 2001.
10. American Thoracic Society: Dyspnea: mechanisms, assessment, and management [consensus statement], Am J Respir Crit Care Med 159:321-340, 1999.
11. Mahler D, Wells C: Evaluation of clinical methods for rating dyspnea, Chest 93:580-586, 1988.
12. ZuWallack RL: Selection criteria and outcome assessment in pulmonary rehabilitation, Monaldi Arch Chest Dis 53:429-437, 1998.
13. National Emphysema Treatment Trial Research Group: A randomized trial comparing lung-volume–reduction surgery with medical therapy for severe emphysema, N Engl J Med 348:2059-2073, 2003.
14. Kinsman RA, Fernandez E, Schocket M et al: Multidimensional analysis of the symptoms of chronic bronchitis and emphysema, J Behav Med 6:339-357, 1983.
15. Guyatt GH, Townsend M, Berman LB et al: Quality of life in patients with chronic air-flow limitation, Br J Dis Chest 81:45-54, 1987.
16. Breslin E, van der Schans C, Breukink S et al: Perception of fatigue and quality of life in patients with COPD, Chest 114:958-964, 1998.
17. Meek PM, Lareau SC, Anderson D: Memory for symptoms in COPD patients: how accurate are their reports? Heart Lung 18:474-481, 2001.
18. ZuWallack R, Lareau S, Meek P: The effect of pulmonary rehabilitation on dyspnea. In Mahler D, O'Donnell D, editors: Lung biology in health and disease 208:Dyspnea, London, 2005, Informa Healthcare, pp 301-320.
19. Borg GA: Psychophysical bases of perceived exertion, Med Sci Sports Exerc 14:377-381, 1982.
20. Hayes M, Patterson D: Experimental development of the graphic rating method, Psychol Bull 18:98-99, 1921.
21. Meek PM, Lareau SC: Critical outcomes in pulmonary rehabilitation: assessment and evaluation of dyspnea and fatigue, J Rehabil Res Dev 40:13-24, 2003.
22. McGavin CR, Gupta SP, McHardy GJ: Twelve-minute walking test for assessing disability in chronic bronchitis, BMJ 1:822-823, 1976.
23. Butland RJ, Pang J, Gross ER et al: Two-, six-, and 12 minute walking tests in respiratory disease, Br Med J 284:1607-1608, 1982.
24. Larson JL, Covey MK, Vitalo CA et al: Reliability and validity of the 12-minute distance walk in patients with chronic obstructive pulmonary disease, Nurs Res 45:203-210, 1996.
25. Singh SJ, Morgan MD, Scott S et al: Development of a shuttle walking test of disability in patients with chronic airways obstruction, Thorax 47:1019-1024, 1992.
26. Singh SJ, Morgan MD, Hardman AE et al: Comparison of oxygen uptake during a conventional treadmill test and the shuttle walking test chronic airflow obstruction, Eur Respir J 7:2016-2020, 1994.
27. Elpern EH, Stevens D, Kesten S: Variability in performance of timed walk tests in pulmonary rehabilitation programs, Chest 118:98-105, 2000.
28. Steele B: Timed walking tests of exercise capacity in chronic cardiopulmonary illness, J Cardiopulm Rehabil 16:25-33, 1996.
29. Sciurba F, Criner GJ, Lee SM, et al for the National Emphysema Treatment Trial Research Group: Six-minute walk distance in chronic obstructive pulmonary disease, Am J Respir Crit Care Med 167:1522-1527, 2003.

30. Guyatt GH, Puglsey SO, Sullivan MJ et al: Effect of encouragement on walking test performance, Thorax 39:818-822, 1984.
31. American Thoracic Society: Guidelines for the six-minute walk test [statement], Am J Respir Crit Care Med 166:111-117, 2002.
32. American Thoracic Society/American College of Chest Physicians: ATS/ACCP statement on cardiopulmonary exercise testing, Am J Respir Crit Care Med 167:211-277, 2003.
33. Selecky PA: Sexuality and the patient with lung disease. In Casaburi R, Petty TL, editors: Principles and practice of pulmonary rehabilitation, Philadelphia, 1993, WB Saunders, pp 382-391.
34. Lareau SC, Meek PM, Roos PJ: Development and testing of a modified version of the Pulmonary Functional Status and Dyspnea Questionnaire (PFSDQ-M), Heart Lung 27:159-168, 1998.
35. Steele BG, Belza B, Cain K et al: Bodies in motion: monitoring daily activity and exercise with motion sensors in people with chronic pulmonary disease, J Rehabil Res Dev 40:45-58, 2003.
36. Steele BG, Holt L, Belza B et al: Quantitating physical activity in COPD using a triaxial accelerometer, Chest 117:1359-1367, 2000.
37. Pitta F, Troosters T, Spruit MA et al: Validation of a triaxial accelerometer to assess various activities in COPD patients [abstract], Am J Respir Crit Care Med 169:A594, 2004.
38. Engelen MPKJ, Schols AMWJ, Baken WC et al: Nutritional depletion in relation to respiratory and peripheral skeletal muscle function in outpatients with COPD, Eur Respir J 7:1793-1797, 1994.
39. Braun SR, Keim NL, Dixon RM et al: The prevalence and determinants of nutritional changes in chronic obstructive pulmonary disease, Chest 86:558-563, 1984.
40. De Benedetto F, Del Ponte A, Marinari S et al: In COPD patients, body weight excess can mask lean tissue depletion: a simple method of estimation, Monaldi Arch Chest Dis 55:273-278, 2000.
41. Openbrier DR, Irwin MM, Rogers RM et al: Nutritional status and lung function in patients with emphysema and chronic bronchitis, Chest 83:17-22, 1983.
42. Fiaccadori E, Del Canale S, Coffrini E et al: Hypercapnic-hypoxemic chronic obstructive pulmonary disease (COPD): influence of severity of COPD on nutritional status, Am J Clin Nutr 48:680-685, 1988.
43. Schols AMWJ, Soeters PB, Dingemans AMC et al: Prevalence and characteristics of nutritional depletion in patients with stable COPD eligible for pulmonary rehabilitation, Am Rev Respir Dis 147:1151-1156, 1993.
44. Baarends EM, Schols AM, Mostert R et al: Peak exercise response in relation to tissue depletion in patients with chronic obstructive pulmonary disease, Eur Respir J 10:2807-2813, 1997.
45. Wouters EF: Nutrition and metabolism in COPD, Chest 117(5 Suppl 1):274S-280S, 2000.
46. Schols AM: Nutrition in chronic obstructive pulmonary disease, Curr Opin Pulm Dis 6:110-115, 2000.
47. Shoup R, Dalsky G, Warner S et al: Body composition and health-related quality of life in patients with obstructive airways disease, Eur Respir J 10:1576-1580, 1997.
48. Prescott E, Almdal T, Mikkelsen KL et al: Prognostic value of weight change in chronic obstructive pulmonary disease: results from the Copenhagen City Heart Study, Eur Respir J 20:539-544, 2002.
49. Schols AM, Slangen J, Volovics L et al: Weight loss is a reversible factor in the prognosis of chronic obstructive pulmonary disease, Am J Respir Crit Care Med 157(6 pt 1):1791-1797, 1998.
50. Wilson DO, Rogers RM, Wright EC et al: Body weight in chronic obstructive pulmonary disease. The National Institutes of Health Intermittent Positive-Pressure Breathing Trial, Am Rev Respir Dis 139:1435-1438, 1989.
51. Landbo C, Prescott E, Lange P et al: Prognostic value of nutritional status in chronic obstructive pulmonary disease, Am J Respir Crit Care Med 160:1856-1861, 1999.
52. Engelen MP, Deutz NE, Wouters EF et al: Enhanced levels of whole-body protein turnover in patients with chronic obstructive pulmonary disease, Am J Respir Crit Care Med 162:1488-1492, 2000.
53. Lareau SC, Insel KC: Patient and family education. In Hodgkin JE, Celli BR, Connors GL, editors: Pulmonary rehabilitation: guidelines to success, ed 3, Philadelphia, 2000, Lippincott Williams & Wilkins, pp 91-102.
54. Bodenheimer T, Lorig K, Holman H et al: Patient self-management of chronic disease in primary care, JAMA 288:2469-2475, 2002.
55. Bourbeau J, Nault D, Dang-Tan T: Self-management and behaviour modification in COPD, Patient Educ Couns 53:271-277, 2004.
56. Bandura A: Self-efficacy: toward a unifying theory of behavioral change, Psychol Rev 84:191-215, 1977.
57. Wigal JK, Creer TL, Kotses H: The COPD Self-Efficacy Scale, Chest 99:1193-1196, 1991.
58. Hopp JW, Lee JW, Hills R: Development and validation of a Pulmonary Rehabilitation Knowledge Test, J Cardiopulm Rehabil 7:273-278, 1989.
59. Farkas SW: Impact of chronic illness on the patient's spouse, Health Social Work 5:39-46, 1980.
60. Zigmond AS, Snaith RP: The Hospital Anxiety and Depression Scale, Acta Psychiatr Scand 67:361-370, 1983.
61. Beck AT, Ward CH, Mendelson M et al: An inventory for measuring depression. Arch Gen Psychiatry 4:561-571, 1961.

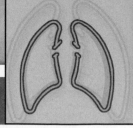

Chapter 3

Pathophysiology of Chronic Obstructive Pulmonary Disease

BARTOLOME R. CELLI

CHAPTER OUTLINE

Definition
Pathophysiology
Airflow Limitation
Hyperinflation
Alteration in Gas Exchange

Control of Ventilation
Respiratory Muscles
Dyspnea
Peripheral Muscle Function
Integrative Approach

PROFESSIONAL SKILLS

On completion of this chapter, the reader will be able to do
the following:

* Gain insight about the anatomic and pathologic lung abnormalities leading to airflow obstruction
* Understand the physiologic changes associated with the development of chronic obstructive pulmonary disease (COPD)
* Relate the pathophysiologic changes to the cardinal symptom of dyspnea
* Review the consequence of exercise and increased ventilatory demands on pulmonary mechanics
* Better comprehend the rationale behind some of the possible forms of treatment of COPD

Chronic obstructive pulmonary disease (COPD) currently ranks as the fourth leading cause of death in the United States.[1] Its prevalence has increased as overall mortality from myocardial infarction and cerebrovascular accident, the two organ systems affected by the same risk factor (namely, cigarette smoking), have decreased. Once diagnosed, COPD is progressive and leads to disability, usually because of dyspnea at a relatively early age (sixth or seventh decade). Limitation to airflow occurs as a consequence of the destruction of lung parenchyma or as a result of alterations in the airway itself. This chapter integrates the pathologic changes of COPD with the known adaptive and maladaptive consequences of those changes. Knowledge of these factors should help us understand the rationale

behind the various therapeutic strategies aimed at decreasing the symptoms and improving the well-being of patients with COPD.

DEFINITION

COPD is a disease state characterized by the presence of airflow obstruction due to emphysema or intrinsic airway disease, classically typified by small airway inflammation and chronic bronchitis. The airflow limitation is generally progressive, may be accompanied by airway hyperactivity, and may be partially reversible. Emphysema is defined pathologically as an abnormal permanent enlargement of the airspaces distal to the terminal bronchioles, accompanied by destruction of their walls, without fibrosis. An enlarged airspace (diameter, >1 cm) is defined as an emphysematous bulla. The pathologic spectrum of bullae is large, ranging from asymptomatic subpleural lesions to giant ones that may compress otherwise normal parenchyma. In most patients with emphysema, the airspace enlargement is variable, with uneven distribution in the site and extent of these bullous changes.[2,3] On the other hand, chronic bronchitis is defined clinically as the presence of chronic predictive cough for 3 months in each of 2 successive years in patients in whom other causes of chronic cough have been excluded. Most patients have a variable degree of airway inflammation, especially of the small airways (<2 mm in diameter), and mucous gland hypertrophy, and up to 30% have airway hyperreactivity. In most patients, both processes coexist. The disease does not affect all portions of the lung to the same degree. This uneven distribution influences the physiologic behavior of different parts of the lung.

PATHOPHYSIOLOGY

Biopsy studies from the large airways of patients with COPD reveal the presence of a large number of neutrophils.[4] This neutrophilic predominance is more manifest in smoking patients who have airflow obstruction than in smoking patients without airflow limitation.[5] Interestingly, biopsy samples of smaller bronchi reveal the presence of a large number of lymphocytes, especially of the CD8[+] type.[6] The same type of cells, as well as macrophages, have been shown to increase in biopsy samples that include lung parenchyma.[6-9] Taken together, these findings suggest that cigarette smoking induces an inflammatory process characterized by intense interaction and accumulation of cells, which are capable of releasing many cytokines and enzymes that may cause injury. Indeed, the level of interleukin-8 is increased in the secretions of patients with COPD. This is also true for tumor necrosis factor and markers of oxidative stress.[8,10,11] In addition, the release of enzymes known to be capable of destroying lung parenchyma, such as neutrophilic elastase and metalloproteinases, by many of these activated cells has been documented in patients with COPD.[12,13] Therefore an increasing body of evidence indicates that the anatomic alterations of COPD, such as airway inflammation and dysfunction as well as parenchymal destruction, could result from altered cellular interactions triggered by external agents such as cigarette or environmental smoke. A schematic representation of these events is shown in Figure 3-1. Whatever the mechanisms, the disease distribution is not uniform, so in a single patient areas of the lung with severe destruction may coexist with less affected areas.

Functionally, COPD is characterized by a decrease in airflow, which is more prominent on

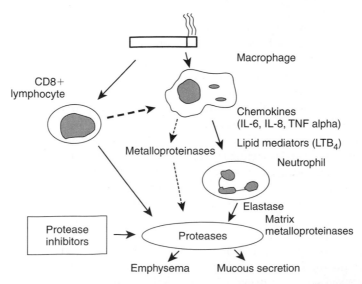

FIGURE 3-1 Schematic representation of the cellular and biologic response to inhalation of noxious agents, such as cigarette smoke. Similar events could occur after inhalation of environmental smoke. The *intermittent lines* represent potentially important interactions. IL-6, interleukin-6; LTB$_4$, leukotriene B$_4$; TNF-α, tumor necrosis factor-α.

maximal efforts. Like the pathologic distribution, the airflow limitation is not uniform in nature. This causes uneven distribution of ventilation and also of blood perfusion.[14,15] This in turn results in arterial hypoxemia (decreased arterial partial pressure of oxygen [Pa_{O_2}]) and, if overall ventilation is decreased, in hypercarbia (increased arterial partial pressure of carbon dioxide [Pa_{CO_2}]). In patients with an important component of emphysema or bullous disease, total lung volume increases, resulting in hyperinflation. Each of these interrelated elements is important in the adaptive changes observed in patients with COPD and helps explain the clinical manifestations of the disease.

The relationship between structure and function in COPD is not well understood. Whether owing to loss of attachments or tethering forces and/or owing to inflammation and mucous secretion, patients with COPD have decreased airflow. Despite this, no good correlation exists between the currently used scoring system for either emphysematous or bronchitic changes and the degree of airflow obstruction. Therefore it is practical to describe the patient by the degree of physiologically determined airflow limitation. At present, the best predictor of morbidity and mortality in COPD is the value of postbronchodilator forced expiratory volume in 1 second (FEV_1).[1,16-19] Because researchers define the obstruction as being only minimally reversible (if airflow limitation is highly reversible, then asthma is considered), it seems desirable to develop a more comprehensive staging system that would allow categorization of the heterogeneous population of patients with COPD for epidemiologic and clinical studies, health resource planning, and prognosis. Such a system incorporating the body mass index (B), degree of obstruction (O), dyspnea (D), and exercise endurance (E), called the BODE Index, has been developed[20] and it facilitates the application of clinical information and recommendations. Indeed, in one report, postrehabilitation improvement in the BODE Index was associated with better survival over time.[21]

The literature on factors that affect mortality in patients with COPD is extensive. The principal variables are age and FEV_1.[15-17] The data are relatively old and by and large precede the advent of low-flow oxygen and mechanical ventilation. The presence of hypoxemia and hypercapnia is also important in that they are predictive of mortality once the patient has moderate to severe airflow limitation. Conversely, death is not the only outcome attributable to COPD, and the impact of COPD on the ability of patients to perform the normal activities of a vocation or daily living is incompletely described by the FEV_1 and arterial blood gases. Even with those limitations, the FEV_1 remains the most important tool with which to classify disease severity in COPD. The Global Initiative for Chronic Obstructive Lung Disease and both the American Thoracic Society and European Respiratory Society stage COPD according to the degree of FEV_1 compromise.[1]

A comprehensive dynamic staging system can be constructed on the basis of available information. The first element should be the postbronchodilator FEV_1, expressed as a percentage of its predicted value. This value is the best single predictor of mortality in patients with COPD. However, it is not until values fall below 50% of predicted that mortality begins to increase.[16] Once patients reach very low values of FEV_1, this measurement has little predictive value, but no other measurements have been thoroughly validated.

The severity of gas exchange derangement obtained in the upright, sitting position while breathing room air is easily categorized as to the presence or absence of significant hypoxemia (or evidence of hypoxic and organ injury) and hypercarbia. Although the degree of hypoxemia has been correlated with mortality in patients with COPD, this relationship is obviated by chronic domiciliary use of supplemental oxygen. Nonetheless a patient with significant hypoxemia represents a complicated medical problem and one likely to require more resources. Similarly, the presence of hypercarbia is recognized as a significant correlate of mortality and a marker of advanced, complicated disease.[18]

The cardinal symptom of COPD is dyspnea.[1,22] This sensation is the consequence of the interaction between cognitive and nonvolitional neural processes and respiratory mechanics including airway obstruction. Dyspnea often limits functional activity and frequently causes the patient to seek medical attention.[23] Because COPD is a chronic disorder that limits a patient's ability to work and, in severe cases, impairs the activities of daily living, a monitoring system that includes some attribute of this limitation is highly desirable. Furthermore, in several studies, dyspnea is an independent predictor of survival.[20,24,25] A practical, simple, and validated instrument to measure dyspnea is the Medical Research

Council Dyspnea Scale, which in its modified version is readily accessible.[1]

In one study, a large number of patients with symptomatic severe COPD who had a uniformly low FEV_1 were evaluated. In this rather homogeneous population, FEV_1 failed to predict survival, whereas the 6-minute walk test was the single most important predictor of mortality in this population.[26] Data from our group[27] and one of the lung volume reduction programs[28] support the predictive value of the 6-minute walking distance. Inclusion of this component is justified.

Perhaps the time has come to integrate our newly acquired knowledge into a more comprehensive staging system. The BODE Index has already proved to be a better predictor of mortality than the FEV_1 and it responds well to interventions such as lung volume reduction.[20,29] Until now, researchers have traditionally tested efficacy of treatment by its impact on lung function (FEV_1). This seems paradoxical because researchers have defined the airflow limitation of COPD as being relatively "fixed" in nature. Under this new staging system it is easy to see how patients who receive therapy that does not alter lung function, such as supplemental oxygen, pulmonary rehabilitation, and noninvasive mechanical ventilation, may improve in this clinical stage. The elements of the staging system are shown in Box 3-1.

AIRFLOW LIMITATION

To move air in and out of the lungs, the bellows must force air through the conducting airways. The resistance to flow is given by the interaction of air molecules with each other and with the internal surface of the airways. Therefore airflow resistance depends on the physical property of the gas and the length and diameter of the airways. For a constant diameter, flow is proportional to the applied pressure. This relationship holds true in healthy individuals for inspiratory flow measured at fixed lung volume, as shown in Figure 3-2. In contrast, expiratory flow is linearly related to the applied pressure only during the early portion of the maneuver. Beyond a certain point, flow does not increase despite further increase in driving pressure. This flow limitation is caused by the dynamic compression of airways as force is applied around them during forced expirations. This can be readily understood in the commonly determined flow-volume expression of the vital capacity. Figure 3-3 shows the flow-volume loop of a healthy individual. It is clear that as effort increases, expiratory flow increases up to a certain point (outer envelope), beyond which further efforts result in no further increase in airflow. During tidal breathing (Figure 3-3, inner tracing) only a small fraction of the maximal flow is used, and therefore flow is not limited under these circumstances.

In contrast, the flow-volume loop of patients with COPD is significantly different, as shown in Figure 3-4. The expiratory portion of the curve

BOX 3-1	Variables Included in a New Staging System for Patients with COPD
Forced expiratory volume in 1 second Timed walked distance Dyspnea rating Nutrition	
COPD, *Chronic obstructive pulmonary disease.*	

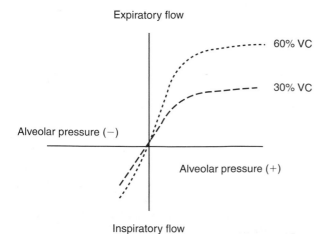

FIGURE 3-2 At a given lung volume (expressed as percent vital capacity [VC]), inspiratory flow is proportional to inspiratory pressure. In contrast, expiratory flow does not increase with increased expiratory pressure as the airways are dynamically compressed by the increased pressure.

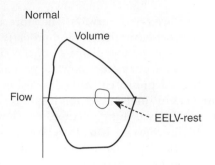

FIGURE 3-3 Flow-volume loop of a healthy individual. Ample flow reserve exists between tidal and forced breathing. EELV, end-expiratory lung volume.

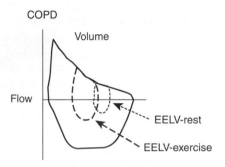

FIGURE 3-4 Flow-volume loop of a patient with chronic obstructive pulmonary disease (COPD). These patients may reach airflow limitation even during tidal breathing. EELV, end-expiratory lung volume.

is concave. This shape is caused by the smaller diameter of the intrathoracic airways, which decreases even more as pressure is applied around them. The flow limitation can be severe enough that maximal flow may be reached even during tidal breathing, as represented in this diagram. A patient with this degree of obstruction (a not uncommon finding in clinical practice) cannot increase flow with increased ventilatory demand. As later reviewed, increased demands can be met only by increasing the respiratory rate, which in turn is detrimental to the expiratory time, a significant problem for patients with COPD.

The precise reason for the development of airflow obstruction in COPD is not entirely clear, but it may likely be multifactorial. In pure emphysema, destruction of the tissue around the airways will decrease the forces that act to keep the airways open.[30] In patients with a component of airway inflammation, the problem is compounded by intrinsic narrowing of the airways.[9,31]

Because airflow obstruction is physiologically evident during exhalation, COPD has been thought to be a problem of "expiration." However, inspiration is also affected because inspiratory resistance is also increased, and, more important, the inability to expel the inhaled air, coupled with parenchymal destruction, leads to hyperinflation.[32]

HYPERINFLATION

As the parenchymal destruction of many patients with COPD progresses, the distal airspaces enlarge. The loss of lung elastic recoil resulting from this destruction increases resting lung volume. In a pervasive way, the loss of elastic recoil and airway attachments narrows even more the already constricted airways. The decrease in airway diameter increases resistance to airflow and worsens the obstruction. Decreased lung elastic recoil therefore is a major contributor to airway narrowing in emphysema.[33,34] Because in most patients the distribution of emphysema is not uniform, portions of lung with low elastic recoil may coexist with portions with more normal elastic recoil. It follows that ventilation to each of these portions will not be uniform. This helps explain some of the differences in gas exchange. It also explains why reduction of the uneven distribution of recoil pressures by procedures that resect more afflicted lung areas results in better ventilation of the remainder of the lung and improved gas exchange.

Increased breathing frequency worsens hyperinflation[35-37] because the expiratory time decreases, even if patients simultaneously shorten their inspiratory time. The resulting "dynamic" hyperinflation is detrimental to lung mechanics and helps explain many of the findings associated with higher ventilatory demand, such as exercise or acute exacerbation. Implementation of techniques, such as pursed lip breathing, that decrease breathing frequency may result in deflation and thereby improve dyspnea.

ALTERATION IN GAS EXCHANGE

The uneven distribution of airway disease and emphysema helps explain the change in blood gases. The lungs of patients with COPD can be considered as consisting of two portions: one more emphysematous and the other more normal. The pressure—volume curve of the emphysematous portion is displaced up and to the left compared with that of the more normal portion (Figure 3-5). At low lung volume the

COPD: Lung Pressure–Volume Curves

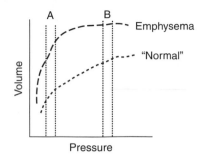

FIGURE 3-5 Volume–pressure relationship in portions of lung with "normal" and "emphysematous" behavior. At low volume (*A*), a small change in pressure results in a larger volume increase in the emphysematous portion. At higher lung volume (*B*), a similar change in pressure results in minimal change in volume in the emphysematous portion, which now behaves as a "stiff" lung. See text for details. COPD, chronic obstructive pulmonary disease.

emphysematous (more compliant) portion undergoes greater volume changes than does the more healthy portion. In contrast, at higher lung volume the emphysematous lung portion is over-inflated and accepts less volume change, per unit of pressure change, than does the healthy portion. Therefore the distribution of ventilation is non-uniform, and, overall, the emphysematous areas of the lung are underventilated compared with the more normal areas. Because perfusion is even more compromised than ventilation in the emphysematous areas, they have a high ventilation:perfusion ratio and behave as dead space. Indeed, this wasted portion of ventilation (dead space volume to tidal volume [V_{DS}/V_T]), corresponding to approximately 0.3 to 0.4 of the tidal breath of a healthy person, has been measured to be much higher in patients with severe emphysema.[38] At the same time, narrower bronchi in other areas may not allow appropriate ventilation to reach relatively well-perfused areas of the lung. This low ventilation-to-perfusion ratio ($\dot{V}/\dot{Q}$) will contribute to venous admixture and hypoxemia.[39,40] The overall result is the simultaneous coexistence of high V_{DS}/V_T regions with regions of low $\dot{V}/\dot{Q}$ match. Both increase the ventilatory demand, thereby taxing even more the respiratory system of these patients.

As ventilatory demand increases, so does the work of breathing, and therefore the patient with COPD must attempt to increase ventilation to maintain an adequate delivery of oxygen.

Alveolar ventilation must also be sufficient to eliminate the carbon dioxide (CO_2) produced. If this does not occur, Pa_{CO_2} will increase. Indeed, the arterial blood gas changes over time in patients with COPD parallel this sequence. Initially Pa_{O_2} progressively decreases, but it is compensated by increased ventilation. When the ventilation is insufficient, the Pa_{CO_2} rises.[41,42] This is consistent with the observation that patients with COPD who have severe hypoxemia and hypercarbia have a poor prognosis.[16]

CONTROL OF VENTILATION

For gas exchange to occur, it is necessary to move air in and out of the lung. This is achieved by the respiratory pump, which is composed of the respiratory centers; the nerves that carry the signals from those centers; the respiratory muscles, which are the pressure-generating structures; and the rib cage and abdomen. These components are linked and ordinarily function in a well-orchestrated manner whereby ventilation goes unnoticed and uses little energy.[43-45]

The central controller or respiratory center is located in the upper medulla and integrates input from the periphery and other parts of the nervous system.[46] The output of this generator is modulated not only by mechanical, cortical, and sensory input but also by the state of oxygenation (Pa_{O_2}), CO_2 concentration (Pa_{CO_2}), and acid-base status (pH). Once generated, the output is distributed by the conducting nerves to the respiratory muscles, which shorten, deform the rib cage and abdomen, and generate intrathoracic pressures. These pressure changes displace volume and air moves in and out, depending on the direction of the pressure changes.

The relation between "drive" and inspiratory pressure or volume is referred to as "coupling." Coupling is usually smooth and occurs with minimal effort. That is the reason breathing is perceived as effortless. Whenever the act of breathing requires effort, this effort is perceived as "work," which is defined as the unpleasant sensation of dyspnea. The interaction between the central drive (controller output) and the final output (ventilation) is complex and involves many components.[47,48] This complexity renders it difficult to ascribe dyspnea to a dysfunction in any portion of the system. The ventilatory control can be assessed at different levels. The simplest is the minute ventilation ($\dot{V}_E$), which reflects the final effectiveness of the ventilatory drive. Further insight can be obtained by measuring the two contributors to $\dot{V}_E$: tidal volume (V_T), represented by the volume of air inhaled in a breath, and respiratory frequency.[43,45]

Analysis of these variables in COPD reveals that as the disease progresses, $\dot{V}_E$ increases.[45,47,48] This is expected because the need to keep oxygen uptake and CO_2 removal constant is challenged by the changes in lung mechanics and ventilation perfusion. The increase in $\dot{V}_E$ is achieved first by an increase in V_T, but as the resistive work owing to airflow obstruction worsens, V_T decreases (Figure 3-6). The respiratory rate responds in a more linear fashion, increasing as the obstruction progresses (Figure 3-7).[49] $\dot{V}_E$ can also be expressed in terms of the mean inspiratory flow rate. This is obtained by relating V_T to the inspiratory time (V_T/T_I) and the fractional duration of inspiration ($T_I/Ttot$). V_T/T_I reflects drive, and $T_I/Ttot$ reflects timing. In COPD, both are altered by the need to increase $\dot{V}_E$. $T_I/Ttot$, which normally has values close to 0.38, shortens somewhat, and V_T/T_I increases more to accommodate the increase in respiratory rate and shortened $T_I/Ttot$.

A relatively noninvasive way to measure central drive is by mouth occlusion pressure measured 0.1 second after the onset of inspiration ($P_{0.1}$).[48] With increased central drive, the increase in $P_{0.1}$ is higher than that of V_T/T_I [50,51] because of airflow impedance that decreases mean inspiratory flow measured at the mouth while air is moving. $P_{0.1}$ is much less affected in COPD as it is measured under conditions of no airflow, because the airway is temporarily obstructed. Mouth occlusion pressure, or $P_{0.1}$, has been shown to increase as the degree of obstruction worsens irrespective of the alteration in arterial blood gases. As shown in Figure 3-8, the central drive increases as the degree of airflow obstruction progresses, reaching its maximum in patients in respiratory failure.[52] The drive is effectively "coupled" to increased V_T in the early stages of obstruction, but V_T actually drops as the work to move air becomes very high. The only alternative is to increase the respiratory rate.

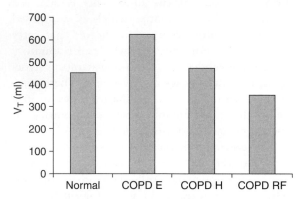

FIGURE 3-6 With progression of airflow limitation, work of breathing increases. To provide the increased oxygen demanded by the breathing pump, tidal volume (V_T) increases in eucapnic (E) patients, begins to decrease as the response fails with hypercapnia (H), and falls, even below the value in normal subjects, in patients with chronic obstructive pulmonary disease (COPD) and respiratory failure (RF).

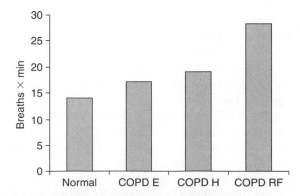

FIGURE 3-7 In patients with chronic obstructive pulmonary disease (COPD), respiratory rate (expressed as breaths per minute) increases as airflow progresses from eucapnia (E) to hypercapnia (H), reaching the highest value in patients in respiratory failure (RF).

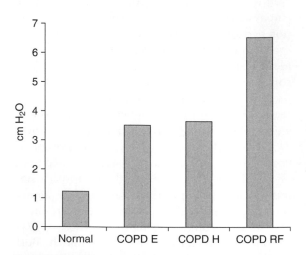

FIGURE 3-8 Mouth occlusion pressure, expressed as centimeters of water at 0.1 second of an occluded tidal breath. This value increases as a function of the progression of airflow limitation and is lower in normal subjects than in eucapnic (E) and hypercapnic (H) individuals, and is highest in patients with chronic obstructive pulmonary disease (COPD) and respiratory failure (RF).

This also occurs, but as determined by the flow limitation characteristics of these patients, this adaptive phenomenon may result in further hyperinflation. As described earlier, hyperinflation displaces diseased portions of lung higher in their pressure—volume relationship. This effectively turns many portions of the lung into "restrictive" tissue. At this point, respiration is less demanding (in terms of work or pressure changes) when a fast and shallower ventilatory pattern is adopted. Indeed, this is the observed breathing strategy in patients with the most severe COPD.[49,53]

RESPIRATORY MUSCLES

As noted previously, breathing depends on the coordinated action of different groups of muscles. The respiratory muscles can be divided into those that help inflate the lungs (inspiratory) and those that have an expiratory action. In addition, there are upper airway muscles (tongue and muscles of the palate, pharynx, and vocal cords), the function of which is to contract at the beginning of inspiration and hold the upper airways open throughout inhalation. Although important in normal function, they play a limited role in pure COPD and are not discussed further in this chapter.

The diaphragm and the other inspiratory muscles are innervated by a wide array of motor neurons that range from cranial nerve 11 (C-11), which provides neuronal input to the sternomastoid, to lumbar roots L2-L3, which innervate abdominal muscles. The respiratory cycle is regulated by a complex series of centrally organized neurons, which maintain rhythmic breathing that usually goes unnoticed and that can be voluntarily overridden by the cortex.

The most important inspiratory muscle is the diaphragm.[54] It is well suited to perform its work because of its anatomic arrangement and histochemical composition. Its long fibers extend from the noncontractile central tendon and are directed down and outward to insert circumferentially in the lower ribs and upper lumbar spine. This concave shape allows the muscle its lifting action as it contracts. The diaphragm can shorten up to 40% between full expiration and end inspiration.[55] During quiet breathing, it accounts for most of the force needed to displace the rib cage. Other inspiratory muscles are also agonists during quiet breathing and contribute to

inspiratory effort: the scalene and parasternal intercostal. Yet other muscles (truly accessory in nature) are not active during quiet breathing in healthy individuals but may contribute to ventilation in situations of increased demand. Muscles such as the sternomastoid, pectoralis minor, latissimus dorsi, and trapezius are some of these truly "accessory" muscles.[44,56] The abdominal muscles are expiratory in action because their contractions decrease lung volume.[57] Inasmuch as they provide tone to the abdominal wall, they help the diaphragm because they contribute to the generation of the gastric pressure needed for diaphragmatic contraction to be effective.

It has been postulated that the automatic and voluntary ventilatory pathways are different and that the respiratory and tonic functions of these muscles are driven from different central nervous areas and integrated at the spinal level. In patients in whom some of these muscles are participating in respiration, to perform nonventilatory work they must maintain a high degree of coordination. Either because of the load or because of competing central integration, muscle function may become dyscoordinated and result in dysfunction. This has been shown to occur in patients with COPD who perform unsupported arm exercise. This type of exercise leads to early fatigue of the muscles involved in arm positioning and to dyssynchrony between the rib cage and the diaphragm—abdomen. This could also be caused by competing outputs of the various driving centers that control rhythmic respiratory and tonic activities of the accessory ventilatory muscles and the diaphragm. This dyssynchrony may be perceived as dyspnea. Its occurrence has been observed in healthy individuals breathing against resistive loads and in patients with COPD breathing during voluntary hyperventilation.[58] Likewise, it has been observed in patients immediately after disconnection from ventilators but before evidence of contractile fatigue, which suggests that dyssynchrony is a consequence of the load and not an indication of fatigue itself. Whatever the reason, this breathing pattern is ineffective and is associated with respiratory muscle dysfunction.[57]

DYSPNEA

Many patients with COPD stop exercising because of dyspnea, and dyspnea is the dominant symptom during acute exacerbations of the disease.[58-60] Studies have shown that in COPD, dyspnea with exercise correlates better with the degree of dynamic hyperinflation than with changes in airflow indices or blood gas exchange.[35-37] Dyspnea also correlates better with respiratory muscle function than with airflow obstruction.[35,61] Studies in healthy individuals have shown that dyspnea increases as the ratio between the pressure needed to ventilate and the maximal pressure that the muscles can generate. Dyspnea also worsens in proportion to the duration of the inspiratory contraction ($T_I/Ttot$) and respiratory frequency. These are also the factors that are associated with electromyographic evidence of respiratory muscle fatigue.[62] Therefore it has been suggested that patients with COPD have dynamic hyperinflation that compromises ventilatory muscle function and that this is the main determinant of dyspnea in these patients. Although respiratory muscle fatigue has been reasonably well documented in patients with COPD experiencing acute decompensation,[63] its presence in stable patients remains in doubt. It is fair to state that the respiratory muscles of patients with severe COPD are functioning at a level closer to the fatigue threshold but are not fatigued. It is possible that restoration of the respiratory muscles to a better contractile state could improve the dyspnea of these patients. Indeed, Martinez and colleagues[64] observed that the factor that best predicted the improvement in dyspnea reported by patients with COPD after lung volume reduction surgery was the lesser dynamic hyperinflation seen during exercise after the procedure. This is consistent with similar reports from other groups[64-67] and the close association between decreased dynamic hyperinflation and dyspnea in patents treated with bronchodilators.[68,69]

Dyspnea in a patient with severe COPD may also be influenced by the resting respiratory drive level and the individual's central output response to various stimuli. In other words, at similar mechanical load and similar levels of respiratory muscle dysfunction, dyspnea may be the result of an individual's central motor output response. This hypothesis is supported by work from Marin and colleagues,[70] who demonstrated that the most important predictor of dyspnea with exercise was the baseline central drive response to CO_2. The importance of this observation lies in the possibility that a group of patients with COPD may manifest increased central drive, and adequate manipulation of this drive may result in decreased dyspnea. Until further studies are completed, this remains just an interesting hypothesis.

PERIPHERAL MUSCLE FUNCTION

Many patients with COPD will stop exercising because of leg fatigue rather than dyspnea. This observation has prompted renewed interest in the function of limb muscles in these patients. Perhaps the most important of these studies are those reported by Maltais and colleagues,[71,72] who performed biopsies of the vastus lateralis before and after lower extremity exercise training in patients with severe COPD. At baseline, patients with COPD have lower levels of the oxidative enzymes citric synthase and 3-hydroxyacyl-CoA-dehydrogenase than do healthy individuals. After exercise, the mitochondrial content of these enzymes increased. This was associated with an improvement in exercise endurance and decreased lactic acid production at peak exercise. These biochemical changes are in line with the observations of several groups, suggesting the presence of a dysfunctional myopathy or even inflammation[73] in patients with COPD. The importance of deconditioning, peripheral muscle dysfunction, and training in COPD is addressed elsewhere in this book (see Chapter 10).

INTEGRATIVE APPROACH

The overall function of the respiratory system in COPD can be represented by the model shown in Figure 3-9. Central to the model is the problem of airway narrowing and hyperinflation. To reverse the model to a normal state, it is necessary to resolve those two problems. Efforts to prevent the disease from developing (smoking cessation) must be associated with methods aimed at reversing airflow obstruction. Indeed, pharmacotherapy, including bronchodilators, antibiotics, and corticosteroids, is given to improve airflow. If this is effective, hyperinflation should consequently decrease. One alternative is to resect those parts of the lungs that are severely diseased, such as has been done in cases of large bullae.[74] Partial resection of less evident emphysematous areas (lung volume reduction surgery) seems effective for a few patients.[75] For most patients, pulmonary rehabilitation through improvement in peripheral muscle function, better coordination of breathing, improved nutrition, and implementation of adequate coping mechanisms remains the best available option.

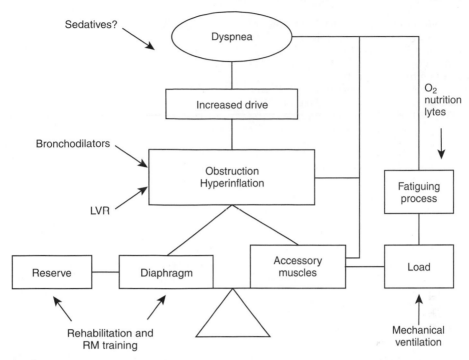

FIGURE 3-9 Schematic model that integrates the various components of breathing in patients with chronic obstructive pulmonary disease (COPD). On the basis of this model, several interventions may be beneficial. See text for details. LVR, lung volume reduction; RM, respiratory muscle.

References

1. Celli BR, MacNee W: Standards for the diagnosis and treatment of COPD, Eur Respir J 23:932-946, 2004.
2. Mitchell RS, Stanford RE, Johnson JM et al: The morphologic features of the bronchi, bronchioles and alveoli in chronic airway obstruction, Am Rev Respir Dis 114:137-145, 1976.
3. Thurlbeck WM: Pathophysiology of chronic obstructive pulmonary disease, Clin Chest Med 11:389-403, 1990.
4. Jeffrey PK: Structural and inflammatory changes in COPD: a comparison with asthma, Thorax 53:129-136, 1998.
5. Keatings VM, Barnes PJ: Granulocyte activation markers in induced sputum: comparison between chronic obstructive pulmonary disease, asthma and normal subjects, Am J Respir Crit Care Med 155:449-453, 1997.
6. Saetta M, Di Stefano A, Turato G: CD8+ T-lymphocytes in peripheral airways of smokers with chronic obstructive pulmonary disease, Am J Respir Crit Care Med 157:822-826, 1998.
7. Finkelstein R, Fraser RS, Ghezzo H et al: Alveolar inflammation and its relation to emphysema in smokers, Am J Respir Crit Care Med 152: 1666-1672, 1995.
8. Yamamoto C, Yoneda T, Yoshikawa M et al: Air-way inflammation in COPD assessed by sputum level of interleukin-8, Chest 112:505-510, 1997.
9. Hogg JC, Chu F, Utokaparch S et al: The nature of small-airway obstruction in chronic obstructive pulmonary disease, N Engl J Med 350:2645-2653, 2004.
10. Barnes PJ: Chronic obstructive pulmonary disease, N Engl J Med 343:269-280, 2000.
11. Pratico D, Basili S, Vieri M, et al: Chronic obstructive pulmonary disease is associated with an increase in urinary levels of isoprostane F_{2a}-111, an index of oxidant stress, Am J Respir Crit Care Med 158:1709-1714, 1998.
12. Finlay GA, O'Driscoll LR, Russell KJ et al: Matrix-metalloproteinase expression and production by alveolar macrophages in emphysema, Am J Respir Crit Care Med 156:240-247, 1997.
13. Vignola AM, Riccobono L, Mirabella A et al: Sputum metalloprotinase-9/tissue inhibitor of metalloprotinase-1 ratio correlates with airflow obstruction in asthma and chronic bronchitis, Am J Respir Crit Care Med 158:1945-1950, 1998.
14. Berend N, Woolcock AJ, Marlin GE: Correlation between the function and the structure of the lung in smokers, Am Rev Respir Dis 119:695-702, 1979.
15. Buist AS, Van Fleet DL, Ross BB: A comparison of conventional spirometric tests and the tests of closing volume in one emphysema screening center, Am Rev Respir Dis 107:735-740, 1973.
16. Fletcher C, Peto R: The natural history of chronic airflow obstruction, BMJ 1:1645-1648, 1977.

17. Anthonisen NR: Prognosis in chronic obstructive pulmonary disease: results from multicenter clinical trials, Am Rev Respir Dis 133:95-99, 1989.

18. Pauwels RA, Buist AS, Calverly PM et al: GOLD Scientific Committee: Global strategy for the diagnosis, management, and prevention of chronic obstructive pulmonary disease. NHLBI/WHO Global Initiative for Chronic Obstructive Lung Disease (GOLD) workshop summary, Am J Respir Crit Care Med 163:1256-1276, 2001. Available at http://www.goldcopd.com (last major revision, November 2006). Retrieved March 18, 2008.

19. Hodgkin JE: Prognosis in chronic obstructive pulmonary disease, Clin Chest Med 11:555-569, 1990.

20. Celli BR, Cote CG, Marin JM et al: The body mass index, airflow obstruction, dyspnea and exercise capacity index in chronic obstructive pulmonary disease, N Engl J Med 350:1005-1012, 2004.

21. Cote CG, Celli BR: Pulmonary rehabilitation and the BODE Index in COPD, Eur Respir J 26:630-636, 2005.

22. Sweer L, Zwillich CW: Dyspnea in the patient with chronic obstructive pulmonary disease, Clin Chest Med 11:417-455, 1990.

23. Mahler DA, Weinburg DH, Wells CK et al: The measurement of dyspnea: contents, interobserver agreement, and physiologic correlates of two new clinical indexes, Chest 85:751-758, 1984.

24. Ries A, Kaplan R, Limberg T et al: Effects of pulmonary rehabilitation on physiologic and psychosocial outcomes inpatients with COPD, Ann Intern Med 122:823-832, 1995.

25. Nishimura K, Izumi T, Tsukino M et al: Dyspnea is a better predictor of 5-year survival than airway obstruction in patients with COPD, Chest 121:1434-1440, 2002.

26. Gerardi D, Lovett L, Benoit-Connors J et al: Variables related to increased mortality following outpatient pulmonary rehabilitation, Eur Respir J 9:431-435, 1996.

27. Pinto-Plata VM, Cote C, Cabral H et al: The 6-minute walk distance: change over time and value as a predictor of survival in severe COPD, Eur Respir J 23:28-33, 2004.

28. Szekely L, Oelberg D, Wright C et al: Preoperative predictors of operative mortality in COPD patients undergoing bilateral lung volume reduction surgery, Chest 111:550-558, 1997.

29. Imfeld S, Bloch KE, Weder W et al: The BODE Index after lung volume reduction surgery correlates with survival, Chest 129:873-878, 2006.

30. Nagai A, Yamawaki I, Takizawa T et al: Alveolar attachments in emphysema of human lungs, Am Rev Respir Dis 144:888-891, 1991.

31. Postma DS, Slinter HJ: Prognosis of chronic obstructive pulmonary disease: the Dutch experience, Am Rev Respir Dis 140:100-105, 1989.

32. Bates DV: Respiratory function in disease, ed 3, Philadelphia, 1989, WB Saunders, pp 172-187.

33. Greaves IA, Colebatch HJ: Elastic behavior and structure of normal and emphysematous lungs postmortem, Am Rev Respir Dis 121:127-128, 1980.

34. Hogg JC, Macklem PT, Thurlbeck WA: Site and nature of airways obstruction in chronic obstructive lung disease, N Engl J Med 278:1355-1359, 1968.

35. O'Donnell SE, Sanil R, Anthonisen NR, et al: Effect of dynamic airway compression on breathing pattern and respiratory sensation in severe chronic obstructive pulmonary disease, Am Rev Respir Dis 135:912-918, 1987.

36. O'Donnell D, Lam M, Webb K: Measurement of symptoms, lung hyperinflation and endurance during exercise in COPD, Am J Respir Crit Care Med 158:1557-1565, 1998.

37. Marin J, Carrizo S, Gascon M et al: Inspiratory capacity, dynamic hyperinflation, breathlessness and exercise performance during the 6 minute walk test in chronic obstructive pulmonary disease, Am J Respir Crit Care Med 163:1395-1400, 2001.

38. Javahari S, Blum J, Kazemi H: Pattern of breathing and carbon dioxide retention in chronic obstructive lung disease, Am J Med 71:228-234, 1981.

39. Rodriguez-Roisin R, Roca J: Pulmonary gas exchange. In Calverly PM, Pride NB, editors: Chronic obstructive pulmonary disease, London, 1995, Chapman & Hall, pp 167-184.

40. Parot S, Miara B, Milic-Emili J et al: Hypoxemia, hypercapnia and breathing patterns in patients with chronic obstructive pulmonary disease, Am Rev Respir Dis 126:882-886, 1982.

41. Begin P, Grassino A: Inspiratory muscle dysfunction and chronic hypercapnia in chronic obstructive pulmonary disease, Am Rev Respir Dis 143:905-912, 1991.

42. Montes de Oca M, Celli BR: Mouth occlusion pressure, CO2 response and hypercapnia in severe obstructive pulmonary disease, Eur Respir J 12:666-671, 1998.

43. Flaminiano L, Celli BR: Respiratory muscle testing, Clin Chest Med 22:661-677, 2001.

44. Roussos CH, Macklem PT: The respiratory muscles, N Engl J Med 307:786-797, 1982.

45. Laghi F, Tobin MJ: Disorders of the respiratory muscles, Am J Respir Crit Care Med 168:10-48, 2003.

46. VonEuler C: On the central pattern generator for the basic breathing rhythmicity, J Appl Physiol 55:1647-1659, 1983.

47. Derenne JP, Macklem PT, Roussos CH: The respiratory muscles: mechanics, control and pathophysiology, Am Rev Respir Dis 119:119-133, 373-390, 1978.

48. Sears TA: Central rhythm and pattern generation, Chest 97:45-47, 1990.

49. Martinez FJ, Couser JI, Celli BR: Factors influencing ventilatory muscle recruitment in patients with chronic airflow obstruction, Am Rev Respir Dis 142:276-282, 1990.

50. Murciano D, Broczkowski J, Lecocguic M et al: Tracheal occlusion pressure: a simple index to monitor respiratory muscle fatigue during acute respiratory failure in patients with chronic obstructive pulmonary disease, Ann Intern Med 108: 800-805, 1988.

51. Milic-Emili J, Grassino AE, Whitelaw WA: Measurement and testing of respiratory drive,

In Hornbein TF, editor: Regulation of breathing (lung biology in health and disease series, vol. 17), New York, 1981, Marcel Dekker, pp 675-743.

52. Sasoon CS, Te TT, Mahutte CR et al: Airway occlusion pressure: an important indicator for successful weaning in patients with chronic obstructive pulmonary disease, Am Rev Respir Dis 135: 107-113, 1987.

53. Loveridge B, West P, Anthonisen NR et al: Breathing patterns in patients with chronic obstructive pulmonary disease, Am Rev Respir Dis 130:730-733, 1984.

54. Rochester DF: The diaphragm contractile properties and fatigue, J Clin Invest 75:1397-1402, 1985.

55. Braun NM, Arora NS, Rochester DF: The force–length relationship of the normal human diaphragm, J Appl Physiol 53:405-412, 1982.

56. DeTroyer A, Estenne M: Functional anatomy of the respiratory muscles, Clin Chest Med 9:175-193, 1988.

57. Sharp JT: The respiratory muscles in emphysema, Clin Chest Med 4:421-432, 1983.

58. Killian K, Jones N: Respiratory muscle and dyspnea, Clin Chest Med 9:237-248, 1988.

59. LeBlanc P, Bowie DM, Summers E et al: Breathlessness and exercise in patients with cardiorespiratory disease, Am Rev Respir Dis 133:21-25, 1986.

60. Girish M, Pinto V, Kenney L et al: Dyspnea in acute exacerbation of COPD is associated with increase in ventilatory demand and not with worsened airflow obstruction, Chest 114:266s, 1998.

61. Killian K, Jones N: Respiratory muscle and dyspnea, Clin Chest Med 1988; 9:237-248.

62. Bellemare F, Grassino A: Forces reserve of the diaphragm in patients with chronic obstructive pulmonary disease, J Appl Physiol 55:8-15, 1983.

63. Cohen C, Zagelbaum G, Gross D et al: Clinical manifestations of inspiratory muscle fatigue, Am J Med 73:308-316, 1982.

64. Martinez F, Montes de Oca M, Whyte R et al: Lung-volume reduction surgery improves dyspnea, dynamic hyperinflation and respiratory muscle function, Am J Respir Crit Care Med 155:2018-2023, 1997.

65. Brantigan OC, Mueller E, Kress MB: A surgical approach to pulmonary emphysema, Am Rev Respir Dis 80:194-202, 1959.

66. Cooper JD, Trulock ER, Triantafillou AN et al: Bilateral pneumonectomy (volume reduction) for chronic obstructive pulmonary disease, J Thorac Cardiovasc Surg 109:116-119, 1995.

67. Knudson RJ, Gaensler E: Surgery for emphysema, Ann Thorac Surg 1:332-362, 1965.

68. Belman M, Botnick W, Shin W: Inhaled bronchodilators reduce dynamic hyperinflation during exercise in patients with chronic obstructive pulmonary disease, Am J Respir Crit Care Med 53:967-975, 1996.

69. O'Donnell DE, Lam M, Webb KA: Spirometric correlates of improvement in exercise performance after anticholinergic therapy in chronic obstructive pulmonary disease, Am J Respir Crit Care Med 160:542-549, 1999.

70. Marin J, Montes De Oca M, Rassulo J et al: Ventilatory drive at rest and perception of exertional dyspnea in severe COPD, Chest 115: 1293-1300, 1999.

71. Maltais F, Simard A, Simard J et al: Oxidative capacity of the skeletal muscle and lactic acid kinetics during exercise in normal subjects and in patients with COPD, Am J Respir Crit Care Med 153:288-293, 1995.

72. Maltais F, LeBlanc P, Simard C et al: Skeletal muscle adaptation of endurance training in patients with chronic obstructive pulmonary disease, Am J Respir Crit Care Med 154:442-447, 1996.

73. Montes de Oca M, Torres SH, De Sanctis J et al: Skeletal muscle inflammation and nitric oxide in patients with COPD, Eur Respir J 26:390-397, 2005.

74. Fitzgerald MX, Keelan PJ, Cugel DW et al: Longterm results of surgery for bullous emphysema, J Thorac Cardiovasc Surg 68:566-587, 1974.

75. National Emphysema Treatment Trial Research Group: A randomized trial comparing lung–volume-reduction surgery with medical therapy for severe emphysema, N Engl J Med 348: 2059-2073, 2003.

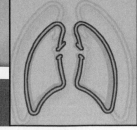

Systemic Effects of Chronic Obstructive Pulmonary Disease

ERNEST SALA • ÀLVAR AGUSTI

CHAPTER OUTLINE

Systemic Effects of Chronic Obstructive Pulmonary Disease
   Systemic Inflammation
   Nutritional Abnormalities and Weight
     Loss
   Skeletal Muscle Dysfunction

   Cardiovascular Effects
   Other Systemic Effects
Clinical Relevance
Potential Therapeutic Options
Conclusion

PROFESSIONAL SKILLS

On completion of this chapter, the reader will be able to do
the following:
* Gain insight about the systemic effects of chronic obstructive pulmonary disease (COPD)
* Assess the relevance of the systemic effects of COPD
* Review the potential therapeutic implications of current and future treatments of the systemic effects of COPD

The 2004 American Thoracic Society/ European Respiratory Society guidelines for chronic obstructive pulmonary disease (COPD) management[1] as well as the latest update of the Global Initiative for Chronic Obstructive Pulmonary Disease guidelines (2006) explicitly recognize that COPD is associated with significant extrapulmonary abnormalities, and that these systemic effects of COPD contribute significantly to the clinical presentation, management, and prognosis of these patients. This chapter describes the main systemic effects of COPD identified to date (Box 4-1), discusses their clinical impact, and comments on some potential therapeutic alternatives. Because systemic inflammation is thought to play a key, albeit probably not exclusive, role in the pathogenesis of many (if not all) these systemic effects, it is discussed first.

SYSTEMIC EFFECTS OF CHRONIC OBSTRUCTIVE PULMONARY DISEASE

Systemic Inflammation

COPD is characterized by an abnormal inflammatory response of the lung parenchyma to the inhalation of particles and toxic fumes, mostly tobacco smoking,[1] that includes increased numbers of neutrophils, macrophages, and T lymphocytes (with a predominance of $CD8^+$ cells), augmented concentrations of proinflammatory cytokines (such as leukotriene B_4, interleukin [IL]-8, and tumor necrosis factor [TNF]-α, among others), and evidence of oxidative stress. Several studies have shown that this inflammatory response is not limited to the lungs but can also be detected in the peripheral blood[2-4] in the form of increased levels of proinflammatory

BOX 4-1	Systemic Effects of Chronic Obstructive Pulmonary Disease

SYSTEMIC INFLAMMATION
- Increased plasma levels of cytokines and increased acute-phase reactants
- Oxidative stress
- Activated inflammatory cells (neutrophils and lymphocytes)

NUTRITIONAL ABNORMALITIES AND WEIGHT LOSS
- Increased resting energy expenditure
- Abnormal body composition
- Abnormal amino acid metabolism

SKELETAL MUSCLE DYSFUNCTION
- Loss of muscle mass
- Abnormal structure and function
- Exercise limitation

CARDIOVASCULAR EFFECTS

OTHER POTENTIAL SYSTEMIC EFFECTS
- Nervous system effects
- Osteoskeletal effects

cytokines and acute-phase reactants, oxidative stress, and activated inflammatory cells.

Several studies have documented increased concentrations of TNF-α and its receptors (TNFR-55 and TNFR-75), several interleukins such as IL-6 and IL-8, C-reactive protein (CRP), lipopolysaccharide-binding protein, Fas, and Fas ligand.[5-8] These abnormalities were seen in patients considered clinically stable but were generally more pronounced during exacerbations of the disease. In this context, however, it is interesting to note that other chronic inflammatory diseases (such as heart failure, acquired immunodeficiency syndrome, and diabetes), and even the normal aging process, are also associated with systemic inflammation.

Other studies have identified the presence of fingerprints of oxidative stress in patients with COPD. Rahman and colleagues[9] determined the antioxidant capacity and the plasma level of lipid peroxidation products in nonsmokers, healthy smokers, and patients with COPD, during both clinically stable periods and exacerbations of the disease. They showed that the former was decreased and the latter increased in smokers and even more so in patients with COPD, particularly during exacerbations.[9] Praticò and colleagues[10] found that urinary levels of isoprostane $F_{2\alpha}$-III, a stable prostaglandin isomer formed by the peroxidation of arachidonic acid, were increased in patients with COPD, again especially during exacerbations of the disease.

Finally, several other studies have demonstrated alterations in circulating neutrophils, lymphocytes, and monocytes in COPD. Burnett and colleagues[11] showed that neutrophil chemotaxis was increased in COPD. Noguera and colleagues reported that the "respiratory burst" (amount of reactive oxygen species produced) of circulating neutrophils was higher in patients with COPD than in nonsmokers or smokers with normal lung function, both under basal conditions and after stimulation in vitro.[12] The same authors showed that the surface expression of several adhesion molecules, particularly Mac-1 (CD11b), was higher in the circulating neutrophils of patients with stable COPD than in healthy control subjects.[13] Interestingly, this difference disappeared during exacerbations of the disease, suggesting neutrophil sequestration in the pulmonary circulation during exacerbations.[13] Circulating lymphocytes have been less well studied than circulating neutrophils in patients with COPD. However, Sauleda and colleagues[14] were able to show activation of circulating lymphocytes in patients with COPD, as compared with healthy nonsmoking control subjects. Finally, De Godoy and colleagues[15] observed that circulating monocytes harvested from patients with COPD and low body weight are capable of producing more TNF-α when stimulated in vitro than those obtained from healthy control subjects. This suggests that an excessive production of TNF-α by peripheral monocytes may play a role in the pathogenesis of weight loss in COPD (discussed later).

Although the evidence discussed earlier strongly supports the presence of systemic inflammation in COPD, several important questions remain. The first concerns whether all patients with COPD have systemic inflammation. To address this question, Mannino, Ford, and Redd[16] used data from the Third National Health and Nutrition Examination Survey to examine the prevalence of increased CRP in COPD. They found that 41% of patients with moderate COPD (forced expiratory volume in 1 second [FEV$_1$] >50%–80% predicted) had a CRP level exceeding 3 mg/L, and 6% had a level exceeding 10 mg/L, whereas 52% of patients with severe COPD (FEV$_1$ <50% predicted) had a CRP level greater than 3 mg/L and 23% had a level greater than 10 mg/L.[16]

Second, because all studies carried out so far are cross-sectional, the longitudinal variation of systemic inflammation is unknown. It is known, however, that systemic inflammation (like pulmonary inflammation) appears to burst during episodes of exacerbation of the disease.[17-20] It is therefore likely that the overall level of systemic inflammation changes with time and, it is hoped, with therapy.

Finally, the origin of systemic inflammation in COPD is unclear. Several potential mechanisms (alone or in combination) could be involved. Tobacco smoking is capable of producing systemic inflammation,[21] but ex-smokers with COPD still present significant systemic inflammation.[4] An alternative explanation is that lung inflammation "spills over" into the systemic circulation or contributes to the priming and activation of various inflammatory cells in their transit through the pulmonary circulation.[2,3] To explore this hypothesis, Vernooy and colleagues[22] compared the levels of a number of inflammatory markers in induced sputum (local inflammation) and plasma (systemic inflammation) in patients with moderate COPD and in smokers with normal lung function. These authors could not find a significant relationship between the levels of these inflammatory markers in the lungs and in the peripheral circulation and concluded that systemic inflammation in COPD was not due to an overflow of inflammatory mediators from the local compartment and that the inflammatory responses in the local and systemic compartments are regulated differently.[22] Another potential mechanism that can contribute to systemic inflammation in COPD is tissue hypoxia, as shown by the relationship between arterial hypoxemia and circulating levels of TNF-α and its soluble receptors sTNFR-55 and sTNFR-75.[23] Skeletal muscle can be another potential site of production of systemic inflammation, particularly during exercise, in patients with COPD[24-26]; however, as discussed later, skeletal muscle is also a target organ of systemic inflammation in these patients.[27]

Nutritional Abnormalities and Weight Loss

Nutritional abnormalities are frequent in patients with COPD, including alterations in caloric intake, basal metabolic rate, intermediate metabolism, and body composition.[28-31] The most obvious clinical expression of these nutritional abnormalities is unexplained weight loss. This is particularly prevalent in patients with severe COPD and chronic respiratory failure, occurring in about 50% of these patients,[29] but it can also be seen in about 10% to 15% of patients with mild to moderate disease.[29] Loss of skeletal muscle mass is the main cause of weight loss in COPD, whereas loss of fat mass contributes to a lesser extent. Importantly, however, alterations in body composition can occur in COPD in the absence of clinically significant weight loss.[28,29]

The causes of nutritional abnormalities are unclear but are probably multiple. Decreased caloric intake does not appear to be prominent in these patients, except during episodes of exacerbation of the disease.[32] In contrast, most patients with COPD exhibit an increased basal metabolic rate, and because this increased metabolic requirement is not met by a parallel increase in caloric intake, weight loss ensues.[32] The cause of the increased basal metabolic rate is also unclear. Traditionally, it has been explained on the basis of the increased work of breathing that characterizes the disease.[33] However, other mechanisms can also contribute, including drugs commonly used in the treatment of COPD (e.g., β_2-agonists),[34] systemic inflammation (as shown by the relationship between metabolic derangement and increased levels of inflammatory mediators in COPD[6]), and tissue hypoxia.[35,36]

Skeletal Muscle Dysfunction

Exercise limitation is a core symptom of COPD. Although this was classically attributed to airflow obstruction, it is now clear that skeletal muscle dysfunction (SMD) is common in these patients and that it can also contribute (often significantly) to limiting their exercise capacity and quality of life.[27,37]

SMD in COPD is characterized by net loss of muscle mass and malfunction of the remaining muscle mass. Several mechanisms can contribute to SMD in COPD (Box 4-2).

Systemic inflammation is likely to be one of the most important causes of SMD in COPD. As discussed earlier, patients with COPD show increased plasma levels of a variety of proinflammatory cytokines, in particular TNF-α.[5-7,38] Also, circulating monocytes harvested from such patients produce more TNF-α in vitro than do those from healthy control subjects,[15] and several authors have now shown increased plasma concentrations of soluble TNF-α receptors.[6,7] TNF-α

can affect muscle cells in a number of ways.[39] In differentiated myocytes studied in vitro, TNF-α activates the transcription factor nuclear factor-κB and induces the expression of a variety of genes, such as those encoding the inducible form of nitric oxide synthase.[39] This can increase NO production and cause protein nitrotyrosination that would facilitate protein degradation through the ubiquitin–proteasome system.[40] Likewise, induction of the inducible form of nitric oxide synthase can also cause contractile failure,[41] thus potentially limiting exercise tolerance in these patients. TNF-α can also induce apoptosis.[39] This has been shown to occur in the skeletal muscle of patients with COPD and weight loss.[40]

The role of systemic inflammation in the pathogenesis of SMD in COPD is further supported by several epidemiologic observations. Yende and colleagues[42] analyzed data from elderly participants in the Health, Aging, and Body Composition Study and found that in COPD, lower quadriceps strength was associated with higher IL-6 and CRP levels.[42] Further, IL-6 levels predicted exercise tolerance. Broekhuizen and colleagues[43] built on the observations by Yende and colleagues,[42] reporting that raised CRP levels in patients with COPD admitted for pulmonary rehabilitation were associated with diminished muscle strength and reduced exercise endurance, work load, 6-minute walking distance (6MWD), increased resting energy expenditure, and health status. Pinto-Plata and colleagues[44] reported that 6MWD, age, and body mass index significantly predicted CRP levels in patients with COPD. The most important, clinically relevant predictor was 6MWD, which decreased with increasing CRP levels.

Other mechanisms that can also contribute to SMD in COPD include sedentarism, tissue hypoxia, smoking, endocrine dysregulation, and drugs used in clinical practice. Patients with COPD often adopt a sedentary lifestyle; physical inactivity causes net loss of muscle mass, reduces the force-generating capacity of muscle, and decreases its resistance to fatigue.[45] Chronic hypoxia suppresses protein synthesis in muscle cells, causes net loss of amino acids, and reduces expression of myosin heavy chain isoforms[46]; the skeletal muscle of patients with COPD and chronic respiratory failure exhibits structural (decrease in type I fibers[47]) and functional[36] alterations proportional to the severity of arterial hypoxemia. Tobacco smoke contains many

---

BOX 4-2   Potential Mechanisms of Skeletal Muscle Dysfunction in Chronic Obstructive Pulmonary Disease

- Sedentary behavior
- Nutritional abnormalities
- Tissue hypoxia
- Systemic inflammation
- Skeletal muscle apoptosis
- Oxidative stress
- Tobacco smoking
- Hormone alterations
- Drugs

---

substances potentially harmful to skeletal muscle; nicotine alters the expression of important growth factors, such as transforming growth factor–β₁, involved in the maintenance of muscular mass[48] and competes with acetylcholine for its receptor at the neuromuscular junction, thus having the potential to affect muscle contraction directly.[49] Patients with COPD often show low levels of testosterone and growth hormone[50] and leptin, all of which can alter muscle mass and function. Finally, some of the drugs used in the treatment of COPD can also interfere with skeletal muscle function, most clearly exemplified by the use of oral steroids.[51-53]

SMD in COPD has two clinically relevant consequences. First, it contributes to weight loss,[29] a poor prognostic factor for these patients.[54] Second, it is one of the main causes of exercise limitation in COPD,[27] profoundly affecting the quality of life of these individuals.[55] Thus appropriate treatment of SMD should be a priority in the clinical management of COPD.[27] At present, this is based mostly on rehabilitation programs, nutritional support, and, perhaps, oxygen therapy.[56-58] However, more specific and effective therapies need to be developed (see the section on potential therapeutic options).

Cardiovascular Effects

COPD increases the risk of cardiovascular disease twofold to threefold.[59] Several studies have shown that endothelial function in COPD is abnormal in both the pulmonary[60] and systemic circulation.[61,62] The mechanisms underlying these abnormalities are unclear, but again, several mechanisms can be conceived, including tobacco smoking (a shared risk factor for both COPD and cardiovascular disease) and, importantly, systemic inflammation.[59] In fact, CRP is a powerful predictor of cardiovascular risk both in healthy individuals[63] and in patients with COPD.[59,64] This may have important therapeutic implications in the management of these patients because anti-inflammatory therapy would be beneficial not only for the chronic inflammatory process in their lungs but also for the prevention of cardiovascular disease (see the section on potential therapeutic options).

Other Systemic Effects

Although much less investigated than the extrapulmonary effects discussed earlier, other organ systems might also be affected in COPD, including the central nervous system and the osteoskeletal system.

Brain energy metabolism is abnormal[65], and depression is highly prevalent in COPD.[66] Likewise, the autonomic nervous system may also be altered in patients with COPD, particularly those with low body weight.[67] It is possible that these abnormalities bear some relationship with the systemic inflammation that occurs in COPD.[68]

On the other hand, the prevalence of osteoporosis is increased in patients with COPD.[69] Because proinflammatory cytokines can alter bone metabolism significantly, excessive osteoporosis in relation to age could also be considered a systemic effect of COPD.[70]

CLINICAL RELEVANCE

The systemic effects of COPD have a profound impact on the clinical management of the disease. Weight loss and skeletal muscle dysfunction limit the exercise capacity of these patients and worsen their quality of life. Also, weight loss is a prognostic factor in patients with COPD that, importantly, is independent of other prognostic indicators, such as FEV_1 or arterial partial pressure of oxygen, that assess the degree of pulmonary dysfunction.[54,71] Thus weight loss identifies a new systemic domain of COPD not considered by the traditional measures of lung function. Accordingly, in addition to the severity of lung disease, the clinical assessment of patients with COPD should take into consideration the extrapulmonary consequences of COPD. On the basis of this concept, Celli and colleagues[72] have proposed a new, multidimensional classification of COPD (the BODE Index) that considers the body mass index (B), the degree of airflow obstruction (O) and functional dyspnea (D), and

exercise capacity (E) as assessed by the 6-minute walk test. The BODE Index predicts the risk of all-cause death and the risk of death from respiratory causes in patients with COPD better than FEV_1.[72] This is the first approximation that assesses the severity of COPD multidimensionally. It is possible that this index will be modified in the future by incorporating other domains that may also be important in patients with COPD, such as the frequency and severity of exacerbations, the type and intensity of inflammation (both at the pulmonary and systemic level), and the degree and reversibility of lung hyperinflation, among others. These possibilities will need to be rigorously tested in future studies.

POTENTIAL THERAPEUTIC OPTIONS

Because the pathogenesis of the systemic effects of COPD is not well understood, specific therapies for them are not yet available. However, given that systemic inflammation is likely to be a key pathogenic mechanism, as discussed earlier, some recommendations can be suggested.

Because smoking causes systemic inflammation in human beings, quitting smoking can reduce it. By decreasing dynamic hyperinflation, bronchodilators have the potential to reduce inflammation. Inhaled steroids can also contribute to this goal, as shown by Sin and colleagues.[73] These authors showed that inhaled fluticasone reduced CRP levels by 50%.[73] Likewise, Pinto-Plata and colleagues[44] reported that CRP levels were lower in patients with COPD treated with inhaled steroids. This effect has the potential to reduce cardiovascular risk in these patients,[59] as shown by Huiart and colleagues[74] in a retrospective study. The TORCH Study has explored the effects of salmeterol and fluticasone (vs. placebo in COPD). Although there is debate about the statistical significance of these effects on the main outcome variable of the study (all-cause mortality), combination therapy proved effective in reducing the number of exacerbations, and the rate of decline of both lung function and health status over a 3-year period.[75] The use of antioxidant agents, such as *N*-acetylcysteine, deserves further study.[76]

Nonpharmacologic therapy also has the potential to influence systemic inflammation in COPD. Oxygen therapy has never been explored formally, but given that tissue hypoxia is a likely

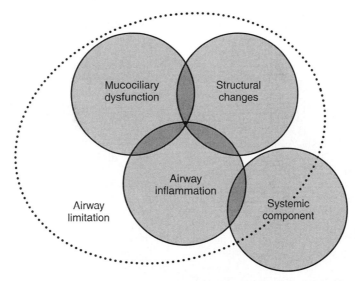

FIGURE 4-1 COPD as a multicomponent disease. *(Modified from Agustí AG: COPD, a multicomponent disease: implications for management, Respir Med 99:670-682, 2005.)*

contributor to systemic inflammation in these patients, oxygen therapy can improve it, thus contributing to its well-established effects prolonging survival in patients with COPD and respiratory failure. Bathon and colleagues[77] failed to show a systemic anti-inflammatory effect of pulmonary rehabilitation. Although nutritional supplementation seems a logical alternative in undernourished patients, a meta-analysis does not support its usefulness.[78] It is possible, however, that the combination of more specific nutritional support with effective anti-inflammatory therapy (and regular exercise training) may provide different results in future.

The role of more specific therapeutic alternatives for systemic inflammation needs to be further explored. For instance, although anti—TNF-α antibodies appear to be useful in other chronic inflammatory diseases,[79] initial results in COPD seem discouraging. Inhibitors of the angiotensin-converting enzyme prevent weight loss in patients with chronic heart failure,[78] but their usefulness in COPD has not been investigated. The potential role of inducible nitric oxide synthase inhibitors may also merit investigation.[80] Finally, it is interesting to note that in the National Emphysema Treatment Trial, the patients who benefited the most (in terms of survival) were those with poor exercise capacity after rehabilitation.[81] Because these patients are likely to have skeletal muscle dysfunction, this observation suggests that skeletal muscle dysfunction (and perhaps other systemic effects of COPD) can be ameliorated by removing diseased lung parenchyma. The mechanisms underlying the improvement are unclear but may be related to the removal of a potential site of systemic inflammation or to the improvement in oxygen transport that occurs after surgery.

CONCLUSION

Available evidence clearly demonstrates that COPD is a multicomponent disease (Figure 4-1) with an important systemic component, that the clinical assessment of these patients must take into account this extrapulmonary component of the disease, and that treatment of these systemic effects can have a significant impact on the prognosis and well-being of individuals with this devastating disease.[82] Better understanding of the cellular and molecular causes of these systemic effects is required to develop novel, more specific, and more effective therapeutic strategies.

References

1. Celli BR, MacNee W, Agustí AG et al: Standards for the diagnosis and treatment of patients with COPD: a summary of the ATS/ERS position paper, Eur Respir J 23:932-946, 2004.
2. Agustí AG, Noguera A, Sauleda J et al: Systemic effects of chronic obstructive pulmonary disease, Eur Respir J 21:347-360, 2003.
3. Wouters EF, Creutzberg EC, Schols AM: Systemic effects in COPD, Chest 121(5 Suppl):127S-130S, 2002.

4. Gan WQ, Man SF, Senthilselvan A et al: Association between chronic obstructive pulmonary disease and systemic inflammation: a systematic review and a meta-analysis, Thorax 59:574-580, 2004.

5. Di Francia M, Barbier D, Mege JL et al: Tumor necrosis factor-alpha levels and weight loss in chronic obstructive pulmonary disease, Am J Respir Crit Care Med 150:1453-1455, 1994.

6. Schols AM, Buurman WA, Staal van den Brekel AJ et al: Evidence for a relation between metabolic derangements and increased levels of inflammatory mediators in a subgroup of patients with chronic obstructive pulmonary disease, Thorax 51:819-824, 1996.

7. Yasuda N, Gotoh K, Minatoguchi S et al: An increase of soluble Fas, an inhibitor of apoptosis, associated with progression of COPD, Respir Med 92:993-999, 1998.

8. Eid AA, Ionescu AA, Nixon LS et al: Inflammatory response and body composition in chronic obstructive pulmonary disease, Am J Respir Crit Care Med 164:1414-1418, 2001.

9. Rahman I, Morrison D, Donaldson K et al: Systemic oxidative stress in asthma, COPD, and smokers, Am J Respir Crit Care Med 154:1055-1060, 1996.

10. Praticò D, Basili S, Vieri M et al: Chronic obstructive pulmonary disease is associated with an increase in urinary levels of isoprostane F2alpha-III, an index of oxidant stress, Am J Respir Crit Care Med 158:1709-1714, 1998.

11. Burnett D, Hill SL, Chamba A et al: Neutrophils from subjects with chronic obstructive lung disease show enhanced chemotaxis and extracellular proteolysis, Lancet 2:1043-1046, 1987.

12. Noguera A, Batle S, Miralles C et al: Enhanced neutrophil response in chronic obstructive pulmonary disease, Thorax 56:432-437, 2001.

13. Noguera A, Busquets X, Sauleda J et al: Expression of adhesion molecules and G proteins in circulating neutrophils in chronic obstructive pulmonary disease, Am J Respir Crit Care Med 158:1664-1668, 1998.

14. Sauleda J, Garcia-Palmer FJ, Gonzalez G et al: The activity of cytochrome oxidase is increased in circulating lymphocytes of patients with chronic obstructive pulmonary disease, asthma, and chronic arthritis, Am J Respir Crit Care Med 161:32-35, 2000.

15. De Godoy I, Donahoe M, Calhoun WJ et al: Elevated TNF-a production by peripheral blood monocytes of weight-losing COPD patients, Am J Respir Crit Care Med 153:633-637, 1996.

16. Mannino DM, Ford ES, Redd SC: Obstructive and restrictive lung disease and markers of inflammation: data from the Third National Health and Nutrition Examination, Am J Med 114:758-762, 2003.

17. Malo O, Sauleda J, Busquets X et al: Inflamación sistémica durante las agudizaciones de la enfermedad pulmonar obstructiva crónica, Arch Bronconeumol 38:172-176, 2002.

18. Dentener MA, Creutzberg EC, Schols AM et al: Systemic anti-inflammatory mediators in COPD: increase in soluble interleukin 1 receptor II during treatment of exacerbations, Thorax 56:721-726, 2001.

19. Drost EM, Skwarski KM, Sauleda J et al: Oxidative stress and airway inflammation in severe exacerbations of COPD, Thorax 60:293-300, 2005.

20. Wedzicha JA, Seemungal TA, MacCallum PK et al: Acute exacerbations of chronic obstructive pulmonary disease are accompanied by elevations of plasma fibrinogen and serum IL-6 levels, Thromb Haemost 84:210-215, 2000.

21. Van Eeden SF, Tan WC, Suwa T et al: Cytokines involved in the systemic inflammatory response induced by exposure to particulate matter air pollutants (PM10), Am J Respir Crit Care Med 164:826-830, 2001.

22. Vernooy JH, Kucukaycan M, Jacobs JA et al: Local and systemic inflammation in patients with chronic obstructive pulmonary disease: soluble tumor necrosis factor receptors are increased in sputum, Am J Respir Crit Care Med 166:1218-1224, 2002.

23. Takabatake N, Nakamura H, Abe S et al: The relationship between chronic hypoxemia and activation of the tumor necrosis factor-alpha system in patients with chronic obstructive pulmonary disease, Am J Respir Crit Care Med 161:1179-1184, 2000.

24. Rabinovich RA, Figueras M, Ardite E et al: Increased tumour necrosis factor-alpha plasma levels during moderate-intensity exercise in COPD patients, Eur Respir J 21:789-794, 2003.

25. Couillard A, Maltais F, Saey D et al: Exercise-induced quadriceps oxidative stress and peripheral muscle dysfunction in patients with chronic obstructive pulmonary disease, Am J Respir Crit Care Med 167:1664-1669, 2003.

26. Koechlin C, Couillard A, Cristol JP et al: Does systemic inflammation trigger local exercise-induced oxidative stress in COPD? Eur Respir J 23:538-544, 2004.

27. American Thoracic Society, European Respiratory Society: Skeletal muscle dysfunction in chronic obstructive pulmonary disease, Am J Respir Crit Care Med 159:2S-40S, 1999.

28. Schols AM: Nutrition in chronic obstructive pulmonary disease, Curr Opin Pulm Med 6:110-115, 2000.

29. Schols AM, Soeters PB, Dingemans AM et al: Prevalence and characteristics of nutritional depletion in patients with stable COPD eligible for pulmonary rehabilitation, Am Rev Respir Dis 147:1151-1156, 1993.

30. Engelen MP, Wouters EF, Deutz NE et al: Effects of exercise on amino acid metabolism in patients with chronic obstructive pulmonary disease, Am J Respir Crit Care Med 163:859-864, 2001.

31. Engelen MP, Schols AM, Does JD et al: Exercise-induced lactate increase in relation to muscle substrates in patients with chronic obstructive pulmonary disease, Am J Respir Crit Care Med 162:1697-1704, 2000.

32. Schols AM, Wouters EF: Nutritional abnormalities and supplementation in chronic obstructive pulmonary disease, Clin Chest Med 21:753-762, 2000.

33. Baarends EM, Schols AM, Slebos DJ et al: Metabolic and ventilatory response pattern to arm elevation in patients with COPD and healthy age-matched subjects, Eur Respir J 8:1345-1351, 1995.

34. Amoroso P, Wilson SR, Moxham J et al: Acute effects of inhaled salbutamol on the metabolic rate of normal subjects, Thorax 48:882-885, 1993.

35. Sridhar MK. Why do patients with emphysema lose weight? Lancet 345:1190-1191, 1995.

36. Sauleda J, García-Palmer FJ, Wiesner R et al: Cytochrome oxidase activity and mitochondrial gene expression in skeletal muscle of patients with chronic obstructive pulmonary disease, Am J Respir Crit Care Med 157:1413-1417, 1998.

37. Gosker HR, Wouters EF, Van der Vusse GJ et al: Skeletal muscle dysfunction in chronic obstructive pulmonary disease and chronic heart failure: underlying mechanisms and therapy perspectives, Am J Clin Nutr 71:1033-1047, 2000.

38. Sauleda J, Noguera A, Busquets X et al: Systemic inflammation during exacerbations of chronic obstructive pulmonary disease: lack of effect of steroid treatment, Eur Respir J 14:359s, 1999.

39. Li YP, Schwartz RJ, Waddell ID et al: Skeletal muscle myocytes undergo protein loss and reactive oxygen-mediated NF-kappaB activation in response to tumor necrosis factor alpha. FASEB J 12:871-880, 1998.

40. Agustí AGN, Sauleda J, Miralles C et al: Skeletal muscle apoptosis and weight loss in chronic obstructive pulmonary disease, Am J Respir Crit Care Med 166:485-489, 2002.

41. Lanone S, Mebazaa A, Heymes C et al: Muscular contractile failure in septic patients: role of the inducible nitric oxide synthase pathway, Am J Respir Crit Care Med 162:2308-2315, 2000.

42. Yende S, Waterer GW, Tolley EA et al: Inflammatory markers are associated with ventilatory limitation and muscle dysfunction in obstructive lung disease in well functioning elderly subjects, Thorax 61:10-16, 2006.

43. Broekhuizen R, Wouters EF, Creutzberg EC et al: Raised CRP levels mark metabolic and functional impairment in advanced COPD, Thorax 61:17-22, 2006.

44. Pinto-Plata VM, Mullerova H, Toso JF et al: C-reactive protein in patients with COPD, control smokers and non-smokers, Thorax 61:23-28, 2006.

45. Roca J, Whipp BJ, Agustí AGN et al: ERS Task Force: Clinical exercise testing with reference to lung diseases: indications, standardization and interpretation strategies, Eur Respir J 10:2662-2689, 1997.

46. Bigard AX, Sanchez H, Birot O et al: Myosin heavy chain composition of skeletal muscles in young rats growing under hypobaric hypoxia conditions, J Appl Physiol 88:479-486, 2000.

47. Jakobsson P, Jorfeldt L, Brundin A: Skeletal muscle metabolites and fibre types in patients with advanced chronic obstructive pulmonary disease (COPD), with and without chronic respiratory failure, Eur Respir J 3:192-196, 1990.

48. Cucina A, Sapienza P, Corvino V et al: Nicotine-induced smooth muscle cell proliferation is mediated through bFGF and TGF-beta 1, Surgery 127:316-322, 2000.

49. Broal P: Main features of structure and function. In Broal P, editor: The central nervous system, New York, 1992, Oxford University Press, pp 5-50.

50. Kamischke A, Kemper DE, Castel MA et al: Testosterone levels in men with chronic obstructive pulmonary disease with or without glucocorticoid therapy, Eur Respir J 11:41-45, 1998.

51. Gayan-Ramirez G, Vanderhoydonc F, Verhoeven G et al: Acute treatment with corticosteroids decreases IGF-1 and IGF-2 expression in the rat diaphragm and gastrocnemius, Am J Respir Crit Care Med 159:283-289, 1999.

52. Decramer M, De Bock V, Dom R: Functional and histologic picture of steroid-induced myopathy in chronic obstructive pulmonary disease, Am J Respir Crit Care Med 153:1958-1964, 1996.

53. Decramer M, Lacquet LM, Fagard R et al: Corticosteroids contribute to muscle weakness in chronic airflow obstruction, Am J Respir Crit Care Med 150:11-16, 1994.

54. Landbo C, Prescott E, Lange P et al: Prognostic value of nutritional status in chronic obstructive pulmonary disease, Am J Respir Crit Care Med 160:1856-1861, 1999.

55. Jones PW: Issues concerning health-related quality of life in COPD, Chest 107(Suppl):187S-193S, 1995.

56. Lacasse Y, Wong E, Guyatt GH et al: Meta-analysis of respiratory rehabilitation in chronic obstructive pulmonary disease, Lancet 348:1115-1119, 1996.

57. Griffiths TL, Burr ML, Campbell IA et al: Results at 1 year of outpatient multidisciplinary pulmonary rehabilitation: a randomised controlled trial, Lancet 355:362-368, 2000.

58. Rennard S, Carrera M, Agustí AG: Management of chronic obstructive pulmonary disease: are we going anywhere? Eur Respir J 16:1035-1036, 2000.

59. Sin DD, Man SF: Why are patients with chronic obstructive pulmonary disease at increased risk of cardiovascular diseases? The potential role of systemic inflammation in chronic obstructive pulmonary disease, Circulation 107:1514-1519, 2003.

60. Dinh-Xuan AT, Higenbottam TW, Clelland CA et al: Impairment of endothelium-dependent pulmonary-artery relaxation in chronic obstructive lung disease, N Engl J Med 324:1539-1547, 1991.

61. Howes TQ, Deane CR, Levin GE et al: The effects of oxygen and dopamine on renal and aortic blood flow in chronic obstructive pulmonary disease with hypoxemia and hypercapnia, Am J Respir Crit Care Med 151:378-383, 1995.

62. Baudouin SV, Bott J, Ward A et al: Short term effect of oxygen on renal haemodynamics in patients with hypoxaemic chronic obstructive airways disease, Thorax 47:550-554, 1992.

63. Bassuk SS, Rifai N, Ridker PM: High-sensitivity C-reactive protein: clinical importance, Curr Probl Cardiol 29:439-493, 2004.

64. de Torres JP, Cordoba-Lanus E, Lopez-Aguilar C et al: C-reactive protein levels and clinically important predictive outcomes in stable COPD patients, Eur Respir J 27:902-907, 2006.

65. Mathur R, Cox IJ, Oatridge A et al: Cerebral bioenergetics in stable chronic obstructive pulmonary disease, Am J Respir Crit Care Med 160:1994-1999, 1999.

66. Wagena EJ, Huibers MJ, Van Schayck CP: Antidepressants in the treatment of patients with COPD: possible associations between smoking cigarettes, COPD and depression, Thorax 56:587-588, 2001.

67. Takabatake N, Nakamura H, Minamihaba O et al: A novel pathophysiologic phenomenon in cachexic patients with chronic obstructive pulmonary disease: the relationship between the circadian rhythm of circulating leptin and the very low—frequency component of heart rate variability, Am J Respir Crit Care Med 163:1314-1319, 2001.

68. Holden RJ, Pakula IS, Mooney PA: An immunological model connecting the pathogenesis of stress, depression and carcinoma, Med Hypotheses 51:309-314, 1998.

69. Incalzi RA, Caradonna P, Ranieri P et al: Correlates of osteoporosis in chronic obstructive pulmonary disease, Respir Med 94:1079-1084, 2000.

70. Engelen MP, Schols AM, Lamers RJ et al: Different patterns of chronic tissue wasting among patients with chronic obstructive pulmonary disease, Clin Nutr 18:275-280, 1999.

71. Schols AM, Slangen J, Volovics L et al: Weight loss is a reversible factor in the prognosis of chronic obstructive pulmonary disease, Am J Respir Crit Care Med 157:1791-1797, 1998.

72. Celli BR, Cote CG, Marin JM et al: The body-mass index, airflow obstruction, dyspnea, and exercise capacity index in chronic obstructive pulmonary disease, N Engl J Med 350:1005-1012, 2004.

73. Sin DD, Lacy P, York E et al: Effects of fluticasone on systemic markers of inflammation in chronic obstructive pulmonary disease, Am J Respir Crit Care Med 170:760-765, 2004.

74. Huiart L, Ernst P, Ranouil X et al: Low-dose inhaled corticosteroids and the risk of acute myocardial infarction in COPD, Eur Respir J 25:634-639, 2005.

75. Calverley PM, Anderson JA, Celli B et al: Salmeterol and fluticasone propionate and survival in chronic obstructive pulmonary disease, N Engl J Med 356:775-789, 2007.

76. Decramer M, Rutten-Van MM, Dekhuijzen PN et al: Effects of N-acetylcysteine on outcomes in chronic obstructive pulmonary disease (Bronchitis Randomized on NAC Cost-Utility Study, BRONCUS): a randomised placebo-controlled trial, Lancet 365:1552-1560, 2005.

77. Bathon JM, Martin RW, Fleischmann RM et al: A comparison of etanercept and methotrexate in patients with early rheumatoid arthritis, N Engl J Med 343:1586-1593, 2000.

78. Ferreira IM, Brooks D, Lacasse Y et al: Nutritional support for individuals with COPD: a meta-analysis, Chest 117:672-678, 2000.

79. Agustí A, Morla M, Sauleda J et al: NF-KB activation and iNOS upregulation in skeletal muscle of patients with COPD and low body weight, Thorax 59:483-487, 2004.

80. Anker SD, Negassa A, Coats AJ et al: Prognostic importance of weight loss in chronic heart failure and the effect of treatment with angiotensin-converting—enzyme inhibitors: an observational study, Lancet 361:1077-1083, 2003.

81. Meyers BF, Yusen RD, Guthrie TJ et al: Results of lung volume reduction surgery in patients meeting a National Emphysema Treatment Trial high-risk criterion, J Thorac Cardiovasc Surg 127:829-835, 2004.

82. Agustí AG: COPD, a multicomponent disease: implications for management, Respir Med 99:670-682, 2005.

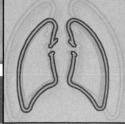

Chapter 5

Dyspnea: Assessment and Management

VIRGINIA CARRIERI-KOHLMAN • DORANNE DONESKY-CUENCO

CHAPTER OUTLINE

Mechanisms of Dyspnea
  Physiologic Mechanisms
  Perception of Dyspnea
Measurement of Dyspnea
  Reasons to Measure Dyspnea
  Timing and Measurement
  Clinical Measurements
  Monitoring Symptoms
  Language of Breathlessness
  Measurement of the Affective
    Dimension of Dyspnea
  Minimal Clinically Important Difference
**Diagnostic Approach to the Patient
  with Dyspnea: Procedures
  and Methods**

Diseases and Clinical States
    Presenting with Dyspnea
Patient History
Physical Examination
Laboratory Evaluation
Symptomatic Treatments for Dyspnea
  Reducing the Sense of Effort and
    Improving Muscle Function
  Decrease Respiratory Drive to Breathe
  Alter Central Perception
  Exercise Training Alone or with
    Pulmonary Rehabilitation
  Exercise Training Is Critical
Conclusion

PROFESSIONAL SKILLS

On completion of this chapter, the reader will be able to do
the following:
* Define dyspnea
* Discuss the physiologic and multifactorial causes of dyspnea
* Identify components of the patient history and physical examination that can be used to differentiate
  the diagnostic cause(s) of dyspnea
* Describe two methods to measure dyspnea: one method that can be used during exercise and one
  method to determine dyspnea with activities of daily living
* Describe a program of strategies that could be used to assist patients in managing acute and chronic
  dyspnea

Despite optimal medical and pharmacologic therapy, at one time or another most individuals with cardiopulmonary disease will experience acute or chronic progressive dyspnea (shortness of breath).[1] Dyspnea may be considered part of the warning system for human beings to know when they are at risk for receiving inadequate ventilation. The symptom attains clinical importance when it occurs at a level of activity that is unacceptably low for the individual.

Dyspnea has been identified as an important outcome and evaluation measure of pulmonary rehabilitation.[2,3]

Dyspnea (Greek *dys*, meaning painful, difficult, and *pneuma*, meaning breath) is a clinical term for shortness of breath or breathlessness. The consensus statement from the American Thoracic Society[4] offers the following definition:

> Dyspnea is a term used to characterize a subjective experience of breathing discomfort that is comprised of qualitatively distinct sensations that vary in intensity. The experience derives from interactions among multiple physiological, psychological, social and environmental factors, and may induce secondary physiological and behavioral responses.

This description extends the more physiologic perspective of the earlier definition of "...difficult or labored breathing rated by the patient himself..."[5] to that of a symptom that may be influenced by psychological and social factors resulting in physiologic and behavioral responses. It also provides evidence that strategies that may be expected to modulate the symptom of dyspnea can target other dimensions of the symptom experience beyond the physiologic domain, including cognitive, emotional, sensory, and behavioral dimensions.

MECHANISMS OF DYSPNEA

Considerable progress has been made in the understanding of the causes of dyspnea.[6] It is clear that dyspnea is not one sensation, but many and that the different types of perceived respiratory sensations relate to some extent to different types of physiologic stimuli from different pathophysiologic changes.[7,8]

In general, three primary categories of breathing discomfort have been identified: (1) *air hunger*—the need to breathe more, that is, unsatisfied inspiration; (2) *work/effort*—the sensation of exerting muscular effort or force in the act of breathing; and (3) *chest tightness*—a sensation usually associated with bronchospasm and asthma.[9-13] *Depth and frequency of breathing*[7] and *unsatisfied inspiration*[9] are two other categories that have been proposed to describe the experience of breathlessness.

Respiratory sensations arise from various stimuli. Broad categories of physiologic stimuli or mechanisms include (1) increased ventilatory demand and drive to breathe, (2) increased ventilatory impedance and required respiratory effort,

and (3) altered central perception of dyspnea.[4] These broad categories encompass obstructive diseases, such as COPD and asthma, and restrictive diseases, such as interstitial lung diseases and obesity. Other physiologic stimuli include exercise, breath holding, and hypoxia. Effort or increased movement of the chest wall is not the only cause for dyspnea, but the respiratory center also must be stimulated for dyspnea to occur.[8] It is still unclear whether there is a final common pathway for these sensations.

Unlike localized sensations, such as touch or pain, which arise from peripheral stimulation, dyspnea is a visceral sensation somewhat analogous to hunger or nausea, sensations that are experienced as a result of central neural activity.[7] The sensation is generated through a complex series of processes involving an individual's conscious awareness of the respiratory motor command to the ventilatory muscles, and the activation of sensory receptors, including chest wall, pulmonary vagal, irritant, and chemoreceptors.[4,11]

Physiologic Mechanisms
Respiratory Muscles
Respiratory muscles and the chest wall play an important role in the generation of dyspnea. Factors that necessitate an increasing motor command to achieve a certain tension in the muscles, such as decreasing muscle force with hyperinflation or increasing muscle weakness, trigger a higher sense of respiratory effort. There is a conscious awareness of the outgoing respiratory motor command to the respiratory muscles.[4] This separate sense of "respiratory effort" has been attributed to a "corollary discharge" from the motor cortex or brain stem respiratory neurons to the sensory cortex.[14,15] It is thought that the brain expects a certain ventilatory response according to the afferent information it receives from the central nervous system. When the response of the respiratory muscles does not match the afferent information coming to the brain, this represents a "mismatch" or "neuroventilatory disassociation,"[16] resulting in the sensation of dyspnea.

Chest Wall Receptors
Projections to the brain of afferent signals from mechanoreceptors in the joints, tendons, and muscles of the chest all shape the type of respiratory sensations. In experimental studies, constraints on lung volume and chest vibration have demonstrated that afferents from intercostal

muscles,[17] and muscle[18] and chest wall receptors[19] all have a prominent role in the generation of dyspnea. Further evidence for this mechanism is the decrease in experimentally induced dyspnea with stimulation of the chest wall with external vibration.[20,21]

Pulmonary Vagal Receptors

Afferent information from pulmonary vagal receptors can stimulate the respiratory center and sensory cortex, which detect reductions in tidal volume that produce air hunger without feedback from chest wall receptors.[22,23] Vagal blockade has been shown to ameliorate dyspnea both in exercise and breath holding.[24,25] Dyspnea associated with bronchoconstriction has also been found to be mediated in part by airway receptors.[26]

Chemoreceptors

Dyspnea can be experienced even in the absence of signals coming from the respiratory muscles. For example, carbon dioxide (CO_2) breathing can elicit dyspnea in experimentally paralyzed normal subjects[27] or in individuals with high-level spinal cord transection.[28] There is evidence that dyspnea may be directly affected by input from chemoreceptors, with studies showing that increased partial pressure of carbon dioxide produces air hunger in subjects paralyzed with neuromuscular blocking agents.[29] Additional evidence of the independent role of chemoreceptors in the generation of dyspnea is provided by studies showing that the administration of oxygen (O_2) reduces dyspnea out of proportion to that expected in the reduction of ventilation,[30] and that the sensation of dyspnea is more intense at a given level of ventilation produced by hypercapnia compared with ventilation achieved by exercise or voluntary hyperventilation.[31]

Perception of Dyspnea
Factors That Affect the Perception of Dyspnea

In the pulmonary rehabilitation setting, it is always important to remember that, as with all symptoms, other factors also influence the individual's perception of dyspnea. Psychosocial factors that influence the perception of dyspnea include cognitive variables such as personality,[32] emotions including anxiety[33,34] and depression,[35-38] attention to the symptom,[39] the meaning of the symptom for the person,[40] and beliefs in coping

strategy effectiveness.[41,42] Social–environmental influences, including prior history with the symptom, the social context in which it is experienced,[43] family support,[44] and symptoms such as fatigue,[45,46] also influence the perception of shortness of breath. Bodily preoccupation, usual level of physical activity, weight, state of nutrition, ethnicity,[47] and medications may also influence the perception of intensity or distress of dyspnea.[7]

Affective Dimension

Laboratory studies of mechanisms and clinical studies of treatments for dyspnea have placed greater emphasis on the sensory dimension of dyspnea. However, dyspnea is not simply a sensation; it is a multidimensional symptom that is shaped by individual perception, appraisal, and interpretation influenced by biopsychosocial factors such as those listed previously. As a subjective symptom rated only by the patient, the relationship between a patient's rating of dyspnea and the severity of the disease varies greatly. Dyspnea, like pain, is associated with affective feelings, such as anxiety, unpleasantness, panic, and depression, as well as with components such as intensity, duration, location, and quality.[33,48,49] Growing evidence of an "unpleasant" or "distressing" dimension of dyspnea is derived from clinical and research observations. These include patients' actual descriptions of affective emotions, such as the anger and anxiety they feel during episodes of shortness of breath,[44,46] the synergistic cycle of anxiety and shortness of breath observed in both acute and chronic clinical situations, the reported influence of anxiety on dyspnea in patients with acute dyspnea,[34] and the ability of patients to differentiate the intensity of experienced dyspnea from the anxiety and distress they are feeling.[48,50]

Techniques for imaging brain function, including positron emission tomography[51-56] and functional magnetic resonance imaging, have been applied to dyspnea perception in healthy subjects and provide more evidence that emotions are triggered when dyspnea is perceived.[57] Despite the use of markedly different methods when healthy volunteers experienced air hunger in the laboratory, strong activation of the anterior insular cortex, a limbic structure, was observed.[53,58,59] This is the first neurologic evidence that emotions are activated when healthy subjects experience air hunger and that there is an affective dimension to the sensation of dyspnea.

MEASUREMENT OF DYSPNEA

Reasons to Measure Dyspnea

Dyspnea is a major symptom that has been recommended as an outcome measure in the evaluation of pulmonary rehabilitation programs.[3] The two primary purposes for measuring dyspnea are to differentiate patients who have less dyspnea from those who have more (discriminative) and to determine whether the dyspnea has changed over time or has responded to new therapies (evaluative).[9] Other reasons for measuring a patient's shortness of breath or perceived dyspnea are as follows:

- Ratings of the subjective symptom of dyspnea provide a different dimension not provided by laboratory physiologic measurements, such as pulmonary function and incremental or endurance exercise tests.[60-62]
- Clinical measurements of dyspnea influence and predict general health status to a greater extent than do physiologic measurements.[63,64]
- Measurements of dyspnea during daily activities and after a paced walk test relate well to quality of life measurements.[65,66]
- A baseline rating of dyspnea can be used to determine the type and intensity of exercise treatments and as a guide for determining an exercise prescription.[67]
- Symptom reduction is a goal and an expected outcome of the pulmonary rehabilitation program; therefore it is important to measure dyspnea at baseline and at the end of the pulmonary rehabilitation program to determine whether the dyspnea has changed over time.[3,68]

Timing and Measurement

In the pulmonary rehabilitation setting, dyspnea is assessed either in "real time" or by recall of the level of dyspnea the patient experiences during activities. The ideal time to assess the impact of dyspnea on the patient's life is during a baseline interview. While taking a dyspnea history, the dimensions of the symptom experience—including persistence or variability of the symptom, the sensations, location, aggravating factors or triggers, individual strategies used to manage shortness of breath, and use of medications for alleviating the symptom—should be determined to help the clinician understand the meaning of the symptom for the individual patient and heighten the patient's awareness of triggers, while reinforcing the strategies that they are using to manage their shortness of breath.[46]

Patients may be unaware of factors that precipitate dyspnea (e.g., altitude, foods, medications, allergens, obesity, or severe weight loss) or relieve their dyspnea (e.g., position, medications, breath control) for them. An initial "dyspnea interview" during the history and physical examination is an excellent time to determine the extent of the consequences of the symptom on functional status, social and role relationships, and quality of life.[46] This also is a time to ask patients about the words they usually use to describe shortness of breath or uncomfortable breathing.

Ideally, real-time dyspnea should be measured at baseline during exercise testing with an incremental or endurance treadmill, cycle ergometer test, or 6-minute or shuttle walk test to assess the level of dyspnea the patient experiences with a specific amount of exercise (work). These exercise tests used to measure the level of dyspnea have been discussed extensively elsewhere.[3,9,69,70] Determining the level of dyspnea during laboratory exercise testing also provides a baseline of symptom severity that can be used to evaluate the patient's progress through the intensive and maintenance phases of the program.

Knowledge about the symptom at baseline can assist the health care provider in formulating an individual treatment plan for each patient. Severity of illness is most often used to determine an exercise prescription; however, the individualized treatment program, including type and modality of exercise, frequency, and level of intensity of exercise, is also determined with consideration of the patient's rating of dyspnea with exercise and daily activities. It has been shown that patients can be taught to remember the intensity of shortness of breath during laboratory exercise testing as a "dyspnea target" to monitor the intensity of their exercise training during walks at home.[71]

Clinical Measurements

Multidimensional instruments used to measure recalled dyspnea during activities, and unidimensional instruments to measure real-time dyspnea during exercise testing, have been extensively described and evaluated for psychometric properties elsewhere[4,72-74]; therefore the discussion of specific instruments in this chapter is limited to situations in which the instrument may be used and a brief description of the unique purpose of the instrument.

There are certain specific measurement issues to keep in mind when deciding the instruments to be used to measure dyspnea or other subjective outcomes of pulmonary rehabilitation. The suggested requirements for a valid clinical dyspnea instrument are that the instrument be a subjective report by the patient, be multidimensional, be simple to use, be responsive to therapy, and have an established minimal clinically important difference.[9] In addition, the American Thoracic Society/European Respiratory Society pulmonary rehabilitation statement recommends that additional technical issues should be considered when selecting a questionnaire to measure outcomes for the rehabilitation setting, including length of time to complete the questionnaire, whether it is completed by the patient or health care provider, cost, complexity of scoring, and whether written permission is needed.[3] It is important to remember that generic measures are typically less responsive than disease-specific measures of outcomes.[75-77]

Clinically the simplest, yet least sensitive, method to measure dyspnea is to ask the patient whether he or she is short of breath with activities. This yes-or-no categorical measurement, which gives no information about the severity or quality of the symptom, is frequently used in the clinical setting to assess dyspnea. More informative for measuring the intensity of dyspnea are the unidimensional scales that have been tested and validated and can be compared with patient outcomes in other programs.

Unidimensional Instruments

Unidimensional instruments are most frequently used during exercise testing to determine the amount and change in dyspnea with an increasing workload. They can also be used by the patient to monitor dyspnea during exercise treatments as part of a log/diary completed after daily walks or activities.[82]

Although the exact stimulus for dyspnea during an exercise test is unknown, the common understanding is that the work or power production, usually measured in watts, O_2 consumption, or both, is the "stimulus" for provoking dyspnea during exertion.[83] Typically the patient points to a number on a scale at discrete measurement times. Mahler and colleagues[84] have reported a continuous method of measuring dyspnea during exercise tests. The advantages of this method include the following: (1) the perception of dyspnea may change throughout the course of exercise rather than at certain set time intervals and (2) the

continuous method enables patients to provide about twice the number of dyspnea ratings. This is important if the patient is able to exercise only for a short period. The validity and responsiveness of this continuous measurement have been established in healthy adults and patients with COPD.[85]

Patients with symptomatic COPD can be taught to use both heart rate and dyspnea to monitor the intensity of daily exercise with one of the unidimensional instruments. Horowitz and colleagues[86,87] have shown that patients with COPD were able to use dyspnea ratings and heart rate to accurately and reliably produce an expected exercise intensity reached in the laboratory.[71]

Two unidimensional instruments have been extensively tested and used for measuring dyspnea during exercise; the Visual Analog Scale (VAS) and the modified Borg Scale. An additional scale, the Numeric Rating Scale (NRS), has not received as much testing[7,88]; however, it is the most frequently used scale in measuring other symptoms such as pain, and given its ease and quality of comprehension by older people, it is expected that this scale will gain more favor in the future.

Visual Analog Scale. The VAS is a vertical or horizontal line most commonly 10 cm or 100 mm in length with anchors to indicate extremes of the sensation. Subjects indicate the intensity of their dyspnea by pointing to or marking a line at the level of their dyspnea.[89,90] Although investigators have used various end points it is recommended that anchors at the bottom and top should be "No Breathlessness" and "Worst Imaginable Breathlessness." Concurrent validity with the modified Borg Scale is high ($r > .90$), indicating that either of these scales can be used to rate dyspnea and the findings can be compared with those of others.[91,92] The VAS is reproducible at the same level of exercise and at maximal exercise[93,94] and is sensitive to treatment effects.[95] Although most clinicians use the vertical VAS, the correlation between a horizontal and vertical VAS is high at $r = .97$, and therefore either could be used.[89] The major advantage of the VAS is that it is more sensitive to changes in dyspnea than is the Borg Scale.

Modified Borg Scale for Breathlessness. The modified Borg Scale for Breathlessness is a 10-point category ratio (CR-10) scale with a nonlinear scaling scheme and descriptive terms to anchor responses (Figure 5-1). It was originally developed for perceived exertion[96,97] and subsequently revised for shortness of breath.[98] This scale is strongly correlated with the VAS ($r = .99$),[91] minute ventilation

Modified Borg Scale	
0	None at all
0.5	Very, very slight (just noticeable)
1	Very slight
2	Slight
3	Moderate
4	Somewhat severe
5	Severe
6	
7	Very severe
8	
9	Very, very severe
10	Maximal (worst possible you can imagine)

FIGURE 5-1 Modified Borg Scale for Breathlessness, with dyspnea descriptors.

0	Not troubled with breathlessness except with strenuous exercise.
1	Troubled by shortness of breath when hurrying or walking up a slight hill.
2	Walks slower than people of the same age due to breathlessness or has to stop for breath when walking at own pace on the level.
3	Stops for breath after walking ~100 m or after a few minutes on the level.
4	Too breathless to leave the house or breathless when dressing or undressing.

FIGURE 5-2 Medical Research Council Breathlessness Scale (MRC).

(r = .98), and O_2 consumption during exercise (r = .95),[99] and is moderately correlated with peak expiratory flow rates and arterial oxygen saturation in patients in the emergency department.[100] Advantages of the modified Borg Scale are that conceptually, with the use of numbers, it is more understandable for older patients than the "open-ended" VAS; that is, the descriptors may help patients in selecting the sensation intensity and direct comparisons between individuals may be more valid. However, the sensitivity of the scale may be blunted by "ceiling effects" triggered by the verbal descriptors and patients may tend to choose the numbers only on the basis of the descriptors. The scale used to measure perceived exertion during exercise in healthy people and in patients during cardiac rehabilitation is similar to the Borg scale for breathlessness shown in Figure 5-1; however, the questions and descriptors are different. Therefore the "perceived exertion" scale should not be used to measure dyspnea.

Medical Research Council Breathlessness Scale. One of the oldest discriminative clinical instruments is the Medical Research Council Breathlessness Scale (MRC). Over the years different versions of this instrument have been published.[73,101] At the present time a five-point scale is used. Patients rate the level of exercise at which they are short of breath, such as at rest or walking on the level with others (Figure 5-2). The MRC has gained favor as a simple discriminative measure of "functional dyspnea" levels[102,103] because it can be used to categorize patients according to the severity of their dyspnea and it is predictive of health-related quality of life[104] and survival.[105] Until recently, the testing of the MRC has been minimal. Earlier studies found the

instrument to have test–retest and inter-rater reliability[106] and content validity.[105,107] The MRC is less than ideal when used as an evaluative instrument, to determine differences between groups or changes in dyspnea with a treatment because the grades are broad and not as discrete; therefore it lacks the sensitivity for small changes with medical treatments or new patient strategies. Celli and colleagues[108] have combined the level of dyspnea measured by the MRC with the body mass index, forced expiratory volume in 1 second expressed as a percentage of the predicted value (FEV_1% predicted), and distance on the 6-minute walk test (6MWT) and constructed the BODE Index, a 10-point scale in which higher scores indicate a higher risk of death. This index has been found to be more predictive of pulmonary rehabilitation outcomes and survival than any of the factors alone.

Multidimensional Instruments

The following questionnaires can be used to measure dyspnea, the impact of dyspnea on daily activities and functional performance, or both (Table 5-1).

Baseline/Transitional Dyspnea Index and Chronic Respiratory Disease Questionnaire. The Baseline/Transitional Dyspnea Index (BDI/TDI) and Chronic Respiratory Disease Questionnaire (CRQ) are evaluative instruments widely used to achieve a more comprehensive assessment of dyspnea and the impact of the symptom on functional status.[9] The BDI/TDI measures functional impairment (the degree to which activities of daily living are impaired), magnitude of effort (the overall effort exerted to perform activities), and the magnitude of task that provokes breathing difficulty. The TDI measures changes in dyspnea compared with a baseline state. The focus is on the activity consequences of the individual's

TABLE 5-1 Clinical Instruments for Measuring the Intensity of Dyspnea			
	Grades	**Year of Publication**	**MCID**
Unidimensional Instruments			
Pneumoconiosis Research Unit Dyspnea Questionnaire	1-4	1952	
Medical Research Council Breathlessness Scale (MRC)	1-5	1959	
Visual Analog Scale (VAS)	1-100 mm	1969	10-20 mm
Oxygen Cost Diagram	mm on line	1978	
WHO Dyspnea Questionnaire	1-4	1982	
ATS Dyspnea Scale	0-4	1982	
Modified Borg Scale for Breathlessness	0, 0.5, 1-10	1982	2 units
Breathlessness component of Breathlessness, Cough, and Sputum Scale (BCSS)		2003	>1 = substantial 0.6 = moderate 0.3 = small
Multidimensional Instruments			
Baseline Dyspnea Index (BDI)	0-12	1984	NA
Transition Dyspnea Index (TDI)	−9 to +9	1984	1 unit
Dyspnea component of Chronic Respiratory Disease Questionnaire (CRQ)	1-5	1987	0.5 unit
UCSD Shortness of Breath Questionnaire (SOBQ)	0-120	1998	5 units
Self-administered computerized BDI/TDI	0-12 (BDI)	2004	1 unit
Self-administered CRQ	1-5	2003	0.5 unit
Pulmonary Functional Status and Dyspnea Questionnaire (PFSDQ, PFSDQ-M)	0-10	1994, 1998	
St. George's Respiratory Questionnaire (SGRQ)	0-100	1991	4 units

ATS, *American Thoracic Society;* MCID, *minimal clinically important difference;* MRC, *Medical Research Council;* NA, *not applicable;* WHO, *World Health Organization.*
Modified from Mahler DA: Mechanisms and measurement of dyspnea in chronic obstructive pulmonary disease, Proc Am Thorac Soc 3:236-238, 2006.

breathlessness.[109] The CRQ is a 20-item self-report questionnaire that measures four dimensions of health status: dyspnea, fatigue, emotional function, and mastery of breathing.[110] For the CRQ dyspnea component, the patient rates the level of dyspnea he/she has with five activities. Both of these instruments have been shown to be valid, reliable, and responsive.[73] The responsiveness of the TDI and the CRQ dyspnea component to treatments for breathlessness including bronchodilator therapy, pulmonary rehabilitation, and inspiratory muscle training has been shown in a number of studies.[111-119] Both of these original instruments were developed as an interview, requiring the time for a health care provider to question the patient. More recently, both instruments have been developed into self-administered instruments so that the dyspnea scores appropriately represent the self-report of the patient. These paper-and-pencil or computerized versions are highly correlated with the previous interview versions.[120-123]

University of California, San Diego Shortness of Breath Questionnaire and Pulmonary Functional Status and Dyspnea Questionnaire. Two other multidimensional instruments are useful in monitoring a patient's symptom trajectory over time and tracking the loss of activities with increasing dyspnea. The University of California, San Diego Shortness of Breath Questionnaire (SOBQ) asks patients to rate their shortness of breath on a 6-point scale, from 0 ("not at all") to 5 ("maximally or unable to do because of breathlessness"), during 21 activities of daily living.[124] Three additional questions ask about fear of harm from overexertion, limitations caused by shortness of breath, and fear caused by shortness of breath.[116] The advantages of the SOBQ are that it has been tested in the large

National Emphysema Treatment Trial,[125] correlates with other measures of shortness of breath such as the dyspnea component of the CRQ, and specifically measures shortness of breath with each activity for the person.

The Pulmonary Functional Status and Dyspnea Questionnaire (PFSDQ) is a self-administered instrument that rates dyspnea with 79 activities in 6 categories: self-care, mobility, eating, home management, social, and recreational.[126] The modified shorter version (the PFSDQ-M) measures dyspnea associated with 10 activities and includes a fatigue component. Dyspnea is also measured, separately from activities, with five items.[127] The shorter PFSDQ-M has moderate test–retest reliability (r = .83), high internal consistency (α = .94), and is responsive to change after pulmonary rehabilitation.[128] The advantages of this instrument are that it is sensitive to small changes in dyspnea with activities and can be used over time to monitor an individual patient's dyspnea with activities.

St. George's Respiratory Questionnaire. A questionnaire that measures health-related quality of life or health status and symptoms, but not specifically the symptom of dyspnea, is the St. George's Respiratory Questionnaire (SGRQ). It is a disease-specific quality of life self-administered questionnaire listing 53 questions measuring 3 areas of illness: symptoms, activity, and impact of disease on daily life. The symptoms category elicits information about four symptoms: cough, sputum, wheeze, and dyspnea. These are combined for a symptoms score.[129] Test–retest reliability of the questionnaire is r = .92,[130] the instrument is responsive to treatments,[131] and thresholds of significant clinical change are reported.[132] Advantages of this instrument are that it is self-administered, has been used extensively, and has computerized scoring. One disadvantage is that dyspnea is not measured as a separate symptom; therefore the dyspnea response to rehabilitation cannot be measured as a separate outcome with this instrument.

Monitoring Symptoms

Dyspnea with changing activities, treatments, or emotional situations can be monitored with a daily log filled out by the patient.[133,134] Diaries or logs may improve adherence to a treatment regimen because they provide the patient with patterns of triggers and symptoms, as well as his or her response to therapies.[134] Daily symptom monitoring also provides more accurate reflection

of symptoms than recall during a weekly or monthly visit.[135] Monitoring dyspnea may result in more appropriate self-regulatory behaviors.[136] Examples of diaries have been published and can be used to develop an ongoing monitoring system for patients.[134]

One instrument that measures daily dyspnea and has had adequate psychometric testing is the Breathlessness, Cough, and Sputum Scale (BCSS), which measures the severity of three respiratory symptoms.[137] Patients evaluate each symptom/item on a five-point Likert-type scale, ranging from 0 to 4, with higher scores indicating a more severe manifestation of the symptom. The BCSS is internally consistent (α = .70 daily and 0.95-0.99 over time), and there is evidence of concurrent, convergent, divergent, and discriminant validity. The instrument was reproducible in a stable situation and responsive to change.[138]

Language of Breathlessness

People use different words to describe their dyspnea, and these descriptors may vary with the type of disease process or ethnicity.[47,78] The variety of words patients use to describe the sensations they feel when they are short of breath has been studied.[78] For example, the three most common phrases chosen from a list of 15 items by 85 patients with COPD were "My breathing requires effort" (85%), "I feel out of breath" (49%), and "I cannot get enough air in" (38%).[9] Mahler, Harver, and Lentine[79] found that patients often chose unique descriptors depending on their diagnosis (e.g., asthma with "work/effort" and "tight"; interstitial lung disease with "work/effort" and "rapid" breathing). Although descriptor choices have been found to be different between health and disease states, as yet there is not sufficient sensitivity or construct validity to support the use of word descriptors and clusters to help determine a diagnosis.[11,80,81] However, when the measurement of descriptors is useful for the clinician or researcher, a standardized instrument to measure various descriptors of dyspnea has been tested and is available for use.[11,12]

Measurement of the Affective Dimension of Dyspnea

In the palliative care phase of the illness trajectory, when the treatment is not expected to bring about changes in the physiologic causes of dyspnea, it is important to measure the anxiety or distress associated with dyspnea in addition to the intensity of the symptom. At the completion of education and exercise training, patients have reported that they have the same shortness of breath but that they are able to control it and therefore have less distress with the symptom in daily life.[139] Rather than the intensity of the symptom, anxiety or distress with dyspnea may decrease after treatments, such as pulmonary rehabilitation or exercise training. Both healthy subjects[140] and patients with COPD who are exercising[50] or completing daily self-reports[141] can distinguish the intensity of their shortness of breath from the anxiety and/or distress it causes them; however, to date there is little consensus as to whether the dimension of anxiety or distress should be measured or what is the most valid method to measure the affective dimension. The VAS and modified Borg Scale have been used to measure the "distress" felt by patients experiencing dyspnea during exercise, by asking the patients to rate their response to the following questions: "How anxious are you about your shortness of breath?" or "How bothersome or distressing is your shortness of breath to you?"[139] Others have been asked to complete daily self-report measures of breathing distress[141] or to rate their anxiety on a VAS anchored by "no anxiety" and "worst possible anxiety."[142] Other investigators have measured state anxiety, defined as "situational anxiety" with the State-Trait Anxiety Inventory,[143] during times that patients with COPD were acutely short of breath.[34,144]

Minimal Clinically Important Difference

A newer measurement concept that should be considered by the clinician is the minimal clinically important difference (MCID), defined as the smallest difference that a patient perceives to be beneficial.[145] This "clinically significant difference" may be larger than a statistically detectable change. Investigators developing instruments to measure dyspnea and health-related quality of life have been at the forefront in determining clinical differences for instruments used in pulmonary rehabilitation. Various approaches are used to determine the MCID, and to date there is not one method that is considered the most valid.[146,147] More important for clinical practice and for measuring outcomes related to dyspnea, the following MCIDs have been recommended for the instruments discussed previously: the threshold for significant clinical change for the Chronic Respiratory Disease Questionnaire (CRQ) is 0.5 unit per question[148-150]; for the UCSD Shortness of Breath Questionnaire (SOBQ) it is 5 units[151]; for the St. George's Respiratory Questionnaire it is 4 points[132,152]; for the TDI, a change of 1 unit is clinically significant[153]; and a mean change greater than 1.0 in the BCSS total score represents substantial symptomatic improvement, changes of approximately 0.6 can be interpreted as moderate, and changes of 0.3 are considered small.[138]

DIAGNOSTIC APPROACH TO THE PATIENT WITH DYSPNEA: PROCEDURES AND METHODS

Diseases and Clinical States Presenting with Dyspnea

The correct diagnosis is important before beginning pulmonary rehabilitation. Although patients with almost any disease may benefit from rehabilitation, it is vital that they are receiving appropriate care for their underlying disease. The diagnostic approach to dyspnea can be thought of in terms of diseases imposing mechanical limitations on the respiratory system, diseases producing increased drive to breathe, and diseases affecting the central perception of the symptom. Many diseases (e.g., asthma) fall into more than one category. Therefore in the diagnostic process one may eventually test for evidence of disease affecting all three categories. As described previously in the discussion of mechanisms, diseases that mechanically interfere with ventilation result in increases in the work and effort of breathing, whether because of narrowing of the airways, changes in the elasticity of the lungs or chest wall, weakened respiratory muscles, or vocal cord dysfunction. If respiration is stimulated (e.g., by acidosis or hypoxia), the increased respiratory drive is perceived centrally by the patient as dyspnea. Abnormalities of ventilation–perfusion matching (e.g., pulmonary emboli) cause dyspnea directly through their secondary physiologic effects (e.g., hypoxemia, bronchospasm, or fall in cardiac output). Any of the emotions or moods that have been cited previously for their relationship to the perception of dyspnea may exaggerate dyspnea from any cause, as well as be the primary cause of dyspnea.

Patient History

Clinical assessment of dyspnea should include a complete history of the symptom as outlined in the previous section. The seven dimensions of a symptom include its temporal onset (acute, sub-acute, or chronic); variability of the symptom; aggravating factors including ambulation, eating, and position; its qualities; any associated symptoms; previous response to medications or other relieving strategies; and its impact on the patient's psychosocial and functional status.[154-156] A history of smoking, underlying lung or cardiac disease or other concurrent medical conditions, allergy history, and details of previous medications or treatments should also be recorded.[157,158]

It is helpful to inquire whether the patient's dyspnea changes with position.[156] *Orthopnea*, difficulty breathing while lying flat, is common with symptomatic congestive heart failure, mitral valvular disease, and superior vena cava syndrome, but rare in people with emphysema, severe asthma, chronic bronchitis, and neurologic diseases. *Platypnea*, difficulty breathing while sitting up and relieved by lying flat, is rare, but it does occur in patients after pneumonectomy, and in patients with cirrhosis, hypovolemia, or some neurologic diseases. *Trepopnea*, in which patients are more comfortable breathing while lying on one side, occurs in people with congestive heart failure or a large pleural effusion.[2,156] Studies have shown that patients universally respond to breathlessness by decreasing their activity to whatever degree necessary. It is therefore helpful to ask about shortness of breath in relation to activities, using the MRC described previously or one of the available multidimensional instruments that measure the level of dyspnea with activities. It is also important to quantify the amount of exercise, or lack thereof, that is needed for the person to become breathless as this will provide a baseline for comparison to assess progression or improvement.[156]

Physical Examination

It is important to remember that dyspnea, like pain, is a subjective experience that may not be evident to the examiner. Often the patient's assessment of dyspnea must be accepted without measurable physical correlates. However, a physical examination may provide vital clues to diagnosis: respiratory rate, body habitus (e.g., cachexia or obesity), posture, use of pursed lips breathing, use of accessory muscles, and emotional state. For example, the health care provider may assume that a patient is short of breath if the individual is tachypneic; however, a rapid respiratory rate is not a measure of dyspnea. Abnormal chest expansion may suggest restriction or severe hyperinflation. Cough on inspiration or expiration may suggest obstructive or interstitial lung disease. Decrease in the intensity of breath sounds may suggest emphysema, pneumothorax, or pleural effusion. Forced expiration may uncover focal or diffuse wheezing. The cardiac examination may suggest pulmonary hypertension (e.g., right ventricular heave, increased pulmonic sound) or right ventricular failure (e.g., jugular venous distention, hepatojugular reflux, pedal edema). Clubbing may be associated with many processes, notably cancer. Lower extremity edema suggests congestive failure if symmetric, and thromboembolic disease if asymmetric.

Laboratory Evaluation

Choice of the appropriate test to diagnose the cause and extent of dyspnea in the rehabilitation setting should be guided by the stage of disease, by the prognosis, by the risk-to-benefit ratios of any test, and by communication with the patient and family. The clinical laboratory is often not helpful in the diagnosis of dyspnea. Anemia may be a clue to occult bleeding or serious systemic problems. Polycythemia may suggest chronic hypoxemia. The white blood cell count differential may indicate infection. Abnormal serum calcium, potassium, magnesium, and phosphate levels may impair the function of the respiratory muscles.[159] Elevation of the sedimentation rate may suggest occult inflammation in the lungs but is insensitive for inflammatory disease of the interstitium.[160] Laboratory testing may reveal unsuspected renal disease or metabolic acidosis. Arterial blood gases may reveal unexpected hypoxemia or hypercapnia.[161]

A newer test, measurement of brain natriuretic peptide (BNP), is finding wide acceptance in the differential diagnosis of acute dyspnea.[162,163] The hormone is secreted by the ventricle in response to elevated ventricular pressure. It is, therefore, usually elevated in patients with left ventricular failure or cor pulmonale and not in patients with exacerbations of obstructive lung disease. It has been shown to be more accurate in the immediate differential diagnosis than echocardiography in recognizing left ventricular dysfunction as a cause of acute dyspnea.[164]

The database should include chest radiographs, spirometry, and an electrocardiogram. If appropriate, radiologic examinations may also include a ventilation–perfusion scan, computed tomography (CT) scan, CT angiogram, magnetic resonance imaging, or an echocardiogram.[7] Classic findings that are of help include hyperinflation, parenchymal infiltration, and pleural disease. Less obvious findings may include early indications of interstitial lung disease (e.g., decreases in lung volume or subtle increases in lung density). Although the yield of "routine" electrocardiography is low, it may reveal previously unsuspected coronary artery disease or even pulmonary hypertension (i.e., signs of right ventricular hypertrophy or strain).

Spiral CT scanning of the chest with iodinated contrast is replacing ventilation–perfusion lung scanning as the screening procedure of choice for the diagnosis of pulmonary embolic disease.[165,166] Gallium and high-resolution CT scanning are sensitive but not specific for occult infectious (e.g., *Pneumocystis carinii*) and inflammatory (e.g., interstitial pneumonitis) lung disease.[167,168] If exercise testing suggests cardiac dysfunction, echocardiography, radionuclide scanning, or even cardiac catheterization (preferably combined with supine exercise) may identify unsuspected wall motion abnormalities, valvular disease, or pulmonary hypertension.[169,170] An echocardiogram may reveal mitral valve prolapse, a rare cause of occult dyspnea, even with normal hemodynamics.[171]

O_2 saturation can be measured noninvasively with a pulse oximeter. Pulse oximeters are reasonably accurate (±3%) at high saturations but less accurate below saturations of about 80%.[172] O_2 saturation also gives no indication as to whether the patient is not getting enough O_2 because of anemia or is retaining CO_2.

Although pulmonary function tests are critical for the diagnosis of dyspnea, the degree of abnormality in tests of respiratory function correlates only moderately with severity of dyspnea.[173] Spirometry, including FEV_1 and forced vital capacity (FVC), are excellent screening tests for both obstructive and restrictive disease, although both may be normal despite significant asthma or interstitial fibrosis. Maximal inspiratory and expiratory measurements can be helpful in assessing respiratory muscle strength but are dependent on patient effort. Measures of maximal expiratory pressure ($r = .35$) and maximal inspiratory pressure (PImax) ($r = .34$) are strongly correlated with the intensity of dyspnea measured by the Baseline Dyspnea Index (BDI). In patients with asthma, FVC ($r = .78$) and FEV_1 ($r = .77$) were

highly related to dyspnea and in interstitial lung disease, PImax ($r = .51$) and FVC ($r = .44$) showed significant correlations with breathlessness.[106] Others have found that maximal voluntary ventilation ($r = .78$), the largest volume in liters that can be breathed per minute by voluntary effort, had the greatest correlation with dyspnea in patients with COPD, with PImax ($r = .51$) and FVC ($r = .44$) again being more related to dyspnea in patients with interstitial lung disease.[174]

Cardiopulmonary exercise tests provide information additional to that gathered from lung function tests that are performed at rest. Cardiopulmonary exercise testing helps in determining whether exercise is limited by the pulmonary or cardiovascular system (or even some unrelated problem such as leg pain or fatigue). In the appropriate setting, an exercise test can distinguish a cardiac or respiratory cause for exercise limitation, quantify functional disability, and assess the response to treatment.[172] The breathing reserve (fraction of maximal ventilation not used at peak exercise) is useful in distinguishing obstructive disease from cardiac disease, even when the cardiac response is similar; in one study[175] the breathing reserve was 49.7% in the chronic heart failure group and 8.4% in the COPD group ($P < .01$). Simpler measures of exercise capacity include the 6- or 12-minute walk test and the shuttle walking test. Those taking the 6- or 12-minute walk test walk as far as they can at their own pace for 6 or 12 minutes on a set course. Walking tests correlate with measures of both dyspnea and exercise capacity.[109] In the shuttle walking test patients walk around two points at a speed that is controlled by an audiotape and progressively increased. Subjects are to continue until they cannot keep up with the tape or have to stop.[172] The shuttle walking test has been validated in comparison with the treadmill exercise test[176] and is a reproducible test of functional capacity in ambulatory patients with advanced cancer.[177] In progressive exercise testing, subjects exercise on either a cycle ergometer or treadmill with increasing workloads while various parameters are continuously measured. Modern exercise systems can provide various degrees of information to help distinguish the organ system that is limiting exercise capacity.[172] This type of assessment can be used to establish a baseline of dyspnea and exercise performance for people entering a pulmonary rehabilitation program, to identify the cause of exertional dyspnea, and to assess the effect of specific interventions or the total program.

If dyspnea is clearly unrelated to exercise, and especially if it increases with medical attention or emotional distress, psychological consultation should be sought.[178,179] Patients with chronic lung disease are prone to anxiety and symptoms of panic, and patients with panic disorder may present with dyspnea as a primary symptom. Because the symptoms of panic attacks and lung disease may overlap, determination of the primary disorder may not always be easy.[180]

SYMPTOMATIC TREATMENTS FOR DYSPNEA

For many patients entering a rehabilitation program, dyspnea still remains an incapacitating symptom after traditional medical treatment strategies have been exhausted. At this phase in the illness trajectory, treatment should focus on the symptom rather than on the disease and particularly on the specific mechanisms contributing to an individual's dyspnea.[3,4,7] Many of the interventions or treatments discussed in this chapter to treat dyspnea are presented exclusively in other chapters in this book. These include education, exercise, ventilatory muscle training, and O_2 therapy. Therefore in this chapter the discussion is limited to empirical observations and controlled clinical trials of specific interventions that focus on dyspnea as an outcome. Strategies are categorized into targeted mechanisms that include the following:

- Reducing the sense of effort and improving respiratory muscle function
- Decreasing respiratory drive to breathe
- Altering central perception
- Instituting exercise training that may target all proposed mechanisms (Box 5-1)[7]

Reducing the Sense of Effort and Improving Muscle Function

Energy Conservation and Activity Modification

Dyspnea and fatigue are related to each other and both are highly related to activity level.[46,181] Conservation of energy, activity modification, and advanced planning of activities decrease the amount of respiratory effort or minute ventilation, metabolic demand, and most probably fatigue. All these changes theoretically will decrease dyspnea. However, there is little scientific study of

---

| BOX 5-1 | Symptomatic Treatment of Dyspnea |

REDUCE SENSE OF EFFORT AND IMPROVE RESPIRATORY MUSCLE FUNCTION
- Energy conservation
- Breathing strategies
- Position
- Correcting obesity or malnutrition
- Inspiratory muscle training
- Respiratory muscle rest
- Medications

DECREASE RESPIRATORY DRIVE
- Oxygen therapy
- Opiates and sedatives
- Exercise conditioning

ALTER CENTRAL NERVOUS SYSTEM FUNCTION
- Education
- Cognitive—behavioral interventions
- Opiates and sedatives

USE EXERCISE TRAINING ALONE OR WITH PULMONARY REHABILITATION
- Enhance self-efficacy and self-confidence in ability to perform
- Improve efficiency of movement
- Desensitize dyspnea with repeated exercise (response shift)

Modified from Stulbarg MS, Adams L: Dyspnea. In Mason RJ, Broaddus VC, Murray JF et al, editors: Murray and Nadel's textbook of respiratory medicine, vol 2, ed 4, Philadelphia, 2005, WB Saunders, p 815.

---

the relationship between energy conservation and dyspnea. A study of the energy used and dyspnea experienced with and without energy conservation techniques by patients with COPD during activities of daily living found that dyspnea was significantly decreased when energy conservation techniques were used. Activities completed by the patients included personal hygiene, putting on and taking off shoes, and storing groceries on high and low shelves.[182]

Clinical practice and descriptive studies suggest that patients who are short of breath use strategies that incorporate energy conservation.[44,136,183] Strategies include the following: pacing activities; slowing down; using good posture and breathing techniques in the performance of any task; replacing hobbies and activities with others that require less effort; and advanced planning of "breathing stations" during activities.[183,184] Patients should be instructed that there is a crucial balance between pacing or resting and quality exercise, that is, the effort used for unnecessary tasks contrasted with energy that is used for a daily exercise program and leisure activities that enhance the efficiency of the muscles and the body.

Patients need help with learning advanced planning skills for almost any activity. Trips should be organized early to allow time to anticipate the availability of O_2, the elevation, the potential for triggers/irritants, the amount of energy needed, and the scheduling of rest periods. Most clinicians suggest a "daily outline," dividing the day into phases with activities and interspersed with scheduled rests. Activities can be substituted that are pleasurable but require less effort. For example, hobbies such as playing cards can be suggested as a less strenuous activity to replace the weekly golf game.

Patients can be taught to avoid unnecessary motions including minimizing steps in any task, avoiding overreaching and bending by arranging equipment closely, sitting and using good posture and body mechanics, planning hardest chores for "best breathing" times, using controlled pursed lips breathing (PLB) in performing any task, using slow smooth movements, and sitting whenever possible. Setting up proper working conditions includes working at proper work height, avoiding clutter in the work area, breaking the job down into steps, and sliding and pushing items rather than lifting. There are recommendations, published by the American Lung Association and others,[185-187] to help patients conserve energy and minimize shortness of breath during activities of daily living. If available, an occupational therapist can be consulted to provide the patient with alternative ways to complete activities of daily living with minimal shortness of breath. Specific guidelines for completing activities of daily living such as grooming, bathing, showering, dressing, sexual activity, meal preparation, and eating[188] are available to use as visual aids when teaching patients and family.[189]

Strategies for Decreasing Dyspnea During Sexual Activity

Patients who are comfortable confiding in a health professional frequently complain of experiencing shortness of breath during sexual activity. As with other activities, patients can be taught strategies to decrease energy expenditure and dyspnea during sexual activity. Suggestions include learning and practicing relaxation techniques; planning a rest period and using inhaled bronchodilators before intimacy; engaging in massage to relax tense muscles; exploring alternative expressions of love; using supplemental O_2; timing sexual relations to take place before meals and after resting; choosing less active positions for the partner with lung disease that do not require supporting the body with arms, or that do not put pressure on the chest or abdomen[190,191] (see Chapter 18 for a complete discussion of this topic).

Breathing Strategies

Pursed Lips Breathing. Clinically, some patients report that using PLB during periods of acute dyspnea or during activities of daily living is the most effective strategy that they have for controlling their shortness of breath. PLB decreases respiratory rate (RR), increases tidal volume (V_T) and vital capacity (VC), improves respiratory muscle recruitment, improves gas exchange, increases efficiency of ventilation, and reduces dyspnea.[192-195] Most notably, a group of investigators measured lung volumes noninvasively and found that PLB significantly reduced dyspnea by decreasing end-expiratory lung volume, caused by decreasing RR and lengthening expiratory time.[196] All of these changes in the pattern of breathing, lung volumes, and oxygenation may reduce the respiratory effort and decrease dyspnea for an individual patient.[192,194,197] Teaching the method of correct PLB, emphasizing a deeper slow breath, relaxed facial muscles, and long exhalation, is a fundamental component of education in pulmonary rehabilitation programs.[3]

Abdominal Breathing. To date, only physiologic measures have been used to investigate the effect of diaphragmatic and abdominal breathing techniques on pulmonary function. In these studies the duration of treatment, type of technique, and length of measurement time varied considerably. Collectively, investigators found an increase in vital capacity and a decrease in RR, functional residual capacity, and O_2 consumption.[198,199] Presumably these changes in lung function would result in a concomitant decrease in dyspnea. In contrast various investigators have studied the effect of diaphragmatic breathing on thoracoabdominal motion and found that this technique increases asynchronous and paradoxic breathing in patients with COPD.[200,201] Focusing on the movement of the lower rib cage, rather than on the abdomen, may minimize paradoxic breathing.[202] The true effect of abdominal and diaphragmatic breathing on dyspnea remains unknown.[203,204]

Alter Breathing Patterns. People who are short of breath have a tendency to take shallow breaths at a rapid rate.[205,206] This type of breathing pattern increases dyspnea, and more important, it may escalate the anxiety or panic associated with increasing shortness of breath.[33,144] Helping the patient practice and develop a pattern of slow, deep breathing becomes even more significant with the evidence that dynamic hyperinflation, with resulting restriction of V_T, is the primary contributor to dyspnea during exercise.[118,207,208] Investigators have found that patients can change their rate and depth of breathing through ventilatory feedback during exercise.[209] Others have suggested that the traditional yoga pranayama technique of 4-4-8 can be modified for patients with COPD to a 4-2-7-0 pattern, that is, a count of 4 during inhalation, a count of 2 while holding the breath, with exhalation to a count of 7 while exhaling and holding the breath for a very short—almost 0—count.[210] The length of inhalation and exhalation can be modified to accommodate the patient's abilities and music or distraction can be added if the patient is unable to count or needs greater relaxation. This pattern of breathing can be practiced in walking and stair climbing to pace inspiration and expiration[211] and has been suggested as a helpful exercise to possibly reduce dynamic hyperinflation. Continual practice of this new breathing pattern, which includes reducing the respiratory rate, prolonging the expiratory time, and using a gentle forced expiration, may ultimately become unconscious and automatic for the patient.

Change Position

One of the first descriptions of people with shortness of breath changing their positions to decrease dyspnea was given in a study in which people with COPD described using "breathing stations." These stations were places where they could rest when they were short of breath.[184] During an acute episode of dyspnea, adults and children with asthma have described standing still, being "motionless," "keeping still," "staying quiet," or finding a "place to sit or lean on."[212] A position that is often helpful in reducing dyspnea for patients is the leaning forward position, either standing or sitting.[213] This postural relief was shown to be due to an improvement in the mechanical efficiency of the diaphragm and optimal functioning of the inspiratory accessory muscles.[214] The important principle for the health care provider working in pulmonary rehabilitation is to allow the patient to assume the position

in which he or she feels more breathing comfort and less shortness of breath, and include the family in these recommendations.

Strategies for Nutrition and Eating

Approximately one third of patients with COPD are underweight. Dyspnea may be increased during meal preparation and eating because of energy requirements for chewing and arm movements, the reduction in airflow while swallowing, and O_2 desaturation.[215,216] In addition, many patients who are chronically short of breath often lose their appetite and desire to eat. Nutrition repletion for cachectic patients can improve respiratory muscle strength and decrease dyspnea, although the clinical effectiveness of this therapy is not clear.[217-221] In contrast, obesity also causes breathlessness. Increased appetite due to corticosteroid use and decreased mobility are two reasons for weight gain. Helping patients to plan meals, constant encouragement to lose weight, weighing the patient at each visit, and referral to a weight loss program, dietitian, or both will help motivate patients to lose weight. Self-care strategies that can be taught to decrease dyspnea during eating are listed in Box 5-2.

Inspiratory Muscle Training

If ventilation limits exercise tolerance, then strengthening the respiratory muscles should improve ventilation and exercise performance, thereby improving dyspnea.[222] The present evidence suggests that the reduction in dyspnea results from the improvement in inspiratory muscle strength, which lowers the inspiratory pressure with each breath related to the maximal

---

BOX 5-2	**Self-Care Strategies for Decreasing Dyspnea During Eating**

- Preparing meals in advance, allowing rest time before eating
- Eating smaller portions more frequently
- Avoiding high-carbohydrate and gas-forming foods
- Assuming a body position that minimizes perceived work of breathing and using pursed-lips breathing
- Using O_2 during meals
- Using liquid supplements between meals to provide nutrition without the work of chewing
- Eating with significant others in a pleasing environment

inspiratory pressure (P_B/Pimax ratio). The effect of inspiratory muscle training (IMT) on respiratory muscle strength and dyspnea is reviewed extensively elsewhere.[223] Although the results of strength training of the inspiratory muscles are inconsistent when the level of inspiratory load has not been optimal or controlled,[224] more recent studies have shown that the use of IMT leads to significant reductions in dyspnea with daily activities.[113,225-230] The inspiratory load must be controlled to ensure training effects with an intermediate load of approximately 30% Pimax or higher.[223] Patients who benefit the most seem to be those who are severely dyspneic, have low exercise tolerance, and have minimal inspiratory muscle strength. Further evidence of benefit was shown in a meta-analysis, which concluded that IMT was of value in those patients with weakness of the respiratory muscles.[231]

Noninvasive Positive Airway Pressure

In a meta-analysis, it was found that noninvasive ventilatory support during exercise relieved dyspnea and improved exercise performance in patients with COPD.[232] Nasal pressure support ventilation for 2 hours for 5 consecutive days also decreased dyspnea at rest in nonintubated patients with COPD.[233] However, the benefits of reduction in dyspnea from chronic use of partial ventilatory support were not found in one controlled 3-week trial of partial ventilatory support, with stable, severely hypercapnic patients with COPD who did not improve their pulmonary function or dyspnea.[234] Patient tolerance of the available devices is a major problem.[235,236]

Bronchodilators

For people with COPD, the intensity of activity-related dyspnea is closely related to the degree of dynamic hyperinflation during exercise.[80,207,237] Bronchodilators reduce small airway smooth muscle tone, thereby improving lung emptying and allowing the dynamically determined end-expiratory lung volume to decline to a level closer to relaxation volume with each breath during exercise. Improvement in dyspnea after bronchodilators has been shown to be related to increased resting inspiratory capacity, enhancing the patient's ability to increase V_T.[117] Short-acting β_2-agonists have been shown to be related to significant reductions in breathlessness during exercise; however, there are no published studies on the effect of these medications on dyspnea with daily activities.[208,238] Seven randomized controlled trials (RCTs) have reported reductions in dyspnea measured by the Transition Dyspnea Index (TDI) after a trial of salmeterol.[239] Both short-acting and long-acting anticholinergic bronchodilators have been shown to decrease dyspnea more than placebo drugs. Randomized clinical trials with large samples have found that long-acting tiotropium bromide decreased dyspnea, measured by the TDI, significantly more than a placebo group and beyond the MCID for the TDI of 1 unit.[111,112,117,240] Three RCTs showed that inhaled corticosteroids generally reduced the severity of dyspnea as measured by the TDI in patients with COPD.[241,242]

Patients need to be encouraged to take an active role in the manipulation of complex medical regimens and action plans. The dosage and frequency of medications may need to be altered without prior contact with their health care provider. Using a combination of written action plans, medical review, and self-monitoring, with the support of the physician and nurse and an objective physiologic measure of lung function, such as a peak flowmeter, patients with asthma can learn to manipulate their dose of bronchodilators, medication regimens, and corticosteroid therapy until they are able to contact their clinician. Controlled studies of medication self-management with patients with asthma have resulted in a decrease in symptoms,[243] decreased resource use,[244] and improved quality of life.[245] Studies of self-management programs for patients with COPD that have included either a prescription or a supply of antibiotics have decreased health care utilization, which might be assumed to be a result of decreased symptoms.[246,247]

Decrease Respiratory Drive to Breathe

Oxygen Therapy

Because dyspnea is so closely related to respiratory drive, treatments that can reduce the drive (e.g., O_2 and opiates) may reduce dyspnea. O_2 can reduce carotid body output[248] and the ventilatory response to exercise.[249-251] Conflicting evidence exists about whether O_2 has a direct central effect on dyspnea apart from its effect on ventilation mediated through the carotid bodies.[30,99,252-254] Beneficial effects of O_2 on dyspnea that are unrelated to reduction in respiratory drive may include effects on ventilatory muscle function[255] and pulmonary artery pressure.[256]

The dose of O_2 should be titrated to prevent desaturation.[257] Higher doses may be more beneficial for dyspnea during exercise.[249,256] Patients need to learn to vary the dose depending on activity and level of symptom. In one systematic review of 19 crossover controlled studies, 14 found significant relief of dyspnea in patients with COPD using various flow rates of ambulatory O_2 (2-6 L/minute) during exercise.[258] Two crossover controlled studies with small samples found significant relief of dyspnea in patients with interstitial lung disease, using the same varied flow rates of ambulatory O_2 during exercise.[259,260]

Patients need to be supported in the therapeutic, behavioral, and emotional tasks needed to manage an O_2 prescription. Despite similarities in medical prescriptions, there is often wide variability in how patients use their O_2. Patients should be asked about their current regimen to assess proper adherence to flow changes with activities. Home safety measures, such as keeping O_2 tubing out of major traffic pathways, and not using oxygen near an open flame or in areas where others are smoking, should be emphasized during pulmonary rehabilitation sessions.

Medications

Opiates and Sedatives. Although most trials of opiates have demonstrated benefits for the treatment of dyspnea,[261-264] longitudinal placebo-controlled outpatient studies have shown inconsistent benefits and some undesirable side effects.[264-268] A systematic review examined 18 randomized double-blind controlled trials and found that in the studies of non-nebulized routes of administration there was statistically strong evidence for a small effect of oral and parenteral opioids for the treatment of breathlessness.[269] This review and others[270] have not found evidence for the use of nebulized opiates for dyspnea management in patients with COPD or cancer.

Although results of controlled studies discourage routine use of opiates for stable outpatients, they may still be appropriate for treatment of dyspnea in carefully selected patients with far advanced disease.[271] It is important to educate such patients about the risks and side effects that they may encounter, so that they and their family may make informed decisions. A dyspnea management plan for palliative care patients is available and includes an algorithm and guidelines for the initiation and titration of opioids for the management of dyspnea. Although not directly used in a pulmonary rehabilitation program, this plan for opiate use in palliative care can be discussed with patients and families with other topics, such as the use of advance directives.[272]

Anxiolytic Therapy. Centrally acting pharmacologic agents have a limited role in the treatment of dyspnea. Although controlled studies of patients with COPD have shown no benefit of anxiolytics,[155,268,273,274] they may still be useful in controlling dyspnea in carefully selected patients when anxiety is known to trigger their dyspnea.[275,276] Buspirone, a nonbenzodiazepine anxiolytic, did decrease dyspnea and improve exercise tolerance in one study with a sample of patients with COPD.[277] It is important to determine whether anxiety or dyspnea is the primary symptom by asking the patient "Which sensation do you feel first?" or "Which sensation triggers the other?"

Antidepressants. Little information is available about antidepressants and dyspnea, but a small case series suggested that sertraline, a serotonin reuptake inhibitor, in doses of 25 to 100 mg/day may be useful in the treatment of dyspnea, even in patients who are not otherwise considered candidates for antidepressant therapy.[278] The mechanism of improvement was not clear but was thought possibly to be related to impact on mood or anxiety. In two cases of dyspnea caused by fibromyalgia, an antidepressant, amitriptyline, was found to be effective for both dyspnea and other symptoms of the disease.[279]

Decrease Afferent Stimuli from Peripheral Receptors

Chest Wall Vibration. Stimulation of the chest wall with external vibration can lessen experimentally induced dyspnea.[20,21] The vibration must be given in phase with inspiration. This form of vibration was found to reduce the breathing discomfort of breath holding but not that of exercise. The value in clinical practice of applying in-phase vibration to the chest wall is still unknown.

Inhaled Opiate Therapy. On the basis of the concept of opiate receptors in the airways, inhalation of opiates has been examined as a way of relieving dyspnea without the side effects of systemic administration. Although earlier studies showed positive results,[280,281] subsequent controlled studies have shown disappointing results for exercise performance and dyspnea.[270,282-284] The findings are contradictory at best, but anecdotal reports are sufficient to justify a trial in patients with terminal illness and intolerance of oral or subcutaneous delivery.[7,285] Optimal doses are uncertain; therefore, individual titration to symptom relief without unacceptable side effects is required.

Fans. People with chronic dyspnea have described their use of fans or fresh air as one strategy for managing dyspnea.[46] In the laboratory, cool air on the face has decreased dyspnea in healthy volunteers in response to hypercapnia and inspiratory resistive loads.[286] Although this modality has not been tested in pulmonary patients, cool air or a fan can be suggested as strategies for managing dyspnea.[287,288]

Alter Central Perception

Education

Although considered essential as a foundation for behavior change and knowledgeable self-management, the effects of education alone for patients with COPD without exercise training are considered minimal.[116,289,290] The few self-management programs for COPD that include only education and limited skills training have not significantly improved symptoms.[291-296] However, empirical evidence has shown that patients with lung disease need information about the pattern of illness expected, medications and O_2, and dyspnea self-management strategies to improve their quality of life and reduce reliance on the health care system. A program of dyspnea management, including relaxation, breathing retraining, pacing self-talk, and panic control without an exercise component, was compared with general health education; neither measure alleviated dyspnea or improved the 6MWT distance.[292] Programs for patients with COPD that have provided self-management education, action plans, prescriptions for antibiotics and steroids, and minimal exercise, such as a home exercise prescription, have shown reductions in health resource use but not in symptoms.[291,293] In contrast, the fact that improvements in dyspnea with activities of daily living and in functioning can be achieved from home-based exercise programs, reinforces the need to include exercise as an integral part of any symptom management program for patients with COPD.[246,297,298]

Interestingly, the positive effects of education programs on outcomes for patients with asthma have been established,[299,300] and two studies of patients with COPD and one of patients with lung cancer contradict the studies cited previously and did find improvement in dyspnea as a result of an education program without exercise. In one study a group of patients received teaching and counseling by a nurse, compared with three other groups of patients (who underwent nonspecific surveillance with psychotherapy, analytic psychotherapy from experienced psychotherapists, and supportive psychotherapy from experienced psychotherapists); the study found that the group treated by the nurse was the only one that experienced a "sustained relief in breathlessness."[301] Eight interactive small-group education-only sessions significantly decreased dyspnea with activity, measured by the CRQ, compared with untreated control subjects.[302] Another group of patients with lung cancer decreased their dyspnea more than a control group after completing a clinic-based program on dyspnea management.[303,304]

The educational component of pulmonary rehabilitation programs continues to include important self-management strategies such as early treatment of exacerbations, breathing techniques, medications, and end-of-life decision making. Regular monitoring of symptoms coupled with a clear individualized action plan for early recognition and treatment of exacerbations negotiated with a primary health care provider are essential educational components. Teaching sessions provide patients with coping and self-care strategies that can be used in the future and enhance their perception of self-efficacy, control, and mastery over their shortness of breath.[40,305-307] In patients with COPD, the increases in self-efficacy for managing dyspnea in varied situations[308] and the feelings of mastery or control of difficulty breathing[3,41,309] have an effect on the perception of dyspnea intensity or distress. Although this finding has not been tested in other pulmonary diseases, it would be expected that this would also be true with patients with other diseases.

Cognitive–Behavioral Strategies

"Self-management" strategies are typically cognitive–behavioral strategies. The cognitive–behavioral strategies presented in this chapter are theorized to alter the perception of dyspnea with or without a concomitant change in the physiologic mechanisms. The theoretical perspectives that provide the foundation for the efficacy of these strategies to modulate dyspnea include social cognitive learning theory,[310] self-management principles,[311] social support,[312] and pathophysiological[313] theories.[307] Most of these strategies do not require a medical prescription. Thus the strategies can be used by a person to manage his or her shortness of breath with varied frequency and "dose" in any situation. Managing the symptoms of a chronic illness on a daily basis requires that patients monitor their physical and emotional status and make appropriate management decisions, adhere to recommended treatment protocols, interact with health care providers, and manage the effects of their illness on emotions, relationships, and ability to function.[314] Self-care strategies learned and used by patients themselves to cope with chronic dyspnea have been described and compared across different pulmonary diseases.[42,44,183] They span every category of intervention that is listed in Box 5-1. People with chronic shortness of breath become excellent "symptom managers." They have a repertoire of management strategies for dyspnea. The patient should be asked to describe the strategies he or she has used in the past and the health care provider can then incorporate them into the self-management program.

Nonspecific effects or the placebo effect can also change the perception of the intensity or distress of dyspnea.[315,316] Several possible mechanisms are suggested as underlying the placebo effect, including expectancy that the treatment will be effective, classic conditioning, motivation, anxiety reduction, endorphin release, and response shift.[315,317-320] Response shift has been described as a change in an individual's perception of a symptom from one of three processes: a change in the person's internal standards of measurement with scale recalibration,[321] reconceptualization or giving new meaning to the symptom, or a change in the person's value system.

Distraction and Attention Coping Strategies. Cognitive–behavioral strategies have been theoretically categorized as distraction or attention strategies. Research has shown that if the symptom is relatively brief, acute distraction is more effective for alleviating distress and increasing tolerance than attention to the stressor.[322] Avoiding the noxious stimulus may provide more benefits than attention strategies if used

early after a crisis or upset. Active distraction, or removing oneself from a noxious physical sensation or from one's own reaction to it, can increase physical tolerance and modify both physiologic arousal and psychological distress. This often facilitates tolerance of and adaptation to the physical stressor.[40] During acute dyspnea, distraction is often effective in the short term because it is difficult to focus on two demands at once. Adults with asthma report using television and distancing themselves from a trigger and other stimuli to distract themselves.[46] Children report various types of distraction, including music and "walking anywhere and looking at things that are good, like flowers and trees."[323]

In general, research findings suggest that using attentional coping strategies (e.g., symptom monitoring and information seeking) to cope with chronic symptoms, such as pain, is associated with better illness adjustment, whereas using coping strategies that avoid the problem (e.g., hoping, praying, ignoring, denial, and attention diversion), results in higher levels of physical and psychological disability and poorer adjustment to illness.[324,325] Over time it is important to encourage patients to concentrate on their breathing and shortness of breath. Especially during acute episodes, patients report they need to concentrate on their breathlessness and become frustrated with suggestions of distraction.[326] Examples of attention strategies include medication regimens, action plans, and integration of breathing techniques into daily activities. The categories of attention and distraction are not mutually exclusive; attention strategies can also provide distraction and vice versa. For instance, planning an outing with a supportive group of people with COPD may be an attention strategy, but it also may provide distraction for the patient.

Relaxation Techniques. It has long been observed clinically that dyspnea and anxiety increase in a summative fashion. Previously this has been primarily a clinical observation, with anxiety increasing with increasing shortness of breath in a synergistic spiral resulting in severe shortness of breath and panic. More recently, anxiety has been associated with increasing or high-level dyspnea in a controlled trial of patients with COPD in an emergency department,[144] in patients with COPD during treadmill exercise,[327] and in patients with cancer.[328] Because they are related, strategies that decrease this anxiety or modulate the level of distress might be expected to reduce dyspnea. Relaxation may have a physiologic effect by reducing the respiratory rate and increasing V_T, thus improving breathing efficiency and dyspnea.[204] One investigator studied the effect of relaxation on dyspnea in 10 patients with COPD compared with a control group that was instructed to relax but not given specific instructions. Although dyspnea was significantly reduced for the relaxation group during treatment sessions, the scores were similar after 4 weeks.[329] In another study, relaxation techniques used by patients with COPD decreased state anxiety and the perception of dyspnea at rest.[330] In these preliminary studies immediate decreases in dyspnea did not persist outside the experimental session. They do provide beginning evidence that teaching a patient a program of relaxation to use when dyspnea increases may modulate dyspnea at the time.

Biofeedback. Technological advances in monitoring body systems represent a rapidly growing area of research, with findings being translated into clinical practice.[331,332] Patients are monitoring physiologic data, such as peak flow rate and heart rate, that are often rapidly transferred to the health care provider. In the near future there will be opportunities to use physiologic data as feedback for patients to use as a monitor of effort and goal attainment. Different types of biofeedback have been shown to reduce respiratory rate, weaning time, and paradoxical breathing, and to increase V_T and airway diameter, but up to this time dyspnea has not been targeted.[333,334] With the emphasis on dynamic hyperinflation as one of the primary mechanisms of dyspnea,[207] there is a heightened focus on helping patients change their breathing patterns.

A group of investigators[209] compared the efficacy of a 6-week, 18-session program of ventilation–feedback combined with cycle exercise, ventilation–feedback only, or exercise only on exercise endurance and breathlessness in 39 patients with COPD. The purpose of the feedback was to train patients to prolong their expiratory time and maintain V_T during exercise. The visual and auditory ventilation–feedback was an indicator of inhalation and exhalation (moving horizontal bar) presented on a screen with an audible alert when the time of expiration was met. After 6 weeks there was a significantly greater change in exercise duration in the group that received feedback during exercise compared with those who received just the ventilatory feedback. The group that received

feedback during exercise also had significant improvements in dyspnea and breathing pattern parameters, including minute ventilation, V_T, frequency, and expiratory time.

Other investigators[335] examined the feasibility and outcomes of a breathing training program designed to change the breathing pattern, using heart rate variability biofeedback and walking with pulse oximetry feedback. The major outcomes germane to this chapter were the intensity and distress accompanying breathlessness measured on the Borg Scale after the 6MWT and dyspnea with activities, measured by the modified Pulmonary Functional Status and Dyspnea Questionnaire (PFSDQ-M). Twenty patients with COPD participated in five weekly sessions of heart rate variability biofeedback, which consisted of a computer display of a pacing stimulus with which they were told to match their breathing. This feedback was then replaced by a signal showing heart rate variability, which the patient was instructed to maximize. This biofeedback and practice was followed by four weekly sessions of walking practice with oximetry and instructions to walk at home. In this observational study the respiratory rate decreased, V_T increased, and significant improvements were found in distance and dyspnea distress after the 6MWT, and in self-reported activity impairments measured by the PFSDQ-M.

Music. Listening to music affects cognitive and emotional processes, which can distract people sufficiently so that they do not attend to internal sensory information to the same extent.[336] Thornby, Haas, and Axen[337] found that at every level of treadmill exercise, perceived "respiratory effort" was lower in patients with COPD while listening to music than while listening to gray noise or silence. In a more recent study of listening to music during a home-walking program, 24 patients with COPD significantly decreased their dyspnea in week 2 after the use of music during home walking. However, over the total 5-week period there were no significant changes in anxiety or dyspnea.[338] Other investigators used a crossover design to measure the effect of music on dyspnea and anxiety experienced by 30 patients with COPD while walking in their home. Subjects walked for 10 minutes without music or for 10 minutes while listening to selected music. There was no significant difference in dyspnea or anxiety levels between when the subject walked with music and when the same subject walked without music.[339]

Guided Imagery. Guided imagery is another method of distraction that can be used in a comfortable position or while exercising. Patients are asked to allow their minds to take them to a desirable scene and focus on something other than their uncomfortable breathing. Clinically, people seem to walk longer and move through greater dyspnea levels when they use some type of guided imagery, such as when thinking about or pretending they are walking in a place they enjoy. However, in both an observational study[340] and an RCT with a sample of 26 patients with COPD,[341] the latter including 13 subjects who practiced guided imagery for six sessions and 13 control subjects, there was no significant change in dyspnea. Dyspnea in both trials was measured at rest, not during exercise.

Acupressure and Acupuncture. The true effect of acupuncture and acupressure on dyspnea cannot be understood from the few published studies with small sample sizes; however, there is enough evidence for some dyspnea relief to continue investigating this "complementary" therapy. Because studies had shown that opiates relieved dyspnea and acupuncture is thought to cause a release of endogenous opiates, Jobst and colleagues[342] hypothesized that acupuncture may relieve dyspnea and compared the effects of "traditional" and "placebo" acupuncture for 13 sessions over 3 weeks in 24 patients with COPD with breathlessness. Both groups improved their dyspnea on two different scales and at the end of the 6MWT, with the acupuncture group having significantly greater improvement than the placebo group.

Filshie and colleagues[343] studied acupuncture in 20 patients with cancer-related breathlessness. Twenty patients received four needles (two in the upper sternum and one in each hand) by an experienced acupuncturist. Needles were left in place for 90 minutes. Seventy percent of the patients reported significantly improved relief in breathlessness, anxiety, and relaxation that peaked at 90 minutes and lasted up to 6 hours. In this uncontrolled study it is not known whether this relief was due to the treatment or to the reassurance of the nurse who observed the patients for 90 minutes.

Maa and colleagues[344,345] published two studies using both acupuncture and acupressure with varying results. With a single-blind crossover design, an acupressure treatment was added to a pulmonary rehabilitation program to determine whether there was added improvement in dyspnea. Thirty-one patients with COPD practiced acupressure daily at home for 6 weeks, alternating with a "sham" acupressure for 6 weeks. Dyspnea measured on a VAS was significantly less during acupressure than during sham acupressure; however, these differences were not seen with the Borg Scale.[344] Later, Maa and colleagues[345] randomly assigned 41 patients with asthma to standard care (SC) alone, SC plus 20 acupuncture treatments, or SC plus self-administered acupressure for 8 weeks. All three groups had a slight improvement in dyspnea measured by the VAS and modified Borg Scale after 8 weeks; however, there were no significant differences within the groups or between the groups.[345]

Positive results were found by a group of Taiwanese investigators[346] who matched and randomly assigned 44 patients with COPD to true or sham acupressure for five 16-minute sessions per week for 4 weeks. The true acupressure group experienced significantly greater improvements in dyspnea, measured by the PFSDQ-M[127] and other outcome variables including 6MWT, state anxiety measured by Spielberger's State-Trait Anxiety Inventory, and O_2 saturation, than did the sham group.

Social Support. The provision of emotional and informational support (education) is proposed to buffer stress in chronic diseases,[347] influence self-management and adaptation to the illness, and improve functioning,[348,349] and may even decrease the number of exacerbations in patients with COPD through improved immune functioning.[350] In one cross-sectional survey, the intensity of recalled dyspnea was related to the number of persons in the social support network and the frequency of contact with others.[351] However, it is important to remember that the same tangible assistance, emotional interactions, or social groups may be helpful for one individual but not for another. The positive effects of social support are determined by an individual's preference for the type, amount, source, timing, and control of support sources.[347,352] Specific social support for a task is more powerful than general support. For example, social support focused on initiation or maintenance of exercise has been found to predict adherence to exercise.[353,354] Vicarious learning from other people who have experienced the same symptom and tested successful strategies to decrease the symptom is a powerful self-efficacy—enhancing experience that allows individuals to develop a shared sense of commonality, acceptance, and normalization.[355,356] Being a member of a group or attending an educational program may support the patient's change in behavior, such as smoking cessation or adherence to an exercise program.[357] Pulmonary rehabilitation programs give patients the opportunity to see that they are not alone and to learn strategies from others. It may be that the component of social support provided in pulmonary rehabilitation programs is one of the major contributors to symptom reduction and quality of life improvement.[358]

On the other hand, some patients with dyspnea prefer to isolate themselves, and they begin to limit their interactions with friends and family.[359] Patients may actually benefit from isolating themselves from others in certain acute situations. Failure of patients with COPD to adequately use withdrawal during acute episodes of shortness of breath was associated with an increase in symptoms and psychological deterioration.[359] People with COPD have suggested that health care providers and family might permit them to withdraw and isolate themselves when experiencing severe dyspnea.[326]

Exercise Training Alone or with Pulmonary Rehabilitation

Comprehensive pulmonary rehabilitation programs typically include many or all of the therapeutic interventions listed in Box 5-1. This combination of interventions has been shown in *all* RCTs to result in improvement in dyspnea during laboratory exercise and with activities of daily living.[3,289,360]

Exercise Training Is Critical

Exercise training appears to be the critical component for improving dyspnea.[3,116,289,361] The goal of exercise training is to transfer and maintain the improvement in performance and dyspnea that is achieved with supervised exercise in the PR program (e.g., treadmill walking, cycling, or both) to activities of daily living. With no definitive studies of a dose response with the outcome of dyspnea, the optimal length of the program continues to be a question.[289,362] A meta-analysis of 14 clinical trials strongly supported pulmonary rehabilitation programs with exercise training for at least 4 weeks for clinically and statistically significant

improvements in dyspnea with activities as measured by the CRQ.[309] Most authors suggest that programs should include a minimum of 20 sessions given at least three times per week.[3] Exercise training alone has been shown to decrease dyspnea.[139,363] Although most exercise studies have used treadmills or cycles, weight training of upper and lower limb muscles may also improve exercise performance and dyspnea.[364] Because upper extremity activity may be particularly troublesome for patients with COPD, training of these muscles may have an important impact on dyspnea with activities of daily living such as grooming.[363,365,366]

Exercise training alone has also been shown to decrease dyspnea.[139,363] Exercise training is thought to improve dyspnea by several mechanisms. Exercise training may result in true conditioning with decreased lactate production and thereby decreased stimulation of ventilation.[367] Increased mechanical efficiency (e.g., longer stride length[368]) may lower O_2 consumption and ventilation for a given activity.[116] Exercise training may decrease dyspnea even when it does not improve exercise performance or mechanical efficiency.[364] Decreases in dyspnea after exercise training that are not accompanied by changes indicative of true "conditioning" may be due to other physiologic factors such as improvement in respiratory and peripheral muscle strength,[369] lower O_2 consumption and ventilation for a given activity,[116] or changes in the pattern of breathing resulting in less dynamic hyperinflation with exercise.[3,118,370] Other theoretical explanations for a decrease in dyspnea after exercise without concomitant physiologic changes include a placebo response,[371] prior ventilatory experience,[372] a more relaxed stride,[373] a practice effect,[94] adaptation to the sensation,[374] or a response shift–type placebo effect.[320,375] One proposed alternative is desensitization or a decrease in dyspnea relative to work resulting from exposure to greater than usual dyspnea in a safe monitored environment. This exposure gives the patient an opportunity to use coping strategies and develop more effective techniques[336] and increases the person's control or self-efficacy for managing the symptom of dyspnea.[41]

People who have chronic dyspnea become skilled in knowing their exercise tolerance relative to the amount of dyspnea they will experience and seem to regulate their activity to keep the level of perceived breathlessness at the same intensity.[128,376] They can be taught to use both heart rate and dyspnea to monitor their level and length of daily exercise.[71,86,87] Patients with COPD were able to use dyspnea ratings and heart rate to accurately and reliably produce an expected exercise intensity reached in the laboratory.[71] They should be encouraged to increase their intensity of exercise while slowly experiencing higher levels of dyspnea, with reminders that it is "OK" to be breathless while exercising. Clinically, one approach to decreasing a patient's perceived dyspnea for a certain activity level has been to encourage ambulation to the point that greater than usual dyspnea occurs, while coaching the patient to use breathing strategies such as PLB. If this procedure is performed in a supportive environment with someone the patient trusts, the patient's distress associated with dyspnea decreases while confidence is gained in the ability to control the symptom through his or her own actions.[377] Coaching maneuvers to decrease the patient's perception of dyspnea while patients are exercising might include setting short-term goals, modeling breathing strategies and relaxation techniques, small incremental increases in workload or duration of exercise, distraction by guided imagery, and feedback of physiologic parameters.[378]

Complementary Types of Exercise

Exercises such as yoga or tai chi may be alternatives to aerobic or endurance training for people who are limited by severe shortness of breath. These exercises may bring about relaxation, calmness, and balance, and may promote changes in the pattern of breathing, including slow and deep breathing. Earlier studies of yoga training that used small samples, with male subjects only, showed promise that yoga training may reduce dyspnea.[379,380] An RCT with a small sample of both males and females found that a program specifically developed for patients with COPD was safe and improved the distress associated with dyspnea, functional status, and peripheral muscle strength.

CONCLUSION

Dyspnea or breathlessness is a subjective complex symptom that must be rated only by the patient. Dyspnea arises from the central processing of information relayed from the respiratory center and integrated within the psychological and intellectual makeup of the individual. It is still unclear whether there is a final common pathway for the sensation, but much has been learned from research in the last 30 years. The experience derives from interactions among multiple physiologic, psychological, social, and environmental factors, and may induce secondary physiologic and behavioral responses. It is clear that dyspnea is not one sensation but many and that nuances of it relate to some extent to the stimulus (i.e., the nature of the physiologic dysfunction). It is exacerbated by stimuli to ventilation, but correlation with physiologic dysfunction is moderate at best.

Dyspnea may be caused by diseases in virtually any organ system, whether because of interference with breathing, increased demand for breathing, or effective weakening of the respiratory pump. Diagnosis of dyspnea requires a comprehensive database that will uncover many of the causes. When the cause is not obvious, a series of studies assessing cardiopulmonary function at rest and with exercise will usually uncover a specific diagnosis. The experience of dyspnea should be assessed before the pulmonary rehabilitation program is instituted, with a "dyspnea history" interview to understand the meaning of the symptom to the patient. There are several standardized questionnaires that can be used to measure recalled dyspnea with activities of daily living. Ratings of dyspnea should also be made by the patient before, during, and after exercise training. Patients can be taught to rate their dyspnea at home during exercise to estimate an exercise goal.

Treatment of dyspnea is most effective when based on a specific diagnosis. When treatment of the underlying disease is inadequate, treatment focused on the symptom per se is just as important. The combination of education about strategies for managing dyspnea, medications, exercise training, O_2, and muscle strengthening in a pulmonary rehabilitation program helps patients control or increase their tolerance, or both, for this disabling chronic symptom (Figure 5-3).

As with other symptoms, the experience of dyspnea is affected by many factors, including education, cultural background, knowledge of the disease, emotional state, bodily preoccupation, previous experience with illness, judgment about the intensity of the activity that brings it on, and involvement in litigation (e.g., alleged industrial injury). Altering the central experience of dyspnea may be the focus of treatment even when physiologic approaches prove inadequate.

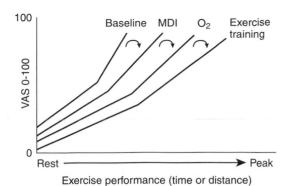

FIGURE 5-3 Relationship between dyspnea and exercise performance, dependent on type and amount of treatment. Shown are the potentially additive effects of various dyspnea treatments on the response to exercise. Bronchodilators, oxygen, and exercise training can each increase the amount of work or exercise individuals can do before reaching their maximal tolerable level of dyspnea. The relative benefit of each of these treatments would vary from individual to individual. Note that the maximal tolerable level of dyspnea tends to stay about the same. MDI, metered dose inhaler; VAS, Visual Analog Scale.

References

1. Pulmonary rehabilitation: joint ACCP/AACVPR evidence-based guidelines. ACCP/AACVPR Pulmonary Rehabilitation Guidelines Panel. American College of Chest Physicians. American Association of Cardiovascular and Pulmonary Rehabilitation, Chest 112:1363-1396, 1997, 2.
2. Mahler DA, O'Donnell DE: Lung biology in health and disease, vol. 208, ed 2: Dyspnea: mechanisms, measurement, and management, Boca Raton, Fla, 2005, CRC Press/Taylor & Francis.
3. Nici L, Donner C, Wouters E et al: American Thoracic Society/European Respiratory Society statement on pulmonary rehabilitation, Am J Respir Crit Care Med 173:1390-1413, 2006.
4. Dyspnea. Mechanisms, assessment, and management: a consensus statement. American Thoracic Society, Am J Respir Crit Care Med 159:321-340, 1999.
5. Comroe JH: Some theories of the mechanisms of dyspnea. In Howell JBL, Campbell EJM, editors: Breathlessness, Oxford, 1966, Blackwell Scientific, pp 1-7.
6. O'Donnell DE, Banzett RB et al: Pathophysiology of dyspnea in chronic obstructive pulmonary disease: a roundtable, Proc Am Thorac Soc 4: 145-168, 2007.
7. Stulbarg MS, Adams L: Dyspnea. editors: In Mason RJ, Broaddus VC, Murray JF, Nadel JA, editors: Murray and Nadel's textbook of respiratory medicine, vol 2, ed 4, Philadelphia, 2005, WB Saunders, pp 815-830.
8. Carrieri-Kohlman V, Stulbarg M: Dyspnea. In Carrieri-Kohlman V, Lindsey A, West C, editors: Pathophysiological phenomena in nursing: human responses to illness, ed 3, St. Louis, 2003, WB Saunders, pp 175-208.
9. Mahler DA: Mechanisms and measurement of dyspnea in chronic obstructive pulmonary disease, Proc Am Thorac Soc 3:234-238, 2006.
10. Demediuk BH, Manning H, Lilly J et al: Dissociation between dyspnea and respiratory effort, Am Rev Respir Dis 146:1222-1225, 1992.
11. Wilcock A, Crosby V, Hughes A et al: Descriptors of breathlessness in patients with cancer and other cardiorespiratory diseases, J Pain Symptom Manage 23:182-189, 2002.
12. Simon PM, Schwartzstein RM, Weiss JW et al: Distinguishable types of dyspnea in patients with shortness of breath, Am Rev Respir Dis 142:1009-1014, 1990.
13. Simon PM, Schwartzstein RM, Weiss JW et al: Distinguishable sensations of breathlessness induced in normal volunteers, Am Rev Respir Dis 140:1021-1027, 1989.
14. Killian KJ, Gandevia S, Summers E et al: Effect of increased lung volume on perception of breathlessness, effort and tension, J Appl Physiol 57:686-691, 1984.
15. Campbell EJM, Gandevia SC, Killian KJ et al: Changes in the perception of inspiratory resistive loads during partial curarization, J. Physiol (London) 309:93-100, 1980.
16. O'Donnell DE, Webb KA: Exertional breathlessness in patients with chronic airflow limitation: the role of lung hyperinflation, Am Rev Respir Dis 148:1351-1357, 1993.
17. Gandevia SC, Macefield G: Projection of low threshold afferents from human intercostal muscles to the cerebral cortex, Respir Physiol 77: 203-214, 1989.
18. Homma I, Obata T, Sibuya M et al: Gate mechanism in breathlessness caused by chest wall vibrations in humans, J Appl Physiol 56:8-11, 1984.
19. Altose MD, Syed I, Shoos L: Effects of chest wall vibration on the intensity of discharge during constrained breathing, Proc Int Union Physiol Sci 17:288, 1989.
20. Nakayama H, Shibuya M, Yamada M et al: In-phase chest wall vibration decreases dyspnea during arm elevation in chronic obstructive pulmonary disease patients [see comments], Intern Med 37:831-835, 1998.
21. Cristiano LM, Schwartzstein RM: Effect of chest wall vibration on dyspnea during hypercapnia and exercise in chronic obstructive pulmonary disease, Am J Respir Crit Care Med 155:1552-1559, 1997.
22. Banzett RB, Lansing RW, Brown R: High level quadriplegics perceive lung volume change, J Appl Physiol 62:567-573, 1987.
23. Manning HL, Shea SA, Schwartzstein RM et al: Reduced tidal volume increases air'hunger' at fixed PCO2 in ventilated quadriplegics, Respir Physiol 90:19-30, 1992.

24. Davies SF, McQuaid KR, Iber C et al: Extreme dyspnea from unilateral pulmonary venous obstruction: demonstration of a vagal mechanism and relief by right vagotomy, Am Rev Respir Dis 136:184-188, 1987.
25. Guz A, Noble MIM, Eisele JH et al: Experimental results of vagal block in cardiopulmonary disease. In Porter R, editor: Breathing: Hering Breuer Centenary Symposium, London, 1970, Churchill, pp 315-329.
26. Taguchi O, Kikuchi Y, Hida W et al: Effects of bronchoconstriction and external resistive loading on the sensation of dyspnea, J Appl Physiol 71:2183-2190, 1991.
27. Gandevia SC, Killian K, McKenzie DK et al: Respiratory sensations, cardiovascular control, kinaesthesia and transcranial stimulation during paralysis in humans, J Physiol (Lond) 470:85-107, 1993.
28. Banzett RB, Lansing RW, Reid MG et al: "Air hunger" arising from increased PCO2 in mechanically ventilated quadriplegics, Respir Physiol 76:53-68, 1989.
29. Banzett RB, Lansing RW, Brown R et al: "Air hunger" from increased PCO2 persists after complete neuromuscular block in humans, Respir Physiol 81:1-17, 1990.
30. Lane R, Cockcroft A, Adams L et al: Arterial oxygen saturation and breathlessness in patients with chronic obstructive airways disease, Clin Sci 72:693-698, 1987.
31. Chonan T, Mulholland MB, Leitner J et al: Sensation of dyspnea during hypercapnia, exercise, and voluntary hyperventilation, Arch Intern Med 150:1604-1613, 1990.
32. Chetta A, Gerra G, Foresi A et al: Personality profiles and breathlessness perception in outpatients with different gradings of asthma, Am J Respir Crit Care Med 157:116-122, 1998.
33. Dudgeon DJ, Lertzman M, Askew GR: Physiological changes and clinical correlations of dyspnea in cancer outpatients, J Pain Symptom Manage 21:373-379, 2001.
34. Gift AG, Plaut SM, Jacox A: Psychologic and physiologic factors related to dyspnea in subjects with chronic obstructive pulmonary disease, Heart Lung 15:595-601, 1986.
35. van Manen JG, Bindels PJ, Dekker FW et al: Risk of depression in patients with chronic obstructive pulmonary disease and its determinants, Thorax 57:412-416, 2002.
36. van Ede L, Yzermans CJ, Brouwer HJ: Prevalence of depression in patients with chronic obstructive pulmonary disease: a systematic review, Thorax 54:688-692, 1999.
37. Janson C, Bjornsson E, Hetta J et al: Anxiety and depression in relation to respiratory symptoms and asthma, Am J Respir Crit Care Med 149:930-934, 1994.
38. Nguyen HQ, Carrieri-Kohlman V: Dyspnea self-management in patients with chronic obstructive pulmonary disease: moderating effects of depressed mood, Psychosomatics 46:402-410, 2005.
39. Meek PM: Influence of attention and judgment on perception of breathlessness in healthy individuals and patients with chronic obstructive pulmonary disease, Nurs Res 49:11-19, 2000.
40. Cioffi D: Beyond attentional strategies: a cognitive—perceptual model of somatic interpretation, Psychol Bull 109:25-41, 1991.
41. Davis AH, Carrieri-Kohlman V, Janson SL et al: Effects of treatment on two types of self-efficacy in people with chronic obstructive pulmonary disease, J Pain Symptom Manage 32:60-70, 2006.
42. Janson-Bjerklie S, Ferketich S, Benner P et al: Clinical markers of asthma severity and risk: importance of subjective as well as objective factors, Heart Lung 21:265-272, 1992.
43. Pennebaker JW: Psychological factors influencing the reporting of physical symptoms. In Stone AA, Turkkan JS, Bachrach CA, Jobe JB et al, editors: The science of self-report: implications for research and practice, Mahwah, NJ, 2000, Lawrence Erlbaum Associates, pp 299-316.
44. Brown ML, Carrieri V, Janson B et al: Lung cancer and dyspnea: the patient's perception, Oncol Nurs Forum 13:19-24, 1986.
45. Meek PM, Lareau SC: Critical outcomes in pulmonary rehabilitation: assessment and evaluation of dyspnea and fatigue, J Rehabil Res Dev 40(5 Suppl 2):13-24, 2003.
46. Janson-Bjerklie S, Kohlman-Carrieri V, Hudes M: The sensations of pulmonary dyspnea, Nurs Res 35:154-159, 1986.
47. Hardie GE, Janson S, Gold WM et al: Ethnic differences: word descriptors used by African-American and white asthma patients during induced bronchoconstriction, Chest 117:935-943, 2000.
48. Price DD, Harkins SW: The affective—motivational dimension of pain: a two stage model, Am Pain Soc J 1:229-239, 1992.
49. Gracely R, McGrath P, Dubner R: Validity and sensitivity of ratio scales of sensory and affective verbal pain descriptors: manipulation of affect by diazepam, Pain 2:19-29, 1978.
50. Carrieri-Kohlman V, Gormley JM, Douglas MK et al: Differentiation between dyspnea and its affective components, West J Nurs Res 18:626-642, 1996.
51. Corfield DR, Fink GR, Ramsay SC et al: Evidence for limbic system activation during CO2-stimulated breathing in man, J Physiol 488:77-84, 1995.
52. Liotti M, Brannan S, Egan G et al: Brain responses associated with consciousness of breathlessness (air hunger), Proc Natl Acad Sci USA 98:2035-2040, 2001.
53. Banzett RB, Mulnier HE, Murphy K et al: Breathlessness in humans activates insular cortex, Neuroreport 11:2117-2020, 2000.
54. Peiffer C, Poline JB, Thivard L et al: Neural substrates for the perception of acutely induced dyspnea, Am J Respir Crit Care Med 163:951-957, 2001.
55. Brannan S, Liotti M, Egan G et al: Neuroimaging of cerebral activations and deactivations associated

with hypercapnia and hunger for air, Proc Natl Acad Sci USA 98:2029-2034, 2001.

56. Parsons LM, Egan G, Liotti M et al: Neuroimaging evidence implicating cerebellum in the experience of hypercapnia and hunger for air, Proc Natl Acad Sci USA 98:2041-2046, 2001.

57. Evans KC, Banzett RB, Adams L et al: BOLD fMRI identifies limbic, paralimbic, and cerebellar activation during air hunger, J Neurophysiol 88:1500-1511, 2002.

58. Evans K, Banzett R, McKay L et al: MRI identifies limbic cortex activation correlated with air hunger in healthy humans, FASEB J 14:A645, 2000.

59. Banzett RB, Moosavi SH: Dyspnea and pain: similarities and contrasts between two very unpleasant sensations, APS Bull 11:1-8, 2001.

60. Nguyen HQ, Altinger J, Carrieri-Kohlman V et al: Factor analysis of laboratory and clinical measurements of dyspnea in patients with chronic obstructive pulmonary disease, J Pain Symptom Manage 25:118-127, 2003.

61. Mahler DA, Harver A: A factor analysis of dyspnea ratings, respiratory muscle strength, and lung function in patients with chronic obstructive pulmonary disease, Am Rev Respir Dis 145:467-470, 1992.

62. Hajiro T, Nishimura K, Tsukino M et al: Analysis of clinical methods used to evaluate dyspnea in patients with chronic obstructive pulmonary disease, Am J Respir Crit Care Med 158:1185-1189, 1998.

63. Ries AL: Impact of chronic obstructive pulmonary disease on quality of life: the role of dyspnea, Am J Med 119(10 Suppl 1):12-20, 2006.

64. Schlecht NF, Schwartzman K, Bourbeau J: Dyspnea as clinical indicator in patients with chronic obstructive pulmonary disease, Chron Respir Dis 2:183-191, 2005.

65. Jones PW, Baveystock CM et al: Relationships between general health measured with the sickness impact profile and respiratory symptoms, physiological measures, and mood in patients with chronic airflow limitation, Am Rev Respir Dis 140:1538-1543, 1989.

66. Curtis JR, Deyo RA, Hudson LD: Pulmonary rehabilitation in chronic respiratory insufficiency. 7. Health-related quality of life among patients with chronic obstructive pulmonary disease, Thorax 49:162-170, 1994.

67. Brolin SE, Cecins NM, Jenkins SC: Questioning the use of heart rate and dyspnea in the prescription of exercise in subjects with chronic obstructive pulmonary disease, J Cardiopulm Rehabil 23:228-234, 2003.

68. Mahler D: Breathlessness in chronic obstructive pulmonary disease. In Adams L, Guz A, editors: Respiratory sensation, New York, 1996, Marcel Dekker, p 242.

69. ATS Committee on Proficiency Standards for Clinical Pulmonary Function Laboratories: ATS statement: guidelines for the six-minute walk test, Am J Respir Crit Care Med 166:111-117, 2002.

70. Sciurba F, Criner GJ, Lee SM et al: Six-minute walk distance in chronic obstructive pulmonary disease: reproducibility and effect of walking course layout and length, Am J Respir Crit Care Med 167:1522-1527, 2003.

71. Mejia R, Ward J, Lentine T et al: Target dyspnea ratings predict expected oxygen consumption as well as target heart rate values, Am J Respir Crit Care Med 159:1485-1489, 1999.

72. Carrieri-Kohlman V, Dudgeon D: Multidimensional assessment of dyspnea. In Booth S, Dudgeon D, editors: Dyspnoea in advanced disease: a guide to clinical management, New York, 2006, Oxford University Press, pp 19-37.

73. Mahler DA: Measurement of dyspnea: clinical ratings. In Mahler DA, O'Donnell DE, editors: Lung biology in health and disease, vol 208, ed 2: Dyspnea: mechanisms, measurement, and management, Boca Raton, Fla, 2005, CRC Press/Taylor & Francis, pp 147-165.

74. Mahler DA: Measurement of dyspnea ratings during exercise. In Mahler DA, O'Donnell DE, editors: Lung biology in health and disease, vol 208, ed 2: Dyspnea: mechanisms, measurement, and management, Boca Raton, Fla, 2005, CRC Press/Taylor & Francis, pp 167-182

75. Guyatt GH, King DR, Feeny DH et al: Generic and specific measurement of health-related quality of life in a clinical trial of respiratory rehabilitation, J Clin Epidemiol 52:187-192, 1999.

76. Berry MJ, Rejeski WJ, Adair NE et al: Exercise rehabilitation and chronic obstructive pulmonary disease stage, Am J Respir Crit Care Med 160:1248-1253, 1999.

77. Ries AL, Kaplan RM, Myers R et al: Maintenance after pulmonary rehabilitation in chronic lung disease: a randomized trial, Am J Respir Crit Care Med 167:880-888, 2003.

78. Schwartzstein RM: Language of dyspnea. In Mahler DA, O'Donnell DE, editors: Lung biology in health and disease, vol 208, ed 2: Dyspnea: mechanisms, measurement, and management, Boca Raton, Fla, 2005, CRC Press/Taylor & Francis, pp 115-146.

79. Mahler DA, Harver A, Lentine T: Descriptors of breathlessness in cardiorespiratory diseases, Am J Respir Crit Care Med 154:1357-1363, 1996.

80. O'Donnell DE, Bertley JC, Chau LK et al: Qualitative aspects of exertional breathlessness in chronic airflow limitation: pathophysiologic mechanisms, Am J Respir Crit Care Med 155:109-115, 1997.

81. O'Donnell DE, Chau L, Webb KA: Qualitative aspects of exertional dyspnea in patients with interstitial lung disease, J Appl Physiol 84:2000-2009, 1998.

82. Donesky-Cuenco D, Janson S, Neuhaus J et al: Adherence to a home walking prescription in patients with chronic obstructive pulmonary disease, Heart Lung 36:348-363, 2007.

83. Mahler D, Fierro-Carrion G, Baird JC: Mechanisms and measurement of exertional dyspnea. In

Weisman I, Zeballos R, editors: Progress in respiratory research, vol 32: clinical exercise testing, Basel, 2002, Karger, pp 72-80.

84. Mahler DA, Mejia-Alfaro R, Ward J et al: Continuous measurement of breathlessness during exercise: validity, reliability, and responsiveness, J Appl Physiol 90:2188-2196, 2001.

85. Harty HR, Heywood P, Adams L: Comparison between continuous and discrete measurements of breathlessness during exercise in normal subjects using a visual analogue scale, Clin Sci (Lond) 85:229-236, 1993.

86. Horowitz MB, Littenberg B, Mahler DA: Dyspnea ratings for prescribing exercise intensity in patients with COPD, Chest 109:1169-1175, 1996.

87. Horowitz MB, Mahler DA: Dyspnea ratings for prescription of cross-modal exercise in patients with COPD, Chest 113:60-64, 1998.

88. Gift AG, Narsavage G: Validity of the Numeric Rating Scale as a measure of dyspnea, Am J Crit Care 7:200-204, 1998.

89. Gift AG: Validation of a vertical visual analogue scale as a measure of clinical dyspnea, Rehabil Nurs 14:323-325, 1989.

90. Aitken RCB: Measurement of feelings using visual analogue scales, Proc R Soc Med 62:989-993, 1969.

91. Lush MT, Janson BS, Carrieri VK et al: Dyspnea in the ventilator-assisted patient, Heart Lung 17:528-535, 1988.

92. Wilson RC, Jones PW: A comparison of the Visual Analogue Scale and modified Borg Scale for the measurement of dyspnoea during exercise, Clin Sci 76:277-282, 1989.

93. Muza SR, Silverman MT, Gilmore GC et al: Comparison of scales used to quantitate the sense of effort to breathe in patients with chronic obstructive pulmonary disease, Am Rev Respir Dis 141:909-913, 1990.

94. Mador MJ, Kufel TJ: Reproducibility of Visual Analog Scale measurements of dyspnea in patients with chronic obstructive pulmonary disease, Am Rev Respir Dis 146:82-87, 1992.

95. Mahler DA, Faryniarz K, Lentine T et al: Measurement of breathlessness during exercise in asthmatics: predictor variables, reliability, and responsiveness, Am Rev Respir Dis 144:39-44, 1991.

96. Borg G: Subjective effort and physical activities, Scand J Rehabil Med 6:108-113, 1978.

97. Borg GA: Psychophysical bases of perceived exertion, Med Sci Sports Exerc 14:377-381, 1982.

98. Burdon JG, Juniper EF, Killian KJ et al: The perception of breathlessness in asthma, Am Rev Respir Dis 126:825-828, 1982.

99. Adams L, Chronos N, Lane R et al: The measurement of breathlessness induced in normal subjects: validity of two scaling techniques, Clin Sci 69:7-16, 1985.

100. Kendrick KR, Baxi SC, Smith RM: Usefulness of the modified 0-10 Borg Scale in assessing the degree of dyspnea in patients with COPD and asthma, J Emerg Nurs 26:216-222, 2000.

101. Fletcher CM, Elmes P, Fairbairn A et al: The significance of respiratory symptoms and the diagnosis of chronic bronchitis in a working population, BMJ 2:257-266, 1959.

102. Celli BR, MacNee W: ATS/ERS Task Force: Standards for the diagnosis and treatment of patients with COPD: a summary of the ATS/ERS position paper, Eur Respir J 23:932-946, 2004.

103. Bestall JC, Paul EA, Garrod R et al: Usefulness of the Medical Research Council (MRC) Dyspnoea Scale as a measure of disability in patients with chronic obstructive pulmonary disease, Thorax 54:581-586, 1999.

104. Hajiro T, Nishimura K, Tsukino M et al: A comparison of the level of dyspnea vs. disease severity in indicating the health-related quality of life of patients with COPD, Chest 116:1632-1637, 1999.

105. Nishimura K, Izumi T, Tsukino M et al: Dyspnea is a better predictor of 5-year survival than airway obstruction in patients with COPD, Chest 121:1434-1440, 2002.

106. Mahler DA, Wells CK: Evaluation of clinical methods for rating dyspnea, Chest 93:580-586, 1988.

107. Mahler DA, Rosiello RA, Harver A et al: Comparison of clinical dyspnea ratings and psychophysical measurements of respiratory sensation in obstructive airway disease, Am Rev Respir Dis 135:1229-1233, 1987.

108. Celli BR, Cote CG, Marin JM et al: The body-mass index, airflow obstruction, dyspnea, and exercise capacity index in chronic obstructive pulmonary disease, N Engl J Med 350:1005-1012, 2004.

109. Mahler DA, Weinberg DH, Wells CK et al: The measurement of dyspnea: contents, interobserver agreement, and physiologic correlates of two new clinical indexes, Chest 85:751-758, 1984.

110. Guyatt GH, Berman LB, Townsend M et al: A measure of quality of life for clinical trials in chronic lung disease, Thorax 42:773-778, 1987.

111. Casaburi R, Mahler DA, Jones PW et al: A long-term evaluation of once-daily inhaled tiotropium in chronic obstructive pulmonary disease, Eur Respir J 19:217-224, 2002.

112. Vincken W, van Noord JA, Greefhorst AP et al: Improved health outcomes in patients with COPD during 1 yr's treatment with tiotropium, Eur Respir J 19:209-216, 2002.

113. Lisboa C, Munoz V, Beroiza T et al: Inspiratory muscle training in chronic airflow limitation: comparison of two different training loads with a threshold device, Eur Respir J 7:1266-1274, 1994.

114. Martinez FJ, de Oca MM, Whyte RI et al: Lung-volume reduction improves dyspnea, dynamic hyperinflation, and respiratory muscle function, Am J Respir Crit Care Med 155:1984-1990, 1997.

115. Reardon J, Awad E, Normandin E et al: The effect of comprehensive outpatient pulmonary rehabilitation on dyspnea, Chest 105:1046-1052, 1994.

116. Ries AL, Kaplan RM, Limberg TM et al: Effects of pulmonary rehabilitation on physiologic and

psychosocial outcomes in patients with chronic obstructive pulmonary disease, Ann Intern Med 122:823-832, 1995.

117. O'Donnell DE, Fluge T, Gerken F et al: Effects of tiotropium on lung hyperinflation, dyspnoea and exercise tolerance in COPD, Eur Respir J 23:832-840, 2004.

118. O'Donnell DE, McGuire M, Samis L et al: The impact of exercise reconditioning on breathlessness in severe chronic airflow limitation, Am J Respir Crit Care Med 152:2005-2013, 1995.

119. Mahler DA, Wire P, Horstman D et al: Effectiveness of fluticasone propionate and salmeterol combination delivered via the Diskus device in the treatment of chronic obstructive pulmonary disease, Am J Respir Crit Care Med 166:1084-1091, 2002.

120. Schunemann HJ, Goldstein R, Mador MJ et al: A randomised trial to evaluate the self-administered standardised chronic respiratory questionnaire, Eur Respir J 25:31-40, 2005.

121. Williams JE, Singh SJ, Sewell L et al: Health status measurement: sensitivity of the self-reported Chronic Respiratory Questionnaire (CRQ-SR) in pulmonary rehabilitation, Thorax 58:515-518, 2003.

122. Mahler DA, Ward J, Fierro-Carrion G et al: Development of self-administered versions of modified Baseline and Transition Dyspnea Indexes in COPD, COPD 1:165-172, 2004.

123. Mahler DA, Waterman LA, Ward J et al: Validity and responsiveness of the self-administered computerized versions of the baseline (BDI) and transition dyspnea indexes, Chest, 132:1283-1290, 2007.

124. Eakin E, Sassi-Dambron D, Ries A et al: Reliability and validity of dyspnea measures in patients with obstructive lung disease, Int J Behav Med 2:118-134, 1995.

125. Ries AL, Make BJ, Lee SM et al: The effects of pulmonary rehabilitation in the National Emphysema Treatment Trial, Chest 128:3799-3809, 2005.

126. Lareau SC, Carrieri-Kohlman V, Janson-Bjerklie S et al: Development and testing of the Pulmonary Functional Status and Dyspnea Questionnaire (PFSDQ), Heart Lung 23:242-250, 1994.

127. Lareau SC, Meek PM, Roos PJ: Development and testing of the modified version of the Pulmonary Functional Status and Dyspnea Questionnaire (PFSDQ-M), Heart Lung 27:159-168, 1998.

128. Lareau SC, Meek PM, Press D et al: Dyspnea in patients with chronic obstructive pulmonary disease: does dyspnea worsen longitudinally in the presence of declining lung function? Heart Lung 28:65-73, 1999.

129. Jones PW, Quirk FH, Baveystock CM: The St George's Respiratory Questionnaire, Respir Med 85(Suppl B):25-31, discussion 33-37, 1991.

130. Jones PW, Quirk FH, Baveystock CM et al: A self-complete measure of health status for chronic airflow limitation: the St. George's Respiratory Questionnaire, Am Rev Respir Dis 145:1321-1327, 1992.

131. Jones PW, Bosh TK: Quality of life changes in COPD patients treated with salmeterol, Am J Respir Crit Care Med 155:1283-1289, 1997.

132. Jones PW: Quality of life measurement for patients with diseases of the airways, Thorax 46:676-682, 1991.

133. Janson-Bjerklie S, Shnell S: Effect of peak flow information on patterns of self-care in adult asthma, Heart Lung 17:543-549, 1988.

134. Burman ME: Health diaries in nursing research and practice, Image J Nurs Sch 27:147-152, 1995.

135. Verbrugge LM: Health diaries, Med Care 18:73-95, 1980.

136. Janson S, Reed ML: Patients' perceptions of asthma control and impact on attitudes and self-management, J Asthma 37:625-640, 2000.

137. Leidy NK, Rennard SI, Schmier J et al: The Breathlessness, Cough, and Sputum Scale: the development of empirically based guidelines for interpretation, Chest 124:2182-2191, 2003.

138. Leidy NK, Schmier JK, Jones MK et al: Evaluating symptoms in chronic obstructive pulmonary disease: validation of the Breathlessness, Cough and Sputum Scale, Respir Med 97(Suppl A):S59-S70, 2003.

139. Carrieri-Kohlman V, Gormley JM, Douglas MK et al: Exercise training decreases dyspnea and the distress and anxiety associated with it: monitoring alone may be as effective as coaching, Chest 110:1526-1535, 1996.

140. Wilson RC, Jones PW: Differentiation between the intensity of breathlessness and the distress it evokes in normal subjects during exercise, Clin Sci 80:65-70, 1991.

141. Meek PM, Lareau SC, Hu J: Are self-reports of breathing effort and breathing distress stable and valid measures among persons with asthma, persons with COPD, and healthy persons? Heart Lung 32:335-346, 2003.

142. Dudgeon DJ, Lertzman M: Dyspnea in the advanced cancer patient, J Pain Symptom Manage 16:212-219, 1998.

143. Spielberger L: STAI manual, Palo Alto, Calif, 1983, Psychologists Consultants Press.

144. Gift AG, Cahill CA: Psychophysiologic aspects of dyspnea in chronic obstructive pulmonary disease: a pilot study, Heart Lung 19:252-257, 1990.

145. Jaeschke R, Singer J, Guyatt GH: Measurement of health status: ascertaining the minimal clinically important difference, Control Clin Trials 10:407-415, 1989.

146. Make B, Casaburi R, Leidy NK: Interpreting results from clinical trials: understanding minimal clinically important differences in COPD outcomes, COPD 2:1-5, 2005.

147. Guyatt GH, Osoba D, Wu AW et al: Methods to explain the clinical significance of health status measures, Mayo Clin Proc 77:371-383, 2002.

148. Juniper EF, Guyatt GH, Willan A et al: Determining a minimal important change in a

disease-specific Quality of Life Questionnaire, J Clin Epidemiol 47:81-87, 1994.

149. Redelmeier DA, Guyatt GH, Goldstein RS: Assessing the minimal important difference in symptoms: a comparison of two techniques, J Clin Epidemiol 49:1215-1219, 1996.

150. Schunemann HJ, Puhan M, Goldstein R et al: Measurement properties and interpretability of the Chronic Respiratory Disease Questionnaire (CRQ), COPD 2:81-89, 2005.

151. Kupferberg D, Kaplan RM, Slymen DJ et al: Minimal clinically important difference for the UCSD Shortness of Breath Questionnaire, J Cardiopulm Rehabil 25:370-377, 2005.

152. Jones PW: Interpreting thresholds for a clinically significant change in health status in asthma and COPD, Eur Respir J 19:398-404, 2002.

153. Witek TJ Jr, Mahler DA: Minimal important difference of the Transition Dyspnoea Index in a multinational clinical trial, Eur Respir J 21: 267-272, 2003.

154. Dudgeon D: Multidimensional assessment of dyspnea. In Portenoy RK, Bruera E, editors: Issues in Palliative Care Research, New York, 2003, Oxford University Press, pp 83-96.

155. Man GCW, Hsu K, Sproule BJ: Effect of alprazolam on exercise and dyspnea in patients with chronic obstructive pulmonary disease, Chest 90:832-836, 1986.

156. Swartz MH: Textbook of physical diagnosis: history and examination, Philadelphia, 2002, WB Saunders.

157. Silvestri GA, Mahler DA: Evaluation of dyspnea in the elderly patient, Clin Chest Med 14:393-404, 1993.

158. Ferrin MS: Acute dyspnea, AACN Clin Issues 8:398-410, 1997.

159. Lewis MI, Belman MJ: Nutrition and the respiratory muscles, Clin Chest Med 9:337-348, 1988.

160. Turner-Warwick M, Burrows B, Johnson A: Cryptogenic fibrosing alveolitis: clinical features and their influence on survival, Thorax 35:171-180, 1980.

161. Strunk BL, Cheitlin MD, Stulbarg MS et al: Right-to-left interatrial shunting through a patent foramen ovale despite normal intracardiac pressures, Am J Cardiol 60:413-415, 1987.

162. Morrison LK, Harrison A, Krishnaswamy P et al: Utility of a rapid B-natriuretic peptide assay in differentiating congestive heart failure from lung disease in patients presenting with dyspnea, J Am Coll Cardiol 39:202-209, 2002.

163. Pesola GR: The use of B-type natriuretic peptide (BNP) to distinguish heart failure from lung disease in patients presenting with dyspnea to the emergency department, Acad Emerg Med 10:275-277, 2003.

164. Logeart D, Saudubray C, Beyne P et al: Comparative value of Doppler echocardiography and B-type natriuretic peptide assay in the etiologic diagnosis of acute dyspnea, J Am Coll Cardiol 40:1794-1800, 2002.

165. Cross JJ, Kemp PM, Walsh CG et al: A randomized trial of spiral CT and ventilation perfusion scintigraphy for the diagnosis of pulmonary embolism, Clin Radiol 53:177-182, 1998.

166. Mayo JR, Remy-Jardin M, Müller NL et al: Pulmonary embolism: prospective comparison of spiral CT with ventilation–perfusion scintigraphy, Radiology 205:447-452, 1997.

167. Santín M, Podzamczer D, Ricart I et al: Utility of the gallium-67 citrate scan for the early diagnosis of tuberculosis in patients infected with the human immunodeficiency virus, Clin Infect Dis 20:652-656, 1995.

168. Witt C, Dörner T, Hiepe F et al: Diagnosis of alveolitis in interstitial lung manifestation in connective tissue diseases: importance of late inspiratory crackles, 67 gallium scan and bronchoalveolar lavage, Lupus 5:606-612, 1996.

169. Caidahl K, Svardsudd K, Eriksson H et al: Relation of dyspnea to left ventricular wall motion disturbances in a population of 67-year-old men, Am J Cardiol 59:1277-1282, 1987.

170. Himelman RB, Stulbarg MS, Kircher B et al: Noninvasive evaluation of pulmonary pressure with exercise by Doppler echocardiography in chronic pulmonary disease, Circulation 79:863-871, 1989.

171. Vavuranakis M, Kolibash AJ, Wooley CF et al: Mitral valve prolapse: left ventricular hemodynamics in patients with chest pain, dyspnea or both, J Heart Valve Dis 2:544-549, 1993.

172. Hancox B, Whyte K: McGraw-Hill's pocket guide to lung function tests, Roseville, NSW, Australia, 2001, McGraw-Hill.

173. Killian KJ, Campbell EJ: Dyspnea and exercise, Annu Rev Physiol 45:465-479, 1983.

174. Epler GR, Sabec FA, Goensler EA: Determination of severe impairment (disability) in interstitial lung disease, Am Rev Respir Dis 121:647-659, 1980.

175. Messner-Pellenc P, Ximenes C, Brasileiro CF et al: Cardiopulmonary exercise testing: determinants of dyspnea due to cardiac or pulmonary limitation, Chest 106:354-360, 1994.

176. Singh SJ, Morgan MD, Hardman AE et al: Comparison of oxygen uptake during a conventional treadmill test and the shuttle walking test in chronic airflow limitation, Eur Respir J 7:2016-2020, 1994.

177. Booth S, Adams L: The shuttle walking test: a reproducible method for evaluating the impact of shortness of breath on functional capacity in patients with advanced cancer, Thorax 56:146-150, 2001.

178. Howell JB: Behavioural breathlessness [see comments], Thorax 45:287-292, 1990.

179. Bass C: Unexplained chest pain and breathlessness, Med Clin North Am 75:1157-1173, 1991.

180. Smoller JW, Pollack MH, Otto MW et al: Panic anxiety, dyspnea, and respiratory disease: theoretical and clinical considerations, Am J Respir Crit Care Med 154:6-17, 1996.

181. Gift AG, Pugh LC: Dyspnea and fatigue, Nurs Clin North Am 28:373-384, 1993.

182. Velloso M, Jardim JR: Study of energy expenditure during activities of daily living using and not using body position recommended by energy

conservation techniques in patients with COPD, Chest 130:126-132, 2006.

183. Carrieri V, Janson-Bjerklie S: Strategies patients use to manage the sensation of dyspnea, West J Nurs Res 8:284-305, 1986.

184. Fagerhaugh SY: Getting around with emphysema, Am J Nurs 73:94-99, 1973.

185. Petty TL, Burns M, Tiep BL: Essentials of pulmonary rehabilitation: a do it yourself guide to enjoying life with chronic lung disease, ed 2, Lomita, Calif, PERF, 2005. Available at http://www.perf2ndwind.org/Essentials.html. Retrieved March 27, 2008.

186. Carter R, Nicotra B, Tucker J et al.: Courage and information for life with chronic obstructive pulmonary disease: the handbook for patients, families and care givers managing COPD, emphysema, bronchitis, Peabody, Mass, New Technology Publishing, 2001.

187. American Association of Cardiovascular and Pulmonary Rehabilitation: Guidelines for pulmonary rehabilitation programs, Champaign, Ill, Human Kinetics, 2004.

188. Carrieri-Kohlman V: Coping strategies for the breathless patient, Eur Respir Rev 12:1-4, 2002.

189. McDonald GJ: VHI PC-Kits: Pulmonary rehabilitation CD-ROM, Tacoma, Wash, 2005, Visual Health Information.

190. Selecky PA: Sexuality in the pulmonary patient. In Hodgkin JE, Celli BR, Connors GL, editors: Pulmonary rehabilitation: guidelines to success, vol 3, Baltimore, 2000, Lippincott Williams & Wilkins, pp 317-334.

191. Tibbals S: Sexuality. In Turner JG, McDonald G, Larter N, editors: Handbook of adult and pediatric respiratory home care, St. Louis, 1994, Mosby-Year Book/Elsevier, pp 332-335.

192. Breslin EH: The pattern of respiratory muscle recruitment during pursed-lip breathing, Chest 101:75-78, 1992.

193. Mueller RE, Petty TL, Filley GF: Ventilation and arterial blood gas changes induced by pursed lip breathing, J Appl Physiol 28:784-789, 1970.

194. Tiep BL, Burns M, Kao D et al: Pursed lips breathing training using ear oximetry, Chest 90:218-221, 1986.

195. Thoman RL, Stoker GL, Ross JC: The efficacy of pursed-lips breathing in patients with chronic obstructive pulmonary disease, Am Rev Respir Dis 93:100-106, 1966.

196. Bianchi R, Gigliotti F, Romagnoli I et al: Chest wall kinematics and breathlessness during pursed-lip breathing in patients with COPD, Chest 125:459-465, 2004.

197. Tiep BL: Reversing disability of irreversible lung disease, West J Med 154:591-597, 1991.

198. Miller WF: A physiologic evaluation of the effects of diaphragmatic breathing training in patients with chronic pulmonary emphysema, Am J Med 17:471-477, 1954.

199. Campbell E, Friend J: Action of breathing exercises in pulmonary emphysema, Lancet 1:325-329, 1955.

200. Sackner MA, Gonzalez HF, Jenouri G et al: Effects of abdominal and thoracic breathing on breathing pattern components in normal subjects and in patients with chronic obstructive pulmonary disease, Am Rev Respir Dis 130:584-587, 1984.

201. Willeput R, Sergysels R: Respiratory patterns induced by bent posture in COPD patients, Rev Mal Respir 8:577-582, 1991.

202. Gigliotti F, Romagnoli I, Scano G: Breathing retraining and exercise conditioning in patients with chronic obstructive pulmonary disease (COPD): a physiological approach, Respir Med 97:197-204, 2003.

203. Dechman G, Wilson CR: Evidence underlying breathing retraining in people with stable chronic obstructive pulmonary disease, Phys Ther 84:1189-1197, 2004.

204. Gosselink R: Controlled breathing and dyspnea in patients with chronic obstructive pulmonary disease (COPD). J Rehabil Res Dev 40(5 Suppl 2):25-33, 2003.

205. Gallo-Silver L, Pollack B: Behavioral interventions for lung cancer-related breathlessness, Cancer Practice 8:268-273, 2000.

206. Kawut SM, Mandel M, Arcasoy SM: Two faces of progressive dyspnea, Chest 117:1500-1504, 2000.

207. O'Donnell DE, Revill SM, Webb KA: Dynamic hyperinflation and exercise intolerance in chronic obstructive pulmonary disease, Am J Respir Crit Care Med 164:770-777, 2001.

208. Belman MJ, Botnick WC, Shin JW: Inhaled bronchdilators reduce dynamic hyperinflation during exercise in patients with chronic obstructive pulmonary disease, Am J Respir Crit Care Med 153:967-975, 1996.

209. Collins E, Fehr L, Bammert C et al: Effect of ventilation-feedback training on endurance and perceived breathlessness during constant work-rate leg-cycle exercise in patients with COPD, J Rehabil Res Dev 40(Suppl 2):35-44, 2003.

210. Sharma V: Personal communication, 2004.

211. Frownfelter D, Massery M: Facilitating ventilation patterns and breathing strategies. In Frownfelter D, Dean E, editors: Cardiovascular and pulmonary physical therapy: evidence and practice, ed 4, St. Louis, 2006, Mosby, pp 377-404.

212. Kohlman-Carrieri V, Janson-Bjerklie S: Strategies patients use to manage the sensation of dyspnea, West J Nurs Res 8:284-305, 1986.

213. Norton LC, Neureuter A: Weaning the long-term ventilator-dependent patient: common problems and management, Crit Care Nurse 9:42-52, 1989.

214. Sharp JT, Drutz WS, Moisan T et al: Postural relief of dyspnea in severe chronic obstructive pulmonary disease, Am Rev Respir Dis 122:201-213, 1980.

215. Schols AM: Nutrition in chronic obstructive pulmonary disease, Curr Opin Pulm Med 6:110-115, 2000.

216. Brug J, Schols A, Mesters I: Dietary change, nutrition education and chronic obstructive pulmonary disease, Patient Educ Couns 52:249-257, 2004.

217. Planas M, Alvarez J, Garcia-Peris PA et al: Nutritional support and quality of life in stable chronic obstructive pulmonary disease (COPD) patients, Clin Nutr 24:433-441, 2005.

218. Goldstein SA, Thomashow B, Askanazi J: Functional changes during nutritional repletion in patients with lung disease, Clin Chest Med 7:141-151, 1986.

219. Efthimiou J, Fleming J, Gomes C et al: The effect of supplementary oral nutrition in poorly nourished patients with chronic obstructive pulmonary disease, Am Rev Respir Dis 137:1075-1082, 1988.

220. Arora NS, Rochester DF: Respiratory muscle strength and maximal voluntary ventilation in undernourished patients, Am Rev Respir Dis 126:5-8, 1982.

221. Maltais F, LeBlanc P, Jobin J et al: Peripheral muscle dysfunction in chronic obstructive pulmonary disease, Clin Chest Med 21:665-677, 2000.

222. Gandevia SC: Neural mechanisms underlying the sensation of breathlessness: kinesthetic parallels between respiratory and limb muscles, Aust N Z J Med 18:83-91, 1988.

223. Lisboa C, Borzone G: Inspiratory muscle training. In Mahler D, O'Donnell DE, editors: Lung biology in health and disease, vol. 208, ed 2: Dyspnea: mechanisms, measurement, and management, Boca Raton, Fla, 2005, CRC Press/Taylor & Francis, pp 321-344.

224. Smith K, Cook D, Guyatt GH et al: Respiratory muscle training in chronic airflow limitation: a meta-analysis, Am Rev Respir Dis 145:533-539, 1992.

225. Harver A, Mahler DA, Daubenspeck JA: Targeted inspiratory muscle training improves respiratory muscle function and reduces dyspnea in patients wth chronic obstructive pulmonary disease, Ann Intern Med 111:117-124, 1989.

226. Lisboa C, Villafranca C, Leiva A et al: Inspiratory muscle training in chronic airflow limitation: effect on exercise performance, Eur Respir J 10:537-542, 1997.

227. Weiner P, Magadle R, Massarwa F et al: Influence of gender and inspiratory muscle training on the perception of dyspnea in patients with asthma, Chest 122:197-201, 2002.

228. de Jong W, van Aalderen WM, Kraan J et al: Inspiratory muscle training in patients with cystic fibrosis, Respir Med 95:31-36, 2001.

229. Sanchez Riera H, Montemayor Rubio T, Ortega Ruiz F et al: Inspiratory muscle training in patients with COPD: effect on dyspnea, exercise performance, and quality of life, Chest 120:748-756, 2001.

230. Patessio A, Rampulla C, Fracchia C et al: Relationship between the perception of breathlessness and inspiratory resistive loading: report on a clinical trial, Eur Respir J 7:587s-591s, 1989.

231. Lotters F, van Tol B, Kwakkel G et al: Effects of controlled inspiratory muscle training in patients with chronic obstructive pulmonary disease: a meta-analysis, Eur Respir J 20:570-576, 2002.

232. van 't Hul A, Kwakkel G, Gosselink R: The acute effects of noninvasive ventilatory support during exercise on exercise endurance and dyspnea in patients with chronic obstructive pulmonary disease: a systematic review, J Cardiopulm Rehabil 22:290-297, 2002.

233. Renston JP, DiMarco AF, Supinski GS: Respiratory muscle rest using nasal BiPAP ventilation in patients with stable severe COPD, Chest 105:1053-1060, 1994.

234. Kossler W, Lahrmann H, Brath H et al: Feedback-controlled negative pressure ventilation in patients with stable severe hypercapnic chronic obstructive pulmonary disease, Respiration 67: 362-366, 2000.

235. Nava S, Ceriana P: Patient–ventilator interaction during noninvasive positive pressure ventilation, Respir Care Clin N Am 11:281-293, 2005.

236. Strumpf DA, Millman RP, Carlisle CC et al: Nocturnal positive-pressure ventilation via nasal mask in patients with severe chronic obstructive pulmonary disease, Am Rev Respir Dis 144:1234-1239, 1991.

237. O'Donnell DE, Sanii R, Dubo H et al: Steady-state ventilatory responses to expiratory resistive loading in quadriplegics, Am Rev Respir Dis 147:54-59, 1993.

238. Oga T, Nishimura K, Tsukino M et al: A comparison of the effects of salbutamol and ipratropium bromide on exercise endurance in patients with COPD, Chest 123:1810-1816, 2003.

239. O'Donnell DE, Mahler DA: Effect of bronchodilators and inhaled corticosteriods on dyspnea in COPD. In Mahler DA, O'Donnell DE, editors: Lung biology in health and disease, vol. 208, ed 2: Dyspnea: mechanisms, measurement, and management, Boca Raton, Fla, 2005, CRC Press/Taylor & Francis, pp 283-300.

240. Brusasco V, Hodder R, Miravitlles M: Health outcomes following treatment for six months with once daily tiotropium compared with twice daily salmeterol in patients with COPD, Thorax 58:399-404, 2003.

241. Calverley PM, Boonsawat W, Cseke Z et al: Maintenance therapy with budesonide and formoterol in chronic obstructive pulmonary disease, Eur Respir J 22:912-919, 2003.

242. Hanania NA, Darken P, Horstman D et al: The efficacy and safety of fluticasone propionate (250 microg)/salmeterol (50 microg) combined in the Diskus inhaler for the treatment of COPD, Chest 124:834-843, 2003.

243. Wilson SR, Starr-Schneidkraut N: State of the art in asthma education: the US experience, Chest 106(4 Suppl):197S-205S, 1994.

244. Lahdensuo A, Haahtela T, Herrala J et al: Randomised comparison of guided self management and traditional treatment of asthma over one year, BMJ 312:748-752, 1996.

245. Gibson P, Powell H, Couglan J et al: Self-management education and regular practitioner review for adults with asthma [review]. Cochrane Database Syst Rev 2003:CD001117. 2003.

246. Bourbeau J, Julien M, Maltais F et al: Reduction of hospital utilization in patients with chronic

obstructive pulmonary disease: a disease-specific self-management intervention, Arch Intern Med 163:585-591, 2003.

247. Monninkhof E, van der Valk P, van der Palen J et al: Effects of a comprehensive self-management programme in patients with chronic obstructive pulmonary disease, Eur Respir J 22:815-820, 2003.

248. Davidson JT, Whipp BJ, Wasserman K et al: Role of the carotid bodies in breath-holding, N Engl J Med 290:819-822, 1974.

249. O'Donnell DE, Bain DJ, Webb KA: Factors contributing to relief of exertional breathlessness during hyperoxia in chronic airflow limitation, Am J Respir Crit Care Med 155:530-535, 1997.

250. Stein DA, Bradley BL, Miller W: Mechanisms of oxygen effects on exercise patients with chronic obstructive pulmonary disease, Chest 81:6-10, 1982.

251. Swinburn CR, Wakefield JM, Jones PW: Relationship between ventilation and breathlessness during exercise in chronic obstructive airways disease is not altered by prevention of hypoxemia, Clin Sci 67:515-519, 1984.

252. Lane R, Adams L, Guz A: The effects of hypoxia and hypercapnia on perceived breathlessness during exercise in humans, J Physiol (Lond) 428:579-593, 1990.

253. Chronos N, Adams L, Guz A: Effect of hyperoxia and hypoxia on exercise-induced breathlessness in normal subjects, Clin Sci 74:531-537, 1988.

254. Ward SA, Whipp BJ: Effects of peripheral and central chemoreflex activation on the isopnoeic rating of breathing in exercising humans, J Physiol 411:27-43, 1989 [published erratum appears in J Physiol (Lond) 1990;420:489].

255. Bye PTP, Esau SA, Levy RD et al: Ventilatory muscle function during exercise in air and oxygen in patients with chronic air-flow limitation, Am Rev Respir Dis 132:236-240, 1985.

256. Dean NC, Brown JK, Himelman RB et al: Oxygen may improve dyspnea and endurance in patients with chronic obstructive pulmonary disease and only mild hypoxemia, Am Rev Respir Dis 146:941-945, 1992.

257. Tiep BL: Long-term home oxygen therapy, Clin Chest Med 11:505-521, 1990.

258. Spathis A, Wade R, Booth S: Oxygen in the palliation of breathlessness. In Booth S, Dudgeon D, editors: Dyspnoea in advanced disease: a guide to clinical management, New York, 2006, Oxford University Press, pp 205-236.

259. Leach RM, Davidson AC, Chinn S et al: Portable liquid oxygen and exercise ability in severe respiratory disability, Thorax 47:781-789, 1992.

260. Swinburn CR, Mould H, Stone TN et al: Symptomatic benefit of supplemental oxygen in hypoxemic patients with chronic lung disease, Am Rev Respir Dis 143:913-915, 1991.

261. Bruera E, MacEachern T, Ripamonti C et al: Subcutaneous morphine for dyspnea in cancer patients, Ann Intern Med 119:906-907, 1993.

262. Bruera E, Macmillan K, Pither J et al: Effects of morphine on the dyspnea of terminal cancer patients, J Pain Symptom Manage 5:341-344, 1990.

263. Light RW, Muro JR, Sato RI et al: Effects of oral morphine on breathlessness and exercise tolerance in chronic obstructive pulmonary disease, Am Rev Respir Dis 139:126-133, 1989.

264. Cohen MH, Anderson AJ, Krasnow SH et al: Continuous intravenous infusion of morphine for severe dyspnea, South Med J 84:229-234, 1991.

265. Woodcock AA, Johnson MA, Geddes DM: Breathlessness, alcohol and opiates. N Engl J Med 306:1363-1364, 1982.

266. Johnson MA, Woodcock AA, Geddes DM: Dihydrocodeine for breathlessness in "pink puffers", Br Med J (Clin Res Ed) 286:675-677, 1983.

267. Eisner N, Luce P, Denman W et al: Effect of oral diamorphine on dyspnea in chronic obstructive pulmonary disease (COPD), Am Rev Respir Dis 141:A323, 1990.

268. Rice KL, Kronenberg RS, Hedemark LL et al: Effects of chronic administration of codeine and promethazine on breathlessness and exercise tolerance in patients with chronic airflow obstruction, Br J Dis Chest 81:287-292, 1987.

269. Jennings AL, Davies AN, Higgins JP et al: Opioids for the palliation of breathlessness in terminal illness, Cochrane Database Syst Rev 2001: CD002066, 2001.

270. Joyce M, McSweeney M, Carrieri Kohlman V et al: The use of nebulized opioids in the management of dyspnea: evidence synthesis, Oncol Nurs Forum 31:551-561, 2004.

271. Robin ED, Burke CM: Single-patient randomized clinical trial: opiates for intractable dyspnea, Chest 90:888-892, 1986.

272. Dudgeon D: Management of dyspnea at the end of life. In Mahler DA, O'Donnell DE, editors: Lung biology in health and disease, vol. 208, ed 2: Dyspnea: mechanisms, measurement, and management, Boca Raton, Fla, 2005, CRC Press/Taylor & Francis, pp 429-461.

273. Woodcock AA, Gross ER, Geddes DM: Drug treatment of breathlessness: contrasting effects of diazepam and promethazine in pink puffers, Br Med J 283:343-346, 1981.

274. Eimer M, Cable T, Gal P et al: Effects of clorazepate on breathlessness and exercise tolerance in patients with chronic airflow obstruction, J Fam Pract 21:359-362, 1985.

275. Mitchell-Heggs P, Murphy K, Minty K et al: Diazepam in the treatment of dyspnoea in the 'Pink Puffer' syndrome, Q J Med 49:9-20, 1980.

276. Greene JG, Pucino F, Carlson JD et al: Effects of alprazolam on respiratory drive, anxiety, and dyspnea in chronic airflow obstruction: a case study, Pharmacotherapy 9:34-38, 1989.

277. Argyropoulou P, Patakas D, Koukou A et al: Buspirone effect on breathlessness and exercise performance in patients with chronic obstructive pulmonary disease, Respiration 60:216-220, 1993.

278. Smoller JW, Pollack MH et al: Sertraline effects on dyspnea in patients with obstructive airways disease, Psychosomatics 39:24-29, 1998.

279. Weiss DJ, Kreck T, Albert RK: Dyspnea resulting from fibromyalgia, Chest 113:246-249, 1998.

280. Young IH, Daviskas E, Keena VA: Effect of low dose nebulised morphine on exercise endurance in patients with chronic lung disease, Thorax 44:387-390, 1989.

281. Farncombe M, Chater S: Clinical application of nebulized opioids for treatment of dyspnoea in patients with malignant disease, Support Care Cancer 2:184-187, 1994.

282. Noseda A, Carpiaux JP, Markstein C et al: Disabling dyspnoea in patients with advanced disease: lack of effect of nebulized morphine, Eur Respir J 10:1079-1083, 1997.

283. Masood AR, Subhan MM, Reed JW et al: Effects of inhaled nebulized morphine on ventilation and breathlessness during exercise in healthy man, Clin Sci (Lond) 88:447-452, 1995.

284. Leung R, Hill P, Burdon J: Effect of inhaled morphine on the development of breathlessness during exercise in patients with chronic lung disease, Thorax 51:596-600, 1996.

285. Chandler S: Nebulized opioids to treat dyspnea [see comments]. Am J Hosp Palliat Care 16:418-422, 1999.

286. Schwartzstein RM, Lahive K, Pope A et al: Cold facial stimulation reduces breathlessness induced in normal subjects, Am Rev Respir Dis 136:58-61, 1987.

287. Simon PM, Basner RC, Weinberger SE et al: Oral mucosal stimulation modulates intensity of breathlessness induced in normal subjects, Am Rev Respir Dis 144:419-422, 1991.

288. Liss HP, Grant BJ: The effect of nasal flow on breathlessness in patients with chronic obstructive pulmonary disease, Am Rev Respir Dis 137:1285-1288, 1988.

289. Troosters T, Casaburi R, Gosselink R et al: Pulmonary rehabilitation in chronic obstructive pulmonary disease, Am J Respir Crit Care Med 172:19-38, 2005.

290. Gallefoss F, Bakke PS, Rsgaard PK: Quality of life assessment after patient education in a randomized controlled study on asthma and chronic obstructive pulmonary disease, Am J Respir Crit Care Med 159:812-817, 1999.

291. Gallefoss F, Bakke PS: Cost–benefit and cost–effectiveness analysis of self-management in patients with COPD: a 1-year follow-up randomized, controlled trial, Respir Med 96:424-431, 2002.

292. Sassi-Dambron DE, Eakin EG, Ries AL et al: Treatment of dyspnea in COPD: a controlled clinical trial of dyspnea management strategies [see comments], Chest 107:724-729, 1995.

293. Watson P, Town G, Holbrook N et al: Evaluation of a self-management plan for chronic obstructive pulmonary disease, Eur Respir J 10:1267-1271, 1997.

294. Zimmerman BW, Brown ST, Bowman JM et al: A self-management program for chronic obstructive pulmonary disease: relationship to dyspnea and self-efficacy, Rehabil Nurs 21:253-257, 1996.

295. Monninkhof EM, Van Der Valk PD, Van Der Palen J et al: Self-management education for chronic obstructive pulmonary disease [review], Cochrane Database Syst Rev 2003:CD002990, 2003.

296. Lorig KR, Sobel DS, Stewart AL et al: Evidence suggesting that a chronic disease self-management program can improve health status while reducing hospitalization: a randomized trial, Med Care 37:5-14, 1999.

297. Hernández MT, Rubio TM, Ruiz FO et al: Results of a home-based training program for patients with COPD, Chest 118:106-114, 2000.

298. Puente-Maestu L, Sanz ML, Sanz P et al: Comparison of effects of supervised versus self-monitored training programmes in patients with chronic obstructive pulmonary disease, Eur Respir J 15:517-525, 2000.

299. Janson SL, Fahy JV, Covington JK et al: Effects of individual self-management education on clinical, biological, and adherence outcomes in asthma, Am J Med 115:620-626, 2003.

300. Ignacio-Garcia JM, Gonzalez-Santos P: Asthma self-management education program by home monitoring of peak expiratory flow, Am J Respir Crit Care Med 151:353-359, 1995.

301. Rosser R, Denford J, Heslop A et al: Breathlessness and psychiatric morbidity in chronic bronchitis and emphysema: a study of psychotherapeutic management, Psychol Med 13:93-110, 1983.

302. Ashikaga T, Vacek PM, Lewis SO: Evaluation of a community-based education program for individuals with chronic obstructive pulmonary disease, J Rehabil 46:23-27, 1980.

303. Bredin M, Corner J, Krishnasamy M et al: Multicentre randomised controlled trial of nursing intervention for breathlessness in patients with lung cancer, BMJ 318:901-904, 1999.

304. Corner J, Plant H, A'Hern R et al: Non-pharmacological intervention for breathlessness in lung cancer, Palliat Med 10:299-305, 1996.

305. Strijbos JH, Koeter GH, Meinesz AF: Home care rehabilitation and perception of dyspnea in chronic obstructive pulmonary disease (COPD) patients, Chest 97(3 Suppl):109S-110S, 1990.

306. Thompson SC: Will it hurt less if I can control it? A complex answer to a simple question, Psychol Bull 90:89-101, 1981.

307. Carrieri Kohlman V: Coping and self-management strategies for dyspnea. In Mahler DA, O'Donnell DE, editors: Lung biology in health and disease, vol. 208, ed 2: Dyspnea: mechanisms, measurement, and management, Boca Raton, Fla, 2005, CRC Press/Taylor & Francis, pp 365-396.

308. Scherer YK, Schmieder LE: The effect of a pulmonary rehabilitation program on self-efficacy, perception of dyspnea, and physical endurance, Heart Lung 26:15-22, 1997.

309. Lacasse Y, Wong E, Guyatt GH et al: Meta-analysis of respiratory rehabilitation in chronic obstructive pulmonary disease [see comments], Lancet 348:1115-1119, 1996.

310. Bandura A: Self-efficacy: the exercise of control, New York, 1997, WH Freeman.

311. Clark NM, Becker MH, Janz NK et al: Self-management of chronic disease by older adults: a review and questions for research, J Aging Health 3:3-27, 1991.

312. Tobin DL, Reynolds RVC, Holroyd KA et al: Self-management and social learning theory. In Holroyd KA, Creer TL, editors: Self-management of chronic disease, Orlando, Fla, 1986, Academic Press, pp 29-58.

313. American Thoracic Society: Standards for the diagnosis and care of patients with chronic obstructive pulmonary disease: ATS statement, Am J Respir Crit Care Med 152:S77-S120, 1995.

314. Von Korff M, Gruman J, Schaefer J et al: Collaborative management of chronic illness, Ann Intern Med 127:1097-1102, 1997.

315. Kwekkeboom K: The placebo effect in symptom management, Oncol Nurs Forum 24:1393-1399, 1997.

316. Turner JA, Deyo RA, Loeser JD et al: The importance of placebo effects in pain treatment and research, JAMA 271:1609-1614, 1994.

317. Moerman DE, Jonas WB: Toward a research agenda on placebo, Adv Mind-Body Med 16:33-46, 2000.

318. Wilson IB: Clinical understanding and clinical implications of response shift. In Schwartz CE, Sprangers MAG, editors: Adaptation to changing health: response shift in quality-of-life research, Washington, DC, 2000, American Psychological Association, pp 159-174.

319. Sprangers MAG, Schwartz CE: Integrating response shift into health-related quality-of-life research: a theoretical model, Social Sci Med 48:1507-1515, 1999.

320. Schwartz CE, Sprangers MAG: Adaptation to changing health: response shift in quality-of-life research, Washington, DC, 2000, American Psychological Association.

321. Hoogstraten J: Influence of objective measures on self-reports in a retrospective pretest–posttest design, J Exp Educ 53:207-210, 1985.

322. Suls J, Fletcher B: The relative efficacy of avoidant and nonavoidant coping strategies: a meta-analysis, Health Psychol 4:249-288, 1985.

323. Carrieri V, Kieckhefer G, Janson-Bjerklie S et al: The sensation of pulmonary dyspnea in school-age children, Nurs Res 40:81-85, 1991.

324. Keefe FJ, Dunsmore J, Burnett R: Behavioral and cognitive–behavioral approaches to chronic pain: recent advances and future directions, J Consult Clin Psychol 60:528-536, 1992.

325. Lazarus RS: The costs and benefits of denial. In Breznitz S, editor: The denial of stress, New York, 1983, International Universities Press, pp 1-30.

326. DeVito AJ: Dyspnea during hospitalizations for acute phase of illness as recalled by patients with chronic obstructive pulmonary disease, Heart Lung 19:186-191, 1990.

327. Carrieri-Kohlman V, Gormley JM, Eiser S et al: Dyspnea and the affective response during exercise training in obstructive pulmonary disease, Nurs Res 50:136-146, 2001.

328. Dudgeon DJ, Kristjanson L, Sloan JA et al: Dyspnea in cancer patients: prevalence and associated factors, J Pain Symptom Manage 21:95-102, 2001.

329. Renfroe KL: Effect of progressive relaxation on dyspnea and state anxiety in patients with chronic obstructive pulmonary disease, Heart Lung 17:408-413, 1988.

330. Gift AG, Moore T, Soeken K: Relaxation to reduce dyspnea and anxiety in COPD patients, Nurs Res 41:242-246, 1992.

331. Gustafson DH, Hawkins R, Pingree S et al: Effect of computer support on younger women with breast cancer, J Gen Intern Med 16:435-445, 2001.

332. Gustafson DH, Robinson TN, Ansley D et al: Consumers and evaluation of interactive health communication applications: the Science Panel on Interactive Communication and Health, Am J Prevent Med 16:23-29, 1999.

333. Sitzman J, Kamiya J, Johnson J: Biofeedback training for reduced respiratory rate in chronic obstructive disease: a preliminary study, Nurs Res 32:218-223, 1983.

334. Holliday JE, Hyers TM: The reduction of weaning time from mechanical ventilation using tidal volume and relaxation biofeedback, Am Rev Respir Dis 141:1214-1220, 1990.

335. Giardino ND, Chan L, Borson S: Combined heart rate variability and pulse oximetry biofeedback for chronic obstructive pulmonary disease: preliminary findings, Appl Psychophysiol Biofeedback 29:121-133, 2004.

336. Haas F, Salazar-Schicchi J, Axen K: Desensitization to dyspnea in chronic obstructive pulmonary disease. In Casaburi R, Petty T, editors: Principles and practice of pulmonary rehabilitation, Philadelphia, 1993, WB Saunders, pp 241-251.

337. Thornby MA, Haas F, Axen K: Effect of distractive auditory stimuli on exercise tolerance in patients with COPD, Chest 107:1213-1217, 1995.

338. Bauldoff GS, Hoffman LA, Zullo TG et al: Exercise maintenance following pulmonary rehabilitation: effect of distractive stimuli, Chest 122:948-954, 2002.

339. Brooks D, Sidani S, Graydon J et al: Evaluating the effects of music on dyspnea during exercise in individuals with chronic obstructive pulmonary disease: a pilot study, Rehabil Nurs 28:192-196, 2003.

340. Moody LE, Fraser M, Yarandi H: Effects of guided imagery in patients with chronic bronchitis and emphysema, Clin Nurs Res 2:478-486, 1993.

341. Louie SW: The effects of guided imagery relaxation in people with COPD, Occup Ther Int 11:145-159, 2004.

342. Jobst K, Chen J, McPherson K et al: Controlled trial of acupuncture for disabling breathlessness, Lancet 2:1416-1419, 1986.

343. Filshie J, Penn K, Ashley S et al: Acupuncture for the relief of cancer-related breathlessness, Palliative Med 10:1447-1452, 1996.

344. Maa SH, Gauthier D, Turner M: Acupressure as an adjunct to a pulmonary rehabilitation program, J Cardiopulm Rehabil 17:268-276, 1997.

345. Maa SH, Sun M, Hsu KH et al: Effect of acupuncture or acupressure on quality of life of patients with chronic obstructive asthma: a pilot study, J Altern Complement Med 9:659-670, 2003.

346. Wu HS, Wu SC, Lin JG et al: Effectiveness of acupressure in improving dyspnoea in chronic obstructive pulmonary disease, J Adv Nurs 45:252-259, 2004.

347. Cohen S, Syme SL: Social support and health, New York, 1985, Academic Press.

348. Graydon JE, Ross E, Webster PM et al: Predictors of functioning of patients with chronic obstructive pulmonary disease, Heart Lung 24:369-375, 1995.

349. Lee RN, Graydon JE, Ross E: Effects of psychological well-being, physical status, and social support on oxygen-dependent COPD patients' level of functioning, Res Nurs Health 14:323-328, 1991.

350. Uchino BN, Cacioppo JT, Keicolt-Glaser JK: The relationship between social support and physiological processes: a review with emphasis on underlying mechanisms and implications for health, Psychol Bull 119:488-531, 1996.

351. Janson-Bjerklie S, Ruma SS, Stulbarg M et al: Predictors of dyspnea intensity in asthma, Nurs Res 36:179-183, 1987.

352. Jacobson DE: Types and timing of social support, J Health Social Behav 27:250-264, 1986.

353. Oka RK, King AC, Young DR: Sources of social support as predictors of exercise adherence in women and men ages 50 to 65 years, Womens Health 1:161-175, 1995.

354. Wilcox S, Castro C, King AC et al: Determinants of leisure time physical activity in rural compared with urban older and ethnically diverse women in the United States, J Epidemiol Commun Health 54:667-672, 2000.

355. Borkman TJ: Understanding self-help/mutual aid, New Brunswick, NJ, 1999, Rutgers University Press.

356. Spiegel D: Living beyond limits, New York, 1993, Times Books.

357. Sobel DS: The cost-effectiveness of mind—body medicine interventions, Prog Brain Res 122:393-412, 2000.

358. California Pulmonary Rehabilitation Collaborative Group: Effects of pulmonary rehabilitation on dyspnea, quality of life, and healthcare costs in California, J Cardiopulm Rehabil 24:52-62, 2004.

359. Dudley DL, Pitts-Poarch AR: Psychological aspects of respiratory control, Clin Chest Med 1:131-143, 1980.

360. ZuWallack R, Lareau SC, Meek PM: The effect of pulmonary rehabilitation on dyspnea. In Mahler DA, O'Donnell DE, editors: Lung biology in health and disease, vol. 208, ed 2: Dyspnea: mechanisms, measurement, and management, Boca Raton, Fla, 2005, CRC Press/Taylor & Francis, pp 301-320.

361. Goldstein RS, Gort EH, Stubbing D et al: Randomised controlled trial of respiratory rehabilitation, Lancet 344:1394-1397, 1994.

362. Carrieri-Kohlman V, Nguyen HQ, Donesky-Cuenco D et al: Impact of brief or extended exercise training on the benefit of a dyspnea self-management program in COPD, J Cardiopulm Rehabil 25:275-284, 2005.

363. Lake FR, Henderson K, Briffa T et al: Upper-limb and lower-limb exercise training in patients with chronic airflow obstruction, Chest 97:1077-1082, 1990.

364. Simpson K, Killian K, McCartney N et al: Randomised controlled trial of weightlifting exercise in patients with chronic airflow limitation, Thorax 47:70-75, 1992.

365. Couser JJ, Martinez FJ, Celli BR: Pulmonary rehabilitation that includes arm exercise reduces metabolic and ventilatory requirements for simple arm elevation, Chest 103:37-41, 1993.

366. Epstein SK, Celli BR, Martinez FJ et al: Arm training reduces the VO2 and VE cost of unsupported arm exercise and elevation in chronic obstructive pulmonary disease, J Cardiopulm Rehabil 17:171-177, 1997.

367. Casaburi R, Patessio A, Ioli F et al: Reductions in exercise lactic acidosis and ventilation as a result of exercise training in patients with obstructive lung disease, Am Rev Respir Dis 143:9-18, 1991.

368. McGavin CR, Gupta SP, Lloyd EL et al: Physical rehabilitation for the chronic bronchitic: results of a controlled trial of exercises in the home, Thorax 32:307-311, 1977.

369. O'Donnell DE, Lam M, Webb KA: Measurement of symptoms, lung hyperinflation, and endurance during exercise in chronic obstructive pulmonary disease, Am J Respir Crit Care Med 158:1557-1565, 1998.

370. O'Donnell DE, Webb KA: Mechanisms of dyspnea in COPD. In Mahler DA, O'Donnell DE, editors: Lung biology in health and disease, vol. 208, ed 2: Dyspnea: mechanisms, measurement, and management, Boca Raton, Fla, 2005, CRC Press/Taylor & Francis, pp 29-58.

371. Moerman D: Meaning, medicine, and the "placebo effect.", Cambridge, 2002, Cambridge University Press.

372. Wilson RC, Oldfield WL, Jones PW: Effect of residence at altitude on the perception of breathlessness on return to sea level in normal subjects, Clin Sci (Lond) 84:159-167, 1993.

373. Belman MJ: Exercise in chronic obstructive pulmonary disease, Clin Chest Med 7:585-597, 1986.

374. Helson H: Adaptation-level theory: an experimental and systematic approach to behavior, New York, 1964, Harper & Row.

375. Gibbons FX: Social comparison as a mediator of response shift, Social Sci Med 48:1517-1530, 1999.

376. Roberts DK, Thorne SE, Pearson C: The experience of dyspnea in late-stage cancer: patients' and nurses' perspectives, Cancer Nurs 16:310-320, 1993.

377. Carrieri-Kohlman V, Douglas MK, Gormley JM et al: Desensitization and guided mastery: treatment approaches for the management of dyspnea, Heart Lung 22:226-234, 1993.

378. Williams SL: Guided mastery treatment of agoraphobia: beyond stimulus exposure, Prog Behav Modif 26:89-121, 1990.

379. Behera D: Yoga therapy in chronic bronchitis, J Assoc Physicians India 46:207-208, 1998.

380. Tandon MK: Adjunct treatment with yoga in chronic severe airways obstruction, Thorax 33:514-517, 1978.

381. Donesky-Cuenco D, Carrieri-Kohlman V, Park SK et al: Safety and feasibility of yoga in patients with COPD [abstract]. Proc Am Thorac Soc 3:A221, 2006.

382. Carrieri-Kohlman V, Donesky-Cuenco D, Nguyen H et al: Efficacy of yoga for self-management of dyspnea in patients with chronic obstructive pulmonary disease (abstract). Paper presented at the North American Research Conference on Complementary and Integrative Medicine, May 24-27, 2006, Edmonton, Alberta, Canada.

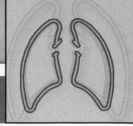

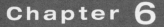

Chapter 6

Education in Pulmonary Rehabilitation

PHILLIP D. HOBERTY • GEORGIANNA G. SERGAKIS • REBECCA J. HOBERTY

CHAPTER OUTLINE

Adult Education
Teaching and Teaching Styles in Adult
   Education
Examples of Facilitating Adult
   Education in Patient and Family
   Education

Characteristics of the Learner in
   Pulmonary Rehabilitation
Outcome Assessment in Pulmonary
   Rehabilitation
Conclusion

PROFESSIONAL SKILLS

On completion of this chapter, the reader will be able to do
the following:
* Understand the principles and application of adult learning in pulmonary rehabilitation
* Explain the four principles of andragogy
* Know the variables that need to be addressed in learning
* List the 12 principles of adult learning
* Understand the characteristics of the patient in pulmonary rehabilitation

*B*ecause patient education is an almost universal component of comprehensive pulmonary rehabilitation, it deserves more than passing consideration. In this chapter, the education of the older adult is emphasized. However, much of it is applicable to the care of any patient with chronic lung disease who, whether a child, teenager, or young adult, has a rich history of personal experiences with medical therapy and health care providers, and with the challenges and limitations of the disease. In this way the more youthful patient has much in common with the older patient in being prepared to start, not with a the proverbial blank slate, but with some existing knowledge, good or bad, and functionality, high or low, on which to build.

The American Thoracic Society/European Respiratory Society statement on pulmonary rehabilitation asserts: "Patient education remains a core component of comprehensive pulmonary rehabilitation, despite the difficulties in measuring its direct contribution to overall outcomes."[1] Although a search of the research literature indicates that the benefits of a pulmonary rehabilitation program are not questioned, research regarding teaching style and education delivery in pulmonary rehabilitation is sparse. Much of the teaching and learning material discussed in this chapter is taken from the literature on nursing, general education, and adult education. The first section of this chapter focuses on the principles of adult learning and their application to patients in pulmonary rehabilitation. The second part is devoted to examining the characteristics of the population usually receiving pulmonary rehabilitation services.

Teaching adults about health has been identified as an important part of health care in a variety of settings.[2] This educational intervention is not limited to the hospital or outpatient setting, nor is it always conducted on a one-to-one basis. The health educator, regardless of what clinical "hat" he or she wears, interacts with the learners on an individual level, as well as in group situations. Pulmonary rehabilitation is often applied to small groups of patients, who start and stop the rehabilitation sessions at the same time. Furthermore, the educational experience may take place at any time and in any setting. This means the facilitator of education in pulmonary rehabilitation may interact with the learner either during time set aside for formal education or at any time during the course of the learner's pulmonary rehabilitation experience. The education literature contends that these educational interactions should take into consideration that the pulmonary rehabilitation client is an adult learner.[3]

ADULT EDUCATION

Adult teaching–learning interactions are multifaceted and diverse. The concept of adult learning theory has been studied extensively for many years. Perhaps the most recognizable concept is that of andragogy. Initially introduced by Knowles in 1973, *andragogy* has been defined as "the art and science of helping adults learn."[4] Knowles later added that principles of adult learning should be added to the basic assumptions of good childhood education. The assumptions made by andragogy are that the adult learner (1) moves, through maturation, from dependency toward self-directedness, (2) relies on past experiences as a rich resource for learning, (3) becomes ready to learn when he or she experiences a need to learn to cope with real-life tasks or situations, and (4) is performance or problem centered and wants knowledge gained to apply immediately to life situations as opposed to postponed application.[4] Adult learners would benefit most in pulmonary rehabilitation educational interactions when the concept of andragogy is

taken into consideration. This construct proposed by Knowles[5] is consistent with the nurse–patient/client relationship found in the patient education literature and contends that "it places more power in the hands of students, it asks students to take responsibility for a good deal of their learning, it involves them, and, perhaps most importantly, it encourages educators to trust them." The result is that andragogy treats patients like adults.[5]

Pulmonary rehabilitation specialists might be thinking of ways in which they have seen these principles "come to life" in their clients' day-to-day program developments. This could be illustrated by clients who ask, "Why should I care about this now?" or who refer back to their personal experiences with each new concept or material that is shared with them. The main point to remember is that the adult learner comes to the education table with a variety of experiences and a breadth of needs and expectations. Adults also have the need to understand the reasoning or rationale behind what they learn.[6] Along with any interaction or introduction of new pulmonary rehabilitation concepts or skills, the health care professional should add *why* the teaching and learning are important.

Adult development and readiness to learn should be considered in patient education with regard to the "teachable moment." The immediacy of application and problem-oriented learning of adult education is relevant to pulmonary rehabilitation education in that the patient educator must determine that the goals of the educational intervention meet the needs of the patient. Although the value of education for the patient may seem self-evident, the pulmonary rehabilitation facilitator should clearly state why and how the information is useful to the client at that particular time.[7] Because adults learn best by active involvement in their learning, activities should be functional and clearly linked to daily activities.[6]

In addition to recommending that Knowles's four principles of andragogy be considered when dealing with adult patients/clients, research also suggests that the educator use certain techniques to create positive attitudes during the learning process. The following are suggestions:

- Share personal experiences or build humor into the interaction, which will build trust and develop the facilitator–learner relationship.
- Openly share a cooperative intention which at best may result in cooperative self-management, to assisting them to learn and participate in their proactive care.

- Be sensitive to and respond to the learner's language and perspective when approaching the learning interaction.
- Share the rationale behind including certain information when discussing disease management and self-care.[8]

The adult educator should reflect on several variables when facilitating the learning interaction: the motivation of the adult learner, content, needs assessment, and outcomes expectation. These variables are important to consider when planning adult education.[9] These are dealt with more thoroughly in the second section of the chapter. Several other variables should be taken into consideration when in an educational situation with an adult: the learner's personal characteristics such as background, goals, learning styles, and attitudes. The general notion of adult education is that it is more learner-centered than teacher-centered.

TEACHING AND TEACHING STYLES IN ADULT EDUCATION

Good patient educators, as good facilitators of learning, encourage active participation on the part of the learner, motivate learners to want to learn, and encourage discussion from various points of view.[10] Good facilitators have extensive knowledge of the subject matter; are organized, enthusiastic, energetic, flexible, and well prepared; and possess good interpersonal skills. A good facilitator of learning uses repetition to clarify difficult subject matter, and gives the learner sufficient opportunity to share ideas and ask questions. It is also important to model desired behaviors and give opportunity for practice while providing feedback.[9]

Creating a supportive and positive learning environment is also paramount when facilitating learning with an adult. Jane Vella,[11] an adult educator, suggests that there are 12 principles the adult educator can follow to facilitate dialogue in the teacher–learner interaction and foster a positive learning environment. These principles reflect the points made in the adult education literature and are consistent with the assumptions in Knowles's andragogy. They are outlined in Box 6-1.

Teaching style refers to the behaviors displayed by the educator over time, situation, and subject matter. It is the observable implementation of the educator's beliefs regarding teaching and learning and general beliefs and values about life.[9]

BOX 6-1	Twelve Principles for Effective Adult Learning

1. Needs assessment: participation of the learners in naming what is to be learned
2. Safety in the environment and the process
3. A sound relationship between teacher and learner for learning and development
4. Careful attention to the sequence of content and reinforcement
5. Praxis: action with reflection or learning by doing
6. Respect for learners as subjects of their own learning
7. Cognitive, affective, and psychomotor aspects: ideas, feelings, actions
8. Immediacy of the learning
9. Clear roles and role development
10. Teamwork: using small groups
11. Engagement of the learners in what they are learning
12. Accountability: how do they know what they know?

From Vella J: Learning to listen, learning to teach, San Francisco, 2002, Jossey-Bass.

Teaching style is often contingent on the educator's likes and dislikes, health, professional affiliation, and experiences. Teaching style includes behaviors related to leading discussion, developing learning opportunities for the patients, planning the rehabilitation subject matter, presenting the information, and leading the patient to new learning experiences.[9] A collaborative teaching–learning mode of working with adults has been supported by the adult education literature.[12] In addition, consistency in one teaching style was found to be more effective than styles that at one point accepted the patient as a collaborative partner in designing and implementing the education, whereas at another point made the patient a passive recipient of the teacher's methods and expectations.

EXAMPLES OF FACILITATING ADULT EDUCATION IN PATIENT AND FAMILY EDUCATION

The following are some practical examples of how a few of the principles of effective adult learning in a pulmonary rehabilitation program might be implemented. Many of the principles might be recognized as practices already in use; others might require a slight adjustment of thinking regarding the role of the pulmonary rehabilitation specialist in the teaching–learning interaction.

Needs assessment: A needs assessment is an essential part of every rehabilitation program. A discussion with learners regarding their personal functional goals for participation should precede their active participation. This will allow the educator, as the facilitator of their learning, to find out what is important to the learners and what they expect to get out of pulmonary rehabilitation. A needs assessment enables the educator to better construct their learning interactions to help them meet their personal goals. It is more than desirable that each patient's goals be congruent with the pulmonary rehabilitation specialist's goals for education. If the patient's goals are unrealistic then the specialist must, jointly with the patient, consider alternatives that are consistent with the patient's potential for fullest function.

Safety in the environment and the process: This principle has little to do with the clients' physical safety (although that is important to consider) and more to do with the learner feeling safe to say and do anything without the fear of embarrassment or humiliation. Building a trusting relationship with the client is important and allows them to find their voice through active participation in the learning process. For example, when introducing a new breathing technique, the educator should ask learners to form small groups and encourage them to discuss their expectations, reservations, and challenges, allowing active participation. Throughout the learning interaction, affirmation of learner contributions should be consistent. One of the biggest violations of the principle of safety is when a learner contributes to the group or individual interaction and the contribution falls flat or "plops," or is left without comment; this "plop" destroys the safety of the learner and discourages further contributions.

A *sound relationship between teacher and learner for learning and development:* Facilitating adult learning involves abandonment of a power relationship between the learner and facilitator. This means that in addition to maintaining safety, the facilitator should be a good listener and invite open communication with the learners. The patient must think that the patient educator is interested in what is said and that he or she is being taken seriously.

Praxis: action with reflection or learning by doing: What differentiates praxis from simple repetitive practice of a new skill is that the learner has the opportunity to practice the skill and then discuss or reflect upon the quality of the skill practice. An example is when a patient, adept at diaphragmatic breathing in a stationary position, applies it to some activity of daily living that can make it meaningful and adaptive. This moves practice to praxis.

Respect for learners as decision makers: This principle might be honored by asking learners before or after a learning interaction: "What else would you feel you need to know about this topic?" Another way to respect the learner as subjects of their own learning is to ask the learner to share more of their thoughts about the learning topic. For example, when presenting inhaled medication administration the learner might be asked, "Which of these inhaled medications presents you with difficulties in taking them or with side effects?" This encourages the learner to participate in making decisions about their learning.

Characteristics of the Learner in Pulmonary Rehabilitation

To design the specific teacher–learner interactions that would make up the educational plan, it is important to know the characteristics of the learner. Susan Bastable[13] has identified several characteristics, which are applied here to the pulmonary rehabilitation setting. Although knowing the characteristics does not guarantee that a great deal of learning will occur, it is certainly more likely if they are taken into account.

Developmental Stage

Developmental stage is a good place to begin and an important consideration in understanding the total learner. This includes physical, cognitive, and psychosocial elements of maturation. The age in years is not synonymous with the developmental stage. This is particularly true as we deal with geriatric patients who may or may not illustrate advanced levels of cognition and problem solving. The same is true for the preadult learner, who may or may not be wise in years. But, for the most part, we deal with middle-aged and older adults in pulmonary rehabilitation. For that reason their usual characteristics are concentrated on here.

Middle-aged adults are experiencing changes due to age. Some may facilitate learning from a history of successful learning in the past, be it in formal education or in alternative or nontraditional settings. Others have a history of frustrations and conflict in dealing with "school" settings. Some may have experienced change in their lives but learned little from it and respond with a knee-jerk reaction opposing change. Physical changes may have a negative influence, such as decreased vision or hearing. Many individuals are experiencing a life-changing event, such as the empty-nest syndrome, that may serve as a stressor in learning or alternatively as a motivator to consider new issues such as health enhancement or maintenance. Much older adults also share some common elements related to their stage in life. Although this age group is rapidly growing and consuming a larger proportion of the overall health care budget, its members are sometimes dismissed as poor learners because their educational level is generally lower and some demonstrate a reluctance to participate in learning because of a combination of physical and psychosocial disabilities. Shortness of breath, denial, and depression all act to decrease the effectiveness of the learning environment. For the most part, these older adults demonstrate a continued ability to learn and comprehend if other attributes are taken into consideration. So, each individual must be approached as such, not allowing the age-related challenges and limitations to overshadow the fundamental learner within.

Motivation

The motivation of the learner to engage in the learning process has been related to a number of factors. In pulmonary rehabilitation individual motivation is key to the whole rehabilitation process. This should be encouraged in all the components of a comprehensive pulmonary rehabilitation program even if the results are small and slow in coming. More specifically, there are some elements that are more closely related to the learning process. Bastable[13] identified a number of components to the motivational assessment of the learner. These include the capacity to learn; the readiness to learn; the presence of facilitating beliefs about self, health, and health care; the expression of a constructive emotional state; the presence of moderate anxiety, which promotes learning; the physical capacity to perform the desired behavior; previous successful experiences; an appropriate physical environment; a variety of social support systems; and a positive teacher–learner relationship. The motivational components should begin to be assessed in the pulmonary rehabilitation intake patient interview and

initial physical evaluation. Additional motivational components require a certain amount of pulmonary rehabilitation exposure and are assessed from the first few rehabilitation sessions. Patients may be motivated in some areas and not in others. For instance, patients may wish to return to functional activities that require moderate exercise (such as grocery shopping). However, they may not be motivated to learn further about the pathophysiology of their lung disease although this is key to understanding and using pharmacologic therapy and thus to improve their functional state.

Compliance

Compliance in the rehabilitation context has to do with the ability to adapt to and follow through with a health-promoting regimen. Why patients are or are not compliant with the instructions given to them is a question that remains basically unanswered. Models of health belief and health promotion provide explanations of how patients make decisions along the lines of actions that encourage a healthy lifestyle and pertain to disease prevention.[14] However, certain elements seem consistent with patients' adherence to behaviors requested of them. In general, the patient must value the more healthy state that rehabilitation may promote and believe that the actions occurring in the rehabilitation process will help attain that state. It is difficult for the patient at the beginning of rehabilitation to envision the better state of living that is possible through participation in and compliance with rehabilitation. One of the values of group sessions in which patients are at different ages or stages of lung disease is that patients may see how others cope with lung disease and how understanding and acceptance occur. Likewise, it is difficult for patients at the beginning of the rehabilitation process to see that the sum of new behaviors will result in a better quality of life. The rehabilitation specialist must serve as a constant coach promoting each new rehabilitation component as worthwhile to the *total* capabilities that the program graduate wants to possess.

Literacy

Although low literacy has been perceived as being a problem confined to developing countries, research and anecdotal evidence points to the fact that low literacy is a significant problem in the United States as well. This is of particular importance in the realm of health literacy, which requires the ability not only to read and understand health care literature, but also to apply the information in following a health care prescription/regimen. Researchers have identified a number of populations that are at increased risk due to poor literacy.[15-19] These may include the following:

- Those in a poor economic state of affairs
- Those who are very old (with age-related changes)
- Immigrants (in increasing number)[16,17]
- Racial minorities
- Educational dropouts
- Those who experience long-term unemployment
- Prison populations
- Inner city residents
- Rural residents
- Populations of some Southern states
- Those with chronic illness (both physical and mental)[18]

Of these, advanced age and lower educational level are the factors most common to the rehabilitation population.[19] For these reasons educational materials used in rehabilitation programs should be printed in a large font and written at a low educational level (fifth or sixth grade). Most people with a low literacy level are reluctant to admit it and tend to withdraw from educational information that they do not understand. It is recommended that all educational material be prepared along those guidelines of readability so that the patients, and not just the health care providers, are able to understand the material. Health care providers become so accustomed to using certain jargon that they sometimes forget that the patient may not understand (and often will not ask about) the terms and expressions.

Socioeconomics

Low social and economic status has been found to predict poor health status and the making of adverse health decisions.[20] For this reason it is important that the rehabilitation provider be aware of these factors when approaching the patient. It used to be that the patients who followed through on physician referrals to pulmonary rehabilitation were generally from middle- and upper-class environments, and had private insurance that often reimbursed for the rehabilitation services. The fact that those of lower economic status are also being referred to pulmonary rehabilitation programs makes it all

the more important that educators be particularly diligent in providing clear information and encouragement. Patients with low socioeconomic status more often have more literacy problems, low self-esteem, low expectations of the components of the health care process, and lower expectations of the end results of rehabilitation.[13]

Cultural Attributes

The difference in cultures is becoming increasingly important because of the influx of immigrants into the United States. Understanding these attributes may make it easier to understand the willingness or reluctance of some groups to accept and follow instructions in rehabilitation. An important element of this is an understanding of the patient's perception of health and illness in general. Also important is the patient's use of alternative remedies, trust in health care providers, willingness to use clinics and hospitals, role of the family in providing health care, and need for spousal, family, and social support. By pursuing these considerations, the health care provider can provide rehabilitation in a manner that does not conflict with these cultural attitudes and beliefs.

Deficits and Disabilities

Hearing, vision, and learning disabilities are common in pulmonary rehabilitation. Sound augmentation may be possible, especially with hearing aids. Many patients who own hearing aids do not use them or use them improperly, so that they get little value from them. The rehabilitation specialist may need to refer such patients to a hearing and speech specialist, who can perform a thorough examination if this seems to be the problem in preventing good communication. Vision difficulties may preclude the use of certain written materials and videotapes as a part of the educational process. This is one reason why few programs can rely on printed or video material to instruct patients in major components of what they are expected to learn. Some of these difficulties may be overcome with corrective lens or contacts. However, many age-related difficulties that are not correctable must be dealt with by finding other means of getting the information to the patient. This may require one-on-one education done in a nonthreatening manner. Finally, learning disabilities generally plague the individual from childhood. They must not be confused with the normal aging process. Input and output disabilities, although obviously different in terms of process, reduce the patient's ability to benefit from rehabilitation and can easily be confused with mental retardation, senility, or lack of native intelligence.

Outcome Assessment in Pulmonary Rehabilitation

Determination of patient outcomes can be seen as a necessary part of patient education, consisting of a continuous loop of assessment, functional goal setting, intervention, and evaluation.[13] Although evaluation can and should occur at any stage of the rehabilitation process, at the end of the rehabilitation program the providers should answer four fundamental questions that represent four levels of program assessment: "Did they like it?", "Did they learn it?", "Did they use it?", and "Was teaching it worth it in the long run?"[14] Answers to these questions will examine outcomes on the basis of both the individual and the program. Assessment often stops after the first level—"Did they like it?"—because of the fear that the use of tests in "Did they learn it?" will cause too much anxiety in patients. The third level of assessment—"Did they use it?"—requires additional time that may translate into additional patient sessions that a program may not have allotted in their schedule.

Patient education that does not translate into changes in knowledge and skills may accomplish little and give an unpleasant answer at the fourth level. Therefore informal ways should be found to assess whether the patient learned and whether the patient put what was learned into use. Careful assessment of verbal comments from patients and observed behaviors may not be useful for research or national pulmonary rehabilitation program certification purposes; however, if consistently applied, they may substitute as evaluations at the second and third levels in the qualitative sense. This may be done through informal questioning and observation during the last few rehabilitation sessions. For the quantitative assessment of outcomes in the health, clinical, behavioral, and service domains, written documentation through progress notes, exercise flow sheets, and pre- and post-testing from 6-minute walk test to quality of life tests is necessary. This is also true for program benchmarking. These latter functions can be facilitated by use of a multicenter database. In future, professional state and national organizations may offer access to databases to help with outcome documentation.

CONCLUSION

By applying what is known and what is being learned, the rehabilitation specialist will be better able to effectively deal with patient differences and forge common goals in rehabilitation. The diligent application of the principles of adult learning, combined with a thorough knowledge of the patient's characteristics, helps in making the patient not only more knowledgeable, but more functional as well.

References

1. Nici L, Donner C, Wouters E et al: ATS/ERS Pulmonary Rehabilitation Writing Committee: American Thoracic Society, European Respiratory Society: statement on pulmonary rehabilitation, Am J Respir Crit Care Med 173:1390-1413, 2006.
2. Redman BK: The practice of patient education: a case study approach, ed 10, St. Louis, 2007, Mosby.
3. Knowles MS: The modern practice of adult education, Englewood Cliffs, NJ, 1980, Prentice Hall.
4. Knowles MS: The adult learner: a neglected species, ed 4, Houston, 1990, Gulf.
5. Milligan F: In defense of andragogy. 2. An educational process consistent with modern nursing's aims, Nurse Educ Today 17:487-493, 1997.
6. Davis LA, Chesbro SB: Integrating health promotion, patient education, and adult education principles with the older adult: a perspective for rehabilitation professionals, J Allied Health 32:106-109, 2003.
7. Gessner BA: Adult education: the cornerstone of patient teaching, Nurs Clin North Am 24:589-595, 1989.
8. Greene DS, Beaudin BP, Bryan MM: Addressing attitudes during diabetes education: suggestions from adult education, Diabetes Educator 17:470-473, 1991.
9. Elliot DL: The teaching styles of adult educators at the Buckeye Leadership Workshop as measured by the principles of adult learning scale [thesis], Columbus, Ohio, 1996, Ohio State University.
10. Seaman DF, Fellenz RA: Effective strategies for teaching adults, Columbus, Ohio, 1989, Merrill.
11. Vella J: Learning to listen, learning to teach, San Francisco, 2002, Jossey-Bass.
12. Conti GJ: Identifying your teaching style. In Galbraith MW, editor: Adult learning methods, Malabar, Fla, 1990, Robert Krieger.
13. Bastable SB: Essentials of patient education, Boston, 2006, Jones and Bartlett.
14. Rankin SH, Stallings KD, London F: Patient education in health and illness, Philadelphia, 2005, Lippincott Williams & Wilkins.

15. Edmunds M: Health literacy: a barrier to patient education, Nurse Practitioner 30:54, 2005.

16. University of Michigan Health System: Available at http://www.med.umich.edu/pteducation/cultcomm2.htm.

17. Cutilli CC: Do your patients understand? Providing culturally congruent patient education, Orthop Nurs 25:218-224, 2006.

18. Harris M, Smith B, Veal A: Printed patient education interventions to facilitate shared management of chronic disease: a literature review, Intern Med J 35:711-716, 2005.

19. Cotugna N, Vickery CE, Carpenter-Haefele KM: Evaluation of literacy level of patient education pages in health-related journals, J Community Health 30:213-219, 2005.

20. Cole MR: The high risk of low literacy, Nurs Spectr 13:16-17, 2000.

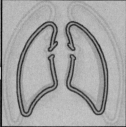

Chapter 7

Pharmacologic Therapy for Chronic Obstructive Pulmonary Disease

BARTOLOME R. CELLI

CHAPTER OUTLINE

Chronic Obstructive Pulmonary Disease
   Multicomponent Disease
   Treatable Disease
Effective Therapy for Respiratory
   Manifestations
   Smoking Cessation and Decreased
      Exposure to Biomass Fuel

Pharmacologic Therapy of Airflow
   Obstruction
   Bronchodilators
   β-Agonists
Exacerbations, Hospitalization,
   and Discharge Criteria
Conclusion

PROFESSIONAL SKILLS

On completion of this chapter, the reader will be able to do
the following:
* Understand the importance of airflow limitation and lung volume in determining the response to pharmacologic therapy
* Review the pharmacologic agents that are being used in patients with chronic obstructive pulmonary disease (COPD)
* Relate the value of pharmacologic therapy in improving dyspnea, functional capacity, and health-related quality of life in patients with COPD
* Review the basic approach to patients during exacerbations
* Better comprehend the rationale behind the value of good pharmacologic control in the prevention of exacerbations

The airflow obstruction of chronic obstructive pulmonary disease (COPD), as defined by the forced expiratory volume in 1 second (FEV_1), is thought to be only partially irreversible.[1,2] This physiologic fact has generated an unjustified nihilistic therapeutic attitude in many health care providers. The evidence accumulated suggests otherwise, and an optimistic attitude toward these patients goes a long way in relieving their fears and misconceptions. In contrast to many other diseases, some forms of interventions, such as smoking cessation,[1,2] long-term oxygen therapy in patients with hypoxemia,[3,4] lung volume reduction surgery in certain patients with inhomogeneous upper lobe emphysema,[5] and perhaps pharmacologic therapy,[6] improve survival, whereas others such as pulmonary rehabilitation,[1,2,3,7] lung transplantation,[8] and bronchodilators[1,2] improve symptoms and the quality of a patient's life once the diagnosis has been established. Table 7-1 summarizes the available therapeutic options for patients with COPD. This chapter reviews the pharmacologic management of COPD.

The overall goals of treatment are to prevent further deterioration in lung function, to alleviate symptoms, and to treat complications as they arise.[1,2] Once COPD has been diagnosed, patients should be encouraged to actively participate in their management. This concept of collaborative management may improve self-reliance and esteem. Although not proven, it may also help improve compliance with treatment. All patients should be encouraged to lead a healthy life and exercise regularly. Preventive care is extremely important at this time and all patients should receive immunizations including pneumococcal vaccine every 5 years and yearly influenza vaccines.[1,2,9,10] An algorithm detailing this comprehensive approach is shown in Figure 7-1.

CHRONIC OBSTRUCTIVE PULMONARY DISEASE

Multicomponent Disease

There is increasing evidence that independent of the degree of airflow obstruction, lung volume is important in the genesis of symptoms and limitations among patients with more advanced disease. A series of elegant studies have demonstrated that dyspnea perceived during exercise, including walking, relates more closely to the development of dynamic hyperinflation than to changes in FEV_1.[11-16] Further, the improvement in exercise brought about by several therapies including bronchodilators, oxygen, lung reduction surgery, and even rehabilitation is more closely related to delaying dynamic hyperinflation than to changing the degree of airflow obstruction.[17,18] Casanova and colleagues[19] showed that hyperinflation, expressed as the ratio of inspiratory capacity to total lung capacity, predicted survival better than the FEV_1. This not only provides us with new insights into pathogenesis, but also opens the door for new imaginative ways to alter lung volume and perhaps affect disease progression.

That COPD may be associated with important systemic expressions in patients with more advanced disease is now accepted.[1,5,20-27] Perhaps as a consequence of a persistent systemic inflammatory state or because of other yet unproven mechanisms such as imbalanced oxidative stress or abnormal immunologic response, the fact is that many patients with COPD may have decreased free fat mass, impaired systemic muscle function, anemia, osteoporosis, depression, pulmonary hypertension, and cor pulmonale, all of which are important determinants of outcome. Indeed, dyspnea measured with a simple tool such as the modified Medical Research Council Scale,[21] the body mass index obtained by dividing the weight in kilograms by the height in meters squared (kg/m^2),[22,23] and the timed walked distance in 6 minutes[24,25] are all better predictors of mortality than the FEV_1. The incorporation of these variables into the multidimensional BODE (*b*ody mass index, airflow *o*bstruction, *d*yspnea, and *e*xercise capacity)

TABLE 7-1   Therapy of Patients with Symptomatic Stable Chronic Obstructive Pulmonary Disease

Improves Survival	May Improve Survival	Improves Patient-Centered Outcomes

Smoking cessation	Pharmacotherapy with salmeterol and fluticasone	Pharmacotherapy
		    Short-acting bronchodilators
		    Long-acting antimuscarinics
		    Long-acting β-agonists
		    Inhaled corticosteroids
		    Theophylline
		    α_1-Antitrypsin for selected patients
		    Antibiotics for selected patients

Lung volume reduction surgery for selected patients	Pulmonary rehabilitation	Oxygen therapy

Noninvasive ventilation for acute or chronic hypercapnic ventilatory failure		Surgery
		    Lung volume reduction
		    Lung transplantation
		    Pulmonary rehabilitation

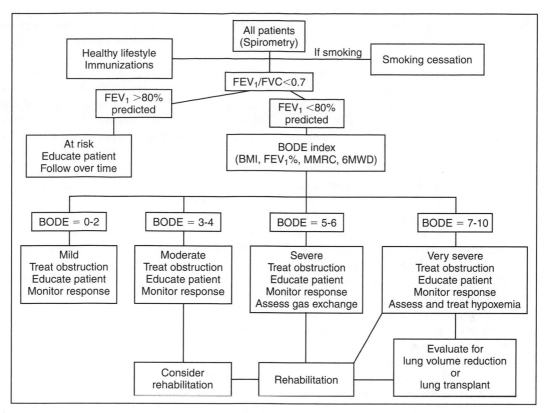

FIGURE 7-1 Algorithm describing the comprehensive management of patients with chronic obstructive pulmonary disease (COPD). 6MWD, 6-minute walk distance; BMI, body mass index; BODE, *b*ody mass index, airflow *o*bstruction, *d*yspnea, and *e*xercise capacity; FEV$_1$, forced expiratory volume in 1 second; FEV$_1$%, FEV$_1$ expressed as a percentage of the predicted value; FVC, forced vital capacity; MMRC, modified Medical Research Council Dyspnea Scale.

Index predicts survival even better. The BODE Index is also responsive to exacerbations[26] and, more important, acts as a surrogate marker of future outcome after interventions,[27,28] thus providing clinicians with a useful tool to help determine the comprehensive severity of disease. Several chapters in this book more amply detail each of these concepts.

On the basis of the multidimensional nature of the disease and the availability of multiple effective therapies, the approach shown in Figure 7-1 may more accurately help clinicians evaluate patients and choose therapies than the current approach using primarily the FEV$_1$ expressed as a percentage of the predicted reference value.

Treatable Disease

Current evidence suggests that besides smoking cessation,[29-32] long-term oxygen therapy in patients with hypoxemia,[3,4] mechanical ventilation in acute respiratory failure, and lung volume reduction surgery for patients with upper lobe emphysema and poor exercise capacity[5] improve survival.

The TORCH (*To*wards a *R*evolution in *C*OPD *H*ealth) Study, involving more than 6000 patients, showed that the combination of salmeterol and fluticasone not only improved lung function and health status but reduced the relative risk of dying over the 3 years of the study by 17.5%.[6] Other therapies such as pulmonary rehabilitation and lung transplantation improve symptoms and the quality of a patient's life once the diagnosis has been established.[1,2,7,8]

EFFECTIVE THERAPY FOR RESPIRATORY MANIFESTATIONS

Once COPD is diagnosed, the patient should be encouraged to actively participate in disease management. This concept of collaborative management may improve self-reliance and esteem. All patients should be encouraged to lead a healthful lifestyle and exercise regularly. Preventive care is extremely important at this time, and all patients should receive immunizations including pneumococcal vaccine and yearly influenza vaccines.[1,3]

Smoking Cessation and Decreased Exposure to Biomass Fuel

As smoking is the major cause of COPD, smoking cessation is the most important component of therapy for patients who still smoke[1,3] and should be recommended to all patients who smoke. Because second-hand smoke is known to damage lung function, limitation of exposure to involuntary smoke, particularly in children, should be encouraged. The factors that cause patients to smoke include the following: the addictive potential of nicotine; conditional responses to stimuli surrounding smoking; psychosocial problems such as depression, poor education, and low income; and forceful advertising campaigns. As the causes that drive patients to smoke are multifactorial, smoking cessation programs should also involve multiple interventions. The clinician should always participate in the treatment of smoking addiction because a physician's advice and intervention and use of appropriate medications including nicotine patch, gum, or inhalers; bupropion; and varenicline help determine successful results.[33,34] The significant burden of COPD in patients exposed to biomass fuel in certain areas of the world should improve by changing to more efficient and less polluting sources of energy.

PHARMACOLOGIC THERAPY OF AIRFLOW OBSTRUCTION

Most patients with COPD require pharmacologic therapy. This should be organized according to the severity of symptoms, the degree of lung dysfunction, and the tolerance of each patient to specific drugs.[1,3] A stepwise approach similar in concept to that developed for systemic hypertension may be helpful because medications alleviate symptoms, improve exercise tolerance and quality of life, and may decrease mortality. Tables 7-2 and 7-3 provide a summary of the evidence supporting the effect of individual and combined therapies on outcomes of importance to patients with COPD. Because most patients with COPD are elderly, care must be taken when prescribing drugs for this population.[35]

Bronchodilators

Several important concepts guide the use of bronchodilators. In some patients changes in the FEV$_1$ may be small, and the symptomatic benefit may be due to other mechanisms such as a decrease in hyperinflation of the lung.[11,13] Some older patients with COPD cannot effectively activate metered dose inhalers, and staff should work with the patient to achieve mastery of the metered dose inhaler. If this is not possible, use of a spacer or nebulizers to facilitate inhalation of the medication will help achieve the desired results. Mucosal deposition in the mouth will result in local side effects (i.e., thrush with inhaled steroids) or general absorption and its consequences (i.e., tremor after β-agonists). Finally, the inhaled route is preferred over oral administration, and long-acting bronchodilators are more effective than short-acting ones.[1,2]

β-Agonists

β-Agonists increase cyclic adenosine monophosphate within many cells and promote airway smooth muscle relaxation. Other nonbronchodilator effects have been observed, but their significance is uncertain. In patients with mild

TABLE 7-2   Effect of Individual Pharmacologic Agents on Outcomes of Importance to Patients with Chronic Obstructive Pulmonary Disease*

	FEV$_1$	Lung Volume	Dyspnea	QoL	AEs	Exercise Endurance	Disease Modifier by FEV$_1$	Mortality	Side Effects
Albuterol	Yes (A)	Yes (B)	Yes (B)	NA	NA	Yes (B)	NA	NA	Some
Ipratropium bromide	Yes (A)	Yes (B)	Yes (B)	No (B)	Yes (B)	Yes (B)	No	NA	Minimal
Long-acting β-agonists	Yes (A)	Yes (A)	Yes (A)	Yes (A)	Yes (A)	Yes (B)	No	NA	Minimal
Tiotropium	Yes (A)	Yes (A)	Yes (A)	Yes (A)	Yes (A)	Yes (A)	NA	NA	Minimal
Inhaled corticosteroids	Yes (A)	NA	Yes (B)	Yes (A)	Yes (A)	NA	No	No	Some
Theophylline	Some (A)	Yes (B)	Yes (A)	Yes (B)	NA	Yes (B)	NA	NA	Important
PDE4 inhibitors	Some (B)	NA	NA	Yes (B)	NA	NA	NA	NA	Some

Level of evidence: A, more than one randomized trial; B, limited randomized trials.
AEs, Adverse events; FEV$_1$, forced expiratory volume in 1 second; NA, not available; PDE4, phosphodiesterase E4; QoL, quality of life.

TABLE 7-3   Effect of Some Combined Pharmacologic Agents on Outcomes of Importance to Patients with Chronic Obstructive Pulmonary Disease*

	FEV$_1$	Lung Volume	Dyspnea	QoL	AEs	Exercise Endurance	Disease Modifier by FEV$_1$	Mortality	Side Effects
Salmeterol + theophylline	Yes (B)	NA	Yes (B)	Yes (B)	NA	NA	NA	NA	Some
Formoterol + tiotropium	Yes (A)	NA	Yes (B)	Yes (B)	NA	NA	NA	NA	Minimal
Salmeterol + fluticasone	Yes (A)	Yes (B)	Yes (A)	Yes (A)	Yes (A)	Yes (B)	Yes	Some	Some
Formoterol + budesonide	Yes (A)	NA	Yes (A)	Yes (A)	Yes (A)	NA	NA	NA	Minimal
Tiotropium + salmeterol + fluticasone	Yes (A)	NA	Yes (B)	Yes (A)	Yes (A)	NA	NA	NA	Some

*Level of evidence: A, more than one randomized trial; B, limited randomized trials.
See Table 7-2 for other abbreviations.

intermittent symptoms it is reasonable to initiate drug therapy with a metered dose inhaler of a short-acting β-agonist as needed for relief of symptoms.[1,2] In patients with persistent symptoms, it is indicated to use long-acting β-agonists,[1,2,11,13,36-39] twice daily. They prevent nocturnal bronchospasm, increase exercise endurance, and improve quality of life. The safety profile of salmeterol in the TORCH Study[6] is reassuring to clinicians who frequently prescribe selective long-acting β-agonists to their patients with COPD.

Anticholinergics

Anticholinergics act by blocking muscarinic receptors, which are known to be functional in COPD. The appropriate dosage of the short-acting ipratropium bromide is 2 to 4 puffs three or four times per day, but some patients require and tolerate larger doses.[1,2] The therapeutic effect is a consequence of a decrease in exercise-induced increased lung inflation or dynamic hyperinflation.[12] The long-acting tiotropium is effective in inducing prolonged bronchodilation[14] and decreased lung volume[15] in patients with COPD. In addition, it improves dyspnea, decreases exacerbations,[40] and improves health-related quality of life when compared with placebo and even with ipratropium bromide. The results of the large UPLIFT (Understanding the Potential Long-term Impacts on Function with Tiotropium) trial evaluating the potential role of tiotropium as a disease-modifying agent[41] will determine its place in the overall armamentarium of treatments for patients with COPD. At present, tiotropium represents a first-line agent for patients with persistent symptoms.

Phosphodiesterase Inhibitors

Theophylline is nonspecific phosphodiesterase inhibitor that increases intracellular cyclic adenosine monophosphate within airway smooth muscle. The bronchodilator effects of these drugs are best seen at high doses, with which there is also a higher risk of toxicity. Its potential for toxicity has led to a decline in its popularity. Theophylline is of particular value for less compliant or less capable patients who cannot use aerosol therapy optimally. The previously recommended therapeutic serum levels of 15 to 20 mg/dl are too close to the toxic range and are frequently associated with side effects. Therefore, a lower target range of 8 to 13 mg/dl is safer and still therapeutic in nature.[1,3] The combination of two or more bronchodilators (theophylline, albuterol, and ipratropium) has some logical rationale because they seem to have additive effects and can result in maximal benefit in stable COPD.[1,2,42] A possible action of theophylline in the gene expression of events central to inflammation in COPD[43] deserves further investigation.

The specific phosphodiesterase E4 inhibitors cilomilast and roflumilast may have anti-inflammatory and bronchodilator effects but less gastrointestinal irritation and thus may prove extremely useful if their theoretical advantages are clinically confirmed. The first 6-month studies show modest bronchodilation effects and some effect on quality of life.[44,45]

Anti-inflammatory Drugs

In contrast to their value in asthma management, anti-inflammatory drugs have not been documented to have a significant role in the routine treatment of patients with stable COPD.[1,2] Cromolyn and nedocromil have not been established as useful agents, although they could possibly be helpful if the patient has associated respiratory tract allergy. One study using monoclonal antibody against interleukin-8[46] and another one against tumor necrosis factor-α[47] failed to detect any response. However, patients were selected according to the degree of airflow obstruction and not on the basis of the presence or level of the specific targeted molecule. The groups of leukotriene inhibitors that have proven useful in asthma have not been adequately tested in COPD, so that a final conclusion about their potential use cannot be drawn.

Corticosteroids

Glucocorticoids act at multiple points within the inflammatory cascade, although their effects in COPD appear more modest compared with bronchial asthma. In outpatients, exacerbations necessitate a course of oral steroids, as discussed later in the book, but it is important to wean patients quickly because the older COPD population is susceptible to complications such as skin damage, cataracts, diabetes, osteoporosis, and secondary infection. These risks do not accompany standard doses of inhaled corticosteroid aerosols, which may cause thrush but pose a negligible risk for other outcomes such as cataracts and osteoporosis. Several large multicenter trials evaluated the role of inhaled corticosteroids in preventing or slowing the progressive course of symptomatic COPD.[48-55] The results of these earlier studies showed minimal if any benefits in the rate of decline of lung function. On the other hand, in the one study where it was evaluated, inhaled fluticasone decreased the rate of loss of health-related quality of life and exacerbations.[6,48] In addition, its regular use was also associated with a decreased rate of exacerbations. Retrospective analyses of large databases suggested a possible effect of inhaled corticosteroids on improving survival[51,52]; this was not confirmed in the TORCH Study, in which the inhaled corticosteroid—only arm did not show improved survival compared with placebo whereas the combination treatment (salmeterol and fluticasone) was significantly more effective than inhaled corticosteroid alone.[6] In

that trial the combination treatment was superior in terms of all outcomes evaluated. This, coupled with the more frequent development of investigator-associated pneumonia among patients receiving inhaled corticosteroid, suggests that inhaled corticosteroid should not be prescribed alone but rather in association with a long-acting β-agonist.[6]

Combination Therapy

All of the studies that have explored the value of combining different agents have shown significant improvements over single agents alone, and it may be time to think of drug combinations as first-line therapy. Initially, the inhaled combination of ipratropium and albuterol proved effective in the management of COPD.[56] More recently, the combination of tiotropium and formoterol, even when administered once daily, was almost as effective as tiotropium administered once daily and the recommended twice per day dose of formoterol.[57] Similarly, the combination of theophylline and salmeterol was significantly more effective than either agent alone. The TORCH Study showed an effect of the salmeterol—fluticasone combination on survival, FEV_1, exacerbation rate, and quality of life compared with placebo and either of the single components,[6] confirming earlier studies evaluating the combination of β-agonists and corticosteroids.[53,54] Another trial compared tiotropium plus placebo, tiotropium plus salmeterol, and tiotropium plus a combination of salmeterol and fluticasone in more than 400 patients.[58] Although the primary outcome, the exacerbation rate, was similar among the groups, the number of hospitalizations, health-related quality of life, and lung function were significantly better in the group receiving tiotropium plus salmeterol and fluticasone.

Pending economic considerations, once symptoms become persistent, therapy should begin with a long-acting antimuscarinic agent such as tiotropium or long-acting β-agonists twice daily. Once a patient reaches an FEV_1 lower than 60% predicted, and continues to be symptomatic, evidence from the TORCH Study supports addition of a combination of inhaled corticosteroid and long-acting β-agonist. Continuation of tiotropium is reasonable, given its effectiveness and safety record. This author believes that all of the trials support the concept that intense and aggressive therapy does modify the course of

COPD, including rate of decline of FEV_1, as was shown in the TORCH Study.[6]

Mucokinetic drugs aim to decrease sputum viscosity and adhesiveness in order to facilitate expectoration. The only controlled study in the United States suggesting a value for these drugs in the chronic management of bronchitis was a multicenter evaluation of organic iodide.[59] This study demonstrated symptomatic benefits. Oral acetylcysteine is favored in Europe for its antioxidant effects. A large trial reported failure to document any substantial benefit.[60] Genetically engineered ribonuclease seems to be useful in cystic fibrosis, but is of no value in COPD.[1,2]

Antibiotics

In patients with evidence of respiratory tract infection, such as fever, leukocytosis, and a change in chest radiograph, antibiotics have proven effective.[61-65] If recurrent infections occur, particularly in winter, continuous or intermittent prolonged courses of antibiotics may be useful.[1,2] The major bacteria to be considered are *Streptococcus pneumoniae*, *Haemophilus influenzae*, and *Moraxella catarrhalis*. The choice of antibiotic will depend on local experience, supported by sputum culture and sensitivities if the patient is moderately ill or needs to be admitted to hospital.[1,2]

α₁-Antitrypsin

Although supplemental weekly or monthly administration of the enzyme α_1-antitrypsin may be indicated in nonsmoking, younger patients with genetically determined emphysema, in practice such therapy is difficult to initiate. There is evidence that the administration of α_1-antitrypsin is relatively safe.[1,3,66,67] Although not entirely clear, the most likely candidates for replacement therapy would be patients with mild to moderate COPD.

Vaccination

Ideally, infectious complications of the respiratory tract should be prevented in patients with COPD by the use of effective vaccines. Thus routine prophylaxis with pneumococcal and influenza vaccines is recommended.[12,68,69]

EXACERBATIONS, HOSPITALIZATION, AND DISCHARGE CRITERIA

Although acute exacerbations are difficult to define and their pathogenesis is poorly understood, impaired lung function can lead to respiratory failure requiring intubation and mechanical ventilation. In addition, repeated exacerbations are associated with poor outcome.[70-75] The purpose of acute treatment is to manage the patient's decompensation and comorbid conditions in order to prevent further deterioration and readmission. Table 7-4 lists the components of the history, physical examination, and laboratory evaluation that should be obtained during a moderate to severe acute exacerbation to assist the formulation of therapy and the decision for hospital admission.[1,2] Figure 7-2 describes an approach to patients with exacerbation of COPD.

Therapy of an exacerbation is based on administration of the same medications that are given to the stable patient, with preference for nebulized medications. In addition, administration of systemic corticosteroids has resulted in improved

---

TABLE 7-4 Emergency Department Evaluation of Exacerbations of COPD

History	Baseline respiratory status, sputum volume, and characteristics, duration and progression of symptoms
	Dyspnea severity, exercise limitations, sleep and eating difficulty, home care resources, home therapeutic regimen
	Comorbid acute or chronic conditions
Physical examination	Evidence of cor pulmonale, tachypnea, bronchospasm, pneumonia
	Hemodynamic instability, altered mentation, respiratory muscle fatigue, excessive work of breathing
Laboratory evaluation	ABG, chest radiograph (PA, Lat), ECG, theophylline level (if outpatient theophylline is used)
	Pulse oximetry monitoring, ECG monitoring
	Additional studies including sputum or blood culture as clinically indicated

ABG, *Arterial blood gas;* ECG, *electrocardiogram;* FEV_1, *forced expiratory volume in 1 second;* Lat, *lateral.;* PA, *posterior–anterior.*

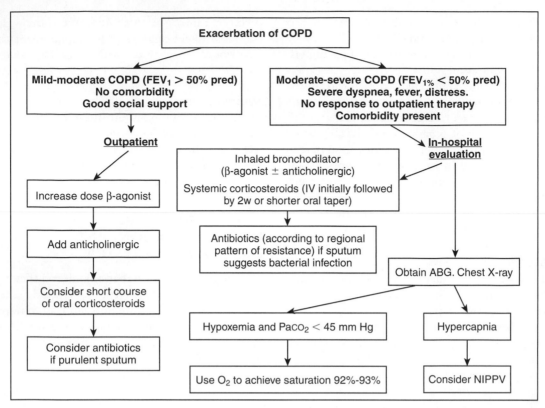

FIGURE 7-2 Algorithm by which to approach a patient with exacerbation of COPD. ABG, arterial blood gas; COPD, chronic obstructive pulmonary disease; FEV_1, forced expiratory volume in 1 second; IV, intravenous; NIPPV, noninvasive positive-pressure ventilation; pred, predicted; $Paco_2$, arterial partial pressure of carbon dioxide.

outcomes.[75-79] If a bacterial infection is suspected, administration of antibiotics based on the local prevalence of bacteria is indicated.[80-84]

Traditionally, the decision to hospitalize a patient derives from subjective interpretation of clinical features, such as the severity of dyspnea, determination of respiratory failure, short-term response to emergency department (ED) therapy, degree of cor pulmonale, and the presence of complicating features such as severe bronchitis, pneumonia, or other comorbid conditions.[1] This approach to decision-making is less than ideal in that up to 28% of patients with an acute exacerbation of COPD discharged from an ED have recurrent symptoms within 14 days. In addition, 17% of patients discharged after ED management of COPD will relapse and require hospitalization. Few clinical studies have investigated patient-specific objective clinical and laboratory features that identify patients with COPD who require hospitalization. General consensus supports the need to hospitalize patients with severe acute hypoxemia or acute hypercarbia; less extreme arterial blood gas abnormalities,

however, do not assist decision analysis. The post-treatment FEV_1 as a percentage of the predicted value, combined with clinical assessment, identifies patients in need of admission. Asymptomatic patients with post-treatment FEV_1 less than 40% predicted have been successfully discharged from the ED; patients with a post-treatment FEV_1 less than 40% predicted accompanied by persistent respiratory symptoms require admission.

Other factors that identify "high-risk" patients include an ED visit within the previous 7 days, the number of doses of nebulized bronchodilators, use of home oxygen, previous relapse rate, administration of aminophylline, and the use of corticosteroids and antibiotics at the time of ED discharge.

Once improved, clinical assessment plans for modifying drug regimens, use of home oxygen, or pulmonary rehabilitation programs should be prepared. How long a patient with COPD should be hospitalized depends at least partially on the existence of a multidisciplinary team that directs respiratory management.

Because of the complex management issues in caring for patients with COPD with impending or frank respiratory failure, physician specialists with extensive experience in and knowledge of COPD should participate in the care of hospitalized patients who have an underlying severe disease, those who require invasive or noninvasive modes of mechanical ventilation, those who have hypoxemia that is unresponsive to an increased fraction of inspired oxygen (0.50) or new-onset hypercarbia, those who require steroids for more than 48 hours to maintain adequate respiratory function, those who undergo thoracoabdominal surgery, or those who require specialized techniques to manage copious airway secretions.

The indications for hospital admission are summarized in Box 7-1. On the basis of expert consensus, these indications reflect the severity of the underlying respiratory dysfunction, the progression of symptoms, the response to outpatient therapies, existence of comorbid conditions, the necessity for surgical interventions that may affect pulmonary function, and the availability of adequate home care. The severity of respiratory dysfunction dictates the need for admission to an intensive care unit. Depending on the resources available within an institution, admission of patients with severe exacerbations of COPD to intermediate or special respiratory care units may be appropriate if personnel, skills, and equipment exist to identify and manage acute respiratory failure successfully.

CONCLUSION

Over the years, knowledge about COPD has increased significantly. Smoking cessation campaigns have resulted in a significant decrease in smoking prevalence in the United States. Similar efforts in the rest of the world should have the same impact. The consequence should be a drop in incidence of COPD in the years to come. The widespread application of long-term oxygen therapy for patients with hypoxemia has resulted in increased survival. During this time, the drug therapy armamentarium has expanded and has been used them to effectively improve dyspnea and quality of life and, perhaps, even to prolong survival. With all these options, a nihilistic attitude toward the patient with COPD is not justified.[84]

BOX 7-1	Indications for Hospitalization of Patients with COPD

1. The patient has an acute exacerbation of COPD characterized by increase dyspnea, cough, and sputum production with one or more of the following features:
   - Symptoms that do not adequately respond to outpatient management
   - Inability of a previously mobile patient to walk between rooms
   - Inability to eat or sleep because of dyspnea
   - Family or physician assessment that the patient cannot manage at home and supplementary home care resources are not immediately available
   - Presence of high-risk comorbid pulmonary (e.g., pneumonia) or nonpulmonary conditions
   - Prolonged, progressive symptoms before emergency room visit
   - Presence of worsening hypoxemia, new or worsening hypercarbia, or new or worsening cor pulmonal
2. The patient has acute respiratory failure characterized by severe respiratory distress, uncompensated hypercarbia, or severe hypoxemia.
3. The patient has new or worsening cor pulmonale unresponsive to outpatient management.
4. Invasive surgical or diagnostic procedures are planned, requiring analgesics or sedatives that may worsen pulmonary function.
5. Comorbid conditions, such as severe steroid myopathy or acute vertebral compression fractures with severe pain, have worsened pulmonary function.

COPD, *Chronic obstructive pulmonary disease.*

References

1. Celli BR, MacNee W: Standards for the diagnosis and treatment of COPD, Eur Respir J 23:932-946, 2004.
2. Global Initiative for Chronic Obstructive Pulmonary Disease: Global strategy for diagnosis, management, and prevention of COPD [GOLD report, 2006 revision]. Available at http://www.goldcopd.com.
3. Continuous or nocturnal oxygen therapy in hypoxemic chronic obstructive lung disease, Nocturnal Oxygen Therapy Trial Group, Ann Intern Med 93:391-398, 1980.
4. Long-term domiciliary oxygen therapy in chronic hypoxic cor pulmonale complicating chronic bronchitis and emphysema. Report of the Medical Research Council Working Party, Lancet 1:681-685, 1981.
5. Fishman A, Martinez F, Naunheim K et al: National Emphysema Treatment Trial Research Group: A randomized trial comparing lung-volume–reduction surgery with medical therapy for severe emphysema, N Engl J Med 348:2059-2073, 2003.
6. Calverley PM, Anderson JA, Celli B et al: TORCH investigators: Salmeterol and fluticasone propionate and survival in chronic obstructive pulmonary disease, N Engl J Med 356:775-789, 2007.

7. Nici L, Donner C, Wouters E et al: ATS/ERS Pulmonary Rehabilitation Writing Committee: American Thoracic Society/European Respiratory Society statement on pulmonary rehabilitation, Am J Respir Crit Care Med 173:1390-1413, 2006.

8. Patterson G, Maurer J, Williams T et al: Comparison of outcomes of double and single lung transplantation for obstructive lung disease, J Thorac Cardiovasc Surg 110:623-632, 1999.

9. Nichol KL, Baken L, Nelson A: Relation between influenza vaccination and outpatient visits, hospitalization, and mortality in elderly persons with chronic lung disease, Ann Intern Med 130:397-403, 1999.

10. Nichol KL, Mendelman PM, Mallon KP et al: Effectiveness of live, attenuated intranasal influenza virus vaccine in healthy, working adults: a randomized controlled trial, JAMA 282:137-144, 1999.

11. Belman MJ, Botnick WC, Shin JW: Inhaled bronchodilators reduce dynamic hyperinflation during exercise in patients with chronic obstructive pulmonary disease, Am J Respir Crit Care Med 153:967-975, 1996.

12. O'Donnell D, Lam M, Webb K: Spirometric correlates of improvement in exercise performance after anticholinergic therapy in chronic obstructive pulmonary disease, Am J Respir Crit Care Med 160:542-549, 1999.

13. O'Donnell D, Voduc N, Fitzpatrick M et al: Effect of salmeterol on the ventilatory response to exercise in chronic obstructive pulmonary disease, Eur Respir J 24:86-94, 2004.

14. O'Donnell D, Flugre T, Gerken F et al: Effects of tiotropium on lung hyperinflation, dyspnea and exercise tolerance in COPD, Eur Respir J 23:832-840, 2004.

15. Celli B, ZuWallack R, Wang S et al: Improvement of inspiratory capacity and hyperinflation with tiotropium in COPD patients with severe hyperinflation, Chest 124:1743-1748, 2003.

16. O'Donnell DE, Sciurba F, Celli B et al: Effect of fluticasone propionate/salmeterol on lung hyperinflation and exercise endurance in COPD, Chest 130:647-656, 2006.

17. Marin J, Carrizo S, Gascon M et al: Inspiratory capacity, dynamic hyperinflation, breathlessness and exercise performance during the 6 minute walk test in chronic obstructive pulmonary disease, Am J Respir Crit Care Med 163:1395-1400, 2001.

18. Martinez F, Montes de Oca M, Whyte R et al: Lung-volume reduction surgery improves dyspnea, dynamic hyperinflation and respiratory muscle function, Am J Respir Crit Care Med 155:2018-2023, 1997.

19. Casanova C, Cote C, de Torres JP et al: Inspiratory-to-total lung capacity ratio predicts mortality in patients with chronic obstructive pulmonary disease, Am J Respir Crit Care Med 171:591-597, 2005.

20. Agustí AG, Noguera A, Sauleda J et al: Systemic effects of chronic obstructive pulmonary disease, Eur Respir J 21:347-360, 2003.

21. Nishimura K, Izumi T, Tsukino M et al: Dyspnea is a better predictor of 5-year survival than airway obstruction in patients with COPD, Chest 121:1434-1440, 2002.

22. Schols AM, Slangen J, Volovics L et al: Weight loss is a reversible factor in the prognosis of chronic obstructive pulmonary disease, Am J Respir Crit Care Med 157:1791-1797, 1998.

23. Landbo C, Prescott E, Lange P et al: Prognostic value of nutritional status in chronic obstructive pulmonary disease, Am J Respir Crit Care Med 160:1856-1861, 1999.

24. Gerardi DA, Lovett L, Benoit-Connors ML et al: Variables related to increased mortality following out-patient pulmonary rehabilitation, Eur Respir J 9:431-435, 1996.

25. Pinto-Plata VM, Cote C, Cabral H et al: The 6-minute walk distance: change over time and value as a predictor of survival in severe COPD, Eur Respir J 23:28-33, 2004.

26. Celli BR, Cote CG, Marin JM et al: The body mass index, airflow obstruction, dyspnea and exercise capacity index in chronic obstructive pulmonary disease, N Engl J Med 350:1005-1012, 2004.

27. Cote CG, Dordelly LJ, Celli BR: Impact of chronic obstructive pulmonary disease exacerbations on patient centered outcomes, Chest 131:696-704, 2007.

28. Imsfeld S, Bloch KE, Weder W et al: The BODE Index after lung volume reduction surgery correlates with survival, Chest 129:835-836, 2006.

29. Kottke TE, Battista RN, DeFriese GH: Attributes of successful smoking cessation interventions in medical practice: a meta-analysis of 39 controlled trials, JAMA 259:2882-2889, 1988.

30. Anthonisen NR, Connett JE, Kiley JP et al: Lung Health Study Group: The effects of smoking intervention and the use of an inhaled anticholinergic bronchodilator on the rate of decline of FEV1: the Lung Health Study, JAMA 272:1497-1505, 1994.

31. Anthonisen NR, Skeans MA, Wise RA et al: Lung Health Study Research Group: The effects of a smoking cessation intervention on 14.5-year mortality: a randomized clinical trial, Ann Intern Med 142:233-239, 2005.

32. Fiore M, Bailey W, Cohen S et al: Treating tobacco use and dependence Rockville, Md, June 2000, U.S. Department Of Health and Human Services.

33. Jorenby DE, Leischow SG, Nides MA et al: A controlled trial of sustained release buproprion, a nicotine patch or both for smoking cessation, N Engl J Med 340:685-691, 1999.

34. Keating GM, Siddiqui MA: Varenicline: a review of its use as an aid to smoking cessation therapy, CNS Drugs 20:945-980, 2006.

35. Chalker R, Celli B: Special considerations in the elderly, Clin Chest Med 14:437-452, 1993.

36. Dahl R, Greefhorst LA, Nowak D et al: Inhaled formoterol dry powder versus ipratropium bromide in chronic obstructive pulmonary disease, Am J Respir Crit Care Med 164:778-784, 2001.

37. Tantucci C, Duguet A, Similowski T et al: Effect of salbutamol on dynamic hyperinflation in chronic obstructive pulmonary disease patients, Eur Respir J 12:799-804, 1998.

38. Rennard SI, Anderson W, ZuWallack R et al: Use of a long-acting inhaled beta2-adrenergic agonist, salmeterol xinafoate, in patients with chronic

obstructive pulmonary disease, Am J Respir Crit Care Med 163:1087-1092, 2001.

39. Ramirez-Venegas A, Ward J, Lentine T et al: Salmeterol reduces dyspnea and improves lung function in patients with COPD, Chest 112:336-340, 1997.

40. Niwehowener D, Rice K, Cote C et al: Prevention of exacerbations of chronic obstructive pulmonary disease with tiotropium, a once daily anticholinergic: a randomized trial, Ann Intern Med 143:317-326, 2005.

41. Decramer M, Celli B, Tashkin D et al: Clinical trial design considerations in assessing long-term functional impacts of tiotropium, J Chron Obstruct Pulmon Dis 1:303-312, 2004.

42. Karpel JP, Kotch A, Zinny M et al: A comparison of inhaled ipratropium, oral theophylline plus inhaled β-agonist, and the combination of all three in patients with COPD, Chest 105:1089-1094, 1994.

43. Barnes PJ, Ito K, Adcock IM: Corticosteroid resistance in chronic obstructive pulmonary disease: inactivation of histone deacetylase, Lancet 363:731-733, 2004.

44. Rabe K, Bateman E, O'Donnell D et al: Roflumilast—an oral anti-inflammatory treatment for chronic obstructive pulmonary disease: a randomized controlled trial, Lancet 366:563-571, 2005.

45. Rennard S, Schachter N, Strek M et al: Cilomilast for COPD: results of a 6-month, placebo controlled study of a potent, selective inhibitor of phosphodiesterase 4, Chest 129:56-66, 2006.

46. Mahler D, Huang S, Tabrizzi M et al: Efficacy and safety of a monoclonal antibody recognizing interleukin-8 in COPD: a pilot study, Chest 126:926-934, 2004.

47. Rennard S, Fogarty C, Kelsen S et al: The safety and efficacy of infliximab in moderate to severe chronic obstructive pulmonary disease, Am J Respir Crit Care Med 175:926-934, 2007.

48. Vestbo J; TORCH Study Group: The TORCH (TOwards a Revolution in COPD Health) survival study protocol, Eur Respir J 24:206-210, 2004.

49. Pauwels R, Lofdahl C, Laitinen L et al: Long-term treatment with inhaled budesonide in persons with mild chronic obstructive pulmonary disease who continue smoking, N Engl J Med 340:1948-1953, 1999.

50. Vestbo J, Sorensen T, Lange P et al: Long-term effect of inhaled budesonide in mild and moderate chronic obstructive pulmonary disease: a randomised trial, Lancet 353:1819-1823, 1999.

51. Sin DD, Tu JV: Inhaled corticosteroids and the risk for mortality and readmission in elderly patients with chronic obstructive pulmonary disease, Am J Respir Crit Care Med 164:580-584, 2001.

52. Soriano JB, Vestbo J, Pride N et al: Survival in COPD patients after regular use of fluticasone propionate and salmeterol in general practice, Eur Respir J 20:819-824, 2002.

53. Calverley PM, Boonsawat W, Cseke Z et al: Maintenance therapy with budesonide and formoterol in chronic obstructive pulmonary disease, Eur Respir J 22:912-919, 2003.

54. Szafranski W, Cukier A, Ramirez A et al: Efficacy and safety of budesonide/formoterol in the management of COPD, Eur Respir J 21:74-81, 2003.

55. Cazzola M, Dahl R: Inhaled combination therapy with inhaled long-acting beta 2-agonist and corticosteroids in stable COPD, Chest 126:220-237, 2004.

56. COMBIVENT Inhalation Aerosol Study Group: In chronic obstructive pulmonary disease, a combination of ipratropium and albuterol is more effective than either agent alone: an 85-day multicenter trial, Chest 105:1411-1419, 1994.

57. Van Noord J, Aumann J, Jasnseens E et al: Comparison of tiotropium once daily, formoterol twice daily and both combined once daily in patients with COPD, Eur Respir J 26:214-222, 2005.

58. Aaron S, Vandemheen KL, Fergusson D et al: Tiotropium in combination with placebo, salmeterol or fluticasone–salmeterol for treatment of chronic obstructive pulmonary disease: a randomized trial, Ann Intern Med 146:545-555, 2007.

59. Petty TL: The National Mucolytic Study: results of a randomized, double-blind, placebo-controlled study of iodinated glycerol in chronic obstructive bronchitis, Chest 97:75-83, 1990.

60. Decramer M, Rutten-van Molken M, Dekhuijzen PN et al: Effects of N-acetylcysteine on outcomes in chronic obstructive pulmonary disease (Bronchitis Randomized on NAC Cost-Utility Study, BRONCUS): a randomised placebo-controlled trial, Lancet 365:1552-1560, 2005.

61. Anthonisen NR, Manfreda J, Warren CPW et al: Antibiotic therapy in exacerbations of chronic obstructive pulmonary disease, Ann Intern Med 106:196-204, 1987.

62. Saint S, Bent S, Vittinghoff F et al: Antibiotics in chronic obstructive pulmonary disease exacerbation: a metanalysis, JAMA 273:957-960, 1995.

63. Stockley R, O'Bryan C, Pie A et al: Relationship of sputum color to nature and outpatient management of acute exacerbation of COPD, Chest 117:1638-1645, 2000.

64. Miravitlles M: Epidemiology of chronic obstructive pulmonary disease exacerbations, Clin Pulm Med 9:191-197, 2002.

65. Adams SG, Melo J, Luther M et al: Antibiotics are associated with lower relapse rates in outpatients with acute exacerbations of COPD, Chest 117:1345-1352, 2000.

66. Dirksen A, Dijkman JH, Madsen F et al: A randomized clinical trial of alpha(1)-antitrypsin augmentation therapy, Am J Respir Crit Care Med 160:1468-1472, 1999.

67. Sandhaus Ralpha-1-Antitrypsin deficiency: new and emerging therapies for alpha1-antitrypsin deficiency, Thorax 59:904-909, 2004.

68. Nichol KL, Baken L, Nelson A: Relation between influenza vaccination and outpatient visits, hospitalization, and mortality in elderly persons with chronic lung disease, Ann Intern Med 130:397-403, 1999.

69. Nichol KL, Mendelman PM, Mallon KP et al: Effectiveness of live, attenuated intranasal influenza virus vaccine in healthy, working adults: a randomized controlled trial, JAMA 282:137-144, 1999.

70. Donaldson GC, Seemungal TA, Bhowmik A et al: Relationship between exacerbation frequency and lung function decline in chronic obstructive pulmonary disease, Thorax 57:847-852, 2002.

71. Connors AF Jr, Dawson NV, Thomas C et al: Outcomes following acute exacerbation of severe chronic obstructive lung disease: the SUPPORT investigators (Study to Understand Prognoses and Preferences for Outcomes and Risks of Treatments), Am J Respir Crit Care Med 154:959-967, 1996.

72. Dewan NA, Rafique S, Kanwar B et al: Acute exacerbation of COPD: factors associated with poor treatment outcome, Chest 117:662-671, 2000.

73. Wedzicha JA: Role of viruses in exacerbations of chronic obstructive pulmonary disease, Proc Am Thorac Soc 1:115-120, 2004.

74. Stockley RA, Bayley D, Hill SL et al: Assessment of airway neutrophils by sputum colour: correlation with airways inflammation, Thorax 56:366-372, 2001.

75. Davies L, Angus RM, Calverley PM: Oral corticosteroids in patients admitted to hospital with exacerbations of chronic obstructive pulmonary disease: a prospective randomised controlled trial, Lancet 354:456-460, 1999.

76. Sayiner A, Aytemur ZA, Cirit M et al: Systemic glucocorticoids in severe exacerbations of COPD, Chest 119:726-730, 2001.

77. Niewoehner DE, Erbland ML, Deupree RH et al: Effect of systemic glucocorticoids on exacerbations of chronic obstructive pulmonary disease, N Engl J Med 340:1941-1947, 1999.

78. Aaron SD, Vandemheen KL, Hebert P et al: Outpatient oral prednisone after emergency treatment of chronic obstructive pulmonary disease, N Engl J Med 348:2618-2625, 2003.

79. Maltais F, Ostinelli J, Bourbeau J et al: Comparison of nebulized budesonide and oral prednisolone with placebo in the treatment of acute exacerbations of chronic obstructive pulmonary disease: a randomized controlled trial, Am J Respir Crit Care Med 165:698-703, 2002.

80. Groenewegen KH, Wouters EF: Bacterial infections in patients requiring admission for an acute exacerbation of COPD: a 1-year prospective study, Respir Med 97:770-777, 2003.

81. Ellis DA, Anderson IM, Stewart SM et al: Exacerbations of chronic bronchitis: exogenous or endogenous infection? Br J Dis Chest 72:115-121, 1978.

82. Wilson R, Jones P, Schaberg T et al: Antibiotic treatment and factors influencing short and long term outcomes of acute exacerbations of chronic bronchitis, Thorax 61:337-342, 2006.

83. Allegra L, Blasi F, de Bernardi B et al: Antibiotic treatment and baseline severity of disease in acute exacerbations of chronic bronchitis: a re-evaluation of previously published data of a placebo-controlled randomized study, Pulm Pharmacol Ther 14:149-155, 2001.

84. Celli BR: Chronic obstructive pulmonary disease: from unjustified nihilism to evidence-based optimism, Proc Am Thorac Soc 3:58-65, 2006.

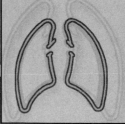

Chapter 8

Aerosol Therapy

ROBERT M. KACMAREK • R. SCOTT HARRIS

CHAPTER OUTLINE

Bronchodilators
  Anticholinergic Therapy
  β₂-Agonists
Corticosteroids
Mucokinetic Agents
  Bland Aerosols
  Mucolytics
Antibiotics

Modes of Aerosol Delivery
  Small-Volume Nebulizers
  Electronic Nebulizers
  Metered Dose Inhalers
  Dry Powder Inhalers
Patient Education
SVNs, MDIs, MDIs with Holding
  Chambers, and DPIs: A Comparison

PROFESSIONAL SKILLS

On completion of this chapter, the reader will be able to do the following:
- Identify the various bronchodilator compounds available and classify their mode of action
- Discuss the appropriate use of corticosteroids in the management of patients with chronic obstructive pulmonary disease (COPD)
- Describe concerns and indications for the use of mucokinetic agents in patients with COPD
- Discuss the appropriate use of antibiotics in this population of patients
- Identify the components of a small-volume nebulizer and discuss its proper use
- Define when spacers and holding chambers should be used and discuss the operation of metered dose inhalers
- Describe the proper use of dry powder inhalers and outline the settings where they may be used
- Contrast the advantages and disadvantages of small-volume nebulizers, metered dose inhalers, and dry powder inhalers

Aerosolization of medications provides an opportunity to deliver high concentrations of a therapeutic agent to lung tissue while keeping bloodstream levels low and thus reducing systemic effects. For this reason, the development of drugs that may be aerosolized, and of techniques designed to improve drug delivery, has intensified. Although bronchodilators remain the most important class of aerosolized medications, anti-inflammatory agents, antibiotics, mucolytics, and immunomodulators delivered directly to the airway all have a role in specific instances.

In patients with chronic obstructive pulmonary disease (COPD), airway mucosal edema, glandular hypertrophy, and airway secretions combine with a loss of airway "tethering," resulting from the destruction of lung parenchyma by emphysema, to produce chronic airflow obstruction. In addition, at least two thirds of these patients have bronchoconstriction contributing to obstructive disease.[1] Increasing obstruction, measured as the drop in forced expiratory volume in 1 second (FEV$_1$), decreasing inspiratory capacity due to hyperinflation, disordered ventilatory mechanics, and gas exchange abnormalities result in decreased functional capacity. The course of the illness is often punctuated by periodic acute exacerbations resulting in significant morbidity and mortality.

Data from the TORCH (TOwards a Revolution in COPD Health) Study indicated a reduction in mortality among patients using the combination of inhaled fluticasone dipropionate and salmeterol.[1] Over a period of 3 years, this study showed that the reduction in mortality in COPD was comparable to the reduction in cardiovascular deaths among patients given statin drugs after a myocardial infarction. It is anticipated that other ongoing clinical trials using other drugs known to reduce COPD exacerbations, such as inhaled tiotropium, will show reduced mortality. In the past, short of providing long-term oxygen therapy to patients with severe hypoxemia, and promoting smoking cessation, nothing else had been shown to alter the disease course. Despite these encouraging results, chronic medical therapy of these patients will still continue to center around improving functional capacity through medications designed to relieve airflow obstruction, reduce hyperinflation, and prevent exacerbations. Although this chapter focuses on patients with COPD as defined by the American Thoracic Society,[2] that is, patients with chronic bronchitis and emphysema, aerosol therapy in other chronic airway diseases, such as asthma, bronchiectasis, and cystic fibrosis, is also briefly discussed.

BRONCHODILATORS

Aerosolized bronchodilators are considered first-line therapy in both the acute and chronic settings for patients with asthma or COPD, although significant differences exist. In general, individuals with asthma are thought to respond better to bronchodilators. Differentiating these diseases in adult smokers with obstructive lung disease can be difficult. At least one third of patients with COPD have a significant bronchodilator response when tested once, whereas more than two thirds will show a bronchodilator response with serial testing.[3] In addition, inhaled bronchodilators may provide substantial subjective benefits in

COPD in the absence of significant changes in expiratory flows. This may be related to reduction of hyperinflation and improved lung mechanics that may be independent of large airway tone. For these reasons, all patients with COPD should receive bronchodilator therapy. Although β-agonists are the most potent bronchodilators in patients with asthma, anticholinergic agents may be better bronchodilators in COPD. In addition, patients with COPD, as a group, are older, have more comorbidity, and may be less able to tolerate adverse systemic effects.[2] In both diseases, bronchodilation is used mainly for symptom control and has not been thought to positively affect the course of the underlying process[4]; however, as mentioned, data concerning patients with COPD who received combination therapy with inhaled corticosteroids and long-acting β$_2$-agonists appear to contradict this.[1] At this time, it is not known which drug of the combination (the steroid or long-acting β-agonist) was most responsible for the improved outcome.

Anticholinergic Therapy

Anticholinergic agents are recommended for all patients with COPD and daily symptoms; they are considered by many to be the bronchodilators of choice for this disease[5] (Table 8-1). Parasympathetic innervation of the airways via branches of the vagus nerve is the primary determinant of resting airway smooth muscle tone. Activation of muscarinic receptors on effector cells, such as airway smooth muscle, submucosal glands, and postsynaptic nerves, by acetylcholine released from presynaptic nerve terminals results in bronchoconstriction and an increase in airway secretions. Parasympathetic innervation predominates in large airways and contributes to the bronchoconstriction produced by diverse stimuli. Cholinergic tone has a circadian rhythm, peaking during the night, and likely contributing to the worsened airflow and oxygen desaturation during sleep that are often seen in chronic obstructive lung disease.[6]

Atropine, the tertiary ammonium alkaloid derived from the nightshade plant (Atropa belladonna), is the classic anticholinergic bronchodilator. In addition to bronchodilation and reduction of all upper and lower airway secretions, atropine can also cause antimuscarinic side effects such as sedation, tachycardia, ileus, bladder dysfunction, and elevated intraocular pressure. Because it is lipid soluble, it is well absorbed through the

TABLE 8-1	Anticholinergic Agents for Inhalation		
Drug	Formulation	Adult Dosage	Peak, Duration (hr)
GLYCOPYRROLATE*			1, 2-6
Robinul	Nebulized (0.2 mg/cc)	1-2 mg every 2-6 hr	
IPRATROPIUM BROMIDE			1-2, 3-8
Atrovent	pMDI (18 µg/inh)	2 inh every 6-8 hr	
Atrovent HFA	pMDI (17 µg/inh)	2 inh every 6-8 hr	
Atrovent, generic	Nebulized (0.02%)	500 µg every 6-8 hr	
TIOTROPIUM BROMIDE			1.5-3, >24
Spiriva HandiHaler	DPI (18 µg/inh)	2 inh once every day	

Glycopyrrolate (Robinul) solution can be used off label for nebulization.
DPI, Dry powder inhaler; HFA, hydrofluoroalkane; inh, inhalation; pMDI, pressurized metered dose inhaler.

airway and oral mucosa, and systemic side effects limit aerosolized use of the drug.

Ipratropium bromide, the synthetic N-isopropyl derivative of atropine, is the main anticholinergic medicine used for aerosolization in the United States, and the only one available in a metered dose inhaler (MDI). Because it is a quaternary ammonium ion, it is poorly absorbed through mucous membranes, and when aerosolized it is remarkably free of systemic adverse effects. Because its peak effect is delayed compared with the intermediate-acting β_2-agonist bronchodilators (90 to 120 minutes), it is inappropriate for use as a "rescue" medication. Peak bronchodilation and length of effect are greater than with intermediate-acting β_2-agonists in patients with COPD.[7] Ipratropium may be nebulized as a 0.02% solution. The standard dose is 500 µg (2.5 cc), usually given three or four times per day. Each MDI canister carries 200 inhalations of 18 µg each. Although the American Thoracic Society recommends a starting dose of 2 to 4 puffs with a spacer three to four times per day, its safety profile allows for up to 8 puffs three or four times per day to be given to patients with chronically severe airflow obstruction or during an exacerbation. Tolerance to the bronchodilator effects of this medication has not been an issue. Ipratropium decreases airway mucous secretion but does not impair ciliary function or have adverse effects on secretion viscosity.[8] Its use relieves dyspnea, improves exercise tolerance, and improves sleep quality in patients with COPD. It does not alter the natural history of the disease and has no role in asymptomatic patients.

Several other synthetic quaternary ammonium anticholinergic agents are available for use around the world, and more selective and longer acting agents are being studied. In the United States, glycopyrrolate is available for nebulization (off-label). This agent, like atropine, is often used to decrease airway or pharyngeal secretions before surgery or endoscopy. Its bronchodilator effect has not been compared directly with that of ipratropium bromide.

The combination of ipratropium and albuterol in an MDI is available in the United States.[9] In addition, ipratropium 0.02% solution is often combined with one of the β_2-agonist solutions for nebulization for acute and chronic therapy in COPD and asthma.[10,11] Combinations may provide additive bronchodilation and are easier to use. For acute exacerbations of COPD or asthma, they have become the standard of care in many institutions. In patients with COPD with adrenergic side effects such as ectopy or tremor, we prefer to limit β_2-agonists to "rescue" therapy, although the combination inhaler is useful in patients desiring simplification of their medication regimen.

Tiotropium, an anticholinergic agent with a much longer duration of action than ipratropium, is available as a dry powder inhaler and is given once daily. It has been shown in large clinical trials of patients with COPD to sustain bronchodilation, improve dyspnea, improve quality of life, and decrease exacerbations when compared with ipratropium given four times daily.[12,13] Tiotropium appears to improve symptoms in patients with COPD, even when there is no measurable change in FEV_1, by reducing lung hyperinflation and increasing inspiratory capacity.[14,15] A large clinical trial (UPLIFT [Understanding Potential Long-term Impacts on Function with Tiotropium]) is underway to evaluate the effect of tiotropium on mortality in COPD.[16]

TABLE 8-2 Short- and Intermediate-Acting β_2-Agonists*

Drug	Formulation	Adult Dosage	Peak, Duration (hr)
ALBUTEROL OR SALBUTAMOL SULFATE			0.5-2, 4-6
Proventil, Proventil HFA, Ventolin, Ventolin HFA, generic	pMDI (90 µg/inh)	2 inh every 4-6 hr PRN	
Ventolin Rotacaps	DPI (200 µg/inh)	1 or 2 capsules every 4-6 hr PRN	
AccuNeb, generic	Nebulized (5 mg/ml)	2.5 mg every 4-6 hr PRN	
BITOLTEROL MESYLATE			0.5-2, 4-6
Tornalate	pMDI (370 µg/inh)	2 inh every 4-6 hr PRN	
	Nebulized (2 mg/ml)	1.5-3.5 mg two or four times daily PRN	
EPINEPHRINE			<1 min, 0.5
Primatene Mist	pMDI (0.22 µg/inh)	1-3 inh every 4-6 hr PRN	
Generic	Nebulized (2.25%)	2-3 mg every 4-6 hr PRN	
ISOETHARINE MESYLATE			5-15 min, 1-4
Bronkometer	pMDI (340 µg/spray)	1 or 2 sprays every 4-6 hr PRN	
Isoetharine hydrochloride	Nebulized (0.1, 0.125, 0.2%)	3-5 mg every 2-4 hr PRN	
ISOPROTERENOL HYDROCHLORIDE			5-15 min, 1-4
Isuprel	Nebulized (0.2 mg/5 ml)	0.5 ml every 2-4 hr PRN	
LEVALBUTEROL HYDROCHLORIDE			0.5-2, 0.5-2
Xopenex HFA	pMDI (45 µg/inh)	2 inh every 4-6 hr PRN	
Xopenex	Nebulized (0.63 mg, 1.25 mg)	0.63 mg or 1.25 mg every 6-8 hr PRN	
METAPROTERENOL			<1, 1-5
Alupent, Metaprel	pMDI (650 µg/inh)	2 or 3 inh every 4-6 hr PRN	
Alupent	Nebulized (50 mg/cc)	15 mg every 4-6 hr PRN	
PIRBUTEROL ACETATE			0.5-2, 4-6
Maxair Autohaler	pMDI (breath actuated)	2 inh every 4-6 hr PRN	
TERBUTALINE			0.5-2, 4-6
Brethine		2 inh every 4-6 hr PRN	

*Listed dose schedule is for standard PRN use. All may be used more frequently temporarily for acute bronchospasm. Metaproterenol and bitolterol have a slightly longer time to action than the other intermediate-acting drugs, which have an initial bronchodilating effect in 5 to 15 minutes (bitolterol is a prodrug metabolized to the active bronchodilator colterol in the liver).
DPI, Dry powder inhaler; HFA, hydrofluoroalkane; inh, inhalation; pMDI, pressurized metered dose inhaler; PRN, as needed.

β_2-Agonists

β_2-Agonists are potent bronchodilators that interact with the β_2-receptors, which are most dense on smooth muscle cells of the smaller airways (Tables 8-2 and 8-3). The activation of adenylate cyclase results in a cyclic adenosine monophosphate—dependent decrease in cytosolic calcium that relaxes airway smooth muscle. In the United States, short-acting (isoproterenol, epinephrine, and isoetharine), intermediate-acting (albuterol, bitolterol, levalbuterol, metaproterenol, pirbuterol, and terbutaline), and long-acting (salmeterol, formoterol, and arformoterol) agents are available.

β-Agonists also increase mucociliary transport and may decrease airway edema.[8]

Intermediate-acting β-agonists are the drugs of choice for acute, symptomatic relief of bronchospasm in all obstructive lung diseases owing to their rapid peak effect (5-15 minutes). Significant side effects of these agents include tremor, palpitations, and anxiety. The cardiac β_1-receptor effects are dose dependent and are decreased with the use of β_2-receptor—selective agents (all except isoproterenol and metaproterenol). Fine tremor is probably a β_2 effect.[8] Hypokalemia and hyperglycemia may also occur.

TABLE 8-3	Long-Acting β_2-Agonists*		
Drug	Formulation	Adult Dosage	Peak, Duration (hr)
ARFORMOTEROL TARTRATE Brovana	Nebulized (15 µg/2 ml)	15 µg every 12 hr	1-3, >12
FORMOTEROL FUMARATE Foradil	DPI (12 µg/inhalation)	1 inhalation every 12 hr	1-3, >12
SALMETEROL XINAFOATE Serevent Diskus	DPI (50 µg/inhalation)	1 inhalation every 12 hr	2-4, ≤12

*Long-acting β_2-agonists are inappropriate for use as "rescue" medication and should be used twice daily for "maintenance" therapy.
DPI, Dry powder inhaler.

As with anticholinergic agents, no evidence exists that bronchodilator therapy with β_2-agonists will alter the natural history of COPD. Intermediate-acting β_2-agonists are recommended for symptomatic relief of bronchospasm in patients with COPD with variable symptoms or during an acute exacerbation. In patients with continuing symptoms, intermediate-acting β_2-agonists are recommended either for daily use up to four times per day or as needed.[2] In asthma, β_2-agonists are clearly the most potent bronchodilators, although much controversy surrounds their use. It has been suggested that chronic use of β-agonists in asthma may result in tolerance to the medication and worsened asthma control.[16,17] The best study to date found no significant difference in subjective or objective asthma control in patients with mild asthma treated with either albuterol that was inhaled four times daily or albuterol as needed.[18] We agree with the recommendation of the authors of this study to use the intermediate-acting drugs as needed in asthma and have adopted this strategy in patients with COPD as well. The higher systemic doses of nebulized versus inhaler-delivered β-agonists may place patients at risk for atrial or ventricular arrhythmias or coronary ischemia. In addition, the pulmonary vasodilator effects of these agents may worsen ventilation-to-perfusion ratio matching and worsen hypoxemia in asthma or COPD. We try to limit nebulized β_2-agonist use to significant acute exacerbations of COPD presenting with bronchospasm.

In the patient with COPD and airway hyperresponsiveness, exercise-induced bronchoconstriction may limit strenuous exercise in the rehabilitation setting. Cool, dry ambient air will worsen this response. Use of 2 puffs of an intermediate-acting β_2-agonist 5 to 10 minutes before beginning exercise should be the treatment of choice for these patients.

The long-acting β_2-agonists salmeterol and formoterol (duration of effect, up to 12 hours) represent the standard of care in the management of chronic asthma and are beginning to find a role in COPD as well. Arformoterol, a long-acting β_2-agonist for nebulization, was approved for use in COPD in the United States. Formoterol and arformoterol have the advantage of faster onset and thus more rapid symptom relief than salmeterol. In asthma, multiple studies have shown that the addition of 1 puff twice daily of salmeterol to inhaled corticosteroid provides better results than doubling the dose of inhaled corticosteroids in patients with suboptimal control.[19,20] In COPD, a body of evidence is accumulating to suggest that long-acting β_2-agonists are safe and effective bronchodilators and may be useful even in patients without a short-term bronchodilator response.[21,22] One well-designed study suggested improved lung function with the use of salmeterol compared with low-dose ipratropium bromide (2 puffs four times per day) in moderate COPD.[22] In patients with COPD requiring multiple daily treatments with intermediate-acting β_2-agonists for symptomatic bronchospasm, the addition of salmeterol, formoterol, or arformoterol to ipratropium or tiotropium bromide is a rational choice.

Levalbuterol, the (R)-isomer of racemic albuterol, is available as a solution for nebulization or as a metered dose inhaler. Whereas this isomer is responsible for β_2-receptor—mediated bronchodilation, the longer lasting (S)-isomer has no intrinsic bronchodilator activity and may be responsible for the tolerance sometimes seen with the use of β_2-agonists in patients with asthma.[23] Initial studies comparing this agent with racemic albuterol showed a modest increase in bronchodilation and mild reduction in tremor and heart rate increase.[24] Two emergency department studies have shown higher emergency department discharge rates, shorter hospital stays, and lower relapse rates with its use.[25,26] There are limited data concerning levalbuterol in COPD. One study examining the bronchodilatory effects of levalbuterol was unable to demonstrate any difference in duration or magnitude of bronchodilation when compared with racemic albuterol or albuterol mixed with ipratropium bromide.[27] Another study demonstrated reduced medication use, shorter hospital stay, reduced costs, and more prolonged therapeutic benefit when compared with racemic albuterol.[28] This study has been criticized for being retrospective, nonrandomized, and unblinded.[29] Although there are some intriguing theoretical advantages to levalbuterol in the prevention of inflammation and paradoxical bronchoconstriction associated with (S)-albuterol, some of which appear to be supported by in vitro and animal data, there is a lack of clinical data supporting its routine use for asthma or COPD.[30,31] For this reason, as well as its higher cost and similar side effects profile to racemic albuterol, we do not routinely use levalbuterol.

CORTICOSTEROIDS

Inhaled corticosteroids are the mainstay of therapy in patients with persistent asthma and have revolutionized treatment of this disease (Tables 8-4 and 8-5). Full discussion of the benefits and side effects of corticosteroids in asthma is beyond the scope of this discussion; it has been the subject of many excellent reviews.[32,33] Several points, however, are worth making:

- Inhaled corticosteroids decrease airway inflammation in asthma, reducing bronchial hyperresponsiveness and improving airflow and overall disease control.
- Current recommendations are to begin therapy with a relatively high dose of one of the available steroids (see Tables 8-4 and 8-5) to achieve control and then slowly taper to the lowest possible dose maintaining control; any change in dose should be made at intervals of 3 months or more.
- As the dose–response curve of the airway effect of inhaled corticosteroids is relatively flat, the addition of other drugs, including salmeterol (discussed earlier), theophylline preparations, and leukotriene inhibitors, to a suboptimal regimen may be preferable to doubling the dose of inhaled steroid.
- Systemic manifestations of inhaled corticosteroids are dose related; because of the flat dose response for efficacy, chronic doses above 2000 µg should be avoided.

The higher potency inhaled steroids, budesonide and fluticasone propionate, have extensive first-pass metabolism and may be preferable. Further comparative studies are needed.[32]

As mentioned previously, the TORCH Study was completed and published in abstract form.[1] It showed a mortality benefit for the combination of fluticasone and salmeterol over placebo (12.6% versus. 15.2%, respectively; P =.52). Interestingly,

TABLE 8-4	Inhaled Corticosteroids	
Drug	**Formulation**	**Adult Dosage**
BECLOMETHASONE DIPROPIONATE		
Beclovent/Vanceril	pMDI (42 µg/puff)	4-8 inh BID
Vanceril double-strength	pMDI (84 µg/puff)	2-4 inh BID
BUDESONIDE		
Pulmicort Turbuhaler	DPI (200 or 400 µg/inh)	1-2 inh BID
FLUNISOLIDE		
Aerobid	pMDI (250 µg/puff)	2-4 inh BID
FLUTICASONE PROPIONATE		
Flovent	pMDI (44, 110, 220 µg/inh)	2-4 inh BID
Flovent Rotadisk	DPI (50, 100, 250 µg/inh)	1 inh BID
MOMETASONE FUROATE		
Asmanex Twisthaler	DPI (220 µg/inh)	1-2 inh BID
TRIAMCINOLONE ACETONIDE		
Azmacort	pMDI (100 µg/inh)	2 inh TID–QID

BID, *Twice daily;* DPI, *dry powder inhaler;* inh, *inhalation;* pMDI, *pressurized metered dose inhaler;* QID, *four times daily;* TID, *three times daily.*

TABLE 8-5	Combination Aerosols	
Drug Combination	Formulation	Adult Dosage
IPRATROPIUM/ALBUTEROL		
Combivent	MDI (18 µg/103 µg per puff)	2 inhalations every 6-8 hr
DuoNeb	Nebulized (0.5 mg/2.5 mg per 3 ml)	0.5 mg/2.5 mg every 6-8 hr
FLUTICASONE/SALMETEROL		
Advair	DPI (100, 250, 500 µg/50 µg)	1 inhalation BID
BUDESONIDE/FORMOTEROL		
Symbicort	DPI (80, 160 µg/4.5 µg)	1 inhalation BID

BID, *Twice daily;* DPI, *dry powder inhaler;* MDI, *metered dose inhaler.*

two other groups using either fluticasone alone or salmeterol alone failed to show any difference relative to placebo. It is important to note that the dose of fluticasone used in the fluticasone-alone study (1,000 µg/day) is a high dose for patients who, with COPD, are likely to be at greater risk for side effects from corticosteroids. The TORCH Study results are consistent with data that have been accumulating regarding the positive effects of steroids and long-acting β-agonists on exacerbations, symptoms, hospitalizations, and quality of life in COPD. Earlier studies documenting the lack of efficacy of long-term, inhaled budesonide on pulmonary function in these patients may have been because of a lack of power or too short a treatment period.[34,35]

At present, it is recommended to prescribe inhaled long-acting β-agonists for those patients with moderate or worse COPD, and inhaled corticosteroids for severe or worse COPD.[5] Because of the new findings previously described, the combination of steroids and long-acting β-agonists may be recommended for patients with less severe COPD in subsequent Global Initiative for Chronic Obstructive Pulmonary Disease treatment guidelines. As always, when to start new medications must be weighed against possible negative side effects.

MUCOKINETIC AGENTS

Retained tracheobronchial mucus contributes to the airflow obstruction of COPD, but large quantities of secreted mucus are uncommon in this disease.[3] Whereas copious sputum production is characteristic of diseases with predominant bronchiectasis, such as cystic fibrosis, patients with COPD rarely cough up more than 60 ml of mucoid sputum per day. Aerosol delivery of agents enhancing mucociliary clearance by reducing the viscosity of mucus (mucokinetic agents) should provide symptomatic relief of airflow obstruction and could theoretically have a positive effect on the degree of chronic airway inflammation and remodeling by limiting contact of infected, inflammatory secretions with the airway mucosa. Trials of mucokinetic therapy in patients with COPD have traditionally been disappointing, although a meta-analysis of oral agents showed a modest beneficial effect on COPD exacerbations.[36] Mucokinetic agents that are delivered directly to the airway include bland aerosols and various drugs and enzymes that interfere with the structure of mucus (mucolytics).

Bland Aerosols

Little clinical evidence suggests that simple humidification, aerosolized water (i.e., mist) or isotonic saline, can significantly "hydrate" respiratory secretions and reduce secretion viscosity.[37] Conversely, the use of bland aerosols or humidification to prevent further desiccation of the airway mucosal surface during administration of aerosolized drugs or high-flow oxygen is clearly warranted.[8] Nebulized hypertonic saline (1.8% to 20%) is an airway irritant that causes cough and mucus hypersecretion; it may be used to facilitate acquisition of sputum specimens for microbiologic tests such as acid-fast smears for tuberculosis or staining for *Pneumocystis* organisms. Again, little evidence suggests that the hypertonic fluid can promote dilution of airway secretions. Reflex cough and bronchospasm limit its use in obstructive lung disease, although data suggest improved sputum rheology and transiently improved sputum clearance in patients with cystic fibrosis treated with hypertonic saline aerosols.[38,39]

Alkalinization of mucus may weaken strand cross-linking and improve mucus viscosity.[8] Aerosolization of a 2% sodium bicarbonate solution has been tried in this regard. Although reported to be safe, bronchospasm and cough produced by the irritant require concurrent β_2-agonist use (must be mixed fresh and used immediately to prevent breakdown of β_2-agonist). No reliable data support the use of alkaline aerosols in COPD.

Mucolytics

Much clinical experience has been had with drugs containing reactive sulfhydryl groups that disrupt disulfide links in mucus proteins and reduce sputum viscosity. Topical acetylcysteine (*N*-acetyl-L-cysteine) rapidly liquefies sputum (maximal at 5 to 10 minutes) when instilled down endotracheal or tracheal tubes or bronchoscopically instilled in patients with tenacious mucous plugs (5 to 10 cc of a 10% to 20% solution). Again, induced bronchoconstriction, severe at times, limits the use of acetylcysteine in patients with obstructive lung disease. In rare cases, we have found it more helpful and bronchospasm less troublesome when the agent is directly instilled through the bronchoscope. We do not recommend its routine use or its use as an aerosol.

Aerosolized recombinant human DNase I has found a role as a mucolytic in patients with cystic fibrosis, in whom significantly increased sputum viscosity is largely a function of excessive amounts of leukocyte and bacterial DNA.[40] DNase I is given daily or twice daily in 2.5-mg doses. DNase has had a beneficial effect in cystic fibrosis, but not in either chronic bronchitis or bronchiectasis.[40,41]

ANTIBIOTICS

As with other aerosolized drugs, direct delivery of antibiotics to the respiratory tract in patients with suppurative lung infection has the theoretical advantage of delivering high local doses of the drug while avoiding systemic toxicity. Aerosol delivery of antibiotics has been limited by fear of inducing antibiotic resistance.

Although aerosolization of β-lactam antibiotics, aminoglycosides, and colistin can decrease the bacterial burden in the airways, controlled outcome trials have been positive only in patients with cystic fibrosis.[42] In these patients, chronically colonized with multidrug-resistant pseudomonal species, aerosolized tobramycin has been most extensively studied. In a 24-week, randomized, controlled trial, use of a tobramycin inhalational formulation via a jet ventilator (300 mg twice daily) resulted in significant clinical improvement without substantial toxic effects.[43] There was a trend toward an increase in aminoglycoside resistance of the airway flora, and this will need to be monitored closely in longer term studies.

Although the role of chronic and acute infection in the pathogenesis of COPD and COPD exacerbations is unclear, and many flares resolve without systemic antibiotics, treatment of acute exacerbations of COPD with antibiotics directed against the classic colonizing flora—*Streptococcus pneumoniae, Haemophilus influenzae*, and *Moraxella catarrhalis*—remains the standard of care. Data suggest that isolates in patients with severe COPD or exacerbations requiring hospitalization are predominantly enteric gram-negative bacteria and *Pseudomonas* species.[44,45] In many patients, exacerbations may be caused by the acquisition of different strains of the same bacteria.[46] With widespread bacterial antibiotic resistance growing, aerosolization of potent antibiotics with systemic toxicity may eventually be considered in COPD exacerbations. At present, aerosolized aminoglycosides or colistin (150 mg twice daily) is occasionally used in chronically ventilated patients with persistent, symptomatic pseudomonal infection unresponsive to systemic therapy or highly resistant to other available agents.

MODES OF AEROSOL DELIVERY

Aerosolized pharmacologic agents can be delivered to the lower respiratory tract of spontaneously breathing patients by the use of small-volume nebulizers (SVNs), metered dose inhalers (MDIs), metered dose inhalers with a spacer or holding chamber (MDIhs), and dry powder inhalers (DPIs).[47] SVNs, MDIs, and MDIhs have been readily available for use in the home for years. More recently, DPIs have gained popularity for aerosol administration in the home as a result of international agreements to eliminate the use of chlorofluorocarbons.[48]

Data,[47,49] like those illustrated in Figure 8-1, indicate that patient response to these three

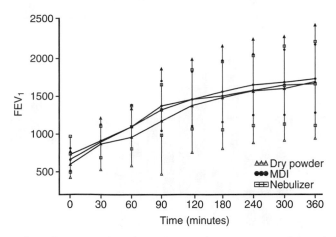

FIGURE 8-1 Absolute changes in forced expiratory volume in 1 second (FEV$_1$) (mean ± SD) following cumulative doses of inhaled albuterol in 27 patients in the emergency department with an FEV$_1$ of less than 30% predicted. Patients (nine in each group) were treated with albuterol via nebulizer (5 mg), metered dose inhaler (MDI) with a spacer or holding chamber (400 µg), and dry power inhaler (DPI) (Rotahaler, 400 µg). All groups received the respective treatments on arrival in the emergency department, every 30 minutes during the first 2 hours, and then hourly until the sixth hour. The total dose of inhaled albuterol administered during the 6-hour treatment was 45 mg of nebulized solution or 3600 µg via MDI and DPI. All groups improved compared with baseline, with no difference between groups.

approaches are similar. All three result in approximately 8% to 12% of delivered drug depositing in the lower respiratory tract.[50] Some of the newer design devices, specifically the hydrofluoroalkane-powered MDIs, claim much higher lung deposition.[51] However, the distribution of the remainder of the delivered drug differs among the three approaches.[48] With SVNs, most of the delivered drug deposits in the apparatus itself, with little drug depositing in the oropharynx and about 20% of the drug lost to the atmosphere.[52] MDIs result in little loss of the drug to the atmosphere; however, about 80% of the drug deposits in the oropharynx.[53] The use of a spacer essentially moves the 80% oropharyngeal deposition to deposition in the spacer.[53] With DPIs, little drug is lost to the atmosphere or deposited in the oropharynx, but about 80% of the drug is deposited in the apparatus.[54]

It should be emphasized that these data greatly depend on technique. Poor technique with any of these devices can result in marked changes in deposition within the respiratory tract.[55,56] Improper techniques are common with all of these devices but especially with MDIs and DPIs.[55,56] When a particular drug is available for delivery by all three techniques, at least theoretically patient response can be expected to be similar with each technique.[54] However, specific issues associated with the use of each of these

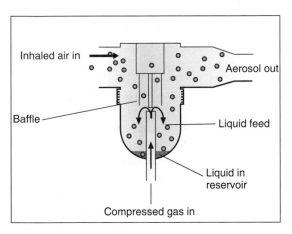

FIGURE 8-2 Schematic of an small-volume nebulizer (SVN). See text for discussion.

techniques can direct the clinician to choose a particular device for a specific patient.

Small-Volume Nebulizers

A typical SVN is illustrated in Figure 8-2.[57] All of these devices operate by use of the jet drag effect. That is, the high velocity of a rapidly flowing gas moving through the narrow outlet of the compressed gas inlet port draws fluid from the liquid reservoir by establishing a subatmospheric pressure lateral to the high-velocity flow. As a result, fluid is drawn up in front of the gas flow. When the gas strikes the fluid it aerosolizes

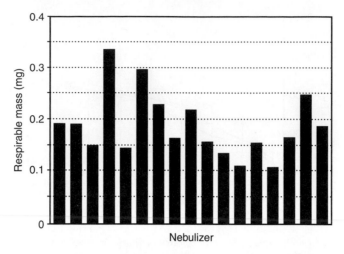

FIGURE 8-3 Respirable mass delivered from 17 small-volume nebulizers (SVNs). Respirable mass represents particles measuring 1 to 5 μm in size delivered to the mouthpiece with simulated spontaneous breathing and 2.5 mg of albuterol in a 4-ml volume placed in the SVN.

the liquid. The large particles are removed from the aerosol by striking the baffle, the walls, and the cap of the SVN.[58] These particles are in turn renebulized. Despite the fact that all SVNs function in this manner, their performance is clearly different. Figure 8-3 illustrates the respirable mass of aerosol produced by 17 different SVNs.[59] In addition, performance of a particular SVN model from the same company may vary from year to year as a result of changes in overall design features. Because of this variability in performance of SVNs, many newer drugs, especially antibiotics, indicate the precise nebulizer that should be used to deliver the drug.[58] SVNs are the only delivery devices that do not come packaged with the specific drug to deliver. MDIs and DPIs are designed specifically for the drug they deliver. As a result, efficacy of a drug delivered by SVN may depend on the SVN used to aerosolize it.

Factors Affecting Function of Small-Volume Nebulizers

In addition to the design of the SVN, several other factors affect the quantity of drug delivered, including gas flow powering the SVN,[59-61] diluent volume,[59-61] the drug solution to be nebulized,[62] the gas used to power the unit,[63] and the temperature of the solution being nebulized.[58]

All SVNs have a dead volume, which is a volume of fluid that will never be nebulized regardless of the solution used, the volume of solution nebulized, or the driving gas flow.[59]

This volume generally varies between about 1 and 1.5 ml. As a result, the smaller the actual volume of solution the greater the percentage of "drug" remaining in the dead volume. In general, about 25% to 30% of the drug placed in the nebulizer remains in the dead volume even if the optimal solution volume is used.[59] As nebulization time continues, the drug tends to concentrate in the dead volume. Increasing driving gas flow decreases the dead volume and also increases the percentage of aerosol particles in the therapeutic range (1 to 5 μm). However, from a practical perspective, the greater the solution volume the longer the treatment time, and the greater the delivered flow the greater the drug volume lost to the room. As a result, on the basis of current data,[59,63] it is recommended that the total drug volume be 4 to 5 ml and the driving gas flow be 6 to 8 L/min. This results in a total treatment time of about 8 to 15 minutes.

Because SVNs are designed to be used with oxygen–nitrogen mixtures, the use of a less dense driving gas (heliox) decreases delivered mass at the specific driving gas flow rate. If heliox is used to power the SVN, driving gas flow should be increased 30% to 40% or set at 8 to 11 L/min.[63]

Temperature and humidity of the nebulized solution and driving gas can affect the size of particles delivered by SVNs and the concentration of the drug in the dead volume.[64,65] Evaporation of water and adiabatic expansion of the driving gas reduce the temperature of the aerosol solution to about 8° to 12° F below atmospheric. The evaporation of water increases the concentration of drug in the nebulizer solution. Because the gas temperature increases once the aerosol leaves the nebulizer, particle size of the aerosol is reduced. Therefore the nebulizer driving gas should ideally be at room temperature and saturated with water vapor. This, of course, is impractical; however, use of a gas compressor instead of compressed gas increases the temperature and humidity of the driving gas. The aerosol solution temperature can be kept more constant if the patient grasps the SVN in the hand during treatment.[59,66]

Delivery Technique of Small-Volume Nebulizers

Box 8-1 outlines the procedure for using an SVN. As indicated earlier, all nebulizers have a dead volume that affects drug delivery. As a result, nebulization should continue until no aerosol is produced. This may require tapping of the sides of the aerosol to force large drops of solution to fall to the bottom of the device. Some have recommended placing a Y piece in the gas delivery tubing so that the patient can control when the drug is nebulized.[60] This markedly reduces the volume of drug lost to the environment but increases nebulization time twofold to threefold and requires significant patient coordination. Patients should be instructed to inspire normally to avoid hyperventilation. However, a periodic deep breath with an inflation hold does increase

retention of the drug in the lower respiratory tract. In addition, care should be exercised to ensure that patients do not breathe through the nose. Some patients may require the use of a nose clip.

Advantages and Disadvantages of Small-Volume Nebulizers

The major advantages of SVNs are their ability to deliver large quantities of drugs without patients having to coordinate aerosol delivery for optimal effect. In addition, nebulization can be performed continuously, they do not release environmental contaminants, and any drug conceivable can theoretically be delivered by SVNs. Important disadvantages of these devices are as follows:

- A pressurized gas source is required to operate the device
- The drug must be mixed before administration
- Contamination is highly probable if the device is not cleaned properly
- Drug is wasted
- SVNs are expensive
- A lengthy administration time (8-12 min) is required.[59]

Of these, the lack of portability (high-pressure gas source) and the need for drug preparation make this approach undesirable for use outside the hospital.

Electronic Nebulizers

As illustrated in Figure 8-4 an increasing variety of devices are available for the administration of aerosol therapy. One is the electronic nebulizer, or modified piezoelectric small-volume nebulizer.[56] This type of device is small, battery operated, and functions on the basis of a modification of historic ultrasonic nebulizer technology.[20] Although these devices are relatively expensive they can be used with any drug in a liquid preparation, are portable, and produce an aerosol of consistent small particle size. At present, they are infrequently used in the management of patients with COPD in the home; however, with improvements in technology and anticipated reduction in cost, their use can only be expected to increase.

Metered Dose Inhalers

Figure 8-5 illustrates the basic operation of a typical MDI.[67] All MDIs are constructed and operate in a similar manner. On actuating the MDI, drug stored in the metering chamber is released as an aerosol through the valve stem. When the metering chamber empties, solution from the tank

BOX 8-1	Technique for Use of a Small-Volume Nebulizer (SVN)

1. Assemble device.
2. Place drug in nebulizer; total solution volume, 4 to 5 ml.
3. Set driving flow to 6 to 8 L/min.
4. Connect patient to SVN via mouthpiece or mask (for some a nose clip may be necessary).
5. Instruct patient to inspire through an open mouth if using a mask or to close lips around mouthpiece.
6. Have patient hold nebulizer upright.
7. Have patient inhale slowly (0.5 L/sec) at normal tidal volumes.
8. Have patient take a periodic deep breath.
9. Continue treatment until no aerosol is produced.
10. Clean nebulizer.

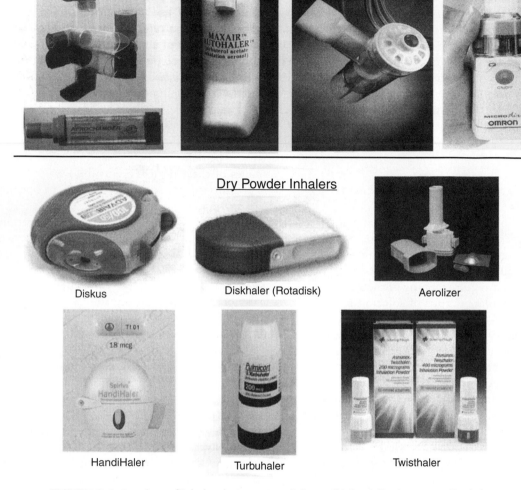

| MDIs, Spacers/ Holding Chambers | Breath-Actuated pMDI | Small-Volume Nubulizers | Modified Piezoelectric Small-Volume Nebulizer |

Dry Powder Inhalers

Diskus   Diskhaler (Rotadisk)   Aerolizer

HandiHaler   Turbuhaler   Twisthaler

FIGURE 8-4 A variety of inhaler devices potentially useful for delivering aerosolized drugs to patients with chronic obstructive pulmonary disease. In addition to small-volume nebulizers and pressurized metered dose inhalers (pMDIs) with a holding chamber or spacer, there are at present six different models of dry powder inhalers available. MDI, metered dose inhaler.

retaining cup enters the metering chamber and solution from the main reservoir enters the tank retaining cup. All of this can take time and requires the stimulation of vigorous shaking. As a result, all manufacturers recommend waiting at least 15 seconds before a second actuation and shaking vigorously before every actuation.[68,69] Vigorous shaking also ensures that the drug is evenly mixed with propellant/surfactant solution.[70]

Inspiring with Metered Dose Inhalers

To maximize drug delivery with an MDI, proper technique must be used. After vigorous shaking

of the canister, the patient should be instructed to exhale to functional residual capacity, place the MDI mouthpiece between wide-open lips, and begin to inhale slowly with inspiratory flows less than 30 L/min.[71] Immediately after the onset of inspiration, the MDI should be actuated while the patient continues to inhale to total lung capacity.[72] After completing a maximal inspiration, patients ideally should hold their breath for about 4 to 10 seconds (Box 8-2).

Patients should be aware of two other issues concerning the use of MDIs: loss of prime and inability to identify how much drug remains

Metered Dose Inhaler

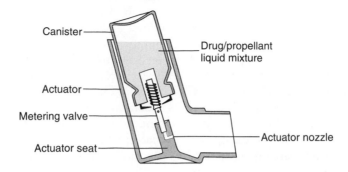

Metering Valve Function

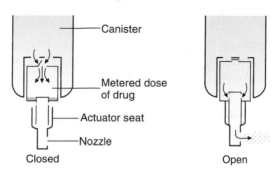

FIGURE 8-5 Components of a metered dose inhaler, including function of the metering valve.

within the canister.[59,71] If an MDI has been sitting for a few days, solution in the metering chamber can either evaporate or drain from it,[73,74] resulting in an inadequate dose of the drug being delivered in the first one or two actuations. As a result, with all new MDIs or MDIs that have not been used for longer than 48 hours, two actuations should be wasted to the room to ensure consistent dosing on every actuation the patient receives.

Most MDIs, when full, can deliver about 200 actuations. Unfortunately, it is impossible to look at an MDI and determine whether 10 or 190 actuations are left in the device. There is no good method of determining the number of actuations left in an MDI. As a result, patients ideally should keep a record of the number of actuations used or at least have determined the date by which the MDI will be empty, based on the number of prescribed doses per day. Unfortunately, the number of actuations in a single MDI varies by manufacturer.

BOX 8-2	Technique for Use of Metered Dose Inhaler (MDI)

1. Warm MDI to body temperature.
2. Uncap mouthpiece and inspect for presence of foreign objects.
3. Assemble apparatus.
4. Shake canister vigorously.
5. Hold canister upright.
6. Breathe out normally.
7. Place mouthpiece at mouth opening.
8. (If using a holding chamber, tightly seal lips around mouthpiece.)
9. Begin to inhale slowly at less than 30 L/min.
10. Actuate MDI (if using a holding chamber, actuate first and then begin to slowly inhale at < 30 L/min).*
11. Continue to inspire to total lung capacity.
12. Hold breath for 4 to 10 seconds or as long as is comfortable.
13. Wait at least 15 seconds before repeating steps 1 through 12 for additional actuations.
14. Recap MDI.

Some spacers have unit-specific instructions.

Advantages and Disadvantages of Metered Dose Inhalers

Use of MDIs has several compelling advantages.[68,70,71] They are convenient, small, lightweight, portable, difficult to contaminate, and inexpensive and do not require any drug preparation. However, the patient must coordinate actuation of the MDI with inspiration, and a high level of pharyngeal deposition of the drug occurs with MDIs.[69-71] It is also easy to increase dosing with MDIs but difficult to deliver large quantities of the drug; not all medications are available in MDIs, and drugs cannot be mixed. Finally, the technique for use of an MDI is more complex then for the other aerosol devices and improper use is common with this device.[55,56]

Spacers and Holding Chambers

The two most important disadvantages to the use of MDIs, coordination and pharyngeal deposition of the drug, can be overcome by the use of spacers or holding chambers.[75] However, it is important to note that no physiologic benefit has been found for the use of spacers or holding chambers. Figure 8-6 illustrates several different types of these devices.[76] Some are small and compact (OptiHaler; Respironics, Cedar Grove, N.J.),

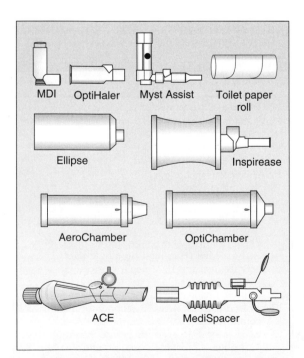

FIGURE 8-6 Various spacers and holding chambers available to deliver aerosol therapy in association with a pressurized metered dose inhaler (MDI).

whereas others are large (InspirEase; Schering-Plough, Kenilworth, N.J.). Most have one-way valves and require less coordination than a simple nonvalved MDI.[59,69] These devices are designed to allow actuation of the drug into the device before the patient inspires. As a result, patients can simply inspire without coordinating actuation during inspiration, and, most important, large aerosol particles deposit in the spacer, not in the oral pharynx. Spacers should always be used when steroids are administered.

Use of spacers and holding chambers is not without concerns. Two specific issues should be addressed when instructing patients about these devices[77]: the development of a static charge on the spacer and avoidance of multiple actuations into the spacer.[78] Over time most spacers develop, on the inner surface of the device, a static charge that attracts aerosol particles to the surface, decreasing the amount of drug delivered. This can be avoided by washing the device in soapy water and allowing it to air dry.[79] Hand drying of the device reestablishes the static charge. There are, however, new chambers on the market that are antistatic.[51]

Spacer-specific instructions should be followed. However, with most of these devices, after the drug is actuated, the patient should immediately inspire from the chamber.[80] The longer the wait, the smaller the respirable mass. In addition, multiple actuations into the spacer should be avoided.[81] More than one actuation into the spacer results in diminished drug delivery.[81]

Breath-Actuated Metered Dose Inhalers

At least one company manufactures a breath-actuated MDI (Figure 8-7).[82] With this device, the patient must generate enough flow (>27 L/min) to trigger the device. If the patient cannot generate sufficient flow, the device will not actuate. In addition, this device is available only with pirbuterol and cannot be used with other MDIs.[69]

Dry Powder Inhalers

DPIs have become increasingly available. In the ambulatory setting, DPIs have been shown to be comparable to SVNs and MDIs.[48,58,71] DPIs create drug aerosols by drawing room air through the powdered drug preparation. The powder contains either micronized (<5 μm in diameter) drug particles bound into loose aggregates or micronized drug particles that are loosely bound to large

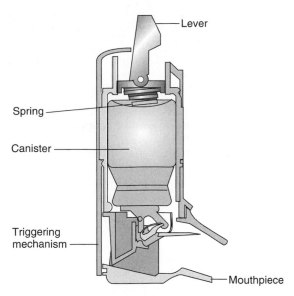

FIGURE 8-7 Schematic illustration of a breath-actuated Maxair Autohaler (pirbuterol inhalation).

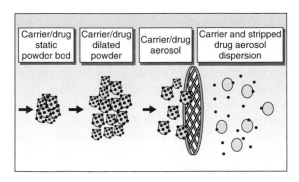

FIGURE 8-8 Aerosolization of a drug with a dry powder inhaler.

(>30 μm in diameter) lactose or glucose particles.[83] Because micronized particles adhere to each other and to most surfaces, the addition of larger carrier particles decreases interparticulate forces so that the powder separates into individual respirable particles more readily.[83] That is, the carrier particles aid flow of the drug from the device and act as fillers by adding bulk to the powder when the drug dose is very small. Usually the drug is stripped from the carrier particles[84] by the energy of the patient's inhalation (Figure 8-8).[85] As a result, release of respirable particles of the drug requires inspiration at relatively high flow rates (>30 L/min).[86,87] Drug particles of 1 to 2 μm are delivered along with large carrier particles (>30 μm) that impact in the pharynx. Two types of DPI are currently available: those in which the drug is packaged in individual doses (in a gelatin capsule or a foil blister) and those that contain a reservoir of drug that is metered with each dose.[88]

Factors Affecting Drug Delivery

Several factors influence drug delivery from DPIs, including manufacturer's design, resistance to airflow, proper assembly of components (loading of drug), accumulation of powder within the device,[48] and humidity.[89] Particle deposition in the device is influenced by electrostatic charge on the particles in the powder and the materials of the DPI device. The overall internal design of the device influences the resistance to gas flow (Figure 8-9)[90] and, as a result, the peak flow required during inhalation. Of primary concern for patients is the correct assembly and priming of the DPI. It is critical for the patient to correctly set up the DPI for use to ensure consistent dosing.

High environmental humidity can be extremely problematic for DPIs.[89,91] High humidity produces clumping of the dry powder, creating larger particles that are not effectively aerosolized and therefore less likely to reach the lung. Devices that contain a single large reservoir of the drug rather than individually packaged doses generally contain a desiccant to prevent clumping by ambient humidity. Use of a desiccant minimizes but does not eliminate the problems of humidity. These devices should not be stored in the bathroom.

Technique for Use of Dry Powder Inhalers

Box 8-3 lists the steps for use of a DPI. First and most important, the DPI must be correctly assembled and primed. As with MDIs, inspiration through a DPI should be from resting functional residual capacity level. The device needs to be placed between the patient's lips and a tight seal created. For most effective use, all inspired gas should move through the device. Because these devices are patient activated, the patient's inspiration produces aerosolization. As discussed, a rapid inspiratory flow of greater than 30 L/min is required. In general, the greater the flow, the greater the percentage of particles in the respirable range.[56] Breath holding after inhalation allows greater time for drug particles to deposit by sedimentation in the airways[48]; however, the need for a breath hold is controversial.[92] It is also important

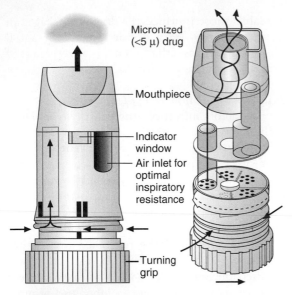

FIGURE 8-9 Components and airflow of the Turbuhaler (AstraZeneca, Westborough, Mass.). The inhaler contains up to 200 doses in its reservoir. A rotating disk below the reservoir has a series of clusters of conical cavities. Turning the grip at the bottom of the device rotates the disk, and plastic scrapers above the closing unit load the dose into a group of conical holes. The inhaler must be held upright during this operation so that a reproducible quantity of drug is fed, by gravity, into the conical cavities. A desiccant in the device protects the drug from moisture. The powder used in this device consists of micronized drug particles, without carrier particles. Because a minute amount of powder is inhaled, the patient may not experience any sensation of receiving a dose. The Turbuhaler does not have a dose counter, but a red sign appears in the dose indicator window when 20 doses remain in the device. When the patient inhales, air enters through channels at the base of the operating unit, passes through the pressure plate, through the cavities in the dosing unit, and into the inhalation channel. Turbulent airflow in the spiral channels disaggregates the particles. The twisting channels cause resistance to inhalation, so inspiratory airflow greater than 30 L/min is needed to obtain an adequate dose. Particles that are poorly entrained are retained in the channels and become re-entrained as smaller particles during subsequent inhalations.

to ensure that patients do not exhale back through the DPI. Exhalation through the device blows drug from the device and adds humidity, reducing the amount of aerosol produced.

Advantages and Disadvantages of Dry Powder Inhalers

DPIs are small, portable, and lightweight drug delivery devices. In addition, DPIs do not contain

---

BOX 8-3 | Technique for Use of a Dry Powder Inhaler (DPI)

1. Assemble apparatus (technique specific for each device).
2. Open capsule (technique specific for each device).
3. Exhale normally to functional residual capacity.
4. Place device mouthpiece in mouth and seal lips around mouthpiece.
5. Hold in proper position (technique specific for each device).
6. Inhale rapidly (>27 L/min) through device.
7. Hold breath for 4 to 10 seconds.
8. Exhale, but never back into the DPI.
9. Repeat process until capsule is empty (technique specific for each device).
10. Rinse mouth after use regardless of drug, but especially when using steroids.
11. Store in a cool dry place, not bathroom.

---

chlorofluorocarbons and do not require patient coordination during inspiration. However, a great deal of patient coordination may be required to set up and prime DPIs. In addition, very high sustained peak flow rates are required for correct use. The presence of high humidity is a clear problem with these devices that can markedly limit their use in certain seasons in parts of the United States.

PATIENT EDUCATION

It is becoming increasingly clear that patient education may be the most important factor determining patient's response.[93] Part of the problem with device-appropriate education is the fact that a given patient with COPD may be receiving aerosolized drugs by a number of different devices, each of which operates uniquely.[55] Box 8-4 from Hess[94] defines the differences in techniques between an MDI and a DPI. It can easily be seen how a patient using both of these devices could easily confuse the approach to be used with each. A number of studies clearly indicate that patient proper use of aerosol therapy devices is poor.[95,96] Some of this problem can be attributed to poor knowledge of the operation of aerosol therapy devices by clinicians.[97,98] Successful rehabilitation programs ensure that a respiratory therapist, knowledgeable concerning all aspects of drug delivery, teaches patients the correct operational technique for each aerosol delivery device used in the home.

SVNs, MDIs, MDIs WITH HOLDING CHAMBERS, AND DPIs: A COMPARISON

A comparison of SVNs, MDIs, MDIs with holding chambers, and DPIs is provided in Table 8-6. As noted, each of these devices has several advantages and disadvantages. On the basis of these ratings, we recommend the use of MDIs, MDIs with holding chambers, or DPIs when available. However, because of legislation regarding chlorofluorocarbons, it can be expected that increasing use of DPIs will occur, unless alternative propellants (hydrofluoroalkane) for MDIs become more widely available.

BOX 8-4	Some of the Differences in Technique between Metered-Dose Inhalers and Dry Powder Inhalers

- Shake the MDI but not the DPI.
- The DPI is breath actuated, whereas most MDIs are press-and-breathe.
- Use a slow flow with the MDI but a fast flow with the DPI.
- A spacer is not used with the DPI.
- A breath hold is more important with an MDI than with a DPI (and more important with an HFA MDI than with a CFC MDI).
- Do not exhale into the DPI.

From Hess DR: Metered-dose inhalers and dry powder inhalers in aerosol therapy, Respir Care 50:1376-1383, 2005.
CFC, *Chlorofluorocarbon;* DPI, *dry powder inhaler;* HFA, *hydrofluoroalkane;* MDI, *metered-dose inhaler.*

TABLE 8-6	Comparison of Advantages and Disadvantages among SVN, MDI, MDI with Holding Chamber, and DPI

Advantages	Disadvantages
SVN	
No patient coordination required	Compressed gas source required
No chlorofluorocarbon release	Easily contaminated
Able to mix drugs easily	Treatment time lengthy
Easy to administer high doses	Drug preparation required
Can administer drugs continuously	Expensive
Little pharyngeal deposition of drug	Lacks portability
	Must carefully clean nebulizer
MDI	
No drug preparation required	Significant patient coordination required
Difficult to contaminate	Patient actuation required
Easily portable	High pharyngeal deposition
Convenient	Difficult to deliver high doses
	Not all medications available
	Some are still chlorofluorocarbon driven
MDI WITH HOLDING CHAMBER	
No drug preparation required	Patient actuation required
Difficult to contaminate	Difficult to deliver high doses
Convenient	Not all medications available
No coordination required	Some are still chlorofluorocarbon driven
Little pharyngeal deposition	Some are large and bulky
	Periodically must clean holding chamber
DPI	
Little coordination required	Some assembly and priming required
Difficult to contaminate	Patient actuation required
Convenient	High inspiratory flow needed
Little pharyngeal deposition	Some medications not available
No chlorofluorocarbons	Difficult to deliver high doses
Highly portable	Must store in a cool, dry place

DPI, *Dry powder inhaler;* MDI, *metered dose inhaler;* SVN, *small-volume nebulizer.*

References

1. Calverley PM, Celli B, Anderson JA et al: The TOwards a Revolution in COPD Health (TORCH) Study: fluticasone propionate/salmeterol improves survival in COPD over three years [abstract], Chest 130:122S, 2006.

2. American Thoracic Society: ATS statement: standards for the diagnosis and care of patients with chronic obstructive lung disease, Am J Respir Crit Care Med 152:78-121, 1995.

3. Anthonisen NR, Wright EC: Bronchodilator response in chronic obstructive pulmonary disease, Am Rev Respir Dis 133:814-819, 1986.

4. Anthonisen NR, Connett JE, Kiley JP et al: Effects of smoking intervention and the use of an inhaled anticholinergic bronchodilator on the rate of decline of FEV_1: the Lung Health Study, JAMA 272:1497-1505, 1994.

5. Global Initiative for Chronic Obstructive Lung Disease (GOLD) 2007: Global strategy for the diagnosis, management and prevention of COPD. Available at http://www.goldcopd.org. Accessed December 9, 2006..

6. Martin RJ, Bartelson BL, Smith P et al: Effect of ipratropium bromide treatment on oxygen saturation and sleep quality in COPD, Chest 115:1338-1345, 1999.

7. Tashkin DP, Ashutosh K, Bleecker ER et al: Comparison of the anticholinergic bronchodilator ipratropium bromide with metaproterenol in chronic obstructive pulmonary disease: a 90-day multi-center study, Am J Med 81:81-90, 1986.

8. Chernow B: The pharmacologic approach to the critically ill patient, ed 3, Baltimore, 1994, Williams & Wilkins.

9. COMBIVENT Inhalation Aerosol Study Group: In chronic obstructive pulmonary disease, a combination of ipratropium and albuterol is more effective than either agent alone: an 85-day multicenter trial, Chest 105:1411-1419, 1994.

10. COMBIVENT Inhalation Solution Study Group: Routine nebulized ipratropium and albuterol together are better than either alone in COPD, Chest 112:1514-1521, 1997.

11. Gross N, Tashkin D, Miller R et al: Inhalation by nebulization of albuterol–ipratropium combination (Dey combination) is superior to either agent alone in the treatment of chronic obstructive pulmonary disease, Respiration 65:354-362, 1998.

12. Casaburi R, Hahler DA, Jones PW et al: A long-term evaluation of once-daily inhaled tiotropium in chronic obstructive pulmonary disease, Eur Respir J 19:217-224, 2002.

13. Vincken W, van Noord JA, Greefhorst AP et al: Improved health outcomes in patients with COPD during 1 year's treatment with tiotropium, Eur Respir J 19:209-216, 2000.

14. Celli B, ZuWallack R, Wang S et al: Improvement in resting inspiratory capacity and hyperinflation with tiotropium in COPD patients with increased static lung volumes, Chest 124:1743-1748, 2003.

15. O'Donnell DE, Fluge T, Gerken F et al: Effects of tiotropium on lung hyperinflation, dyspnoea and exercise tolerance in COPD, Eur Respir J 23: 832-840, 2004.

16. Decramer M, Celli B, Tashkin DP et al: Clinical trial design considerations in assessing long-term functional impacts of tiotropium in COPD; the UPLIFT Trial, COPD 1:303-312, 2004.

17. Nelson HS, Weiss ST, Bleecker ER et al: The Salmeterol Multicenter Asthma Research Trial: a comparison of usual pharmacotherapy for asthma or usual pharmacotherapy plus salmeterol, Chest 129:15-26, 2006.

18. Drazen JM, Israel E, Boushey HA et al: Comparison of regularly scheduled with as-needed use of albuterol in mild asthma: Asthma Clinical Research Network, N Engl J Med 335:841-847, 1996.

19. van Noord JA, Schreurs AJ, Mol SJ et al: Addition of salmeterol versus doubling the dose of fluticasone propionate in patients with mild to moderate asthma, Thorax 54:207-212, 1999.

20. Condemi JJ, Goldstein S, Kalberg C et al: The addition of salmeterol to fluticasone propionate versus increasing the dose of fluticasone propionate in patients with persistent asthma: Salmeterol Study Group, Ann Allergy Asthma Immunol 82:383-389, 1999.

21. Cazzola M, Matera M: Should long-acting beta 2-agonists be considered an alternative first choice option for the treatment of stable COPD? Respir Med 93:227-229, 1999.

22. Mahler DA, Donohue JF, Barbee RA et al: Efficacy of salmeterol xinafoate in the treatment of COPD, Chest 115:957-965, 1999.

23. Nelson HS, Bensch G, Pleskow WW et al: Improved bronchodilation with levalbuterol compared with racemic albuterol in patients with asthma, J Allergy Clin Immunol 102:943-952, 1998.

24. Levalbuterol for asthma: Med Lett Drugs Ther 41:51-53, 1999.

25. Nowak R, Emerman C, Hanrahan JP et al: A comparison of levalbuterol with racemic albuterol in the treatment of acute severe asthma exacerbations in adults, Ann Emerg Med 24:259-267, 2006.

26. Schrech DM, Babin S: Comparison of racemic albuterol and levalbuterol in the treatment of acute asthma in the ED, Ann Emerg Med 23:842-847, 2005.

27. Datta D, Vitale A, Lahiri B et al: An evaluation of nebulized levalbuterol in stable COPD, Chest 124:844-849, 2003.

28. Truitt T, Witko J, Halpern M: Levalbuterol compared to racemic albuterol: efficacy and outcomes in patients hospitalized with COPD or asthma, Chest 123:128-135, 2003.

29. Hendeles L, Hartzema A, Truitt T: Levalbuterol is not more cost-effective than albuterol for COPD, Chest 124:1176, 2003.

30. Ameredes BT, Calhoun WJ: (R)-Albuterol for asthma: pro [a.k.a. (S)-albuterol for asthma: con], Am J Respir Crit Care Med 174:965-969, 2006.

31. Barnes PJ: Treatment with (R)-albuterol has no advantage over racemic albuterol, Am J Respir Crit Care Med 174:969-972, 2006.

32. Barnes PJ: Efficacy of inhaled corticosteroids in asthma, J Allergy Clin Immunol 102:531-538, 1998.

33. Kamada AK, Szefler SJ, Martin RJ et al: Issues in the use of inhaled glucocorticoids: the Asthma Clinical Research Network, Am J Respir Crit Care Med 153:1739-1748, 1996.

34. Pauwels RA, Lofdahl CG, Laitinen LA et al: Long-term treatment with inhaled budesonide in persons with mild chronic obstructive pulmonary disease who continue smoking: European Respiratory Society Study on Chronic Obstructive Pulmonary Disease, N Engl J Med 340:1948-1953, 1999.

35. Vestbo J, Sorensen T, Lange P et al: Long-term effect of inhaled budesonide in mild and moderate chronic obstructive pulmonary disease: a randomised controlled trial, Lancet 353:1819-1823, 1999.

36. Poole PJ, Black PN: Mucolytic agents for chronic bronchitis, Oxford, 1999, The Cochrane Library.

37. Ziment I: Pharmacologic therapy of obstructive airway disease, Clin Chest Med 11:461-486, 1990.

38. Elkins MR, Robinson M, Rose BR et al: A controlled trial of long-term inhaled hypertonic saline in patients with cystic fibrosis, N Engl J Med 354:229-240, 2006.

39. Donaldson SH, Bennett WD, Zeman KL et al: Mucus clearance and lung function in cystic fibrosis with hypertonic saline, N Engl J Med 354:241-250, 2006.

40. Fuchs HJ, Borowitz DS, Christiansen DH et al: Effect of aerosolized recombinant human DNase on exacerbations of respiratory symptoms and on pulmonary function in patients with cystic fibrosis: the Pulmozyme Study Group, N Engl J Med 331:637-642, 1994.

41. Wills PJ, Wodehouse T, Corkery K et al: Short-term recombinant human DNase in bronchiectasis: effect on clinical state and in vitro sputum transportability, Am J Respir Crit Care Med 154:413-417, 1996.

42. Itozaku G, Weinstein R: Aerosolized antimicrobials: another look, Crit Care Med 26:5-6, 1998.

43. Ramsey BW, Pepe MS, Quan JM et al: Intermittent administration of inhaled tobramycin in patients with cystic fibrosis, N Engl J Med 340:23-26, 1999.

44. Soler N, Torres A, Santiago E et al: Bronchial microbial patterns in severe exacerbations of chronic obstructive pulmonary disease (COPD) requiring mechanical ventilation, Am Rev Respir Crit Care Med 157:1498-1505, 1998.

45. Eller J, Ede A, Schaberg T et al: Infective exacerbations of chronic bronchitis: relation between bacteriologic etiology and lung function, Chest 113:1542-1548, 1998.

46. Sethi S, Evans N, Grant BJ et al: New strains of bacteria and exacerbations of chronic obstructive pulmonary disease, N Engl J Med 347:465-471, 2002.

47. Raimondi AC, Schottlender J, Lombardi D et al: Treatment of acute severe asthma with inhaled albuterol delivered via jet nebulizer, metered dose inhaler with spacer, or dry powder, Chest 97:24-28, 1997.

48. Dhand R, Fink J: Dry powder inhalers, Respir Care 44:940-951, 1999.

49. Dolovich MB, Ahrens RC, Hess DR et al: Device selection and outcomes of aerosol therapy: evidence based guidelines: American College of Chest Physicians/American College of Asthma, Allergy and Immunology, Chest 127:335-377, 2005.

50. Pauwels R: Inhalation device, pulmonary deposition and clinical effect of inhaled therapy [review], J Aerosol Med 10:S17-S21, 1997.

51. Geller DE: Comparing clinical features of the nebulizer, metered-dose inhaler, and dry powder inhaler, Respir Care 50:1313-1321, 2005.

52. Lewis RA, Fleming JS: Fractional deposition from a jet nebulizer: how it differs from a metered dose inhaler, Br J Dis Chest 79:361-367, 1985.

53. Newman DP, Pavia D, Moren F et al: Deposition of pressurized aerosols in the human respiratory tract, Thorax 36:52-55, 1981.

54. Lipworth BJ, Clark DJ: Lung delivery of salbutamol by breath activated pressurized aerosol and dry powder inhaler devices, Pulmon Pharmacol Ther 10:211-214, 1997.

55. Fink JB, Rubin BK: Problems with inhaler use: a call for improved clinician and patient education, Respir Care 50:1360-1374, 2005.

56. Rau JL: Practical problems with aerosol therapy in COPD, Respir Care 51:158-172, 2006.

57. Newman SP: Aerosol generators and delivery systems, Respir Care 36:939-951, 1991.

58. Hess DR: Aerosolized medication delivery. In Branson RD, Hess DR, Chatburn RL, editors: Respiratory care equipment, Philadelphia, 1999, Lippincott Williams & Wilkins, pp 133-156.

59. Hess D, Fisher D, Williams P et al: Medication nebulizer performance: effects of diluent volume, nebulizer flow and nebulizer brand, Chest 110:498-505, 1996.

60. Clay MM, Pavia D, Newman SP et al: Assessment of jet nebulizers for lung aerosol therapy, Lancet 2:592-594, 1983.

61. Loffert DT, Ikle D, Nelson HS: A comparison of commercial jet nebulizers, Chest 106:1788-1793, 1994.

62. Coates AL, MacNeish CF, Meisner BR: The choice of jet nebulizer, nebulizing flow, and addition of albuterol affects the output of tobramycin aerosols, Chest 111:1206-1212, 1997.

63. Hess DR, Acosta FL, Ritz R et al: Effect of helix on nebulizer function, Chest 115:184-189, 1999.

64. Newman SP, Pellow PGD, Clarke SW: In vitro comparison of DeVilbiss jet and ultrasonic nebulizers, Chest 92:991-994, 1987.

65. Phipps PR, Gonda I: Droplets produced by medical nebulizers: some factors affecting their size and solute concentration, Chest 97:1327-1332, 1990.

66. Fink J: Aerosol drug therapy. In Wilkins RL, Stoller JK, Scanlan CL, editors: Egan's fundamentals of respiratory care, ed 8, St. Louis, 2003, Mosby, pp 683-714.

67. Rau JL Jr: Respiratory care pharmacology, ed 6, St. Louis, 2002, Mosby.

68. Byron RR: Performance characteristics of pressurized metered dose inhalers in vitro, J Aerosol Med 10:S3-S6, 1997.

69. Hess D, Daugherty A, Simmons M: The volume of gas emitted from five metered dose inhalers at three levels of fullness, Respir Care 37:444-447, 1992.

70. Berg E: In vitro properties of pressurized metered dose inhalers with and without spacer devices, J Aerosol Med 8:S3-S11, 1995.

71. Kacmarek RM, Hess D: The interface between patient and aerosol generator, Respir Care 36:952-976, 1991.

72. Hess D: Aerosol therapy, Respir Clin North Am 1:235-263, 1995.

73. Shultz RK: Drug delivery characteristics of metered dose inhalers, J Allergy Clin Immunol 96:284-287, 1995.

74. Everard ML, Devadason SG, Summers BG: Factors affecting total and "respirable" dose delivered by a salbutamol metered dose inhaler, Thorax 50:746-749, 1995.

75. Guidry GG, Brown WD, Stogner SW: Incorrect use of metered dose inhalers by medical personnel, Chest 101:31-33, 1992.

76. Wilkes W, Fink J, Dhand R: Selecting an accessory device with a metered-dose inhaler: variable influence of accessory devices on fine particle dose, throat deposition, and drug delivery with asynchronous actuation from a metered-dose inhaler, J Aerosol Med 14:351-360, 2001.

77. Newman SP: Principles of metered-dose inhaler design, Respir Care 50:1177-1190, 2005.

78. Clark DJ, Lipworth BJ: Effects of multiple actuations, delayed inhalation and antistatic treatment on the lung bioavailability of salbutamol via a spacer device, Thorax 57:981-986, 1996.

79. Wildhaber JH, Devadason SG, Hayden MJ et al: Electrostatic charge on a plastic spacer device influences the delivery of salbutamol, Eur Respir J 9:1943-1946, 1996.

80. Barry PW, O'Callaghan C: The effect of delay, multiple actuations, and spacer static charge on the in vitro delivery of budesonide from the Nebuhaler, Br J Clin Pharmacol 40:76-78, 1995.

81. Barry PW, O'Callaghan C: The effect of delay, multiple actuations and spacer static change on the in-vitro delivery of budesonide from the Nebuhaler, Br J Clin Pharmacol 40:76-78, 1995.

82. Newman DP, Weisz AWB, Talau N et al: Improvement of drug delivery with a breath activated pressurized aerosol for patients with poor inhaler technique, Thorax 46:712-716, 1991.

83. Ganderton D: The generation of respirable clouds from coarse powder aggregates, J Biopharm Sci 3:101-105, 1992.

84. Dolovich M, Rheim R, Rashid F et al: Measurement of the particle size and dosing characteristics of a radiolabelled albuterol—sulphate lactose blend used in the SPIROS dry powder inhaler. In Dalby RN, Byron P, Farr S, editors: Respiratory drug delivery V: program and proceedings, Buffalo Grove, Ill, 1996, Interpharm Press/CRC, pp 332-345.

85. Dalby RN, Hickey AJ, Tiano SL: Medical devices for the delivery of therapeutic aerosols to the lungs. In Hickey AJ, editor: Lung biology in health and disease, vol 94: inhalation aerosols: physical and biological basis for therapy, New York, 1996, Marcel Dekker, pp 441-473.

86. Hansen OR, Pederson S: Optimal inhalation technique with terbutaline Turbuhaler, Eur Respir J 2:637-639, 1989.

87. Pedersen S, Hansen OR, Fuglsang G: Influence of inspiratory flow rate upon the effect of a Turbuhaler, Arch Dis Child 65:308-310, 1990.

88. Atkins PJ: Dry powder inhalers: an overview, Respir Care 50:1304-1312, 2005.

89. Maggi L, Bruni R, Conte U: Influence of moisture on the performance of a new dry powder inhaler, Int J Pharm 177:83-91, 1999.

90. Crompton GK: Delivery systems. In Kay AB, editor: Allergy and allergic diseases, London, 1997, Blackwell Science, pp 1440-1450.

91. Jashnani RN, Byron PR, Dalby RN: Testing of dry powder aerosol formulations in different environmental conditions, Int J Pharm 113:123-130, 1994.

92. Pedersen S: Delivery systems in children. In Barnes PJ, Grunstein MM, Leff AR, Woolcock AJ, editors: Asthma, Philadelphia, 1997, Lippincott-Raven, pp 1915-1929.

93. Rau JL: Determinants of patient adherence to an aerosol regimen, Respir Care 50:1346-1356, 2005.

94. Hess DR: Metered-dose inhalers and dry powder inhalers in aerosol therapy, Respir Care 50:1376-1383, 2005.

95. Melani AS, Zanchetta D, Barbato W et al: Inhalation technique and variables associated with misuse of conventional metered-dose inhalers and newer dry powder inhalers in experienced adults, Ann Allergy Asthma Immunol 93:439-449, 2004.

96. McFadden ER Jr: Improper patient technique with metered dose inhalers: clinical consequences and solutions to misuse, J Allergy Clin Immunol 96:278-283, 1995.

97. Guidny GG, Brown WD, Stogner SW et al: Incorrect use of metered dose inhalers by medical personnel, Chest 101:31-33, 1992.

98. Interiano B, Guntupalli KK: Metered-dose inhalers: do health care providers know what to teach? Arch Intern Med 153:81-85, 1993.

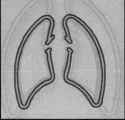

Chapter 9

Therapeutic Oxygen

BRIAN L. TIEP • RICK CARTER

CHAPTER OUTLINE

Oxygen Transport
Scientific Basis for Long-Term Oxygen
   Therapy
Clinical Signs of Hypoxia
Measuring Arterial Oxygenation
Hazards, Pitfalls, and Cautions
Role of Oxygen in the Medical Regimen
Oxygen During Sleep
Oxygen During Exercise
Ambulatory Oxygen During Exercise
Exercise Oxygen as a Therapeutic
   Modality

Physiologic Criteria for Prescribing
   Long-Term Oxygen Therapy
Oxygen Prescription
Oxygen Systems
Oxygen Delivery Methods
   Intermittent (Pulsed) Flow Devices
   Reservoir Cannulas
   Transtracheal Catheters
Humidification
Patient Education and Exercise Training
Therapeutic Oxygen in Pulmonary
   Rehabilitation

PROFESSIONAL SKILLS

On completion of this chapter, the reader will be able to do
the following:

- Understand the physiology of oxygen (O_2) therapy during rest, sleep, and exertion
- Have a working knowledge of O_2 systems, both stationary and portable
- Conceptualize O_2 as more than supplementation; rather, as a therapeutic intervention with many
  potential benefits

The history of oxygen (O_2) both mirrors and tracks the progress of medical science and chemistry over the past 300 years. Joseph Priestley, who has been credited for discovering O_2 in the late 1700s, described it as a possible treatment, as well as an article of luxury.[1] Today O_2 is largely regarded as supplemental, from which it may be inferred that it is *replacement therapy*, that is, replacing that which was removed by lung disease. O_2 is considered protective because hypoxia is damaging to the body's machinery. In the early years oxygen was prescribed as a therapy for a

variety of disorders from pneumonia to gout. Thomas Beddoes and his able assistant, Sir Humphry Davy, established the Pneumatic Institution in Bristol, England during the 1800s.[2] They administered O_2 as a primary therapy to treat many conditions. Although they were not necessarily practicing evidence-based medicine, they did set forth a path of exploration that eventually established the role of oxygen in modern medicine.

Hyperbaric oxygen notwithstanding, clinicians are coming full circle in regarding O_2 as a therapy, particularly in the context of pulmonary rehabilitation. Studies have appeared that support the view that oxygen may be administered as a therapeutic adjunct to improve the patient's physiologic response to exercise and ability to function in life. The concept of therapeutic O_2 encompasses both its supplemental role as a primary or adjunctive therapy. The role of O_2 in addressing medical issues depends on its application, the goal of therapy, and the pathophysiology involved. The widened concept of therapeutic O_2 now encompasses administering O_2 to patients who are not hypoxemic.

Categorization of these concepts is helpful in understanding and designing an approach to administering O_2 to patients. This chapter addresses the therapeutic administration of O_2 in both contexts: as supplementation and protection from the ravages of tissue hypoxia, as well as an enabling therapy administered within the restorative fabric of a pulmonary rehabilitation program.

OXYGEN TRANSPORT

O_2, in its essential role in metabolic processes, must make its way from the atmosphere to each living cell. It must be taken up and incorporated into the scheme of high-energy metabolism.[3] The pathway of O_2 transport is sequential—powered through pressure gradients (i.e., lung, capillary, and cell), conveyed in chemical attachment to hemoglobin, propelled by the cardiovascular system through multiple interfaces, and eventually arriving at the cell, where it moves into the mitochondria and is used in cellular respiration and energy production. Throughout this pathway the risk of malfunction lurks.

The partial pressure of oxygen in the arteries (Pa_{O_2}) is determined by the fraction of inspired oxygen (Fi_{O_2}) in the atmosphere breathed, alveolar ventilation, ventilation—perfusion matching, and diffusion of O_2 across the alveolar—capillary membrane.[4] Arterial O_2 saturation is determined by these factors plus the ability of hemoglobin to bind and transport O_2 to the tissues. Other influencing factors include cardiac output, tissue capillary distribution, and the uptake and use of O_2 by the mitochondria. A defect in any of these physiologic links is likely to impede oxygen from reaching its final destination and prevent it from being optimally used in cellular metabolism.

Chronic hypoxia impairs cellular function and may progress to cellular necrosis. Initially, cell survival will be prolonged by means of anaerobic glycolysis, a process that is short-lived.[5] Cells can function temporarily in this anaerobic environment, albeit inefficiently and uncomfortably. Meanwhile, there is a buildup of lactate in the cells and eventually in the circulation in the form of lactic acidosis. A return to oxidative metabolism must occur without delay if the cells are to survive and function optimally. The clinician must be vigilant for signs of tissue hypoxia.

SCIENTIFIC BASIS FOR LONG-TERM OXYGEN THERAPY

Whereas the discovery of O_2 occurred in the late 1700s, proof that long-term oxygen therapy (LTOT) is clinically efficacious appeared only in 1980 with results from the Medical Research Council (MRC) study[6] and the National Institutes of Health Nocturnal Oxygen Therapy Trial (NOTT).[7] These controlled multicenter trials clearly demonstrated increased survival with O_2 therapy in a time- and dose-dependent relationship (Figure 9-1). The British MRC study randomly assigned patients with hypoxemia to receive LTOT for 15 hours/day (including the hours of sleep) versus no oxygen. After 4 years, 19 of 42 patients undergoing O_2 therapy died as compared with 30 of 45 control patients, who received no oxygen.[6] Thus there was a 21% survival advantage in the oxygen therapy group as compared with control subjects with respect to mortality.

The NOTT, performed in North America on a similar population of 203 hypoxemic patients with

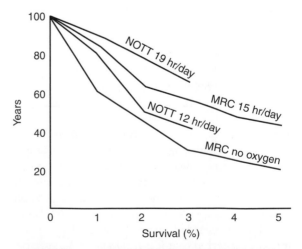

FIGURE 9-1 Combined results of the Medical Research Council (MRC) Study and Nocturnal Oxygen Therapy Trial (NOTT), demonstrating the dose-response benefit for patients using oxygen for an increasing number of hours per day.

chronic obstructive pulmonary disease (COPD), randomly assigned patients to receive O_2 for 12 hours/day (including the hours of sleep) or 24 hours/day. Patients in the 12-hours/day nocturnal group fully complied, whereas the continuous group averaged 19 hours of oxygen use per day. Survival was 1.94 times better for the continuous versus the nocturnal oxygen therapy group, with a significant survival difference noted at 12 months.[7] Given the similarity of the patient populations in these two studies, the results are often combined to deliver a unified message. Survival is poor if patients with hypoxemia are denied O_2. If they receive oxygen part of the time survival is improved but the best survival accrues through continuous oxygen therapy. Thus survival is correlated with the number of hours per day of oxygen use. See Figure 9-1.

CLINICAL SIGNS OF HYPOXIA

Clinicians should always be watchful for signs of tissue hypoxia. Signs indicative of tissue hypoxia differ, based on the affected tissue and local circulation. Hypoxic manifestations of specific tissues and organ systems will often characterize a failure in the function of those tissues. In the lungs, hypoxemia causes the following:
- Pulmonary vasoconstriction that manifests as right heart failure
- Bronchospasm
- Respiratory muscle dysfunction
- Eventual respiratory failure[8]
Cardiac muscle hypoxia may present as:
- Tachycardia and a reduction in stroke volume due to loss of cardiac contractility
- Atrial or ventricular arrhythmias
- Congestive heart failure[8]

Brain tissue hypoxia may first present as a loss of short-term memory, followed by euphoria and impaired judgment.[9] Psychomotor function falters and more severe cerebral hypoxia induces cerebral edema, a life-threatening event.[10] Alimentary tissue hypoxia may manifest as an impairment of gastric or intestinal motility or as alterations in gastric acidity.[11] Some of the manifestations of tissue hypoxia may be created or modified by the coexistence of hypercarbia.

MEASURING ARTERIAL OXYGENATION

No clinical sign accurately or promptly assesses for a deficiency in arterial oxygenation. Cyanosis is a late finding and may indicate the presence of 5 g of deoxygenated hemoglobin per 100 ml of blood. This is a variable sign that will occur earlier in the polycythemic patient or late to never if the patient is anemic. Arterial blood gas (ABG) measurement is the "gold standard" for blood O_2, as well as carbon dioxide (CO_2) and acid–base status. Arterial sampling is safe and standardized. Sources of error include improper sample site, sampling of venous rather than arterial blood, poor specimen handling (e.g., air leaks to sampled blood), or inadequate blood gas analyzer calibration.

A commonly used noninvasive alternative to the ABG is pulse oximetry. Pulse oximetry reflects arterial oxygen saturation and is noted as SpO_2 (SaO_2 is the notation used when measured by ABG). Pulse oximetry compares two wavelengths of light transmitted through the finger, earlobe, or other body area. It computes the saturation from the comparison of oxygenated blood (red band) with deoxygenated blood (infrared band).[12] SpO_2 correlates with SaO_2 with a 1% to 2% error when the saturation is in the 85%+ range when carboxyhemoglobin is minimal.[13] The greatest advantage of pulse oximetry over the ABG is the ability to noninvasively track saturation over time and thereby assess trends. This is particularly useful for exercise and sleep studies as well as when titrating supplemental O_2.

HAZARDS, PITFALLS, AND CAUTIONS

O_2 therapy is safe, lifesaving, and enabling. However, some caution is warranted. Oxygen in metabolism largely breaks down to CO_2 and water (H_2O). However, a small portion of O_2 does not submit to this complete breakdown. Intermediate breakdown products include oxidants or other highly reactive O_2 species that damage the airways and alveoli, as well as other tissues, initiating inflammatory responses and fibrosis. As a protective mechanism the body synthesizes antioxidant enzymes such as catalase and superoxide dismutase, which empowers the completion of the metabolic breakdown while offering a level of protection to the tissue. However, as the concentration of O_2 increases, particularly above 50%, this protective system may be overwhelmed, leaving the ventilatory tract vulnerable to oxidation and inflammation. Investigators have questioned whether low-flow O_2 therapy can be damaging.[14] In an uncontrolled study that examined lung biopsy specimens of patients receiving LTOT and who died of other causes, some fibrotic changes were detected.[15] However, the NOTT and MRC study demonstrated a net positive and life-preserving effect of long-term O_2.[6,7]

There is concern that O_2 therapy can lead to absorptive atelectasis and areas with a low ventilation-to-perfusion ratio ($\dot{V}/\dot{Q}$).[16] This is of particular concern after surgery, when administering oxygen may promote $\dot{V}/\dot{Q}$ mismatch, thereby increasing the need for supplemental oxygen. This is not usually a ground for concern in patients receiving LTOT. Again, long-term studies have failed to confirm these speculated negative effects.[6,7] Thus supplemental O_2 remains a positive therapy for which there is no alternative treatment.

Oxygen therapy equipment is designed to be operated by the patient and family safely and effectively. However, some caution should prevail. Patients should never smoke in the presence of O_2 equipment and particularly when O_2 is flowing through the nasal cannula.[17] Lighting a cigarette with O_2 flowing through the nasal cannula has been known to cause a devastating and sometimes fatal fire that blazes up the nasal passages. Compressed O_2 cylinders have occasionally been tipped over, causing the valve to break off and turning the O_2 cylinder into a missile capable of penetrating a concrete wall. This fortunately is a very rare event. Liquid O_2 during transfilling may leak and cause freezing burns if the liquid O_2 comes in contact with the skin. Also, O_2 in high concentration (>40%) may support rapid combustion and stoke an intensely hot fire. Again, with common sense and thoughtful care, these disasters are avoidable.

In the past, clinicians were concerned about the possibility that administering O_2 would lead to CO_2 narcosis and respiratory acidosis and that the patient would simply stop breathing and die. Early studies by Bigelow and colleagues[18] showed that CO_2 retention is rare and usually does not lead to CO_2 narcosis or respiratory acidosis. Sassoon, Hassell, and Mahutte[19] and Aubier and colleagues[20] demonstrated that when patients retained CO_2, they did not decrease their minute ventilation—a finding inconsistent with respiratory drive suppression. Actually patients showed an increase in their dead space—to—tidal volume (V_D/V_T) ratio and a widening $\dot{V}/\dot{Q}$ mismatch.

On occasion, respiratory drive suppression does occur. Robinson and colleagues[21] observed a reduction in ventilation in some patients during an exacerbation. CO_2 retainers tended to be patients with lower room air Sao_2 receiving hyperoxic O_2 flows. This suppressed hypoxic vasoconstriction restricts perfusion. The combined reduction in ventilation and $\dot{V}/\dot{Q}$ mismatch may result in CO_2 retention with or without significant respiratory acidosis. Dunn, Nelson, and Hubmayr[22] showed that ventilator-dependent patients receiving hyperoxic mixtures had an increase in the CO_2 recruitment threshold. V_D/V_T increased, whereas CO_2 elimination remained constant. In general, titrating O_2 flow to a target Sao_2 of 92% will maintain adequate oxygenation and minimize the likelihood of CO_2 retention and respiratory acidosis. If respiratory acidosis does occur, then ventilatory support should be considered.

The kidneys of many patients with advanced COPD are able to compensate for chronic hypercapnia by producing bicarbonate; in this way the patients maintain their acid–base balance. In such cases chronic CO_2 retention serves an adaptive function that spares the patient from excessive work of breathing. Chronic hypercapnia need not be an ominous prognostic sign in these patients.[23] Any adverse consequences of hypercapnia are related to acute acidosis. Acute changes in acid–base balance can be detected by ABG and the clinician should pay attention to the clinical signs such as decreased alertness or excessive sleepiness. As a general rule, correction of hypoxemia must supersede concerns about CO_2 retention.

ROLE OF OXYGEN IN THE MEDICAL REGIMEN

O_2 therapy is only one element of an interactive multicomponent care plan for patients with COPD. Exercise, airway hygiene, bronchodilation and minimization of hyperinflation all have a direct salutary impact on oxygen transport. In addition, optimization of cardiovascular function is essential, especially in the presence of comorbidities. There is no substitute for O_2 therapy in the hypoxemic patient. As is noted in a later section, oxygen is an important adjunct in maximizing the physiologic response to exercise. Moreover, it is crucial that pulmonary mechanics and gas exchange variables function as efficiently as possible to maximize the effectiveness of oxygen. In pulmonary rehabilitation, pursed lips breathing retraining not only slows exhalation and minimizes hyperinflation but actually increases arterial oxygenation.[24]

OXYGEN DURING SLEEP

We generally spend 8 hours, more or less, per night in slumber. It is common for people with normal lungs to slow their breathing during sleep and exhibit mild transient desaturations. In the patient with COPD whose arterial oxygenation is borderline while awake, it is not unusual for the SaO_2 to dip below 90% during sleep. Desaturations are most often associated with REM sleep but can occur at any stage. Consequences of significant desaturations can include the following: pulmonary hypertension, systemic hypertension, cardiac arrhythmias, derangement of sleep architecture promoting daytime somnolence, and increased morbidity and mortality.[25] In a subgroup of patients with COPD with nocturnal O_2 desaturation, O_2 therapy has been shown to prevent or reverse some of these complications.[26]

The mechanisms for nocturnal O_2 desaturation in patients without evidence of obstructive sleep apnea may include hypoventilation largely due to reduction in tidal volume,[27] alveolar hypoventilation, increased V_D/V_T, or exaggerated $\dot{V}/\dot{Q}$ mismatch. Studies that examined predictors of nocturnal oxygen desaturation have yielded variable results, perhaps because of differences in the populations studied. One study demonstrated that sleep desaturation could be predicted by daytime SaO_2, which also was correlated with elevated $PaCO_2$.[28] Patients with both hypercapnia and hypoxemia while awake are most likely to desaturate at night.[29] The tendency to desaturate at night is not always predictable by daytime blood gases, suggesting involvement of sleep dynamics.[30]

In practice it is common to prescribe the daytime O_2 setting for sleep. Because patients receiving oxygen therapy are likely to desaturate more during sleep, the daytime setting is often insufficient. Many of these patients will end up spending more than 30% of the night with an SaO_2 less than 90%.[31,32] In the NOTT, the daytime O_2 setting was increased by 1 L/minute for sleep.[7] More recent studies have shown that 50% of patients with COPD who are receiving LTOT with corrected daytime saturation require the 1-L/minute increase to maintain nocturnal saturation and reduce sleep disturbances, for example, arousals. This confirms the wisdom of the early NOTT investigators.

Patients with COPD with no sign of obstructive sleep apnea (OSA) and adequate daytime SaO_2 may undergo sleep desaturations of 9% to 21%.[30] These patients are in a group referred to as *nocturnal-only desaturators*. Disease severity, CO_2 retention, and high body mass index were all predictive of nocturnal-only desaturation.[33,34] Further, patients who desaturate during sleep also tend to have hypercarbia, as well as severely impaired pulmonary mechanics. There is evidence that these patients can benefit from nocturnal O_2.[26] Higher mortality rates among nocturnal-only desaturating patients and daytime SaO_2 greater than 90% has been demonstrated in retrospective studies.[25] However, well-controlled studies of nocturnal-only desaturating patients failed to detect an improvement in clinical course in spite of the fact that there was a small reduction in pulmonary artery pressure.[35] In a large multicenter trial involving patients with daytime hypoxemia between 55 and 60 mm Hg, nocturnal O_2 therapy did not reduce the evolution of pulmonary hypertension, prevent the onset of further hypoxemia, or improve survival.[35] Nevertheless, it is reasonable to be concerned about this patient population. Certainly, in patients with signs of pulmonary hypertension and cor pulmonale with adequate daytime saturations, it is logical to perform overnight oximetry and prescribe O_2 for sleep.

Some patients have both COPD and OSA, often referred to as *overlap syndrome*.[36] Both COPD and OSA may predispose patients to fragmented sleep and impaired quality of life. It is tempting to think that OSA is more common among patients with COPD, but this may not be the case.[37] Both conditions are common. The prevalence of COPD in patients with OSA is 11%.[37] The prevalence of OSA in a selected group of patients with COPD was 20%.[38] Factors that explain this finding are influenced by the demographics of overweight smokers with hypertension. OSA may hasten the onset of respiratory failure in COPD. One study showed a higher incidence of pulmonary hypertension.[37]

It is generally recommended that patients with overlap syndrome be treated for their OSA.[39] Polysomnography is not recommended for across-the-board screening—rather for evaluation of patients suspected of having OSA. Look for signs of upper airway obstruction because it could both affect sleep quality and contribute to OSA.[31]

OXYGEN DURING EXERCISE

O_2 is administered during exercise to protect against cellular hypoxia, enhance the ability to perform at a higher work rate, or augment the patient's ability to derive physiologic benefit from exercise training. An increase in the oxygen flow setting is usually required to accommodate a higher work rate. The higher oxygen requirement during exercise is not only necessary for the increased rate of metabolism but also for the change in dynamics in the lung. There is a decrease in red cell transit time at the alveolar capillaries; $\dot{V}/\dot{Q}$ matching is altered, often to the disadvantage of successful O_2 transport; and end-expiratory lung volume is elevated, increasing the work of breathing and V_D/V_T. During exercise a reduction in diffusing capacity may become a limiting factor. Understanding these physiologic variables is a key to prescribing successful oxygen therapy, particularly in association with an exercise program.

An exercise training program that enables and supports an active lifestyle is an essential component of a successful pulmonary rehabilitation program.[40] A normal cardiopulmonary response to submaximal exercise is characterized by an increase in Pa_{O_2} coupled with a lowering of Pa_{CO_2}. Both the pulmonary and cardiovascular systems are fully capable of accommodating to nearly maximal levels of exercise in their ability to supply O_2 to exercising muscle. The diffusing capacity of the lung and capillary blood flow are able to more than double.[41] Under resting conditions, even patients with significant lung disease are not limited by their lung diffusing capacity or by red cell transit time.[42] However, during exercise, the effectiveness of alveolar–capillary oxygen transport is challenged by a marked decrease in red cell transit time, as well as by $\dot{V}/\dot{Q}$ mismatch. Both conditions conspire to limit O_2 supply to exercising muscle.

The immediate effects of administering O_2 during exercise include a reduction in hyperinflation, the capacity to exercise longer and at a higher work rate, the ability to achieve a greater physiologic response to exercise, a reduction in transient increases in pulmonary vasoconstriction as reflected in pulmonary artery pressure and pulmonary vascular resistance, a reduction in dyspnea for a given work rate, and the prevention of tissue hypoxia during exercise. O_2 improves the ability to exercise in a dose-dependent fashion up to an FI_{O_2} of 50%.[43] Patients who train on O_2 are able to perform at higher work rates while breathing room air than those who train on room air.[44]

The major ventilatory limitation to exercise in the patient with COPD is dynamic hyperinflation. The mechanism seems to be related to the minute ventilation, more specifically to breath rate. Rapid breathing does not allow time for lungs to empty before taking in the next breath.[45] O_2 may reduce the breath rate for a given work rate by suppressing carotid body activity (sympathetic drive).[46] In fact, exercise training also reduces the breath rate for a given work rate.[45] Thus exercise training and O_2 are mutually beneficial in enabling the patient to exercise longer and harder while reducing dyspnea and leg fatigue. If exercise O_2 were to be administered to prevent exercise desaturation, it would be given as a supplement or replacement with the setting adjusted for that goal. If O_2 is administered to enable the patient to exercise at a higher level or to augment the training effect of exercise, it is a specific therapy that may require a higher setting.

AMBULATORY OXYGEN DURING EXERCISE

Ambulatory O_2 either prevents or limits the extent of exercise desaturation. With all other factors in place this ensures adequate oxygenation of exercising muscle. Ambulatory oxygen has been shown to improve quality of life in a randomized study.[47] In a study comparing a portable oxygen system with the same system delivering room air, there was an immediate improvement in exercise performance, but no long-term increase in exercise performance or quality of life was observed.[48] To date, no study has convincingly demonstrated a survival benefit from portable O_2; however, an adequately powered study has yet to be performed.[49] Other studies have supported the concept of protecting exercising muscle from cellular hypoxia.[50] It is also known that cardiac arrhythmias may be provoked during hypoxemic episodes,[51] although little is known about arrhythmias during exercise in patients with COPD. Because the ability to be active is limited by hypoxemia, clinical judgment should prevail in the direction of providing O_2 to prevent hypoxia in exercising muscle.

EXERCISE OXYGEN AS A THERAPEUTIC MODALITY

O_2 as a therapeutic modality to augment the restorative benefits of a pulmonary rehabilitation program is an emerging concept. Not all studies have lent support to this concept. Rooyackers and colleagues[52] showed no benefit of training with O_2 versus training on room air. At the same time they reported a reduction in dyspnea. However, if a reduction in dyspnea translates into a reduction in breath rate, it would be reasonable to expect that their patients would be able to exercise at a higher work rate. Exercise training at a higher intensity is known to achieve a greater physiologic response. Again, on the negative side, Garrod, Paul, and Wedzicha[53] found that O_2 during a pulmonary rehabilitation program did not increase exercise capacity. A key difference between the foregoing studies and those that follow is that more recent studies involve exercise at a higher work rate. Somfay and colleagues[43] demonstrated a dose-dependent reduction in hyperinflation and improvement in endurance as the F_{IO_2} increases to 50%. These results were consistent with the early findings by Cotes and Gilson,[54] who also found a dose-dependent effect. O'Donnell, D'Arsigny, and Webb[55] determined that O_2 ameliorated exercise dyspnea by reducing hyperinflation and decreasing lactate levels. Emtner and colleagues[44] discovered that patients who train on O_2 are able to exercise to a higher work rate and lower breathing rate with less hyperinflation and greater endurance. Peters, Webb, and O'Donnell[56] demonstrated that the combination of exercise, bronchodilators, and O_2 reduces dynamic hyperinflation. Maltais and colleagues[57] found that administering 75% oxygen improved blood flow to the lower extremities, which supports the concept of a circulatory factor in O_2 transport. Thus O_2 has independent, as well as collaborative, therapeutic benefits for patients in pulmonary rehabilitation.

PHYSIOLOGIC CRITERIA FOR PRESCRIBING LONG-TERM OXYGEN THERAPY

Patients are evaluated for LTOT by measuring their Pa_{O_2} as recommended by the American Thoracic Society and European Respiratory Society COPD guidelines.[58] ABGs are recommended for initial measurement because of their greater accuracy and because they provide a wider

---

BOX 9-1	Arterial Blood Gas or Sa_{O_2} Indications for Home Oxygen Therapy

A. Continuous O_2 therapy
 1. $Pa_{O_2} \leq 55$ mm Hg or $Sa_{O_2} \leq 88\%$
 2. $Pa_{O_2} = 56$ to 59 mm Hg or $Sa_{O_2} = 89\%$ with
   a. Dependent edema from CHF or
   b. Cor pulmonale or pulmonary hypertension or Hct $> 56\%$
B. Nocturnal O_2 only
 1. $Pa_{O_2} \leq 55$ mm Hg or $Sa_{O_2} \leq 88\%$ during sleep or drop in $Sa_{O_2} > 5\%$ with signs or symptoms of hypoxemia
C. Exercise O_2 only
 1. $Pa_{O_2} \leq 55$ mm Hg or $Sa_{O_2} \leq 88\%$

CHF, *Congestive heart failure;* Hct, *hematocrit;* O_2, *oxygen;* Pa_{O_2}, *arterial partial pressure of oxygen;* Sa_{O_2}, *arterial oxygen saturation*

---

clinical picture that includes Pa_{CO_2} and acid–base status. This is particularly important if hypercapnia or acidosis is suspected. Box 9-1 lists indications for home O_2 therapy.

Patients who become hypoxemic during an exacerbation (but were not hypoxemic before that exacerbation) may eventually recover to the point that they no longer meet the physiologic criteria for LTOT. It is thus recommended that the need for LTOT be reassessed during rest and exercise in 60 to 90 days after clinical stability is realized. If the patient no longer meets the established criteria, the O_2 can be discontinued. On the other hand, patients who become hypoxemic through the natural progression of the disease may also improve with O_2 to the point that they do not meet the criteria for LTOT. This improvement is thought to be due to a reparative effect of their O_2 therapy.[59] It is generally recommended that these patients continue O_2 supplementation even if they do not meet the criteria for LTOT after retesting. This recommendation is based on the concept that O_2 is reparative, and as such, it may be harmful to withdraw O_2, thereby allowing progression of the disease to reinstate itself.

OXYGEN PRESCRIPTION

Patients are initially evaluated for LTOT on the basis of an ABG along with a concomitant Sp_{O_2} via pulse oximetry to establish a reliable baseline relationship.[58] All of the flow adjustments for oxygenation are then made, using Sp_{O_2} readings as a guide. If hypercapnia is a concern, further initial adjustments should be made on the basis of the ABG. The O_2 setting should be titrated to ensure an adequate SpO_2 greater than 90% during the usual physiologic conditions of life: rest, exercise, and sleep. A reasonable target SpO_2 is 92% (Figure 9-2).

OXYGEN SYSTEMS

Three different sources are available for home O_2: compressed gas, liquid, or O_2 concentrators. Each has advantages and disadvantages and specific application. O_2 concentrators are largely

designated to be stationary O_2 sources in the home. They are plug-in devices that use a zeolite filter to separate room air O_2 from nitrogen. They are inexpensive, operate at low pressures, and are reliable. Compressed gas O_2 is stored under pressure (usually 2200 psi) and can be easily stored for long periods. O_2 cylinders are inexpensive and provide reliable sources of oxygen. Liquid oxygen is created by supercooling room air to nearly absolute 0° C (or −273° F). Oxygen is fractionally distilled from the O_2–nitrogen mixture and stored in a thermos-like container called a Dewar flask. The advantage of liquid O_2 is its ability to store nearly 1,000 gaseous liters of O_2 in a

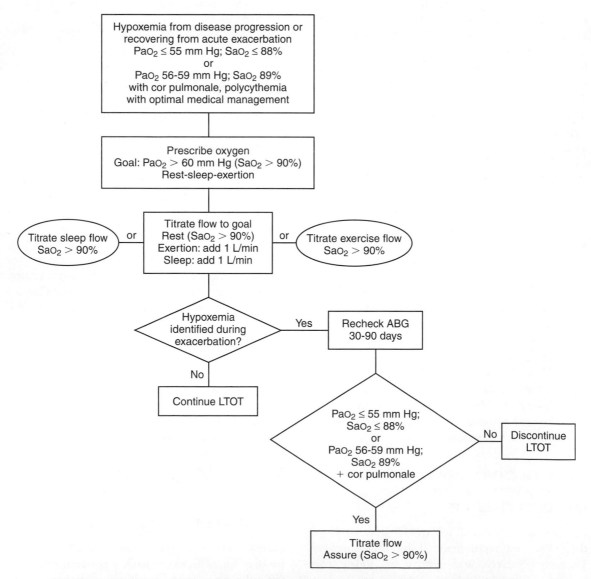

FIGURE 9-2 American Thoracic Society and European Respiratory Society flow diagram for prescribing long-term oxygen therapy. ABG, arterial blood gases; LTOT, long-term oxygen therapy; PaO_2, arterial partial pressure of oxygen; SaO_2, arterial oxygen saturation as measured by ABG.

1–liter liquid volume, making it an excellent source of portable O_2. Its disadvantages include its higher cost and the fact that most units must vent to the atmosphere—which limits the life of a refill.

At present, all O_2 systems have stationary and portable components. Concentrators are largely stationary, but new portable concentrators have become available and are now acceptable sources of O_2 on some airlines. They vary in weight from 6 to 16 lb, the latter having a continuous flow feature. Their greatest advantage is that they are self-contained systems independent of an outside O_2 source. There are also O_2 concentrators that refill portable O_2 cylinders; this enables patients to be free from home deliveries and to use highly portable O_2 containers. Liquid oxygen is available as a very portable system weighing as little as 3.5 lb. Compressed cylinders are now available as 4-lb systems, but these do not last as long as liquid O_2 between refills. However, multiple small containers can be stored and transported.

OXYGEN DELIVERY METHODS

O_2 is administered via continuous flow or intermittent flow, using reservoir devices or transtracheal catheters. By far the most commonly prescribed delivery device is the dual-pronged nasal cannula. It is generally well tolerated once patients accept their need for O_2 and the benefits of using it.

O_2 is most commonly administered via continuous flow. However, continuous flow is inefficient given that O_2 is delivered throughout the breath cycle; this wastes most of the O_2 flow. As a consequence of this inefficiency continuous flow delivery does not lend itself to portable systems.

To provide O_2 that is lightweight and portable, three solutions have been developed: intermittent (pulsed) flow devices, reservoir cannulas, and transtracheal catheters.[60] These devices vary in efficiency from 2:1 to 7:1 versus continuous flow and are fundamental to the development of portable lightweight delivery systems with wide usage range.[61]

Intermittent (Pulsed) Flow Devices

Intermittent (pulsed) flow delivery devices sense the beginning of inhalation and rapidly deliver a pulse of O_2. For the delivery pulse to be included in alveolar–capillary gas exchange, the pulse must begin immediately on initiation of inhalation and finish just before the last 150 ml of inhalation (anatomic dead space).[62-65] The devices that meet those specifications may improve upon the efficiency of O_2 delivery by a factor of 7:1 as compared with continuous flow. There are many devices available with different delivery volumes, timing, flow settings, and efficacies.[66] Most will oxygenate the lungs while the patient is at rest, but many will be unable to maintain adequate saturation during exercise (exertion).[67]

During exercise there is not only an increase in the metabolic requirement for O_2 but also additional pathophysiologic variables that contribute to exercise hypoxemia. There is a further widening of $\dot{V}/\dot{Q}$ mismatch, higher V_D/V_T, diffusion impairment, and a decrease in red cell transit time through the alveolar capillaries. Pulsed delivery devices often fail to maintain adequate saturation at the usual settings. Larger delivery pulses and better-timed devices may be required.[68] Some patients must use a reservoir cannula or transtracheal catheter, which are more effective during exercise.[69] The only way to ensure adequate O_2 delivery during exercise is to test the patient during exercise while titrating O_2 delivery.

Most activities of daily living are carried out in short bursts. This requires that patients increase and decrease their O_2 setting many times throughout the day, which is rather impractical. A pulse delivery device with a built-in activity sensor makes these changes automatically to maintain saturation.[70] This innovation may signal the further development of devices that track each patient's lifestyle and ensure appropriate O_2 delivery to them.

Reservoir Cannulas

Reservoir cannulas (Oxymizer and fluidically controlled Pendant; CHAD Therapeutics) store O_2 during exhalation, accumulating an O_2 bolus for the next inhalation.[71,72] The efficiency of these devices varies from 2:1 to 4:1 or even higher when using pursed lips breathing.[73] They are inexpensive disposable devices that are reliable and work well with any O_2 source. They can be used during exercise and sleep.[74] Reservoir cannulas are particularly effective for oxygenating lungs in patients who are difficult to oxygenate or require high flow oxygen.[75] Their disadvantage is that they tend to be large and more noticeable (improvements are on the immediate horizon).

Transtracheal Catheters

Transtracheal catheters deliver O_2 directly into the trachea.[76] There is a significant cosmetic advantage to this arrangement; other physiologic advantages include a reduction in work of breathing and the ability to deliver higher flow for ventilation and treatment of OSA.[77,78] They also improve the efficiency of O_2 delivery by 2:1 to 3:1. Disadvantages include their higher cost and the requirement for surgical placement. They can be supplied by continuous flow or intermittent pulsed flow O_2 sources.[79]

HUMIDIFICATION

In the hospital setting it is common to humidify O_2, coming from the wall outlet, through a bubble humidifier. Studies that evaluated standard bubble humidifiers in patients receiving flows up through 4 L/minute have found no difference in nasal drying and patients could not subjectively distinguish between dry and humidified O_2.[80] These results are not surprising given the low vapor output of bubble humidifiers and the fact that O_2 contributes only a small portion of inspiratory flow. Also, as the inspired gas is raised to body temperature the room temperature humidification drops even further. Actually, the nasal mucosa is an excellent source of humidification at body temperature, raising the humidity of the inhaled air and O_2 close to the point of saturation.

Transtracheal delivery presents a different set of challenges. The nasal mucosa humidifier is bypassed. Thus the most important source of moisture is missing. At higher transtracheal flows, there is a risk of mucous ball formation at the end of the catheter. At flows greater than 5 L/minute or more, patients may benefit from heated and humidified O_2.

PATIENT EDUCATION AND EXERCISE TRAINING

LTOT is prescribed with laudable physiologic and clinical goals of preventing tissue hypoxia, facilitating better function, and boosting exercise performance. Clinicians regard O_2 as enabling, whereas patients may view O_2 as disabling. The first goal of education would be a meeting of the minds. The clinician must show concern and understanding for the patient's viewpoint, and the patient must understand that O_2 is a therapy rather than

a sign of impending disability and death. The patient must accept the O_2 and use it appropriately and safely. When patients embrace their portable O_2 along with an active lifestyle, the clinical course of the disease may be turned into a positive direction. Education is a continuing and nurturing process that helps patients through the various bumps and hurdles of life.

THERAPEUTIC OXYGEN IN PULMONARY REHABILITATION

Patients in a pulmonary rehabilitation program undergo comprehensive multifaceted training to restore them to their highest level of function. Those who require O_2 to prevent tissue hypoxia are prescribed oxygen during rest, sleep, and exercise to help ensure adequate tissue oxygenation (Figure 9-3). Those who are not hypoxemic during rest or exercise, but will undergo high-intensity exercise training, will likely benefit from therapeutic O_2 targeted to maximize their physiologic response to exercise.[43,44] Because both exercise training and O_2 reduce dynamic hyperinflation, exercise training and oxygen could be considered cotherapeutic.

In addition, within the fabric of pulmonary rehabilitation patients are prescribed bronchodilators including tiotropium. These bronchodilators decrease dynamic hyperinflation and improve exercise performance. Combining tiotropium with O_2 has amplified that effect.[56] Combining O_2 with helium (heliox) has also been shown to diminish hyperinflation.[81]

In addition, pursed lips breathing both alone and with O_2 increases oxygenation and reduces dynamic hyperinflation.[24] Thus within the pulmonary rehabilitation setting, multiple approaches both alone and in combination are known to reduce ventilatory impediments to exercise and, thus, enable higher intensity training to improve O_2 transport and functional performance while decreasing dyspnea and leg fatigue.

Given all of these findings and the role played by O_2, oxygen can now be regarded as a therapy within the pulmonary rehabilitation program rather than as simply protective against hypoxemia. If O_2 is considered a primary therapy, it is likely that clinicians will modify how O_2 delivery is prescribed to meet specific physiologic goals. During rest and sleep, the goal is to prevent tissue hypoxia and therefore a setting that ensures a Sao_2 of 90% to 92% will meet that requirement. However, during exertion,

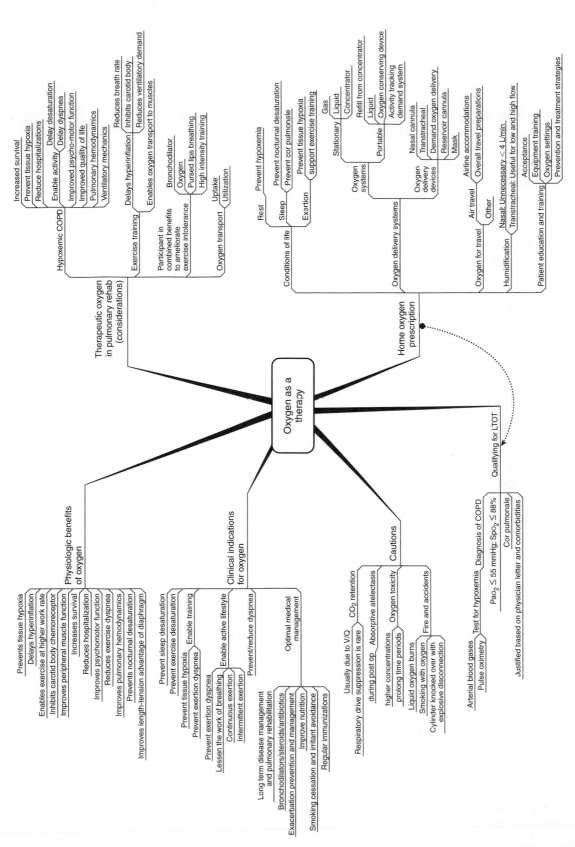

FIGURE 9-3 Summary of oxygen as a therapy in pulmonary rehabilitation. CO_2, carbon dioxide; COPD, chronic pulmonary obstructive disease; LTOT, long-term oxygen therapy; PaO_2, arterial partial pressure of oxygen; SpO_2, arterial oxygen saturation as measured by pulse oximetry; $\dot{V}/\dot{Q}$, ventilation-to-perfusion ratio.

the goal may be to enable more activity that is less encumbered by dyspnea. Hence, the SaO_2 goal may be higher, say, 95%. If O_2 is administered to maximize the intensity of exercise training, clinicians may be prescribing therapeutic O_2 settings up to an FIO_2 of 50%.[43]

Although these are important clinical considerations, the current state of knowledge requires a stronger physiologic foundation. At present, however, O_2 can be regarded as part of the exercise equipment in its restorative role in pulmonary rehabilitation. In presenting this concept to the patient, it is important for the patient to understand that it is not a grave prognostic sign—rather, the O_2 is being prescribed as a therapeutic enabler.

References

1. Petty TL: Historical highlights of long-term oxygen therapy, Respir Care 45:29-36, 2000.
2. Tiep B: History of oxygen in medicine. In Tiep B, editor: Portable oxygen therapy: including oxygen conserving methodology, Mt. Kisco, NY, 1991, Futura Publishing.
3. Leach RM, Treacher DF: ABC of oxygen: oxygen transport. 2. Tissue hypoxia, BMJ 317:1370-1373, 1998.
4. West JB: Gas exchange. In West JB, editor: Respiratory physiology: the essentials, Philadelphia, 2005, Lippincott Williams & Wilkins, pp 49-56.
5. Wasserman K, Stringer WW, Casaburi R et al: Determination of the anaerobic threshold by gas exchange: biochemical considerations, methodology and physiological effects, Z Kardiol 83(suppl 3):1-12, 1994.
6. Long term domiciliary oxygen therapy in chronic hypoxic cor pulmonale complicating chronic bronchitis and emphysema, Report of the Medical Research Council Working Party, Lancet 1:681-686, 1981.
7. Continuous or nocturnal oxygen therapy in hypoxemic chronic obstructive lung disease: a clinical trial. Nocturnal Oxygen Therapy Trial Group, Ann Intern Med 93:391-398, 1980.
8. Alpert JS: Pulmonary hypertension and cardiac function in chronic obstructive pulmonary disease, Chest 75:651-652, 1979.
9. Fix AJ, Daughton D, Kass I et al: Cognitive functioning and survival among patients with chronic obstructive pulmonary disease, Int J Neurosci 27:13-17, 1985.
10. Fix AJ, Golden CJ, Daughton D et al: Neuropsychological deficits among patients with chronic obstructive pulmonary disease, Int J Neurosci 16:99-105, 1982.
11. Gutierrez G, Palizas F, Doglio G et al: Gastric intramucosal pH as a therapeutic index of tissue oxygenation in critically ill patients, Lancet 339:195-199, 1992.
12. Carter R: Oxygen and acid—base status: measurement, interpretation, and rationale for oxygen therapy. In Tiep BL, editor: Portable oxygen therapy: including oxygen conserving methodology, Mt. Kisco, NY, 1991, Futura Publishing, pp 136-138.
13. Ralston AC, Webb RK, Runciman WB: Potential errors in pulse oximetry. I. Pulse oximeter evaluation, Anaesthesia 46:202-206, 1991.
14. Jenkinson SG: Oxygen toxicity, New Horizons 1:504-511, 1993.
15. Petty TL, Stanford RE, Neff TA: Continuous oxygen therapy in chronic airway obstruction: observations on possible oxygen toxicity and survival, Ann Intern Med 75:361-367, 1971.
16. Benoît Z, Wicky S, Fischer JF et al: The effect of increased FIO(2) before tracheal extubation on postoperative atelectasis, Anesth Analg 95:1777-1781, 2002.
17. West GA, Primeau P: Nonmedical hazards of long-term oxygen therapy, Respir Care 28:906-912, 1983.
18. Bigelow DB, Petty TL, Levine BL et al: The effect of oxygen breathing on arterial blood gases in patients with chronic airway obstruction living at 5,200 feet, Am Rev Respir Dis 96:28-34, 1967.
19. Sassoon CS, Hassell KT, Mahutte CK: Hyperoxic-induced hypercapnia in stable chronic obstructive pulmonary disease, Am Rev Respir Dis 135:907-911, 1987.
20. Aubier M, Murciano D, Fournier M et al: Central respiratory drive in acute respiratory failure of patients with chronic obstructive pulmonary disease, Am Rev Respir Dis 122:191-199, 1980.
21. Robinson TD, Freiberg DB, Regnis JA et al: The role of hypoventilation and ventilation—perfusion redistribution in oxygen-induced hypercapnia during acute exacerbations of chronic obstructive pulmonary disease, Am J Respir Crit Care Med 161:1524-1529, 2000.
22. Dunn WF, Nelson SB, Hubmayr RD: Oxygen-induced hypercarbia in obstructive pulmonary disease, Am Rev Respir Dis 144:526-530, 1991.
23. Aida A, Miyamoto K, Nishimura M et al: Prognostic value of hypercapnia in patients with chronic respiratory failure during long-term oxygen therapy, Am J Respir Crit Care Med 158:188-193, 1998.
24. Tiep BL, Burns M, Kao D et al: Pursed lips breathing training using ear oximetry, Chest 90:218-221, 1986.
25. Kimura H, Suda A, Sakuma T et al: Nocturnal oxyhemoglobin desaturation and prognosis in chronic obstructive pulmonary disease and late sequelae of pulmonary tuberculosis. Respiratory Failure Research Group in Japan, Intern Med 37:354-359, 1998.
26. Fletcher EC, Luckett RA, Goodnight-White S et al: A double-blind trial of nocturnal supplemental oxygen for sleep desaturation in patients with chronic obstructive pulmonary disease and a daytime PaO2 above 60 mm Hg, Am Rev Respir Dis 145:1070-1076, 1992.
27. Becker HF, Piper AJ, Flynn WE et al: Breathing during sleep in patients with nocturnal desaturation, Am J Respir Crit Care Med 159:112-118, 1999.

28. Thomas VD, Vinod KS, Gitanjali B: Predictors of nocturnal oxygen desaturation in chronic obstructive pulmonary disease in a south Indian population, J Postgrad Med 48:101-104, 2002.

29. Plywaczewski R, Sliwinski P, Nowinski A et al: Incidence of nocturnal desaturation while breathing oxygen in COPD patients undergoing long-term oxygen therapy, Chest 117:679-683, 2000.

30. Mohsenin V, Guffanti EE, Hilbert J et al: Daytime oxygen saturation does not predict nocturnal oxygen desaturation in patients with chronic obstructive pulmonary disease, Arch Phys Med Rehabil 75:285-289, 1994.

31. Hawrylkiewicz I, Palasiewicz G, Plywaczewski R et al: [Effects of nocturnal desaturation on pulmonary hemodynamics in patients with overlap syndrome (chronic obstructive pulmonary disease and obstructive sleep apnea)], Pneumonol Alergol Pol 68:37-43, 2000.

32. Fletcher EC, Donner CF, Midgren B et al: Survival in COPD patients with a daytime PaO2 greater than 60 mm Hg with and without nocturnal oxyhemoglobin desaturation, Chest 101:649-655, 1992.

33. De AG, Sposato B, Mazzei L et al: Predictive indexes of nocturnal desaturation in COPD patients not treated with long term oxygen therapy, Eur Rev Med Pharmacol Sci 5:173-179, 2001.

34. Fletcher EC, Luckett RA: The effect of positive reinforcement on hourly compliance in nasal continuous positive airway pressure users with obstructive sleep apnea, Am Rev Respir Dis 143:936-941, 1991.

35. Chaouat A, Weitzenblum E, Kessler R et al: A randomized trial of nocturnal oxygen therapy in chronic obstructive pulmonary disease patients, Eur Respir J 14:1002-1008, 1999.

36. Flenley DC: Breathing during sleep, Ann Acad Med Singapore 14:479-484, 1985.

37. Chaouat A, Weitzenblum E, Krieger J et al: Association of chronic obstructive pulmonary disease and sleep apnea syndrome, Am J Respir Crit Care Med 151:82-86, 1995.

38. Fischer J, Raschke F: [Incidence of obstructive sleep apnea syndrome in combination with chronic obstructive respiratory tract disease], Pneumologie 47(supp. 4):731-734, 1993.

39. Nicholson D, Tiep B, Jones R et al: Noninvasive positive-pressure ventilation in chronic obstructive pulmonary disease, Curr Opin Pulm Med 4:66-75, 1998.

40. Tiep BL: Disease management of COPD with pulmonary rehabilitation, Chest 112:1630-1656, 1997.

41. Hadeli KO, Siegel EM, Sherrill DL et al: Predictors of oxygen desaturation during submaximal exercise in 8,000 patients, Chest 120:88-92, 2001.

42. Owens GR, Rogers RM, Pennock BE et al: The diffusing capacity as a predictor of arterial oxygen desaturation during exercise in patients with chronic obstructive pulmonary disease, N Engl J Med 310:1218-1221, 1984.

43. Somfay A, Porszasz J, Lee SM et al: Dose—response effect of oxygen on hyperinflation and exercise endurance in nonhypoxaemic COPD patients, Eur Respir J 18:77-84, 2001.

44. Emtner M, Porszasz J, Burns M et al: Benefits of supplemental oxygen in exercise training in nonhypoxemic chronic obstructive pulmonary disease patients, Am J Respir Crit Care Med 168:1034-1042, 2003.

45. Porszasz J, Emtner M, Goto S et al: Exercise training decreases ventilatory requirements and exercise-induced hyperinflation at submaximal intensities in patients with COPD, Chest 128:2025-2034, 2005.

46. Somfay A, Porszasz J, Lee SM et al: Effect of hyperoxia on gas exchange and lactate kinetics following exercise onset in nonhypoxemic COPD patients, Chest 121:393-400, 2002.

47. Eaton T, Garrett JE, Young P et al: Ambulatory oxygen improves quality of life of COPD patients: a randomised controlled study, Eur Respir J 20:306-312, 2002.

48. McDonald CF, Blyth CM, Lazarus MD et al: Exertional oxygen of limited benefit in patients with chronic obstructive pulmonary disease and mild hypoxemia, Am J Respir Crit Care Med 152:1616-1619, 1995.

49. Fujii T, Kurihara N, Otsuka T et al: [Relationship between exercise-induced hypoxemia and long-term survival in patients with chronic obstructive pulmonary disease], Nihon Kyobu Shikkan Gakkai Zasshi 35:934-941, 1997.

50. Payen JF, Wuyam B, Levy P et al: Muscular metabolism during oxygen supplementation in patients with chronic hypoxemia, Am Rev Respir Dis 147:592-598, 1993.

51. Weitzenblum E, Chaouat A, Charpentier C et al: Sleep-related hypoxaemia in chronic obstructive pulmonary disease: causes, consequences and treatment, Respiration 64:187-193, 1997.

52. Rooyackers JM, Dekhuijzen PN, van Herwaarden CL et al: Training with supplemental oxygen in patients with COPD and hypoxaemia at peak exercise, Eur Respir J 10:1278-1284, 1997.

53. Garrod R, Paul EA, Wedzicha JA: Supplemental oxygen during pulmonary rehabilitation in patients with COPD with exercise hypoxaemia, Thorax 55:539-543, 2000.

54. Cotes JE, Gilson JC: Effect of oxygen on exercise ability in chronic respiratory insufficiency: use of portable apparatus, Lancet 270:872-876, 1956.

55. O'Donnell DE, D'Arsigny C, Webb KA: Effects of hyperoxia on ventilatory limitation during exercise in advanced chronic obstructive pulmonary disease, Am J Respir Crit Care Med 163:892-898, 2001.

56. Peters M, Webb K, O'Donnell DE: Combined physiological effects of bronchodilators and hyperoxia on exertional dyspnea in normoxic COPD, Thorax 61:559-567, 2006.

57. Maltais F, Simon M, Jobin J et al: Effects of oxygen on lower limb blood flow and O2 uptake during exercise in COPD, Med Sci Sports Exerc 33:916-922, 2001.

58. American Thoracic Society/European Respiratory Society Task Force: Standards for the diagnosis and management of patients with COPD

[Internet], version 1.2, New York, 2004 [updated September 8, 2005], American Thoracic Society. Available from http://www.thoracic.org/sections/copd. Retrieved April 2, 2008.

59. O'Donohue WJ Jr: Effect of oxygen therapy on increasing arterial oxygen tension in hypoxemic patients with stable chronic obstructive pulmonary disease while breathing ambient air, Chest 100:968-972, 1991.

60. Hoffman LA: Novel strategies for delivering oxygen: reservoir cannula, demand flow, and transtracheal oxygen administration, Respir Care 39:363-377, 1994.

61. Tiep B: Portable oxygen therapy with oxygen conserving devices and methodologies, Monaldi Arch Chest Dis 50:51-57, 1995.

62. Tiep B: The basis for improving the efficiency of oxygen delivery. In Tiep B, editor: Portable oxygen therapy: including oxygen conserving methodology, Mt. Kisco, NY, 1991, Futura Publishing, pp 221-232.

63. Tiep BL, Nicotra MB, Carter R et al: Low-concentration oxygen therapy via a demand oxygen delivery system, Chest 87:636-638, 1985.

64. Tiep BL, Carter R, Nicotra B et al: Demand oxygen delivery during exercise, Chest 91:15-20, 1987.

65. Carter R, Tashkin D, Djahed B et al: Demand oxygen delivery for patients with restrictive lung disease, Chest 96:1307-1311, 1989.

66. McCoy R: Oxygen-conserving techniques and devices, Respir Care 45:95-103, 2000.

67. Bower JS, Brook CJ, Zimmer K et al: Performance of a demand oxygen saver system during rest, exercise, and sleep in hypoxemic patients, Chest 94:77-80, 1988.

68. Tiep BL, Barnett J, Schiffman G et al: Maintaining oxygenation via demand oxygen delivery during rest and exercise, Respir Care 47:887-892, 2002.

69. Arlati S, Rolo J, Micallef E et al: A reservoir nasal cannula improves protection given by oxygen during muscular exercise in COPD, Chest 93:1165-1169, 1988.

70. Tiep BL, Murray R, Barnett M et al: Auto-adjusting demand oxygen delivery system that minimizes SaO2 swings between rest and exertion, Chest 126(supp. 4):763S, 2004.

71. Soffer M, Tashkin DP, Shapiro BJ et al: Conservation of oxygen supply using a reservoir nasal cannula in hypoxemic patients at rest and during exercise, Chest 88:663-668, 1985.

72. Carter R, Williams JS, Berry J et al: Evaluation of the pendant oxygen-conserving nasal cannula during exercise, Chest 89:806-810, 1986.

73. Tiep BL, Burns M, Hererra J: A new pendant oxygen-conserving cannula which allows pursed lips breathing, Chest 95:857-860, 1989.

74. Hagarty EM, Skorodin MS, Stiers WM et al: Performance of a reservoir nasal cannula (Oxymizer) during sleep in hypoxemic patients with COPD, Chest 103:1129-1134, 1993.

75. Collard P, Wautelet F, Delwiche JP et al: Improvement of oxygen delivery in severe hypoxaemia by a reservoir cannula, Eur Respir J 2:778-781, 1989.

76. Heimlich HJ, Carr GC: The micro-trach: a seven-year experience with transtracheal oxygen therapy, Chest 95:1008-1012, 1989.

77. Christopher KL: Transtracheal oxygen catheters, Clin Chest Med 24:489-510, 2003.

78. Christopher KL, VanHooser DT, Jorgenson SJ et al: Preliminary observations of transtracheal augmented ventilation for chronic severe respiratory disease, Respir Care 46:15-25, 2001.

79. Yaeger ES, Goodman S, Hoddes E et al: Oxygen therapy using pulse and continuous flow with a transtracheal catheter and a nasal cannula, Chest 106:854-860, 1994.

80. Campbell EJ, Baker MD, Crites-Silver P: Subjective effects of humidification of oxygen for delivery by nasal cannula: a prospective study, Chest 93:289-293, 1988.

81. Casaburi R, Porszasz J: Reduction of hyperinflation by pharmacologic and other interventions, Proc Am Thorac Soc 3:185-189, 2006.

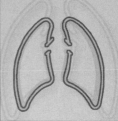

Chapter 10

Exercise in the Rehabilitation of Patients with Respiratory Disease

BARTOLOME R. CELLI

CHAPTER OUTLINE

Physical Reconditioning
  General Principles
  Physiologic Adaptation to Training
Lower Extremity Exercise
  Do All Patients Benefit?
  Type of Training

Upper Extremity Exercise
  Unsupported Arm Exercise
  Effect of Arm and Leg Training
  Practical Training of the Upper
    Extremities
Conclusion

PROFESSIONAL SKILLS

On completion of this chapter, the reader will be able to do
the following:
* Understand the effect and role of leg and arm training and give practical recommendations
* List important factors that contribute to decreased exercise in patients with chronic obstructive pulmonary disease
* Understand principles that apply to training patients with severe pulmonary problems

Patients with chronic respiratory diseases decrease their overall physical activity because any form of exercise will often result in debilitating dyspnea. The progressive deconditioning associated with inactivity initiates a vicious cycle in which dyspnea increases, at ever lower physical demands (Figure 10-1). With time, the patients will also adopt a breathing pattern (shallow and rapid) that is detrimental to overall gas exchange, thus worsening their symptoms. In general, physical reconditioning is a broad therapeutic concept that has unfortunately been equated with simple lower extremity exercise training. This chapter reviews the current knowledge regarding exercise conditioning in much broader terms. The effect and role of leg and arm training are critically analyzed, and practical recommendations are given. Ventilatory muscle training is not

reviewed because it is addressed in Chapter 11 in this book.

Current knowledge about exercise conditioning has been obtained from patients with intrinsic lung disease, such as emphysema, bronchitis, bronchiectasis, cystic fibrosis, and acute respiratory failure. Little is known about reconditioning in patients with pure "pump failure," such as those with degenerative neuromuscular diseases (e.g., myasthenia gravis, postpolio syndrome, or kyphoscoliosis). There is every reason to believe that in these patients, physical exercise could worsen rather than improve their overall function and sensation of well-being. Conversely, pure breathing retraining, such as slow deep breathing, could have a more universal application as long as extra loads are not placed on already weakened and dysfunctional respiratory muscles. As is

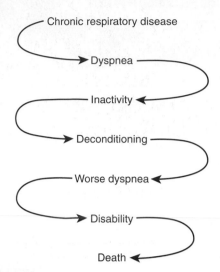

FIGURE 10-1 Respiratory disease is associated with progressive development of dyspnea at an even lower exercise level. This leads to progressive inactivity, which in turn induces further deconditioning and ever-increasing dyspnea at lower exercise intensity. This "vicious cycle" can be reversed with exercise training.

reviewed in Chapter 11, patients with symptomatic pump failure may benefit more from ventilatory assistance and resting than from further training.

PHYSICAL RECONDITIONING

Exercise conditioning is the most important factor in the rehabilitation of patients with symptomatic respiratory disease. It is important to understand the principles and components of exercise training to adequately incorporate them in the treatment of these patients.

General Principles

The short- and long-term effects of systematic exercise conditioning have been the subject of extensive investigation. In healthy individuals, it is known that participation in and completion of well-designed exercise training programs result in several objective changes:
- Increased maximal oxygen (O_2) uptake, primarily owing to increases in blood volume, hemoglobin level, and heart stroke volume, with improvement in the peripheral use of oxygen
- Increased muscular strength and endurance (the consequence of specific training), resulting primarily from enlargement of muscle fibers, improved blood and energy supply, and change in the enzymes that help energy formation

- Improved muscle coordination
- Change in body composition, with increased muscle mass and loss of adipose tissue
- Improved sensation of well-being
- The possibility of improved chances of survival

In patients with obstruction to airflow, participation in a similar program will result in different outcomes depending on the severity of the obstruction. Patients with mild to moderate disease will, as a rule, manifest the same findings as healthy persons, whereas, as is discussed later, patients with the severe form will be able to increase exercise endurance and improve their sensation of well-being with little if any increase in maximal O_2 uptake. Several studies have shown outcome improvement different from the specific effects of training on exercise performance in these patients, including improved muscle enzyme content, less dyspnea for similar work level, decreased lactic acid production at isowork, decreased ventilatory demand for any given work, and improvement in activities of daily living and health-related quality of life. Once the benefits are achieved, little information is available regarding the effect of maintenance programs on any of the outcomes, including exercise performance.

The most important factors thought to contribute to exercise limitation in patients with chronic obstructive pulmonary disease (COPD) are as follows:
- Alterations in pulmonary mechanics
- Dysfunction of the respiratory muscles
- Peripheral muscle dysfunction
- Abnormal gas exchange
- Alterations in cardiac performance
- Malnutrition
- Development of dyspnea

Other factors are less well characterized, including active smoking and polycythemia.

Physiologic Adaptation to Training

To train patients with severe pulmonary problems, several principles that apply to exercise training must be understood:
- Specificity of training
- Intensity, frequency, and duration of the exercise load
- Detraining effect

Specificity of Training

Specific training is beneficial only for the trained muscle or muscle group, and the effect depends on the stimulus applied. Thus use of high-resistance, low-repetition stimulus (weight lifting) increases muscle strength, whereas low-resistance, high-repetition stimulus increases muscle endurance. Strength training is achieved by increasing myofibrils in certain muscle fibers, whereas endurance training increases the number of capillaries and enzymatic mitochondrial content in the trained muscles.

The training is specific to the trained muscle. Clausen and colleagues[1] trained subjects in various arm or leg exercises and observed that the decreased heart rate observed for arm muscle training could not be transferred to the leg group and vice versa. Davis and Sargeant[2] showed that if training was completed for one leg, the beneficial effect could not be transferred to exercise involving the untrained leg. Belman and Kendregan[3] confirmed these findings in patients with COPD. They examined the effect of 6 weeks of training in eight patients who trained only their arms and seven patients who trained only their legs. They observed improved exercise only for the exercise for which the patients trained.

Intensity, Frequency, and Duration of the Exercise Load

Intensity, frequency, and duration of the exercise load affect the degree of training effect. Athletes will usually train at maximal or near-maximal levels to rapidly achieve the desired effects. Conversely, middle-aged nonathletes may require less intense exercise. Siegel, Blonquist, and Mitchell[4] showed that training sessions of 30 minutes close to three times per week for 15 weeks significantly improved maximal O_2 uptake if the heart rate was raised above 80% of the predicted maximal rate. In patients with chronic lung disease, the issue of exercise intensity and duration has been studied by various authors, as is reviewed later, but it seems that the greater the number of sessions and the more intense the sessions (as a function of maximal performance), the better the results.

In their work, Belman and Kendregan[3] exercised patients at 30% of maximum, and after 6 weeks of training four times weekly in which the load was increased as tolerated, they observed significant improvement in endurance time in 9 of the 15 patients. It is possible that the relatively low training level (30% of maximum) may help explain why six of their patients failed to increase their endurance time. In contrast,

Niederman and colleagues[5] started the exercise at 50% of maximal cycle ergometer level and increased its intensity on a weekly basis, and observed endurance improvement in most patients. Clark, Cochrane, and Mackay[6] randomized 48 patients with severe COPD to training (n = 32) and control (n = 16). The training consisted of low-intensity aerobic exercise and isolated conditioning of peripheral muscles, including shoulder circling, abdominal exercise, wall press-up, quadriceps, and step-up exercise. The exercises were supervised in the hospital once weekly and were carried out daily at home for a total of 12 weeks. The trained group showed significant improvement in whole-body endurance, decreased ventilation for similar O_2 uptake, and decreased breathlessness.

Other authors have used higher starting exercise levels and have achieved higher endurance.[6-9] The best study in this regard is that by Casaburi and colleagues,[10] who studied 19 patients with COPD who could achieve anaerobic threshold (moderate COPD with a forced expiratory volume in 1 second [FEV_1] of 1.8 ± 0.53 L [mean ± SD]) before and after randomly assigned low-intensity (50% of maximal) or high-intensity (80% of maximal) exercise. The authors showed that the high-intensity training program was more effective than the low-intensity program. They also observed a drop in ventilatory requirement for exercise after training that was proportional to the drop in lactate at a given work rate. It therefore seems that training is achieved if the intensity of exercise is at least 50% of maximum and that it can be increased as tolerated. Conversely, any exercise is better than none, and indeed good results have been shown even for patients with moderate exercise performance when tested.[5,11,12] Some benefits have also been obtained when using interval training,[13,14] that is to say, intermittent increase in load interspaced with periods of lower load.

The number of exercise sessions is also a matter of debate.[3,15] In general, as the number of sessions is increased, so is the change in observed endurance time.[16,17] Because exercise cessation results in a loss of the training effect, the optimal plan should involve an intense training phase and a maintenance phase. The latter is difficult to implement and results in the frequently observed failure to maintain and preserve the beneficial effects achieved through training. Unfortunately, only a limited number of studies have addressed this important issue. Foglio and colleagues[18] evaluated 35 patients with asthma and 26 patients with COPD before and immediately after discharge from an inpatient rehabilitation program and after 1 year of follow-up. Treatment improved muscle strength, exercise tolerance, dyspnea, and health-related quality of life. The improvement decreased with time but was maintained above baseline at 1-year follow-up. More studies are needed to verify this important finding. In an important study, Cote and Celli[19] observed lasting benefits over 2 years in 115 patients who completed pulmonary rehabilitation.

Detraining Effect

The detraining effect principle is based on observations that the effect achieved by training is lost after the exercise is stopped. Saltin and colleagues[20] showed that bed rest in healthy subjects resulted in a significant decrease in maximal O_2 uptake within 21 days of resting. It took 10 to 50 days for the values to return to those seen before resting. Keens and colleagues[21] examined ventilatory muscle endurance after training in healthy subjects who had undergone ventilatory muscle training. Within 1 month of having stopped training, the subjects had lost the training effect that they had achieved. Therefore it seems important to continue to train, but the minimal practical and effective timing of maintenance training remains to be determined. Ries and colleagues[22] showed that after 12 weeks of intense exercise training, a once-a-month maintenance program maintained the benefit achieved for at least 1 year. In a subsequent report, the same authors confirmed these preliminary finding and indicated the need for more frequent maintenance if the benefits of training were to be maintained.[23]

Our exercise program is based on the data and concepts developed in the previous sections of this chapter. Patients are exercised at 70% of the maximal work achieved in a test day. This work is increased on a weekly basis as tolerated by the patient. The goal is to complete 24 sessions, typically in an outpatient setting with sessions held three times weekly. The program may be completed more quickly if the patient is in the hospital because the sessions occur at least on a daily basis. Each session lasts 30 minutes if tolerated; otherwise, it is begun as guided by the patient's symptoms and no further load is provided until

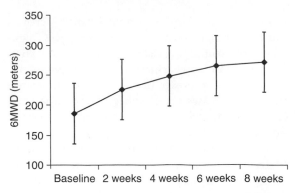

FIGURE 10-2 After initiation of a high-intensity training program, it takes 8 to 10 weeks for the patient to be able to maintain the targeted load for 25 to 30 minutes. 6MWD, 6-minute walk distance.

the patient can complete the 30 minutes of the session. Typically, it takes 6 to 8 weeks of high-intensity training to reach the targeted load (Figure 10-2). In those settings in which metabolic measurements are not possible, the perception of dyspnea, using a Borg visual analog scale, can substitute for a target work rate. This has been shown in a series of studies of patients with COPD.[24,25] It is appealing to use dyspnea and not heart rate as the target by which to train patients with lung disease because breathlessness constitutes their most important complaint. The study by Mejia and colleagues[25] supports this concept and provides a useful, inexpensive, and rather accurate way to prescribe exercise in the simplest of settings.

LOWER EXTREMITY EXERCISE

Many uncontrolled studies have shown that the inclusion of leg exercise in the training of patients with lung disease is beneficial.[26-30] This has been confirmed in a series of controlled trials.

Cockcroft, Saunders, and Berry[31] randomized 39 patients with dyspnea who were younger than 70 years and not receiving O_2 therapy to (1) a treatment group that spent 6 weeks in a rehabilitation center, where they underwent gradual endurance exercise training, and (2) a control group that received medical care but was given no special advice to exercise. The control group served as such for 4 months and was then admitted to the rehabilitation center for 6 weeks. Just like the treated patients, they were instructed to exercise at home afterward. Thirty-four patients completed the program. After rehabilitation, only 2 of the 16 control patients manifested improvement in dyspnea and cough, whereas 16 of the 18 patients included in the treatment group manifested improvement in these symptoms. More important, treated patients showed significant improvement in 12-minute walk distance and in peak oxygen uptake $\dot{V}o_2$ compared with control subjects.

Sinclair and Ingram[32] randomized 33 patients with chronic bronchitis and dyspnea to two groups. The 17 patients in the treatment group exercised by climbing up and down on two 24-cm steps twice daily. Exercise time was increased to tolerance. Patients exercised at home and were evaluated by the treatment team weekly. The control group did not exercise, but all its members were reassessed after 6 months. The degree of airflow obstruction did not change in either group. Similarly, no improvement in strength of the quadriceps, minute ventilation, and heart rate occurred. In contrast, performance on the 12-minute walk test significantly increased in patients who were trained.

O'Donnell, Webb, and McGuire[33] compared breathlessness, 6-minute walk distance, and cycle ergometer work between two age-matched groups of patients with moderate COPD. The endurance exercise—trained group (n = 23) achieved significant reduction in dyspnea scores and increased the distance walked as well as the cycle ergometry work compared with the control group (n = 13). This trial is important in that it not only documented increased endurance but for the first time evaluated the patient's perception of dyspnea, which is the most problematic symptom and the one leading to physical limitation. Since those initial studies, several trials have documented the beneficial effect of lower extremity exercise.[34-39] Perhaps the most important one is the study by Ries and colleagues.[22] In this study, 119 patents were randomized to an educational support group (n = 62) or to a similar educational program with the addition of walking exercise two times weekly for 8 weeks (n = 57). At 2 months, and still seen at 4, 6, and 12 months, the patients who exercised manifested increased exercise endurance, less dyspnea with exercise, less dyspnea with activities of daily living, and a non-statistically significant increase in survival. This landmark study establishes the pivotal role of lower extremity exercise in the proven benefit of pulmonary rehabilitation. The results of several studies are summarized in Table 10-1.

TABLE 10-1	Controlled Studies of Rehabilitation with Exercise in Patients with COPD			
Study	**No. of Patients**	**Duration**	**Course (wk)**	**Results**
Cockcroft, Saunders, and Berry[31]	18 T	Daily	16	↑ 12MWD, ↑ $\dot{V}o_2$
	16 C	—	—	No change
Sinclair and Ingram[32]	17 T	Daily	40	↑ FVC, ↑ 12MWD
	16 C	—	—	No change
O'Donnell, Webb, and Maguire[33]	23 T	Daily	8	↑ FVC, ↑ 12MWD, ↓ Dyspnea
	13 C	—	—	No change
Reardon et al[35]	10 T	Twice weekly	6	↓ Dyspnea
	10 C	—	—	No change
Ries et al[22]	57 T	Daily	8	↑ Exercise capacity, ↓ Dyspnea, ↑ Self-efficacy
	62 C	Daily education	8	No change
Wykstra et al[36]	28 T	Daily at home	12	↑ Exercise capacity, ↑ HRQoL
	15 C	—	—	No change
Goldstein et al[34]	45 T	Daily	24	↑ 6MWD, $\dot{V}o_2$ ↓ Dyspnea
	44 C	None	24	No change
Strijbos et al[37]	15 OP	Twice weekly	12	↑ 4MWD, ↑ work, ↓ Dyspnea
	15 Home	Twice weekly	12	↑ 4MWD, ↑ work, ↓ Dyspnea
	15 C	None	12	No change
Wedzicha et al[38]	30 Ex, MRC grade 5	NA (home)	8	No change
	30 C, MRC grade 5	NA (home)	8	No change
	33 Ex, MRC grade ¾	NA (hospital)	8	↑ WD, ↑ HRQoL
	33 C, MRC grade ¾	NA (hospital)	8	No change

4MWD, *4-minute walk distance;* 6MWD, *6-minute walk distance;* 12MWD, *12-minute walk distance;* C, *control subjects;* COPD, *chronic obstructive pulmonary disease;* Ex, *exercise;* FVC, *forced vital capacity;* HRQoL, *health-related quality of life;* MRC, *Medical Research Council Dyspnea Scale;* NA, *not available;* OP, *outpatient;* T, *treated;* $\dot{V}o_2$, *peak oxygen uptake.*

Numerous trials that have used patients as their own control subjects have shown similar results, with significantly increased exercise endurance. The mechanism by which this improvement occurs remains a matter of debate. Some studies[7,30] have demonstrated a drop in heart rate at a similar work level, a hallmark of a training effect for the specific exercise. This is perhaps related to a decrease in exercise lactate level as suggested by at least two studies.[10,40] The patients showed a reduction in exercise lactic acidosis and ventilation after training. Furthermore, the reduction was proportional to the intensity of the training. A 12% decrease occurred in the lactic acidosis rise in patients trained at the low work rate (50% of maximum) and a 32% decrease occurred in those trained at the high work rate (80% of maximum). Other studies have failed to document either an increase in maximal O_2 uptake or a decrease in heart rate or lactate at a similar work level. The most important study in this group is that by Belman and Kendregan,[3] which failed to show a decrease in heart rate at the same work load as represented by the $\dot{V}o_2$. These authors went further and analyzed muscle biopsy sample oxidative enzyme content before and after training. They observed no change in this parameter. Interestingly, nine of the treated patients improved their exercise endurance. As stated previously, it is possible that this study used too low a training effort; training was started at 30% of the maximum achieved during their testing. That this may be so is supported by two studies from Maltais and colleagues.[41,42] They first showed that muscle biopsy samples from the legs of patients with COPD had a decreased content of oxidative enzymes in their mitochondria. Subsequently, and extremely important for those who believe in physiologic training, the mitochondrial enzymatic content significantly increased after exercise training. In that same group of patients they also documented a delay of onset of the lactase threshold after training. Since those initial studies there have been more controlled trials, all supporting the beneficial effect of exercise in rehabilitation.[43,44]

The evidence, indicating that exercise of the lower extremities of patients with COPD is beneficial, is now so strong that it has been categorized as type A. Figure 10-3 shows the average change in two important physiologic variables from some of these studies. It is interesting to note

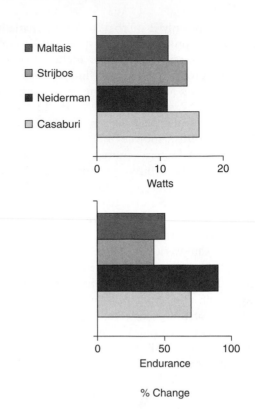

FIGURE 10-3 Improvement in work rate (watts) and exercise endurance time in selected series of exercise training in patients with chronic obstructive pulmonary disease (COPD). Little difference in outcome occurred despite differences in the training programs. The studies indicated include Maltais and colleagues,[41,42] Strijbos and colleagues,[37] Niederman and colleagues,[5] and Casaburi and colleagues.[45]

that the average improvement in outcomes, such as walking distance or exercise endurance, was similar whether high-intensity training,[10,42] lower intensity training,[5] or even home training[37] was used.

Do All Patients Benefit?

Whether all patients benefit is an important question because many patients with the most severe COPD do not exercise to the intensity required to reach anaerobic threshold or to induce cardiovascular training. Most studies to date suggest a benefit that is independent from the degree of impairment. Niederman and colleagues[5] exercised 33 patients with different degrees of COPD (FEV$_1$ range, 0.33-3.82 L). After training, there was no correlation between the degree of airflow obstruction in these patients and their observed improvement. In other words, patients with very low FEV$_1$ were as likely to improve as were patients with high FEV_1. Similarly, ZuWallack and colleagues[11] evaluated 50 patients with COPD (FEV_1 range, 0.38-3.24 L) before and after exercise training. They observed an inverse relationship between the baseline 12-minute walk distance and $\dot{V}o_2$ and the observed improvement. They concluded that patients with poor performance on either the 12-minute walk distance or the maximal exercise test are not necessarily poor candidates for an exercise program. Casaburi and colleagues[45] reported the effect, on 15 men and 10 women with severe COPD (FEV_1, 0.93 ± 0.27 L), of leg training at close to 80% of maximum. After training three times weekly for 6 weeks, a 77% improvement in the duration of a submaximal test, an improvement in O_2 kinetics, and a decrease in minute ventilation at the same work level were seen. Also, the respiratory rate decreased and tidal volume increased. From these data it seems prudent to conclude that most patients capable of undergoing leg exercise endurance training will benefit from a program that includes leg exercise. This overall principle is contradicted by a randomized trial of pulmonary rehabilitation in patients with COPD who were stratified on the basis of the perception of dyspnea, using the Medical Research Council (MRC) Dyspnea Scale. In that rather complex trial, patients with the most severe dyspnea (MRC = 5) failed to improve after exercise training, whereas patients with less dyspnea (MRC = ¾) did show improvement in exercise performance.[38] Of note, patients in the most severe group were treated at home, whereas those with less dyspnea were supervised at a rehabilitation institute, so it is possible that the exercise program was not the same for all groups. Nevertheless, this study is important in that it suggests that some patients may be too ill to benefit from exercise training. Certainly, more research is needed to clarify this important issue.

Type of Training

The type of exercise training to be prescribed and the testing modality are also subject to debate. Various studies have used different training techniques. Most studies include walking as both a measurement of exercise tolerance and of the training program, whereas others have relied on more precise methods, such as the cycle ergometer or treadmill.

The classic timed walk (6- or 12-minute walking distance), in which the distance walked over 6 or 12 minutes is recorded, is good for patients

with moderate to severe COPD but may not be taxing enough for patients with a lesser degree of airflow obstruction.[46] The 6-minute walk distance has been found to be a reliable, inexpensive, and a useful test. In at least two studies, the timed walk distance test has been shown to predict overall survival among patients with severe COPD.[47,48] Singh and colleagues[49] have reported a good correlation between the O_2 uptake measured during cycle ergometry and the "shuttle walking" test. This test progressively increases the demands on the patient being tested, thereby proving to be useful in patients with a lesser degree of airflow limitation.

Stair climbing has been evaluated, and it has been shown that $\dot{V}o_2$ can be estimated from the number of steps climbed during a symptom-limited test.[50] Several studies have used treadmill testing, step testing, or both, even though the training has been done with the patient walking. O_2 uptake is higher for stair climbing or treadmill testing than for the more commonly used leg ergometry, presumably because the former uses more body muscles than does leg cycling. Leg ergometry has become popular in its use as a testing device and has been the training apparatus for most of the more recent studies. The apparatus is smaller than the treadmill, and with relatively inexpensive units in the market, it is possible to place several together and to train groups of patients simultaneously.

Most of the studies quoted relied on either in-hospital or outpatient hospital training. Little information exists regarding implementation of such programs at home. In a unique report, O'Hara and colleagues[51] enrolled 14 patients with moderate COPD (FEV_1, 1.17 ± 0.76 L) in a home exercise program. The authors randomized the patients to daily walking while carrying a lightweight backpack (2.6 ± 0.5 kg) or the same backpacking regimen with additional weight lifting and limb-strengthening exercises. These included wrist curls, arm curls, partial leg squats, calf raises, and supine dumbbell presses. The initial load was 4.3 ± 0.9 kg and was increased weekly by 1.2 ± 0.5 kg for 6 weeks to reach 10.4 ± 2.6 kg by the last week. The weight lifters performed 10 repetitions 3 times, avoiding dyspnea, breathholding, and fatigue, for a total time of 30 minutes daily. Patients documented their exercises in a diary. Health care personnel visited the patients on a weekly basis. After training, all weight lifters had reduced their minute ventilation during bicycle ergometry compared with control subjects. Furthermore, the weight-trained patients showed a 16% increase in exercise endurance. This study suggests that exercise training can be achieved at home with relatively inexpensive programs, with the beneficial consequence of no hospital visits. This initial report is supported by more recent data that supervised exercise at home achieves the same outcomes as those obtained in the hospital.[36,37]

In our pulmonary rehabilitation program, testing is completed with an electrically braked ergometer, whereas the training is done with a mechanically controlled ergometer; subjects train either as outpatients or as inpatients depending on their condition. Box 10-1 describes the practical details of our training program. The training must be tailored to each individual and to the available training equipment. The experience in less developed countries (as discussed elsewhere in this book) confirms that it is not necessary to have expensive equipment to successfully implement an exercise program for symptomatic patients with respiratory disease.

Although not all possible outcomes have been determined in every trial, it is possible to obtain a picture of the most important benefits of lower extremity exercise. The average changes reported[5,6,10,11,22,23,31-39] until now are summarized in Figure 10-4. Most studies report a large improvement in walk distance or submaximal exercise endurance. This occurs with more modest, but still significant, increases in work rate or O_2 uptake. This is likely due to changes in the enzymatic content of muscle mitochondria such as citric synthase and 3-hydroxyacyl-CoA dehydrogenase. This change in enzyme content is associated with decreased lactate production and ventilatory requirement at similar work load.[42] The overall consequence is a consistent improvement in exercise performance.

BOX 10-1	Training Method for Leg Exercise

1. Train at 60% to 80% of maximal work capacity.*
2. Increase work every fifth session as tolerated.
3. Monitor dyspnea and heart rate.
4. Increase work after 20 to 30 minutes of submaximal targeted work is achieved.
5. Aim for 24 sessions.

Work capacity as determined by an exercise test, not necessarily by evaluating heart rate. It is possible to substitute work capacity for dyspnea (see text for discussion).

UPPER EXTREMITY EXERCISE

Most of the knowledge about exercise conditioning in patients undergoing rehabilitation is derived from programs emphasizing leg training. This is unfortunate because the performance of many everyday tasks requires not only the hands but also the concerted action of other muscle groups that partake in upper torso and arm positioning. Some muscles of the upper torso and shoulder girdle serve both respiratory and postural functions. Muscles such as the upper and lower trapezius, latissimus dorsi, serrfatus anterior, subclavius, and pectoralis minor and major possess both thoracic and extrathoracic anchoring points. Depending on the anchoring point they may help position the arms or shoulder or, if given an extra thoracic fulcrum (such as fixing the arms in a supported position), they may exert a pulling force on the rib cage. It has been shown that in patients with chronic airflow obstruction, as severity worsens, the diaphragm loses its force-generating capacity and the muscles of the rib cage become more important in the generation of inspiratory pressures.[52] When patients perform unsupported arm exercise, some of the shoulder girdle muscles must decrease their participation in ventilation, and if the task involves complex purposeful arm movements, the pattern of ventilation may be affected.

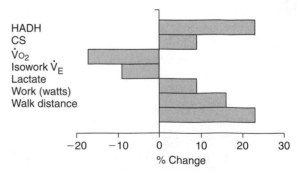

FIGURE 10-4 Lower extremity exercise training results in a large increase in exercise endurance (walk distance), with a lesser but significant increase in work (watts) and oxygen uptake ($\dot{V}o_2$). Exercise training increases the mitochondrial content of citric synthase (CS) and 3-hydroxyacyl-CoA dehydrogenase (HADH). After training, a decrease occurs in the generation of lactate and ventilation at any given work load (isowork $\dot{V}_E$). Data are the average of results from references 5, 6, 10, 11, 22, 23, and 31-39.

Unsupported Arm Exercise

Tangri and Woolf[53] used a pneumobelt to study breathing patterns in seven patients with COPD while they performed simple activities of daily living such as tying their shoes and brushing their teeth. The patients had an irregular and a rapid pattern of breathing with the arm exercise. After the exercise, the patients breathed faster and deeper, which according to the authors was done to restore the blood gases to normal.

The ventilatory response to unsupported arm exercise has been explored, and it has been compared with the response to leg exercise in patients with severe chronic lung disease.[54] Arm exercise resulted in dyssynchronous thoracoabdominal excursion that was not caused solely by diaphragmatic fatigue. The dyspnea that was reported by the patients was associated with a dyssynchronous breathing pattern. It was concluded that unsupported arm exercise could shift work to the diaphragm and in some way lead to dyssynchrony. To test this hypothesis, pleural pressure versus gastric pressure plots (with a gastric and endoesophageal balloon) have been used. The changes, as well as the ventilatory response, have been evaluated to unsupported arm exercise, and they have been compared with leg cycle ergometry in healthy subjects and in patients with airflow obstruction.[55,56] Increased diaphragmatic pressure excursion with arm exercise and alterations in the pattern of pressure generation were documented, with more contribution by the diaphragm and abdominal muscles of respiration and less contribution by the inspiratory muscles of the rib cage. Patients can also have dynamic hyperinflation, as has been documented for lower extremity exercise. These findings have been confirmed in studies not only of patients with COPD but also of patients with cystic fibrosis.[57,58]

Our knowledge of ventilatory response to arm exercise was based on arm cycle ergometry. It is known that at a given work load in healthy subjects, arm cranking is more demanding than leg cycling, as shown by higher $\dot{V}O_2$, minute ventilation ($\dot{V}_E$), heart rate, blood pressure, and lactate production.[59-63] At maximal effort, however, $\dot{V}O_2$, $\dot{V}O_E$, cardiac output, and lactate levels are lower during arm than leg cycle ergometry. Little is known about the metabolic and ventilatory cost of simple arm elevation. Some reports underscore the importance of arm position in ventilation. Banzett and colleagues[64] showed that arm bracing increases the capacity to sustain maximal ventilation compared with lifting the elbows from the braced position. Others have shown a decrease in the maximal attainable work load and increases in O_2 uptake and ventilation at any given work load when healthy subjects exercised with their arms elevated.[65,66] The metabolic and respiratory consequence of simple arm elevation was evaluated in patients with COPD.[67] Elevation of the arms to 90° in front of them results in a significant increase in $\dot{V}O_2$ and peak carbon dioxide update $\dot{V}CO_2$. Concomitant increases occurred in heart rate and $\dot{V}_E$. When ventilatory muscle recruitment patterns were evaluated with the use of continuous recording of gastric pressure and pleural pressure, the contribution to ventilation by the different muscle groups shifted, toward increased diaphragmatic and abdominal muscle use. This suggests that if the arms are trained to perform more work or if the ventilatory requirement is decreased for the same work, the patient's capacity to perform arm activity should improve.

Effect of Arm and Leg Training

Several studies have used both arm and leg training and have shown that the addition of arm training results in improved performance, and that the improved performance is for the most part task specific. In their study, Belman and Kendregan[3] showed a significant increase in arm exercise endurance after exercise training. Lake and colleagues[68] randomized patients to arm exercise, leg exercise, and arm and leg exercise. There were increases for arm ergometry in the arm group and for leg ergometry in the leg group, and increased improvement in sensation of well-being when both exercises were combined. Ries, Ellis, and Hawkins[69] studied the effect of two forms of arm exercise, gravity resistance and modified proprioceptive neuromuscular facilitation, and compared them with no arm exercise in a group of 45 patients with COPD who were involved in a comprehensive, multidisciplinary pulmonary rehabilitation program. Although only 20 patients completed the program, they showed improved performance on tests that were specific for the training. The patients reported a decrease in fatigue in all tests performed. It is worth pointing out that in the study by Keens and colleagues[21] a group of patients with cystic fibrosis underwent upper extremity training consisting of swimming and

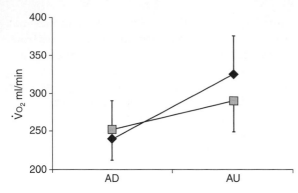

FIGURE 10-5 Oxygen uptake ($\dot{V}o_2$) in 18 patients with chronic obstructive pulmonary disease with arms down (AD) or arms up (AU), before *(diamonds)* and after *(squares)* rehabilitation. $\dot{V}o_2$ increases from baseline during arm elevation. After arm training, the increase in $\dot{V}o_2$ with arms up is significantly lower than previously.

canoeing for 1.5 hours daily. At the end of 6 weeks, upper extremity endurance increased, but, most important, maximal sustainable ventilatory capacity had an increase similar to that obtained with ventilatory muscle training. This suggests that ventilatory muscles could be trained by using an arm exercise training program.

Because simple arm elevation results in a significant increase in $\dot{V}_E$, $\dot{V}o_2$, and $\dot{V}co_2$, 14 patients with COPD were studied before and after 8 weeks of three times weekly, 20-minute sessions of unsupported arm and leg exercise as part of a comprehensive rehabilitation program to test whether arm training decreases ventilatory requirement for arm activity.[70] A 35% decrease in the rise of $\dot{V}o_2$ and $\dot{V}co_2$ was brought about by arm elevation (Figure 10-5). This was associated with a significant decrease in $\dot{V}o_E$. Because the patients also trained their legs, it was inconclusive whether the improvement was caused by the arm exercise. To answer this question, a study of 25 patients with COPD randomized to either unsupported arm training (11 patients) or resistance breathing training (14 patients) was completed. After 24 sessions, arm endurance increased only for the unsupported arm training group and not for the resistance breathing training group. Interestingly, maximal inspiratory pressure increased significantly for both groups, indicating that by training the arms, ventilatory muscle training could be induced for those

muscles of the rib cage that hinge on the shoulder girdle.[71]

Practical Training of the Upper Extremity

On the basis of the information available, arm exercise has been recommended as an essential component of pulmonary rehabilitation programs.[72,73] As seen in Boxes 10-2 and 10-3, the methods for supported and unsupported arm vary in their implementation. Arm ergometry is performed for 20 minutes per session. It is started at 60% of the maximal work achieved in the exercise test. The work is increased weekly as tolerated. Dyspnea and heart rate are monitored. Maximal work capacity is defined as the watts that the patient is capable of achieving. If the limiting symptom is dyspnea at minimal work, the patient exercises at 60% of the work that makes him or her stop. In patients with the most severe disease, monitoring the heart rate is unreliable because these patients may be tachycardic even at rest and may not show any significant increase with exercise. In these patients, dyspnea may be a more reliable index to follow. In contrast, unsupported arm exercise training is achieved by having the patient lift a dowel (750 g in weight) to shoulder level at the same rhythm as the patient's breathing rate. The sequence is repeated for 2 minutes, with a 2-minute resting period. The exercises are repeated for 30 minutes. Dyspnea and heart rate are monitored. The load is increased by 250 g weekly as tolerated. The goal is to complete 24 sessions.

Martinez and colleagues[74] compared unsupported arm training with arm ergometry training in a randomized clinical trial. Total endurance time improved significantly for both groups, but unsupported arm training decreased O_2 uptake at the same work load compared with arm cranking training. They concluded that arm exercise against gravity may be more effective in training patients for activities that resemble those of daily living.

An increasing body of evidence indicates that upper extremity exercise training results in improved performance for arm activities (Table 10-2). There is also a drop in the ventilatory requirements for similar upper extremity activities. All this should result in an improvement in the capacity of the patients to perform activities of daily living.

TABLE 10-2   Controlled Studies of Arm Exercise in Patients with COPD

Study	No. of Patients	Course (wk)	Duration	Type	Results
Keens et al[21]	7 Arms	4	1.5 hr daily	Swimming/canoeing	↑ VMT (56%)
	4 VMT	4	15 min daily	VMT	↑ VME (52%)
	4 Control subjects	—		VMT	↑ VME (22%)
Belman and Kendregan[3]	8 Arms	6	20 min 4 times per wk	Arm Ergometry	↑ Arm cycle No ↑ PFT
	7 Legs	6	20 min 4 times per wk	Cycle Ergometry	↑ Leg cycle No ↑ PFT
Lake et al[68]	6 Arms	8	1 hr 3 times per wk	Several types	No change in $P_{I}max$, VME
	6 Legs	8	1 hr 3 times per wk	Walking	No change in $P_{I}max$, VME
	7 Arms and legs	8	1 hr 3 times per wk	Combined	No change in $P_{I}max$, VME
Ries, Ellis, and Hawkins[69]	8 Gravity resistance arms	6	15 min daily	Low resistance, high repetition	↑ Arm endurance, ↓ Dyspnea
	9 Neuromuscular facilitation	6	15 min daily	Weight lifts	↑ Arm endurance, ↓ Dyspnea
Epstein et al[71]	11 Control subjects	6	—	Walk	No change
	13 Arms	8	30 min daily	UAE	↓ $\dot{V}o_2$ and $\dot{V}_E$ for arm elevation, ↑ $P_{I}max$
	10 VMT	8	30 min daily	VMT	↑ $P_{I}max$ and VME
Martinez et al[74]	18 UAE	10	30 min 3 times per wk	UAE	↑ Work, ↓↓ Isowork $\dot{V}o_2$
	17 Ergometry	10	30 min 3 times per wk	Arm ergometry	↑ Work, ↓ Isowork $\dot{V}o_2$

COPD, Chronic obstructive pulmonary disease; PFT, pulmonary function tests; $P_{I}max$, maximal inspiratory pressure; $\dot{V}_E$, minute ventilation; UAE, unsupported arm exercise; VMT, ventilatory muscle training; VME, ventilatory muscle endurance; $\dot{V}o_2$, peak oxygen uptake.

TABLE 10-3 Work of Breathing, Exercise Endurance, and Maximal Transdiaphragmatic Pressure Before and After Pulmonary Rehabilitation

Rehabilitation	Endurance Time (sec)	$\int$ Pes·dt (cm H_2O · min^{-1})	Pdimax (cm H_2O)
Before	434	288	48
After	512*	219*	52

*P < .05.

Pdimax, *Maximal transdiaphragmatic pressure;* $\int$ Pes · dt, *work of breathing as estimated by the pressure–time index calculated from continuous recording of endoesophageal pressure.*

TABLE 10-4 Evidence Benefits of Exercise Training in Patients with COPD

Type of Training	Outcome	Type of Evidence*
Lower extremity	Improves exercise performance, dyspnea, and health-related quality of life	A
Upper extremity	Improves arm exercise endurance and decreases O_2 uptake during arm elevation	B

A, evidence obtained from large controlled trials; B, evidence obtained from smaller controlled trials.
COPD, *Chronic obstructive pulmonary disease;* O_2, *oxygen.*

BOX 10-2 Training Method for Supported (Ergometric) Arm Exercise Training

1. Train at 60% of maximal work capacity.*
2. Increase work every fifth session as tolerated.
3. Monitor dyspnea and heart rate.
4. Train for as long as tolerated up to 30 minutes.

Work capacity as determined by an exercise test, not necessarily by evaluating heart rate (see text for discussion).

BOX 10-3 Training Method for Unsupported Arm Training

1. Dowel (weight = 750 g).
2. Lift to shoulder level for 2 minutes; rate equal to breathing rate.
3. Rest for 2 minutes.
4. Repeat sequence as tolerated for up to 32 minutes.
5. Monitor dyspnea and heart rate.
6. Increase weight (250 g) every fifth session as tolerated.

CONCLUSION

Exercise training is the most important component in the rehabilitation of patients with obstructive airway disease. Table 10-3 shows the recommendation provided by the American College of Chest Physicians/American Association of Cardiovascular and Pulmonary Rehabilitation evidence-based guidelines for pulmonary rehabilitation[72] and endorsed by the statement on pulmonary rehabilitation by the American Thoracic Society.[73] The benefits of lower and upper extremity exercise are multiple and seem to persist for at least 1 year after an 8- to 12-week program (Table 10-4). Because exercise can be performed by physically able patients regardless of age[75] or disease severity,[5,9] it should be the cornerstone of any program. Future research will clarify the issues of optimal duration and frequency of training so that the benefits last even longer.

References

1. Clausen JP, Clausen K, Rasmussen B et al: Central and peripheral circulatory changes after training of the arms or legs, Am J Physiol 225:675-682, 1973.
2. Davis CT, Sargeant AJ: Effects of training on the physiological responses to one and two legged work, J Appl Physiol 38:377-381, 1975.
3. Belman MJ, Kendregan BA: Exercise training fails to increase skeletal muscle enzymes in patients with chronic obstructive pulmonary disease, Am Rev Respir Dis 123:256-261, 1981.
4. Siegel W, Blonquist G, Mitchell JH: Effects of a quantitated physical training program on middle-aged sedentary man, Circulation 41:19-29, 1970.
5. Niederman MS, Clemente PH, Fein A et al: Benefits of a multidisciplinary pulmonary rehabilitation program: improvements are independent of lung function, Chest 99:798-804, 1991.
6. Clark CJ, Cochrane L, Mackay E: Low intensity peripheral muscle conditioning improves exercise tolerance and breathlessness in COPD, Eur Respir J 9:2590-2596, 1996.

7. Mohsenifar Z, Horak D, Brown H et al: Sensitive indices of improvement in a pulmonary rehabilitation program, Chest 83:189-192, 1983.
8. Holle RH, Williams DB, Vandree JC et al: Increased muscle efficiency and sustained benefits in an outpatient community hospital-based pulmonary rehabilitation program, Chest 94:1161-1168, 1988.
9. Zack M, Palange A: Oxygen supplemented exercise of ventilatory and nonventilatory muscles in pulmonary rehabilitation, Chest 88:669-675, 1985.
10. Casaburi R, Patessio A, Ioli F et al: Reductions in exercise lactic acidosis and ventilation as a result of exercise training in patients with obstructive lung disease, Am Rev Respir Dis 143:9-18, 1991.
11. ZuWallack RL, Patel K, Reardon JZ et al: Predictors of improvement in the 12-minute walking distance following a six-week outpatient pulmonary rehabilitation program, Chest 99:805-808, 1991.
12. Normandin EA, McCusker C, Connors M et al: An evaluation of two approaches to exercise conditioning in pulmonary rehabilitation, Chest 121:1085-1091, 2002.
13. Gosselink R, Troosters T, Decramer M: Effects of exercise training in COPD patients: interval versus endurance training, Eur Respir J 12:2S, 1998.
14. Vogiatzis I, Nanas S, Roussos C: Interval training as an alternative modality to continuous exercise in patients with COPD, Eur Respir J 20:12-19, 2002.
15. Make BJ, Buckolz P: Exercise training in COPD patients improves cardiac function, Am Rev Respir Dis 143:80A, 1991.
16. Carrieri-Kohlman V, Nguyen HQ, Donesky-Cuenco D et al: Impact of brief or extended exercise training on the benefit of a dyspnea self-management program in COPD, J Cardiopulm Rehabil 25:275-284, 2005.
17. Ringbaek TJ, Broendum E, Hemmingsen L et al: Rehabilitation of patients with chronic obstructive pulmonary disease: exercise twice a week is not sufficient! Respir Med 94:150-154, 2000.
18. Foglio K, Bianchi L, Brulette G et al: Long-term effectiveness of pulmonary rehabilitation in patients with chronic airways obstruction, Eur Respir J 13:125-132, 1999.
19. Cote CG, Celli BR: Pulmonary rehabilitation and the BODE Index in COPD, Eur Respir J 26:630-636, 2005.
20. Saltin B, Blomquist G, Mitchell JH et al: Response to exercise after bed rest and after training, Circulation 38(5 suppl):VII1-VII78, 1968.
21. Keens TG, Krastins IR, Wannamaker EM et al: Ventilatory muscle endurance training in normal subjects and patients with cystic fibrosis, Am Rev Respir Dis 116:853-860, 1977.
22. Ries AZ, Kaplan R, Linberg T et al: Effects of pulmonary rehabilitation on physiologic and psychosocial outcomes in patients with chronic obstructive pulmonary disease, Ann Intern Med 122:823-827, 1995.
23. Ries AL, Kaplan RM, Myers R et al: Maintenance after pulmonary rehabilitation in chronic lung disease, Am J Respir Crit Care Med 167:880-888, 2003.
24. Horowitz MB, Littenberg B, Mahler D: Dyspnea ratings for prescribing exercise intensity in patients with COPD, Chest 109:1169-1175, 1997.
25. Mejia R, Ward J, Lentine T et al: Target dyspnea ratings predict expected oxygen consumption as well as target heart rate values, Am J Respir Crit Care Med 159:1485-1498, 1999.
26. Moser KM, Bokinsky GC, Savage RT et al: Results of comprehensive rehabilitation programs, Arch Intern Med 140:1596-1601, 1980.
27. Beaumont A, Cockcroft A, Guz A: A self-paced treadmill walking test for breathless patients, Thorax 40:459-464, 1985.
28. Christie D: Physical training in chronic obstructive lung disease, BMJ 2:150-151, 1968.
29. Hughes RL, Davidson R: Limitations of exercise reconditioning in COPD, Chest 83:241-249, 1983.
30. Paez PN, Phillipson EA, Mosangkay M et al: The physiologic basis of training patients with emphysema, Am Rev Respir Dis 95:944-953, 1967.
31. Cockcroft AE, Saunders MJ, Berry G: Randomized controlled trial of rehabilitation in chronic respiratory disability, Thorax 36:200-203, 1981.
32. Sinclair DJ, Ingram CG: Controlled trial of supervised exercise training in chronic bronchitis, BMJ 1:519-521, 1980.
33. O'Donnell DE, Webb HA, McGuire MA: Older patients with COPD: benefits of exercise training, Geriatrics 48:59-66, 1993.
34. Goldstein RS, Gork EH, Stubing D et al: Randomized trial of respiratory rehabilitation, Lancet 344:1394-1398, 1994.
35. Reardon J, Awad E, Normandin E et al: The effect of comprehensive outpatient pulmonary rehabilitation on dyspnea, Chest 105:1046-1048, 1994.
36. Wykstra PJ, Van Altens R, Kran J et al: Quality of life in patients with chronic obstructive pulmonary disease improves after rehabilitation in house, Eur Respir J 7:269-274, 1994.
37. Strijbos J, Postma D, Van Altena R et al: A comparison between out-patient hospital-based pulmonary rehabilitation programs and a home-care pulmonary rehabilitation program in patients with COPD, Chest 109:366-372, 1996.
38. Wedzicha J, Bestall J, Garrod R et al: Randomized controlled trial of pulmonary rehabilitation in severe chronic obstructive pulmonary disease patients, stratified with the MRC Dyspnea Scale, Eur Respir J 12:363-369, 1998.
39. Griffiths TL, Burr ML, Campbell IA et al: Results at 1 year of outpatient multidisciplinary pulmonary rehabilitation: a randomized controlled trial, Lancet 355:362-368, 2000.
40. Woolf CR, Suero JT: Alterations in lung mechanics and gas exchange following training in chronic obstructive lung disease, Chest 55:37-44, 1969.
41. Maltais F, Simard A, Simard J et al: Oxidative capacity of the skeletal muscle and lactic acid kinetics during exercise in normal subjects and in patients with COPD, Am J Respir Crit Care Med 153:288-293, 1995.

42. Maltais F, Leblanc P, Simard C et al: Skeletal muscle adaptation to endurance training in patients with chronic obstructive pulmonary disease, Am J Respir Crit Care Med 154:442-447, 1996.

43. Green RH, Singh SJ, Williams J et al: A randomised controlled trial of four weeks versus seven weeks of pulmonary rehabilitation in chronic obstructive pulmonary disease, Thorax 56:143-145, 2001.

44. Troosters T, Gosselink R, Decramer M: Short- and long-term effects of outpatient rehabilitation in patients with chronic obstructive pulmonary disease: a randomized trial, Am J Med 109:207-212, 2000.

45. Casaburi R, Porszarz J, Burns M et al: Physiologic benefits of exercise training in rehabilitation of patients with severe chronic obstructive pulmonary disease, Am J Respir Crit Care Med 155:1541-1551, 1997.

46. McGavin CR, Gupta SP, McHardy GJ: Twelve minute walking test for assessing disability in chronic bronchitis, BMJ 1:822-823, 1976.

47. Gerardi D, Lovett L, Benoit-Connors J et al: Variables related to increased mortality following outpatient pulmonary rehabilitation, Eur Respir J 9:431-435, 1996.

48. Pinto-Plata V, Girish M, Taylor J et al: Natural decline in the six minute walking distance (6MWD) in COPD, Eur Respir J 24:28-33, 2004.

49. Singh S, Morgan M, Hardman A et al: Comparison of oxygen uptake during a conventional tread-mill test and the shuttle walking test in chronic airflow limitation, Eur Respir J 7:2016-2020, 1994.

50. Pollock M, Roa J, Benditt J et al: Stair climbing (SC) predicts maximal oxygen uptake in patients with chronic airflow obstruction, Chest 104:1378-1383, 1993.

51. O'Hara WJ, Lasachuk BP, Matheson P et al: Weight training and backpacking in chronic obstructive pulmonary disease, Respir Care 29:1202-1210, 1984.

52. Martinez FJ, Couser J, Celli BR: Factors influencing ventilatory muscle recruitment in patients with chronic airflow obstruction, Am Rev Respir Dis 142:276-282, 1990.

53. Tangri S, Woolf CR: The breathing pattern in chronic obstructive lung disease, during the performance of some common daily activities, Chest 63:126-127, 1973.

54. Celli BR, Rassulo J, Make B: Dyssynchronous breathing associated with arm but not leg exercise in patients with COPD, N Engl J Med 314:1485-1490, 1968.

55. Celli BR, Criner GJ, Rassulo J: Ventilatory muscle recruitment during unsupported arm exercise in normal subjects, J Appl Physiol 64:1936-1941, 1988.

56. Criner GJ, Celli BR: Effect of unsupported arm exercise on ventilatory muscle recruitment in patients with severe chronic airflow obstruction, Am Rev Respir Dis 138:856-867, 1988.

57. Alison J, Regnis J, Donnelly P et al: End expiratory lung volume during arm and leg exercise in normal subjects and patients with cystic fibrosis, Am J Respir Crit Care Med 158:1450-1458, 1998.

58. Alison J, Regnis J, Donnelly P et al: End-expiratory lung volume during arm and leg exercise in normal subjects and patients with cystic fibrosis, Am J Respir Crit Care Med 158:1450-1458, 1998.

59. Bobbert AC: Physiological comparison of three types of ergometry, J Appl Physiol 15:1007-1014, 1960.

60. Steinberg J, Astrand PO, Ekblom B et al: Hemodynamic response to work with different muscle groups, sitting and supine, J Appl Physiol 22:61-70, 1967.

61. Davis JA, Vodak P, Wilmore JH et al: Anaerobic threshold and maximal power for three modes of exercise, J Appl Physiol 41:549-550, 1976.

62. Reybrouck T, Heigenhouser GF, Faulkner JA: Limitations to maximum oxygen uptake in arm, leg and combined arm-leg ergometry, J Appl Physiol 38:774-779, 1975.

63. Martin TW, Zeballos RJ, Weisman IM: Gas exchange during maximal upper extremity exercise, Chest 99:420-425, 1991.

64. Banzett R, Topulus G, Leith D et al: Bracing arms increases the capacity for sustained hyperpnea, Am Rev Respir Dis 138:106-109, 1988.

65. Dolmage TE, Maestro L, Avendano M et al: The ventilatory response to arm elevation of patients with chronic obstructive pulmonary disease, Chest 104:1097-1100, 1993.

66. Maestro L, Dolmage T, Avendano MA et al: Influence of arm position in ventilation during incremental exercise in healthy individuals, Chest 98:113s, 1990.

67. Couser J, Martinez F, Celli B: Respiratory response to arm elevation in normal subjects, Chest 101:336-340, 1992.

68. Lake FR, Hendersen K, Briffa T et al: Upper limb and lower limb exercise training in patients with chronic airflow obstruction, Chest 97:1077-1082, 1990.

69. Ries AL, Ellis B, Hawkins RW: Upper extremity exercise training in chronic obstructive pulmonary disease, Chest 93:688-692, 1988.

70. Couser J, Martinez F, Celli B: Pulmonary rehabilitation that includes arm exercise reduces metabolic and ventilatory requirements for simple arm elevation, Chest 103:37-38, 1993.

71. Epstein S, Celli B, Martinez F et al: Arm training reduces the VO2 and VE cost of unsupported arm exercise and elevation in chronic obstructive pulmonary disease, J Cardiopulm Rehabil 17:171-177, 1997.

72. Ries A, Carlin B, Carrieri-Colman V et al: Pulmonary rehabilitation: joint ACCP/AACVPR evidence-based guidelines, Chest 112:1363-1396, 1997.

73. Nici L, Donner C, Wouters E et al: ATS/ERS Pulmonary Rehabilitation Writing Committee: American Thoracic Society/European Respiratory Society statement on pulmonary rehabilitation, Am J Respir Crit Care Med 173:1390-1413, 2006.

74. Martinez FJ, Vogel PD, DuPont DN et al: Supported arm exercise vs. unsupported arm exercise in the rehabilitation of patients with chronic airflow obstruction, Chest 103:1397-2002, 1993.

75. Couser J, Guthman R, Abdulgany M et al: Pulmonary rehabilitation improves exercise capacity in elderly patients with COPD, Chest 107:730-734, 1995.

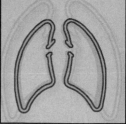

Chapter 11

Inspiratory Muscle Training

JAMES A. MURRAY • DONALD A. MAHLER

CHAPTER OUTLINE

Diagnosis of Inspiratory Muscle
  Weakness
Rationale for Inspiratory Muscle
  Training
Types of Inspiratory Muscle Training
Review of Published Studies
Outcomes
  Respiratory Muscle Function
  Dyspnea Related to Activities of Daily
    Living

Health Status
Exercise Performance
Studies of Inspiratory Muscle Training
  Combined with Exercise Training
Candidate Selection for Inspiratory
  Muscle Training
Exercise Prescription Guidelines for
  Inspiratory Muscle Training
What Outcomes Should Be Measured
Conclusion

PROFESSIONAL SKILLS

On completion of this chapter, the reader will be able to do
the following:
- Understand the rationale for inspiratory muscle training (IMT)
- Describe the results of randomized controlled studies of IMT in patients with chronic obstructive pulmonary disease
- Prescribe specific training goals or targets for the frequency, intensity, and duration of IMT

The thorax is a complex assembly of muscles and bony structures. Like other skeletal muscles, the respiratory muscles contract to generate tension and create negative pressure within the pleural space. The primary muscle of inspiration is the diaphragm, which acts in concert with the external intercostals, and other muscles of the chest to rhythmically contract and relax to reshape the thoracic cavity, and provide the tidal volume of each breath.

The capacity of any muscle to perform work is a function of the demands placed on the muscle (amount of force and velocity of shortening), and the capacity of the muscle to respond to these demands (fiber type, oxidative capacity, capillary density, biochemical milieu, innervation, and mechanical advantage). In many patients with chronic obstructive pulmonary disease (COPD), the relationship between the demand placed on the inspiratory muscles and the capacity to perform this work is abnormal. Inspiratory muscle weakness has been demonstrated in patients with COPD[1,2] and has been associated with subcellular changes in the diaphragm.[3] Although patients with COPD have been shown to have structural changes that render the diaphragm more resistant to fatigue,[4] biopsy specimens from patients with mild to moderate COPD have demonstrated reduced force generation per cross-sectional area.[5]

Any muscle, including the respiratory muscles, can develop fatigue if the load is excessive. Respiratory muscle fatigue is considered a process that is reversible by rest, whereas respiratory muscle weakness persists despite rest. From a functional standpoint, weakness and fatigue may coexist, and varying levels of ventilatory muscle weakness can lower the threshold to fatigue, which can develop with even relatively small increases in the work of breathing. In patients with COPD, inspiratory muscle weakness may occur as a result of the combined effects of malnutrition, hypercapnia, hypoxemia, increased work of breathing, the use of corticosteroids, and so on.

DIAGNOSIS OF INSPIRATORY MUSCLE WEAKNESS

The diagnosis of inspiratory muscle weakness depends on testing in the pulmonary function laboratory, with appropriate equipment as part of the initial evaluation for pulmonary rehabilitation, or both. This condition should be considered on the basis of a reduced vital capacity on spirometry and reductions in other lung volumes (i.e., restrictive lung disease). However, decreases in maximal inspiratory mouth pressure (PImax) occur before decreases in lung volumes can be identified because the relationship between vital capacity and PImax is curvilinear.[6] Therefore PImax and maximal expiratory mouth pressure (PEmax) should be measured when respiratory muscle weakness is suspected in individuals with unexplained breathlessness, orthopnea, or a diagnosis of neuromuscular disease (e.g., amyotrophic lateral sclerosis and myasthenia gravis).

PImax and PEmax are volitional tests that estimate respiratory muscle strength, are simple to perform, and are well tolerated by patients. The method for measuring PImax and PEmax is important to review for the subject to produce the highest possible values that are reproducible.[7] The relationship between the tension generated by the respiratory muscles and the pressure produced in the thorax or mouth is complex. Maximal strength of any skeletal muscle is dependent on optimal length. If the strength of the respiratory muscles is measured at optimal length (i.e., at residual volume), the actual mouth pressure represents the pressure generated by the respiratory muscles

(Pmus) plus the passive elastic recoil pressure of the respiratory system (Prs). If PImax is measured at the optimal length of the vertical muscle fibers of the diaphragm, (residual volume), then Prs may be as high as -30 cm H_2O. At functional residual capacity (FRC), however, Prs is zero, and therefore mouth pressure truly represents Pmus. In patients with COPD who are severely hyperinflated (increased residual volume and FRC), a low PImax value may partly reflect the shortened inspiratory muscle fiber length rather than reduced muscle strength.

PEmax also varies markedly with lung volume. If PEmax is measured at total lung capacity, which is the optimal length of expiratory muscles, then Prs may be as high as $+40$ cm H_2O, which contributes to the measured PEmax value. At FRC Prs is zero so that mouth pressure truly represents Pmus. Therefore when reporting PImax and PEmax, it is important to indicate the lung volume(s) at which they are measured. Despite these considerations, significant decreases in PImax and PEmax reflect global respiratory muscle strength and are useful for clinical evaluation of suspected weakness.

The interpretation of the results depends on comparison of measured values with predicted normal values for PImax and PEmax.[7] A value for PImax of at least -80 cm H_2O usually excludes clinically important inspiratory muscle weakness.[7] Values for PImax that are less negative may represent inspiratory muscle weakness, poor effort, technical artifact as a consequence of an air leak around the mouth, or the significant variation seen in PImax in healthy subjects. Although no single number has been consistently used to define the presence of respiratory muscle weakness, the lower the measured PImax, the more likely there is to be impairment. In selected cases diaphragm muscle strength can be assessed by phrenic nerve stimulation to eliminate possible problems due to poor effort and/or technical issues.[7]

RATIONALE FOR INSPIRATORY MUSCLE TRAINING

The rationale for inspiratory muscle training (IMT) is that increasing the strength or endurance of the respiratory muscles can improve clinical outcomes (i.e., reduce the severity of dyspnea) and enhance the ability of individuals to perform daily activities. However, an extremely high training load has the potential to contribute to inspiratory muscle fatigue. It is therefore important for IMT to provide an adequate, but not excessive, stimulus or load to achieve a training response.

In 1976 Leith and Bradley[8] demonstrated that inspiratory muscle strength and endurance could be specifically increased in healthy individuals with training. These investigators proposed that IMT might be useful in three conditions: for individuals wishing to enhance their sports performance; for persons who must be physically active with imposed ventilatory loads (such as respiratory equipment required by firefighters, miners, and divers); and for patients with respiratory disease in whom ventilatory loads are increased, ventilatory capacity is reduced, or both.[8] Over the subsequent decades IMT has been evaluated in numerous populations including endurance athletes[9-11] and patients with chronic respiratory disease (asthma, cystic fibrosis, and COPD),[12-14] chronic heart failure,[15] chronic cervical spinal cord injury,[16] and muscular dystrophy.[17] In addition, IMT has been investigated in patients before cardiothoracic surgery[18] and to assist weaning from mechanical ventilatory support.[19]

This chapter discusses IMT as a treatment option or as a component of pulmonary rehabilitation for patients with COPD. As already stated, respiratory muscle weakness is a recognized factor that contributes to dyspnea and reduced exercise performance in this population.[20,21] As a consequence, most randomized controlled studies of IMT have focused on symptomatic individuals with COPD.

TYPES OF INSPIRATORY MUSCLE TRAINING

Skeletal muscles can be trained specifically for strength and endurance.[22] As a general principle, strength training requires high workloads with few repetitions, whereas endurance training incorporates low to moderate workloads with a high number of repetitions. The same principles of training apply to IMT, and most IMT programs incorporate a combination of strength and endurance training

In general, there are two types of inspiratory muscle training: inspiratory resistance breathing and sustained hyperpnea. Of these, the use of inspiratory resistance is the more common

approach for IMT. Both flow-resistive loading and threshold loading provide inspiratory resistance to breathing. Flow-resistive load training consists of decreasing the size of the aperture through which the patient is to breathe. The smaller the aperture, the greater the resistance on inspiration. An example is the PFlex device (Respironics HealthScan, Cedar Grove, N.J.). However, one of the limitations of flow-resistive loading is that patients can decrease the amount of inspiratory work by simply breathing slower and thereby reducing the inspiratory resistance.

At present, threshold loading is the most common method used in IMT trials. This technique typically incorporates a spring-loaded valve so that a target level of inspiratory effort is required to overcome the resistance and initiate airflow. An advantage of threshold loading is that inspiratory load can be established at a desired percentage of the PImax. Two examples of threshold loading include the Threshold IMT (Respironics HealthScan) (Figure 11-1) and the POWERbreathe device (Gaiam, Southam, Warwickshire, United Kingdom) (Figure 11-2).

Another method of IMT is sustained hyperpnea, in which the patient achieves maximal sustainable ventilation for a period of time, usually about 15 minutes.[23] However, this method of endurance training typically requires close monitoring to avoid hypocapnia. Supplemental carbon dioxide (CO_2) typically is added to inspired air to maintain isocapnia. This type of endurance training generally requires an experienced technician at a medical facility. However, Scherer and colleagues[24] developed a home device for respiratory muscle endurance training that consisted of tubing connected to a rebreathing bag and a sideport for fresh air that did not require the addition of CO_2.

REVIEW OF PUBLISHED STUDIES

The following criteria were used to select relevant studies of IMT for review and analysis:
- Randomized trial that included treatment and control groups
- Use of an appropriate inspiratory muscle training device
- Selection of an adequate training stimulus (i.e., overload principle of training)
- Inclusion of physiologic (e.g., inspiratory muscle strength and exercise capacity) and clinical (dyspnea ratings, health status, or both) outcomes

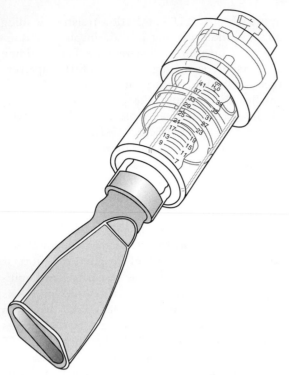

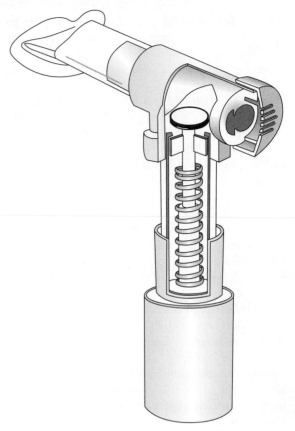

FIGURE 11-1 Diagram of Threshold inspiratory muscle trainer (IMT). The device consists of a spring-loaded one-way valve that provides resistance. The level of resistance can be adjusted manually to provide the desired inspiratory training intensity. In general, the initial training intensity should be more than 30% of maximal inspiratory mouth pressure (PImax).

FIGURE 11-2 Diagram of POWERbreathe device. The instructions recommend that the patient inhale 30 breaths through the device at each training session twice per day. Once the patient is able to complete 30 breaths with ease, then the tension knob should be turned to the right to increase the training load.

Fifteen randomized controlled trials of IMT were identified that met these criteria[24-38] (Table 11-1). In addition, six studies that included IMT combined with general exercise training[39-44] were evaluated (Table 11-2).

The training characteristics (frequency, intensity, and duration) of IMT programs have varied considerably among these various studies. Specific features include the following:

- Frequency: 3 to 7 days/week
- Intensity: The intensity has generally been quantified as a percentage of PImax. Training programs have ranged from 10% (low) to 60% (high) of PImax. The initial training intensity is typically increased over time. Although various inspiratory resistance devices have been used, the most commonly used training device in these studies has been the Threshold IMT (described previously). One study (Scherer and colleagues[24]) used hyperpnea training
- Duration: 5 to 12 weeks. Of the six studies in which IMT was combined with general exercise training (see Table 11-2), the duration varied

from a 4-week inpatient pulmonary rehabilitation program to a 6-month outpatient program.

OUTCOMES

Respiratory Muscle Function

Of the 15 randomized controlled trials listed in Table 11-1, PImax or maximal sustainable inspiratory mouth pressure (PIsmax) (i.e., the heaviest load sustained by the patient for a predetermined period) was measured as a physiologic outcome in all studies except in the study by Pardy and colleagues.[25] Significant increases have been observed in PImax or in PIsmax in the majority of these investigations of IMT. PImax improved by +17% to +48% in the training groups compared with baseline values. To achieve this training response the workload for IMT was more than 30% of the baseline PImax. The control groups in these studies

TABLE 11-1 Randomized Controlled Trials of Inspiratory Muscle Training

Study	Patients	Training Program	Outcomes
Pardy et al[25] Age: 62 yr	9 T	15 min twice per day for 2 mo at an intensity "heralding fatigue"	↑ 12MWD; ↑ exercise endurance
Duration: 8 wk	8 C	General exercise and weight lifting	No changes
Larson et al[26] Age: 64 yr	10 T	30% P$_{I}$max: 15 min/day for first week; 30 min/day thereafter	↑ P$_{I}$max (25%); ↑ 12MWD
Duration: 8 wk	12 C	Same except at 15% P$_{I}$max	↑ P$_{I}$max (14%); no change in 12MWD
Harver, Mahler, and Daubenspeck[27] Age: 63 yr	10 T	15 min twice per day with gradual increase in resistance	↑ P$_{I}$max (32%); ↑ TDI (+3.5 units)
Duration: 8 wk	9 C	Same except sham training with minimal resistance	↑ P$_{I}$max (12%); ↑ TDI (+0.3 unit)
Guyatt et al[28] Age: 66 yr	43 T	10 min five times per day with resistance increased as tolerated	P$_{I}$max (+0.1 cm H$_2$O); no change in 6MWD
Duration: 12 wk	39 C	Same except sham training with minimal resistance	P$_{I}$max (+0.9 cm H$_2$O); no change in 6MWD
Lisboa et al[29] Age: 70 yr	10 T	30% P$_{I}$max: 15 min twice per day with load increased as tolerated	↑ P$_{I}$max (31%); ↑ TDI (+3.8 units)
Duration: 5 wk	10 C	Same except sham training at 12% P$_{I}$max	↑ P$_{I}$max (11%); ↑ TDI (+0.6 unit)
Preusser, Winningham, and Clanton[30] Age: 65 yr	12 T	52% P$_{I}$max: 5 min per session at week 1 to 18 min per session at week 12, three times per week	↑ P$_{I}$max (35%); ↑ 12MWD
Duration: 12 wk	10 C	22% P$_{I}$max: same schedule	↑ P$_{I}$max (12%); ↑ 12MWD
Lisboa et al[31] Age: 62 yr	10 T	30% P$_{I}$max: 30 min/day, 6 days/wk	↑ P$_{I}$max (34%); ↑ TDI (+3.8 units); ↑ 6MWD
Duration: 10 wk	10 C	10% P$_{I}$max: same schedule	↑ P$_{I}$max (19%); ↑ TDI (+1.7 units); no change in 6MWD
Scherer[24] Age: 69 yr Duration: 8 wk	15 T	Hyperpnea training via home device (tube and rebreathing bag): 15 min, twice per day	↑ Sustained ventilation; ↑ respiratory muscle endurance; ↑ 6MWD; ↑ physical component of SF-12
	15 C	Incentive spirometer: same schedule	
Riera et al[32] Age: 67 yr Duration: 6 mo	10 T	Trained at 60% to 70% of P$_{I}$smax for 30 min/day, 6 days/wk	↑ P$_{I}$smax and P$_{I}$max; ↑ shuttle walk test; improved dyspnea and health status
	10 C	No training	No changes
Covey et al[33] Age: 66 yr	12 T	30% to 60% P$_{I}$max for 30 min/day	↑ P$_{I}$max; ↑ dyspnea domain of CRQ
Duration: 4 mo	15 C	Received education	No changes
Weiner et al[34] Age: 63 yr	8 T	15% to 60% P$_{I}$max for 1 hr/day, 6 days/wk	↑ P$_{I}$max; ↑ 6MWD; ↑ BDI (used at follow-up)
Duration: 3 mo	8 C	Same except at fixed resistance of 7 cm H$_2$O	No changes
Weiner et al[35] Age: 65 yr Duration: 12 mo after 3 mo of IMT in both groups	16 T	15% to 60% P$_{I}$max for 30 min/day, 3 to 6 days/wk for initial 3 mo and continued as maintenance for 12 mo	At 12 mo: ↑ P$_{I}$max; ↑ 6MWD; ↑ TDI
	16 C	Same except at fixed resistance of 7 cm H$_2$O as maintenance for 12 mo	At 12 mo: ↓ P$_{I}$max; ↓ 6MWD; ↓ TDI
Beckerman et al[36] Age: 67 yr	21 T	Gradual increase to 60% P$_{I}$max, 15 min twice per day, 6 days/wk	↑ P$_{I}$max; ↑ 6MWD; ↑ health status
Duration: 1 yr	21 C	Training with "very low load": same schedule	No changes
Koppers et al[37] Age: 56 yr Duration 5 wk	18 T	"Tube breathing" for 15 min twice per day, 7 days/wk	↑ P$_{I}$smax; ↑ health status; ↑ exercise endurance; ↓ dyspnea during exercise
	18 C	Incentive flowmeter set to 5% P$_{I}$max	No significant changes

Continued

TABLE 11-1 Randomized Controlled Trials of Inspiratory Muscle Training—cont'd

Study	Patients	Training Program	Outcomes
Hill et al[38] Age: 68 yr Duration: 8 wk	16 T	Maximal load tolerable for each 2-min work interval; seven cycles of 2 min of IMT followed by 1 min of rest (total of 21 min, 3 days/wk)	↑ PImax (29%); ↑ 6MWD; ↑ health status (+0.8 for CRQ total score)
	17 C	10% PImax: same schedule	↑ PImax (8%); no change in 6MWD; ↑ health status (+0.4 for CRQ total score)

6MWD, *6-minute walk distance;* 12MWD, *12-minute walk distance;* BDI, *Baseline Dyspnea Index;* C, *control group;* CRQ, *Chronic Respiratory Disease Questionnaire;* IMT, *inspiratory muscle training;* PImax, *maximal inspiratory mouth pressure;* PIsmax, *maximal sustainable mouth pressure for 45 seconds;* SF-12, *SF-12 Health Survey;* T, *training group;* TDI, *Transition Dyspnea Index (measures change from baseline state).*

TABLE 11-2 Randomized Trials of Inspiratory Muscle Training and Exercise Training

Study	Patients	Training Program	Outcomes
Goldstein et al[39] Age: 66 yr Duration: 4 wk	6 T	43% PImax for 15 min twice per day for 10 min, and increased to a target of 20 min, 5 days/wk	↑ Respiratory muscle endurance; ↑ 6MWD
	5 C	Treadmill walking and IMT at 38% PImax according to same schedule	↑ 6MWD
Dekhuijzen, Folgering, and van Herwaarden[40] Age: 59 yr Duration: 10 wk	20 T	Target flow with added resistance at 70% PImax held for 3 sec for 15 min twice per day with load increased based on response	↑ PImax*; ↑ 12MWD*
	20 C	Cycle ergometry and walking, but no IMT	↑ PImax; ↑ 12MWD
Weiner et al[41] Age: 65 yr Duration: 6 mo	12 T	15% to 80% PImax: 15 min three times per week	↑ PImax; ↑ respiratory muscle endurance*; ↑ 12MWD*; ↑ cycle endurance time*
	12 C	Cycle ergometry and sham IMT	↑ 12MWD; ↑ cycle endurance time
Wanke et al[42] Age: 56 yr Duration: 8 wk	21 T	Strength IMT: 12 maximal static inspiratory efforts Endurance IMT: 70% maximal transdiaphragmatic pressure for 10 min/day	↑ PImax *; ↑ respiratory muscle endurance*; ↑ maximal power output*; ↑ $\dot{V}o_2$ max*
	21 C	Cycle ergometry, but no IMT	
Berry et al[43] Age: 69 yr Duration: 12 wk	8 T 9 C	15% to 80% PImax Walking and sham IMT at 15% PImax	No ↑ in PImax
Larson et al[44] Age: 67 yr Duration: 4 mo	14 T	30% to 60% of PImax: 30 min/day, 5 days/wk	↑ PImax; ↑ peak exercise
	14 C	Cycle ergometry, but no IMT	↑ Peak exercise

P < .05 compared with control group.
6MWD, *6-minute walk distance;* 12MWD, *12-minute walk distance;* C, *control group (exercise with sham IMT or no IMT);* PImax, *maximal inspiratory mouth pressure;* T, *training group (exercise plus inspiratory muscle training);* $\dot{V}o_2$ *maxPA200, maximal oxygen uptake.*

received either sham or minimal resistance "training" and exhibited increases of +3% to +19% in PImax. These small to modest changes are consistent with either learning from repeated testing or a response to a low training load.

Koppers and colleagues[37] studied endurance training via tube breathing. As expected, PIsmax increased significantly with 5 weeks of training (training group: +6 cm H_2O vs. control group: −3 cm H_2O of sustainable inspiratory pressure; $P < .001$), whereas there was no difference in PImax between the groups.

Dyspnea Related to Activities of Daily Living

The intensity of dyspnea is inversely related to the strength of the inspiratory muscles in both healthy subjects and patients with COPD.[45-48] This relationship suggests that augmentation of inspiratory muscle strength may reduce the severity of breathlessness.

In general, the majority of studies that have measured breathlessness related to activities of daily living have shown benefits with IMT (see Table 11-1). For example, Harver, Mahler, and Daubenspeck[27] reported an improvement in the Transition Dyspnea Index (TDI) of +3.5 ± 2.5 units after 8 weeks of IMT, whereas the TDI was +0.3 ± 1.0 in the control group ($P < .05$). In two different studies Lisboa and colleagues[29,31] showed that patients who underwent IMT had significant and clinically meaningful increases in the TDI: +3.8 ± 2.2 and +3.8 ± 0.6 units compared with increases of +0.6 ± 1.6 and +1.7 ± 0.6 units, respectively, in the sham groups (trained at 12% and 10% of PImax, respectively) ($P < .05$). Furthermore, the changes in PImax associated with IMT were correlated significantly with the changes in the TDI in the training groups.[27,29] Riera and colleagues[32] showed that the TDI improved by +4.7 ± 0.6 units in the training group, but a minimal effect was observed (+0.2 ± 0.1 units) in the control group after 6 months of IMT.

In a 3-month trial of IMT, Weiner and colleagues[34] used the Baseline Dyspnea Index (BDI) at the start and at follow-up to investigate changes in breathlessness with activities of daily living. The training group increased the BDI from 5.2 ± 0.8 to 7.3 ± 1.0 ($P < .01$), whereas there was no change in the control group. In a subsequent investigation of maintenance IMT, Weiner and colleagues[35] demonstrated that the training group maintained the improvement in dyspnea

after 1 year (TDI, +1.7 ± 0.2 units) compared with 3 months (TDI, +1.6 ± 0.2 units). In contrast, the control group exhibited a decline in the TDI over the same time period (from +1.8 ± 0.2 at 3 months to +0.3 ± 0.1 units at 1 year) ($P < .05$).

Covey and colleagues[33] reported that IMT (starting intensity was 30% of PImax and increased as tolerated to 60% of PImax) for 16 weeks reduced dyspnea related to activities of daily living as measured with the Chronic Respiratory Disease Questionnaire (CRQ) compared with an educational control group (+4.3 vs. −1.1 units; $P = .018$). These various studies show consistent benefits for relief of breathlessness during daily activities with IMT.

Health Status

Various studies show consistent improvements in health status with IMT. Beckerman and colleagues[36] reported that scores on the St. George's Respiratory Questionnaire improved (i.e., lower values) in the training group compared with both the baseline state ($P < .05$) and the control group ($P < .01$) after 6 months of IMT. This difference was maintained for an additional 6 months of IMT. Hill and colleagues[38] measured health status with the CRQ and found improved scores for dyspnea and fatigue domains but not for mastery and emotional function, compared with the changes observed in the sham-IMT group ($P < .05$). Riera and colleagues[32] found that each of the four domains of the CRQ improved with IMT; the changes exceeded the minimal clinically important difference and was significantly different compared with the control group.

In a study of respiratory muscle endurance training, Koppers and colleagues[37] showed significant improvements in the CRQ total score in the training group compared with baseline ($P = .001$), but the difference between training and control groups did not achieve statistical significance ($P = .07$).

Exercise Performance

IMT has been shown to improve exercise performance. For example, Pardy and colleagues[25] and Larson and colleagues[26] demonstrated increases in the 12-minute walk distance after IMT. Both Beckerman and colleagues[36] and Hill and colleagues[38] demonstrated statistically significant increases in the 6-minute walk distance in the training groups compared with the control groups (an increase of 72 m and 32 m, respectively; $P < .05$). Riera and colleagues[32] showed a difference of 93 m (95% confidence interval, 58-128 m) in the shuttle walk distance in the IMT group compared with the control group ($P <.05$). Weiner and colleagues[34] demonstrated increases in the 6-minute walk distance in the IMT group (276 ± 44 to 347 ± 47 m; $P <.05$) but no significant increase in the control group.

Neither Guyatt and colleagues[28] nor Preusser, Winningham, and Clanton[30] showed any differences in timed walk distance between the training and control groups. However, the IMT groups in these two studies did not achieve significant improvements in PImax. Most likely, the training load was inadequate to achieve the anticipated benefits in respiratory muscle strength and the corresponding exercise performance.

STUDIES OF INSPIRATORY MUSCLE TRAINING COMBINED WITH EXERCISE TRAINING

Several studies have examined the efficacy of IMT combined with general exercise training (see Table 11-2).[39-44] In the study by Goldstein and colleagues,[39] IMT was part of a 4-week inpatient pulmonary rehabilitation program. The training group achieved an increase in inspiratory muscle endurance, but no change in PImax or exercise tolerance. This study was limited by the small sample size (six patients in the training group and five in the control group). In studies from the Netherlands,[40] Israel,[41] and Austria,[42] investigators showed significant improvements in PImax and in exercise performance in the training group (IMT plus exercise) compared with the control group. However, neither dyspnea nor health status was measured in these studies. Berry and colleagues[43] showed that IMT combined with lower extremity exercise resulted in greater improvements in walk distance compared with a control group, but there were no differences in PImax or exercise capacity with combined IMT and exercise training compared with the group that performed only exercise training. Larson and colleagues[44] compared respiratory muscle strength, exercise performance, and dyspnea during exercise testing in four groups: health education, IMT, home-based cycle ergometry, and IMT combined with home-based cycle ergometry. In the IMT plus exercise group there was a modest increase in PImax, but the combination of home exercise plus IMT did not produce additional benefits in exercise performance and exercise-related symptoms.

These six studies (see Table 11-2) are limited by two major factors. First, none of the studies required patients to have inspiratory muscle weakness as an inclusion criterion. Thus it is uncertain whether IMT would benefit patients with normal respiratory muscle strength. In a meta-analysis of studies that compared exercise training versus exercise plus IMT, Lotters and colleagues[49] found that patients with inspiratory muscle weakness improved significantly more compared with patients without inspiratory muscle weakness. Accordingly, it is probably important to require inspiratory muscle weakness as an inclusion criterion for trials of IMT.

Second, clinical outcomes, particularly dyspnea related to activities of daily living and health status, were not measured in any of the studies. Only Larson and colleagues[44] and Berry and colleagues[43] included any symptom assessment (i.e., breathlessness ratings during exercise testing) as secondary outcomes. In contrast, the majority of randomized controlled trials of IMT as the sole intervention included patient-centered outcomes (see Table 11-1).

CANDIDATE SELECTION FOR INSPIRATORY MUSCLE TRAINING

On the basis of the results provided in Tables 11-1 and 11-2, it is reasonable to consider IMT for an individual patient with COPD who has the following characteristics:
- Severe dyspnea with activities
- High-level motivation
- Reduced inspiratory muscle strength (PImax)
- Moderate to severe respiratory impairment, but not "end-stage" COPD with severe hyperinflation and flattened diaphragm

These features are consistent with the recommendations of the evidence-based clinical practice guidelines presented by the American College of Chest Physicians and the American Association of Cardiovascular and Pulmonary Rehabilitation.[14,50]

EXERCISE PRESCRIPTION GUIDELINES FOR INSPIRATORY MUSCLE TRAINING

The optimal IMT program has not been established. However, studies of IMT that demonstrated clinical improvements have included components of both strength and endurance training using inspiratory resistive loads (see Table 11-1).

On the basis of these data the following training goals are recommended when using a targeted inspiratory resistance device:

- Frequency: at least 5 days/week
- Intensity: more than 30% Pimax as the initial training intensity (the intensity can be adjusted on the basis of the patient's ability to achieve the duration goal)
- Duration: 30 minutes/day (15 minutes twice per day or continuous)

If the Threshold IMT is used, an inspiratory pressure can be selected for training based on the target intensity (i.e., a percentage of the individual's Pimax). As noted previously, a training intensity greater than 30% Pimax appears to be the minimal threshold to achieve increases in inspiratory muscle strength and clinical benefits. Belman, Thomas, and Lewis[51] demonstrated that the work of breathing was higher at a respiratory frequency of 30 breaths/minute with resistive breathing either through a fixed orifice or through a threshold valve compared with a frequency of 15 breaths/minute. Thus a high respiratory frequency will increase the training stimulus.

Alternatively, a respiratory muscle strength training program may be instituted. For example, Redline, Gottfried, and Altose[52] instructed seven healthy individuals to perform sustained maximal inspiratory efforts (i.e., 20 maneuvers per day) and found that subjects increased their Pimax by 51% over 6 to 18 weeks. Moreover, they found that the intensity of respiratory sensation during loaded breathing was reduced after inspiratory strength training but returned to baseline levels by 8 weeks after cessation of training. Hill and colleagues[38] compared outcomes in patients who performed IMT at the highest tolerable inspiratory threshold load (101% of baseline Pimax) three times per week for 8 weeks with those in patients who underwent sham IMT (10% Pimax). With the high-intensity IMT, the changes in Pimax (increase, 29%), maximal threshold pressure (increase, 56%), 6-minute walk distance (increase, 27 m), as well as dyspnea (increase, 1.4 units) and fatigue (increase, 0.9 unit) domains on the CRQ, were significantly greater than those that occurred in the sham IMT group.

WHAT OUTCOMES SHOULD BE MEASURED

Both physiologic and clinical outcomes should be measured at baseline, as well as during and at completion of a trial of IMT. For example,

Pimax should be monitored because inspiratory muscle strength should increase if the training stimulus is appropriate. It is recommended that dyspnea related to activities of daily living and health status be measured to evaluate the anticipated clinical benefits of IMT. Exercise performance may also be assessed, based on the objectives of the IMT program.

CONCLUSION

In summary, published randomized controlled trials support the use of IMT in patients with COPD who have inspiratory muscle weakness and complain of exertional breathlessness (see Table 11-1). The most likely reason that IMT has not been incorporated into guideline recommendations for the treatment of COPD is that these data are limited by modest numbers of patients studied at single institutions. The 2007 evidence-based clinical practice guidelines published by the American College of Chest Physicians and the American Association of Cardiovascular and Pulmonary Rehabilitation states that "IMT be considered in selected patients with COPD who have decreased inspiratory muscle strength and breathlessness despite optimal medical therapy."[50]

The clinical benefits of IMT demonstrated in numerous randomized controlled trials (see Table 11-1) indicate that a multicenter, randomized controlled trial should be performed to more completely investigate the role of IMT in patients with COPD. This study should include appropriate statistical power, be designed to examine the type(s) of patients who might benefit (i.e., phenotypes) from IMT, and investigate different methods (intensity and duration) of training.

References

1. Begin P, Grassino A: Inspiratory muscle dysfunction and chronic hypercapnia in chronic obstructive pulmonary disease, Am Rev Respir Dis 143:905-912, 1991.
2. Polkey MI, Kyroussis D, Hamnegard CH et al: Diaphragm strength in chronic obstructive pulmonary disease, Am J Respir Crit Care Med 154:1310-1317, 1996.
3. Orozco-Levi M, Gea J, Lloreta JL et al: Subcellular adaptation of the human diaphragm in chronic obstructive pulmonary disease, Eur Respir J 13:371-378, 1999.
4. Levine S, Kaiser L, Leferovich J et al: Cellular adaptations in the diaphragm in chronic obstructive pulmonary disease, N Engl J Med 337:1799, 1997.

5. Ottenheijm CAC, Heunks LMA, Sieck GC et al: Diaphragm dysfunction in chronic obstructive pulmonary disease, Am J Respir Crit Care Med 172:200-205, 2005.

6. DeTroyer A, Borenstein S, Cordier R: Analysis of lung volume restriction in patients with respiratory muscle weakness, Thorax 35:603-610, 1980.

7. American Thoracic Society, European Respiratory Society: ATS/ERS statement on respiratory muscle testing, Am J Respir Crit Care Med 166:518-624, 2002.

8. Leith DE, Bradley M: Ventilatory muscle strength and endurance training, J Appl Physiol 41:508-516, 1976.

9. Boutellier U: Respiratory muscle fitness and exercise endurance in healthy humans, Med Sci Sports Exerc 30:1169-1172, 1998.

10. Holm P, Sattler A, Fregosi RF: Endurance training of respiratory muscles improves cycling performance in fit young cyclists, BMC Physiol 4:9, 2004.

11. Gething AD, Williams M, Davies B: Inspiratory resistive loading improves cycling capacity: a placebo controlled trial, Br J Sports Med 38:730-736, 2004.

12. Weiner P, Azgad Y, Ganam R et al: Inspiratory muscle training in patients with bronchial asthma, Chest 102:1357-1361, 1992.

13. Sawyer EH, Clanton TL: Improved pulmonary function and exercise tolerance with inspiratory muscle conditioning in children with cystic fibrosis, Chest 104:1490-1497, 1993.

14. Ries AL, Bauldoff GS, Carlin BW et al: Pulmonary rehabilitation: joint ACCP/AACVPR evidence-based clinical practice guidelines, Chest 131:4S-42S, 2007.

15. Cahalin LP, Semigran MJ, Dec GW: Inspiratory muscle training in patients with chronic heart failure awaiting cardiac transplantation: results of a pilot clinical trial, Phys Ther 77:830-838, 1997.

16. Rutchik A, Weissman AR, Almenoff PL et al: Resistive inspiratory muscle training in subjects with chronic cervical spinal cord injury, Arch Phys Rehabil 79:293-297, 1998.

17. Wanke T, Toifl K, Merkle M et al: Inspiratory muscle training in patients with Duchenne muscular dystrophy, Chest 105:475-482, 1994.

18. Nomori H, Kobayashi R, Fuyuno G et al: Preoperative respiratory muscle training: assessment in thoracic surgery patients with special reference to postoperative pulmonary complications, Chest 105:1782-1788, 1994.

19. Aldrich TK, Karpel JP, Uhrlass RM et al: Weaning from mechanical ventilation: adjunctive use of inspiratory muscle resistive training, Crit Care Med 17:143-147, 1989.

20. Killian KJ, Jones NL: Respiratory muscles and dyspnea, Clin Chest Med 9:237-248, 1988.

21. O'Donnell DE: Exertional breathlessness in chronic respiratory disease. In Mahler DA, editor: Lung biology in health and disease, Vol. III: dyspnea, New York, 1998, Marcel Dekker, pp 97-148.

22. Belman MJ, Botnick WC, Nathan SD et al: Ventilatory load characteristics during ventilatory muscle training, Am J Respir Crit Care Med 149:925-929, 1994.

23. Levine S, Weiser P, Gillen J: Evaluation of a ventilatory muscle endurance training program in the rehabilitation of patients with chronic obstructive pulmonary disease, Am Rev Respir Dis 133:400-406, 1986.

24. Scherer TA, Spengler CM, Owassapian D et al: Respiratory muscle endurance training in chronic obstructive pulmonary disease, Am J Respir Crit Care Med 162:1709-1714, 2000.

25. Pardy RL, Rivington RN, Despas PJ et al: Inspiratory muscle training compared with physiotherapy in patients with chronic airflow limitation, Am Rev Respir Dis 123:421-425, 1981.

26. Larson JL, Kim MJ, Sharp JT et al: Inspiratory muscle training with a pressure threshold breathing device in patients with chronic obstructive pulmonary disease, Am Rev Respir Dis 138:689-696, 1988.

27. Harver A, Mahler DA, Daubenspeck JA: Targeted inspiratory muscle training improves respiratory muscle function and reduces dyspnea in patients with chronic obstructive pulmonary disease, Ann Intern Med 111:117-124, 1989.

28. Guyatt G, Keller J, Singer J et al: Controlled trial of respiratory muscle training in chronic airflow limitation, Thorax 47:598-602, 1992.

29. Lisboa C, Munoz V, Beroiza KT et al: Inspiratory muscle training in chronic airflow limitation: comparison of two different training loads with a threshold device, Eur Respir J 7:1266-1274, 1994.

30. Preusser BA, Winningham ML, Clanton TL: High- vs low-intensity inspiratory muscle interval training in patients with COPD, Chest 106:110-117, 1994.

31. Lisboa C, Villafranca C, Leiva A et al: Inspiratory muscle training in chronic airflow limitation: effect on exercise performance, Eur Respir J 10:537-542, 1997.

32. Riera HS, Rubio TM, Ruiz FO et al: Inspiratory muscle training in patients with COPD, Chest 120:748-756, 2001.

33. Covey MK, Larson JL, Wirtz SE et al: High-intensity inspiratory muscle training in patients with chronic obstructive pulmonary disease and severely reduced function, J Cardiopulm Rehabil 21:231-240, 2001.

34. Weiner P, Magadle R, Beckerman M et al: Comparison of specific expiratory, inspiratory, and combined muscle training program in COPD, Chest 124:1357-1364, 2003.

35. Weiner P, Magadle R, Beckerman M et al: Maintenance of inspiratory muscle training in COPD patients: one year follow-up, Eur Respir J 23:61-65, 2004.

36. Beckerman M, Magadle R, Weiner M et al: The effects of 1 year of specific inspiratory muscle training in patients with COPD, Chest 128:3177-3182, 2005.

37. Koppers RJH, Vos PJE, Boot CRL et al: Exercise performance improves in patients with COPD due to respiratory muscle endurance training, Chest 129:886-892, 2006.

38. Hill K, Jenkins SC, Phillippe DL et al: High-intensity inspiratory muscle training in COPD, Eur Respir J 27:1119-1128, 2006.

39. Goldstein R, DeRosie J, Long S et al: Applicability of a threshold loading device for inspiratory muscle testing and training in patients with COPD, Chest 96:564-571, 1989.

40. Dekhuijzen PNR, Folgering HTM, van Herwaarden CLA: Target-flow inspiratory muscle training during pulmonary rehabilitation in patients with COPD, Chest 99:128-133, 1991.

41. Weiner P, Azgad Y, Ganam R: Inspiratory muscle training combined with general exercise reconditioning in patients with COPD, Chest 102:1351-1356, 1992.

42. Wanke T, Formanek D, Lahrman H et al: Effects of combined inspiratory and cycle ergometer training on exercise performance in patients with COPD, Eur Respir J 7:2205-2211, 1994.

43. Berry MJ, Adair NE, Sevensky KS et al: Inspiratory muscle training and whole-body reconditioning in chronic obstructive pulmonary disease, Am J Respir Crit Care Med 153:1812-1816, 1996.

44. Larson JL, Covey MK, Wirtz SE et al: Cycle ergometer and inspiratory muscle training in chronic obstructive pulmonary disease, Am J Respir Crit Care Med 160:500-507, 1999.

45. O'Donnell D, Bertley J, Chau L et al: Qualitative aspects of exertional breathlessness in chronic airflow limitation, Am J Respir Crit Care Med 155:109-115, 1997.

46. Mahler D, Faryniarz K, Tomlinson D et al: Impact of dyspnea and physiologic function on general health status in patients with chronic obstructive pulmonary disease, Chest 102:395-401, 1992.

47. Leblanc P, Bowie D, Summers E et al: Breathlessness and exercise in patients with cardiorespiratory disease, Am Rev Respir Dis 133:21-25, 1986.

48. El-Manshawi A, Killian K, Summers E et al: Breathlessness during exercise with and without resistive loading, J Appl Physiol 61:896-905, 1986.

49. Lotters F, van Tol B, Kwakkel G et al: Effects of controlled inspiratory muscle training in patients with COPD: a meta-analysis, Eur Respir J 20:570-577, 2002.

50. Ries AL, Bauldoff GS, Carlin BW et al: Pulmonary rehabilitation: joint ACCP/AACVPR evidence-based clinical practice guidelines, Chest 131(5 suppl):4S-42S, 2007.

51. Belman MJ, Thomas SG, Lewis MI: Resistive breathing training in patients with chronic obstructive pulmonary disease, Chest 90:662-669, 1986.

52. Redline S, Gottfried SB, Altose MD: Effects of changes in inspiratory muscle strength on the sensation of respiratory force, J Appl Physiol 70:240-245, 1991.

Chapter 12

Physical and Respiratory Therapy for the Medical and Surgical Patient

REBECCA CROUCH

CHAPTER OUTLINE

Interdisciplinary Approach to Pulmonary Rehabilitation
Patient Evaluation
Pulmonary Function Testing
Graded Exercise Testing
Six-Minute Walk Test
Physical Therapy and Respiratory Therapy Evaluation
Patient Medical History from Referring Physician
Evaluation Parameters Unique to the Surgical Pulmonary Rehabilitation Patient
Preoperative Goals
Incisions

Inpatient Postoperative Goals
Exercise Limitations After Surgery
Outpatient Postoperative Goals
Infection Control
Organ Rejection Detection
Planning an Individualized Pulmonary Rehabilitation Program
Oxygen
Designing the Exercise Program
Patient Training
Setting Practical Goals and Facilitating Achievement
Facilitating a Lifestyle Change
Conclusion

PROFESSIONAL SKILLS

On completion of this chapter, the reader will be able to do the following:
- Describe the collaborative roles of physical therapists and respiratory therapists in pulmonary rehabilitation
- Describe the evaluation tools used for patients undergoing medical and surgical pulmonary rehabilitation
- Define the exercise components of a comprehensive rehabilitation program for patients undergoing medical and surgical pulmonary rehabilitation

INTERDISCIPLINARY APPROACH TO PULMONARY REHABILITATION

The history of the physical therapist (PT) and respiratory therapist (RT) caring for patients with pulmonary disease is an interesting journey that closely parallels the beginnings of pulmonary rehabilitation itself. Miss Winifred Linton, an English nurse, initially treated traumatic respiratory complications during World War I. After the war, she entered physical therapy training and began to teach localized breathing exercises to other PTs and surgeons at the Royal Brompton

Hospital in London. Her work continued through the 1940s and during World War II.[1]

A few PTs in the United States were instructed in chest physical therapy techniques and began to use and teach them during the polio epidemic of the 1940s. In the 1960s, the concept of inhalation therapy was developing with the use of artificial airways, positive-pressure ventilators, and supplemental oxygen (O_2).

Coinciding with these chest physical therapy and inhalation therapy techniques of the 1960s was the concept of pulmonary rehabilitation. Medical rehabilitation for neurologic and traumatic injuries had been recognized since 1923, when the American College of Radiology and Physiotherapy was founded. In 1937, the American Medical Association recognized the American Congress of Physical Therapy, which continued to foster the concept of rehabilitation. In the 1950s, Dr. Alvan Barach and colleagues at Goldwater Memorial Hospital in New York City were using supplemental O_2, diaphragmatic breathing exercises, and progressive ambulation to treat the large population of patients with chronic lung disease.[2]

In the 1970s, PTs were providing pulmonary therapy in acute care settings.[1] Respiratory therapists, no longer called "inhalation therapists," would initially treat the patient with lung disease with intermittent positive-pressure breathing followed by the PT performing chest physical therapy, breathing exercises, range of motion (ROM), strengthening exercises, and progressive ambulation. The RT and PT would often work together, administering intermittent positive-pressure breathing in conjunction with breathing exercises, assisting with positioning during chest physical therapy (postural drainage and percussion), teaching the patient bed mobility and sitting for a more effective cough, assisting with sit to stand activity and transfers from bed to chair, and ultimately teaching progressive ambulation with supplemental O_2 and/or bagging for ventilator-dependent patients.

The rehabilitation of patients with pulmonary disease is a collaborative process that may involve a variety of health care professionals.[3-6] The advantage of an interdisciplinary team is that it allows each professional to assess, train, and treat the patient in their specialty discipline. The educational backgrounds of multiple disciplines highlight areas for cooperation and overlapping skills. The blending of talents from these disciplines works extremely well to begin the process of treating, teaching, mobilizing, and rehabilitating the patient with lung disease in acute care and rehabilitation settings.[7-11] The ultimate goal is to evaluate and treat individuals disabled by pulmonary disease. These individuals often have complex medical, psychosocial, and physical disabilities. The team goals are to aid the patient in achieving a higher functional level, an improved sense of well-being, and greater independence. These goals are especially challenging and require a group of health care professionals who possess special talents and can view each patient's needs from a unique perspective.

Communication and documentation are equally important in pulmonary rehabilitation. In a true "interdisciplinary" team approach, health care professionals from several specialties conduct separate assessments of the patient but, through documentation and communication, converge to set goals, plan treatment, and evaluate progress.

The nucleus of the interdisciplinary team is the patient and his or her family.[5,8] The Joint Commission has placed the utmost importance on identifying the goals of the patient as well as the team's short- and long-term goals.[6,12] Objective progress toward those goals must be demonstrated; therefore, team communication, coordination, and documentation are vital.[13]

PATIENT EVALUATION

Diagnostic testing needed for the physical therapy or respiratory therapy evaluation of the patient undergoing pulmonary rehabilitation starts with understanding the disease process and the physiologic impact of the disease through pulmonary diagnostic and exercise testing.

Pulmonary Function Testing

Pulmonary function tests provide the key information that defines the diagnostic classification and degree of impairment caused by diseases affecting the lung.[14] The failure of the respiratory system to effectively ventilate sufficient air to support gas exchange and ultimately the metabolic activity of the muscles results in the primary cause of functional limitations in patients with respiratory diseases. Measuring lung function by spirometry, lung volume, and diffusion studies is essential for a clear diagnostic assessment before starting pulmonary rehabilitation.[15] These studies provide the objective data that support the need for pulmonary rehabilitation. They enable clinicians to define the degree of airway obstruction and to measure response to bronchodilators, amount of lung distention caused by hyperinflation, "lung stiffness" present in restrictive diseases, and gas exchange impairments. Pulmonary function test results provide clinicians with insights into the underlying cause and degree of lung tissue impairment that patients must work against to breathe. Understanding spirometry, lung volume, and diffusion test results is essential to see into the patient's disabling ineffectiveness to breathe at rest and during activity.

Graded Exercise Testing

One of the primary reasons patients with pulmonary disease seek medical attention is because of shortness of breath with physical exertion.[16,17] This complaint offers a puzzling picture for the physician, who must determine if the cause of dyspnea is of cardiac or pulmonary origin. Although pulmonary function tests are helpful in the determination of airway flow dynamics and ventilatory capacities, they do not provide information about potential ventilatory limitations or cardiac abnormalities during physical exertion. The American College of Sports Medicine[16] cited the following indications to perform exercise testing with patients with pulmonary disease:

- Cause of breathlessness unclear despite results from pulmonary function tests
- Patient's severity of breathlessness disproportionate to objective data
- Coexistence of both cardiac and respiratory diseases
- Cause of exercise limitation or dyspnea uncertain
- Evaluation needed for exercise-induced O_2 desaturation
- Exercise prescription

The pulmonary exercise protocol may use either a cycle ergometer or a treadmill. The advantages and disadvantages of cycle ergometry versus treadmill for exercise testing are listed in Table 12-1. The exercise test protocol should be progressive, with equal stages of speed and grade. Small and short-duration exercise stages are preferable to larger and less frequent increases. Measurements of interest during the pulmonary exercise test include not only the workload (e.g., watts, metabolic equivalents [METs], or kilopond-meters per minute

TABLE 12-1	Advantages and Disadvantages of Bicycle Ergometry and Treadmill for Graded Exercise Testing
Bicycle Ergometry	**Treadmill**
ADVANTAGES	
Simple	Familiar
Inexpensive	Natural movement
Portable	Similar to exercise training
Ease of monitoring vital signs and ECG	Preferred method for obtaining maximal $\dot{V}o_2$
Work of breathing eased by stabilizing and elevating the chest when propping the arms on the handlebars	
DISADVANTAGES	
Local muscle fatigue (quadriceps)	Expensive
Unaccustomed to riding	Noisy
Lower maximal $\dot{V}o_2$	Large
Speed dependent	Not easily portable
	Needs electrical source
	Difficult to obtain vital signs and ECG at high intensities

ECG, *Electrocardiogram;* $\dot{V}o_2$, *volume of oxygen consumed per minute.*

[kpm/min]) but specific cardiovascular and ventilatory parameters, rate of perceived exertion, Borg Scale, and arterial blood gases or arterial oxygen saturation (Sao_2).[16]

Cardiovascular measurements should include the electrocardiogram, blood pressure, and heart rate. Ventilatory measurements are extremely useful in exercise testing of patients with pulmonary disease. It is important to measure expired ventilation per minute, respiratory rate, tidal volume, volume of O_2 consumed per minute, and volume of carbon dioxide (CO_2) produced per minute. Subjective symptoms may be rated during the test by means of a Borg or Visual Analog Scale. The testing protocol should be low level and increase by approximately 0.5 MET per stage.[17-19]

Determination of gas exchange can provide pertinent information before beginning a pulmonary rehabilitation program. Although arterial blood gases (e.g., arterial partial pressure of oxygen [Pao_2] and carbon dioxide [$Paco_2$]) have been standardly measured in the past, noninvasive oximeters are capable of detecting O_2

desaturation within ±3% to 5% confidence level. If CO_2 retention is suspected, the measurement of arterial blood gases with and without exertion is warranted to make accurate supplemental O_2 adjustments.[16-20]

Six-Minute Walk Test

The 6-Minute Walk Test (6MWT) has become the "gold standard" of exercise testing for the patient population with pulmonary disease and is a widely reported outcome measure for pulmonary rehabilitation.[21] Many clinicians use the 6MWT as a simple, inexpensive, and efficient evaluation tool. Specific policy and procedures for the 6MWT, ranging from what equipment is used to what is said to the patient, must be followed when administering the test (Box 12-1). A sample 6MWT documentation flowsheet can be seen in Figure 12-1. Numerous outcome measures can be derived from the 6MWT (e.g., percentage of the predicted 6-min walk distance, miles per hour walked, METs, and target heart rate) (Box 12-2).

Physical Therapy and Respiratory Therapy Evaluation

Electronic medical documentation (EMD) has become commonplace within medical practice. Many medical disciplines now record all patient interactions, using EMD. A system of electronic documentation facilitates accessibility of all caregivers to the current plan and intervention of each health care provider. Each care facility usually has individualized documentation templates. The following discussion highlights evaluative points to consider when designing a clinic-specific template.

The physical therapy evaluation (Figure 12-2) and the respiratory therapy evaluation (Figure 12-3) begin with a thorough history that is essential to establishing rapport and to beginning to form a treatment plan for the patient. Comprehensive medical records should be attained before the patient starts the program, but if they are unavailable a verbal account from the patient or family is helpful. The pulmonary diagnosis and onset followed by a

---

BOX 12-1	Six-Minute Walk Test Policy and Procedure

PURPOSE

To provide a protocol for all pulmonary rehabilitation staff to follow when performing the 6-minute walk test (6MWT) evaluation. This protocol will allow maximal patient safety and consistency among team members by avoiding variances in technique. The 6MWT better reflects activities of daily living than other walk tests. It helps to measure functional status of the patient.

Absolute Contraindications
- Unstable angina during the previous month
- Myocardial infarction during the previous month

Relative Contraindications
- Resting heart rate greater than 120 beats per minute
- Resting systolic blood pressure greater than 180 mm Hg
- Resting diastolic blood pressure greater than 100 mm Hg
- Resting systolic blood pressure less than 80 mm Hg
- Resting diastolic blood pressure less than 50 mm Hg (asymptomatic or as directed by referring physician for 6MWT)
- Angina
- Resting Borg Scale score greater than 6
- Dizziness
- Nausea
- Resting oxygen (O_2) saturation level less than 80% while breathing O_2 or room air

Other Safety Issues
- If available, results from a resting electrocardiogram done during the previous 6 months should also be reviewed before testing.
- Stable exertional angina is *not* an absolute contraindication, but patients with these symptoms should perform the test *after using* their antiangina medication (verify that such patients have taken their antiangina medication); rescue nitrate medication should be readily available.

Required Equipment
- Countdown timer (or stopwatch)
- Mechanical lap counter
- Two small orange cones to mark the start and stop points of the patient's walk
- Chairs set up strategically around the walk track for patients to sit in if needed
- Six-Minute Walk Test documentation form on a clipboard
- Source of O_2 with nasal cannula ready for emergency or if patient uses O_2 for activity/walking as prescribed by physician
- Sphygmomanometer
- Stethoscope
- Cutaneous pulse oximeter with finger or forehead probe availability
- Quick-acting β_2-bronchodilator for emergency use

Continued

BOX 12-1 | **Six-Minute Walk Test Policy and Procedure—cont'd**

- Rescue nitroglycerin for chest pain (follow MD direction)
- Aspirin
- Distance marker to determine last lap distance
- Borg Scale, 0-10 points
- Walker with wheels, if indicated

Staff performing the test should know the emergency response routine if the patient falls or experiences cardiac arrest:

- Know the location of the crash cart.
- Have a wheelchair available, to assist the patient if necessary during or after the test.

Patient Preparation

- Comfortable clothing should be worn.
- Appropriate walking shoes should be worn.
- Patients should use their usual walking-assistive devices during the test, as they use at home (e.g., cane or walker).
- Consumption of a light meal is acceptable before the test.
- Patients should not have exercised vigorously within 2 hours of the beginning of the test.
- Each patient's usual medical regimen should be followed the day of the test (e.g., medications, inhalers, breathing treatments).

POLICY

- If the patient arrives without O_2 *but* has it prescribed at a certain liter flow, provide the patient with O_2 according to the doctor's O_2 order.
- If the patient's resting oxygen saturation is greater than or equal to 88% and the patient does *not* use O_2 at home, have the patient perform the 6MWT without supplemental O_2.
- If the patient's resting O_2 saturation is less than 88% on room air, perform the 6MWT while the patient receives continuous O_2 at 2 L/minute via nasal cannula.
- *Wait* 10 minutes after any change in O_2 delivery to start the walk test.
- *Do not* use pulsed O_2 for the 6-Minute Walk Test. (An O_2 prescription walk test will be done to titrate O_2 or to verify adequacy of the pulsed O_2 system the patient is using at home; this is a separate test from the pre/post 6-min walk.)
- *Do not titrate O_2 during the walk test*; leave it at the liter flow prescribed by the referring doctor or at the 2-L/minute flow at which the patient started, as per protocol.
- *Do not walk with the patient or behind them.*
- *No* warming up before the test should be done.
- Only one patient should be undergoing a 6MWT at a time.
- Abnormal results, adverse symptoms, or both, documented on the 6MWT should be faxed/called to the referring physician for advice.

Reasons for Stopping the 6MWT*

- Chest pain
- Intolerable dyspnea, (i.e., Borg Scale score greater than or equal to 7)
- Leg cramps
- Staggering
- Diaphoresis
- Pale or ashen appearance

PROCEDURE

1. Have the patient sit on a chair, located near the starting position of their 6MWT. Complete the first half of the 6MWT documentation worksheet and 0-minute data.
2. Place the pulse oximeter with carrying strap on the patient so that the strap rests on one shoulder and the pulse oximeter is on the opposite side of the patient, above their hip. *Do not* have the patient hold or stabilize the oximeter; make sure the oximeter does not interfere with the patient's stride. Minimize motion artifact.
3. Place the finger probe on the patient, and tell the patient that he or she *does not* have to hold his or her hand upright when walking. If it was initially determined that the patient's circulation is poor, use a forehead probe.
4. Adjust the pulse oximeter to continuous read mode for the entire test.
5. *Do not walk* the track with the patient to note the 3-minute/6-minute data points. Gather the data points as quickly as possible when the patient passes by.
6. Make sure the oximetry readings are stable before recording; note pulse regularity and whether the oximeter signal quality is acceptable.
7. Prepare the clipboard with the 6MWT documentation form and set the lap counter to zero and the timer to 6 minutes. Place one orange cone at the starting point of the walk test. Have the second cone ready to place where the patient stops at the end of the 6MWT.
8. Show the Borg Scale to patients before the test and *explain* its meaning. State that the Borg Scale has no right or wrong answer. Its purpose is to grade their level of shortness of breath. Level 0 represents no breathing difficulty, and at level 10 they are in the emergency department because of their difficulty in breathing. Tell patients you will also use this 0-10 scale to rate their pain level, with 0 indicating no pain and 10 indicating pain sufficient for admittance to the emergency department.
9. When documenting the 3- and 6-minute Borg Scale and pain levels of patients, remind them of their last stated levels.

BOX 12-1	Six-Minute Walk Test Policy and Procedure—cont'd

10. Patient instructions:
    - *The object of this test is to walk as far as possible in 6 minutes. You will walk around the track. Six minutes is a long time to walk. You will be exerting yourself. You may feel out of breath or become exhausted. You are permitted to slow down, to stop, and to rest as necessary. You may use any of the chairs placed around the track to sit and rest if you have to but resume walking as soon as you are able. I will be asking you for your Borg Scale and pain level readings at the 3- and 6-minute marks. I will also be looking at the oximeter to determine your O_2 saturation reading and heart rate. You are not to try to read the oximeter while walking. That is our job. Do not talk to anyone during the test, but tell us if you have any sudden symptoms and when we ask you your Borg Scale and pain levels.*
    - *You will be walking the track as many times as you can. Now I'm going to show you.* (Demonstrate by walking one lap.)
    - *I am going to use this counter to keep track of the number of laps you complete. I will click it each time you return to this starting point. Remember that the object is to walk as far as possible in 6 minutes, but don't run or jog.*

    Note to staff: If all the 0-minute data points have been obtained, from patient, the test can proceed.
    - *Are you ready for the 6-Minute Walk Test?*
11. Position the patient at the starting line. The therapist should also stand near the starting line during the entire test, unless the patient needs help. *Do not walk with the patient.* When telling the patient to *start*, begin the timer and carefully observe the patient as he or she walks, looking for symptoms, gait issues, and so on.
12. The staff performing the test should not talk to anyone during the walk. Use an even tone of voice while expressing the standard phrases of encouragement. Watch the patient. Do not become distracted and lose count of the laps. Each time the patient returns to the starting line, click the lap counter once. Let the participant see you do it; *exaggerate* the click, using body language, like using a stopwatch at a race.
13. What to tell the patient during the test:
    - After the first minute, tell the patient the following (in even tones): *You are doing well. You have 5 minutes to go.*
    - When the timer shows 4 minutes remaining., tell the patient the following: *Keep up the good work. You have 4 minutes to go.*
    - When the timer shows 3 minutes remaining, tell the patient the following: *You are doing well. You are halfway done.*
    - When the timer shows 2 minutes remaining, tell the patient the following: *Keep up the good work. You have only 2 minutes left.*
    - When the timer shows 1 minute remaining, tell the patient the following: *You are doing well. You have only 1 minute to go.*
    - When the timer is 15 seconds from completing, say the following: *In a moment I'm going to tell you to stop. When I do, just stop right where you are and I will come to you.*
    - When the timer rings (or buzzes), say the following: *Stop!*

    Walk over to the patient. Take the wheelchair if the patient looks exhausted. Mark the spot where the patient stopped by placing an orange cone on the floor. Record the 6-minute data.

    Congratulate the patient for making a good effort and offer a drink of water while the patient recovers.

    Do not use other words of encouragement (or body language to speed up the patient).
    - If the patient stops walking during the test and needs a rest, say this: You can sit and rest if you like, then continue walking whenever you feel able.
14. Do not stop the timer. If the patient or therapist stops the walk test before the 6 minutes are up, monitor patient, keep timer going, document length of rest time or stop. Take a wheelchair over for the patient to sit on.
15. Have the patient proceed to the nearest chair. Determine the patient's blood pressure and proceed with recovery data collection.
16. Record the number of laps from the counter and use the distance marker to determine the last lap distance. Record.
17. When the patient has returned to resting parameters and shows no new symptoms, the patient may leave. At this time do the calculation on the 6MWT form.
18. *Enter* the 6MWT date.

DOCUMENTATION FORM
See Figure 12-1.

REFERENCES
American Association of Cardiovascular and Pulmonary Rehabilitation: Guidelines for pulmonary rehabilitation programs, ed 3, Champaign, Ill, 2004, Human Kinetics.
ATS Committee on Proficiency Standards for Clinical Pulmonary Function Laboratories: ATS statement: guidelines for the six-minute walk test, Am J Respir Crit Care Med 166:111-117, 2002.
Enright PL: The six-minute walk test, Respir Care 48:783-785, 2003.

Adapted from the Pulmonary Rehabilitation Program, INOVA Fairfax Hospital (Falls Church, Va.).

Date _____

6 min. walk type:
____ initial
____ discharge
____ maintenance
____ other, _____

Approp. shoes? ____ Y ____ N, _____ **Age:** _____

Bronchodilator last used:
____ Not prescribed
____ Not used today
____ Used, time _____
Name _____

Recent med changes: _____ No _____ Yes
(i.e., prednisone dose, on antibiotics?)

_____

Pre walk symptoms:
____ cough   ____ leg cramps   ____ chest pain
____ sputum   ____ fatigue   ____ chest pressure
____ wheezing ____ other, _____

Orthopedic issues: _____

O_2 walk system: ____ No ____ Yes

Fall risk: ___ N ___ Y,
why _____

Peripheral circulation:
____ good   ____ poor
____ neuropathy
____ gait
____ balance
____ other, _____

____ raynaurds
____ scleraderma
other, _____

O_2 flow type:
_____ liquid
_____ cyclinder

O_2 delivery device:
_____ cannula
_____ oxymizer
_____ non-rereather
_____ Venti mask ___ %
_____ other, _____

_____ cont flow
_____ pulsed

How O_2 transported?
_____ pushed
_____ pulled
_____ carried
_____ staff carried
_____ no O_2 used
_____ other, _____

MMRC dyspnea scale
____ Grade 0
____ Grade 1
____ Grade 2
____ Grade 3
____ Grade 4

Oximeter probe site:
____ finger ____ forehead
____ other, _____

Borg scale 0 no problem – 10 ER	***Pain scale 0 no pain – 10 ER***

0 Min	**3 Min**	**6 Min**	**Post/recovery:**
O_2lpm ____ FIO_2 ____	O_2lpm ____ FIO_2 ____	O_2lpm ____ FIO_2 ____	O_2lpm ____ FIO_2 ____
Spo_2 % ____	Spo_2 % ____	Spo_2 % ____	Spo_2 % ____
HR ____	HR ____	HR ____	HR ____
BORG ____	BORG ____	BORG ____	BORG ____
Pain ____	Pain ____	Pain ____	Pain ____
RR ____		RR ____	RR ____
B/P ____		B/P ____	B/P ____
BS, phase, area: _____			BS, phase, area: _____
#1 Rest time _____	#2 Rest time _____	#3 Rest time _____	= **Total rest time** _____
Ht. _____	Wt. _____	IBW _____	BMI _____

IBW Male lbs = [50 +(2.3 (ht. in inches − 60)] 2.2   **IBW Female lbs** = [45.5 +(2.3 (ht. in inches − 60)] 2.2

Actual total distance (ft.) _____ = _____ laps (114 ft.) + _____ ft.

Predicted distance: _____ ft.   **% predicted:** _____

Men 6MWD reference equations in healthy male adults:
[3,740 ft. − (5.61 × BMI) − (6.94 × age)] − 501 ft. for the lower limit of normal

Women 6MWD reference equations in healthy female adults:
[3,337 ft. − (6.24 × BMI) − (5.83 × age)] − 456 ft. for the lower limit of normal

MPH _____ = {ft. walked (10)} / 5280

METS _____ = [(MPH)(26.83 meters/min)(0.1 ml/kg/min) + 3.5 ml/kg/min] / 3.5ml/kg/min

MMRC _____

BODE index _____   ☐ **Restrictive diag. BODE not applicable**

THR range _____

Check formula used
_____ Standard formula THR =(220 − age) × (70-75%) or other %
_____ Karvonen's formula THR low end = HRR × .70 + RHR
                              THR high end = HRR × .75 + RHR

Calculations:

220 − age = Max Perceived Heart Rate **(MPHR)**
MPHR − resting HR = Heart Rate Reserve **(HRR)**

During walk symptoms:
____ wheezing   ____ fatigue
____ sputum   ____ chest pain
____ cough   ____ chest pressure
____ leg cramps ____ other,

Other comments: _____
_____
_____
_____

Supportive devices used during walk:
____ None   ____ cane
                    ____ walker w/wheels
                    ____ walker no wheels
                    ____ other, _____

Staff signature: _____

_____

FIGURE 12-1 Sample 6-Minute Walk Test documentation flowsheet.

BOX 12-2	Formulas for Calculating Functional Levels from the 6-Minute Walk Test

AVERAGE 6-MINUTE WALK SPEED

Calculating the average walking speed from the 6-Minute Walk Test can provide valuable information about gait and stride limitations when considering a target speed for the exercise program (i.e., free walking, treadmill). Using the average 6-minute walk speed as a beginning target for exercise training may be a comfortable gait speed for the patient. Further increases in work when using the treadmill may be accomplished by adding elevation, speed, or both during the exercise.

$$\text{Speed} = \frac{\text{total distance}}{\text{time}} \times 0.01136$$

where distance is measured in feet. The constant 0.01136 is a conversion factor for turning "feet per minute" into "miles per hour": 60 minutes/hour divided by 5,280 ft/mile = 0.01136.

Example: 863 ft; three rests of 30 seconds each; total walking test time, 6 minutes:

$$\frac{863}{6} = 143.833 \times 0.01136 = 1.63 \, \text{mph}$$

In addition to making a baseline evaluation of a "comfortable speed" for walking on the treadmill, a more important purpose of the 6-Minute Walk Test is its use as a functional evaluation that can be performed at the initiation of rehabilitation and before discharge as an objective outcome measure. Comparing total distance, heart rate, O_2 saturation, and rate of perceived dyspnea can provide a measure of the effectiveness of exercise training on the functional level of the patient.

MET LEVEL CALCULATION

One MET is the level of energy expenditure required at rest, and it has been standardized on the basis of O_2 consumption as 3.5 ml of O_2 per kilogram per minute:

$$\text{METs} = \frac{(\text{mph})(26.83 \, \text{m/min})(0.1 \, \text{ml/kg/min}) + (3.5 \, \text{ml/kg/min})}{3.5 \, \text{ml/kg/min}}$$

Example: If the average 6-minute walk speed is 1.63 mph:

$$\text{METs} = \frac{(1.63 \, \text{mph})(26.83 \, \text{m/min})(0.1 \, \text{ml/kg/min}) + (3.5 \, \text{ml/kg/min})}{3.5 \, \text{ml/kg/min}}$$

In this case METs = 2.25.

Note: MET levels may be used to evaluate the functional expectations of performing various self-care activities in the home. Calculated MET levels provide target work levels of activity for exercise prescription on equipment other than the treadmill (such as bikes and rowers).

MET, *Metabolic equivalent;* O_2, *oxygen.*

summary of other pertinent medical histories allows the therapist to establish a historical background for the rehabilitation patient's present respiratory and functional difficulties, with its impact on daily activities of living. A list of current medications used, and those discontinued and why, is valuable.[22,23] The initial evaluation is essential for developing an individualized treatment plan, establishing realistic goals that involve the patient as the most important member of the team, and justifying the skilled level of intervention by physical therapy or respiratory therapy.

The smoking history, including pack-years of smoking and secondhand smoke exposure, is asked not only to assess the current smoking status and exposure but also to note the presence of smoking in the distant or near past.[24] The therapist should note prior level of function,

medications, and O_2 use and view the information in terms of their musculoskeletal and functional ramifications, as well as their clinical effects. If the patient undergoing pulmonary rehabilitation has been receiving prolonged systemic steroid therapy, he or she is at risk for the development of musculoskeletal complications (e.g., osteoporosis and proximal muscle weakness). The pulmonary rehabilitation history will allow the therapist to evaluate the types of exercises and equipment the patient may already be familiar with and to assess the patient's current exercise habits and capacities.

Assessing the pulmonary rehabilitation participant's psychosocial status and motivation will help the therapist adjust the educational training and treatment approach to a level that is most receptive to the patient. Understanding the family

Pulmonary Rehabilitation Physical Therapy Evaluation

Subjective:

Pulmonary rehabilitation history: 70 yo man with COPD, osteoarthritis, obstructive sleep apnea. S/P AVR (mechanical) 1996. Type II DM, peripheral neuropathy, multiple patellar surgeries both knees. No previous pulmonary therapy. Was previously a member of CFL fitness.

Past medical history:
CA prostate, s/p radiation and medications
Valve replacement AVR 1996
DM (oral meds)
HTN (controlled with meds)
Musculoskeletal pathology knees, OA left hip, bilat. shoulder bursitis/tendonitis

Medications:
Diabetic meds:
Coumadin therapy
See browser for complete list of medications.

Bone density test: Not tested
Pulmonary hygiene: None
Home exercise program:
Household walking
Does very little. States his wife doesn't let him do much.

Prior level of function: Very limited. Air Force retiree.
Equipment: None
Social/family status: Lives in Durham with his wife.
Signs of abuse/neglect:
There were no signs of abuse or neglect noted.

Cough: None
Oxygen use:
At rest: None
With exercise: None
For sleep: None
Pt uses BiPAP during sleep.

Tobacco history: Cigarette smoker quit: 1972
Greatest functional difficulties:
Walking inclines
Stair climbing

Patient goals:
Return to community activities
Resume household chores

Pain: Patient reported pain level since injury/surgery or in the past 4 weeks: Current pain = 2/10, best = 0/10, worst = 10/10, using a number scale.
Location: Bilat. shoulders shaft of humerus. Left hip, right foot
Character: Burning-ache-sharp-throbbing
Duration: Intermittent
Associated symptoms: None

Examination:

Mental status:
Alert and oriented
Motivated

Posture/skin/physical characteristics:
Multiple incisional scars both knees
Bilat. LE peripheral neuropathy R>L.

Edema: Ankles pitting 1+

Breathing pattern:
Diaphragmatic: Fair
Accessory muscle use: Absent
Pursed lips: Good

Auscultation: Clear throughout
Range of motion:
UE limited but functional. Slight shoulder flexion, ER, abduction limitation due to pain.
LE limited but functional. Decreased IR, flexion, adduction left>right hip.
Hamstring length: 60 degrees.

Strength: Impaired in the following areas:
Bilat. UE 3+/5 due to pain with resistance. LLE prox. 3+/5 due to pain. RLE 4/5.

Gait:
Antalgic
Slow

Foot type: Overpronator pt. given shoe list. Large bilat. hallus valgus. Skin looks good. Pt. has pedicure periodically to cut nails.

Special tests:
6-minute walk
Resting vitals:
FIO_2: 0 liters
SpO_2: 99%
HR: 90 bpm
BP: 124/60 mm Hg
Exercise vitals:
FIO_2: 0 liters
SpO_2: 99%
HR: 124 bpm
BP: 140/90 mm Hg
Total distance completed: 1200 feet
DOE: 6/10
Effort: 3/10
Rest breaks required: 0
Assistive device: None, but gait antalgic for right foot and left hip.
Additional comments: Will improve gait with assistive device.

Other:
Today's treatment: Pt. performed with therapist demonstration and supervision: Pt. was instructed in pursed lip breathing, diaphragmatic breathing with verbal and tactile cues.
Orientation session to exercise therapy.

Assessment:

Consult MD about hip pain. Recommend rolling walker or cane for decrease wt. bearing left hip.
Problem list:
Limited ROM
Decreased mobility (transfers, ambulation)
Pain
Decreased strength
Decreased functional level (ADLs, self care)

Precautions:
Hypertension
Musculoskeletal: OA left hip, shoulders, peripheral neuropathy both feet right>left.
Cardiac
Diabetes

FIGURE 12-2 Example of a pulmonary rehabilitation physical therapy evaluation form.

Rehab potential: Good

Goals:

Goal 1: The patient will perform independent diaphragmatic and pursed lip breathing with no verbal or tactile assistance.
Time frame: 2 weeks

Goal 2: The patient will be independent in performing household duties, e.g., cooking, cleaning, bedmaking.
Time frame: 4-6 weeks

Goal 3: The patient will ambulate 20-30 minutes with pain <5/10 in joints using an assistive device.
Time frame: 4-6 weeks

Goal 4: The patient will increase range of motion to shoulders with normal flexion and abduction.
Time frame: 4-6 weeks

Plan: _____

Treatment will include:
Breathing retraining
Progressive ambulation

Strengthening
Stretching
Home exercise program
Footwear education
Monitor blood glucose

Plan of care: Continue PT: 4-5 times per week for 1 month
ICD-9 Diagnosis: 715.09: General osteoarthrosis; 496.:Chr airway obstruct nec
Physician's medicare certification: _____, MD, certifies the reviewed Plan of Care, and PT/OT is necesssary on an outpatient basis, and that services will be furnished while the patient is under my care, and that the plan established is certified from: 11-13-07 through12-13-07.

_____
Therapist

_____
Date

FIGURE 12-2, cont'd Example of a pulmonary rehabilitation physical therapy evaluation form.

dynamics and enlisting the help and cooperation of family members may enhance the benefits of pulmonary rehabilitation and facilitate the formation of more realistic and achievable goals by the therapist, the patient, and the family. The therapist's goal should *always* be to facilitate the participant's individual level of success and a positive attitude about his or her accomplishments in pulmonary rehabilitation.[5]

The therapist's pulmonary assessment should include an evaluation of the breathing pattern. Particular attention to the strength and coordination of the diaphragm muscle is a key component in the evaluation. The use of accessory breathing muscles is prevalent among patients undergoing pulmonary rehabilitation and should be noted (Table 12-2). Patterns of holding the breath and pacing of breathing during movement are important to document. In addition, knowledge of and proficiency in using pursed lips breathing are observed.[20,25-29]

At the same time as the breathing pattern is being assessed, the therapist may observe chest mobility. Over time, postural abnormalities are inevitable in patients with chronic pulmonary disease. Lung hyperinflation leads to rib cage enlargement or "barrel chest" and diaphragmatic flattening. Joint mobility at the rib attachments to the sternum and vertebrae becomes limited, with a loss in overall rib cage mobility during respiration. In the patient with restrictive lung disease, fibrosis leads to an inability to adequately expand the lungs, causing abnormal breathing patterns with shortness of breath.

While the therapist is observing the breathing pattern and chest mobility, it is also appropriate to observe other abnormalities such as rib retractions, clubbing of the digits (Figure 12-4), and skin variations such as rashes or calluses over the elbows or feet. Upper extremity and trunk observations are best performed with the patient's upper body clothing removed.

Prolonged steroid use may result in Cushing's syndrome (e.g., muscle atrophy, redistribution of fat from the extremities to the face and trunk), extensive bruising, and skin tears. Other adverse effects the therapist should be aware of with long-term steroid use include the development of osteoporosis, diabetes, behavioral changes, peptic ulcers, and glaucoma.[22,23]

Assessing the patient's cough history and mechanics as well as auscultating the chest may indicate the need for pulmonary hygiene. Auscultation of the chest allows the quality of air movement within the lungs to be assessed. Listening with a stethoscope over the full area of the thorax overlying the lung tissue while the patient breathes in deeply with an open mouth will provide a full inspiratory and expiratory breath sound assessment. Wheezes indicating bronchoconstriction or airway collapse, and crackles, indicating excessive mucus and inflammation in the

Pulmonary Rehabilitation Assessment–6 Min. Walk

Date: _____ Start time: _____ End time: _____   Total time: _____ Staff Sig.: _____

Referral diagnosis: _____
What lung disease do you understand you have?
_____

Chief complaint: _____
Duration of onset of pulm symptoms: ___ yr(s) ___ mo(s)
Referring pulm. MD: _____
    Primary MD: _____
Medical history: Age: _____
No Yes   TB exposure N Y TB skin test, when _____
           Skin test results: Neg. Post., Tx done _____
           _____
No Yes   Cardiac problems: what _____
No Yes   Hypertension
No Yes   Diabetes, meds? _____ onset _____
No Yes   Gastrointestinal problems
           _____ reflux
           _____ hiatal hernia
No Yes   Osteoporosis
No Yes   Orthopedic problems: _____
No Yes   Hx of falls?: When/how treated?
No Yes   Sinus problems / Postnasal drip (circle)
No Yes   Allergies / Rhinitis (circle)
No Yes   Psychiatric disorder, specify _____
No Yes   Hx of ATOH or substance abuse, not smoking
No Yes   Diag or tx of mood or anxiety disorder
No Yes   Lung related childhood illnesses:
           List: _____
_____   Other _____

Do you have a DMV placard? Y N   **Qualify?** N Y

Symptoms:
N Y Cough, freq _____
N Y Sputum, color _____vol. _____
              consistency _____ freq _____
N Y Wheeze, onset/cause _____
N Y Fluid retention, where _____
              when _____
N Y Dyspnea, onset/cause _____
N Y Sleeping problems, # hrs/night _____
N Y Extra pillows # _____
N Y Pain, location _____ level _____ (0-10)
              Cause _____
Vaccines: flu _____ (yr), pneumonia ____ (yr)
____ Warning signal, infection prevention training

Smoking history: N Y quit date _____
____ packs × ____ years = ____ pack years

Second hand smoke: N Y, who _____

BIPAP/CPAP: N Y vendor_____
cm H$_2$O _____   O$_2$ N Y   lpm _____
sleep study? _____ device (pillows, mask) _____

MMRC Dyspnea index: (Circle one)
0 - not troubled with breathlessness except with strenuous
    exercise
1 - troubled by shortness of breath when hurrying on the
    level or walking up a slight hill
2 - walks slower than people of the same age on the level
    because of breathlessness or has to stop for breath
    when walking at own pace on the level
3 - stops for breath after walking about 100 yards or after
    a few minutes on the level
4 - too breathless to leave the house or breathless when
    dressing or undressing

Allergies:
Food: _____ Meds: _____ Other: _____

Occupation:
Retirement/disability date: _____

Occupational exposures:
____ farm/ranch ____pottery ____welding ____gas/fumes
____ chemicals ____ sand blasting ____dust ____quarry
____ asbestos ____ mines/foundry

Variables affecting learning: N Y vision, ____ glasses
____ other: _____ **N Y** hearing aid **N Y** language _____
N Y ethnic/cultural diver. _____
              other: _____

Respiratory infections past year:
___ infections/year, antibiotic use: _____
_____

Hospitalizations past year:
___ admissions/past yr (hosp/ER etc.) when _____
why _____ problem _____
Stress management:
stressors: _____
relaxation techniques? _____

Aerosol therapy: N Y hand held nebulizer
vendor: _____ medications: _____
freq prescribed vs. use: _____/_____

Breathing retraining:
____ Patient uses accessory muscles
              ____ Pursed lip breathing training
              ____ Diaphragm breathing training

Oxygen therapy: N Y vendor _____
Stationary system: _____ liq. _____ conc.
              ____ cyclinders, what _____
Portable system: __ pulsedose __ liq. __cyclinder __other__
l/m ordered: rest _____ ex. _____ sleep _____
l/m used: rest _____ ex. _____ sleep _____

FIGURE 12-3 Example of a pulmonary rehabilitation respiratory therapy evaluation form.

Inhaler/diskus:

#1 ordered _____

Freq. used _____

#2 ordered _____

Freq. used _____

#3 ordered _____

Freq. used _____

_____ Diskus/inhaler use training

uses holding chamber	N Y	needs training	Y N
uses peak flow	N Y	needs training	Y N
uses acapella valve	N Y	needs training	Y N

Current functional activity level:

Issues: _____

Difficulty with ADL's (showering, etc.) Y   N   What: _____

Patient's functional goals: _____   _____

Fluid intake: (# glasses/day)

_____ water _____ coffee _____ soda _____ tea _____ milk

_____ juice _____ beer _____ wine _____ hard liquor

Nutrition: appetite ____ good ____ poor ____ other, _____

special diet N Y, _____ salt use N Y, _____

multi vit. use N Y, _____ other issues: _____

Oral medications: see medication sheet

Stairs at home: N Y, # stairs vs flights _____

Objective: (See timed distance walk test for additional objective data BS, BP, BORG, etc.)

N Y, edema where: ___ pedal ___ ankle ___ pre-tibial ____   N Y clubbing   N Y cyanosis: Where _____

Spirometry: Date done: _____

FVC_1 pre/post % Pred. _____

FEV_1 Pre/post % Pred. _____

FEF_{25-75} 1./sec. pre/post % Pred. _____

Lung volume: Date done: _____

TLC % Pred. _____ RV % Pred. _____

Chest X-ray: Date done: _____

Result _____

D_{LCO}: Date done: _____ % Pred. _____

Timed distance walk test: See attached documentation form

Assessment:

1. _____   4. _____

2. _____   5. _____

3. _____   6. _____

Plan:

1. follow through with MD pulm. rehab. orders   6. _____

2. _____   7. _____

3. _____   8. _____

4. _____   9. _____

5. _____   10. _____

Staff sig.: _____

FIGURE 12-3, cont'd Example of a pulmonary rehabilitation respiratory therapy evaluation form.

airways, are the typical abnormal breath sounds that will be noted on auscultation. Crackles may also be present in fibrotic changes in lung tissue. Fluid in the lungs, common in congestive heart failure, will also be heard as high-pitched wheezes or high-pitched crackles. Normal, clear aeration in all lung fields will rarely be found in the patient being evaluated for pulmonary rehabilitation but may be the case with patients with chest wall deformities or primary pulmonary hypertension.

Distant and decreased but clear breath sounds of the hyperinflated lung tissue of the patient with emphysema is common, as are Velcro-like lung sounds in the patient with fibrosis.

Auscultation of wheezes and crackles, when considered together with a history of symptoms that include a chronic cough with sputum production, is a clear indication for an intensive bronchial hygiene regimen, which may include postural drainage therapy, directed cough, and positive airway

TABLE 12-2	Muscles of Respiration	
	Inspiration	**Expiration**
Normal	Diaphragm	Passive process (relaxation of the diaphragm and external intercostals)
	External intercostals	
Accessory	Sternocleidomastoid	Internal intercostals
	Scalenes	Abdominal muscles
	Serratus anterior	Rectus abdominis
	Pectoralis major	Obliquus externus abdominis
	Pectoralis minor	Transversus abdominis
	Trapezius (upper, middle, lower)	
	Erector spinae	

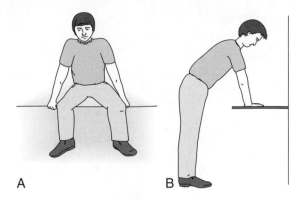

FIGURE 12-5 Postures that assist inspiratory efforts of patients with pulmonary disease.

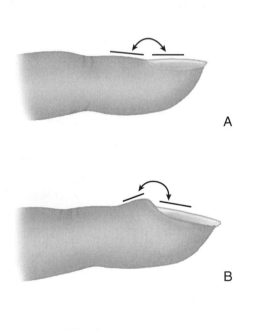

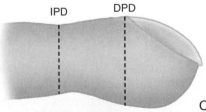

FIGURE 12-4 Digital clubbing. **A,** Normal digit configuration. **B,** Mild digital clubbing with increased hyponychial angle. **C,** Severe digital clubbing; with clubbing the depth of the finger at the base of nail (distal phalangeal depth [DPD]) is greater than the depth of the interphalangeal depth (IPD).

pressure adjuncts. Excessive wheezing on inspiration and expiration may indicate an ineffective bronchodilator prescription.

The musculoskeletal and functional assessment should begin with a gross manual muscle test of the upper and lower extremities and trunk. The ROM and flexibility evaluation must target key areas such as the shoulders, cervical spine, hamstrings, and gastrocnemius muscle. The cervical spine and shoulders lose ROM as a result of poor posture and accessory muscle use. The lower extremity musculature typically loses ROM because of disuse.

Poor posture and pulmonary disease frequently develop simultaneously. The loss of chest wall mobility, the assumption of propping postures (e.g., professorial position) (Figure 12-5), and the use of accessory breathing muscles in the cervical and shoulder girdle may lead to abnormal upper body postures. Scoliosis and kyphotic postures are associated with restrictive lung diseases.

All patients undergoing pulmonary rehabilitation should be questioned about pain. Fortunately, pulmonary diseases usually are not associated with pain; however, most patients will describe pain from other sources. The older age group diagnosed with chronic pulmonary disease often experiences pain from musculoskeletal causes (e.g., osteoarthritis of the cervical and lumbosacral spine, knees, hips, and shoulders). Those who have used systemic corticosteroids for prolonged periods and in higher doses may experience pain from vertebral compression fractures.

A key functional element for all patients with pulmonary disease is the ability to walk. The therapy assessment must identify any gait abnormalities and their origin (e.g., musculoskeletal, neurologic, or deconditioning). Several ambulatory assistive devices are now available to help patients with pulmonary disease reinitiate ambulation or raise their ambulatory training to a higher functional level.

Reviewing the objective PT and RT evaluation results will identify problems to be addressed during the rehabilitation program. Short- and long-term goals should be patient centered, realistic, and measurable. The treatment plan must be individualized and based on all objective test data and observations.

Assessment of dyspnea,[30] cough, sputum, wheezes, edema, fatigue, hemoptysis, postnasal drainage, heart burn, chest pain, swallowing problems, and nocturnal breathing difficulties can be accomplished with simple yes or no questions and asking for explanations of the onset, frequency, and impact these problems have on the patient's daily life. Classification of dyspnea (i.e., Borg Scale) is important documentation that provides quick, "at a glance" information to rate the degree of disability that the patient encounters on a routine basis.[30] Dependent edema with a history of heart disease is an important sign that may indicate the presence of pulmonary congestion and the need for diuretics.

Patient Medical History from Referring Physician

The therapist will find certain information from the physician helpful in planning an individualized pulmonary rehabilitation program. The medical history is invaluable in gathering information about the patient's pulmonary and nonpulmonary diagnoses. In addition to the medical history, a list of medications will allow the therapist to form ideas and questions to ask during the evaluation. Having a complete and current medical history and a medication list from the physician can save a significant amount of time during the rehabilitation interview.

The physician's interpretation of diagnostic tests is beneficial in making plans regarding O_2 needs, medication training, and determination of the patient's status in the course of his or her disease (e.g., mild, moderate, or severe pulmonary disease). The physician may suggest additional diagnostic tests other than the standard tests that are done before beginning the rehabilitation program. Some diagnostic tests may clarify cardiac-like symptoms, whereas others may warrant adjustments in medication dosages.

The physician's recommended precautions are worthwhile to the therapist. No one wants to overlook a potentially harmful medication, concomitant disease, allergic reaction, or activity restriction and place the patient at risk for injury or exacerbation.

The physician's plan should consider all potential medication alterations, additional diagnostics, outside referrals, and medical options available to improve that patient's disease management. As a primary player on the rehabilitation team, the therapist looks to the physician for input based on his or her medical expertise and experience in the treatment of patients with pulmonary disease at all levels of the disease process. With this information, the therapist can begin to form ideas and plans about the type of program that will be most appropriate for the participant.

EVALUATION PARAMETERS UNIQUE TO THE SURGICAL PULMONARY REHABILITATION PATIENT

Rehabilitating the pulmonary patient undergoing a surgical intervention can be challenging and exciting. Although many of the rehabilitation principles are the same for medical and surgical pulmonary rehabilitation, unique considerations exist for surgical rehabilitation.

Preoperative Goals

Fortunately, most patients with pulmonary disease who require surgical intervention are not hospitalized before surgery. Consequently, this time is a window of opportunity to participate in pulmonary rehabilitation. The therapist must not expect significant central cardiopulmonary changes (i.e., heart and lung physiologic conditioning) in the patient's functional abilities; however, peripheral adaptations are common in this population.[18] Preoperative goals for the pulmonary rehabilitation participant include the following:

- Maximize function: This includes walking (with or without an assistive device) and the ability to move comfortably.
- Reduce all musculoskeletal impairments and function: Work with the patient to improve muscle strength, flexibility, and posture.
- Improve the ability to perform the activities of daily living: This includes such things as bathing, shaving, dressing, cooking, and cleaning.

- Decrease sensitization to dyspnea: Help the patient identify the causes of dyspnea and begin to exert greater self-control.
- Improve breathing and cough techniques: Teach breathing retraining, chest physical therapy, and cough techniques.
- Improve activity endurance: Increase the participant's ability for *sustained* activity while performing aerobic activities such as walking, bicycling, or arm ergometry.
- Optimize medication use: Review all medications and check for accurate use.
- Educate: Instruct the patient and family about their pulmonary disease and review lifestyle changes that may occur after surgery.
- Provide psychosocial support: Pulmonary rehabilitation offers a support network for participants and family members who have similar diagnoses and are facing similar life events.[31]

Incisions

Therapists must be familiar with the surgical procedures used in lung transplantation and lung volume reduction surgery (LVRS).[32] Three types of incisions are commonly used for lung transplantation. For single-lung transplantation, a unilateral thoracotomy is preferred. The incision is posterolateral, cutting between the fourth and fifth intercostal spaces. On occasion, a portion of rib is resected to allow for better access to the lung. The latissimus dorsi, lower trapezius, intercostals, rhomboids, and serratus anterior muscles are incised, allowing for greater access to remove and replace the lung.[20,33]

For double-lung transplantation, the surgeon may use a clamshell incision. This is a horizontal incision above the level of the diaphragm. The pectoralis major and pectoralis minor muscles are incised. On occasion, the surgeon may choose to use bilateral posterolateral thoracotomies for a double-lung transplant. This procedure is usually by surgeon preference or occurs when the viability of both donor lungs is not known simultaneously.

Two types of incisions may be used for LVRS. The median sternotomy is a vertical incision along the sternal midline from the sternal notch distally below the xiphoid process. No muscles are incised and the sternum is closed with stainless steel staples or sutures. A thoracoscopic procedure may be used for LVRS or lung tumor resection. Two or three small incisions are made to allow for the insertion of a thoracoscope. Using the thoracoscope, the surgeon has the ability to visualize and resect lung tissue.[31,33-35]

Inpatient Postoperative Goals

Within 12 to 24 hours of surgery, the therapist should begin acute postoperative treatment. The treatment plan and goals of this period are as follows:

- Aggressive pulmonary hygiene therapy: Postural drainage therapy is necessary to mobilize secretions; it is important to consider that in certain surgical cases, the lung is denervated and the patient may not be able to sense secretions that have moved cephaloid.
- Review breathing and directed cough techniques: In this patient population, the therapist must think of breathing retraining in a different way. The therapist is actually retraining the diaphragm muscle, which now has a more normal environment in which to work; in the same sense, the rib cage and chest wall may now assume a more typical configuration. These changes, of course, do not happen quickly, but normal patterns of breathing and movement must be encouraged and taught at this early stage.
- Maintain joint range of motion (ROM) and muscle strength: The patient will be reluctant to move voluntarily; the upper extremities and chest will be painful and stiff, but progressive ROM and movement must be encouraged while the patient is adequately medicated for pain.
- Initiate self-care and activities of daily living: Bed mobility, supine to sit, and sit to stand activities will allow the patient to begin bathing and dressing tasks.
- Progressive ambulation and cardiopulmonary conditioning: Ambulation within the room or in the hall with or without an assistive device is an essential element of early postoperative rehabilitation. In some cases, a treadmill or stationary bicycle may be moved into the patient's room to facilitate cardiopulmonary endurance training. Cardiopulmonary parameters to monitor while conditioning the patient include Sao_2 and the use of supplemental O_2, heart rate, blood pressure, respiratory rate, and the rate of perceived exertion.

Exercise Limitations After Surgery

After lung transplantation or LVRS, the patient should not lift more than 5 to 10 1b with the upper extremities for 6 to 8 weeks. Other upper body activities to avoid for the same period are trunk twisting, trunk bending, abdominal curl-ups, and arm ergometry. Swim strokes should be avoided for 3 months after surgery. The patient can usually resume driving after 6 weeks, or earlier with their physician's approval.

Outpatient Postoperative Goals

When patients are ready to leave the hospital, the pulmonary rehabilitation program must adopt a different set of objectives in the rehabilitative process. Many patients describe this period as both exhilarating and frustrating. For the first time in a long while, they can breathe without a struggle. Breathing is not the primary focus of every movement; however, their bodies cannot keep up with the level at which their lungs can perform, and nagging musculoskeletal aches and pains in the lower extremities may hamper them. Thus the challenge for the pulmonary rehabilitation specialist is to gradually teach and guide the patient through an activity program that will achieve his or her highest functional level. The postoperative outpatient objectives are as follows:

- To decrease incisional pain: Moist heat, ice, positioning, or transcutaneous electrical nerve stimulation may be used for postoperative incisional pain control.
- To increase strength and mobility: The level of postoperative strength depends on the preoperative strength and the length of hospitalization; mobility is highly influenced by pain and pain control.
- To achieve good breathing and cough techniques: This is a continuation of the training that was initiated before surgery.
- To improve stamina: The body must be trained to match the work that the lungs can now perform.
- To adjust and titrate O_2: Postoperatively, some patients who underwent LVRS and lung transplantation may continue to require O_2. As the lungs and the body recuperate, the need for supplemental oxygen may be titrated down or possibly eliminated in certain patients; it is an unrealistic expectation to assume that all postsurgical patients with disease will no longer require supplemental oxygen either at rest or with exercise.
- To assist with adjustments to a new and different lifestyle: It is important for the therapist to understand and help the patient adjust to potential changes in family dynamics, relationships with friends, and societal demands (e.g., return to work, a switch from disabled to "normal"). The patient should be encouraged to adopt a healthy lifestyle that includes a smoke-free environment, regular exercise, and compliance with medication and nutritional regimens.[31,34]

Infection Control

With a postoperative lung transplantation population in the rehabilitation program, special consideration must be given to infection control. Simple steps are usually most effective at keeping the spread of bacteria under control. Probably the most effective way to maintain good infection control is by regular hand washing by all the patients and staff. Many excellent antibacterial soaps are available, and, when needed, the waterless antibacterial soaps are adequate until water is available. Maintaining a 3-ft distance from someone who has an upper respiratory tract infection is advised, especially when coughing is present. Patients should be reminded to cover their nose and mouth when they cough or sneeze.

Making clean linens accessible to all staff and participants is prudent. Equipment used by patients with known infections must be isolated and cleaned with an antibacterial solution before other participants use those same pieces of equipment. Examples of types of equipment that may be isolated include oximeters, dumbbells, cuff weights, Thera-Bands, timers, exercise mats, stationary bicycles, and others. Masks, gloves, and gowns are occasionally used depending on the circumstances.[31]

Organ Rejection Detection

Pulmonary rehabilitation program staff are excellent resources for recognizing early signs of organ rejection. All staff members must be knowledgeable about these warning signs and be able to distinguish between general complaints of fatigue, soreness, and actual troublesome indicators. A decrease in the forced expiratory volume in 1 second, shortness of breath, lower Sao_2 levels, and fever may be early signs of rejection that can be identified by the pulmonary rehabilitation staff.[31]

PLANNING AN INDIVIDUALIZED PULMONARY REHABILITATION PROGRAM

The team approach to pulmonary rehabilitation brings the expertise of many clinical disciplines to work toward the effective treatment of the whole patient. Understanding the multiple needs of the patient justifies the skills of each discipline. As patients progress through the diagnostic testing, team evaluation, education training, and therapy sessions, their individual needs are identified and addressed. Each patient will receive an accurate diagnosis from the physician. The most appropriate medications to treat his or her condition will be ordered. The patient should be prescribed the medical regimen that is best suited for that condition to address the primary respiratory diagnosis and any comorbid conditions. The patient will receive instruction in the proper use of all medications, including respiratory care interventions of aerosols, bronchial hygiene, and oxygenation to optimize respiratory function. Physical therapy assessments for addressing musculoskeletal and neuromuscular efficiency will be performed to develop exercises aimed at improving strength and endurance for enhancing physical function.[36] Occupational therapy involvement dovetails with physical and respiratory therapy to identify the limited strength, breathing impairments, or anxiety/panic that impacts the routine daily tasks for household and personal care needs. Nutritional services address the individual dietary and weight management issues that can have a significant effect on breathing. Counseling services are justified on an individual or group basis to deal with psychosocial issues involving the patient and family and to assist in long-term coping and end-of-life decisions. Often, home medical equipment and pharmacy personnel are consulted to assist in providing the best equipment or prescription recommendations for a particular patient's needs.

These services all provide patients with the well-rounded instruction and training for developing a balanced lifestyle that will help them optimize their lung health and enable them to manage the symptoms of their disease, participate in social activities, and cope with the day-to-day goal of living life to the fullest within the limitations of their condition.

Oxygen

The indications for O_2 therapy in the treatment of hypoxemia are critical to understand. Hypoxemia is a low blood oxygen level and results in constriction of the pulmonary capillary bed, increased pulmonary artery pressure, right-sided heart failure, cardiac arrhythmia, and eventually death. Hypoxemia also results in impaired cognitive function owing to lack of sufficient oxygen to the brain. Correcting hypoxemia with supplemental O_2 is essential to avoid these untoward effects. Pao_2 less than 55 mm Hg or Sao_2 less than 88% is the indication for supplemental oxygen by Medicare and most insurance carriers. Monitoring Spo_2 (oxygen saturation as determined by pulse oximetry) during exercise, sleep, and rest is effective in assessing the patient's needs for specific oxygen prescription flow rates during these activities. Estimating Pao_2 at altitude, using nomograms for "educated guesses," or performing a high-altitude simulation test is beneficial in modifying the O_2 prescription for airline flight (estimated at an altitude of 5000 to 8000 ft) or when patients visit or vacation at mountain elevations.

A complete O_2 prescription provides the patient with directives for use with rest, exercise, and sleep. It states the O_2 system the patient needs, continuous or intermittent flow, and the delivery device required. Some patients who are hypoxemic (Pao_2 < 55 mm Hg) at rest will require O_2 continuously. They may need adjustments to increase the liter flow for exercise and to decrease the flow rate during sleep to maintain Spo_2 greater than 90%. Getting the best home oxygen stationary and portable system to meet the patient's needs can be a difficult endeavor in light of the current cutbacks in reimbursement for home oxygen by Medicare. Clinically, the best system for the patient will be one that maintains Sao_2 above 90% during all phases of daily life and allows mobility, and can be operated by the patient with the least amount of manual dexterity and fear.

Evaluating the patient's ability to ambulate with the type of portable system supplied is important. Some considerations include the weight of the tank, and the ability of the patient to maneuver carts, carry shoulder bags, and transfill the tank. Choice of a continuous flow or O_2-conserving device, whichever best meets the patient's needs, is required during the evaluation.

The O_2-conserving device offers the potential to carry O_2 in a small-capacity reservoir and provides a longer duration of use for each tank. During exercise or other activities requiring increased ventilatory needs, O_2-conserving devices may not meet the oxygenation demands of the patient. Testing the system prescribed during ambulation and with exercise may require adjustments in the liter flow to maintain SpO_2 greater than 90%. This is an important assessment that must be done to document the ability of the O_2 system to meet the patient's needs.

Some patients may require high-flow oxygen at rest or with exercise sessions to maintain adequate oxygenation. Using the lowest fraction of inspired oxygen (FIO_2) to maintain the SpO_2 greater than 90% is the best method of titrating O_2 to the patient's needs. Patients with pulmonary fibrosis or pulmonary hypertension may even require high-flow oxygen through a nonrebreather mask delivering up to 100% pure oxygen to overcome the gas exchange impairments in their lungs.[37] Creative use of oxygen delivery equipment may be needed to meet a patient's inspiratory FIO_2 needs. The goal is always adequate oxygenation to keep the patient safe.

Designing the Exercise Program

Evidence indicates that the individual with chronic obstructive pulmonary disease (COPD) may have changes in the pathophysiology of peripheral muscles. Compared with age-matched healthy people, the patient with COPD has 70% to 80% less muscle strength. Patients also have been found to have a greater number of less efficient type IIB (fast twitch) muscle fibers.[38,39]

These peripheral changes may contribute to a disease-related myopathy represented by a lack of mechanical efficiency, early muscle fatigue, and poor exercise stamina.

Other physiologic principles that should be considered when designing the exercise training program include the following:

- For a given workload, upper extremity work demands more energy than lower extremity work and is accompanied by a higher ventilatory demand.[9]
- Upper body training is more likely to exacerbate breath holding, an asynchronous breathing pattern, and shortness of breath.[36,40,41]
- Exercise benefits are muscle and task specific: Strength and endurance gains cannot be expected

in one muscle group (e.g., upper extremities) from training activities performed by a separate muscle group (e.g., lower extremities).[9,42]

These principles are the foundation for pulmonary rehabilitation exercise training and their implementation will ensure a sound and evidence-based program of exercise training.[9-11,41]

There are three basic components to exercise training with pulmonary rehabilitation patients: Strength training, flexibility and stretching, and endurance training. Each of these components is discussed separately.

Strength Training

Strength training programs for pulmonary rehabilitation programs are most effective when they are simple, practical, and widely applicable. Increasing strength and local muscle endurance improves the pulmonary patient's ability to perform functional activities, decreases local muscle fatigue, and enhances body image.[9,43,44] Each strength training regimen must be individually prescribed on the basis of the initial physical therapy evaluation. Using the objective findings of diagnosis, medical history, muscle strength, and joint ROM, a safe and successful strength training program may be initiated with essentially all pulmonary rehabilitation participants. In general, these programs are received enthusiastically by most individuals.

Many patients with pulmonary disease describe disabling dyspnea with upper extremity activity. Consequently, self-care activities such as bathing, dressing, shaving, hair grooming, and household chores such as lifting pots and pans, lifting clothes from the washer and dryer, and preparing food, become exhausting tasks that are dreaded. Several clinical studies have demonstrated that patients with pulmonary disease can train successfully with upper body resistive work, which promotes improved respiratory muscle function, less fatigue, and less dyspnea.[44-46]

Dumbbells, cuff weights, Thera-Bands, and weight machines may be used for strength training. The program for upper and lower extremities should begin with light weights and advance first by increasing repetitions. This method of progression facilitates the experience of almost immediate success. It also allows the muscles to adapt gradually to the additional demand while avoiding soreness and injury.

A strength program that begins with weights that feel "challenging but not easy or too difficult" is readily accepted by the patient. Repetitions begin with one set of 10 and progress to one set of 20 repetitions. Once the patient is able to perform 20 repetitions while using the guideline of being challenging on two separate days, the weight is increased by small increments (1 to 5 lb) and the repetitions are dropped back to one set of 10. The same progression pattern is used to gradually increase the repetitions and weight for all muscle groups. As an upper limit, the patient should not exceed his or her body weight on any strength training machine. If muscle or joint pain is experienced with strength training, the weight is initially dropped. Conservative treatment of the pain is initiated, which may include ice, moist heat, rest, splinting for joint support, elevation, or transcutaneous electrical nerve stimulation. If the pain continues, that particular strengthening exercise is discontinued until the pain and/or inflammation subsides.

Simple strengthening exercises using one's body weight may also be used effectively in a pulmonary rehabilitation program. Examples of these include stair climbing, toe raises, squats, and lunge steps. Exercises to challenge and improve balance and coordination may be used without additional equipment. Examples of balance exercises include standing hip rotation in clockwise and counterclockwise directions; standing unilateral hip hiking; standing unilateral toe pointing to the front, side, and back; and quadruped arm and leg extension.

Flexibility and Stretching

Most patients with chronic pulmonary disease have reduced joint and muscle flexibility caused primarily by inactivity and postural changes. Stretching exercises should be included in all pulmonary rehabilitation activity programs to increase joint ROM, improve muscle flexibility, discourage injuries, improve posture, and decrease stiffness.[9,10] In the pulmonary rehabilitation population, specific areas of the body require attention. As a result of prolonged postural abnormalities, the cervical, thoracic, and lumbar spines; shoulders; and rib cage typically present with limited ROM. In the lower extremities, the hamstring and gastrocnemius muscles are often limited in ROM.

These muscles may be stretched in many different ways, but the most effective position for stretching these areas is supine. To assume the supine position, the therapist must instruct the patient in how to get up from and down to the floor, especially when stretching classes are taught in a group setting. Even though this activity may be difficult for the patient who is stiff and deconditioned, it is an extremely beneficial, functional, and important task to master. The only patients who should be excluded from learning this activity are those with severe osteoarthritis of the knees, or other musculoskeletal abnormalities that the therapist has determined would absolutely prohibit this task. Osteoporosis, shortness of breath, and O_2 use are *not* contraindications for learning standing-to-floor/supine activity.

Other simple pieces of equipment may be used for stretching. An "over the door" pulley system is frequently used for shoulder and rib cage stretching. Pulleys are particularly effective for postoperative chest incision stretching. Wand exercises with a dowel that is approximately 3 ft long may also be used for shoulder and rib cage mobility. An incline board easily accomplishes bilateral stretching of the gastrocnemius and soleus muscles and the Achilles tendons. The stretches should be held continuously for 20 to 30 seconds for 3 to 5 repetitions.

Endurance Training

Substantial evidence shows that lower extremity exercise training has both physiologic and psychological benefit for patients with pulmonary disease.[9,10] The exercise prescription for lower extremity endurance training may be based on the initial graded exercise test, using an initial intensity of 50% of the maximal workload for most rehabilitation participants. Examples of the equipment used for lower extremity endurance training include upright fixed handlebar stationary bicycles, recumbent bicycles, a recumbent stair stepper, and an upright reciprocal moving handlebar bicycle.

Upper extremity endurance training has been found to improve arm function in patients with pulmonary disease.[9,10] An upright reciprocal moving handlebar bicycle using the arms only, upper body ergometers, a recumbent stair stepper using the arms only, and continuous rhythmic arm movements with or without a wand are examples of upper extremity endurance exercise modalities. An initial workload of 25% of the maximal workload achieved on the exercise test is recommended for upper extremity endurance training. Patients with osteoporosis should avoid arm ergometry because of an increased risk of "wear and tear" on the thoracic vertebrae.[47,48]

Ambulation is a necessary mode of training for patients with pulmonary disease because it is the basis of locomotion and is involved in many activities of daily living.[17,18,42] Modes of ambulation may include level-surface walking with or without an assistive device and treadmill ambulation. The importance of level surface walking must not be ignored in the population with pulmonary disease. Ambulation training on level surfaces must include rolling or carrying one's own portable O_2 system if needed, propelling one's body over a surface, and supporting the body weight. Although the treadmill simulates these conditions, the total energy expenditure is measurably less. Consequently, it is important that all pulmonary rehabilitation programs include level-surface walking as part of the exercise protocol.

Pulmonary patients with mild or moderate disease may have the ability to expand their exercise regimen by using other types of equipment. Stair steppers, rowing machines, cross-country machines, and swimming offer a strenuous challenge to those patients who require a higher intensity of endurance training.

Paced Breathing with Exercise

With all forms of exercise, the patient with pulmonary disease must be instructed in a paced breathing pattern. The patient should be instructed to inspire at rest and exhale during the more difficult phase of the exercise. The most effective breathing pattern encourages inhalation through the nose and exhalation through pursed lips. If the patient has difficulty and becomes anxious by an inability to accomplish this pattern of breathing, the therapist may instruct the patient to "simply pace the breathing with a comfortable pattern of inhalation and exhalation while performing exercise." All patients should be strongly encouraged *never to hold their breath* with activity. Breath holding is a common response of pulmonary patients to strenuous movement; however, this action only intensifies dyspnea, O_2 hunger, and physical distress.

Patient Training

They may forget what you said, but they will never forget how you made them feel.

Carl W. Buehner

Patient education takes patience. Lecturing that simply presents information "at" program participants is not teaching. Education implies that a person is learning and is involved in the process of assimilating the information presented.

In pulmonary rehabilitation, all members of the team must constantly maintain their role as health educators during therapy sessions as they interact with patients and family members. Whether in a formal lecture setting in a classroom or while coaching a patient through a series of upper extremity exercises in the gym, team members should always be looking for the "teachable moment" when the pupil is ready to learn.

Many different situations can be created that will facilitate learning. Simply giving patients and family members a booklet or brochure about the management of their disease will be ineffective. Education involves the presenting of information so that it can be retained, and it should also focus on *training* in skills that are essential to self-care and management of the disease. Box 12-3 provides common topics addressed in education and training sessions in pulmonary rehabilitation.[9]

Improved retention of and adherence to an established treatment plan constitute the goal of all educational and exercise training methods used in pulmonary rehabilitation. Training to improve adherence can be accomplished by providing patients and family members with only the essential information required to understand the need for performing these skills. Obtaining feedback on barriers in their day-to-day life that may prevent them from performing the prescribed treatments is important. Counseling the patient

---

BOX 12-3 Common Educational Topics in Pulmonary Rehabilitation

- Anatomy and physiology of the lung
- Pathophysiology of lung disease
- Airway management
- Breathing retraining strategies
- Energy conservation and work simplification techniques
- Medications
- Self-management skills
- Benefits of exercise and safety guidelines
- Exercise modifications
- Oxygen therapy
- Environmental irritant avoidance
- Respiratory and chest therapy techniques
- Symptom management
- Psychological factors: Coping, anxiety, depression, panic control
- Stress management
- End-of-life planning
- Smoking cessation
- Travel/leisure/sexuality
- Nutrition

and family to develop practical solutions to overcome these barriers will promote adherence to prescribed therapy. Asking group participants who have mastered a skill to share their expertise with a fellow member of the group will promote peer motivation and is a teaching method resulting in the greatest learning and retention.

Setting Practical Goals and Facilitating Achievement

The SMART acronym is a good tool for developing individual patient goals. Goals that are *s*pecific, *me*asurable, *a*ppropriate, *r*ealistic, and *t*imely (SMART) will enable the team members to help patients accomplish effective progress in an efficient manner. Performance of a specific task or skill with decreasing need for tactile or verbal cues is a typical manner in which goals are stated and progress is measured. The skill should be one that is reasonable and medically necessary and appropriate to the patient's condition. Taking into consideration the patient's level of function will help in developing goals that are attainable and realistic and can be achieved in a time span that is likely to demonstrate progress. The first 2 weeks of patient training in breathing control, use of medications, bronchial hygiene therapy, and exercise skills should demonstrate increasing independence with diminishing need for repeated individual instruction and cues. Nearly total independence in performing these and other techniques as previously listed should be accomplished by the time of discharge.

In the facility, many environmental considerations are essential to successful program participation. Handicapped parking and easy accessibility will ensure that patients feel accommodated and will encourage attendance at each scheduled session. Ensuring patient comfort and convenience in getting into the facility will decrease their frustration and anxiety about the walk to the center and their ability to participate in the therapy once they find their way. A program schedule that lists days, dates, and times for group sessions for education and exercise training will provide participants with a calendar of events showing when attendance is expected. Written instructions explaining exercises and appropriate clothing and footwear will keep the guesswork to a minimum for people who may have last exercised in high school gym class 45 years ago. (See the sample program schedule in Figure 12-6.)

Group size is an important consideration in planning a program schedule. Too large a group will not allow the individual attention required for training in the varied skills needed for managing chronic lung disease. A group large enough to promote camaraderie and peer motivation can be accomplished with four to six people. Staffing resources will vary depending on patient acuity, if billing the treatment session one to one or for a group.[6]

FACILITATING A LIFESTYLE CHANGE

Once the patient with pulmonary disease has completed the basic pulmonary rehabilitation program, he or she should be encouraged to maintain and expand on the lifestyle changes that have been initiated. In a healthy population, the physical conditioning effects of an exercise program take approximately 3 to 6 months. In a pulmonary population that is frequently deconditioned and older, conditioning adaptations may take twice as long.[42,46] With this fact in mind, the therapist must counsel the participant to set gradual, realistic goals for pulmonary rehabilitation.[49]

It is important that the patient understand that noticeable changes in one's physical abilities and sense of dyspnea will come about in subtle ways after approximately 2 to 4 weeks of rehabilitation. When the therapist has carefully explained this phenomenon, most patients can sustain their motivation and effort during those first few grueling, exhausting weeks. The therapist should expect the patient to express feelings of doubt, discouragement, and even anger during this time when immediate gains are not obvious and the participant may be verbally and nonverbally expressing the question, "Is it worth all this effort?" In these situations, the therapist must be prepared to give realistic data and time lines concerning expectations and progress. Simultaneously, the therapist must offer optimistic and positive comments about the patient's progress so far and anecdotes about other patients with similar diagnoses who have had successful outcomes. Ultimately, enlisting the assistance of other rehabilitation participants who have successfully completed the rehabilitation program and have moved beyond it to a true lifestyle change while managing their disease will have a profound impact on the novice rehabilitation participant.

Every participant who completes the basic pulmonary rehabilitation program should leave with an *individualized* home exercise program

10 Week Pulmonary Rehabilitation Schedule, 3 Times a Week
Mon/Wed 1:00 PM to 3:30 PM and Friday 9:00 AM to 10:00 AM

Name: _____

Notes:
- Remember to bring your inhalers, and any mid day medications
- Eat a late breakfast, or an early light lunch. Please feel free to bring a snack

Week 1: Monday	**Wednesday**	**Friday**
1:00 PM Therapeutic exercise	1:00 PM Therapeutic exercise	9:00-10:00 AM Therapeutic exercise
2:30 PM SGRQ/orientation	2:30 PM Lung anatomy/ physiology breathing retraining	

Week 2: Monday	**Wednesday**	**Friday**
1:00 PM Therapeutic exercise	1:00 PM Therapeutic exercise	9:00-10:00 AM Therapeutic exercise
2:30 PM Lung disease	2:30 PM Lung disease (cont.)	

Week 3: Monday	**Wednesday**	**Friday**
1:00 PM Therapeutic exercise	1:00 PM Therapeutic exercise	9:00-10:00 AM Therapeutic exercise
2:30 PM Lung medications	2:30 PM Lung medications Part 2	

Week 4: Monday	**Wednesday**	**Friday**
1:00 PM Therapeutic exercise	1:00 PM Therapeutic exercise/ STAIRS	9:00-10:00 AM Therapeutic exercise
2:30 PM Oxygen therapy/ sleep disorders	2:30 PM Nutrition	

Week 5: Monday	**Wednesday**	**Friday**
1:00 PM Therapeutic exercise/ STAIRS	1:00 PM Therapeutic exercise/ STAIRS	9:00-10:00 AM Therapeutic exercise
2:30 PM Diagnostic testing	2:30 PM Preventing infection/ airway clearance	

Week 6: Monday	**Wednesday**	**Friday**
1:00 PM Therapeutic exercise/ STAIRS	1:00 PM Therapeutic exercise/ STAIRS	9:00-10:00 AM Therapeutic exercise
2:30 PM Panic control	2:30 PM Relaxation techniques	

Week 7: Monday	**Wednesday**	**Friday**
1:00 PM Therapeutic exercise	1:00 PM Therapeutic exercise	9:00-10:00 AM Therapeutic exercise
2:30 PM Emotional and social well-being	2:30 PM Energy conservation	

Week 8: Monday	**Wednesday**	**Friday**
1:00 PM Therapeutic exercise	1:00 PM Therapeutic exercise	9:00-10:00 AM Therapeutic exercise
2:30 PM Community resources	2:30 PM Advance directives	

Week 9: Monday	**Wednesday**	**Friday**
1:00 PM Therapeutic exercise	1:00 PM Therapeutic exercise Thera-Bands	9:00-10:00 AM Therapeutic exercise Thera-Bands
2:30 PM Review	2:30 PM Benefits of exercise	

Week 10: Monday	**Wednesday**	**Friday**
*6 Min Walk Test Appointments**	1:00 PM Therapeutic exercise	9:00-10:00 AM Therapeutic exercise
	2:30 PM HAD/SGRQ/ Knowledge test	Home recommendations Graduation

FIGURE 12-6 Example of a pulmonary rehabilitation schedule showing 10 weeks of exercise and education.

Pulmonary Rehab Program

Home Exercise Program

For: **John Doe**   Date: **August 17, 2007**   HX: **COPD, osteoporosis**

Breathing exercises: Do diaphragmatic and pursed lip breathing twice daily for 5 minutes each session.

Floor exercises: Do 4-5 times/week. Gradually increase repetitions to a maximum of 20 repetitions. Once you have achieved 20 reps, increase your weights by 1 lb. Oxygen: 6 LPM (oxymizer)   Cuff weights: **0 lb** Dumbbells: **0 lb**   Thera-Bands: Yellow

Osteoporosis precautions: Do not use arms on Airdyne or Nustep equipment. No arm ergometry. No twisting of the trunk or forward trunk flexion. Keep back straight when bending over (kneel down instead).

Strength training: Use Thera-Bands and dumbbells and cuff weights to simulate the Cybex equipment if you do not have access to this equipment. Remember to breathe properly-**don't hold your breath!!!** Increase your repetitions to 20 then increase the weight by 1 to 5 lb. and advance the color of your Thera-Band. Oxygen: 6 LPM (oxymizer)

Bike: Cateye @ Level 2 **for 10 minutes, level 1 for 10 minutes. (Average mileage = 2.75-3.66).** Heart rate should be 96-108 bpm. Oxygen: 15 LPM (partial rebreather mask)

Walking: Make walking a daily activity (5-7 times/week). Keep a record of time and distance for each walk. See the progressive walking schedule below, for the next 8 weeks. Oxygen: 15 LPM (partial rebreather mask) Use a 4-wheeled walker.

Walking program

Weeks	Distance (miles)	Time (minutes)
1-2	1.0 mile	27 min
3-4	1.0 mile	25 min
5-6	1.0 mile	24 min
7-8	1.0 mile	23 min

The walking program should be done on a flat surface. The treadmill can be used as an addition to your program, but not a substitute to ground surface walking.

FIGURE 12-7 Examples of pulmonary rehabilitation home exercise program.

(Figure 12-7). Patients respond best to specific guidelines based on modes, frequency, and duration of exercise achieved in the last few days of the rehabilitation program. The therapist may add a schedule for gradual advancement of the exercises for those highly motivated participants or as a bridge of instruction until a solid maintenance regimen can be established.

Graduation from the basic pulmonary rehabilitation program should be recognized as a significant accomplishment by the staff. A graduation ceremony or party, diplomas, and written or verbal acknowledgment among peers are effective ways to celebrate the participant's completion of the program.

Near the conclusion of the program, the staff should provide information and resources regarding continuation of involvement. Maintenance or graduate pulmonary rehabilitation programs and other low-level or nonintimidating exercise programs may be suggested.[50] Members of a maintenance exercise and follow-up program form a close support network for each other and encourage continued activity compliance by organizing telephone trees, holiday parties, travel opportunities, and scholarship fund-raising events. Local "better

Pulmonary Rehab Program

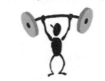

Home Exercise Program

For: <u>**Jane Doe**</u>   Date: <u>**August 17, 2007**</u>   HX: <u>**COPD**</u>

Breathing exercises: Do diaphragmatic and pursed lip breathing twice daily for 5 minutes each session.

Floor exercises: Do 4-5 times/week. Gradually increase repetitions to a maximum of 20 repetitions. Once you have achieved 20 reps, increase your weights by 1 lb. Oxygen: 3-4 LPM   Cuff weights: **2 lb**   Dumbbells: **2 lb**   Thera-Bands: Green

Strength training: Use Thera-Bands and dumbbells and cuff weights to simulate the Cybex equipment if you do not have access to this equipment. Remember to breathe properly-**don't hold your breath!!!** Increase your repetitions to 20 then increase the weight by 1 to 5 lb. and advance the color of your Thera-Band. Oxygen: 3-4 LPM

Bike: Cateye @ Level 2 **for 17 minutes, and Level 1 for 3 minutes. (Average mileage = 3.5-4.0 miles).** Heart rate should be 126-132 bpm. Oxygen: 4-6 LPM

Walking: Make walking a daily activity (5-7 times/week). Keep a record of time and distance for each walk. See the progressive walking schedule below, for the next 8 weeks. Oxygen: 6 LPM You may use a rolling walker.

Walking program

Weeks	Distance (miles)	Time (minutes)
1-2	1.0 mile	22 min
3-4	1.0 mile	21 min
5-6	1.5 miles	32 min
7-8	1.5 miles	31 min

The walking program should be done on a flat surface. The treadmill can be used as an addition to your program, but not a substitute to ground surface walking.

FIGURE 12-7, cont'd For legend see opposite page.

breathers" clubs are excellent avenues to stay in touch with others who have similar diagnoses. For the pulmonary transplantation population, the opportunity exists to participate in athletic events such as the biannual Transplant Olympics sponsored by the National Kidney Foundation.

CONCLUSION

PTs and RTs have a long history of providing care to the patient with pulmonary disease. Because of their educational background, they provide a unique approach to treating these patients; combined with other health care providers, each may complement the other to offer an unparalleled pulmonary rehabilitation program. The process of evaluating the physical and respiratory care

needs of the medical and surgical pulmonary patient are specific and used to directly plan the appropriate treatment intervention in the rehabilitation setting. With thoughtful instruction, compassion, and skill, therapists may navigate the way for a successful lifestyle change among the pulmonary rehabilitation population.

References

1. Frownfelter D: Introduction. In Frownfelter D, editor: Chest physical therapy and pulmonary rehabilitation: an interdisciplinary approach, Chicago, 1978, Year Book, pp xvii-xx.
2. Barach A: The treatment of pulmonary emphysema in the elderly, J Am Geriatr Soc 4:884-887, 1956.
3. Ries A, Squier H: The team concept in pulmonary rehabilitation. In Fishman AP, editor: Lung biology

in health and disease, vol. 91: pulmonary rehabilitation, New York, 1996, Marcel Dekker, pp 55-65.

4. Southard D, Cahalin LP, Carlin BW et al: Clinical competency guidelines for pulmonary rehabilitation professionals: American Association of Cardiovascular and Pulmonary Rehabilitation position statement, J Cardiopulm Rehabil 15:173-178, 1995.

5. Hilling L, Smith J: Pulmonary rehabilitation, Cardiopulmonary physical therapy, ed 3, St. Louis, 1995, Mosby, pp 445-470.

6. American Association of Cardiovascular, & Pulmonary Rehabilitation: Program management, Guidelines for pulmonary rehabilitation programs, ed 3, Champaign, Ill, 2004, Human Kinetics, pp 93-106.

7. Fishman AP: Foreward. In Fishman AP, editor: Lung biology in health and disease, vol. 91: pulmonary rehabilitation, New York, 1996, Marcel Dekker, pp xxv-xxvii.

8. Petty T: Pulmonary rehabilitation: a personal historical perspective. In Casaburi R, Petty T, editors: Principles and practice of pulmonary rehabilitation, Philadelphia, 1993, WB Saunders, pp 1-8.

9. Nici L, Donner C, Wouters E et al: American Thoracic Society/European Respiratory Society statement on pulmonary rehabilitation, Am J Respir Crit Care Med 173:1390-1413, 2006.

10. Ries AL, Bauldoff GS, Carlin BW et al: Pulmonary rehabilitation: joint ACCP/AACVPR evidence-based clinical practice guidelines, Chest 131:4-42, 2007.

11. Ries AL, Make BJ, Lee SM et al: The effects of pulmonary rehabilitation in the National Emphysema Treatment Trial, Chest 128:3799-3809, 2005.

12. The Joint Commission: Chronic obstructive pulmonary disease certification. Available at www.jointcommission.org/CertificationPrograms/COPD. Retrieved December 2007.

13. Jenkins SC, Cecins NM, Collins GB: Outcomes and direct costs of a pulmonary rehabilitation service, Physiother Theory Pract 17:67-76, 2001.

14. Sadowsky SH: Pulmonary diagnostic tests and procedures. In Hillegass EA, Sadowsky HS, editors: Essentials of cardiopulmonary physical therapy, ed 2, Philadelphia, 2001, WB Saunders, pp 421-447.

15. American Association of Cardiovascular and Pulmonary Rehabilitation: Selection and assessment of the pulmonary rehabilitation candidate. In Guidelines for pulmonary rehabilitation programs, ed 3, Champaign, Ill, 2004, Human Kinetic, pp 11-20.

16. American College of Sports Medicine: Clinical exercise testing. In ACSM's Guidelines for exercise testing and prescription, ed 7, Philadelphia, 2006, Lippincott Williams & Wilkins, pp 93-112.

17. American Association of Cardiovascular, & Pulmonary Rehabilitation: Exercise assessment and training. In Guidelines for pulmonary rehabilitation programs, ed 3, Champaign, Ill, 2004, Human Kinetics, pp 31-42.

18. American Association of Cardiovascular, & Pulmonary Rehabilitation: Disease-specific approaches in pulmonary rehabilitation. In Guidelines for pulmonary rehabilitation programs, ed 3, Champaign, Ill, 2004, Human Kinetics, pp 67-91.

19. Hammon WE: History. In Frownfelter D, Dean E, editors: Cardiovascular and pulmonary physical therapy: evidence and practice, ed 4, St. Louis, 2006, Mosby, pp 137-149.

20. Watchie J: Cardiopulmonary physical therapy, Philadelphia, 1995, WB Saunders.

21. ATS Committee on Proficiency Standards for Clinical Pulmonary Function Laboratories: ATS statement: guidelines for the six-minute walk test, Am J Respir Crit Care Med 166:111-117, 2002.

22. Laack SJ, Prancan AV: Respiratory and cardiovascular drug actions. In Frownfelter D, Dean E, editors: Cardiovascular and pulmonary physical therapy: evidence and practice, ed 4, St. Louis, 2006, Mosby, pp 785-796.

23. Ciccone C: Respiratory drugs. In Pharmacology in rehabilitation, ed 4, Philadelphia, 2007, FA Davis, pp 397-413.

24. Cohen SB, Pare PD, Man SFP et al: The growing burden of chronic obstructive pulmonary disease and lung cancer in women: examining sex differences in cigarette smoke metabolism, Am J Respir Crit Care Med 176:113-120, 2007.

25. Wolfson MR, Shaffer TH: Respiratory physiology: structure, function, and integrative responses to intervention with special emphasis on the ventilatory pump. In Irwin S, Tecklin JS, editors: Cardiopulmonary physical therapy: a guide to practice, ed 4, St. Louis, 2004, Mosby, pp 39-81.

26. Dean E: Cardiopulmonary anatomy. In Frownfelter D, Dean E, editors: Cardiovascular and pulmonary physical therapy: evidence and practice, ed 4, St. Louis, 2006, Mosby, pp 53-72.

27. Stackowicz DM, Moffat M, Frownfelter D et al: Impaired ventilation, respiration/gas exchange, and aerobic capacity/endurance associated with airway clearance dysfunction (pattern C). In Moffat M, Frownfelter D, editors: Cardiovascular/pulmonary essentials: applying the preferred physical therapists practice patterns, Thorofare, NJ, 2007, SLACK, pp 83-112.

28. McNamara S: Clinical assessment of the cardiopulmonary system. In Frownfelter D, Dean E, editors: Cardiovascular and pulmonary physical therapy: evidence and practice, ed 4, St. Louis, 2006, Mosby, pp 211-227.

29. Hillegass E: Assessment procedures. In Hillegass EA, Sadowsky HS, editors: Essentials of cardiopulmonary physical therapy, ed 2, Philadelphia, 2001, WB Saunders, pp 610-646.

30. Mahler DA, Harver A: Clinical measurement of dyspnea. In Mahler DA, editor: Dyspnea, Mount Kesco, NY, 1990, Futura, pp 75-100.

31. Crouch R, Schein R: Integrating psychosocial services for lung volume reduction and lung transplantation patients into a pulmonary rehabilitation program, J Cardiopulm Rehabil 17:16-18, 1997.

32. Hillegass EA, Sadowsky HS: Cardiovascular and thoracic interventions. In Hillegass EA, Sadowsky HS, editors: Essentials of cardiopulmonary physical therapy, ed 2, Philadelphia, 2001, WB Saunders, pp 452-473.

33. Scherer SA: The transplant patient. In Frownfelter D, Dean E, editors: Cardiovascular and pulmonary physical therapy: evidence and practice, ed 4, St. Louis, 2006, Mosby, pp 719-733.

34. Versluis-Burlis T, Downs A: Thoracic organ transplantation: heart, heart–lung, and lung. In Hillegass EA, Sadowsky HS, editors: Essentials of cardiopulmonary physical therapy, ed 2, Philadelphia, 2001, WB Saunders, pp 477-508.

35. Forsythe J, Cooley K, Greaver B: Adaptation of a weight management program for a potential lung transplant candidate, Prog Transplant 10: 234-238, 2000.

36. Novitch R, Thomas H: Rehabilitation in chronic interstitial disease. In Fishman AP, editor: Lung biology in health and disease, vol. 91: pulmonary rehabilitation, New York, 1996, Marcel Dekker, pp 683-700.

37. Storer TW: Exercise in chronic pulmonary disease: resistance exercise prescription, Med Sci Sport Exerc 33(suppl 7):S680-S692, 2001.

38. Richardson RS, Leek BT, Gavin TP, et al: Reduced mechanical efficiency in chronic obstructive pulmonary disease but normal peak VO2 with small muscle mass contraction, Am J Respir Crit Care Med 169:89-96, 2004.

39. Celli B, Rassulo J, Make B: Dyssynchronous breathing during arm but not leg exercise in patients with chronic airflow obstruction, N Engl J Med 314:1485-1489, 1986.

40. Cullen DL, Rodak B: Clinical utility of measures of breathlessness, Respir Care 47:986-993, 2002.

41. Verrill D, Barton C, Beasley W et al: The effects of short-term and long-term pulmonary rehabilitation on functional capacity, perceived dyspnea, and quality of life, Chest 128:673-683, 2005.

42. American College of Sports Medicine: General principles of exercise prescription. In Guidelines for exercise testing and prescription, ed 7, Philadelphia, 2006, Lippincott Williams & Wilkins, pp 133-165.

43. Swisher AK: Not just a lung disease: peripheral muscle abnormalities in cystic fibrosis and the role of exercise to address them, Cardiopulm Phys Ther J 17:9-14, 2006.

44. Ries A, Ellis B, Hawkins R: Upper extremity exercise training in chronic obstructive pulmonary disease, Chest 93:688-692, 1988.

45. Lake F, Henderson K, Briffa T et al: Upper-limb and lower-limb exercise training in patients with chronic airflow obstruction, Chest 97:1077-1082, 1990.

46. American College of Sports Medicine: Other clinical conditions influencing exercise prescription. In Guidelines for exercise testing and prescription, ed 7, Philadelphia, 2006, Lippincott Williams & Wilkins, pp 205-231.

47. Caplan-Shaw CE, Arcasoy SM, Lederer DJ et al: Osteoporosis in diffuse parenchymal lung disease, Chest 129:140-146, 2006.

48. Gold DT, McClung MR, Shipp KM: The changing face of osteoporosis, ed 2, Durham, NC, 2005, Duke University School of Medicine, Program in Women's Health.

49. Bowen JB, Votto JJ, Thrall RS et al: Functional status and survival following pulmonary rehabilitation, Chest 118:697-703, 2000.

50. Heppner PS, Morgan C, Kaplan RM et al: Regular walking and long-term maintenance of outcomes after pulmonary rehabilitation, J Cardiopulm Rehabil 26:44-53, 2006.

Chapter 13

Occupational Therapy to Promote Function and Health-Related Quality of Life

SUSAN COPPOLA • WENDY WOOD

CHAPTER OUTLINE

Occupation
    Relationship to Health-Related
        Quality of Life and Function
Therapeutic Process
    Multidimensional Functional
        Assessment

Intervention
    Therapeutic Groups
    Documentation of Intervention
Conclusion

PROFESSIONAL SKILLS

On completion of this chapter, the reader will be able to do
the following:
* Understand the relationship of occupation to health-related quality of life as the ultimate outcome
  of occupational therapy in pulmonary rehabilitation
* Understand how therapeutic occupations can enhance function relative to the World Health
  Organization's dimensions of participation, activity, and body functions and structures and service
  recipients' subjective views and experiences
* Relate the functional dimensions of participation, activity, and body functions and structures to the
  sequence and content of functional assessment and intervention in occupational therapy
* Explain evidence-based principles that should guide the selection of therapeutic occupation to be
  used in treatment and the construction of holistic and comprehensive total treatment programs
* Understand how to incorporate common therapeutic procedures and techniques in pulmonary
  rehabilitation within therapeutic occupations
* Understand how to run therapeutic groups focused on daily living skills and occupational projects

This chapter addresses pulmonary rehabilitation from the perspective of occupational therapy. It begins by discussing the field's core construct of *occupation*. To ensure a shared interdisciplinary language, the chapter proceeds by bridging the idea of occupation to commonly used terms within the rehabilitation field, specifically function as now defined by the World Health Organization (WHO, Geneva, Switzerland)[1] and health-related quality of life (HRQL).

The occupational therapy therapeutic process is next presented, including strategies for assessment and intervention pertaining to those areas of occupational functioning that people with pulmonary disorders deem vital to a high quality of life. This chapter has two purposes: (1) to offer clinical guidelines to occupational therapists in pulmonary rehabilitation that are consistent with contemporary standards of best possible practice in occupational therapy and (2) to facilitate interdisciplinary understanding of the specific contributions of the occupational therapist as a vital team member in pulmonary rehabilitation.

Throughout this chapter, it is understood that the involvement of occupational therapists in pulmonary rehabilitation unfolds in many different treatment contexts across the continuum of care, from inpatient medical facilities and outpatient clinics to the institutional living environments, private homes, schools, workplaces, and communities of persons with pulmonary disorders. Accordingly, approaches to assessment and intervention described herein, as well as views of legitimate treatment goals, methods, and outcomes, are offered as vital guidelines to the practice of occupational therapy in pulmonary rehabilitation no matter where or when that practice occurs. At the same time, shifts in the functional capacities of patients across the differing contexts of care often require that the focus of treatment shift within the scope of these guidelines. It is recognized as well that the "natural" environments of home, school, community, and workplace can be far more conducive to delivering robust programs of occupational therapy than medical facilities, which offer only a limited range of treatment spaces. Across the continuum of care, therefore, occupational therapists are encouraged to implement these guidelines in ways that are resourceful, creative, flexible, and responsive to the current occupational needs of patients.

OCCUPATION

The construct of occupation is the fundamental concern in the practice of occupational therapy.[2] Although the term is used colloquially in the sense of paid work, "occupation" as used by occupational therapists refers to human activities that meaningfully fill time in the stream of daily life, calling forth the use of physical, emotional, and cognitive capacities in the context of a person's environment. Occupations are expressions of core motivations, culture, and identity. Thus occupations imbue people's everyday habits and routines—as well as their infrequent yet personally significant events, rituals, and celebrations—with shape, meaning, and purpose.

Put another way, it might be said that occupation is as vital to people's lives as breathing is to their bodies. Like breathing, moreover, one's obligatory, productive, restful, leisurely, and celebratory occupations are often accomplished in relatively fluid, taken-for-granted fashions—at least, that is, until a change in life circumstances, such as the onset of debilitating medical conditions. Thus, people seek the services of health professionals in pulmonary rehabilitation not only out of fundamental concerns about survival but also out of fundamental concerns that they might continue to have, or might once again have, lives worth living especially with less shortness of breath. If we listen, we hear their occupational identities: the meticulous homemaker, proficient gardener, avid reader, competent professional, devoted grandparent, expert golfer, and loyal church volunteer, all vital cues to successful programs of occupational therapy. Simultaneously, the meticulous homemaker may have become so physically deconditioned that making a bed requires that the balance of the day be spent recovering; the expert golfer may have given up hope of ever again playing nine holes; and the loyal church volunteer may have become homebound out of embarrassment in having to rely on portable oxygen (O_2) in public. When valued undertakings such as these become compromised, or are cut altogether from the fabric of daily life, a spiraling cycle of losses in self-esteem, identity, hopefulness, functional capacity, and family and societal participation often ensues.

It is, accordingly, the work of occupational therapists in pulmonary rehabilitation to engage patients in collaborative processes that place the precise occupations that both challenge and are deemed important by patients and their loved ones at the center of clinical intervention.[3,4] Jackson and colleagues[5] described a therapeutic program of occupational therapy for older adults dedicated to empowering people to actively select and experience individualized patterns of occupations that are simultaneously health promoting and personally satisfying. As applied to pulmonary rehabilitation, effective programs may be limited in focus and duration as well as broad. Yet, no matter where in this range a program falls, its effectiveness is gauged by the degree to which patients achieve a sense of control over their symptoms (e.g., dyspnea, fatigue, weakness), their identities, and their lives by incorporating therapeutic strategies within those occupations that they want and need to do.[6] Thus the "proof" of occupational therapy is in how people learn to "do" life differently in their homes and communities, to the betterment of their health and satisfaction.

Relationship to Health-Related Quality of Life and Function

The emphasis of occupational therapy on every-day occupations is congruent with contemporary emphasis on HRQL as a critical outcome of health care and rehabilitation in general[1,7-9] and of pulmonary rehabilitation in particular.[10-14] More specifically, being able to carry out person-ally valued life activities despite adverse health conditions is commonly viewed as one of several core elements of HRQL, a position that current research of both well and disabled persons strongly supports.[15-19] Furthermore, experiences of a good quality of life are increasingly acknowl-edged as being highly subjective and individual-istic in nature.[20] Thus as Browne, Hannah, and O'Boyle[20] noted with respect to quality of life, "It is of little use, for example, to observe that on average, the mobility of a sample of patients improved following an intervention, without knowing whether this domain is as important [to those patients] as other domains that may have disimproved." Hence, it is possible to affect "function" favorably while having no favorable impact on HRQL whatsoever, perhaps explaining why treatment areas traditionally favored by reha-bilitation professionals, such as basic movement or self-care skills, have often not brought about better lives for those who have undergone exten-sive rehabilitation.[20-22] To understand how occu-pational therapy programs improve function in ways that also enhance HRQL, it is helpful to review the current views of the WHO on function and disablement.

The WHO[1] revised its 1980 International Classification of Impairments, Disabilities, and Handicaps to account more fully for environmen-tal (social and physical) influences on ablement and also to better represent the complex, varied, and dynamic nature of the disablement process. The new WHO classification, the International Classification of Functioning, Disability, and Health (ICF) (Figure 13-1), has shifted away from terminology that emphasizes the negatives of incapacity and toward terminology that emphasizes meaningful activity and social participation.

Whereas the previous classification system defined function as consisting of the three dimen-sions of impairment, disability, and handicap, the ICF defines function in positive terms, describing the dimensions as body functions and structures, activities, and participation.[1] The ICF addresses function at the level of the body, with problems at this level defined as impairments. Impairments are abnormalities in physiologic or psychological functions or body structures. Also using more positive language, function at the level of the person is now described as activity, not disability. Activity refers to how people are able to perform activities of everyday life, from basic physical functions such as grasping, moving a leg, or hear-ing to complex physical and mental activities such as driving a car, playing a piano, or planning and cooking a meal. Problems of activity perfor-mance are called activity limitations. The ICF addresses function at the level of society as

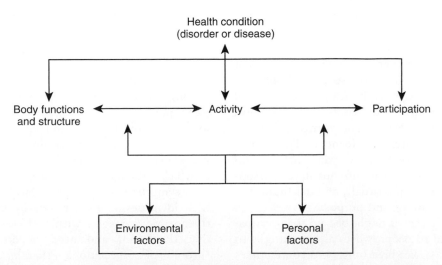

FIGURE 13-1 WHO International Classification of Impairments, Activities, and Participation.

participation, not handicap. Participation, the most significant dimension of function, arises from a complex interplay of health conditions, body functions and structures, activities, and contextual factors that together influence the degree to which people participate in society to their own satisfaction. Participation restrictions arise when involvement in life situations is limited in a manner or extent relative to the individual's desired level of participation.

As well as embracing terminology that speaks to human potential, the ICF emphasizes that simple, unidirectional, causal relationships do not exist between adverse health conditions and the three functional dimensions of body, activity, and participation. Instead, multiple pathways involving many mutually interacting variables, all of which are influenced by the contexts in which people "do" their lives, are viewed as potentially able to impact function profoundly. Emphasis on this complex nexus of factors and processes stems from a now large body of evidence showing that people with identical medical diagnoses, or similar health conditions, vary greatly in their actual functional capacities. That the ICF highlights personal factors and the environment as significant contributors to function comes as no surprise to clinicians who have worked with people trying to live their lives with a disability.

With respect to pulmonary rehabilitation, for example, although a diagnosis of emphysema may account for why a 60-year-old woman performs poorly on a pulmonary function test (functional dimension of body), neither her diagnosis nor her test performance is especially predictive of whether she carries out activities in her home (functional dimension of activity) or successfully works in a paid job (functional dimension of participation). Likewise, improving function with respect to her pulmonary impairments may very well *not* improve function with respect to her activities or social participation. That is, being able to perform daily activities at home may depend far more on learning how to integrate, within basic habits and routines, adaptations to single activities and also to ways of balancing the energy demands of multiple activities than on improved physiologic function alone. In turn, improved function in home activities may bear no relationship to improved function at work if the woman's place of employment exposes her to poor air quality. Finally, even if this woman were unable to function independently in the home or

at work after intensive rehabilitation, her HRQL may still have been greatly improved if therapy enabled her to participate once again in her most enjoyed activities as a grandmother and bridge club member (functional dimension of participation). As this example illustrates, processes of disablement not only are unique to individuals and the particulars of their life situations but defy reductions to simple causal relationships between illness, body functions and structures, activity performance, and participation.

Occupation, as used by occupational therapists in both language and as a therapeutic medium, bears a specific relationship to each of the ICF's three dimensions of function, with specific clinical implications for improving function in ways that promote HRQL. Just as the term "occupation" overlaps with colloquial use of the term "activity," so too does occupation encompass the more complex mental and physical activities within the activity dimension of the ICF. For example, activities such as cooking a meal or driving a car are regarded as occupations because they are purposeful, entail conscious perceptions of doing, tap many different skill areas simultaneously for their execution, and are also typically imbued with personal and sociocultural meanings. Conversely, basic functions that the ICF also calls activities, such as grasping, moving a leg, remembering, and hearing, are viewed as discrete component functions embedded within the "doing" of occupations[23] but not as occupations per se. Keeping this distinction in mind, this chapter departs somewhat from ICF terminology by using activity and occupation interchangeably to denote the complex "doing" experiences of people as whole beings. At the same time, as evidence reviewed later in this chapter suggests, occupation can influence basic physical functions and impairments favorably, such as when enriched rounds of daily activities promote both psychological well-being and physical conditioning. Likewise, occupation is a key vehicle by which identity and social participation can be enhanced as when, say, playing the guitar is a source of personal pride and also the center of many songfests with family and friends.

Table 13-1 summarizes the previous discussion of occupation and its relationship to current WHO definitions, with examples relevant to pulmonary rehabilitation. As shown, occupation substantially overlaps with the functional dimension of participation and with complex mental

TABLE 13-1 Relationship of Occupation to World Health Organization International Classification of Functioning, Disability, and Health

Terminology	WHO Definition	Occupation	Examples of Problems in Pulmonary Rehabilitation
Health condition	Disease or disorder of the body		COPD, asthma, ALS, major depression
Body functions and structures	Function at the level of the *body*; *impairment* is a loss or abnormality of bodily structures or function	Influence of function	Compromised pulmonary function, muscle weakness, anxiety, decreased range of motion, memory deficit
Activities	Function at the level of the *person*; activities may be limited in nature, duration, and quality; activities may range from basic movements to complex tasks	Occupation	Basic movements: difficulties in lifting, breathing, or walking; Complex activities: difficulties in bathing, dressing, shopping, homemaking, or performing leisure interests and hobbies
Participation	Function at the level of *society*; refers to the outcome of complex relationships among health conditions, body functions and structures, and activities in context of persons' lived environments; context includes social, physical, and attitudinal features of environments that serve to facilitate or limit participation; participation can be restricted in nature, duration, and quality	Influence on function	Belief that assistive equipment is stigmatizing or symbolizes personal weakness; inaccessible physical environments in homes or places of work secondary to stairs, long distances, or challenging terrain; lack of knowledge of others about the effects of perfumes, humidity, or temperature on persons with pulmonary dysfunction

ALS, Amyotrophic lateral sclerosis; COPD, chronic obstructive pulmonary disease.
Data from International Classification of Functioning, Disability and Health (ICF). Available at: http://www.who.int/classifications/icf/en/. Retrieved January 2008.

and physical activities within the functional dimension of activity. Directional arrows are used to show that occupation can potentially influence function favorably regarding (1) basic physical functions in the dimension of activity, (2) body functions and structures, and (3) participation.

THERAPEUTIC PROCESS

The therapeutic process of occupational therapy begins with a multidimensional functional assessment, proceeds to a series of interventions and ongoing evaluation of the effectiveness of those interventions, and concludes with evaluation of achieved outcomes pertaining to function and HRQL leading to discharge. This process unfolds within occupational therapy's domain of practice as defined in *Occupational Therapy Practice Framework: Domain and Process*, published by the American Occupational Therapy Association.[24] Occupational therapists pay particular attention to self-care activities (e.g., bathing, toileting, bed mobility, and emergency response), work and productive activities (e.g., child and elder care, housekeeping, shopping, transportation, cooking, and management of money, household, and medication needs), and play and leisure activities (e.g., creative play, sports, and recreational and hobby interests). To ensure that the unique occupational concerns of patients are addressed, the occupational therapist acts throughout the therapeutic process as an expert educator, coach, ally, and advocate who empowers patients and their significant others as full collaborators in therapy.[25,26]

Multidimensional Functional Assessment

Effective and efficient intervention is more likely to ensue if the assessment has clearly delineated core problem areas and opportunities for improvement. Thus this chapter emphasizes the assessment process of occupational performance issues as fundamental to best practice.[27] A sample occupational therapy evaluation form serves as a summary and a guide to the reader on the sequence and content of this section on functional assessment (Figure 13-2).

Before conducting actual assessments of a patient's functional status, the occupational therapist prepares by collecting background information from the medical record and through discussion with the pulmonary rehabilitation team members.[3] Information pertaining to medical diagnosis, medical history, medical precautions, documented impairments, and social and vocational history is especially important. Medical diagnosis is required for insurance reimbursement for occupational therapy, which serves as a clue to the types of impairments that the patient may experience. Onset of diagnoses indicates whether an acute problem or a chronic condition exists for which the patient may have already made many effective adaptations. Medical history includes secondary physical and psychological diagnoses that may limit occupational performance, nutritional issues, and past and present use of medications and O_2. Medical precautions indicate needed constraints in basic movements and activities. Data on impairments such as forced expiratory volume, endurance tests, and 6-minute walk data allow the occupational therapist to anticipate the patient's general level of physical capacity. When available, information pertaining to social and vocational history begins to paint a picture of the patient's culture, values, environment, and lifestyle. Educational level will guide the selection of written instructional materials for use in therapy and will also influence the extent to which a patient may or may not benefit from such materials.

After pertinent background information has been obtained, direct assessment of the patient is undertaken with respect to the functional ICF dimensions of participation, activities, and body functions and structures. To understand sequencing of assessment across these dimensions, rationales underlying top-down approaches are next described. Table 13-2 shows how the ICF classification system organizes functional assessment with respect to each dimension.

Assessing Occupational Performance

Functional assessment in occupational therapy begins by ascertaining people's self-perceived capabilities, satisfactions, and dissatisfactions regarding how well they are functioning in the occupations that are central to their family, school, work, or community lives.[27,28] This approach to functional assessment begins with the total contexts and meanings of occupational performance in everyday life and then proceeds to direct assessments of performance abilities in occupations previously identified by the patient (or family) as especially problematic and important. Last, and only when necessary, is a more detailed evaluation of distinct body functions

Name _____ Medical record #_____ Age _____ Date _____

Diagnosis _____ Onset _____ Precautions_____

Pertinent medical history, medications, oxygen:

Social, vocational, and educational history:

Participation

Extent of participation in:	Routines and time use patterns:	Environmental barriers/resources:	Goals and belief in ability to change:
Activities of daily living			
Leisure and social			
Work and productive			

Activity performance

Problem activities:	Difficulty, duration, assistance, outlook:	Strategies and breathing patterns:
1)	1)	
2)	2)	
3)	3)	
4)	4)	

Body functions and structures, impairments and strengths affecting activity performance

Physical:	Cognitive:	Psychological:
Dyspnea:		
Activity tolerance: MET level:		
Strength:		
Range of motion:		
Other:		

FIGURE 13-2 Sample occupational therapy assessment form. MET, table of metabolic equivalent values.

and structures that directly impede activity performance conducted. Thus each phase of the assessment approach is designed to inform, delimit, and focus the next phase, thereby generating a fine-grained yet comprehensive picture of patients' occupational performance capacities.

This approach to functional assessment has several advantages:

• By first ascertaining the perspectives of patients and their significant others, a foundation of mutual respect that empowers service recipients as collaborators in therapy is immediately established.[27]

TABLE 13-2	Occupational Therapy Multidimensional Functional Assessment Organized According to International Classification of Functioning, Disability, and Health Dimensions of Function: Participation, Activities, and Body Functions and Structures	
Dimension of Function	**Measurement of Dimension and Assessment Goals**	**Evaluation Methods and Tools**
Participation	Determine impact of health conditions and of social and physical environment on everyday lifestyle, particularly social and productive activities	Interview
		Canadian Occupational Performance Measure School Function Assessment Functional Status Questionnaire
	Identify important activities for performance-based assessment	Activity configuration
		Activity checklist Environmental assessment
Activities	Determine ability to perform specific activities relative to difficulty, assistance needed, duration limits, and outlook on activity	Activity analysis
		Metabolic equivalent table Rate of perceived dyspnea Rate of perceived exertion
	Determine areas of strength that enable performance	Functional Independence Measure (FIM)
	Determine which impairments should be evaluated in depth	WeeFIM
		Assessment of Motor and Process Skills
Body functions and structures	Determine degree of severity, location, or duration of impairments that impede activities and social participation	Endurance: 6- or 12-Minute Walk Test
		Strength: manual muscle test, grip strength
	Determine whether the impairment can be remediated or whether it should be compensated for	Range of motion: goniometry
		O_2 saturation: pulse oximetry
	Determine areas of strength	Visual perception, cognitive performance, and motor control tools

Data from International Classification of Functioning, Disability, and Health (ICF). Available at: http://www.who.int/classifications/icf/en/. Retrieved January 2008.

- Therapists can avoid imposing their own treatment regimens that patients may evaluate as having been irrelevant once they actually experience their postdischarge lives (see, for example, DeJong[22] and Klein[29]).
- Patients often assume that what occupational therapists evaluate is what occupational therapists treat.[28] If occupational therapists focus initially on measuring impairments, then a false message is tacitly yet powerfully conveyed that treatment can and will "fix" those impairments. Although remediation of impairments such as muscle weakness or low endurance may be an element of treatment, patients need to understand that occupational therapy's greatest contribution to their postdischarge lives consists of helping them learn how to enact patterns of occupation in ways that promote their health and well-being.
- The top-down approach is cost-effective and time-efficient because it guides the therapist to evaluate and treat only those occupational issues that, from patients' perspectives, adversely affect their quality of life.

First Phase: Dimension of Participation

The first phase of functional assessment targeting participation is accomplished primarily through interview of the patient and, ideally, important others (e.g., family, friends, caregivers, colleagues, and teachers) in the patient's life. If the patient has stopped a valued occupation or reports impoverished rounds of occupations day in and day out, the therapist seeks to uncover the real reasons why. Because processes of disablement cannot be reduced to simple causal relationships, a multiplicity of social, cognitive, emotional, physical, and contextual dynamics are considered. For example, a person may stop doing volunteer work not because of any recent decline in physical capacity but because of embarrassment (an emotional issue) about chronic wheezing and coughing (a physical issue) in public (a social issue). In this phase of assessment, therefore, the occupational therapist explores the patient's involvement with meaningful occupations across multiple life contexts to reveal his or her personal characteristics, motivations, values, and beliefs about possibilities for healthful change. In addition, to whatever degree is possible, the occupational therapist evaluates the social and physical contexts of the patient's life.

Initial interview questions about participation and barriers to participation are geared to the patient's functional, educational, and literacy level: How have breathing problems affected your ability to do the things you want to do? What are the most challenging things for you to do? What is the most important thing that you do or would like to do? What makes your spirit soar? What are you looking forward to? What would you be doing if you did not have breathing problems? How is your day and week typically organized? How do family, friends, and coworkers respond to your breathing problems? These questions illuminate who the patient is as a person and their lived experience of having a disability. In addition to informal interviews, several standardized tools have been published that address participation, initiating a top-down approach.

The Canadian Occupational Performance Measure (COPM)[27] is recommended as a standardized interview tool that can function as a valid outcome measure of occupational therapy with both adults and children. Using this structured interview tool, therapists ask the patient to identify activities that he or she wants or needs to do. Using a scale from 1 to 10, the patient rates how well he or she is able to perform each activity and corresponding levels of satisfaction with performance. A list of five goal areas is generated from these responses to target subsequent interventions to the most critical areas of need identified by the patient. As long as the patient can

communicate concerns and desires, or knowledgeable proxies are available to respond to the COPM questions, it is an effective data-gathering tool with very debilitated patients and those with mild difficulties alike.

The School Function Assessment[30,31] is a standardized criterion-referenced tool that guides goal setting and treatment planning in the school environment. The School Function Assessment identifies both the strengths and the problems of a child with respect to his or her active participation in school activities within the classroom, science laboratory, playground, resource room, school bus, cafeteria, and restroom, among other contexts. In the interest of implementing pragmatic and sustainable solutions, the tool is designed to foster adult teamwork and interdisciplinary understanding of a child's unique constellation of abilities and difficulties across multiple performance contexts.

The Functional Status Questionnaire[32] is a standardized, self-administered screening tool that targets participation. The questions identify general physical, psychological, and social role functions in the past month as well as satisfaction levels. In addition to being an appropriate tool with which to initiate a comprehensive top-down functional assessment, the Functional Status Questionnaire can be used to screen individuals to determine whether they might benefit from occupational therapy.

The activity configuration is a nonstandardized written schedule of the patient's typical day or week. This tool uncovers temporal rhythms of the person's life, social contacts, and habits.[33] In addition, the activity configuration can reveal adaptive strategies that the patient presently uses, ineffectively uses, or altogether fails to use regarding the management of the energy demands of everyday activities. Because energy level, dyspnea, and activity opportunities and demands can vary greatly from day to day, a weeklong activity configuration is useful for revealing whether or to what degree effective adaptive strategies are typically implemented.

Occupational therapists may also wish to use activity checklists, which can ascertain patients' perspectives regarding ability and interest in certain activities. A good example is the Activity Card Sort.[34] A well-designed checklist can add efficiency to the interview by clarifying problem activities for the patient. A checklist can also aid thoroughness by serving as an activity inventory for the therapist and patient to consider. If given in advance of interviewing, the occupational therapist should be aware that patients may have difficulty completing the checklist. Checklists can frustrate people with limited literacy, vision, writing, or information-processing abilities. Checklists have also been found to frustrate patients with very mild or very severe limitations.

Assessing Social and Physical Contexts of Participation. Assessment of the environment targets physical and social enablers and barriers that influence participation.[35] The extent to which the occupational therapist is able to evaluate a patient's actual life environments during initial assessment is greatly influenced by the therapist's work setting. Occupational therapists who see patients in medical facilities are most constrained in this regard, with access limited to important caregivers or family members who are present during assessment. Nevertheless, the therapist is advised to learn as much as possible about the ethics and values that motivate family members. Dimensions of the social environment include expectations that important others have regarding the patient's performance; their attitudes about the patient's capacities, weaknesses, and potential, and their willingness to adapt, assist with, or back away from helping with occupations that are important to the patient.[36]

For example, it would be a waste of the patient's and the occupational therapist's time, and of health care dollars, to insist that a woman with chronic obstructive pulmonary disease perform her self-care activities independently if (1) the woman prefers to be helped by her husband and (2) her husband regards such assistance as an expression of love and also deserved care for all the years in which she subjugated her needs to his. A more fruitful course of action would instead be for the occupational therapist to ascertain the patient's and her husband's perspectives on other areas of occupational functioning that each agrees are troubling. Doing so might reveal, for instance, that increasing "home-boundness" and withdrawal from long-standing activities with family and friends are of concern to both husband and wife. Alternatively, the occupational therapist may come to "see" that although both are satisfied with their interdependence in her self-care, the husband does not support his wife in using her abilities in other daily activities. In either scenario, the occupational

therapist would strive to find acceptable "hooks" for intervention in which both husband and wife agree that she can more actively take charge of her life and he can safely and guiltlessly be less consumed with her care. Such "hooks" may include greater independence in self-care, resumption of responsibility for feeding the dog and cat, among other possibilities that have the potential to enhance function within context of the family system. In addition, the occupational therapist can educate both husband and wife about the progressive debilitation that can occur if helping where no help is needed occurs.

Occupational therapists who work in schools, places of work, private homes, or institutional living environments are in the advantageous position of immediately being able to assess how the physical contexts of daily life influence an individual's usual patterns of participation. Conversely, occupational therapists who work in medical facilities often must rely on descriptions provided by the patient or family members, delaying evaluation until it becomes feasible to travel to relevant settings. When such direct evaluations are not possible, photographs and drawings are used.

Regardless of whether an occupational therapist can assess the patient's everyday physical environments directly or must rely on secondary accounts, the occupational therapist seeks to understand how various qualities of the physical environment influence a patient's abilities and motivations for activity. These qualities include distances that must be traveled to carry out activities in and outside of the home and layout of the living space, including object availability, that is, furnishings, obstructions, and lighting. The investigation attends to issues of efficiency and safety, especially regarding falls, as well as to the patient's willingness to make home modifications. A recommended strategy for obtaining this information is to study typical pathways, including entryways and safe exits, and then to examine each activity space used. The occupational therapist also explores how air quality (e.g., temperature, humidity, pollution, odors, and airborne compounds such as perfumes, cleaning agents, and coatings) influences participation in the different occupational contexts of home, school, work, and community. In so doing, the occupational therapist ascertains possibilities for modifying air quality.

Second Phase: Dimension of Activity

Whereas the first phase of assessment relies mainly on interview approaches to obtain information, the second phase of assessment relies mainly on performance-based assessments of function in single occupations and multiple occupations over time. Insisting that someone do a task that he or she rarely does compromises the clinical validity and utility of generated data while also risking alienating that person from occupational therapy, as suggested by narratives written by people who have undergone occupational therapy. Hence, to whatever degree is possible, patients are observed in those occupations they previously identified as high priorities for intervention. Occupational therapists working in medical facilities are once again most challenged in this regard and must strive to make available to patients possibilities for participating in a wide range of human occupations, or, alternatively, to simulate the demands of real-life activities as closely as possible. Likewise, to whatever degree is pragmatically feasible, patients are to be encouraged to perform priority occupations at the same times and places, and in the same ways, as they usually do. Determining such things as whether someone stands or sits to groom, dresses in the bathroom or bedroom, uses a microwave or conventional oven, gardens in plots or in elevated planters, drives a car or uses public buses, or shops with a scooter or walker is critical. Because patients in medical facilities do activities in unfamiliar spaces with unfamiliar objects, their occupational therapists must also ascertain how observed performances depart (for better or worse) from those typically manifested in everyday environments.[37]

Another principle guiding selection of activities for performance-based assessment concerns the varying metabolic demands of different activities and, hence, the endurance of patients with respect to engaging in single activities as well as a round of multiple activities.[38-41] Occupational therapists can consult tables of metabolic equivalent (MET) values to help select activities of varying energy demands that fall within patients' priority lists of problematic occupations. METs are scaled from 1 to 10 on the basis of the amount of O_2 consumed in the metabolic process to carry out a particular activity. One MET is the amount of energy used when a person is at rest. Thus, the endurance of a person who demonstrated hypoxemia and dyspnea when grooming (1.5 METs) would be much more compromised than that of a person who did not exhibit such symptoms until doing housework (3 to 4 METs) (Table 13-3). In addition to gauging tolerance for single activities, MET tables can help occupational therapists establish a baseline of endurance across multiple activities of varying energy demands. Ideally, during initial assessment or soon thereafter, patients enact some segment of their daily routines, encompassing activities at different MET levels (e.g., showering [2 to 3 METs], followed by grooming [1.5 METs], followed by dressing [3 to 4 METs]). Less ideally but still productive of much clinically useful information, patients perform activities out of their usual sequence during the assessment (e.g., ironing [2 to 3 METs], followed by bed making [3 to 4 METs], followed by sewing [1.5 to 2.0 METs]).

A final guiding principle for this phase of assessment concerns the occupational therapist's adoption of a conservative approach to intervening in the patient's performance. The patient is thus first given the opportunity to perform the activity as he or she normally would. While always ensuring safety, the occupational therapist intervenes only if and when problems arise and only then in incremental fashions corresponding to the nature of those problems, progressing from the least to the highest levels of verbal and physical assistance. This measured approach is particularly effective in revealing the patient's maximal functional capacity. As next described, the ways in which the patient responds to the physical, cognitive, and psychological demands of an activity are also clearly revealed.[42] By analyzing such responses, the occupational therapist can further home in on adaptive strategies that enable, and the nature of impairments that constrain, the patient's occupational performance.

Responses to Physical Demands. To gauge the patient's endurance and general activity tolerance, the occupational therapist keeps in mind the average MET values of activities as published in MET tables, in addition to the specific strength and speed demands of those activities as actually enacted by patients during assessment.[43] For example, ironing with a heavy iron or quickly or while standing is more demanding of energy than is ironing with a light iron or slowly or while sitting. Also, use of the upper extremities is typically more taxing than the same amount of work done by the lower extremities.[44,45] In addition to

TABLE 13-3 Metabolic Equivalent Values for Some Occupational Performance Areas

MET Level (O$_2$ Consumed) [Level of Activity]	Self-Care Activities	Work and Productive Activities	Play and Leisure Activities
1.5-2.0 METs (4-7 ml/ kg/min) [very light/ minimal]	Eating	Desk work	Playing cards
	Shaving, grooming	Typing	Sewing
	Getting in and out of bed	Writing	Knitting
	Standing		
2-3 METs (7-11 ml/kg/ min) [light]	Showering in warm water	Ironing	Level bicycling (8 km/hr or 5 mph)
	Level walking (3.25 km/hr or 2 mph)	Light woodworking	Billiards
		Riding lawn mower	Bowling
			Golfing with power cart
3-4 METs (11-14 ml/kg/ min) [moderate]	Dressing, undressing	Cleaning windows	Bicycling (10 km/hr or 6 mph)
	Walking (5 km/hr or 3 mph)	Making beds	Fly-fishing (standing in waders)
		Mopping floors	Horseshoe pitching
		Vacuuming	
		Bricklaying	
		Machine assembly	
4-5 METs (14-18 ml/kg/ min) [heavy]	Showering in hot water	Scrubbing floors	Bicycling (13 km/hr or 8 mph)
	Walking (5.5 km/hr or 3.5 mph)	Hoeing	Table tennis
		Raking leaves	Tennis (doubles)
		Light carpentry	
5-6 METs (18-21 ml/kg/ min) [heavy]	Walking (6.5 km/hr or 4 mph)	Digging in garden	Bicycling (16 km/hr or 10 mph)
		Shoveling light earth	Canoeing (6.5 km/hr or 4 mph)
			Ice- or roller-skating (15 km/hr or 9 mph)
6-7 METs (21-25 ml/kg/ min) [very heavy]	Walking (8 km/hr or 5 mph)	Snow shoveling	Bicycling (17.5 km/hr or 11 mph)
		Splitting wood	Light downhill skiing
			Ski touring (4 km/hr or 2.5 mph)

km/hr, *Kilometers per hour;* MET, *metabolic equivalent;* ml/kg/min, *milliliters of oxygen consumed per kilogram body weight per minute;* mph, *miles per hour;* O$_2$, *oxygen.*

From Kohlmeyer K: *Evaluation of sensory and neuromuscular performance components.* In Neistadt ME, Crepeau EB, editors: *Willard and Spackman's occupational therapy,* ed 9, Philadelphia, 1998, Lippincott, p 225.

these considerations, the occupational therapist watches for whether and how other common physical impairments in pulmonary disorders, such as dyspnea, fatigue, or limitations in upper extremity strength and range of motion, affect performance.[46] If the patient experiences distress or if medical history or precautions indicate, the occupational therapist monitors the patient's heart rate, O$_2$ saturation rate, respiratory rate, or blood pressure before, during, and after the activity.[47] Table 13-4 offers general guidelines for monitoring vital signs in response to activity.

Another useful test, referred to as the Talk Test, simply assesses whether the patient is able to talk during the activity, knowing that the patient is at a maximal exertion level if he or she is unable to speak. Speaking can be measured as being able to have a conversation versus saying only a word at a time. Such monitoring gauges the severity of various physiologic impairments relative to actual occupational performance, thereby providing contextually valid data that are extremely useful to patients and therapists alike.

TABLE 13-4 Common Vital Signs Used to Monitor Physical Response to Activity*

Vital Sign	Evaluation	Normal Value	Abnormal Value
Pulse heart rate (HR)	Index and first finger at radial or carotid artery; measured as beats per min: 15 sec × 4	Rate, 60-100; avg., 75. *Note*: Even rhythm and strength	Rate: >100—tachycardia <60—bradycardia
Respiratory rate (RR)	Observe rise/fall of abdomen/chest; listen; observe for distress and patterns (breath holding, recruitment of accessory muscles, irregular rate)	12-22 breaths per min	Tachypnea, bradypnea (rare)
Blood pressure (BP)	Sphygmomanometer; seated, supine, and standing; measured as mm Hg	Systolic: 90-140 (avg., 120)	Hypertension
		Diastolic: 60-90 (avg., 80)	Hypotension
Arterial blood gases (ABGs)	Pao_2—Partial pressure of oxygen in arterial blood	75-100 mm Hg on room air, age dependent	Hypoxemia
	Sao_2—Amount of oxygen bound to hemoglobin (oximeter)	>95%	Hypoxemia
	Cao_2—Total content of oxygen in arterial blood (A-line)	16-20 ml/dl blood	Decreased tissue oxygenation

*The physician sets guidelines for individual patients.

For example, if the occupational therapist observes abnormal breathing patterns such as breath holding, forced exhalation, or gasping, then more measured assessment of how underlying physiologic impairments impact performance ought to be undertaken.[3] Pulse oximetry monitoring can be used to offer continuous information about oxygenation and heart rate during occupational performance for patients at risk for hypoxemia. A portable pulse oximeter consists of a finger, ear, or forehead probe attached to a small monitor, which enables use of the device during most activities. Normal O_2 saturation values are 95 to 100%; a reading below 90% is a sign of hypoxemia. Oxygen saturation readings can offer early warnings that an activity should be modified or stopped, or if the patient is using supplemental oxygen the oxygen would need to be titrated to more than 90% saturation during the activity. If decreasing the activity does not resolve the hypoxemia then use of breathing strategies, or shifts in body position such as propping on elbows, may be helpful. Of interest during assessment is how closely the patient's reported symptoms (e.g., shortness of breath, Borg Scale[48]) match changes in oxygenation and pulse, indicating the patient's ability to assess his or her status. If the symptoms and readings do not match, the patient may need a pulse oximeter to ensure safety and may also benefit from biofeedback training with the oximeter.

In addition to the previously mentioned objective measures, it is important that the occupational therapist determine the patient's subjective experience of the activity's difficulty. Borg[48] developed a scale with which patients can rate their perceived levels of dyspnea and exertion during an activity, using verbal anchors to assist in ratings (Table 13-5). An alternative subjective rating scale ranges from 6 to 20, with 6 being no effort and 20 being the maximal effort possible to complete the activity.[46] The 6-to-20 scale is useful for teaching patients to self-monitor heart rate for 6 seconds because of easier mathematical conversions. The counted number between 6 to 20 over a 6-second time interval is then multiplied by 10. A score of 6 has been found to often correlate with a heart rate of 60 beats per minute, and so on up the scale with 20 correlating with 200 beats per minute.

Responses to Psychological Demands. Various psychological dynamics in the patient's occupational experience are also carefully tuned into during performance-based assessment. A vicious cycle of dyspnea and anxiety can interfere with performance, leading a patient to avoid a particular activity after discharge. Thus it can be beneficial for this negative cycle to arise briefly during assessment to observe the patient's awareness and response. The patient is asked about feelings of satisfaction and dignity associated with performance. Motivation for treatment is likely to be enhanced if the patient is dissatisfied with

TABLE 13-5 Instructions for Evaluating Perceived Dyspnea and Perceived Exertion

1. Patient identifies an activity that is important and problematic and then performs that activity.
2. The patient is shown the following 10-point scales and asked to rate perceptions of dyspnea and exertion.
3. Descriptive terms in the scales serve as verbal anchors to assist the patient in rating.
4. To evaluate outcomes, retest using the same activity, rating scales, and instructions.

Note: If assessing for change in activity performance, the patient uses newly acquired energy conservation and breathing strategies in the retest session. If assessing for impairment of endurance, the original activity is replicated.

Perceived Dyspnea Scale

Instructions: "How would you rate your shortness of breath during the activity? On a scale of 0 to 10, with 0 being no shortness of breath and 10 being shortness of breath so severe that you must stop and rest, what number best indicates your experience of shortness of breath?"

My shortness of breath is:

0	None
0.5	Very slight, just noticeable
1	
2	Mild
3	Moderate
4	Somewhat heavy
5	Strong, heavy
6	
7	Severe
8	
9	
10	Very, very severe; I must stop and rest

Perceived Exertion Scale

Instructions: "Rate how hard you were working (or the amount of physical effort) during the activity. On a scale of 0 to 10, with 0 being no effort and 10 being your maximal possible effort, what number best indicates your level of effort?"

My level of effort is:

0	None
0.5	Very slight
1	Slight
2	Mild
3	Moderate
4	Somewhat strong
5	Strong, heavy
6	
7	Very strong
8	
9	
10	Very, very strong, almost the maximum possible

Adapted from Borg GA: Psychophysical bases of perceived exertion, Med Sci Sports Exerc 14:377, 1982.

performance or if receiving assistance is humiliating or unacceptable. If a large discrepancy exists between the performance as observed by the occupational therapist and the patient's subjective experience, the therapist is directed toward working with possible strategies to promote awareness and coping. At all times, frustration tolerance must be monitored so the occupational therapist can intervene to prevent new experiences of failure. Ultimately, effective intervention helps patients achieve a sense of control over the uncertainty that pulmonary dysfunction brings to a person's day-to-day life.[3,6]

Responses to Cognitive Demands. Persons with pulmonary disorders may present with cognitive deficits owing to hypoxemia and given comorbidity with other conditions such as traumatic brain injury, stroke, late-stage Parkinson's disease, alcoholism, schizophrenia, major depression, or dementia, among others. Although secondary diagnoses affecting cognition are often well documented, undocumented problems may still exist, such as when, for example, a patient

incurred a mild brain injury during a recent fall or is in the earliest stages of dementia. The occupational therapist is thus always alert for cognitive deficits in the context of occupational performance. To the extent possible given the cognitive demands of any one assessment activity, the occupational therapist observes the patient's attention span, immediate and short-term memory, organizational and sequencing skills, abilities to follow written or verbal instructions, decision-making capacities, and effectiveness in solving problems. As importantly, the occupational therapist watches for whether and how the patient uses adaptive strategies to accomplish the activity. Because such strategies suggest personal strengths with respect to cognitive processing, learning capabilities, and adaptability,[46] they can be expanded on in subsequent interventions. For example, it may become apparent while watching a patient dress that he takes frequent rest breaks, effectively uses a reacher, but demonstrates poor breathing techniques. In this case, the occupational therapist is cued to build on pacing strategies that are acceptable to the patient and to teach breathing strategies. Use of a reacher also clues the occupational therapist about the person's openness to assistive equipment in other occupations.

Standardized Performance-Based Assessments. Not all occupations that patients identify as high priorities can be assessed with standardized evaluation tools. For example, a city dweller's ability to use public transportation while reliant on portable O_2 may be the most daunting obstacle that person faces in overcoming his or her spiraling social isolation, withdrawal from valued activities, and propensities to cancel outpatient appointments. Although perhaps not immediately able to be assessed, it is nonetheless critical that occupational therapists address capacities in those less routine activities that often prove to be the weakest link in a person's overall quality of life. The previously mentioned approach to performance-based assessment can be used to generate objective measures of functional capacity regarding public transportation use, as well as any other occupational endeavor, be it horseback riding, mall walking, or gardening.

When, however, the occupational needs of patients overlap with the content area of psychometrically sound, performance-based assessment tools, it is wise to use the established validity and reliability of such tools. Occupational therapists have access today to several good criterion-referenced tools that target the performance areas of self-care, work and productive activities (including driving), and play and leisure.[49] Two well-established tools commonly used by occupational therapists that address basic self-care activities are the Functional Independence Measure (FIM)[50] and the WeeFIM.[51] The FIM and WeeFIM measure burden of care relative to assistance for adults and children, respectively. The FIM has been used to measure progress in persons with pulmonary disorders.[14] A recommended tool for instrumental activities of daily living such as homemaking activities is the Assessment of Motor and Process Skills (AMPS).[52] Because the AMPS allows patients to choose from among 56 possible evaluation activities and then perform chosen activities as typically undertaken, it powerfully instills a patient-centered approach to assessment and treatment. Also, through the use of two subscales that analyze motor and cognitive processing in the context of one activity, the AMPS allows occupational therapists to predict abilities in other activities of

comparable difficulty. Because it is beyond the scope of this chapter to provide a more comprehensive overview of standardized assessments, readers are referred to contemporary textbooks in occupational therapy.[27,53,54]

Documenting Occupational Performance. Activity performance is described in terms of levels of assistance, difficulty, duration, and outlook. The patient's level of needed verbal and physical assistance with an occupation is the most common objective measure of functional capacity. When a standardized assessment has not been used, levels of assistance are typically described by the percentage of the activity the patient actually performed, as follows: independent, supervised or verbal cueing, minimal assistance (patient does approximately 75% of the activity), moderate assistance (patient does approximately 50% of the activity), maximal assistance (patient does approximately 25% of the activity), and dependent (patient does little or none of the activity). These levels of assistance are contained in the Medicare guidelines for occupational therapy.[55] Difficulty with an activity can be documented as changes in heart rate, respiration rate, breathing patterns, O_2 saturation levels, and blood pressure before, during, and after activities. Occupational therapists can track the patient's ability to continue with an activity, or duration, as another gauge of endurance and activity tolerance. Duration is measured by describing the length of time the patient is able to persist in an activity, as in a man tolerating washing his face while sitting on the edge of the hospital bed for 1 minute. Because the patient's position, materials used, pace, and environmental context will influence duration, these factors should be described as well. Again regarding activity tolerance, the patient's perceived dyspnea, exertion, and experience of difficulty are important to document, as are psychological responses, or outlook. Finally, to make all of these measures optimally meaningful regarding endurance issues, metabolic demands of the activities used for assessment should be noted (Figure 13-3).

Third Phase: Dimension of Body Functions and Structures

Evaluation of body functions and structures refers to various measurements of specific functions out of the context of occupational performance. In a top-down approach, body functions and structures are evaluated in a conservative and streamlined fashion on the basis of several principles: (1) Only body functions and structures that have already been directly observed to impede occupational performance are considered relevant for further evaluation. (2) Only impairments that require more finely grained measurements to guide intervention than that already obtained in the context of activity performance are evaluated. Evaluating endurance with an ergometer may, after all, produce no new clinically useful data—and also less contextually valid data—than that already obtained in the context of having the patient make a bed or prepare breakfast. (3) Efficiency and comprehensiveness in evaluating body functions and structures are balanced across the interdisciplinary pulmonary rehabilitation team. By not duplicating evaluations of physical or respiratory therapy, the program becomes more cost-effective and patients are protected from undue frustrations in having to do the same tests over again. Thus, collaborations with the rehabilitation team to include psychologists and speech and language pathologists about cognitive, psychological, and communication problems that arise during occupational performance are oftentimes vital. Moreover, when physical impairments can be capably evaluated by either occupational or physical therapists, occupational therapists may wish to "pass the baton" to their colleagues in physical therapy to free their own time for grappling with patients' various occupational challenges as thoroughly as possible. This is an especially critical issue in light of current cost-containment measures. Ultimately, a comprehensive pulmonary rehabilitation program uses teamwork to integrate assessments by all involved professionals across multiple domains of function.[56] With these caveats in mind, occupational therapists may be called on to evaluate impairments in upper body strength, range of motion, coordination, praxis, and sensation. Occupational therapists may also evaluate swallowing difficulties, or dysphagia, that arise from muscle weakness or shortness of breath.[57]

Upper body and proximal muscle weaknesses, common limitations of patients with pulmonary conditions, arise from multiple causes. Many patients have pulmonary problems associated with generalized weakness from neuromuscular diseases such as multiple sclerosis and amyotrophic lateral sclerosis. For patients with chronic pulmonary diseases, trunk, hip, and shoulder

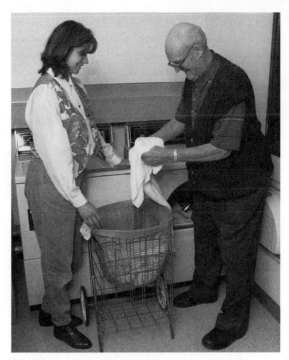

FIGURE 13-3 Occupational therapist observes performance of everyday activities. Assessment of impairments, such as shoulder range of motion, is done only when problems interfere with performance of important activities.

weakness can be caused by chronic steroid use.[58] Upper body weakness results from fatigue of the accessory muscles of respiration, propping on elbows to support the trunk, general debilitation, and posturing shoulders in adduction and elevation to expand the capacity of the lungs.[59] Further upper body weakness results from disuse of arms because of paucity of daily occupations such as carrying groceries, sweeping the floor, or playing sports.

Measurement of strength is done by manual muscle testing. Instead of testing individual muscles, general movement strength is measured and rated on a scale from 0 to 5, from absent to normal. Movements that are often weak are shoulder flexion, external rotation, and abduction. The trunk should be supported when testing the upper extremity to isolate potential weakness areas. Trunk support can be provided by a chair with a back or by lying supine. Trunk strength is measured by first determining whether the patient can sit unsupported and whether that position can be maintained during perturbations in each direction—forward, backward, and to each side. Accessory muscles of respiration may be strong as a result of compensation for compromised lung capacity. Hand and finger strength is measured by dynamometer and pinch meter.

Range of motion limitations are often associated with weakness because they are caused by many of the same factors and are worsened by poor strength. Decreased movement of the shoulders, neck, and trunk results from posturing of the shoulders in elevation and adduction to increase lung space. Posturing leads to a lack of arm swing during ambulation and neck stiffness that can, in turn, be particularly problematic for driving. Tight hip extensors limit the ability to reach the feet, which is worsened by fear or discomfort of flexing forward at the hips. Arthritis and osteoporosis often contribute to musculoskeletal problems of older adults with pulmonary dysfunction. The focus of occupational therapy is not to regain normal range of motion and strength but to improve or compensate for those limitations adequate to perform significant daily activities. Thus a complete manual muscle test and goniometric evaluation is rarely needed. Gross functional range of motion can be efficiently tested by asking the patient to reach with both hands to toes, the small of the back, back of the head, and then raise arms overhead.

Finally, occupational therapists may engage patients in the 6-Minute Walk Test (see Chapter 12).[60] These tests offer objective baselines of endurance relative to estimated MET levels. As needed, upper extremity dowel exercises and upper body ergometers can also be used to reveal breathing strategies and delineate tolerance for upper body exercise.[10]

Outcomes of Multidimensional Functional Assessment

The first phase of assessment, addressing the ICF functional dimension of participation, brings immediate clarity to the occupational needs, problems, and issues of individual patients and their significant others. As concluded by Fisher,[61] this phase of assessment is "critical, and ... must occur, even under the pressures of cost containment, reduced duration of care, [and] staff cuts, ... [as it] results in overall outcomes being enhanced and overall costs reduced." The second phase of assessment, addressing the ICF functional dimension of activities, produces a wealth of clinically useful information pertaining to the performance capacities of patients in valued occupations, including how impairments constrain performance and how areas of strengths might later be applied to

resolve other problems. The third phase of assessment, addressing the ICF functional dimension of body functions and structures, refines understanding of specific deficit areas. The outcome of this multidimensional assessment process is a list of measurable and doable goals generated in collaboration with the patient and his or her significant others, with specific intervention processes and time frames for accomplishing those goals. Table 13-6 offers examples of treatment goals and intervention for body functions and structures, activities, and participation. As next described, on the basis of these goals, individualized programs are implemented to help people learn how to "do" valued occupations in ways that favorably influence their day-to-day functioning and HRQL in postdischarge environments.

Intervention

In determining the best intervention for persons with pulmonary disorders, it is helpful to consider a variety of evidence-based principles that can guide both the selection of specific activities for use as therapy as well as the construction of total treatment programs that, given available time and resources, are as comprehensive and holistic as possible.[10-12,62] With this bigger picture in mind, occupational therapists can then attend to the more technical and procedural aspects of treatment in ways that are most likely to produce valuable outcomes pertaining to function and HRQL.

Evidence-Based Principles of Intervention

A growing body of evidence suggests that therapeutic occupations are more efficacious in promoting function and HRQL than are clinically contrived tasks and exercises. For instance, contrived tasks such as dowel rod exercises or cone stacking often fail to produce sufficient gains to meet the functional challenges of real-life activities in real-life contexts.[63] Likewise, traditional methods of prescribing exercise have been found to be largely ineffective in improving the cardiovascular fitness and overall activity levels of persons with sedentary lifestyles.[64] Conversely, therapeutic programs designed to support participation of adults and older adults with various adverse health conditions in meaningful occupations have been associated with improved cardiovascular fitness, postural stability, emotional well-being, and social participation among other gauges of HRQL.[15,65,66]

TABLE 13-6 Occupational Therapy Outcomes and Interventions Relative to International Classification of Functioning, Disability, and Health Dimensions of Function

Descriptive Terms	Functional Outcomes: Sample Treatment Goals	Intervention Examples
Participation:	*Patient will:*	Increase awareness of environmental barriers and individual's rights to access under the Americans with Disabilities Act
Outcome is described in terms of engagement, participation, or occupation; occupational therapy intervention links to an outcome at the level of participation	Return to half-time work as a bank teller	
	Participate in senior center activity programs three times per week	Modify physical environment; educate caregivers, family, employers, teachers, or other people who influence the patient's social and physical world
	Resume leisure Participation of playing cards Participate in all aspects of public school program, including recess Engage in extended family gatherings Participate in church activities	
Activities: Ability to perform specific activities that are important to participation	*Patient will:* Use energy conservation strategies during homemaking activities to cook a family meal and then have the energy to sit with the family to eat	Education and training: Activity grading
	Use assistive devices to bathe and dress self with minimal assistance	Breathing strategies
	Spontaneously use breathing techniques during yard work task to sustain the activity for 30 min with only mild shortness of breath	Energy conservation techniques
		Assistive equipment Activity modification Environmental modification Assertiveness Relaxation
Body functions and structures: Impairments are addressed if they are remediable and if they enable the patient to perform an important activity	*Patient will:* Tolerate 10 min of upper extremity exercise on the ergometer set at zero resistance	Graded tasks to increase endurance Upper extremity strengthening program
	Increase strength in shoulder flexion and abduction to 4/5 ("good") Increase shoulder range of motion to 150° flexion and 70° external rotation	Range of motion exercises

Data from International Classification of Functioning, Disability and Health (ICF). Available at http://www.who.int/classifications/icf/en/. Retrieved January 2008.

In light of such evidence, best possible practices in occupational therapy today are often described as occupation-centered and client-centered.[67,68] In occupation-centered and client-centered approaches, engagement in real-life occupations is used as the most efficacious medium to treat deficit component areas of function, maximize strength, and generalize abilities across multiple social and physical contexts. Two inherent qualities of everyday occupations are exploited as treatment mechanisms: purposefulness and meaningfulness. As described by Pierce,[69] additional therapeutic qualities of activities are that they are (1) appealing to the person being treated on face value alone; (2) congruent with his or her goals; and (3) intact, meaning what that person actual does, or will do, in his or her everyday environment of living.

By directly matching therapy activities to previously identified occupational needs and issues, occupational therapists can use the treatment mechanisms of purposefulness, meaningfulness, appeal, and goal congruence. The quality of intactness can also be readily used when working with patients in their homes, schools, workplaces, or communities. In addition, even if based in medical facilities, occupational therapists can take advantage of as many existing occupationally enriched spaces as patients can safely access, for example, not just patients' rooms but rehabilitation kitchens and apartment areas, gift shops, public cafeterias, outside parks, and nearby restaurants, post offices, shops, and public transportation stops. In the experience of the authors, occupational therapists in medical facilities have also created occupationally enriched treatment spaces such as handyman work stations, occupation rooms, or home office areas. The quality of intactness also requires that patients' important others be substantively involved in treatment, just as they were in assessment. In addition to exploiting these treatment mechanisms, efficacious treatment programs couple didactic teaching with immediate experiential learning.

To incorporate all of these principles within a cohesive program of occupational therapy during a pulmonary rehabilitation program, occupational therapists can involve patients in daily living activities that are typically completed, start to finish, in one treatment session (e.g., basic self-care tasks, cooking a meal, writing a letter on a computer, or cleaning a room). In addition, occupational therapists can use individualized occupational projects that span multiple treatment sessions, involve outside "homework," require action in multiple physical and social contexts, and culminate in some kind of production, be it a physical object, social event, or both. The extent and number of occupational projects for any one patient can be geared to the number of available treatment sessions; occupational projects have been effectively used by the authors in as short a period as 1-week inpatient rehabilitation stays. Examples of projects undertaken by inpatients include planning and carrying out an outdoor family picnic; using the Internet to research an art history topic and then presenting a talk to the hospital staff; planning and carrying out a trip to the mall to buy glasses; and, for an intubated man with severe pulmonary dysfunction and physical disabilities, adapting the layout of his hospital room, and procuring a tape recorder and headphones, so he could listen to talking books and music without having to call for assistance. Occupational projects can be especially therapeutic because they build a momentum to therapy over sessions, imparting a narrative story line rife with risks, challenges, uncertain outcomes, and multiple possibilities of personal triumph: inherent qualities of therapeutic occupation that are believed to have strong treatment effects. Occupational projects also can help occupational therapists manage their time efficiently, as what to do does not have to be decided anew at each treatment session and special events or trips can be planned in advance.

Incorporating Therapeutic Procedures and Techniques in Occupational Performance

Having ascertained the critical occupations and occupational projects that will constitute the core of patients' individualized treatment programs, occupational therapists then help patients learn how to incorporate relevant therapeutic strategies, techniques, and adaptations into their "doing" of activities. Especially relevant interventions for pulmonary rehabilitation include activity grading, breathing techniques, energy conservation, assertiveness and relaxation training, assistive device use, and modification of activities and the environment.

Activity Grading. Activity grading is a therapeutic strategy used by occupational therapists to promote progressively greater functioning that patients can also be taught to apply to their everyday lives. The purpose of activity grading is to provide a level of challenge that will help people progress in needed skill areas while not overwhelming them. To do so, selected therapeutic occupations are progressively modified, usually regarding their levels of physical challenge pertaining to experienced difficulty, required physical assistance, or duration of time able to be tolerated. For example, a severely debilitated patient may begin light grooming such as face washing for 1 minute while in bed with the head of the bed elevated. Each day the patient may do this task for longer periods and in progressively more challenging positions, from seated in a chair with a back, to seated in a chair without a back, and, finally, to standing. In addition to grading the physical demands of an activity, occupational therapists can grade activities socially. That is, relative independence varies as a function of the social context in which an activity is undertaken. Generalizing highest levels of competence across differing expectations, needs, patience, and attitudes of different caregivers can be critical to maintaining functional gains long term. Hogan[47] offers an excellent description of activity grading for a ventilator-assisted man as he moved from an inpatient program to his home and community.

Breathing Techniques. The teaching of breathing techniques begins with awareness and ends when patients view the techniques as tools that they own and control. In other words, occupational therapists want to avoid the kind of situation that occurred to one of the authors when she asked participants in a group to describe when they exhaled during an activity. Members of the group quietly looked at each other until one patient said, jokingly but earnestly, "Whenever the therapist tells us to!" Patients vary in their levels of awareness with respect to the influence of talking, concentrating, and body position on breathing patterns. During these activities, the occupational therapist asks the patient to observe and reflect on changes in breathing, to begin developing a sense of awareness and then control. Individualization of instruction coupled with immediate practice in selected therapeutic occupations is needed if healthful breathing techniques are to become habitual.

Pursed lips breathing and diaphragmatic breathing are recommended breathing strategies for patients with lung disease. Pursed lips breathing has been shown to improve gas exchange and respiratory muscle recruitment (Box 13-1).[70-74] Another possible benefit of pursed lips breathing is that it helps keep airways open by maintaining positive airway pressure. Although many patients intuitively teach themselves this strategy, coaching by occupational therapists coupled with practice helps overcome tendencies to use inefficient breathing patterns such as breath holding during strenuous activities and, instead, to continue pursed lips breathing before becoming short of breath. The practice of exhaling during the most strenuous part of an activity is

taught as part of pursed lips breathing training (Figure 13-4).

Research on diaphragmatic breathing has not produced evidence of its benefits on O_2 levels.[71] However, the clinical literature and anecdotal accounts suggest that diaphragmatic breathing does reduce dyspnea for some patients with lung disease.[71,75] The benefit of this technique seems to lie in the management of the stress and anxiety components of dyspnea; it may also

---

BOX 13-1	Breathing Techniques and Training Process

PURSED LIPS BREATHING
Used to reduce dyspnea during activities.
1. Initial instruction is in relaxed position, seated or supine.
2. Patient closes mouth and slowly and deeply inhales through the nose.
3. Exhalation is through pursed lips, parted at the center, as in whistling.
4. Prolong the exhalation phase to twice the length of the inspiration phase.
5. Practice pursed lips breathing during an activity, which may be washing one's face for a very debilitated patient or vacuuming for another.
6. Practice exhaling during the most strenuous part of a task, such as lifting an object or bending forward.
7. Practice techniques in a variety of familiar activities, as well as in moments of anxiety, until they are automatic.

DIAPHRAGMATIC BREATHING
Used to retrain muscles of breathing for improved efficiency and to promote relaxation.
1. Place the patient in a supine or seated position.
2. Place one hand on the abdomen just below the rib cage and the other hand on the chest.
3. Patient observes the rise and fall of the abdominal wall during inspiration and expiration, respectively.
4. Therapist explains the relationship between movement of the abdominal wall and the contraction (descending) of the diaphragm during inspiration and the patient's control of this action.
5. Patient then practices consciously relaxing to expand the abdominal wall during inspiration; this can be done for up to an hour several times per day and whenever relaxation is needed.
6. Diaphragmatic breathing may be done in conjunction with or before progressive muscle relaxation.
7. Stronger pressure or a weight can be placed on the abdomen (ideally when supine) to improve strength.
8. Diaphragmatic breathing can be done in conjunction with pursed lips breathing.

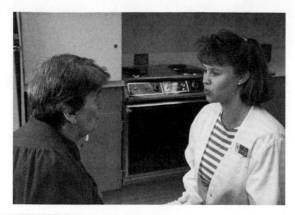

FIGURE 13-4 Occupational therapist must reinforce techniques including pursed lips breathing during activity.

influence perception of dyspnea.[71] Although further evidence is needed to explain and substantiate the effects of breathing training, many patients report that pursed lips and diaphragmatic breathing reduce dyspnea, improve relaxation, improve efficiency or coordination of breathing, and improve functional performance. In practice, occupational therapists systematically observe patient responses to breathing techniques to determine which patients benefit and document those results. Stress management and perception of control of breathing are legitimate benefits of breathing techniques that influence functional performance.

Energy Conservation

Common sense is genius dressed in its working clothes.
                                        Ralph Waldo Emerson

An extremely important dimension of occupational therapy has to do with helping patients learn how to balance satisfactory rounds of occupations over time. The activity configuration discussed previously in this chapter reveals both effective and problematic habits and routines. For example, compressing activities into the morning can lead to experiences of severe fatigue in the afternoon; similarly, overdoing one day can cause fatigue for several subsequent days. Some people learn how to adapt to such experiences by consciously planning their time use over a week or month, regularly interspersing periods of activity with periods of rest, or conserving energy for the most valued activities. Others lack such proactive strategies, living a moment-by-moment existence with choice of activity subjugated to immediate opportunities and energy level. With this information as a baseline, the occupational

therapist helps the patient devise an *occupational plan*, that is, activity schedules that ensure engagement in priority activities and minimize fatigue and frustration. Spontaneity, flexibility, and fun—all valued elements of a good day—are validated by being included in the development of such plans.[76] An effective tool to help patients devise and then implement their plans is an occupational journal. By keeping journals of usual routines and habits before trying to make substantive changes, patients grow more consciously aware of the effect that particular activities and their overall patterns of activity have on their physical conditioning and psychological well-being.

As with breathing techniques, the teaching of energy conservation strategies begins with awareness and ends when patients view the strategies as tools that they own and control. Energy conservation strategies are common sense strategies that are not so common. Principles of efficiency enable patients to simplify their work and still accomplish what they set out to do. Box 13-2 contains a list of energy conservation principles geared to patients at high reading and motivation levels. Occupational therapy programs should have an array of written information, including simpler lists, that focus on a few practical suggestions. Patients often benefit minimally from long lists of general principles, instead needing activity-specific recommendations such as "let your dishes air dry" or "place a chair in the bathroom for grooming." Therapeutic occupation provides a vehicle for practicing energy conservation principles, promoting learning and practical application. The occupational therapist can also model the use of language that is responsive to patients' expressions, concerns, and values yet evidences a stance of personal empowerment: "How can I outsmart this shortness of breath problem, and still go to the baseball game?" "I fatigue easily, so I will decide what is most important for me to do with that limited energy." "I am purchasing energy for the afternoon activity by resting this morning." "I am an efficiency expert." Once energy conservation strategies are part of a patient's routine activities, they are easily generalized to new activities. Ultimately, learning how to incorporate effective energy conservation strategies into everyday life relegates the presence of pulmonary impairments to a lower level of importance than that of human will and agency.

BOX 13-2	Energy Conservation Principles and Strategies

1. Limit the amount of work
   - Prioritize activities
   - Eliminate unnecessary tasks
   - Delegate responsibilities
   - Request assistance
2. Plan ahead and work according to the plan
   - Allow sufficient time to complete activities
   - Incorporate rest breaks into the plan
   - Collect materials before you start
3. Organize your environment
   - Place frequently used items within easy reach
   - Organize the kitchen by function
   - Eliminate clutter
4. Position yourself for comfort and efficiency
   - Sit when possible
   - Use proper body mechanics and posture
   - Wear comfortable clothing and supportive footwear
5. Take control of your time
   - Pace yourself to avoid rushing
   - Spread activities over the day or week
   - Plan rest breaks
   - Rest before you are exhausted
6. Let tools do the work
   - Use assistive devices such as reachers
   - Use convenience items such as a microwave and an electric can opener
   - Keep scissors and knives sharp
7. Tend to your mental hygiene
   - Stay relaxed
   - Use activities to take your mind off worries
   - Get plenty of sleep
   - Use relaxation techniques
   - Have some fun in every day

Occupational therapists should be aware that patients are sometimes confused when encouraged on the one hand to use activities and conditioning exercises to build and maintain their endurance and, on the other hand, to work smarter rather than harder, using energy conservation strategies. As expressed by one patient, "Now who do we listen to, the physical therapist who tells us to exert ourselves, or the occupational therapist, who tells us to conserve our energy?" Patients must clearly understand not only the need for balance of exertion and rest, but when to emphasize one or the other. For patients who do not maintain exercise programs after completion of a pulmonary rehabilitation program, it is especially important that they view an active lifestyle as sustaining of their functional capacities.

Relaxation and Assertiveness Training. Keys to enacting energy conservation principles include assertiveness and the ability to manage stress. Interpersonal relationships become complicated by disability and needs for assistance. Assertiveness training encompasses (1) validation of the patient's worth and right to express needs and opinions, (2) understanding the importance of honest and clear communication, and (3) skill training with the timing, words, and body language of assertive communication. Group settings offer role play opportunities, for example, telling someone their perfume is problematic. Ideally, practice of communication skills occurs with important others who are present for treatment.

Persons with lung disease often experience anxiety and may benefit from relaxation training.[57] Like assertiveness training, the occupational therapist first affirms the patient's right to relaxation and a sense of inner peace and points out the benefits of relaxation to performance and well-being. Techniques of relaxation include guided imagery, muscle relaxation, and breathing retraining. Many disciplines teach relaxation and stress management. When the occupational therapist teaches or reinforces these techniques, the focus is on enabling the patient to engage in important daily life routines and occupations.

Assistive Devices. Assistive devices that enable physical performance can vary from simple long-handled shoehorns to complex computerized environmental control systems. Assistive devices such as calendar systems and computers can also augment cognitive performance. Bombarded with advertisements for energy-saving devices of varying quality, many patients have grown enamored of them, whereas others are put off. The occupational therapist's expertise in assistive devices can guide patients to make wise consumer decisions about which items will in fact be useful. The occupational therapist considers small differences in weight, size, grip, or the actual functioning of particular devices that can greatly alter their utility given a particular person's abilities and limitations. Also considered are subtle problems in motor planning, visual perception, learning ability, and frustration tolerance that can significantly influence a patient's capability with various devices. Symbolic meanings that assistive devices can hold are also important to consider. To one person, a reacher may be seen as a stigmatizing sign of personal weakness or incompetence; to another, it may symbolize mastery over disabilities. The occupational therapist further considers the patient's tolerance for using gadgets, for storing gadgets in their homes, and, of course, financial resources for purchasing gadgets. In summary, physical, psychological, and cognitive capacities relative to personal preference and financial resources guide recommendations of assistive devices.

Activity and Environmental Modification. Table 13-7 offers a variety of specific suggestions to improve performance and safety for sample activities. Activity-specific recommendations incorporate energy conservation principles, environmental modification, assistive devices, and alternative techniques. Because patients vary in the amount of guidance needed to select and implement effective strategies, these suggestions should not be taken as a one-size-fits-all approach. Organizing the home for efficiency and safety, including management of O_2 equipment, is an important function of home-based occupational therapy. An example is arranging living space to prevent falls that might be caused by tripping over the oxygen tubing. For patients who need guidance, the occupational therapist collaborates with the patient and significant other to target modifications that are both doable and personally acceptable.

Therapeutic Groups

One distinct advantage of working in medical facilities is being able to offer therapeutic groups to patients with pulmonary disorders. Occupational therapists have used therapeutic groups as a cornerstone of treatment since the early 1900s.[78] Therapeutic groups are excellent vehicles for assessment and intervention, as well as for building support and sharing information among patients. Groups can be experienced as more fun and interesting for participants than are individual sessions. When participants discuss problems of daily living with one another, they can receive empathy and praise for their clever adaptations from those with firsthand knowledge. Strategies suggested by peers and sanctioned by occupational therapists also seem more doable and legitimate. Moreover, groups are excellent vehicles for combining didactic information with immediate experiential learning.

In creating therapeutic groups, it is important that occupational therapists distinguish between treating aggregates of people together in a group from groups that are truly therapeutic. Groups become therapeutic when the dynamics of the group process are used to promote patient-initiated learning and greater functional capacities. Groups that serve to place patients in relatively passive and subservient roles can violate principles of adult learning and fail to be therapeutic. In therapeutic groups, the occupational therapist plays a facilitative role, one that encourages interaction and exchange of information among group members. In so doing, the therapist validates the importance of continued involvement in peer networks for learning and support after discharge.

In constructing a group, it is useful to attend to issues of group membership. Although effective groups can vary in size from 3 to 12 members, 7 or 8 members offer an ideal balance of richness and manageability. Family members and significant others should be encouraged to attend groups. Groups may consist of particular ages or stages of disease. Children with asthma, older adults, or individuals awaiting lung transplantation may be able to relate better to others in similar circumstance. However, groups that effectively mix these populations can offer rich intergenerational support, hope, and wisdom.

Two types of therapeutic groups used by the authors are recommended: (1) daily living groups that focus on problematic aspects of daily living and (2) occupational project groups. In *daily living groups*, participants identify their most problematic aspects of daily living. Identified problems can be written on a board to help the group select priorities for discussion. Subsequent discussion addresses each problem activity, acknowledging psychosocial and physical issues and generating lists of solutions that participants have used. The occupational therapist facilitates this discussion by ensuring inclusion of all participants, endorsing key responses, and adding new information as appropriate. After discussion, experiential learning on breathing strategies, relaxation, energy conservation, or adaptive equipment use is undertaken. These minilessons can be led by the occupational therapist or by a patient participant. Ideally, such learning is undertaken relative to the demands (actual or as closely simulated as possible) of problematic activities just discussed. Once problem areas have been addressed through informal sharing and experiential learning, the occupational therapist summarizes key principles generated by participants. Principles of energy conservation, such as planning ahead, using equipment, and sitting to work, often top the list. It is often useful at this point to provide a handout on these principles,

TABLE 13-7	Modifications for Specific Activities	
Activity	Modifications	Prevention and Safety
Showering	Plan ahead by collecting all materials before starting; select a time when energy is high and ample time is available for the activity	Use chair, grab bars, and nonskid surface to prevent falls
	Minimize steam by using a well-ventilated room with an exhaust fan, avoiding very hot water, and turning on cold water first	Avoid getting into the tub unless someone is available to help with getting out
	Use assistive devices such as a shower chair, handheld shower head, long bath sponge, and soap on a rope; occupational therapists recommend specific types of shower chairs and grab bar locations for the individual	Install an emergency call system for problems
	Minimize effort for drying by use of a heat lamp, absorbent bathrobe, and slippers	
Dressing	Collect clothing in advance, possibly the evening before	Avoid rushing by allowing sufficient time to dress
	Sit to dress, in a chair with arms and a firm back	Put on all lower body clothing up to the knees, then stand up once to pull up over hips and fasten; if someone assists you to stand, this will save time
	Have any assistive devices used kept near the dressing location	
	Dress in segments, first upper body (rest), lower body (rest), then accessories	
	Set a comfortable room temperature; avoid chill by remaining covered, or replace one clothing item at a time	
	Use easy-to-manage clothing (e.g., slip-on or Velcro shoes, loose socks, stretch or sweat pants, front button or loose pullover shirts and sweaters, loose-fitting dress, clip-on tie, a cape instead of a coat)	
	Minimize fastener frustration: use Velcro, elastic, zippers, large buttons	
	Use assistive devices: dressing stick, reacher, long-handled shoehorn, elastic shoelaces, sock aid	
Job	Modify work schedule, location, tasks, or equipment	Identify a job that offers flexibility of hours and allows for graded tasks
	Develop skills in areas for employment that require less physical activity	Find work that is satisfying and mentally challenging
	Increase value to employer and colleagues by identifying one's unique and creative contributions to the work setting	Develop collegial relationships that promote effective interdependence and helpfulness
	Use rights granted under the Americans with Disabilities Act (1990), which requires that employers make reasonable accommodations for workers with identified disabilities	
Shopping	Prepare a shopping list arranged by the order in which items are found in the store	Stores are increasingly aware of the needs of older and disabled shoppers; get to know local retail personnel so that they will know your needs
	Use a shopping cart or motorized scooter	Be aware of your rights under the Americans with Disabilities Act for access to public services
	Shop frequently for fewer items or have assistance managing bags to the car and into the house	

Continued

TABLE 13-7 Modifications for Specific Activities—cont'd

Activity	Modifications	Prevention and Safety
	Have grocery bags packed with items to be refrigerated or frozen together so that they can be put away at home first, allowing a rest before the other bags need unpacking	
	Have bags packed light	
	Buy items in smaller containers and condensed forms such as frozen juice	
	Shop at times when the stores are not crowded and lines are short	
Golf	Plan optimal time of day for play, based on energy level and congestion at the golf course	Have a call system if out alone
	Use assistive devices: golf cart, wheeled club carrier	
	Hire a caddy	
	Find a course with rest benches	
	Play every other hole or nine holes	
	Have partner drive the ball and you putt	
Sexual intercourse	Identify times when rested, relaxed, and not hurried	Recognize that all individuals are sexual beings and accept one's desires for intimacy and sexual engagement
	Set temperature, ventilation, and humidity for comfort	Seek information about any sexual restrictions that may apply to medical condition
	Have an empty stomach	Open dialog with sexual partner about desires, physical limitations, and strategies for engaging in intercourse
	Use pillows for support	Recognize that the respiratory rate may increase with sexual response
	Seek position with minimal energy expenditure, such as side lying	
	Avoid positions that put pressure on chest or diaphragm	
	Maintain some awareness of breathing patterns so strategies can be used as needed, trying not to let that conscious attention to breathing detract from sexual engagement	

mentioning how many were generated by the group. The focus is shifted to how these principles can be generalized to new occupations and situations. Participants are given resources to obtain equipment, services, or support groups. In closing, participants are commended for their independent problem-solving and willingness to engage in the process of peer learning and support.

The aforementioned sequence is offered as a general guideline, as each therapeutic group is of course unique. A group may need to spend considerable time on a key issue, such as how to explain an invisible disability to others, the importance of having fun each day, or coping with anxiety. The occupational therapist must trust the group's ability to identify the most salient topics, facilitating a positive, problem-solving atmosphere. Participants may also vary a great deal in the amount of personal information they are comfortable sharing. Some may find the group a safer context for disclosing difficulties compared with individual sessions. Although it should not be assumed that verbal engagement is an indicator of learning, it is wise to follow up after the group session with persons who seem particularly quiet, angry, or sad. Subsequent individual sessions may be arranged for patients whose questions and problems cannot be addressed sufficiently in the group format. Issues that arise in the group can be shared with the interdisciplinary team to learn how best to assist the patient.

Occupational project groups are organized, as the name suggests, around an occupational project of the group's choosing. An effective format is to have projects that are 1 week in duration. In these groups, participants decide on a fairly substantial project—usually involving travel outside of the health care facility—that will be planned, enacted, and then reviewed over the course of six consecutive group sessions. An important part of the projects is their inclusion of family and important others as well as access to the community. For example, completed weeklong occupational projects in the authors' experiences have included organizing a food drive for a local homeless shelter, putting on a magic show for family and hospital staff, organizing a potluck dinner for family and significant others, shopping in malls, eating at restaurants, and visiting flea markets and museums. In a 6-day per week schedule, these projects were determined on a Monday, planned Tuesday through Thursday, enacted on Friday, and reviewed on Saturday. Tasks related to the project address individual treatment goals and can be carried over into individual therapy sessions. For example, preparing a food item for the potluck meal becomes a vehicle for learning energy conservation and breathing strategies. Tasks can also consist of "practice homework" outside of therapy sessions, as when patients make phone calls to determine distance demands of the upcoming event or work on pursed lips breathing when posting flyers announcing the event. Typically, the event itself requires a longer session and, in the authors' experience, is especially rich—for patients and therapists alike—when it involves multiple members of the interdisciplinary team.

Documentation of Intervention

Whether describing short- or long-term goals, narrative accounts of responses to intervention, or functional status at discharge, documentation of occupational therapy services is required at the level of occupational performance, and not impairments. Accordingly, relevant physiologic, musculoskeletal, or cognitive impairments, manifested as dyspnea, increased heart rate, reduced O_2 saturation levels and range of motion, or lack of problem-solving skills, are objectively described in the context of occupational performance. As important, in terms of documenting functional status in the ICF[1] dimensions of activities and participation, are (1) adaptive strategies or modified activity approaches that promote performance of valued activities, (2) environmental adaptations that reduce the physical demands of

valued activities, (3) occupational plans that enable a richer round of personally satisfying activities, (4) social influences on occupational performance, and (5) subjective experiences of occupational performance. Documentation by the occupational therapist is valuable to communicate with the pulmonary rehabilitation team the patient's goals and planned treatment program. This documentation also allows the other disciplines of physical and respiratory therapy to not duplicate services but expand on other areas of occupational importance.

CONCLUSION

The purpose of occupational therapy in pulmonary rehabilitation is to help persons learn how to do the necessary and also spirit-enhancing occupations of their lives in ways that promote greater functional capacities and life satisfaction.[79] Occupational therapists thus strive to improve function in ways that directly enhance HRQL and promote a sense of control over symptoms that would limit their engagement with life. A multidimensional functional assessment determines status regarding the dimensions of social participation, activity performance, and body functions and structures. To obtain outcomes of improved participation in meaningful life occupations, individualized programs target the particular occupational issues and concerns of individual patients and their important others. As the link between health and participation in meaningful occupations becomes clearer, occupational therapists will increase in availability and visibility on comprehensive pulmonary rehabilitation teams.

References

1. World Health Organization: International Classification of Functioning, Disability and Health (ICF). Available at http://www.who.int/classifications/icf/en/. Retrieved January 2008.
2. Clark F, Wood W, Larson E: Occupational science: occupational therapy's legacy for the 21st century. In Neistadt ME, Crepeau EB, editors: Willard and Spackman's occupational therapy, ed 9, Philadelphia, 1998, Lippincott, p 13.
3. American Association of Cardiovascular and Pulmonary Rehabilitation: Selection and assessment of the pulmonary rehabilitation candidate, Guidelines for pulmonary rehabilitation programs, ed 3, Champaign, Ill, 2004, Human Kinetics, pp 11-20.

4. Lorenzi CM, Cilione C, Rizzardi R et al: Occupational therapy and pulmonary rehabilitation of disabled COPD patients, Respiration 71:246-251, 2004.

5. Jackson J, Carlson M, Mandel D et al: Occupation in lifestyle redesign: the Well Elderly Study occupational therapy program, Am J Occup Ther 52:326, 1998.

6. Chan SCC: Chronic obstructive pulmonary disease and engagement in occupation, Am J Occup Ther 58:408-415, 2004.

7. Muldoon MF, Barger SD, Flory JD et al: What are quality of life measurements measuring? BMJ 316:542, 1998.

8. Robnett RH, Gliner JA: Qual-OT: a quality of life assessment tool, Occup Ther J Res 15:198, 1995.

9. Jette A: Using health-related quality of life measures in physical therapy outcomes research, Phys Ther 73:528, 1993.

10. Ries AL, Bauldoff GS, Carlin BW et al: Pulmonary rehabilitation: joint ACCP/AACVPR evidence-based clinical practice guidelines, Chest 131:4S-42S, 2007.

11. Donner CF, Muir JF: Rehabilitation and Chronic Care Scientific Group of the European Respiratory Society: Selection criteria and programmes for pulmonary rehabilitation in COPD patients, Eur Respir J 10:744-757, 1997.

12. Nici L, Donner C, Wouters E et al: American Thoracic Society/European Respiratory Society statement on pulmonary rehabilitation, Am J Respir Crit Care Med 173:1390-1413, 2006.

13. Rodrigues JC, Ilowite JS: Pulmonary rehabilitation in the elderly patient, Clin Chest Med 14:429, 1993.

14. Rashbaum I, Whyte N: Occupational therapy in pulmonary rehabilitation: energy conservation and work simplification techniques, Phys Med Rehabil Clin N Am 7:325, 1996.

15. Clark F, Azen S, Zemke R et al: Occupational therapy for independent-living older adults: a randomized controlled study, JAMA 278:1321, 1997.

16. Yerxa E: Health and the human spirit for occupation, Am J Occup Ther 52:412, 1998.

17. Hasselkus E: Occupation and well-being in dementia: the experience of day care staff, Am J Occup Ther 52:423, 1998.

18. Jackson J: The value of occupation as the core of treatment: Sandy's experience, Am J Occup Ther 52:466, 1998.

19. Kane RA, Caplan AL, Urv-Wong EK et al: Everyday matters in the lives of nursing home residents: wish for and perception of choice and control, J Am Geriatr Soc 45:1093, 1997.

20. Browne JP, Hannah MM, O'Boyle CA: Conceptual approaches to the assessment of quality of life, Psychol Health 12:737, 1997.

21. Radomski MV: Nationally speaking: there is more to life than putting on your pants, Am J Occup Ther 49:487, 1995.

22. DeJong B: Independent living: from social movement to analytic paradigm, Arch Phys Med Rehabil 60:435, 1979.

23. American Occupational Therapy Association: Uniform terminology for occupational therapy, Am J Occup Ther 48:1047, 1994.

24. Occupational Therapy Practice Framework: domain and process, Am J Occup Ther 56:609-639, 2002.

25. Law M: Client-centered occupational therapy, Thorofare, NJ, 1998, Slack, p 25.

26. Egan M, Dubouloz CJ, von Zweck C et al: The client-centred, evidence-based practice of occupational therapy, Can J Occup Ther 65:136, 1998.

27. Law M, Baum C, Dunn W, editors: Measuring occupational performance: supporting best practice in occupational therapy, Vol 2, Thorofare, NJ, 2005, Slack.

28. Trombly CA: Anticipating the future: assessment of occupational function, Am J Occup Ther 47:253, 1993.

29. Klein BS: Slow dance: a story of stroke, love and disability, Toronto, 1997, Alfred A. Knopf Canada.

30. Coster WJ, Deeny T, Haltiwanger J et al: The School Function Assessment: standardized version. Boston, 1998, Boston University Press.

31. Coster W: Occupation-centered assessment of children, Am J Occup Ther 52:337, 1998.

32. Jette AM, Davies AR, Cleary PD et al: The Functional Status Questionnaire: reliability and validity when used in primary care, J Gen Intern Med 1:143-149, 1986 [published erratum appears in J Gen Intern Med 1986;1:427].

33. Sandland CJ, Singh SJ, Curcio A et al: A profile of daily activity in chronic obstructive pulmonary disease, J Cardiopulm Rehabil 25:181-183, 2005.

34. Baum MC, Edwards DF: The Washington University Activity Card Sort. San Antonio, Tx, 2001, Harcourt Assessment.

35. Corcoran M, Gitlin L: The role of the physical environment in occupational performance. Occupational therapy: enabling function and well-being, Thorofare, NJ, 1997, Slack, p 336.

36. McColl MA: Social support and occupational therapy. In Occupational therapy: enabling function and well-being, Thorofare, NJ, 1997, Slack, p 410.

37. Pitta F, Troosters T, Spruit MA et al: Characteristics of physical activities in daily life in chronic obstructive pulmonary disease, Am J Respir Crit Care Med 171:972-977, 2005.

38. Kohlmeyer K: Evaluation of sensory and neuromuscular performance components. In Neistadt ME, Crepeau EB, editors: Willard and Spackman's occupational therapy, ed 9, Philadelphia, 1998, Lippincott, p 223.

39. Atchison B: Cardiopulmonary diseases. In Trombly CA, editor: Occupational therapy for physical dysfunction, ed 4, Baltimore, 1995, Williams & Wilkins, p 875.

40. Brannon FJ, Foley MW, Starr JA et al: Cardiopulmonary rehabilitation: basic theory and application, ed 2, Philadelphia, 1993, F.A. Davis.

41. Trombly CA: Cardiopulmonary rehabilitation. In Trombly CA, editor: Occupational therapy for physical dysfunction, ed 3, Baltimore, 1989, Williams & Wilkins.

42. Crepeau EB: Activity analysis: a way of thinking about occupational performance. In Neistadt ME, Crepeau EB, editors: Willard and Spackman's

occupational therapy, ed 9, Philadelphia, 1998, Lippincott, p 135.

43. Minor MA: Promoting health and physical fitness. In Christianson C, Baum C, editors: Occupational therapy: enabling function and well-being, Thorofare, NJ, 1997, Slack, pp 256-287.

44. Berry MJ, Walschalger SA: Exercise training and chronic obstructive pulmonary disease: past and future research directions, J Cardiopulm Rehabil 18:181, 1998.

45. Celli BR: The clinical use of upper extremity exercise, Clin Chest Med 15:339, 1994.

46. Boissoneau CA: Breath of life: occupational therapy with ventilator assisted and pulmonary patients in a rehabilitation program, OT Practice 2:28-34, 1997.

47. Hogan BM: Pulse oximetry for an adult with a pulmonary disorder, Am J Occup Ther 49:1062, 1994.

48. Borg GA: Psychophysical bases of perceived exertion, Med Sci Sports Exerc 14:377, 1982.

49. Sewell L, Singh SJ, Williams JE et al: Can individualized rehabilitation improve functional independence in elderly patients with COPD? Chest 128:1194-1200, 2005.

50. UDS Data Management Service: Guide for the uniform data set for medical rehabilitation (adult FIM), version 4.0, Buffalo, NY, 1993, State University of New York at Buffalo.

51. Msall ME, DiGaudio K, Duffy LC et al: WeeFIM: normative sample of an instrument for tracking functional independence in children, Clin Pediatr 44:431, 1994.

52. Fisher A: The assessment of instrumental activities of daily living motor skill: an application of the many-faceted Rasch analysis, Am J Occup Ther 47:319, 1993.

53. Duncan EA: Foundations for practice in occupational therapy, ed 4, Edinburgh, Churchill Livingstone, 2005.

54. Davis S: Rehabilitation: the use of theories and models in practice, Edinburgh, Churchill Livingstone, 2005.

55. Health Care Financing Administration, Department of Health and Human Services: Medical review of part B intermediary outpatient occupational therapy (OT) bills (DHHS transmittal No. 1424), Washington DC, U.S. Government Printing Office, 1989.

56. Corsello PR: Selection and assessment of the chronic respiratory disease patient for pulmonary rehabilitation. In Hodgkin JE, Celli BR, Connors JL, editors: Pulmonary rehabilitation: guidelines to success, ed 3, Philadelphia, 2000, Lippincott, p 31.

57. Walsh LR: Occupational therapy as part of a pulmonary rehabilitation program. In Occupational therapy in health care, vol. 3, No. 1: Occupational therapy for the energy deficient patient, New York, 1986, Hayworth Press, p 65.

58. Bowyer SL, LaMothe ML, Hollister JR: Steroid myopathy: incidence and detection in a population with asthma, J Allergy Clin Immunol 76:234, 1985.

59. Strunk RE, Mascia AV, Lipkowitz MA et al: Rehabilitation of a patient with asthma in the outpatient setting, J Allergy Clin Immunol 87:601, 1991.

60. ATS Committee on Proficiency Standards for Clinical Pulmonary Function Laboratories: ATS statement: guidelines for the six-minute walk test, Am J Respir Crit Care Med 166:111-117, 2002.

61. Fisher A: Uniting practice and theory in an occupational framework: 1998 Eleanor Clark Slagle lecture, Am J Occup Ther 52:509, 1998.

62. American Association of Cardiovascular and Pulmonary Rehabilitation: Patient education and skills training. In Guidelines for pulmonary rehabilitation programs, ed 3, Champaign, Ill, 2004, Human Kinetics, pp 21-29.

63. Lin K, Wu C, Tickle-Degnan L et al: Enhancing occupational performance through occupationally embedded exercise: a meta-analytic review, Occup Ther J Res 17:25, 1997.

64. Dunn AL, Marcus BH, Kampert JB et al: Comparison of lifestyle and structured interventions to increase physical activity and cardiorespiratory fitness, JAMA 281:327, 1999.

65. Gray JM: Putting occupation into practice: occupation as ends, occupation as means, Am J Occup Ther 52:354, 1998.

66. Clark F: Occupation embedded in real life: interweaving occupational science and occupational therapy: 1993 Eleanor Clarke Slagle lecture, Am J Occup Ther 47:1067, 1993.

67. Holm MB, Rogers JC, Stone RG: Person–task environment interventions: decision-making guide. In Neistadt ME, Crepeau EB, editors: Willard and Spackman's occupational therapy, ed 9, Philadelphia, 1998, Lippincott, p 471.

68. Wood W, editor: Special issue: occupation-centered practice and education, Am J Occup Ther 52:313-496, 1998.

69. Pierce D: The issue is: what is the source of occupation's treatment power? Am J Occup Ther 52:490, 1998.

70. Breslin EH: The pattern of respiratory muscle recruitment during pursed-lips breathing in COPD, Chest 101:75, 1992.

71. Breslin EH: Breathing retraining in chronic obstructive pulmonary disease, J Cardiopulm Rehabil 15:25, 1995.

72. Tiep BL, Burns M, Kao D et al: Pursed lips breathing training using ear oximetry. Chest 90:218-221, 1986.

73. Spahija J, de Marchie M, Grassino A: Effects of imposed pursed-lips breathing on respiratory mechanics and dyspnea at rest and during exercise in COPD. Chest 128:640-650, 2005.

74. Bianchi R, Gigliotti F, Romagnoli I et al: Chest wall kinematics and breathlessness during pursed-lip breathing in patients with COPD, Chest 125:459-465, 2004.

75. Berzins GF: An occupational therapy program for the chronic obstructive pulmonary disease patient, Am J Occup Ther 24:81, 1970.

76. Ludwig FM: The unpackaging of routine in older women, Am J Occup Ther 52:168, 1998.

77. Velloso M, Jardim JR: Study of energy expenditure during activities of daily living using and not using body position recommended by energy conservation techniques in patients with COPD, Chest 130:126-132, 2006.
78. Schwartzberg SL: Group process. In Neistadt ME, Crepeau EB, editors: Willard and Spackman's occupational therapy, ed 9, Philadelphia, 1998, Lippincott, p 120.
79. Kaplan RM, Ries AL: Quality of life as an outcome measure in pulmonary diseases, J Cardiopulm Rehab 25:321-331, 2005.

Chapter 14

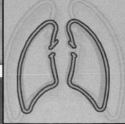

Nutritional Assessment and Support

ANNEMIE SCHOLS

CHAPTER OUTLINE

Rationale for Nutritional Support
Nutritional Assessment
  Weight Indices
  Weight Loss
  Body Composition
Causes of Weight Loss and Muscle Wasting
  Energy and Substrate Metabolism
  Dietary Intake

Nutritional Intervention to Maintain or Improve Energy Balance
Muscle Atrophy
Muscle Metabolism
Practical Implementation of Nutritional Support

PROFESSIONAL SKILLS

On completion of this chapter, the reader will be able to
do the following:
- Know how to assess nutritional status in chronic obstructive pulmonary disease (COPD)
- Know the effects of weight loss and muscle wasting in COPD on physical performance, morbidity, and mortality
- Have insight into the causes of a negative energy balance and a negative protein balance
- Be able to position the various strategies to improve nutritional status in COPD

The association between weight loss and chronic obstructive pulmonary disease (COPD) has been recognized since the late 19th century. In the 1960s several studies already reported that a low body weight and weigh loss are negatively associated with survival in COPD.[1] Nevertheless, therapeutic management of weight loss and muscle wasting in patients with COPD has gained interest only more recently because it was generally considered as a terminal progression in the disease process and therefore inevitable and irreversible. Furthermore, weight loss has even been suggested as an adaptive mechanism to decrease oxygen (O_2) consumption. Studies have challenged this attitude and showed that weight loss and muscle wasting are associated with poor prognosis independent of, or at least not closely correlated with, the degree of lung function impairment.[2,3] Moreover, in advanced COPD, weight gain after nutritional support was associated with decreased mortality.[4]

The renewed interest in nutritional support as therapy in COPD runs parallel to changing concepts in the disease management, not only aiming predominantly at the primary organ failure but also at the systemic consequences of the disease including skeletal muscle weakness and wasting.

RATIONALE FOR NUTRITIONAL SUPPORT

The most prominent symptoms of COPD are dyspnea and impaired exercise capacity. Research has shown that besides airflow obstruction and loss of alveolar structure, skeletal muscle weakness is an important determinant of these symptoms.[5] Peripheral skeletal muscle dysfunction is partly determined by skeletal muscle wasting in COPD and partly by decreased muscle oxidative metabolism.[5] Muscle mass is a strong predictor of muscle strength and, indeed, patients with COPD and muscle wasting were characterized by more pronounced muscle weakness compared with nondepleted patients.[6] Several studies have also shown that body weight and, in particular, fat-free mass (FFM), an indirect measure of muscle mass, are significant determinants of cycle exercise capacity and exercise response.[7,8] Patients with depleted FFM were characterized by lower peak O_2 consumption, a lower peak work rate, and early onset of lactic acid compared with non-depleted patients. These findings suggest that the functional consequences of nutritional depletion relate not only to muscle wasting per se, but also to alterations in muscle morphology and metabolism. Muscle wasting specifically affects muscle fiber type II cross-sectional area in COPD.[9] Furthermore, studies in other diseases and experimental models have shown altered levels of glycolytic and oxidative enzymes[10,11] and depletion of energy-rich substrates such as phosphocreatine and glycogen[12,13] after hypoenergetic feeding. Nutritional depletion not only decreases peripheral muscle mass and function, but also affects respiratory muscle mass and strength.[14] The functional consequences of depletion of FFM are furthermore reflected in decreased health status as measured by the disease-specific St. George's Respiratory Questionnaire.[15]

Weight loss is a predictor for outcome of acute exacerbations as illustrated by an increased risk for nonelective hospital readmission[16] among patients who had experienced weight loss during or immediately after recovery from a severe acute exacerbation. Furthermore, a longitudinal study revealed that frequent exacerbators were characterized by a greater decline in FFM than infrequent exacerbators.[17] In different COPD populations with varying disease severity, a low body mass index (BMI) and weight loss were associated with an increased mortality risk.[2,4] After adjustment for the effect of age, gender, smoking, and resting lung function, a cutoff point for BMI of 25 kg/m² was identified below which mortality risk was substantially increased.[4] Remarkably, overweight patients with moderate to severe COPD even had a lower mortality risk than normal-weight patients.[2,4] This could be explained by the fact that depletion of FFM is not only associated with weight loss, but so-called hidden loss of FFM may also occur in normal-weight patients with a relatively increased fat mass. Indeed, studies of various COPD populations have consistently shown that FFM is a predictor of mortality in COPD independent of BMI.[18,19]

NUTRITIONAL ASSESSMENT

On the basis of the relationship between nutritional status and outcome, the following screening measures of nutritional status are recommended (Figure 14-1).

Weight Indices

On the basis of BMI, patients can be characterized as underweight, normal weight, and overweight. Underweight is normally defined as a body mass index less than 20 kg/m².[20]

Weight Loss

There are limitations to weight for height indices. Underweight patients are not necessarily in a poor nutritional state. This was illustrated for patients with COPD by the fact that underweight patients with a relative preservation of FFM had comparable muscle strength and exercise performance as normal-weight subjects with a normal FFM.[21] The adverse effects of involuntary weight loss, however, are well described, and progressive weight loss will ultimately lead to underweight and depletion of FFM. Therefore recent involuntary weight loss should be considered in nutritional screening and followed up, particularly for patients with a BMI less than 25 kg/m².[4] Commonly used criteria include weight loss greater than 10% of usual body weight in the past 6 months or greater than 5% in the past month.

Body Composition

Weight is a rather global measure of nutritional depletion because it does not take body composition into consideration. Weight can be simply divided into fat mass and FFM. The FFM consists of water (approximately 73%), protein, and minerals. Water is distributed intracellularly in the body cell

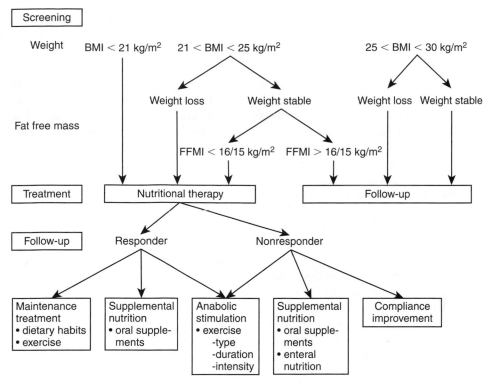

FIGURE 14-1 Flowchart: nutritional screening and therapy. BMI, body mass index; FFMI, fat-free mass index.

mass and extracellularly. The largest single tissue of the body cell mass is muscle mass. In the absence of shifts between the water compartments, FFM is a useful measure of the body cell mass and thus of muscle mass. Depletion of FFM in COPD is defined as an FFM less than 16 kg/m² (males) or 15 kg/m² (females). This value is based on a linear gender-specific relationship between FFM and body weight (in the absence of obesity), using a cutoff point for the BMI of 21 kg/m². One study suggests that the value for male patients may be very strict and could be elevated to 17 kg/m².[19] On the basis of measurement of body weight and FFM, patients with COPD can be classified in three wasting categories: (1) cachexia: underweight and low FFM; (2) semistarvation: underweight and relative preservation of FFM; (3) sarcopenia: normal weight and depletion of FFM. From a diagnostic perspective body composition analysis is of particular importance to diagnose sarcopenia, because the proportion of underweight stable patients with COPD who are experiencing semistarvation appears to be low, particularly in advanced disease.

Bioelectrical impedance analysis is a relatively easy, inexpensive, and noninvasive method to assess FFM and has been used and validated

extensively in COPD.[21,22] Dual-energy x-ray absorptiometry allows measurement of lean tissue mass, bone, and fat mass not only at the whole body level, but also at the various regions (trunk, arm, leg).[23]

In clinically stable patients with moderate to severe COPD, depletion of FFM has been reported in 20% of outpatients[24] and in 35% of those eligible for pulmonary rehabilitation.[25] There is no clear relationship between measures of nutritional status and airflow obstruction, but weight loss per se and underweight are associated with decreased diffusing capacity and are observed more frequently in patients with emphysema than in patients with chronic bronchitis.[26] The difference in body weight between the two COPD subtypes is merely a difference in fat mass and is responsive to therapies targeted at reducing the adverse effects of hyperinflation (i.e., lung volume reduction surgery and noninvasive ventilation).

CAUSES OF WEIGHT LOSS AND MUSCLE WASTING

To be able to judge the need for and the effectiveness of nutritional therapy, as well as the optimal nutritional support strategy, insight is needed into the underlying mechanisms and factors contributing to overall weight loss and specific tissue wasting in COPD. Weight loss and, in particular, loss of fat mass occur if energy expenditure exceeds dietary intake. Loss of muscle mass is a complex process involving changes in the control of substrate and protein metabolism as well as changes in muscle cell turnover. Impaired protein metabolism may result in muscle atrophy when protein degradation exceeds protein synthesis. Few studies have yet examined protein metabolism in patients with COPD. There are indications that cachectic patients with COPD are characterized by accelerated protein breakdown, but this is unclear for sarcopenic patients with COPD.[27,28] At the cellular level, increased apoptosis of muscle cells has been demonstrated in the skeletal muscle of severely cachectic patients with COPD, whereas this observation was not confirmed in a sarcopenic group.[29,30] This could implicate involvement of different mechanisms in loss of muscle mass in the absence or presence of weight loss, subsequently requiring different therapeutic strategies.

Energy and Substrate Metabolism

Total energy expenditure can be divided into different components. The basal metabolic rate is usually the largest component of total energy expenditure. Physical activity–induced thermogenesis can vary substantially between different individuals. Other components of total energy expenditure include diet-induced thermogenesis, drug-induced thermogenesis, and thermoregulation. By measuring gas exchange in patients under awake, relaxed conditions after an overnight fast, it is possible to conveniently measure the so-called resting energy expenditure (REE). The REE comprises the sleeping basal metabolic rate and the energy cost of arousal.

On the basis of the assumption that the REE is the major component of total energy expenditure in sedentary persons, several studies have measured the REE in COPD. After adjustment for the metabolically active FFM, the REE was found to be elevated in COPD.[31] Whereas in healthy control subjects FFM could explain up to 84% of the individual variation in REE, in patients with COPD, FFM could account for only 43%.[31] Other factors therefore have been considered, such as work of breathing, hormone levels, drug therapy, and inflammation. A likely but difficult-to-measure cause of the increased

metabolic rate in patients with COPD is the increasing respiratory muscle work, because the energy cost of increasing ventilation is higher in patients with advanced disease than in healthy control subjects of comparable age and gender.

Maintenance bronchodilating treatment for many patients consists of inhaled β-agonists. Two weeks of salbutamol increased REE by less than 8% in healthy males.[32] Acute inhalations of clinical doses of salbutamol, on the other hand, have been shown to increase the REE in healthy subjects in a dose-dependent way up to 20%.[33] High doses of nebulized salbutamol are commonly administered during acute disease exacerbations.

Systemic inflammation may also contribute to hypermetabolism and increased protein turnover. Several studies provided clear evidence for the involvement of C-reactive protein and markers of the tumor necrosis factor (TNF) system in the pathogenesis of tissue depletion. Elevated levels of TNF-α in (stimulated) plasma and of soluble TNF receptors were found in patients with COPD,[34,35] particularly those experiencing weight loss. Furthermore, several studies showed a relationship between C-reactive protein and resting metabolic rate.[36,37] Despite methodologic difficulties in measuring total daily energy expenditure, several studies focused attention on the activity-related energy expenditure in patients with COPD. Using the doubly labeled water ($^2H_2O^{18}$) technique to measure total daily energy expenditure (TDE), it was demonstrated that some patients with COPD have a significantly higher TDE compared with healthy subjects.[38,39] The cause of an increased activity-related TDE is yet unclear but could be related to the observed decreased mechanical efficiency during leg exercise.[40] Part of this increased O_2 consumption during exercise can be explained by inefficient ventilation during increased ventilatory demand, especially under conditions of dynamic hyperinflation. Furthermore, impaired oxidative phosphorylation during exercise in COPD may contribute, because anaerobic metabolism is less efficient than aerobic metabolism.

Besides impaired oxidative phosphorylation during exercise, studies have also shown decreased muscle oxidative capacity in patients with moderate to severe COPD,[41,42] resulting from a shift in muscle fibers from type I (oxidative) to type II (glycolytic) fibers.[43] In addition, the oxidative capacity within intermediary type IIa fibers is also reduced.[44] Peroxisome proliferator–activated receptors (PPARs) are key regulators of mitochondrial biogenesis and hence of skeletal muscle oxidative capacity. More specifically, they are involved in the regulation of proteins implicated in the uptake, handling, and oxidation of fatty acids,[45] but the clinical implications are yet unclear. PPAR expression is reduced in the skeletal muscle of patients with COPD.[45]

Limited data are available regarding carbohydrate and fat metabolism in COPD. These data are needed to judge whether specific nutrients may modulate the regulation of fatty acid metabolism and in this way improve oxidative metabolism at rest or in response to exercise. This in turn may aid in maintaining energy balance and optimizing body composition, and may also provide supportive therapy during rehabilitation to improve exercise capacity.

Dietary Intake

Hypermetabolism can explain why some patients with COPD lose weight despite an apparent normal to even high dietary intake.[46] Nevertheless, it has been shown that dietary intake in weight-losing patients is lower than in weight-stable patients both in absolute terms and in relation to the measured REE.[46] This is quite remarkable because the normal adaptation to an increase in energy requirements in healthy men is an increase in dietary intake. The reasons for a relatively low dietary intake in COPD are not completely understood. It has been suggested that patients with COPD eat suboptimally because chewing and swallowing change breathing pattern and decrease arterial O_2 saturation. Furthermore, gastric filling in these patients may reduce the functional residual capacity and lead to an increase in dyspnea. The role of leptin in energy homeostasis is intriguing. This adipocyte-derived hormone represents the afferent hormonal signal to the brain in a feedback mechanism regulating fat mass. In addition, leptin has a regulatory role in lipid metabolism and glucose homeostasis, and increases thermogenesis. Furthermore, leptin has effects on T cell–mediated immunity. Few data have been reported on leptin metabolism in COPD. Circulating leptin correlates well with BMI and fat percentage, as expected, but significantly lower values were observed compared with healthy subjects.[47] In experimental studies administration of endotoxins or cytokines produced a prompt increase in serum leptin levels.[48] In patients with COPD a positive association was demonstrated between leptin and soluble TNF-receptor 55 in emphysematous patients as well as during acute exacerbations.[49,50] Leptin as well as soluble TNF-receptor 55 were in turn inversely related to dietary intake in absolute terms as well as when adjusted for the REE.[49,50] The exact regulation of leptin in COPD needs further exploration. Another factor of interest in evaluating dietary intake is the influence of psychological dysfunctioning such as anxiety, depression, and appetite. Although no systematic studies are available, limited physical abilities, financial constraints, and lack of supportive care should also be considered as factors that may interfere with dietary intake.

NUTRITIONAL INTERVENTION TO MAINTAIN OR IMPROVE ENERGY BALANCE

The first clinical trials to investigate the effectiveness of nutritional intervention consisted of nutritional supplementation by means of oral liquid supplements. All short-term studies (2 to 3 weeks)[50,51] showed a significant increase in body weight and respiratory muscle function. This short-term effectiveness is probably related partly to repletion of muscle water and potassium besides reconstitution of muscle protein nitrogen.[52] Only one study addressed the immune response to short-term nutritional intervention in nine patients with advanced COPD.[53] Refeeding and weight gain were associated with a significant increase in absolute lymphocyte count and with an increase in reactivity to skin test antigens after 21 days of refeeding.

Significant improvements[54,55] in respiratory and peripheral skeletal muscle function, and also in exercise capacity and health-related quality of life, were observed in one inpatient study and one outpatient study after 3 months of oral supplementation by about 1000 kcal daily. In other outpatient studies, however, despite a similar nutritional supplementation regimen, the average weight gain was less than 1.5 kg in 8 weeks.[56-58] Besides noncompliance and biological characteristics, the poor treatment response may be attributed at least partly to inadequate assessment of energy requirements and to the observation that the patients were taking supplements instead of their regular meals.

Despite the positive outcome of nutritional repletion in a controlled setting, the progressive character of weight loss in COPD demands appropriate feeding strategies to allow sustained outpatient nutritional intervention. To be able to provide a sufficient energy supply the effect of an aggressive nutritional support regimen was studied in patients with severe COPD and weight loss not responding to oral supplementation.[59] Over a prolonged interval of 4 months, nocturnal enteral nutrition support via percutaneous endoscopic gastrostomy tube was provided. The treated group had nightly enteral feeding adjusted to maintain a total daily caloric intake greater than two times the measured resting metabolic rate for sustained weight gain. Despite the magnitude of the intervention, a mean weight gain of only 3.3% (0.2 kg/week) was seen in the treated group. Weight gain appeared to be limited by the magnitude of the required caloric intake and by significant shifting of caloric intake between oral and enteral intake. The majority of the increase in body weight was fat mass, and no significant improvement of physiologic function was observed. The limited therapeutic impact of isolated aggressive nutrition support could be related to the absence of a comprehensive rehabilitative strategy or to the fact that the selected patients were not only in a hypermetabolic state but also hypercatabolic.[60] Other means to improve therapeutic outcome are to tailor nutritional supplementation to physical activity pattern and to decrease the portion size of dietary supplements.[61,62]

From a functional point of view, and perhaps also to stimulate appetite, it is advised to combine nutritional support with exercise if possible. The effects of a daily nutritional supplement as an integrated part of a pulmonary rehabilitation program indeed resulted in significant weight gain (0.4 kg/week), despite a daily supplementation that was much less than in most previous outpatient studies.[60] The combined treatment of nutritional support and exercise not only increased body weight but also resulted in a significant improvement in FFM and respiratory muscle strength. The clinical relevance of treatment response was shown in a post hoc survival analysis of this study demonstrating that weight gain and increase in respiratory muscle strength were associated with significantly increased survival rates.[4] On Cox regression analysis weight gain during the rehabilitation period remained a significant predictor of mortality independent of baseline lung function and other risk factors including age, sex, smoking, and resting arterial blood gases.

Most studies have investigated the effects of nutritional supplementation in clinically stable patients. Anamnestic data, however, indicate that in some patients weight loss follows a stepwise pattern, associated with acute (infectious) exacerbations. During an acute exacerbation energy balance is often temporarily negative because of a further increase in REE, but particularly because of a temporarily dramatic decrease in dietary intake.[63] Furthermore, these patients may have an increased risk for protein breakdown that may limit the effectiveness of nutritional supplementation.[64] Factors contributing to weight loss and muscle wasting during an acute exacerbation include an increase in symptoms, more pronounced systemic inflammation, alterations in leptin metabolism, and the use of high doses of glucocorticoids. Two studies showed positive effects of nutritional support during hospitalization for an acute exacerbation, particularly in the restoration of protein balance.[64,65] More research is needed to evaluate the relative effectiveness of nutritional support during acute exacerbation versus immediately afterward, during the recovery phase.

MUSCLE ATROPHY

Several studies have investigated in patients with COPD the effects of exercise training and pharmacologic anabolic stimuli to promote protein synthesis. Both resistance exercise[66] and a combined strength and endurance exercise approach[67] resulted in gain of muscle mass. Anabolic steroids, testosterone, and growth hormone also showed a variable but overall positive effect on muscle mass.[68-70] These studies illustrate that stimulation of protein synthesis is a feasible therapeutic strategy. Insulin-like growth factor (IGF)-I is an important mediator of anabolic pathways in skeletal muscle cells. Binding of IGF-I to its receptor initiates a signal transduction cascade that promotes mRNA translation and consequently increases protein synthesis. It was shown that high-intensity exercise stimulated muscle IGF-I mRNA and protein expression in COPD. Optimizing protein intake may stimulate protein synthesis per se, but may also enhance the efficacy of anabolic drugs as well as physiologic stimuli such as resistance exercise. Amino acids are the building blocks of protein and several studies have to date reported an abnormal plasma amino acid pattern in COPD. Of interest are the consistently reduced plasma levels of branched-chain amino acids in underweight patients with COPD and in those with low muscle mass.[71] In particular, leucine is an interesting nutritional substrate because it not only serves as a precursor, but also activates IGF-I—mediated signaling pathways that enhance activity and the synthesis of proteins involved in mRNA translocation to up-regulate protein synthesis in skeletal muscle.

The anabolic response after tailored (nutritional) rehabilitation and pharmacologic stimulation is soon reversed when the anabolic stimulus is terminated. Some patients with COPD do not respond at all in terms of improvement of FFM.[72] Muscle wasting in COPD may be the result of a perpetuating systemic inflammatory response, as studies in experimental models have demonstrated cachexia-inducing effects of proinflammatory cytokines such as TNF-α, interleukin-1, and interleukin-6. Furthermore, cross-sectional studies provide evidence for inflammation as a trigger for muscle atrophy, and systemic inflammation appeared to discriminate patients with a poor therapeutic response to a standardized and controlled clinical rehabilitation program from so-called responders.[73] As increased levels of multiple inflammatory mediators have been reported in COPD, the relevant question concerns which of these should be targeted to prevent muscle atrophy in patients with COPD. On the basis of the available data in the literature a logical choice might be to use an anti—TNF-α antibody as a therapeutic agent. A large multicenter trial investigated the effects of infliximab during 24 weeks of treatment, but in general it did not show beneficial effects.[74] Post hoc analysis revealed that subjects who were younger or cachectic showed improvement in 6-minute walk distance. It may, however, be more effective to modulate at a level at which many stimuli of atrophy converge, that is, activation of nuclear factor (NF)-κB in skeletal muscle. Evidence to support such a strategy is provided by studies revealing that NF-κB activation in skeletal muscle is required for the induction of muscle loss by a number of stimulants of atrophy,[75-77] whereas induction of NF-κB specifically in skeletal muscle is sufficient to induce atrophy.[75] Importantly, inactivation of muscular NF-κB was also documented to stimulate muscle differentiation,[75,78,79] promote muscle regeneration, and increase muscle strength.[77] Alternatively, strategies to increase local IGF-I may also exert inflammatory signal—suppressive effects.[80] This strategy would positively modulate muscle mass by overcoming the suppressive effects of inflammation on muscle regeneration, as well as by stimulating muscle growth via IGF-I signaling.

MUSCLE METABOLISM

Positive effects of pulmonary rehabilitation, in particular of endurance exercise training on oxidative enzymes and exercise capacity, illustrate that decreased muscle oxidative capacity in COPD is at least partly reversible. A randomized clinical trial involving patients with COPD participating in a pulmonary rehabilitation program furthermore showed that polyunsaturated fatty acids markedly enhanced exercise capacity compared with placebo.[81] These positive effects might be explained by modulating effects on PPAR content and activity in skeletal muscle, as polyunsaturated fatty acids are natural ligands of the PPARs. Importantly, there is experimental evidence that PPARs can also exert anti-inflammatory effects in airways and muscle cells, thereby not limiting their promising beneficial effects on the pathogenesis of COPD to the extrapulmonary manifestations of the disease, but expanding it to the level of the primary organ dysfunction.[82,83]

PRACTICAL IMPLEMENTATION OF NUTRITIONAL SUPPORT

On the basis of the current insights concerning the relationship between nutritional depletion and outcome in COPD, a flowchart for nutritional screening and therapy is presented. Simple screening can be performed on the basis of repeated measurements of body weight. Patients are characterized by body mass index (BMI = weight/height squared) and the presence or absence of involuntary weight loss. Nutritional supplementation is indicated for underweight patients (BMI <21 kg/m^2). Involuntary weight loss in patients with a BMI less than 25 kg/m^2 should be treated to prevent further deterioration; involuntary weight loss in patients with a BMI greater than 25 kg/m^2 should be monitored to assess whether it is progressive. If possible, measurement of FFM as an indirect measure of muscle mass may provide more detailed screening of patients, because this allows identification of the sarcopenic subgroup that, even despite a normal body weight, should be considered for diet therapy specifically to stimulate protein synthesis. Depending on the underlying cause of the energy imbalance (decreased dietary intake or increased nutritional requirements), initial nutritional therapy may involve adaptations of the dietary behavior and food pattern followed by implementation of nutritional supplements. Nutritional support should be given as energy-dense supplements well divided during the day to avoid loss of appetite and adverse metabolic and ventilatory effects resulting from a high caloric load. When feasible, the patients should be stimulated to follow an exercise program. For the severely disabled cachectic patients unable to perform exercise training, even simple strength maneuvers combined with activities of daily living training and energy conservation techniques may be effective. Exercise not only improves the effectiveness of nutritional therapy, but also stimulates appetite. After 4 to 8 weeks, therapy response can be determined. If weight gain and functional improvement are noted, the caregiver and the patient must decide whether more improvement by a similar strategy is feasible or whether maintenance is the aim. It may then also be worthwhile to add or alter the exercise training program. If the desired response is not noted, it may be necessary to identify compliance issues. If compliance is not the problem, more calories may be needed as supplements or by enteral routes. Screening of nutritional status in relation to functional status can be done by the chest physician during hospitalization for an acute exacerbation or during outpatient follow-up. The chest physician can consult the dietitian for insight concerning the cause and treatment of impaired energy balance in weight-losing subjects and the physiotherapist for the type and intensity of an exercise program. The respiratory nurse or a nutrition therapist can play a valuable role in hospital and home care of patients with chronic lung disease during regular visits or phone calls. They can monitor compliance and the weight course during diet therapy, give advice on meals and nutritional symptoms in the home setting to patient and family, and provide feedback to the other caregivers. Despite an optimal implementation of nutritional therapy as part of an integrated treatment approach to COPD, it should be recognized that even then a subgroup of patients may not reach the intended effect because of an underlying mechanism of weight loss that cannot be reversed simply by caloric supplementation. Potential reversibility by means of specific nutrients (nutriceuticals) or pharmaceuticals will be a major focus of future research in this field.

References

1. Vandenbergh E, Van de Woestijne KP, Gyselen A: Weight changes in the terminal stages of chronic obstructive pulmonary disease, Am Rev Respir Dis 95:556-566, 1967.

2. Wilson DO, Rogers RM, Wright EC et al: Body weight in chronic obstructive pulmonary disease: the National Institutes of Health Intermittent Positive-pressure Breathing Trial, Am Rev Respir Dis 139:1435-1438, 1989.

3. Gray Donald K, Gibbons L, Shapiro SH et al: Nutritional status and mortality in chronic obstructive pulmonary disease, Am J Respir Crit Care Med 153:961-966, 1996.

4. Schols A, Slangen J, Volovics L et al: Weight loss is a reversible factor in the prognosis of chronic obstructive pulmonary disease, Am J Respir Crit Care Med 157:1791-1797, 1998.

5. Skeletal muscle dysfunction in chronic obstructive pulmonary disease. A statement of the American Thoracic Society and European Respiratory Society, Am J Respir Crit Care Med 159:S1-S40, 1999.

6. Bernard S, LeBlanc P, Whittom F et al: Peripheral muscle weakness in patients with chronic obstructive pulmonary disease, Am J Respir Crit Care Med 158:629-634, 1998.

7. Palange P, Forte S, Onorati P et al: Effect of reduced body weight on muscle aerobic capacity in patients with COPD, Chest 114:12-18, 1998.

8. Baarends EM, Schols AM, Mostert R et al: Peak exercise response in relation to tissue depletion in patients with chronic obstructive pulmonary disease, Eur Respir J 10:2807-2813, 1997.

9. Gosker HR, Engelen MP, van Mameren H et al: Muscle fiber type IIX atrophy is involved in the loss of fat-free mass in chronic obstructive pulmonary disease, Am J Clin Nutr 76:113-119, 2002.

10. Russell DM, Walker PM, Leiter LA et al: Metabolic and structural changes in skeletal muscle during hypocaloric dieting, Am J Clin Nutr 39:503-513, 1984.

11. Layman DK, Merdian-Bender M, Hegarty PVJ et al: Changes in aerobic and anaerobic metabolism in rat cardiac and skeletal muscles after total or partial dietary restrictions, J Nutr 111:994-1000, 1981.

12. Pichard C, Vaughan C, Struk R et al: Effect of dietary manipulations (fasting, hypocaloric feeding, and subsequent refeeding) on rat muscle energetics as assessed by nuclear magnetic resonance spectroscopy, J Clin Invest 82:895-901, 1988.

13. Bissonnette DJ, Madapallimatam A, Jeejeebhoy KN: Effect of hypoenergetic feeding and high-carbohydrate refeeding on muscle tetanic tension, relaxation rate, and fatigue in slow- and fast-twitch muscles in rats, Am J Clin Nutr 66:293-303, 1997.

14. Rochester DF, Braun NM: Determinants of maximal inspiratory pressure in chronic obstructive pulmonary disease, Am Rev Respir Dis 132:42-47, 1985.

15. Shoup R, Dalsky G, Warner S et al: Body composition and health-related quality of life in patients with obstructive airways disease, Eur Respir J 10:1576-1580, 1997.

16. Pouw EM, Ten Velde GP, Croonen BH et al: Early non-elective readmission for chronic obstructive pulmonary disease is associated with weight loss, Clin Nutr 19:95-99, 2000.

17. Hopkinson NS, Tennant RC, Dayer MJ et al: A prospective study of decline in fat free mass and skeletal muscle strength in chronic obstructive pulmonary disease, Respir Res 8:25, 2007.

18. Schols AM, Broekhuizen R, Weling-Scheepers CA et al: Body composition and mortality in chronic obstructive pulmonary disease, Am J Clin Nutr 82:53-59, 2005.

19. Vestbo J, Prescott E, Almdal T et al: Body mass, fat-free body mass, and prognosis in patients with chronic obstructive pulmonary disease from a random population sample: findings from the Copenhagen City Heart Study, Am J Respir Crit Care Med 173:79-83, 2006.

20. Evans W, Morley JE, Mitch WE et al: Cachexia and wasting disease: a new definition, Lancet (in press).

21. Schols A, Wouters EFM, Soeters PB et al: Body composition by bioelectrical-impedance analysis compared with deuterium dilution and skinfold anthropometry in patients with chronic obstructive pulmonary disease, Am J Clin Nutr 53:421-424, 1991.

22. Steiner MI, Barton RL, Singh SL et al: Bedside methods versus dual energy X-ray absorptiometry for body composition measurement in COPD, Eur Respir J 19:626-631, 2002.

23. Engelen MPKJ, Schols AMWJ, Heidendal GAK et al: Dual-energy X-ray absorptiometry in the clinical evaluation of body composition and bone mineral density in patients with chronic obstructive pulmonary disease, Am J Clin Nutr 68:1298-1303, 1998.

24. Engelen MPKJ, Schols AMWJ, Baken WC et al: Nutritional depletion in relation to respiratory and peripheral skeletal muscle function in out-patients with COPD, Eur Respir J 7:1793-1797, 1994.

25. Schols AMWJ, Soeters PB, Dingemans AMC et al: Prevalence and characteristics of nutritional depletion in patients with stable COPD eligible for pulmonary rehabilitation, Am Rev Respir Dis 147:1151-1156, 1993.

26. Engelen MPKJ, Schols AMWJ, Lamers RJS et al: Different patterns of chronic tissue wasting among patients with chronic obstructive pulmonary disease, Clin Nutr 18:275-280, 1999.

27. Rutten EP, Franssen FM, Engelen MP et al: Greater whole-body myofibrillar protein breakdown in cachectic patients with chronic obstructive pulmonary disease, Am J Clin Nutr 83:829-834, 2006.

28. Doucet M, Russell A, Leger B: Muscle atrophy and hypertrophy signaling in patients with chronic obstructive pulmonary disease, Am J Respir Crit Care Med 176:261-269, 2007.

29. Agusti AG, Sauleda J, Miralles C: Skeletal muscle apoptosis and weight loss in chronic obstructive pulmonary disease, Am J Respir Crit Care Med 166:485-489, 2002.

30. Gosker HR, Kubat B, Schaart G et al: Myopathological features in skeletal muscle of patients with chronic obstructive pulmonary disease, Eur Respir J 22:280-285, 2003.

31. Creutzberg EC, Schols AM et al: Prevalence of an elevated resting energy expenditure in patients with chronic obstructive pulmonary disease in relation to body composition and lung function, Eur J Clin Nutr 52:396-401, 1998.

32. Wilson SR, Amoroso P, Moxham J et al: Modification of the thermogenic effect of acutely inhaled salbutamol by chronic inhalation in normal subjects, Thorax 48:886-889, 1993.

33. Amoroso P, Wilson SR, Moxham J et al: Acute effects of inhaled salbutamol on the metabolic rate of normal subjects, Thorax 48:882-885, 1993.

34. De Godoy I, Donahoe M, Calhoun WJ et al: Elevated TNF-alpha production by peripheral blood monocytes of weight-losing COPD patients, Am J Respir Crit Care Med 153:633-637, 1996.

35. Di Francia M, Barbier D, Mege JL et al: Tumor necrosis factor-alpha levels and weight loss in chronic obstructive pulmonary disease, Am J Respir Crit Care Med 150:1453-1455, 1994.

36. Schols AMWJ, Buurman WA, Staal van der Brekel AJ et al: Evidence for a relation between metabolic derangements and elevated inflammatory mediators in a subgroup of patients with chronic obstructive pulmonary disease, Thorax 51:819-824, 1996.

37. Broekhuizen R, Wouters EF, Creutzberg EC et al: Elevated CRP levels mark metabolic and functional impairment in advanced COPD, Thorax 61:17-22, 2006.

38. Baarends EM, Schols AM, Pannemans DL et al: Total free living energy expenditure in patients with severe chronic obstructive pulmonary disease, Am J Respir Crit Care Med 155:549-554, 1997.

39. Slinde F, Ellegard L, Gronberg AM: Total energy expenditure in underweight patients with severe chronic obstructive pulmonary disease living at home, Clin Nutr 22:159-165, 2003.

40. Baarends EM, Schols A, Akkermans MA et al: Decreased mechanical efficiency in clinically stable patients with COPD, Thorax 52:981-986, 1997.

41. Maltais F, Simard AA, Simard C et al: Oxidative capacity of the skeletal muscle and lactic acid kinetics during exercise in normal subjects and in patients with COPD, Am J Respir Crit Care Med 153:288-293, 1996.

42. Jakobsson P, Jorfeldt L, Henriksson J: Metabolic enzyme activity in the quadriceps femoris muscle in patients with severe chronic obstructive pulmonary disease, Am J Respir Crit Care Med 151:374-377, 1995.

43. Gosker HR, Zeegers M, Wouters FM et al: Muscle fibre type shifting in the vastus lateralis of patients with COPD is associated with disease severity: a systematic review and meta-analysis, Thorax 62:944-949, 2007.

44. Gosker ERJ, Gosker HR, van Mameren H et al: Skeletal muscle fibre-type shifting and metabolic profile in patients with chronic obstructive pulmonary disease, Eur Respir J 19:617-626, 2002.

45. Remels AH, Schrauwen P, Broekhuizen R et al: Expression and content of PPARs is reduced in skeletal muscle of COPD patients, Eur Respir J 30:245-252, 2007.

46. Schols AM, Soeters PB, Mostert R et al: Energy balance in chronic obstructive pulmonary disease, Am Rev Respir Dis 143:1248-1252, 1991.

47. Takabatake N, Nakamura H, Abes S: Circulating leptin in patients with chronic obstructive pulmonary disease, Am J Respir Crit Care Med 159:1215-1219, 1999.

48. Grunfeld C, Zhao C, Fuller J et al: Endotoxin and cytokines induce expression of leptin, the ob gene product, in hamsters, J Clin Invest 97:2152-2157, 1996.

49. Schols A, Creutzberg E, Buurman W et al: Plasma leptin is related to pro-inflammatory status and dietary intake in patients with COPD, Am J Respir Crit Care Med 160:1220-1226, 1999.

50. Wilson DO, Rogers RM, Sanders MH et al: Nutritional intervention in malnourished patients with emphysema, Am Rev Respir Dis 134:672-677, 1986.

51. Whittaker JS, Ryan CF, Buckley PA et al: The effects of refeeding on peripheral and respiratory muscle function in malnourished chronic pulmonary disease patients, Am Rev Respir Dis 142:283-288, 1990.

52. Russell DM, Prendergast PJ, Darby PL et al: A comparison between muscle function and body composition in anorexia nervosa: the effect of refeeding, Am J Clin Nutr 38:229-237, 1983.

53. Fuenzalida CE, Petty TL, Jones ML et al: The immune response to short-term nutritional intervention in advanced chronic obstructive pulmonary disease, Am Rev Respir Dis 142:49-56, 1990.

54. Rogers RM, Donahoe M, Constatino J: Physiologic effects of oral supplemental feeding in malnourished patients with chronic obstructive pulmonary diseases: a randomized control study, Am Rev Respir Dis 146:1511-1517, 1992.

55. Efthimiou J, Fleming J, Gomes C et al: The effect of supplementary oral nutrition in poorly nourished patients with chronic obstructive pulmonary disease, Am Rev Respir Dis 137:1075-1082, 1988.

56. Otte KE, Ahlburg P, D'Amore F et al: Nutritional repletion in malnourished patients with emphysema, JPEN J Parenter Enteral Nutr 13:152-156, 1989.

57. Knowles JB, Fairbarn MS, Wiggs BJ et al: Dietary supplementation and respiratory muscle performance in patients with COPD, Chest 93:977-983, 1988.

58. Lewis MI, Belman MJ, Dorr Uyemura L: Nutritional supplementation in ambulatory patients with chronic obstructive pulmonary disease, Am Rev Respir Dis 135:1062-1067, 1987.

59. Donahoe M, Mancino J, Costatino J et al: The effect of an aggressive support regimen on body composition in patients with severe COPD and weight loss [abstract], Am J Respir Crit Care Med 149:A313, 1994.

60. Budweiser S, Heinemann F, Meyer K et al: Weight gain in cachectic COPD patients receiving noninvasive positive-pressure ventilation, Respir Care 51:126-132, 2006.

61. Broekhuizen R, Creutzberg EC, Weling-Scheepers CA et al: Optimizing oral nutritional drink supplementation in patients with chronic obstructive pulmonary disease, Br J Nutr 93:965-971, 2005.

62. Goris AHC, Vermeeren MAP, Wouters EFM et al: Energy balance in depleted ambulatory patients with chronic obstructive pulmonary disease: the effect of physical activity and oral nutritional supplementation, Br J Nutr 89:725-729, 2003.

63. Vermeeren MAP, Schols AMWJ, Quaedvlieg FCM et al: The influence of an acute disease exacerbation on the metabolic profile of patients with chronic obstructive pulmonary disease, Clin Nutr 13(Suppl 1):38-39, 1994.

64. Saudny Unterberger H, Martin JG et al: Impact of nutritional support on functional status during an acute exacerbation of chronic obstructive pulmonary disease, Am J Respir Crit Care Med 156:794-799, 1997.

65. Vermeeren MA, Creutzberg EC, Schols AM et al; on behalf of the COSMIC Study Group: Prevalence of nutritional depletion in a large out-patient population of patients with COPD, Respir Med 100:1349-1355, 2006.

66. Bermard S, Whittom F, Leblanc P et al: Aerobic and strength training in patients with chronic obstructive pulmonary disease, Am J Respir Crit Care Med 159:896-901, 1999.

67. Franssen FM, Broekhuizen R, Janssen PP et al: Effects of whole-body exercise training on body composition and functional capacity in normal-weight patients with COPD, Chest 125:2021-2028, 2004.

68. Schols AMWJ, Soeters PB, Mostert R et al: Physiologic effects of nutritional support and anabolic steroids in patients with chronic obstructive pulmonary disease: a placebo-controlled randomized trial, Am J Respir Crit Care Med 152:1268-1274, 1995.

69. Creutzberg EC, Casaburi R: Endocrinological disturbances in chronic obstructive pulmonary disease, Eur Respir J Suppl 46:76s-80s, 2003.

70. Ferreira I, Brooks D, Lacasse Y et al: Nutritional intervention in COPD: a systematic overview, Chest 119:353-363, 2001.

71. Engelen MP, Schols AM: Altered amino acid metabolism in chronic obstructive pulmonary disease: new therapeutic perspective? Curr Opin Clin Nutr Metab Care 6:73-78, 2003.

72. Bolton CE, Broekhuizen R, Ionescu AA et al: Cellular protein breakdown and systemic inflammation are unaffected by pulmonary rehabilitation in COPD, Thorax 62:109-114, 2007.

73. Creutzberg EC, Schols AMWJ, Weling-Scheepers CAPM et al: Characterization of nonresponse to high caloric oral nutritional therapy in depleted patients with chronic obstructive pulmonary disease, Am J Respir Crit Care Med 161:745-752, 2000.

74. Rennard SI, Fogarty C, Kelsen S et al: The safety and efficacy of infliximab in moderate to severe chronic obstructive pulmonary disease, Am J Respir Crit Care Med 175:926-934, 2007.

75. Cai D, Frantz JD, Tawa NE et al: IIKbeta/NF-kappaB activation causes severe muscle wasting in mice, Cell 119:285-298, 2004.

76. Hunter RN, Kandarian SC: Disruption of either Nfkb1 or the Bc13 gene inhibits skeletal muscle atrophy, J Clin Invest 114:1504-1511, 2004.

77. Mourkioti F, Kratsios P, Luedde T et al: Targeted ablation of IIK2 improves skeletal muscle strength, maintains mass and promotes regeneration, J Clin Invest 116:2945-2954, 2006.

78. Guttridge DC, Albanese C, Reuther JY et al: NF-κB controls cell growth and differentiation through transcriptional regulation of cyclin D1, Mol Cell Biol 19:5785-5799, 1999.

79. Langen RC, Schols AM, Kelders MC et al: Inflammatory cytokines inhibit myogenic differentiation through activation of nuclear factor-κB, FASEB J 15:1169-1180, 2001.

80. Pelosi L, Giancinti C, Nardis C et al: Local expression of IGF-1 accelerates muscle regeneration by rapidly modulating inflammatory cytokines and chemokines, FASEB J 21:1393-1402, 2007.

81. Broekhuizen R, Wouters EFM, Creutzberg EC et al: Polyunsaturated fatty acids improve exercise capacity in chronic obstructive pulmonary disease, Thorax 60:376-382, 2005.

82. Birrell MA, Patel HJ, McCluskie K et al: PPAR-gamma agonists as therapy for diseases involving airway neutrophilia, Eur Respir J 24:18-23, 2004.

83. Patel HJ, Belvisi MG, Bishop-Bailey D et al: Activation of peroxisome proliferator-activated receptors in human airway smooth muscle cells has a superior anti-inflammatory profile to corticosteroids: relevance for COPD therapy, J Immunol 170:2663-2669, 2003.

Complementary Alternative Medicine for Patients with Chronic Lung Disease

JAMES A. PETERS • CHERYL D. THOMAS-PETERS

CHAPTER OUTLINE

Botanicals and Herbal Preparations
  Echinacea
  Ginseng
  Astragalus Root
  Boswellia
  Licorice
Nutritional Intervention for the
    Treatment of Chronic Obstructive
    Pulmonary Disease
  Consumption of Fruits and
    Vegetables, and Antioxidants
  Vitamin C
  Antioxidant Supplementation
  Zinc

  Magnesium
  Vitamin D
  Coenzyme Q10
  Omega-3 Fatty Acids
Mind–Body Relaxation and Manual
  Therapies
  Exercise
  Hypogonadism and Muscle Weakness
  Yoga
  Acupressure Therapy
  Manual Therapies
  Biofeedback Treatment for Asthma
Conclusion

PROFESSIONAL SKILLS

On completion of this chapter, the reader will be able
to do the following:
* Define complementary alternative medicine (CAM)
* Recognize the prevalence of CAM use among patients with chronic obstructive pulmonary disease (COPD)
* Identify five botanicals that have been claimed to benefit patients with COPD
* Recognize three benefits of fruit and vegetable intake for patients with COPD
* Discuss antioxidants and select vitamin supplementation advantages for patients with lung disease
* Recognize the emerging role of vitamin D_3 in lung function
* Identify benefits of coenzyme Q10 in the patient with COPD
* Recognize the contributory role of hypogonadism and loss of lean body mass
* Identify one or more benefits patients with COPD may receive from exercise, yoga, acupressure, manual therapy, and biofeedback modalities

The respiratory system is wonderfully unique among all the organ systems. It is responsible for interfacing both with the external environment and the internal environment of the body. Releasing carbon dioxide (CO_2) gas and taking up oxygen (O_2) constitute the most vital function of the body. After only minutes of this process not working, we face death.

Any condition that hinders or affects the free exchange of gas between the blood, lungs, and atmosphere greatly affects the function of other organ systems in the body and the quality of the life one lives. For patients with respiratory disease it is the dyspnea, the work of breathing, the lack of energy, and the overall loss of quality of life that drive them to look for anything that might improve their situation.

Complementary alternative medicine (CAM), also known as "alternative" medicine, includes vitamin, mineral, plant or herbal, naturopathic, and homeopathic preparations and some aromatherapy products.[1] The term includes those treatments for disease or prevention that are considered more "natural" and include most modalities other than prescription medications and surgery.[1] Physicians readily agree with some treatments, such as proper nutrition and exercise, but they typically refer patients to other professionals for further instruction in these modalities. The use of nutritional supplements such as vitamins and minerals is frequent in CAM treatments and is more commonly recognized as reasonable, and thus is not likely to result in opposition. However, research studies have not been supportive of the use of isolated vitamin supplements.[2,3]

Lung function screening, risk factor reduction, early diagnosis, and appropriate medical interventions have greatly improved chronic lung disease outcomes; both patients and health professionals wish to do the most good with the least likelihood of adverse events. However, every medication has side effects, and although many are well tolerated some medications create new health symptoms. The interest in alternative and complementary medicine has continued to expand because it is thought that a more natural approach to treatment is synonymous with better health and fewer side effects. However, despite this perception, health professionals typically wait for clinical trials and evidence-based studies before they are likely to recommend alternative treatments to what is commonly considered current practice guidelines for respiratory conditions. Because there is a paucity of well-based clinical studies on many of the promoted alternative therapies, physicians typically have not pursued these therapies further. The problem is, our patients typically have proceeded with many of the alternative therapies, based on their own reading or health food store recommendations, despite research support.

It is in this setting that we review treatments other than, or in addition to, the well-known and accepted medicines. Patients simply want to feel better. For diseases that do not have cures, but are simply managed, patients and physicians are hopeful and optimistic that better treatments are on the way. There is always the lure that an unknown cure might just be available and if it is promoted as natural, there is no harm in trying it. A survey of patients with chronic obstructive pulmonary disease (COPD) in 2004[1] found that 41% of patients were using some form of CAM, most commonly multivitamins and minerals. It was found that patients used CAM to promote general well-being, to minimize drug side effects, to help compensate for nutritional deficiencies, and to decrease their disease burden. It was noted in this study that safety was more of a concern than efficacy. Other important reasons for use of CAM by patients is that many CAM treatments are more congruent with their own philosophical orientations, beliefs, and values toward health and life.

Patients with chronic and terminal conditions appear to be eager to experiment with different treatment options, including CAM. One survey found that two of five patients with moderate to severe COPD were using CAM preparations in conjunction with their existing treatments.[1] Most people think that CAM treatments are safe because they are natural, which increases their appeal to patients. The concern is that patients with COPD often have multiple comorbidities that require complex medication regimens.[4] The high availability of CAM from health food stores and supermarkets could be a concern for the safety of patients with COPD. The great concern is the potential for adverse events in patients who do not disclose information relating to their intake of CAM preparations to their mainstream health professionals.[1,5] Mainstream health care providers are often uninformed about the use of CAM preparations by their patients. Physicians' knowledge about CAM is often limited, making discussions with patients difficult.[1,6] The Expert Committee on Complementary Medicines in the Health System (Canberra, Australia) recommends that medical practitioners include questions about the use of CAM when taking a patient history, and include CAM in adverse drug reaction reports.[7] Health professionals need to be more accepting of CAM use and increase their basic knowledge about the commonly used CAM preparations. This may help to improve the communication between patients and mainstream health professionals on CAM issues, and potentially improve optimal treatment outcomes.

Table 15-1 summarizes the use of key vitamins, minerals, antioxidants, and botanicals for their possible role in the treatment of patients with COPD. Evidence-based studies were reviewed regarding CAM and COPD. The following sections provide more detail and explanations regarding specific findings about the benefits and the questionable or still unknown benefits of various entities that are used by patients or have been studied to determine efficacy.

BOTANICALS AND HERBAL PREPARATIONS

Echinacea

There are many conflicting studies as to the efficacy of echinacea for respiratory conditions. One study[8] looked at echinacea for the prevention and treatment of the common cold. Researchers did not find that any of the three types of echinacea at 900 mg/day had significant effects on whether volunteers became infected with the cold virus or on the severity or duration of the symptoms among those who developed colds. Critics of this study think that the dosage used was too low.

The Natural Medicines Comprehensive Database does not recommend echinacea because of the lack of clear evidence for prevention or treatment of colds and flu.[9] In 2006, the Cochrane Database of Systematic Reviews published a review of 16 different studies of echinacea for preventing and treating the common cold.[10] Many consumers and physicians are not aware that products available under the term *echinacea* differ appreciably in their composition. This is due

---

TABLE 15-1 Complementary Alternative Medicine Therapies for Patients with Chronic Obstructive Pulmonary Disease

Botanical or Herbal Preparation	Traditional Use	Typical Dosage and Administration
Echinacea: Echinacea root (*Echinacea purpurea*)	Echinacea fresh root (*Echinacea angustifolia, E. purpurea, Echinacea pallida*) is indicated for acute viral or bacterial infection (colds, flu, bronchitis, septicemia, *Streptococcus, Staphylococcus*). Echinacea is also used for acute rhinitis, sinusitis, tonsillitis, otitis media, and laryngitis	Capsules: up to nine 300- to 400-mg capsules per day
Panax ginseng or Asian ginseng (extract G115)	Improves pulmonary function in the treatment of severe, chronic respiratory disease; has an additive effect when combined with antibiotic treatment for respiratory tract infection; strengthens the immune system	Extract (acute): 40 to 60 drops every 2 to 3 hr Glycerite: 60 to 80 drops every 2 to 3 hr Capsules: 200 mg/day (standard dosage)
Astragalus	Strengthens the immune system Useful for chronic lung deficiency	Dried root, powder: 1 to 2 g daily for up to 3 mo Tea: 2 teaspoons root to 16 oz water per day Extract: 40 to 60 drops twice daily
Boswellia	Useful for allergic rhinitis, sore throat; acts as a stimulant and respiratory antiseptic; may be helpful for asthma and to decrease dyspnea	For bronchial asthma: 300 mg three times daily
Licorice	An expectorant, antiviral, immune stimulator, antispasmodic, and anti-inflammatory; it is suggested that it heals the lung from dry, irritating cough	Capsules: up to six 400- to 500-mg capsules per day for not more than 4 to 6 wk *Note:* Excess licorice can elevate blood pressure by increased potassium loss

TABLE 15-1 **Complementary Alternative Medicine Therapies for Patients with Chronic Obstructive Pulmonary Disease—cont'd**

Nutritional Supplementation	Traditional Use	Typical Dosage
Zinc	Patients with chronic bronchitis have been found to have low zinc status. Supplementation normalized plasma zinc levels and resulted in outcomes of improved general health status. Immune stimulating	20 to 50 mg/day (standard dosage); >50 mg/day may adversely affect copper metabolism
Vitamin C	Improves immune function and helps with chronic bronchitis, colds, and flu; may be helpful in exercise-induced asthma; possibly inhibits histamine release	Nonsmokers: 60 mg/day Smokers: 100 mg/day *Note:* Up to 250 to 500 mg one to two times per day may be optimal
Coenzyme Q10	Improves immune function; it is a lipophilic antioxidant present in all tissues; precursor to energy production in mitochondria	Oil-based soft gel: 50 mg/day for best absorption; take with food *Note:* Increase dosage to 60 to 90 mg/day if taking statins; optimal dosage may be 100 to 200 mg/day
Fish oils/omega-3 fatty acids	Has anti-inflammatory action Commonly used in asthma treatment	Dosage: 500-mg capsule two or three times per day; 1000 to 1500 mg/day
Multivitamins and mineral supplementation	No evidence shows prevention of colds and flu Some studies show benefit in decreasing days of respiratory infection in the elderly. Evidence is variable to date, but none show harm.[75]	Daily multivitamin/minerals come predominantly from derivatives of food sources (e.g., vitamin E as D-α-tocopherol with mixed tocopherols)
Magnesium	May be protective for those with asthma or chronic airflow obstruction; appears to improve lung function; may decrease bronchospasm	Magnesium gluconate (form least likely to cause diarrhea): supplement 200 to 400 mg/day. Monitor red blood cell magnesium levels; keep in middle range or higher
Vitamin D$_3$ (cholecalciferol)	Immune system regulator; useful in the treatment of asthma and infectious disease; there is a strong relationship between serum concentrations of vitamin D and lung function	Supplement as necessary to maintain optimal serum vitamin D levels: 50 to 80 ng/ml (25-hydroxyvitamin D) Typically 1000 to 2000 units/day after loading dose
Quercetin	Used to treat asthma, respiratory allergies, and allergic rhinitis; mast cell stabilizer: decreases histamine release	600-mg capsule twice per day as needed

Data from Natural Medicines Comprehensive Database: Natural medicines in clinical management of colds and flu. Available at www.therapeuticresearch.net. Retrieved July 18, 2008, and Kuhn MA, Winston D: Herbal therapy & supplements: a scientific & traditional approach, Philadelphia, 2001, Lippincott.

mainly to the use of variable plant material and extraction methods and to the addition of other components. The authors conclude that echinacea preparations tested in clinical trials differ greatly in their effects and outcomes. There is some evidence that preparations based on the aerial parts of *Echinacea purpurea* might be effective for the early treatment for colds in adults, but results are not consistent. Beneficial effects of other echinacea preparations may exist, but have not been shown in independently replicated, rigorous randomized trials.[10,11]

Ginseng

Ginseng is a root that has been used to treat patients with various illnesses for the last 2000 years. There are three primary, but different types of ginseng: Asian (also known as *Panax ginseng* or ginseng extract G115), American, and Siberian. The majority of benefits appear to be associated with Asian ginseng. In evaluating reports on ginseng it is important to note the type of ginseng that was used in the study.

P. ginseng might have immunostimulant effects, anti-inflammatory effects, and antioxidant effects.[12] Some clinical evidence suggests that *P. ginseng* might protect against colds and improve response to the flu vaccine. When *P. ginseng* is given at 100 mg/day 4 weeks before influenza vaccination and continued for 8 weeks after, there is a reduction in the incidence of contracting a cold or flu. The mechanism is unknown, but *P. ginseng* might increase natural killer cell activity and the antibody response to vaccination.[13] There is not enough evidence to recommend *P. ginseng* for this use, but it is a well-tolerated treatment. Insomnia is the most common complaint. The safety of long-term use is unknown. It is recommended that patients limit use to 3 months.[13]

Researchers looked at CAM treatments in patients with COPD.[1] Among the various CAM preparations, only *P. ginseng*, used in combination with ongoing respiratory medications, has proven clinical efficacy in COPD.[14] Ginseng's potential for interactions with common drugs such as warfarin, digoxin, nifedipine, loop diuretics, and monoamine oxidase inhibitors may override its potential benefits.[15] Preclinical evidence shows some immune-stimulating activity.[11] Ginseng use has shown significant improvement in pulmonary function testing with supplementation of ginseng extract G115 at 100 mg twice per day for 3 months with patients with moderately to severe COPD, with no side effects noted.[14]

Astragalus Root

One Cochrane Database review looked at Astragalus as an immune system stimulator. It noted that some preclinical trials showed intriguing immune activity. The herb has satisfactory safety profiles. It has been found useful for chronic lung deficiency as well.[16] The margin of safety for this herb is good, but more research is needed to demonstrate any clear value in using it to improve resistance to infections.[11]

Boswellia

Boswellia is used for allergic rhinitis, sore throats, as a stimulant, and a respiratory antiseptic. There is some preliminary evidence that taking boswellia extract might help asthma. It may improve forced expiratory volume in 1 second (FEV_1), reduce the number of asthma attacks, and decrease dyspnea.[17] The use of *Boswellia serrata* gum resin extract, 300 mg three times a day, in a randomized, double-blind, controlled trial showed a significant improvement in 70% of the patients, with improvements in lung function and decreases in asthma symptoms.[18] Boswellia has been shown to work via selective leukotriene synthesis inhibition of the 5-lipoxygenase pathway.[19]

Licorice

Licorice sweet root has been shown in some small studies to inhibit the production of O_2 free radicals by neutrophils. It is also a mild anti-inflammatory and has antiarthritic activity. It also may enhance the immune system. It has been used as an expectorant, antispasmodic, anti-inflammatory, and immune stimulant. Hippocrates noted this botanical as an expectorant for asthma and dry coughs and as a carminative.[16,20]

NUTRITIONAL INTERVENTION FOR THE TREATMENT OF CHRONIC OBSTRUCTIVE PULMONARY DISEASE

Consumption of Fruits and Vegetables, and Antioxidants

A 20-year study of COPD mortality in middle-aged men suggests protective effects of fruit and possibly vitamin E intake against COPD signs and symptoms. No effect was observed for intake of vitamin C, beta carotene, vegetables, and fish.[21] Low intake of oranges and other fruit juices, which are the largest sources of vitamin C, were associated with deficits in forced vital capacity and FEV_1 in boys.[22]

Fruit and vitamin E intake is associated with reduced prevalence of phlegm production for 3 months or more per year. The most beneficial combination of dietary components may be found in natural foodstuffs, particularly fresh fruit.[23] Foods and nutrients that include fruits and vegetables; antioxidant vitamins such as vitamin C, vitamin E, beta carotene and other carotenoids, and vitamin A; fatty acids; and some minerals such as sodium, magnesium and selenium could offer protection for several lung diseases associated with oxidative stress linked to oxidant insults such as cigarette smoke, air pollutants, and infections. Studies suggest that vitamin C in particular, and to some extent antioxidant vitamins, exert a protective effect against lung disease. Several interventional studies have not been conclusive. High intakes of fresh fruit and some vegetables appear to have a beneficial effect on lung health. Consumption of these foods on a daily basis should be recommended. Supplementation of vitamin C and other antioxidants could be proposed for subjects with additional oxidative stress challenge, such as exposure to high levels of air pollution. Vitamin A and zinc supplementation also showed benefit to impaired immune system function.[24]

Greater problems are seen in respiratory allergies and infections when there are higher intakes of sodium, omega-6 fatty acids, and trans-fats. Benefits are found, however, with adequate hydration and diets high in omega-3 fatty acids (e.g., fish, almonds, walnuts, and pumpkin and flax seeds), onions, and fruits and vegetables (at least five servings per day).[24]

Safe herbs, such as boswellia and gingko, may be used singly as adjuncts to a comprehensive plan of care if the patient and practitioner have an interest in trying them while staying alert for drug–herb interactions. There are no long-term studies to date looking at these herbs in asthma treatment. The use of L-carnitine and coenzyme Q10 in patients with COPD needs further study.[24]

Further research is needed to establish whether supplementation with probiotics during the first year of life or after antibiotic use decreases the risk of asthma and allergic rhinitis.[25]

Patients with asthma need to monitor their bronchodilator use and peak flowmeter measurements to step up their medical treatment in a timely manner. Patients welcome physician guidance when exploring the breadth of treatments available today. The patient–physician partnership is empowering to patients who are serious about regaining their function and health.[25]

The epidemiologic evidence that eating fish, fruit, and vegetables exerts a beneficial effect on indicators of asthma and COPD is increasing. Epidemiology studies in the general adult population suggest that high fish intake has a beneficial effect on lung function, but the relationship with respiratory symptoms and asthma or COPD is less evident. Experimental studies have not shown an improvement in asthma severity after supplementations with fish oil. Several studies showed a beneficial association between fruit and vegetable intake and lung function, but the relationship with respiratory symptoms and the clinically manifested disease was less convincing. The effectiveness of dietary supplementation in open population samples is often not demonstrated. There is a need for future studies on the relationship between diet and respiratory disease.[26]

Longitudinal data support the hypothesis that fresh fruit consumption, particularly fruit high in vitamin C, is related to a lower prevalence of asthma symptoms and higher lung function. Consumption of fish has also been shown to improve asthma symptoms and higher lung function.[2] There is much evidence to justify the promotion of a healthy diet, high in fruits, vegetables, and whole grain foods and low in alcohol and fatty foods, as set out in existing guidelines for the prevention of cardiovascular disease and cancer and to promote respiratory health in both children and adults.[2,27]

Vitamin C

Data from the second National Health and Nutrition Examination Survey (NHANES II), involving more than 9000 people, revealed that bronchitis was less frequent when serum vitamin C levels were higher. Vitamin C has produced conflicting results in many studies and has been the subject of controversy for at least 60 years; however, it continues to be widely sold and used as a preventive therapeutic agent for this common ailment. A review article on vitamin C (ascorbic acid) intake in the prevention and treatment of the common cold found that routine megadose prophylaxis is not justified for community use.[28] Evidence shows, however, that it could be justified in persons exposed to brief periods of severe physical exercise and/or cold environments.

Vitamin C plays a role in respiratory defense mechanisms; however, dosages of 4 g daily at the onset of cold symptoms showed no benefit, with equivocal results seen at dosages of 8 g daily.[28] Combining high dosages of vitamin C (2 g/day) with zinc supplements, preferably the nasal zinc gel, at the onset of upper respiratory tract infection can shorten the duration of symptoms.[24] At this time there are no good clinical research data examining the use of vitamin C in patients with allergic rhinitis.

A comparison of lung function as it relates to blood levels of copper, selenium, vitamin C, and vitamin E in the general population shows that higher levels of serum vitamin C and selenium appear to be associated with a higher FEV_1. Copper levels, however, were associated with a lower FEV_1.[29] Dietary vitamin C in young smokers has been shown to reduce cough and wheezing, purportedly because of its antioxidant effects.[30]

An increase to 40 mg/day of vitamin C is correlated with a 20-ml increase in FEV_1.[2] Although this effect is modest, these authors conclude that over 20 to 30 years, it could have a meaningful impact on the rate at which pulmonary function declines, particularly in symptomatic subjects.[2] It is thought that vitamin C inhibits histamine release and promotes vasodilation by increasing prostacyclin production.[31]

Antioxidant Supplementation

The underlying pathophysiology of asthma is airway inflammation with altered T-cell immune response. In asthma, the immune system is overactive. It is not known why asthmatics have this out-of-balance immune activity, but genetics, viruses, fungi, heavy metals, nutrition, and pollution all can be contributing factors. Plant lipid sterols have been shown to dampen T-cell activity. Antioxidant nutrients, especially vitamins C and E, selenium, and zinc, appear to be important in asthma treatment. Vitamins B_6 and B_{12} also may be necessary in asthma treatment. Omega-3 fatty acids from fish, the flavonoid quercetin, and botanicals *Tylophora asthmatica*, *B. serrata*, and *Petasites hybridus* all address the inflammatory component. Physical modalities, including yoga, massage, biofeedback, acupuncture, and chiropractic can also be of help.[32] A large randomized controlled study of 1616 subjects concluded that vitamin E appears to be a stronger correlate of lung function than other antioxidant vitamins.[33]

A prospective study on diet and decline of lung function in the general population suggested that a high dietary intake of vitamin C, or foods rich in this vitamin, may reduce the rate of loss of lung function in adults and help to prevent COPD. This study showed no association with intake of magnesium, or vitamin A or E, and improved lung function.[34] In addition to vitamin C being protective, adequate intake of antioxidants and avoidance of increasing waist circumference could also help preserve lung function.[35]

A large study of 29,133 participants in 1997,[3] showed that supplementation with α-tocopherol (50 mg/day) and beta carotene (20 mg/day) for 5 to 8 years did not prevent the development of symptoms related to COPD, but a diet rich in foods containing α-tocopherol and beta carotene, such as fruits and vegetables and seeds and whole grains, offered some protection even among elderly, long-term smokers. The most effective way to prevent COPD remains smoking cessation and increasing fruits and vegetables rich in antioxidants.[3]

The third National Health and Nutrition Examination Survey (NHANES III)[36] examined antioxidant nutrients and pulmonary function. Higher levels of antioxidant nutrients were associated with better lung function. Each of the dietary and serum antioxidant nutrients was significantly associated with pulmonary function (FEV_1). Serum beta carotene was less positively associated with pulmonary function (FEV_1) in smokers than in nonsmokers. Selenium had a stronger positive association with pulmonary function (FEV_1) in smokers. The conclusion from this survey was that higher antioxidant nutrients (both serum levels and dietary levels) are associated with better lung function.[36]

Zinc

Some studies show that patients with chronic bronchitis have low serum zinc status. Zinc supplementation can normalize plasma zinc levels and result in improved general health status.[37] A review article looking at several clinical trials studying the efficacy of zinc against the common cold supports the value of zinc in reducing the duration and severity of symptoms of the common cold when administered within 24 hours of the onset of common cold symptoms. Additional clinical and laboratory evaluations are recommended to further determine the role of zinc in the prevention and treatment of the common cold, and to determine the biochemical mechanisms of zinc in relieving symptoms of cold and flu.[38]

Magnesium

Magnesium is involved in a wide range of biological activities, including some that may protect against the development of asthma and chronic airflow obstruction. A study published in 1994 in the *Lancet*[39] tested the hypothesis that high dietary magnesium intake is associated with better lung function and reduced airway hyperreactivity and wheezing in a random sample of 2633 adults. This study concluded that low magnesium intake may be involved in the etiology of asthma and COPD.[39] Alternative practitioners frequently recommend magnesium supplementation for patients with asthma. Some success has been seen with aerosolized magnesium sulfate as a bronchodilator. It works, but is not as effective as salbutamol alone.[40] When magnesium sulfate is combined with salbutamol there are mixed results: no improvement in benefits over salbutamol alone, in one study that monitored peak expiratory flow rate end points,[41] and significant improvement in another in which FEV_1 was the end point.[42] These differences appear to be due to the specific end points that were measured. Adding 2 g of magnesium, administered intravenously, to the standard emergency department asthma protocol treatment resulted in significantly improved FEV_1 after 4 hours versus placebo administered intravenously.[43] A Cochrane Database review concluded that routine use of magnesium does not improve outcomes but, if used in patients with severe exacerbation magnesium, has benefit and is safe.[44]

Maintaining magnesium levels in the middle to upper normal range would seem to be prudent. Red blood cell magnesium levels may guide the use of magnesium replacement, as this is more reflective of tissue levels than serum levels.

Vitamin D

Vitamin D is known as the sunshine vitamin because it is synthesized from cholesterol in skin that is exposed to the energy from sunlight. It undergoes several transformations in the liver and the kidney before vitamin D_3, also called cholecalciferol, the active form of vitamin D, is achieved. Vitamin D_2, ergocalciferol, is a form of vitamin D that is used in some supplements and prescriptions, but it has only one quarter the activity of vitamin D_3. Vitamin D_2 has greater potential for toxicity. There are some calls for the abandonment of vitamin D_2 with recommendations to only use vitamin D_3.[45] Vitamin D is also referred to as D-hormone [1,25(OH)2D_3], because many of its actions are hormonal in nature.

Vitamin D or D-hormone is an important immune system regulator that appears to inhibit the development of autoimmune disease including experimental inflammatory bowel disease, rheumatoid arthritis, multiple sclerosis, and type 1 diabetes. D-hormone is a selective regulator of the immune system, and the outcome of D-hormone treatment depends on the nature (e.g., infectious disease, asthma, and autoimmune disease) of the immune response.[46] NHANES III reported the relationship between serum 25-hydroxyvitamin D and pulmonary function. This study found a strong relationship between serum concentrations of 25-hydroxyvitamin D and lung function. After adjusting for age, gender, height, body mass index, ethnicity, and smoking history, those with the highest quintile had a greater mean FEV_1 (by 126 ml) and a greater mean forced vital capacity (by 172 ml) than those who were in the lowest quintile.[47] The goal is to maintain upper normal ranges of serum D-hormone levels (25-hydroxyvitamin D). We recommend measurement at least annually, and supplementation with D_3 if necessary, to maintain that goal. Those low in 25-hydroxyvitamin D will need initial loading doses of 6000 to 8000 units of vitamin D_3 (depending on how low they are initially) on a daily basis for 4 to 6 weeks because of the uptake in the fatty tissue first before free levels of vitamin D_3 become available. After the loading dose, 1000 to 2000 units of vitamin D_3 per day for maintenance will usually be required; this of course, guided by serum level determinations. Vitamin D use is considered to have a high safety profile.[48]

Coenzyme Q10

Coenzyme Q10 (CoQ10), also known as ubiquinone or ubidecarenone, is an enzyme found within the mitochondria and is a necessary factor in the respiratory transport chain that ultimately creates adenosine triphosphate (ATP) in the body for energy. Bronchial asthma is a chronic inflammatory disease of the respiratory system, characterized by disturbances in the balance between oxidants and antioxidants in the lungs. It has been suggested that CoQ10 supplementation exerts a beneficial effect on the antioxidative imbalance in patients with bronchial asthma, providing a rationale for supplementation.[49,50] Another study suggested that CoQ10 has favorable effects on the muscular energy metabolism of patients with chronic lung disease who experience hypoxemia at rest or during exercise, and that with CoQ10 supplementation there is a decrease in lactate production.[51] One small study found a significant increase in O_2 uptake (6% greater) with exercise training in patients with COPD who had been supplemented with CoQ10 at 50 mg daily.[52] Chronic administration of corticosteroids has been shown to result in mitochondrial dysfunction and oxidative damage of mitochondrial and nuclear DNAs. Patients with corticosteroid-dependent bronchial asthma have lower CoQ10 concentrations, which may contribute to antioxidant imbalance and oxidative stress. Supplementation with CoQ10 is able to decrease the amount of steroid required.[53] This has important implications for the care of patients with COPD and may help reduce steroid-related side effects by allowing for lower dosing.

CoQ10 is recognized as improving immune function. This lipophilic antioxidant is present in all tissues and is a precursor to energy production in mitochondria. Overall, there are more positive results than negative, but further research is needed. The oil-based soft gel is recommended for better absorption. CoQ10 supplementation should be taken with food. Taken with piperine (black pepper), absorption can increase by 30%. Drug interaction has been noted with warfarin; monitor the INR (international normalized ratio) carefully. HMG-CoA reductase inhibitors, that is, statin drugs, decrease the absorption of CoQ10 and can lower body levels of this important enzyme. Increase supplementation by a minimum of 60 to 90 mg/day or more as the replacement dosage if these medications are being taken.

Omega-3 Fatty Acids

Omega-3 fatty acid, α-linolenic acid, is an essential fat needed by the body for numerous functions. The crucial end products of α-linolenic acid metabolism are eicosapentaenoic acid and docosahexaenoic acid. The Agency for Healthcare Research and Quality (Rockville, Md.) evidence report/technology assessment reviewed 31 articles that looked at the health effect of omega-3 fatty acids in asthma. Its report concluded that omega-3 fatty acid supplementation alone has not been found to provide significant asthma-related benefits and that more research is needed to adequately delineate the role of omega-3 supplementation in respiratory disease.[2,54]

Research looking at omega-3 fatty acids and smoker-related COPD found that the prevalence of COPD was inversely related to docosahexaenoic acid, but not to eicosapentaenoic acid. Docosahexaenoic acid may have a role in preventing and treating COPD and other chronic inflammatory conditions of the lung. Omega-3 fatty acids might be useful in preventing and treating respiratory diseases in which chronic inflammation plays a significant role.[55]

MIND–BODY RELAXATION AND MANUAL THERAPIES

Considerable research has looked at the role of CAM therapies in the management of asthma. One review examined 15 studies on mind–body relaxation, manual therapies, and diet. The authors concluded that more research is needed to determine the efficacy of CAM therapies in asthma management.[56] In motivated patients, mind–body interventions such as yoga, hypnosis, and biofeedback-assisted relaxation and breathing exercises are beneficial for stress reduction in general and may be helpful in further controlling asthma. Massage of children with asthma showed some benefit. Patients with COPD in these review studies showed benefits from exercise, pulmonary rehabilitation, and increased caloric intake from protein and fat.[25]

A systematic review of published articles on CAM and bronchial asthma concluded that there was insufficient support for the use of homeopathy, air ionizers, manual therapy, or acupuncture for asthma.[57] There may be some role, especially in individual cases, for some of these modalities but studies have not been conclusive as to the general applicability of these therapies to all patients in general. The use of antioxidant dietary supplementation and some natural anti-inflammatory and immunomodulatory remedies may hold the most promise. Breathing exercises improved lung function and quality of life in various studies. Psychotherapy-related methods such as relaxation, hypnosis, autogenic training, and biofeedback might have a small effect in selected cases, but have not proven to be superior to placebo. More well-designed randomized controlled trials are needed to allow firm conclusions.[58]

Exercise

Patients with COPD often have limited exercise tolerance as their chief complaint. Dysfunction of ambulatory muscles appears to contribute to exercise intolerance in these patients. Rehabilitative programs of exercise training have been shown to increase exercise tolerance. Endurance training and resistance exercise can increase tolerance substantially. Endurance and strength training can lead to significant improvement in muscle strength in elderly patients with COPD. Yet, this improvement in muscle strength does not translate into additional improvement in quality of life, exercise performance, or quadriceps fatigability compared with that achieved by endurance exercise alone.[59]

Respiratory muscle endurance training can specifically increase endurance and strength of the respiratory muscles beyond that achieved by endurance training alone in patients with COPD. This improvement is associated with increase in exercise performance in patients with COPD.[59,60] Home-based respiratory muscle endurance training, by means of breathing through tubes that create resistance, leads to significant improvement of endurance exercise capacity, a reduction in perception of dyspnea, and an improvement in quality of life in patients with moderate to severe COPD.[61] Inspiratory muscle training relieves dyspnea, increases the capacity to walk, and improves health-related quality of life in patients with COPD.[62]

Hypogonadism and Muscle Weakness

Muscle wasting can be significant in patients with COPD. Strategies to increase caloric intake have met with limited success. It has been found that exercise intolerance and quadriceps muscle weakness in elderly men with COPD is related to low circulating levels of testosterone.[63] The use of anabolic agents to stimulate muscle building and help with lean body mass retention has shown some possibilities for cachectic patients. A study of 85 hypogonadal men with COPD showed that administering replacement testosterone doses for 10 weeks increased lean body mass and leg muscle strength. Resistance training of the legs along with testosterone supplementation resulted in increased lean body mass and a 26.8% increase in strength.[64] Low muscle mass is a predictor of mortality in COPD; effects of these anabolic interventions on survival should be investigated further. Further studies are needed in women with COPD as well.[64]

Yoga

Evaluation of yoga exercises in patients with bronchial asthma shows significant improvements in lung function and eosinophil count along with patient reports of feeling better and having more comfortable breathing. Yoga appears to act at both physical and mental levels. Yoga training for 6 months improved lung function, strength of inspiratory and expiratory muscles, as well as skeletal muscle strength and endurance.[65] Results of yoga studies on lung function showed significant improvement in hand grip strength and endurance, maximal inspiratory and expiratory pressures, FEV_1, and flow rates.[65-67] The practice of yoga exercises and breathing techniques offers performance gain for patients with COPD in a manner different from standard aerobic and resistance training exercises. This may be a suitable alternative for those who find it difficult to engage in traditional exercise programs.

Acupressure Therapy

Acupressure is the technique of directing controlled amounts of focused pressure to specific trigger point areas on the body. In the right hands, this therapy can relieve muscle spasms and pain, and can help achieve better musculoskeletal function. Acupressure has shown improvement in perceived symptoms of dyspnea and anxiety in patients with COPD and who have undergone prolonged mechanical ventilation.[68] Acupressure could be used as a nursing or respiratory therapist intervention to promote relaxation and relieve dyspnea in patients with COPD.[69] Clinically significant improvements in quality of life have been measured when standard care of patients with COPD was supplemented with acupuncture or acupressure.[70] Acupressure therapy appears to be consistently recommended in evidence-based medicine as a treatment option for patients with COPD.

Manual Therapies

Various manual therapies with similar mechanisms of action are commonly used to treat patients with asthma. Manual therapy practitioners are also varied, including physiotherapists, respiratory therapists, and chiropractic and osteopathic physicians. A Cochrane Database review of 68 articles on manual therapy as a treatment for asthma concluded that there is insufficient evidence to support the use of manual therapies for patients with asthma. There is a need for randomized controlled trials that examine the effects of manual therapies on clinically relevant outcomes.[71]

However, specific studies have shown beneficial outcomes from chiropractic spinal manipulative therapy in a pediatric population in addition to optimal medical management. Three months of chiropractic therapy showed persistent patient-reported quality of life and asthma symptom improvements for up to 1 year later, yet no significant changes in lung function were found.[72]

Adult patients with chronic asthma receiving chiropractic spinal manipulation two times weekly for 4 weeks or sham treatments in a 4-week crossover study showed beneficial findings. Nonspecific bronchial hyperreactivity improved by 36%, and patient-rated asthma severity decreased by 34% compared with baseline.[73] Again, standard lung function measures did not change during the study. There appears to be some other mechanism by which these patients benefit. Further studies are warranted.

Biofeedback Treatment for Asthma

Biofeedback treatment for asthma involving heart rate variability may prove to be a useful addition to traditional asthma treatment and may help to reduce dependence on steroid medications. Those receiving biofeedback treatments used less medication, with improvement averaging one full level of asthma severity, with measures from forced oscillation pneumography, and there was also improvement in pulmonary function.[74] A study evaluating the effectiveness of respiratory resistance biofeedback training with 15 adult subjects with asthma led to the conclusion that it may not be an effective technique for the treatment of bronchial asthma in adults. Biofeedback studies and asthma have shown variable effectiveness. Those who receive the most benefit are those who are susceptible to the treatment. Not all patients can make it work for them. Effectiveness of treatment is more on a case-by-case basis. For some patients this may prove to be a valuable treatment addition.

Box 15-1 reviews CAM therapies involving nutritional and lifestyle interventions used to treat respiratory conditions.

CONCLUSION

There is a great need for further research into specific CAM treatments for patients with COPD. The current research findings on CAM treatments for COPD are summarized in this chapter.

There are conflicting findings on the use of specific CAM treatments for patients with COPD. Many of the review articles referenced here indicate that it is difficult to isolate specific botanical or nutrient interventions. The findings most consistent with improvement in lung function describe diets high in antioxidant-rich fruits and vegetables along with endurance and resistance exercise on a regular basis. The most promising single botanical appeared to be *P. ginseng* (or Asian ginseng) for the improvement of anti-inflammation, and for its antioxidant effects and immune stimulation, all leading to an improvement in lung function. In addition, there are a few nutrient supplements that show much promise in current research. These nutrients include vitamin D for its obvious lung function improvements and also for its multiple effects of increasing muscle strength and improving immune function. Vitamin C has consistently shown benefit for its antioxidant ability and lung function protection, and for its important role in strengthening immune function. In the current literature, yoga and acupressure show promise for improving asthma conditions and lung function in the elderly, adults, and children.

Many other botanical supplements, nutritional supplements, and CAM therapies reviewed in this chapter do not show conclusive evidence of effectiveness, but at the same time do not appear to be harmful. On the basis of their mechanism of action or some promise shown in small study designs, these agents may be worth considering on a case-by-case basis for some patients who are difficult to manage. The current findings again bring us back to the basics of good nutrition, consisting of whole foods and high intakes of fruits and vegetables, and increased exercise and water intake, along with CAM therapies such as supplementation of nutrients, botanicals, and psychophysical modalities that, on the basis of current research, appear to be beneficial for the patient with COPD.

Approximately 41% of patients with COPD use some form of CAM intervention. It is important for health professionals to ask their patients if they are using any CAM preparations or treatments. Having some knowledge of alternative treatments fosters an accepting and open dialogue in which all treatment issues can be discussed. In addition, knowing the prescribed and self-prescribed treatments that patients may be using puts the health care provider in a better position

---

BOX 15-1 | **Complementary Alternative Medicine Therapies Involving Diet and Lifestyle Recommendations for Treatment of Respiratory Disease**

- Drink plenty of good-quality water.
- Obtain sufficient calories to maintain normal weight.
- Avoid refined foods when possible.
- Increase intake of antioxidant-rich, fresh fruits and vegetables versus isolated extracted nutrient supplementation.
- Increase "whole plant–based diet"; minimize animal products including dairy.
- Test vitamin D levels (25-hydroxyvitamin D) regularly to maintain upper optimal levels.
- Be cautious of excess salt intake.
- Avoid alcohol, soft drinks, and chronic use of caffeine- and sugar-containing beverages.
- Reduce dietary arachidonic acid, which can lead to inflammatory mediators (leukotrienes) and precipitate asthma attack; diet should be low in meat, eggs, shellfish, vegetable oils (omega-6), and dietary fat.
- Reduce excess carbohydrate load, especially refined carbohydrates (may increase insulin secretion and inflammation). Excess refined sugars can increase CO_2 production and work of breathing in patients with COPD (proper amounts of carbohydrate are crucial for anaerobic work and oxygenation via increased 2,3-diphosphoglycerate).
- Minimize food additives, coloring, and preservatives (aspartame, dyes, and monosodium glutamate).
- Address allergy issues and potential immune-triggering events.
- Make sure that the home is free of any mold or mildew problems.
- Limit the use of carpet whenever possible.
- Take steps to purify whole house air with high-efficiency particulate air filters or electrostatic filters with ozone traps.
- Use hypoallergenic bedding and wash bedding frequently.
- If in a hypogonadal state, consider the use of hormone replacement therapy to improve muscle building and retention and weight management.
- Adhere to a daily exercise program.
- Consider yoga for the treatment of respiratory disease and improved pulmonary function.
- For patients with COPD undergoing pulmonary rehabilitation, commit to endurance exercise training and consider respiratory muscle endurance training.
- Consider the use of acupressure for the treatment of respiratory disease.
- Consider the use of heart rate variability biofeedback for the treatment of asthma.
- Establish a self-management program, including initiation of home peak flow monitoring.
- Wear unrestrictive clothing, allowing free movement of the chest and abdomen for optimal breathing.
- Get adequate sleep, preferably 7 to 9 hours per night.

---

to effectively guide a patient's course of care. Helping the patient avoid potential interactions with current medications and treatments, and being able to advise as to what modalities are most likely to be of benefit, results in better patient care.

References

1. George J, Loannides-Demos LL, Santamaria NM et al: Use of complementary and alternative medicines by patients with chronic obstructive pulmonary disease, Med J Aust 181:248-251, 2004.
2. Romieu I, Trenga C: Diet and obstructive lung diseases, Epidemiol Rev 23:268-287, 2001.
3. Rautalahti M, Virtamo J, Haukka J et al: The effect of alpha-tocopherol and beta-carotene supplementation on COPD symptoms, Am J Respir Crit Care Med 156:1447-1452, 1997.
4. Dolce JJ, Crisp C, Manzella B et al: Medication adherence patterns in chronic obstructive pulmonary disease, Chest 99:837-841, 1991.
5. Drug interaction facts, St. Louis, Mo, 2003, Facts & Comparison, a division of Wolters Kluwer Health.
6. Winslow LC, Shapiro H: Physicians want education about complementary and alternative medicine to enhance communication with their patients, Arch Intern Med 162:1176-1181, 2002.
7. Expert Committee on Complementary Medicines in the Health System: Complementary medicines in the Australian health system. Available at www.tga.gov.au/docs/pdf/cmreport.pdf. Retrieved July 18, 2008.
8. Turner RB, Bauer R, Woelkart K et al: An evaluation of *Echinacea angustifolia* in experimental rhinovirus infections, N Engl J Med 353:341-348, 2005.
9. Natural Medicines Comprehensive Database: Natural medicines in clinical management of colds and flu. Available at www.therapeuticresearch.net. Retrieved July 18, 2008.

10. Linde K, Barrett B, Wolkart K et al: Echinacea for preventing and treating the common cold, Cochrane Database Syst Rev 1:CD000530, 2006.
11. Block KI, Mead MN: Immune system effects of echinacea, ginseng, and astragalus: a review, Integr Cancer Ther 2:247-267, 2003.
12. Kiefer D, Pantuso T: Panax ginseng. Am Fam Physician 68:1539-1542, 2003.
13. Scaglione F, Cattaneo G, Alessandria M et al: Efficacy and safety of the standardized ginseng extract G115 for potentiating vaccination against the influenza syndrome and protection against the common cold, Drugs Exp Clin Res 22:65-72, 1996.
14. Gross D, Shenkman Z, Bleiberg B et al: Ginseng improves pulmonary functions and exercise capacity in patients with COPD, Monaldi Arch Chest Dis 57:242-246, 2002.
15. Drug interaction facts: herbal supplements and food, St. Louis, Mo, 2003, Facts & Comparison, a division of Wolters Kluwer Health.
16. Winston D: Herbal therapeutics: specific indications for herbs & formulas, ed 8, Broadway, NJ, 2003, Herbal Therapeutics Research Library.
17. Natural Medicines Comprehensive Database: Natural medicines in clinical management of colds and flu. Available at www.therapeuticresearch.net. Retrieved July 18, 2008.
18. Gupta I, Gupta V, Parihar A et al: Effects of *Boswellia serrata* gum resin in patients with bronchial asthma: results of a double-blind, placebo-controlled, 6-week clinical study, Eur J Med Res 3:511-514, 1998.
19. Ammon HP, Safayhi H, Mack T et al: Mechanism of antiinflammatory actions of curcumine and boswellic acids, J Ethnopharmacol 38:113-119, 1993.
20. Kuhn MA, Winston D: Herbal therapy & supplements: a scientific & traditional approach, Philadelphia, 2001, Lippincott.
21. Waldo IC, Tabak C, Smit HA et al: Diet and 20-year chronic obstructive pulmonary disease mortality in middle-aged men from three European countries, Eur J Clin Nutr 56:638-643, 2002.
22. Gilliland FD, Berhane KT, Li YF et al: Children's lung function and antioxidant vitamin, fruit, juice, and vegetable intake, Am J Epidemiol 158:576-584, 2003.
23. Kelly Y, Sacker A, Marmot M: Nutrition and respiratory health in adults: findings from the Health Survey for Scotland, Eur Respir J 21:664-671, 2003.
24. Romieu I: Nutrition and lung health, Int J Tuberc Lung Dis 9:362-374, 2005.
25. Jaber R: Respiratory and allergic disease: from upper respiratory tract infections to asthma, Prim Care 29:231-261, 2002.
26. Smit HA, Grievink L, Tabak C: Dietary influences on chronic obstructive lung disease and asthma: a review of the epidemiological evidence, Proc Nutr Soc 58:309-319, 1999.
27. Denny S, Thompson RL, Margetts BM: Dietary factors in the pathogenesis of asthma and chronic obstructive pulmonary disease, Curr Allergy Asthma Rep 3:130-136, 2003.
28. Douglas RM, Hemilä H, D'souza R et al: Vitamin C for preventing and treating the common cold, Cochrane Database Syst Rev 4:CD000980, 2004 [update in Cochrane Database Syst Rev 3: CD000980, 2007].
29. Pearson P, Britton J, McKeever T et al: Lung function and blood levels of copper, selenium, vitamin C and vitamin E in the general population, Eur J Clin Nutr 59:1043-1048, 2005.
30. Omenaas E, Fluge O, Buist AS et al: Dietary vitamin C intake is inversely related to cough and wheeze in young smokers, Respir Med 97:134-142, 2003.
31. Rakel D: Integrative medicine, Philadelphia, 2003, WB Saunders.
32. Miller A: The etiologies, pathophysiology, and alternative/complementary treatment of asthma, Altern Med Rev 6:20-47, 2001.
33. Schunemann HJ, Grant BJ, Freudenheim JL et al: The relation of serum levels of antioxidant vitamin C and E, retinol an carotenoids with pulmonary function in the general population, Am J Respir Crit Care Med 16:1246-1255, 2001.
34. McKeever TM, Scrivener S, Broadfield E et al: Prospective study of diet and decline in lung function in a general population, Am J Respir Crit Care Med 165:1299-1303, 2002.
35. Chen R, Tunstall-Pedoe H, Bolton-Smith C et al: Association of dietary antioxidants and waist circumference with pulmonary function and airway obstruction, Am J Epidemiol 153:157-163, 2001.
36. Hu G, Cassano PA: Antioxidant nutrients and pulmonary function: the third National Health and Nutrition Examination Survey (NHANES III), Am J Epidemiol 151:975-981, 2000.
37. Tadzhiev FS: Trace elements in the pathogenesis and treatment of chronic bronchitis (a clinico-experimental study), Ter Arkh 63:68-70, 1991.
38. Hulisz D: Efficacy of zinc against common cold viruses: an overview, J Am Pharm Assoc 44:594-603, 2004.
39. Britton J, Pavord I, Richards K et al: Dietary magnesium, lung function, wheezing, and airway hyperreactivity in a random adult population sample, Lancet 344:357-362, 1994.
40. Meral A, Coker M, Tanac R: Inhalation therapy with magnesium sulfate and salbutamol sulfate in bronchial asthma, Turk J Pediatr 38:169-175, 1996.
41. Aggarwal P, Sharad S, Handa R et al: Comparison of nebulised magnesium sulphate and salbutamol combined with salbutamol alone in the treatment of acute bronchial asthma: a randomised study, Emerg Med J 23:358-362, 2006.
42. Hughes R, Goldkorn A, Masoli M et al: Use of isotonic nebulised magnesium sulphate as an adjuvant to salbutamol in treatment of severe asthma in adults: randomised placebo-controlled trial, Lancet 361:2114-2117, 2003.
43. Silverman RA, Osborn H, Runge J et al: IV magnesium sulfate in the treatment of acute severe asthma: a multicenter randomized controlled trial, Chest 122:489-497, 2002.

44. Rowe BH, Bretzlaff JA, Bourdon C et al: Magnesium sulfate for treating exacerbations of acute asthma in the emergency department, Cochrane Database Syst Rev 2:CD001490, 2000.

45. Houghton LA, Veith R: The case against ergocalciferol (vitamin D2) as a vitamin supplement, Am J Clin Nutr 84:694-697, 2006.

46. Cantorna MT, Mahon BD: D-hormone and the immune system, J Rheumatol Suppl 76:11-20, 2005.

47. Black PN, Scragg R: Relationship between serum 25-hydroxyvitamin D and pulmonary function in the third National Health and Nutrition Examination Survey, Chest 128:3792-3798, 2005.

48. Hollis BW, Wagner CL: Assessment of dietary vitamin D requirements during pregnancy and lactation, Am J Clin Nutr 79:717-726, 2004.

49. Gazdik F, Gvozdjáková A, Nádvorníková R et al: Decreased levels of coenzyme Q10 in patients with bronchial asthma, Allergy 57:811-814, 2002.

50. Gazdik F, Gvozdjáková A, Horváthová M et al: Levels of coenzyme Q10 in asthmatics, Bratisl Lek Listy 103:353-356, 2002.

51. Fujimoto S, Kurihara N, Hirata K et al: Effects of coenzyme Q10 administration on pulmonary function and exercise performance in patients with chronic lung disease, Clin Investig 71(Suppl 8):S162-S166, 1993.

52. Satta A, Grandi M, Landoni CV et al: Effects of ubidecarenone in an exercise training program for patients with chronic obstructive pulmonary diseases, Clin Ther 13:754-757, 1991.

53. Gvozdjáková A, Kucharská J, Bartkovjaková M et al: Coenzyme Q10 supplementation reduces corticosteroids dosage in patients with bronchial asthma, Biofactors 25:235-240, 2005.

54. U.S. Department of Health and Human Services: Health effects of omega-3 fatty acids on asthma (AHRQ publication No. 04-E013-2, March 2004), Rockville, Md, 2004, U.S. Department of Health and Human Services. Available at http://www.ahrq.gov/downloads/pub/evidence/pdf/o3asthma/o3asthma.pdf. Retrieved October 4, 2007.

55. Shahar E, Boland LL, Folsom AR et al: Docosahexaenoic acid and smoking-related chronic obstructive pulmonary disease, Am J Respir Crit Care Med 159:1790-1795, 1999.

56. Markham AW, Wilkinson JM: Complementary and alternative medicines (CAM) in the management of asthma: an examination of the evidence, J Asthma 41:131-139, 2004.

57. Gyorik SA, Brutsche MH: Complementary and alternative medicine for bronchial asthma: is there new evidence? Curr Opin Pulm Med Jan 2004; 10(1):37-43.

58. Mador MJ, Bozkanat E, Aggarwal A et al: Endurance and strength training in patients with COPD, Chest 125:2036-2045, 2004.

59. Mador MJ, Deniz O, Aggarwal A et al: Effect of respiratory muscle endurance training in patients with COPD undergoing pulmonary rehabilitation, Chest 128:1216-1224, 2005.

60. Weiner P, Magadle R, Beckerman M et al: Specific expiratory muscle training in COPD, Chest 124:468-473, 2003.

61. Koppers RJ, Vos PJ, Boot CR et al: Exercise performance improves in patients with COPD due to respiratory muscle endurance training, Chest 129:886-892, 2006.

62. Sanchez RH, Montemayor RT, Ortega RF et al: Inspiratory muscle training in patients with COPD, Chest 120:748-756, 2001.

63. Van Vliet M, Spruit MA, Verleden G et al: Hypogonadism, quadriceps weakness, and exercise intolerance in chronic obstructive pulmonary disease, Am J Respir Crit Care Med 172:1105-1111, 2005.

64. Casaburi R, Bhasin S, Cosentino L et al: Effects of testosterone and resistance training in men with chronic obstructive pulmonary disease, Am J Respir Crit Care Med 170:870-878, 2004.

65. Mandanmohan JL, Udupa K, Bhavanani AB: Effect of yoga training on handgrip, respiratory pressure, and pulmonary function, Indian J Physiol Pharmacol 47:387-392, 2003.

66. Sathyaprabha TN, Murthy H, Murthy BT: Efficacy of naturopathy and yoga in bronchial asthma: a self-controlled matched scientific study, Indian J Physiol Pharmacol 45:80-86, 2001.

67. Birkel DA, Edgren L: Hatha yoga: improved vital capacity of college students, Altern Ther Health Med 6:55-63, 2000.

68. Tsay SL, Wang JC, Lin KC et al: Effects of acupressure therapy for patients having prolonged mechanical ventilation support, J Adv Nurs 52:142-150, 2005.

69. Wu HS, Wu SC, Lin JG et al: Effectiveness of acupressure in improving dyspnoea in chronic obstructive pulmonary disease, J Adv Nurs 45:252-259, 2004.

70. Maa SH, Sun MF, Hsu KH et al: Effect of acupuncture or acupressure on quality of life of patients with chronic obstructive asthma: a pilot study, J Altern Complement Med 9:659-670, 2003.

71. Hondras MA, Linde K, Jones AP: Manual therapy for asthma, Cochrane Database Syst Rev 18:CD0001002, 2005.

72. Bronfort G, Evans RL, Kubic P et al: Chronic pediatric asthma and chiropractic spinal manipulation: a prospective clinical series and randomized clinical pilot study, J Manipulative Physiol Ther 24:369-377, 2001.

73. Nielson NH, Bronfort G, Bendix T et al: Chronic asthma and chiropractic spinal manipulation: a randomized clinical trial, Clin Exp Allergy 25:80-88, 1995.

74. Lehrer PM, Vaschillo E, Vaschillo B et al: Biofeedback treatment for asthma, Chest 126:352-361, 2004.

Chapter 16

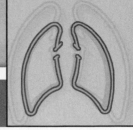

Medical Management of Tobacco Dependence: Concepts and Treatment Objectives

DAVID P. L. SACHS

CHAPTER OUTLINE

**Tobacco Dependence, Nicotine
 Addiction, and Nicotine Withdrawal**
**Pulmonary Consequences of Tobacco
 Use**
 Chronic Obstructive Pulmonary
  Disease
 Bronchogenic Carcinoma
 Interstitial Lung Disease
 Asthma
**Medications for Treating Tobacco
 Dependence**
Controller Medications: First Line
 $\alpha_4\beta_2$ Nicotinic Receptor Partial
  Agonists
 Dopaminergic–Noradrenergic
  Reuptake Inhibitors
 Nicotinic Receptor Agonists
Controller Medications: Second Line
 α_2-Adrenergic Agonists
 Noradrenergic–Serotonergic Reuptake
  Inhibitors
Rescue Medications: First Line
 Nicotinic Receptor Agonists
 Combination Medications
Drug Interactions
 Effect of Stopping Smoking
 Controller Medications: First Line
 Rescue Medications
Side Effects

Controller Medications: First Line
Rescue Medications
Cardiac and Vascular Safety: Controller
 and Rescue Nicotine Medications
Controller Medications: Second Line
**Tobacco-Dependence Medication Use
 During Pregnancy**
**Duration of Tobacco-Dependence
 Medication Use**
**Ineffective Medications for Treating
 Tobacco Dependence**
 Selective Serotonin Reuptake Inhibitors
 Anxiolytics
Behavioral Intervention
 Counseling
 Residential Treatment Programs
**Managing Nicotine Addiction:
 Pharmacotherapy to Eliminate
 Nicotine Withdrawal**
**Medical Record: Tobacco Use
 and Exposure History**
Diagnosis Coding: ICD-9 and CPT
Cost-effectiveness
Conclusion
Appendix 1: Resources
Appendix 2: Case Examples: Treatment
**Appendix 3: Pragmatic Method to
 Initiate Tobacco-Dependence
 Medications**

Professional Skills

On completion of this chapter, the reader will be able to do
the following:

* Explain why tobacco dependence is a severe, life-threatening, chronic medical disease that requires
 long-term medical treatment and management, often for the life of the patient

◆ Explain the difference between psychological dependence and nicotine addiction and why both must be treated during smoking cessation

◆ Describe the fundamental pharmacotherapeutic principles governing rational medical management of tobacco dependence

◆ Explain the difference between Controller and Rescue Medications for treating tobacco dependence and how to individualize treatment through medication combination, dosage, and behavioral intervention

◆ Record patients' tobacco use and exposure history properly in the medical record

◆ Establish appropriate medical diagnoses (ICD-9 diagnostic codes) for symptoms and appropriate medical services (CPT) codes for proper and accurate insurance claims submission

◆ Understand the cost-effectiveness of treating tobacco dependence with pharmacotherapy and intensive physician involvement

TOBACCO DEPENDENCE, NICOTINE ADDICTION, AND NICOTINE WITHDRAWAL

Physicians can effectively diagnose and treat tobacco dependence in their office, if they regard it as a chronic, relapsing, life-threatening medical disease that requires long-term medical management and repeated intervention.[1-4] Advances in basic neurosciences show that cigarette smoking is neither a "lifestyle problem" nor a habit but is a true physical dependence on tobacco. Tobacco dependence is a chronic medical disease, as are diabetes, hypertension, hyperlipidemia, and asthma,[2-5] which generally needs long-term or even lifelong treatment.[4-6] Without the use of both pharmacotherapy and counseling support, at least 45% of all cigarette smokers attempting to quit on their own—"cold turkey"—relapse within 7 days, and 55% to 65% relapse within 14 days.[7,8] Relapse occurs secondary to physically caused nicotine withdrawal symptoms (such as difficulty in concentrating, short-temperedness, depression, mood swings, or cigarette craving; Table 16-1) and the disruption those symptoms have on the patient's life.[9] At a minimum, pharmacotherapy reduces nicotine withdrawal symptoms and can cut the high, 7- and 14-day relapse rates by 50%.[2,10-20]

For a patient to be tobacco dependent, two independent processes must occur.[5] First, the ultrahigh doses of nicotine in cigarette smoke must activate CNS (central nervous system) genetic systems, creating the cellular substrate for nicotine dependence. This activation typically occurs after the "experimenting" smoker—usually a preteen or adolescent—smokes even as few as one cigarette per day for 10 days. CNS sensitivity and responsiveness to nicotine are genetically determined.[21-39] About 10% of cigarette smokers lack the requisite genes and have no physiologic nicotine dependence. The other 90% of experimental smokers become physically dependent on nicotine. The second prerequisite for tobacco dependence is the development of classic conditioned responses to cigarettes, for example, having a cigarette after a meal or while starting the car.

In the tobacco-dependent patient, nicotine, as delivered by tobacco smoke, causes profound and, for many patients, irreversible changes in the CNS. Like many other addicting drugs, nicotine crosses the blood–brain barrier by both active and passive transport and activates multiple brain circuits,

TABLE 16-1 Common Physiologically Induced Nicotine Withdrawal Symptoms

Symptom	Frequency of Occurrence (%)*
Anxiety	87%
Irritability, frustration, or anger	80%
Depression/depressed mood (with a history of depression)	75%[124]
Depression/depressed mood (without a history of depression)	31%[124]
Difficulty in concentrating	73%
Increased appetite or weight gain	73%
Restlessness	71%
Craving for cigarettes	62%
Nocturnal awakenings	24%
Headache	N/A
Constipation	N/A

*Frequency of occurrence measured when cigarette smokers stopped smoking "cold turkey".

N/A, Not available.

Note: All the symptoms except headache and constipation are included as nicotine withdrawal symptoms in the current version of the American Psychiatric Association's Diagnostic and Statistical Manual of Mental Disorders, ed 4, also known as DSM-IV,[150] or the predecessor version, DSM-IIIR.[151] Although headache and constipation are not included in these manuals as nicotine withdrawal symptoms, they are regarded by many clinical experts as such. All of these symptoms show a beneficial dose–response effect, being relieved by all tobacco dependence medications, including Controller and Rescue Medications.

including the acetylcholine, norepinephrine, serotonin, vasopressin, and β-endorphin neurotransmitter systems.[40] Most important, nicotine activates the brain's mesolimbic dopaminergic system—the pleasure—reward system.[40-42] These activated systems improve concentration, reaction time, learning, and memory, reinforcing addiction.[40-42] The rapid onset and short half-life (about 2 hours) of nicotine further increase addiction.[43,44]

The severity of physical nicotine dependence varies from mild (about 10% of cigarette smokers) to severe (also about 10% of cigarette smokers). It can be measured easily in a clinical practice setting with the Fagerström Test for Nicotine Dependence (FTND),[45] a physiologically validated linear scale from 0 to 10. Each 1-point increase on the FTND scale corresponds to an approximately 10% increase in physical nicotine dependence. As with blood pressure in hypertension, a higher FTND score at initial assessment requires correspondingly more intense and longer treatment.

Nicotine withdrawal occurs when the nicotine molecule is no longer available to bind into CNS nicotinic receptors, particularly the $\alpha_4\beta_2$ nicotinic receptor.[46,47] Animal studies show nicotine withdrawal to be of pathophysiologic, not psychological, origin.[48] When nicotine-dependent patients abruptly stop tobacco use (cold turkey), most will experience physically caused nicotine withdrawal[49-51] (see Table 16-1). Average weight gain in successful quitters is 3 to 4 kg, but up to 10% report weight gain of 13 kg or more.[52,53] Withdrawal symptoms peak within 48 to 72 hours,[51] gradually declining over the next 6 months,[49] but last for years to life in some patients.

Practice Concepts and Principles

1. Tobacco dependence is a chronic, relapsing, life-threatening medical disease, with a defined neuropathologic basis, and must be treated as such.
2. Short-term medical treatment should not be expected to produce a "cure" any more than 6-week use of a long-acting β_2-agonist would produce a cure for asthma.
3. Anticipate relapse more than once before the patient is able to stop tobacco use permanently.
4. Cigarette smoking is not a habit or a "lifestyle" choice.
5. Disabling, physically caused nicotine withdrawal symptoms, although generally declining 6 months after a person stops smoking, can last a lifetime, in the absence of adequate and appropriate medical treatment.

PULMONARY CONSEQUENCES OF TOBACCO USE

Chronic Obstructive Pulmonary Disease

In their Global Initiative for Chronic Obstructive Lung Disease (GOLD) guidelines meta-analysis, the National Heart, Lung, and Blood Institute and the World Health Organization concluded that cigarette smoke was the predominant pathogen causing approximately 90% of all chronic obstructive pulmonary disease (COPD) cases among cigarette users, including emphysema and chronic bronchitis.[54] For those who had never smoked, secondhand smoke exposure was the major COPD pathogen.[54]

Is COPD Self-inflicted?

Many physicians and most tobacco users regard the occurrence of any tobacco-induced disease, including COPD, as self-inflicted and clearly the smoker's own fault. This conclusion is *not* supported by the scientific facts that now support our knowledge of the biology of nicotine addition.[40-42] Once the casual cigarette user shifts from an occasional cigarette every few days to even as few as one or two every day, the ultrahigh nicotine doses delivered ultrafast to the CNS induce permanent neuronal changes.[6] Once brain structure and function are permanently altered by the nicotine in tobacco smoke—generally occurring after only 10 days of daily tobacco use—that person has a physical addiction, making it much more difficult, if not impossible, to quit smoking without appropriate treatment. The potency of this physical addiction means that patients really don't have the "choice" of whether or not to smoke. However, they can choose effective treatment that will enable them to quit.

Bronchogenic Carcinoma

Similarly, cigarette smoke, through direct exposure or as secondhand smoke, is the primary pathogen causing approximately 90% of all bronchogenic carcinoma,[55] which is also not "self-inflicted."

Interstitial Lung Disease

Tobacco smoke is also the primary pathogen underlying a large number of the interstitial lung diseases.

Asthma

Direct tobacco smoke exposure or secondhand smoke exposure will aggravate pre-existing asthma, thereby resulting in increased asthma morbidity and mortality.

MEDICATIONS FOR TREATING TOBACCO DEPENDENCE

The fundamental goal in tobacco dependence treatment is to suppress nicotine withdrawal symptoms as completely as possible, to minimize relapse risk.[5] This result can usually be achieved with adequate doses and combinations of the currently available tobacco-dependence medications (Table 16-2).

Five fundamental pharmacologic categories, or classes, of medications are available to treat tobacco dependence. Effectiveness varies widely across medication class, and not all drugs that are effective are approved by the U.S. Food and Drug Administration (FDA) for this indication. Instead of simply grouping medications by these five mechanisms of action, however, dividing them into two descriptive groups—Controller and Rescue Medications—Clarifies appropriate function and use. Controller Medications take time (4 to 6 hours to 1 week) to reach peak levels in the brain and to clear, once the patient stops using them. Rescue Medications have a fast onset (a few seconds to minutes) and so can provide rapid relief when the patient experiences breakthrough nicotine withdrawal symptoms, such as an unexpected, severe cigarette craving.

TABLE 16-2 Medications for Treating Tobacco Dependence

Drug	Available Dosages	Usual Adult Maintenance Dosage	Frequent or Severe Adverse Effects*	Approved (FDA) and/or Recommended (PHS, Sachs)[†]
CONTROLLER MEDICATIONS: FIRST LINE				
α₄β₂ Nicotinic Receptor Partial Agonists				
Varenicline (Chantix)	0.5- and 1.0-mg tablets	1 mg twice per day	Nausea, vomiting, constipation, flatulence, abnormal dreams, headache, xerostomia, weight gain	FDA, Sachs
Dopaminergic–Noradrenergic Reuptake Inhibitors				
Bupropion HCl (immediate acting)	75- and 100-mg tablets	100 mg three times per day	Insomnia, xerostomia, headache, all generally mild and transient. Seizure incidence in long-term, antidepression, safety surveillance studies was 0.4% for the immediate-acting formulation and 0.1% for the sustained-release formulation. Seizure has not occurred, even with daily use of 300 mg up to 1 yr, in the >2500 study participants double-blindly randomized to an active bupropion SR formulation in tobacco dependence treatment trials. Exceeding rare incidence rate of Stevens-Johnson syndrome, hyperanxiety state, and elevated hepatic enzymes. *General caution:* Bupropion	PHS-1, Sachs (bupropion HCl)
Bupropion SR (Wellbutrin SR, Zyban)	100-, 150-, and 200-mg sustained-release tablets	150 mg twice per day		PHS-1, Sachs (Wellbutrin SR); FDA, PHS-1, Sachs (Zyban)
Bupropion XL (Wellbutrin XL)[‡]	150- and 300-mg extended-release tablets	300 mg once daily in the morning		Sachs (bupropion XL)

Continued

TABLE 16-2	Medications for Treating Tobacco Dependence—cont'd

Drug	Available Dosages	Usual Adult Maintenance Dosage	Frequent or Severe Adverse Effects*	Approved (FDA) and/or Recommended (PHS, Sachs)[†]
			should not be administered in conjunction with an MAO inhibitor	
Nicotinic Receptor Agonists				
Nicotine transdermal (NicoDerm CQ, Novartis generic)	7, 14, and 21 mg/24 hr	1 patch/day[¶]	Pruritus at the patch site; insomnia; bizarre dreams; ~2.5%	FDA, PHS-1, Sachs
(Nicotrol)[§,‖]	5, 10, and 15 mg/16 hr	1 patch/day	incidence of cutaneous hypersensitivity reaction caused by 24-hr wear cycle. Neither nicotine overdose nor cardiac events increase with use of transdermal nicotine in conjunction with cigarette smoking beyond that seen with cigarette smoking, alone	FDA, PHS-1, Sachs

CONTROLLER MEDICATIONS: SECOND LINE (OPTIONS IF FIRST-LINE MEDICATIONS NOT TOLERATED)

Drug	Available Dosages	Usual Adult Maintenance Dosage	Frequent or Severe Adverse Effects*	Approved (FDA) and/or Recommended (PHS, Sachs)[†]
α_2-Adrenergic Agonists				
Clonidine HCl (Catapres)	0.1- and 0.2-mg tablets	0.2 or 0.3 mg twice per day	*From tobacco-dependence trials: Dose*	PHS-2, Sachs**
Clonidine transdermal (Catapres-TTS)	0.1, 0.2, and 0.3 mg/day/ 1-wk patch	1 patch/wk delivering 0.2-0.3 mg/day	*related*—Decreased heart rate; decreased systolic blood pressure; decreased diastolic blood pressure; xerostomia; drowsiness; spacey feeling; dizziness; postural hypotension. *Not necessarily dose-related*—Nausea; vomiting. *With transdermal only*—Pruritus; erythema; edema; vesicles; blisters, all at the patch application site, only	PHS-2, Sachs**
Noradrenergic–Serotonergic Reuptake Inhibitor				
Nortriptyline HCl (Aventyl, Pamelor)	25- and 75-mg capsules	25 mg 3-4 times per day	*From tobacco-dependence trials*: constipation; xerostomia; lightheadedness; tremor; blurred vision. *From antidepression trials*: rash; weight gain; xerostomia; lightheadedness; tremor; constipation; blurred vision;	PHS-2, Sachs

| TABLE 16-2 | Medications for Treating Tobacco Dependence—cont'd |

Drug	Available Dosages	Usual Adult Maintenance Dosage	Frequent or Severe Adverse Effects*	Approved (FDA) and/or Recommended (PHS, Sachs)[†]
			impotence; decreased libido; urinary retention; tachycardia; pedal edema; chest pain; shortness of breath; headache; agitation; nausea; vomiting; dizziness; insomnia; hyperhidrosis. *General caution:* Nortriptyline should not be administered in conjunction with an MAO inhibitor	

RESCUE MEDICATIONS: FIRST LINE

Nicotinic Receptor Agonists

Drug	Available Dosages	Usual Adult Maintenance Dosage	Frequent or Severe Adverse Effects*	Approved (FDA) and/or Recommended (PHS, Sachs)[†]
Nicotine-β-cyclodextrin sublingual tablet[‡,††]	2-mg tablet	2 mg 8 to 16 times daily	Hiccups; nausea; dyspepsia	Sachs
Nicotine nasal spray (Nicotrol NS)	0.5 mg/spray; 1 dose = 2 sprays	1 dose 8 to 40 times daily	Minor burning and stinging of the nasal mucosa; minor throat irritation; cough; sneeze; increased lacrimation; rhinorrhea; nausea. (*Note:* All these side effects generally last only a few seconds)	FDA, PHS-1, Sachs
Nicotine oral inhaler (Nicotrol Inhaler)	4-mg cartridge	4-16 cartridges per day	Minor mouth irritation; throat irritation; cough	FDA, PHS-1, Sachs
Nicotine polacrilex gum (Nicorette)[||]	2 and 4 mg/piece	8-24 pieces per day	Side effects generally result from improper chewing technique and include indigestion, nausea, flatulence, unpleasant taste, hiccups, sore mouth, sore throat, sore jaw	FDA, PHS-1, Sachs
Nicotine polacrilex lozenge (Commit)[||]	2 and 4 mg/lozenge	8-20 lozenges per day	Heartburn, hiccup, and nausea, due to swallowed nicotine; headache	FDA, Sachs

COMBINATION MEDICATIONS

Drug	Available Dosages	Usual Adult Maintenance Dosage	Frequent or Severe Adverse Effects*	Approved (FDA) and/or Recommended (PHS, Sachs)[†]
Bupropion SR + nicotine transdermal	150-mg Bupropion SR + 15-mg nicotine/16 hr *or* 21-mg nicotine/24 hr	See previous entries	Bizarre dreams; insomnia; nausea; patch-site erythema or pruritus	FDA, PHS-1, Sachs
Bupropion SR + nicotine medication	See previous entries	See previous entries	Insomnia; xerostomia; side effects specific to the specific nicotine medication	PHS-1, Sachs

Continued

TABLE 16-2 Medications for Treating Tobacco Dependence—cont'd

Drug	Available Dosages	Usual Adult Maintenance Dosage	Frequent or Severe Adverse Effects*	Approved (FDA) and/or Recommended (PHS, Sachs)[†]
Nicotine transdermal+ nicotine nasal spray	See previous entries	See previous entries	Nasal irritation; pruritus and skin irritation at the patch site[‡‡]	PHS-1, Sachs
Nicotine transdermal+ nicotine oral inhaler	See previous entries	See previous entries	Throat irritation and pruritus at the patch site[‡‡]	PHS-1, Sachs
Nicotine transdermal+ nicotine polacrilex gum	See previous entries	See previous entries	Indigestion, nausea, flatulence, unpleasant taste, hiccups, sore mouth, sore throat, sore jaw; pruritus and skin irritation at the patch site[‡‡]	PHS-1, Sachs

FDA, *FDA approved for the treatment of tobacco dependence; MAO, monoamine oxidase; NS, nasal spray; PHS-1, PHS 2000 recommended for first-line treatment, as stated in the Public Health Service, Clinical practice guideline: treating tobacco use and dependence, 2000; PHS-2, PHS 2000 recommended for second-line treatment, as stated in the Public Health Service, Clinical practice guideline: treating tobacco use and dependence, 2000; Sachs, recommended by David P.L. Sachs, MD, as clinically safe, effective, and useful; SR, sustained release; TTS, transdermal therapeutic system; XL, extended release.*
Adverse effects listed are those reported in tobacco-dependence treatment trials, unless otherwise indicated because some side effects frequently associated with a given drug (e.g., impotence with nortriptyline) did not occur significantly more often for active drug than under placebo drug conditions.
[†]*FDA approved and/or recommended by the Public Health Service and/or Dr. David P.L. Sachs for tobacco dependence treatment.*
[‡]*Peer-reviewed, published studies not available by the 12/31/98 deadline for review and consideration by the Clinical Practice Guideline Committee. On the basis of the quality of the published, randomized, double-blind, placebo-controlled clinical trials now available, this medication would likely meet first-line treatment criteria.*
[§]*See specific label for details regarding dose up-titration.*
[‖]*Available without prescription, over the counter.*
[¶]*Wearing the 24-hour patch for 16 hours yields the same dosage as a 16-hour patch.*
**Efficacy data are much less convincing for clonidine than for any of the first-line medications or for nortriptyline.*
[††]*Available in some European countries.*
[‡‡]*No additive or synergistic side effects; side effects are similar in incidence and severity to those seen with individual medications.*

CONTROLLER MEDICATIONS: FIRST LINE

α4β2 Nicotinic Receptor Partial Agonists

Varenicline

Varenicline tartrate, in a sustained-release oral tablet (Chantix; Pfizer, Inc., New York, N.Y.), is the second non-nicotine medication after bupropion sustained release (see Bupropion Sustained Release section, under Dopaminergic–Noradrenergic Reuptake Inhibitors) to gain FDA approval for treating tobacco dependence[56,57] and the first such new medication since 1997.[58] It is the first tobacco-dependence medication that is a product of deliberate drug development.

Mechanism of Action. Centrally acting, varenicline binds with high affinity and selectivity, providing low-to-moderate levels of dopamine release to suppress nicotine withdrawal symptoms while simultaneously blocking nicotine itself from binding to the α4β2 nicotinic acetylcholine receptor (see Figure 16-2).[59] Consequently, there is minimal, if any, pharmacologic reward if the tobacco-dependent patient smokes a cigarette while taking varenicline. The extent of withdrawal symptom suppression has not yet been determined.

Pharmacokinetics. Varenicline is rapidly absorbed across the gastric mucosa, reaching a peak plasma concentration in about 4 hours.[60] With daily dosing, varenicline attains serum steady state and reaches maximal brain concentration after 4 days. Varenicline has a half-life of 17 hours and is excreted virtually unchanged by the kidneys.[60] There is no liver metabolism.

Clinical Trials. Three randomized, double-blind, placebo-controlled clinical trials demonstrated the effectiveness of varenicline for treating tobacco dependence.[18,19,61] The first and second trials also showed its significant superiority to bupropion sustained release (SR),[18,19] using an identical, double-dummy design to compare the effects of sustained-release varenicline (2 mg/day) against bupropion SR (300 mg/day) and placebo tablets for both medications (Figure 16-1 and Table 16-3). After 12 weeks of treatment, continuous nonsmoking rates were 18%, 30%, and 44%[19] and 18%, 30%, and 44%[18] for placebo, bupropion SR, and varenicline, respectively, and each pairwise comparison within each study was significant ($P \leq .001$).[18,19] Nine months after treatment had stopped, the continuous nonsmoking rates were 8%, 16%, and 22% ($P < .001$ for

varenicline vs. placebo but $P = .057$ for varenicline vs. bupropion)[19] and 10%, 15%, and 23% ($P < .001$ for varenicline vs. placebo and $P = .004$ for varenicline vs. bupropion).[18]

Using 7-day point-prevalence nonsmoking data, which more realistically reflect the realities of medical practice, at the end of the 12-week treatment period, 21%, 36%, and 50%[19] and 21%, 36%, and 50%[18] had stopped smoking for placebo, bupropion SR, and varenicline, respectively ($P < .001$ for all pairwise comparisons).[18,19] Nine months after treatment had ended, 14%, 23%, and 28% ($P < .001$ varenicline vs. placebo and $P = .13$ varenicline vs. bupropion)[19] and 17%,

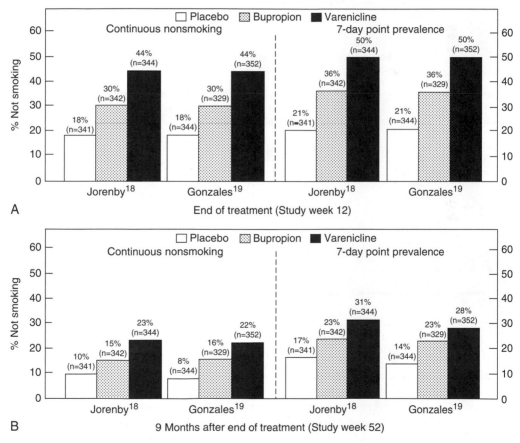

FIGURE 16-1 Side-by-side data from two independent, head-to-head trials comparing varenicline (Chantix) versus bupropion SR (Zyban) versus placebo.[18,19] These trials were randomized, double-blind, double-dummy, placebo-controlled trials. The total number of participants in the study by Jorenby and colleagues was 1027, and the total number of participants in the study by Gonzales and colleagues was 1025. **A,** The end of 12-week treatment outcome results. The percentage of subjects who had successfully stopped smoking was identical across both independent studies, whether using the continuous, no-slip-allowed definition of treatment effectiveness or the 7-day point prevalence definition. Using the continuous nonsmoking definition, varenicline was significantly ($P < .001$) and 1.47-fold more effective than bupropion SR, which in turn was significantly ($P = .001$) and 1.67-fold more effective than placebo tablets; varenicline was 2.44-fold more effective than placebo ($P < .001$). Results and comparative differences were similar using the 7-day point prevalence nonsmoking definition. **B,** The 9-month outcome results from the end of treatment (Study Week 12) through the study end (study week 52).

TABLE 16-3 Effectiveness of Varenicline and Bupropion for Tobacco-Dependence Treatment: Objectively Validated Nonsmoking Rates[18, 19]

Study	Evaluated at:	Medication	Continuous Nonsmoking Rate (%)*	7-Day Point-Prevalence Nonsmoking Rate (%)
Jorenby et al study[18] (N = 1027)	End of treatment (study week 12)	Varenicline SR (2 mg/day) (n = 344)	44[†,‡]	50[§]
		Bupropion SR (300 mg/day) (n = 342)	30[¶]	36[§]
		Placebo (n = 341)	18	21
	1 yr after TQD (9 mo off-treatment)	Varenicline SR (2 mg/day) (n = 344)	23[†,¶]	31[†,**]
		Bupropion SR (300 mg/day) (n = 342)	15[††]	23[‡‡]
		Placebo (n = 341)	10	17
Gonzales et al study[19] (N = 1025)	End of treatment (study week 12)	Varenicline SR (2 mg/day) (n = 352)	44[§]	50[§]
		Bupropion SR (300 mg/day) (n = 329)	30[§]	36[§]
		Placebo (n = 344)	18	21
	1 yr after TQD (9 mo off-treatment)	Varenicline SR (2 mg/day) (n = 352)	22[†,§§]	28[†,§§]
		Bupropion SR (300 mg/day) (n = 329)	16[¶]	23[‡‡]
		Placebo (n = 344)	8	14

SR, *Sustained release;* TQD, *Target Quit Date.*
Continuous nonsmoking, no slips allowed.
[†]P <.001 for varenicline versus placebo.
[‡]P <.001 for varenicline versus bupropion.
[§]P <.001 for all pairwise comparisons.
[||]P =.001 for bupropion versus placebo.
[¶]P =.004 for varenicline versus bupropion.
[**]P =.05 for varenicline versus bupropion.
[††]P =.08 for bupropion versus placebo.
[‡‡]P <.05 for bupropion versus placebo.
[§§]P ≥.06 for varenicline versus bupropion.

23%, and 31% ($P \leq .05$ for all pairwise comparisons)[18] had stopped smoking. As with any chronic medical disease, after short-term treatment stopped, many patients (approximately 40% in the varenicline- and bupropion-treated groups[18,19]) experienced treatment failure (i.e., relapsed to cigarette smoking), within 9 months.

Although bupropion significantly suppressed weight gain 12 weeks after the Target Quit Date (by 40%; 1.27 kg), patients treated with varenicline who stopped smoking gained the same amount of weight as the placebo-treated patients: 2.89 kg versus 3.15 kg ($P > .6$).[18]

The third trial, a 6-month maintenance study, examined the benefit of a second 12 weeks of treatment (double-blind) for those who had successfully stopped smoking after the first 12 weeks (open-label) of varenicline treatment, approximately 1210 (63%) of 1927 study patients (Table 16-4). Although this study design was strongly criticized in an accompanying editorial,[62] it answers a real-world medical question that physicians face each day, confirming that 12 additional weeks of varenicline treatment provided further treatment benefit and reduced relapse.[61] Varenicline more than doubled the time to first lapse during the double-blind phase (weeks 12 to 24): 87 days for placebo versus 198 days for varenicline ($P <.001$).[61] At the end of the second 12 weeks of treatment, the continuous nonsmoking rates were 50% and 71% (placebo and varenicline, respectively; $P <.001$).[61] After 24 more weeks off study drug,

TABLE 16-4 Effectiveness of 6-Month Varenicline Tobacco-Dependence Treatment to Prevent Relapse: Objectively Validated Smoking Cessation Rates[61]

Number of Participants	Evaluated at:	Medication	Continuous Nonsmoking Rate (%)*
Open-label phase study weeks 1-12: (N_1 = 1927)	End of open-label phase (12 wk)	Varenicline (1 mg, twice daily)	64%
Double-blind phase study weeks 13-52: (N_2 = 1210; 63% of N_1)	End of treatment (6 mo)	Varenicline (1 mg, twice daily) (n = 603)	71%[†]
		Placebo (n = 607)	50%
	1 yr after TQD (6 mo off-treatment)	Varenicline (1 mg, twice daily) (n = 603)	44%[‡]
		Placebo (n = 607)	37%

TQD, *Target Quit Date.*
Continuous nonsmoking, no slips allowed.
†P <.001 (vs. placebo).
‡P =.02 (vs. placebo).

more varenicline-treated patients, not surprisingly, had relapsed than those who received placebo for the second 12-week treatment period: 38% (varenicline) versus 26% (placebo). The nature of a chronic disease dictates that when treatment is stopped, symptoms return. Despite that, varenicline-treated participants had significantly better continuous nonsmoking rates from week 12 through week 52 than did those treated with placebo: 44% versus 37% (varenicline vs. placebo, respectively; P =.02).[61]

Dosage. Varenicline should be started at least 7 days *before* the Target Quit Date to allow for adequate steady-state CNS levels.[56] The recommended dosage of varenicline is 0.5 mg once daily for 3 days, increasing to 0.5 mg twice daily for days 4 to 7, and finally increasing to the maintenance dose of 1 mg twice daily for the first 12 weeks of treatment. Patients who have been effectively treated during the first 12 weeks should continue varenicline treatment for at least a second 12-week cycle.

A 3-month course of varenicline significantly improves tobacco dependence treatment, increasing smoking cessation rates at the end of treatment and 9 months thereafter as well as reducing nicotine withdrawal symptoms. Varenicline reduces relapse when used for 6 months rather than 3 months; however, as would be expected when treating a chronic disease with a short-term course of medication, relapse is substantial and significant after stopping varenicline, suggesting that many patients will need treatment for longer than 6 months if they are to remain free of tobacco use. The FDA label does not limit the total duration of use.[63]

There are no currently published guidelines for optimally reducing varenicline dose. The clinical trials abruptly terminated the dose at the end of the active treatment phase. Some clinical experts use a tapering process that is the reverse of the increasing dose titration used during the first 2 weeks of varenicline treatment. With this approach, tapering should be increased to the previous dose if nicotine withdrawal symptoms appear.

Varenicline is 30% more effective than bupropion. Whether varenicline alone is more effective than any of the nicotine medications is not known. Varenicline has not been tested in combination with any other tobacco dependence medications.

Practice Concepts and Principles

Varenicline is the most effective monotherapy for tobacco dependence.
6. Use of varenicline, 2 mg/day for 12 weeks, significantly improves smoking cessation rates compared with either bupropion SR or placebo use for 12 weeks.
7. Use of varenicline, 2 mg/day for 6 months, significantly improves smoking cessation rates compared with only 12 weeks of use.
8. Use of varenicline, 2 mg/day for 12 weeks, does not suppress weight gain compared with placebo. In contrast, use of bupropion SR, 300 mg/day, suppresses weight gain by about one third.
9. Some patients will need continuous varenicline treatment of indefinite duration to provide effective treatment.

Dopaminergic–Noradrenergic Reuptake Inhibitors

Bupropion Sustained Release

There is presently only one medication in this inhibitor category: bupropion sustained release (SR). It was launched in the United States in 1997[58] and was the first non-nicotine medication for tobacco dependence treatment.

Mechanism of Action. Bupropion SR is a centrally acting weak dopamine and norepinephrine reuptake inhibitor (see Figure 16-2). It has no effect on the CNS serotonin system and has no serotonin reuptake inhibition properties.[64]

Pharmacokinetics. Bupropion SR is absorbed across the gastric mucosa, reaching peak plasma levels after 3 hours. Absorption is unaffected by food intake. Steady-state serum levels are thought to occur after about 7 days. While bupropion SR has a serum half-life of 21 hours, it has several therapeutically active metabolites that have much longer half-lives of 3 to 4 weeks. Bupropion is hepatically metabolized.

Clinical Trials. In five randomized, double-blind, placebo-controlled studies, bupropion SR significantly improved cessation rates[12,65-68] (Table 16-5). Although relapse was substantial in the first study after the end of treatment (7 weeks), there was still a significant dose–response relationship 12 months after the Target Quit Date.[12] The same study also documented a significant, orderly, inverse relationship between bupropion SR dose and weight gain. The 300-mg dose suppressed weight gain by 50%, compared with placebo, with the other two doses intermediate between the 300-mg and placebo doses.[12] A second 10-week combination trial comparing bupropion SR with transdermal nicotine showed significantly different nonsmoking rates at the end of the 10-week treatment period.[65] Although relapse was considerable, 9.5 months after short-term medication treatment was stopped, those who had been treated with either combination therapy or bupropion alone were significantly more likely to remain nonsmoking than those who had been treated with either transdermal nicotine alone or placebo.[65]

A third relapse prevention trial showed that long-term bupropion use more than doubled the median number of days to relapse: 65 days (placebo) versus 166 days (bupropion SR) ($P = .021$).[66] During the second year, when patients were off all study medication, the effectiveness of bupropion persisted through month 18. A fourth short-term trial showed bupropion SR to be safe and effective in treating lower income African Americans.[67] Bupropion SR was also shown, in a fifth trial, to be effective in retreating smokers who had previously used bupropion SR but had subsequently relapsed, increasing the continuous nonsmoking rate more than fivefold at the end of the 6-week treatment phase.[68]

Relapse about 10.5 weeks after treatment end is considerable with all short-term studies,[12,65,67,68] further supporting the conclusion that many patients require long-term treatment.

Dosage. Like varenicline, bupropion SR must be started 7 to 14 days *before* the Target Quit Date to allow for adequate, steady-state CNS levels. Typically, patients start with 150 mg each morning, for 3 days, increasing to the maintenance dose of 150 mg every 12 hours. Patients who have been effectively treated for the initial 7 weeks should continue bupropion treatment for at least a total of 1 year. The FDA label does not limit the total duration of use and states in the Maintenance subsection under the Dosage and Administration section (p. 1649): "Nicotine dependence is a chronic condition. Some patients may need continuous treatment."[69]

Only the sustained-release formulation of bupropion hydrochloride, under the brand name Zyban, is approved by the FDA for the treatment of tobacco dependence. Bupropion is also sold generically in two different formulations: immediate acting and sustained release, and as a branded product with multiple formulations: Wellbutrin (bupropion hydrochloride immediate acting), Wellbutrin SR (bupropion hydrochloride sustained release, identical to Zyban), and Wellbutrin XL (bupropion hydrochloride extended release). Although only Zyban is approved by the FDA for tobacco-dependence treatment, all of the cited bupropion formulations should be equally effective. The immediate-acting formulation, which should be given as 100 mg, three times daily, has been tested in randomized, double-blind trials and is effective for tobacco dependence.[70-72] The extended release formulation, which should be given as 300 mg once daily in the morning, has not been tested for tobacco-dependence treatment to date. Most clinical experts use all three dosage formulations interchangeably, in equivalent daily doses, depending on patient needs and compliance.

There are no currently published guidelines for optimally reducing bupropion dose. The clinical trials abruptly terminated the dose at the end of the active treatment phase. Some clinical experts use a tapering process that is the reverse of the

TABLE 16-5   Effectiveness of Bupropion SR for Tobacco Dependence Treatment: Five Randomized, Double-blind Clinical Studies

Number of Participants	Evaluated at:	Medication	Percentage Not Smoking (%)	P Value
1. DOSE–RESPONSE STUDY[12]				
N = 615	6 wk (end of treatment)	Bupropion SR (300 mg/day) (n = 156)	44%*	<.001[†]
		Bupropion SR (150 mg/day) (n = 153)	39%	
		Bupropion SR (100 mg/day) (n = 153)	29%	
		Placebo (n = 153)	19%	
	1 yr	Bupropion SR (300 mg/day) (n = 156)	23%	=.02[†]
		Bupropion SR (150 mg/day) (n = 153)	23%	
		Bupropion SR (100 mg/day) (n = 153)	20%	
		Placebo (n = 153)	12%	
2. COMBINATION STUDY[65]				
N = 893	8 wk (end of treatment)	Bupropion SR (300 mg/day) plus nicotine patch (21 mg/24 hr) (n = 245)	66%*	≤.005
		Bupropion SR (300 mg/day) (n = 244)	58%	
		Nicotine patch (21 mg/24 hr) (n = 244)	42%	
		Placebo (n = 160)	33%	
	1 yr	Bupropion SR (300 mg/day) plus nicotine patch (21 mg/24 hr) (n = 245)	36%	<.001[‡]
		Bupropion SR (300 mg/day) (n = 244)	30%	
		Nicotine patch (21 mg/24 hr) (n = 244)	16%	
		Placebo (n = 160)	16%	
3. RELAPSE PREVENTION STUDY[66]				
Open-label phase (N_1 = 784)	6 wk	Bupropion SR (300 mg/day) (n = 784)	59%*	N/A
Double-blind phase (N_2 = 429; 55% of N_1)	12 wk	Bupropion SR (300 mg/day) (n = 214)	82%	=.003
		Placebo (n = 215)	69%	
	6 mo	Bupropion SR (300 mg/day) (n = 214)	68%	=.003
		Placebo (n = 215)	54%	
	1 yr (end of treatment)	Bupropion SR (300 mg/day) (n = 214)	55%	=.008
		Placebo (n = 215)	42%	
	2 yr (1 yr off study drug)	Bupropion SR (300 mg/day) (n = 214)	42%	>.05
		Placebo (n = 215)	40%	
4. LOW SES AFRICAN AMERICAN STUDY[67]				
N = 600 lower income African Americans	1 wk	Bupropion SR (300 mg/day) (n = 300)	36%*	<.001
		Placebo (n = 300)	16%	
	3 wk	Bupropion SR (300 mg/day) (n = 300)	31%	<.001
		Placebo (n = 300)	14%	
	6 wk (end of treatment)	Bupropion SR (300 mg/day) (n = 300)	36%	<.001
		Placebo (n = 300)	19%	

Continued

TABLE 16-5   Effectiveness of Bupropion SR for Tobacco Dependence Treatment: Five Randomized, Double-blind Clinical Studies—cont'd

Number of Participants	Evaluated at:	Medication	Percentage Not Smoking (%)	P Value
	6 mo	Bupropion SR (300 mg/day) (n = 300)	21%	=.02
		Placebo (n = 300)	14%	
5. BUPROPION RE-TREATMENT STUDY[68]				
N = 450 tobacco-dependent patients previously treated with bupropion SR but relapsed	6 wk	Bupropion SR (300 mg/day) (n = 226)	41%*	≤.002
		Placebo (n = 224)	13%	
	12 wk (end of treatment)	Bupropion SR (300 mg/day) (n = 226)	32%	≤.002
		Placebo (n = 224)	11%	
	6 mo	Bupropion SR (300 mg/day) (n = 226)	21%	≤.002
		Placebo (n = 224)	10%	

N/A, *Not available;* SES, *socioeconomic status;* SR, *sustained release;* TQD, *Target Quit Date.*
Note: *Participants were nondepressed, predominantly white, cigarette-smoking patients, unless otherwise specified.*
Note: *The first week of treatment was pre-TQD for all studies. The evaluation points refer to the time period after the Target Quit Date.*
*All nonsmoking percentages for this study are 7-day point-prevalence nonsmoking rates.
†*Linear-trend P value.*
‡P < .001 for all combinations except for bupropion SR versus bupropion SR plus transdermal nicotine, where P = .22 and transdermal nicotine versus placebo, where P = .84.

increasing dose titration used during the first 2 weeks of bupropion treatment. Because of the long half-life of bupropion's active metabolites, however, each dose reduction should be 4 to 6 weeks in duration. Tapering should be increased to the previous dose if nicotine withdrawal symptoms appear.

Practice Concepts and Principles

10. Use of bupropion SR (sustained release), 300 mg/day (given as 150 mg, two times daily) for 7 weeks, significantly improves smoking cessation rates compared with placebo use for 7 weeks.
11. Use of bupropion SR, 300 mg/day for 1 year, significantly improves smoking cessation rates compared with only 7 weeks of use.
12. Use of bupropion SR, 300 mg/day for 7 weeks, suppresses weight gain by 50% compared with placebo. When used for 1 year, weight gain remains significantly suppressed compared with placebo, without weight gain rebound when bupropion SR is discontinued.
13. Bupropion immediate acting, 300 mg/day (given as 100 mg 3 times daily), and bupropion extended release, 300 mg/day (given as 300 mg each morning), also provide effective tobacco-dependence treatment.
14. Some patients will need continuous bupropion treatment of indefinite duration to provide effective treatment.

Nicotinic Receptor Agonists
Nicotine

Although varenicline is a partial nicotinic receptor agonist, nicotine is the only presently available nicotine receptor agonist (Figure 16-2). It was first made available in the United States in 1984 as nicotine polacrilex gum (Nicorette and others), a Rescue Medication. Nicotine comes in only one Controller Medication delivery system, the nicotine patch, and five Rescue Medication delivery systems (see the discussion of nicotine medication delivery systems in the section on first-line Rescue Medications). Transdermal nicotine (i.e., the nicotine patch) delivers nicotine to the CNS, reaching a peak serum level (arterial and venous) 4 to 8 hours after application, depending on the specific patch brand used.[73] Most clinical experts regard the highest strength patch ("Step 1") within each brand or generic (15 mg/16 hr or 21 mg/24 hr) to have identical therapeutic efficacy. Transdermal nicotine is typically started on the patient's Target Quit Date.

The nicotine patch, when used alone, independent of the level of counseling support provided, doubles to triples smoking cessation rates compared with placebo.[3] As noted elsewhere, pharmacotherapy and counseling support, provided by a physician or health-care professional, each independently improves treatment outcome.[3] Particularly over the first year, longer, more intensive, and more frequent outpatient office visits increase the absolute percentage of effectively treated and tobacco-free patients. Even standard-dose nicotine patch pharmacotherapy will improve treatment effectiveness by twofold to threefold.

Practice Concepts and Principles
15. All first-line Controller Medications significantly: <ul><li>Improve tobacco-dependence treatment outcome,</li><li>Reduce physically-caused nicotine withdrawal symptoms by twofold to threefold during a short-term treatment course (6-12 weeks),</li><li>Improve smoking cessation rates by twofold to threefold at the end of a short-term treatment course (6-12 weeks), and</li><li>Improve smoking cessation rates by twofold to threefold 1 year after Target Quit Date, even although active medication treatment stopped 9 or more months before.</li></ul>

CONTROLLER MEDICATIONS: SECOND LINE

α_2-Adrenergic Agonists
Clonidine
Clonidine (Catapres and Catapres-TTS) may improve smoking cessation rates relative to placebo, but data are mixed.[74,75] Clonidine should be started several weeks before the Target Quit Date, with the dose adjusted up to the highest tolerable dose before side effects—usually hypotension or orthostasis—occur. The dosage generally starts at 0.1 mg twice daily, slowly increasing to a maximal total daily dosage of 0.3 to 0.5 mg/day. *When clonidine is discontinued, the dose should be gradually reduced over 2 to 4 days to avoid possible rebound hypertension, agitation, confusion, and/or tremor.* No clonidine preparation has been systematically tested with any combination of nicotine medications (Controller or Rescue), bupropion SR, or varenicline.

Noradrenergic–Serotonergic Reuptake Inhibitors
Nortriptyline
Nortriptyline HCl (Aventyl and Pamelor) significantly improves smoking cessation rates relative to placebo by two- to threefold.[76,77] Therapy must be initiated 10 to 28 days before the Target Quit Date to allow nortriptyline to reach CNS steady-state levels. The dosage generally starts at 25 mg/day, slowly increasing to a maximum of

75 to 100 mg/day. The longer nortriptyline is used, the better the treatment results (smoking cessation rates): 12 months of use is nearly three times more effective than short-term use for only 3 months, significantly boosting 1-year nonsmoking rates from 20% to 56% (P =.009).[20]

RESCUE MEDICATIONS: FIRST LINE

Nicotinic Receptor Agonists
Nicotine
In addition to the nicotine patch Controller Medication, nicotine is also available as four different types of Rescue Medications, each with different pharmacokinetics: nicotine, nasal spray, oral inhaler, polacrilex gum, and polacrilex lozenge (see Table 16-2). A fifth Rescue Medication, the nicotine sublingual tablet, is available in some European countries, Australia, and New Zealand. All these systems deliver nicotine to the CNS at a substantially lower dose and at a substantially slower rate than tobacco cigarettes.

The nicotine oral inhaler, polacrilex gum, polacrilex lozenge, and sublingual tablet are intermediate in CNS nicotine medication delivery speed (faster than a nicotine patch, slower than nicotine nasal spray) but sufficiently rapid acting to serve as effective Rescue Medications. Peak arterial nicotine level occurs 20 to 30 minutes after use.

Each of these four nicotine delivery systems has its own maximal arterial nicotine concentration (Cmax), time to maximal arterial nicotine concentration (tmax), and arterial–venous nicotine difference ($[a–v]D_{nic}$). The cigarette delivers nicotine to the brain and all end-organs the most rapidly (arterial tmax = 7 seconds) and with the highest concentration (arterial Cmax = 150 to 250 ng of nicotine per milliliter of blood, $[a–v]D_{nic}$ = 180).

The nicotine oral inhaler, surprisingly, delivers its nicotine via the oral buccal mucosa and not the tracheobronchial tree, let alone at the alveolar level,[78] and there is virtually no arterial–venous nicotine gradient ($[a–v]D_{nic} \approx 0$); thus, the venous and arterial tmax and Cmax are equal: about 20 minutes and 10 ng of nicotine per milliliter of blood, respectively. The nicotine oral inhaler uses 4-mg cartridges; however, as with the nicotine polacrilex gum, which is provided in 2- and 4-mg doses, the amount of nicotine actually absorbed varies widely across patients.[79,80] In addition, patients must take 100 to 200 puffs on the

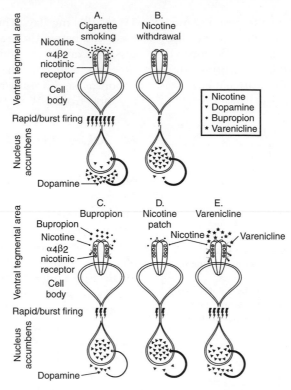

FIGURE 16-2 Schematized dopaminergic neurons in the mesolimbic dopaminergic pathway, extending from the ventral tegmental area (VTA) to the nucleus accumbens. (Not shown are the presynaptic neurons [in the VTA] that contain the normal ligand, acetylcholine, and the postsynaptic neuron [in the nucleus accumbens] that contains the dopamine D_2 receptor sites, into which dopamine binds to activate the next, downstream neuron, which then radiates to the prefrontal cortex.) **A,** Representation of the extremely high density of nicotine molecules (*solid circles*) that flood into the synaptic cleft in the VTA. Nicotine, with a much higher binding affinity, pushes the normal ligand, acetylcholine, out of the way and binds into the $\alpha_4\beta_2$ nicotinic receptor. Nicotine causes considerably more rapid/burst firing of the neuron than acetylcholine could produce, leading to an exuberant discharge of dopamine (*solid inverted triangles*) in the nucleus accumbens. The more dopamine that is released into the postsynaptic cleft, and the longer it remains there, the greater the probability that dopamine will bind into a D_2 receptor in the postsynaptic neurons of the nucleus accumbens, which then radiate to the prefrontal cortex. By this mechanism, nicotine in tobacco smoke produces an intense rush of pleasure. Similarly, nicotine stimulates and enhances cognitive function in the locus ceruleus. After a short period of time, dopamine is recycled back into the distal dopaminergic neuron, in the nucleus accumbens, and repackaged in vesicles for reuse. **B,** The drastically reduced state of rapid/burst firing and dopamine release in the dopaminergic neuron when a tobacco-dependent person attempts to stop cigarette use "cold turkey." Although the presynaptic neuron in the VTA does release acetylcholine, it is incapable of activating the receptor because nicotine from tobacco smoke had desensitized the $\alpha_4\beta_2$ nicotinic receptor sites. Dopamine reuptake occurs at the normal speed, for the little dopamine that is discharged into the synaptic cleft in the nucleus accumbens. **C,** Bupropion (*solid diamonds*) increases dopamine concentration in the distal portion of the dopaminergic neuron, in the synaptic cleft of the nucleus accumbens. As shown by the thinner *semicircular arrow,* bupropion substantially slows dopamine reuptake into the dopaminergic neuron. For some people (about one third), bupropion also exhibits a secondary mechanism of action: it binds into the $\alpha_4\beta_2$ nicotinic receptor site, serving as a partial antagonist to nicotine (shown by the nicotine molecules ricocheting off $\alpha_4\beta_2$ nicotinic receptor sites already occupied by bupropion molecules). **D,** Nicotine (as in **A**), around the proximal end of the dopaminergic neuron in the VTA. However, the standard-dose nicotine patch bathes these regions with approximately 10^3 to 10^6 fewer nicotine molecules than when the person was smoking cigarettes. Thus, standard-dose transdermal nicotine will produce some activation of the dopaminergic neuron, but the rapid/burst firing is substantially less than in (**A**) and about one third less than with the typical therapeutic dose of bupropion (**C**). The nicotine patch has no effect on dopamine reuptake. **E,** The mechanism of action of varenicline. Varenicline (*solid stars*) is a partial agonist of the $\alpha_4\beta_2$ nicotinic receptor site, with much higher binding affinity than nicotine. Varenicline produces about 60% of the rapid/burst firing and subsequent dopamine release that cigarette smoking does. Unlike bupropion, it has no effect on dopamine reuptake at the distal end of the dopaminergic neuron. The ability of varenicline to competitively keep nicotine out of the $\alpha_4\beta_2$ nicotinic receptor site is shown by the nicotine molecules ricocheting off of those receptor sites that are occupied by varenicline.

inhaler during the first 30 to 45 minutes after the cartridge is activated, because most of the nicotine in the cartridge will vaporize into the ambient air within 1 to 2 hours.

The nicotine nasal spray, by far the fastest of all the nicotine medications, is the most effective Rescue Medication, delivering a peak arterial nicotine level to the CNS in only 5 minutes.[81] However, it is still substantially slower than the cigarette, which produces a peak arterial CNS level within 5 to 7 seconds after taking one puff.[81] Each spray delivers 0.5 mg of nicotine (approximately 20% of the nicotine delivered by a cigarette) to the nasal mucosa and turbinates. Its arterial Cmax is approximately 20 ng of nicotine per milliliter of blood, with an arterial tmax of 6 minutes, and an $[a-v]D_{nic}$ of approximately 10.[81] One dose equals 1 spray in each nostril, equivalent to 1 mg of nicotine. Unlike the previously described nicotine delivery systems, the patient will feel a definite beneficial effect from nicotine generally within 60 to 90 seconds after administering one dose.[82,83]

The nicotine polacrilex lozenge, available in the United States since late 2002 in 2- and 4-mg doses, actually delivers more nicotine than the gum because the entire dose is delivered as the lozenge dissolves completely. The 2-mg dose significantly doubles the smoking cessation rate for low-dependent patients, and the 4-mg dose significantly doubles to triples the smoking cessation rate for high-dependent patients.[84] (*Note:* Despite extensive searches of the National Library of Medicine's electronic database and specific queries to the manufacturers, only venous—no arterial—pharmacokinetic data were found for nicotine polacrilex gum or nicotine polacrilex lozenges.)

As with the nicotine patch, each of these four systems doubles to triples the smoking cessation rate when used as monotherapy, *independent* of any physician counseling or support provided. More frequent physician support and longer office visits improve treatment results with any of these Rescue Medications, in direct proportion to the increase.[2] For example, office visits of 15 to 20 minutes (rather than 5 minutes) scheduled 3 to 5 days after the target quit date, then every 3 to 4 weeks for the next several months, and then every 3 months for the first year correspondingly improve results. Allowance should also be made for in-between visits to medically manage new problems or concerns. Controlled clinical trials do not allow us to determine whether or not

certain Rescue Medications might particularly benefit a specific type of patient, such as a highly nicotine-dependent patient or a patient with an underlying depression. When used as monotherapy, any of the Rescue Medications appear equally effective.

Practice Concepts and Principles

16. All Rescue Medications significantly improve smoking cessation rates compared with placebo.
17. The frequency of physician support and office visit duration directly correlate with improved treatment results.

Combination Medications

Most patients will benefit from a combination of a Controller Medication, such as the nicotine patch, and a Rescue Medication, such as the nicotine oral inhaler, which the patient can use on an ad libitum basis to help attenuate sudden, situational, and/or severe nicotine withdrawal symptoms such as break-through anxiety or cigarette craving.[85,86] In addition, taking advantage of the different pharmacokinetic and pharmacodynamic properties of nicotine and non-nicotine medications to provide individualized, combination pharmacotherapy produces the most effective results.[85,86] Unfortunately, no combination trials of varenicline plus any other medication have yet been published. Nonetheless, the pivotal varenicline clinical trials discussed earlier in this chapter suggest that varenicline as monotherapy produces similar treatment outcome results to those achieved by combination treatment with bupropion SR plus standard-dose nicotine patch.[18,65]

The FDA has approved only one combination for tobacco-dependence treatment: Zyban + a nicotine transdermal product. Simultaneous use of a nicotine Controller (i.e., the patch) + a nicotine Rescue Medication (e.g., nicotine nasal spray), although not approved by the FDA, effectively quadruples to sextuples smoking cessation rates during and after treatment.[87-90]

All published studies comparing various nicotine medication combinations show such combinations to be significantly and twofold to threefold more effective than any single, effective medication alone.[87-90] Thus any pairwise medication combination is fourfold to sixfold more effective than treatment that does not use medication at all.

The published combination studies also show such combinations to be safe.[87-90]

Because of its rapid absorption and delivery, nicotine nasal spray can be especially helpful as a Rescue Medication for handling sudden urges or crises, when used in conjunction with the nicotine patch (a Controller) to provide a steady-state plasma level.[88] This approach was validated in an excellent 6-year randomized, double-blind, placebo-controlled study in which subjects used the nicotine patch for 3 months + an active or a placebo nicotine nasal spray for 1 year (Table 16-6). The active combination improved treatment results at 3 months (the end of active nicotine patch treatment), at 6 months (midway during the double-blind phase), and at 1 year (the end of the double-blind active versus placebo nicotine nasal spray treatment phase).[88] Moreover, 6 years after the Target Quit Date, or 5 years after all treatment had ended, those who had received the active nicotine patch for 3 months + an active nicotine nasal spray for 1 year did significantly better than those who had received the active nicotine patch + the placebo nicotine nasal spray.[88] Thus those who had received the combination of active nicotine nasal spray + transdermal nicotine did 1.4-fold better at 3 months, 1.9-fold better at 6 months, 2.5-fold better at 1 year, and 1.8-fold better at 6 years than those who had received only the Controller Medication, the nicotine patch, for 3 months.[88] Because each of these two medications alone is two or three times more effective than placebo, the combination of active nicotine nasal spray + transdermal nicotine was four to six times more effective than no medication at all.

Most clinical experts typically use combinations of two Controllers, bupropion SR and the nicotine patch, plus one or more nicotine Rescue Medications to fully suppress nicotine withdrawal symptoms during the first few weeks or months of treatment. The Public Health Service *Clinical Practice Guideline* recommends two types of combinations as first-line therapy: either the Controllers bupropion SR + a nicotine patch or the Controller nicotine patch + any of the nicotine Rescue Medications (nicotine nasal spray, nicotine oral inhaler, nicotine polacrilex gum, or nicotine polacrilex lozenge).[3]

All published studies to date show combination pharmacotherapy to be safe, even when using nicotine patch doses up to 56 mg of nicotine per day and accompanied by ad libitum nicotine oral inhaler.[91,92] Personal communication directly to me (from L.H. Ferry, 2000)[93] and separately to E.C. Westman (as described in Green and colleagues[92]), as well as my extensive clinical experience with more than 10,000 patients over the past 15 years (unpublished data), show that combination pharmacotherapy with three or more medications is safe, when the combinations and dosages are adjusted to achieve adequate suppression of nicotine withdrawal symptoms. Using the algorithm of adjusting medication doses upward to suppress nicotine withdrawal symptoms as completely as possible, I have used nicotine medication doses as high as 100 mg/day

| TABLE 16-6 | Improved Tobacco-Dependence Treatment Effectiveness Using a Combination of Controller Medication (Nicotine Patch) and Rescue Medication (Nicotine Nasal Spray)[88] |

Evaluated at:	Medication Conditions*	Continuous Nonsmoking (No Slips Allowed) (%)[†]
3 mo (end of nicotine patch treatment)	Nicotine patch plus active NNS	37%
	Nicotine patch plus placebo NNS	25%
6 mo (midway through nicotine nasal spray double-blind phase)	Nicotine patch plus active NNS	31%
	Nicotine patch plus placebo NNS	16%
1 yr (end of nicotine nasal spray treatment)	Nicotine patch plus active NNS	27%
	Nicotine patch plus placebo NNS	11%
6 yr (5 yr after end of nicotine nasal spray treatment)	Nicotine patch plus active NNS	16%
	Nicotine patch plus placebo NNS	9%

NNS, *Nictoine nasal spray.*
Note: *Treatment groups received either active nicotine patch (for 3 months) and active nicotine nasal spray (for 1 year) or active nicotine patch (for 3 months) and placebo nicotine nasal spray (for 1 year).*
Total N = 237 study participants: active nicotine nasal spray (NNS), n = 118; placebo NNS, n = 119.
†P =.004, Kaplan-Meier log-rank test, for the entire survival curve.

from multiple medication sources (Controller + multiple Rescue Medications).

In the most extensive and robust outpatient study to date, Bars and colleagues[85, 86] unequivocally showed that combinations of up to two Controller Medications (nicotine patch + bupropion SR) and up to two Rescue Medications (nicotine nasal spray + nicotine oral inhaler) could be used safely together and that such combinations substantially improved tobacco dependence treatment results, including smoking cessation rates.

Varenicline completely blocks nicotine from being able to bind to central nicotinic receptors, thus eliminating the therapeutic effect of *any* Rescue Medication. No clinical trials have been conducted with any of these combinations. *Use of any of the nicotine Rescue Medications with varenicline is not recommended at this time.*

A limited clinical trial, reported only in the fine print of the physician's prescribing information, was conducted with varenicline + the NicoDerm patch (another Controller Medication).[63] No efficacy data and only some of the adverse event data were reported. Of the participants receiving the active combination, 40% dropped out because of severe nausea, whereas only 3% of those receiving double-blinded placebo for varenicline + active NicoDerm patch dropped out secondary to nausea. Therefore use of varenicline and a nicotine patch is not recommended at this time because of increased adverse effects and the reduced therapeutic effect of nicotine.

The two Controllers, varenicline + bupropion, have not been tested together either but, theoretically, should be more effective than either alone, without an increased incidence of side effects. Nonetheless, until data are available showing safe and effective use, varenicline should not be routinely used with bupropion.

Practice Concepts and Principles

18. Nicotine medication combinations are significantly and twofold to threefold more effective than any single effective medication alone.
19. The combination of Controller Medications bupropion SR + nicotine patch can be used safely and effectively together to improve withdrawal symptom control and smoking cessation rates.
20. The Controller Medication bupropion SR, with or without nicotine patch, + any combination of nicotine Rescue Medications can be used safely and effectively together to further improve nicotine withdrawal symptom control and smoking cessation rates.
21. Varenicline + bupropion SR should be more effective than either listed previously; however, clinical trial efficacy and safety data are not now available.
22. Varenicline should not be more effective if used with nicotine Controller or Rescue Medications; however, clinical trial efficacy data are not now available.
23. The combination of varenicline + nicotine patch (Controller) increased drop-out rate by tenfold resulting from adverse events in the only clinical safety trial to date testing this combination.

Recommendations

1. Optimal cessation rates for physician-directed treatment of tobacco-dependent patients are achieved with at least one Controller Medication, such as bupropion SR or transdermal nicotine, plus at least one Rescue Medication, such as nicotine nasal spray, nicotine oral inhaler, nicotine polacrilex gum, or nicotine polacrilex lozenge.

- The FDA has approved the use of both Controller Medications, bupropion SR and transdermal nicotine, together. Use of both Controller Medications does not preclude the use of one or more Rescue Medications.

2. Varenicline, the most recently released Controller Medication, is also excellent and appears to produce results equivalent to those produced by the combination of bupropion SR + transdermal nicotine. However, there are no known Rescue Medications that can be used safely and effectively with varenicline, so it should be used only as monotherapy.

3. The treating physician should provide regular follow-up office visits to assess treatment effectiveness and side effects, to change medications or dosages to improve treatment results, and to monitor disease complexity. Follow-up visits should be scheduled with criteria similar to those used for other chronic disease states, such as asthma and COPD.

DRUG INTERACTIONS

Effect of Stopping Smoking

Stopping smoking produces profound physiologic changes, altering pharmacodynamics and pharmacokinetics of some commonly used drugs such as insulin, warfarin, thyroxin, and theophylline.[63] Even if the patient is taking combination pharmacotherapy for tobacco dependence, the physician should carefully monitor medication dosages for conditions other than tobacco dependence and adjust them if necessary.[63]

Controller Medications: First Line
Varenicline
Varenicline has no clinically meaningful drug–drug interactions, in part because varenicline is not hepatically metabolized and has negligible effect on the cytochrome P450 system. Excretion of varenicline in the kidney occurs via the renal organic cation transporter OCT2. Cimetidine, an OCT2 inhibitor, reduces varenicline clearance, producing a 29% increase in serum varenicline level.[63] Although coadministration of varenicline (1 mg twice daily) with transdermal nicotine (21 mg/24 hours) did not affect nicotine pharmacokinetics, nausea, headache, vomiting, dizziness, dyspepsia, and fatigue occurred more frequently with the combination than with transdermal nicotine alone. The combination caused 36% premature discontinuance, compared with only 6% in the transdermal nicotine + placebo for varenicline group.[63] Varenicline does not affect warfarin, digoxin, metformin, or bupropion pharmacokinetics.[63]

Bupropion
Only six cases of panic symptoms and psychotic reactions have been reported in patients concurrently taking bupropion and fluoxetine.[94] Millions of patients have safely used bupropion and a selective serotonin reuptake inhibitor (SSRI) concomitantly. One psychotic reaction has been reported with concomitant use of amantadine. Carbamazepine increases the metabolism and decreases the antidepressant effect of bupropion. Bupropion is contraindicated for patients taking a monoamine oxidase inhibitor.

Nicotine
Transdermal nicotine poses no greater risk for interactions with other drugs than that which the patient was exposed to while using tobacco. The greater and more clinically relevant risk is that described previously in the paragraph about the effect of stopping smoking).

Rescue Medications
Nicotine Rescue Medications (nicotine nasal spray, oral inhaler, polacrilex gum, and polacrilex lozenge) do not pose greater drug–drug interaction risk than what the patient has already been exposed to while using tobacco. However, the prescribing physician should closely monitor doses of other medications that nicotine affects. Because the total dose of nicotine delivered via the systemic arterial circulation to the end-organ by these medication systems—even when used in combination and in higher-than-standard doses—is generally 80% to 90% less than from cigarettes (see the discussion of nicotine medication delivery systems in the section on first-line Rescue Medications), dosages of many prescription medications, such as insulin or thyroxin, may need to be adjusted. Multiple nicotine medications have been used in combination in controlled clinical trials without showing any clinically relevant adverse drug interactions.

Practice Concepts and Principles

24. Adverse drug–drug interactions from any of the three Controller Medications or four Rescue Medications with other drugs the patient is taking are generally negligible.
25. Because the high dose of nicotine from tobacco smoke affects hepatic metabolism of many commonly used medications, such as insulin or thyroxin, the treating physician should always closely monitor the therapeutic effect of these medications and adjust doses appropriately after the patient has stopped cigarette use, even if the patient is treated with a nicotine medication (Controller or Rescue).
26. Bupropion SR can be safely used in combination with other antidepressants such as selective serotonin reuptake inhibitors but not with monoamine oxidase inhibitors.

SIDE EFFECTS

Controller Medications: First Line
Varenicline
Varenicline was generally well tolerated, producing few adverse events of clinical consequence. The most frequently occurring adverse events were nausea (29%), abnormal dreams (13%), headache (14%), constipation (9%), vomiting (6%), flatulence (6%), and xerostomia (6%).[18] All these adverse events occurred more frequently with varenicline than with placebo ($P \leq .05$), except for headache (13%), which was significantly greater ($P < .05$) only when compared with bupropion SR (8%).[18] Seizures did not occur in any patient in either of the active treatment groups

(varenicline or bupropion SR) or the placebo group. (*Note:* P values were not provided in the original publications. I computed them with my statistician A. G. Bostrom from the data in the article. Nausea was generally mild to moderate in intensity in about 75% of patients; it is dose dependent[63] but attenuates with longer varenicline use. Side effects that caused premature treatment discontinuation during the 6-month-use study included nausea (3%),[19,61] headache (1%), insomnia (1%), depression (1%), and fatigue (1%).[61] In a separate, 1-year safety study reported in the manufacturer's prescribing information, 36% of patients treated with varenicline (1 mg twice daily) discontinued it as a result of adverse events, mainly nausea, compared with 6% of placebo-treated patients.[63] Taking varenicline with food, however, appears to reduce the incidence and severity of nausea.

In February 2008, the FDA added a warning that depressed mood, agitation, changes in behavior, suicidal ideation, and suicide have been reported in patients attempting to quit smoking while using varenicline. Clinicians should monitor patients for changes in mood and behavior when prescribing this medication.

Fear of weight gain prevents many tobacco-dependent patients from seriously considering stopping smoking, and weight gain is a major cause of relapse. Unlike bupropion SR[12,65,66] and most nicotine medications,[11,94] varenicline does not reduce weight gain after stopping smoking.[18,19,61] Patients who stop smoking with 12 weeks of varenicline treatment can expect to gain 2.89 kg,[18] which is not significantly different than with placebo ($P > .6$),[18,19,61] but is significantly more than with bupropion SR, 1.88 kg ($P < .02$).[18]

Bupropion SR

In all five of the bupropion SR tobacco dependence clinical trials, more than 2500 men and women were randomized to active bupropion SR. There were no seizures,[12,66,67,95] nor did seizures occur in the two more recent large-scale, head-to-head, bupropion–varenicline trials.[18,19] (*Note:* In all seven of these trials, potential study participants were excluded if they met any of the following criteria: previous or current history of seizure, brain surgery, severe head trauma, alcoholism, bulimia, or anorexia nervosa; or were taking a medication known to lower seizure threshold.) Side effects that did occur were generally mild, decreasing with continued bupropion use, and of little

clinical significance.[12,65-67] Insomnia (30% to 50%) and xerostomia (dry mouth) (15%) were significantly and positively associated with mean bupropion metabolite concentration.[96] Insomnia that occurs when bupropion SR is taken every 12 hours can frequently be controlled by taking the evening dose 8 hours after the first dose, or by switching to the XL formulation, which is taken only once daily, in the morning. Sedation, decreased libido, and impotence occurred no more often in bupropion SR-treated patients than in those given placebo.[12,65,66] There was no difference in dropout rates due to adverse events between any of the treatment conditions, including placebo, in any of these five studies. In the 1-year relapse prevention study, there were no significant differences in adverse event rates between the bupropion- and placebo-treated subjects throughout the entire 12 months of treatment.[66]

Nicotine

Nicotine patch is usually well tolerated without side effects of major clinical significance. The only significant side effects that caused some patients to discontinue nicotine patch use were pruritus at the patch site, insomnia, and bizarre dreams.[11,98,99] Each patch uses a different adhesive, so switching brands may reduce skin irritation. Removing the transdermal patch at bedtime, after wearing it for about 16 hours, usually minimizes or eliminates bizarre dreams and sleep disturbances.

Practice Concepts and Principles
27. **All three Controller Medications are generally well tolerated, without serious adverse events.**
28. **In tobacco-dependence clinical trials, no seizures occurred with the use of bupropion SR.**
29. **Bupropion SR does not increase sedation, decrease libido, or cause impotence.**

Rescue Medications
Nicotine

All nicotine Rescue Medications are generally well tolerated and are without side effects of major clinical significance. Dropout due to side effects from nicotine nasal spray in clinical trials was low (about 5%) and did not differ between active and placebo nasal spray groups. Neither nicotine polacrilex lozenge nor nicotine sublingual tablet causes side effects of any clinical significance.

Practice Concepts and Principles

30. All four Rescue Medications are generally well tolerated, without medically serious adverse events.

Cardiac and Vascular Safety: Controller and Rescue Nicotine Medications

The nicotine patch, nasal spray, polacrilex gum, polacrilex lozenge, and inhaler are extraordinarily safe medications,[98,100-103] even when used in individualized, higher than "standard" dosages[104-107] or when the patient is using multiple nicotine medications.[85-92,93] None causes or increases the risk of myocardial infarction[98] even when used with concomitant cigarette smoking.[87,89,90,98,101,107-109] None causes or increases the risk of neoplastic disorders,[100,102] stroke,[99,101,108] or peripheral vascular disease.[98,100-102]

Nicotine does not activate the clotting cascade or facilitate thrombogenesis.[101] The FDA approved the nicotine patch for over-the-counter sale in 1996. One study documented that patients with known coronary artery disease, who had already had a myocardial infarction, had significant *improvement* in myocardial hypoperfusion from transdermal nicotine therapy, *even although they continued to smoke.*[110] Improved myocardial perfusion, despite significantly higher serum nicotine levels from tobacco smoke plus transdermal nicotine, resulted from the significant reduction in carboxyhemoglobin level. Short-term[109] and long-term[108] use of nicotine medications by ex-smokers may even have a cardioprotective effect. Nicotine polacrilex gum has been safely used for up to 14.5 years, at an average of 10 pieces/day, with a *reduction* in hospitalizations for cardiac events[108] and a significant 46% reduction in all-cause mortality.[111]

Practice Concepts and Principles

31. In all combination nicotine medication trials, there was no occurrence of significant cardiac side effects, even in those groups that were smoking while using two or more active nicotine medications.

32. All published studies to date show improved cardiac safety, with a reduction in cardiac events, for patients continuously using nicotine medications, even over many years, and even in the presence of continued cigarette use.

Controller Medications: Second Line

Clonidine

Side effects for clonidine tablets are similar to those seen when clonidine is used for treatment of hypertension, generally are mild, diminish with continued therapy, and include xerostomia (dry mouth) (40%), drowsiness (33%), dizziness (16%), sedation (10%), and constipation (10%).[2]

Nortriptyline

Side effects for nortriptyline are similar to those seen when nortriptyline is used for treatment of depression and include sedation, xerostomia (dry mouth) (64% to 78%), blurred vision (16%), urinary retention, lightheadedness (49%), and tremor (23%).[2] See Table 16-2 for more details.

TOBACCO-DEPENDENCE MEDICATION USE DURING PREGNANCY

The consensus among most recognized, tobacco-dependence clinical experts is that tobacco dependence should be treated during pregnancy and, preferably, before conception. Understandably, there are very few (only three) clinical trials evaluating effectiveness of any tobacco-dependence medications in pregnant cigarette users. In balance, though, results from two of the papers were not significantly different between treatment conditions; the trends favored pharmacotherapy to improve stopping smoking among pregnant women. Cigarette smoking puts both the mother and the fetus at substantial increased medical risk during pregnancy. Moreover, a child born to a mother who smoked during pregnancy is now well-documented to have increased risk for a large number of medical, developmental, and psychosocial problems. Because of the severity of the medical consequences of continued tobacco using during pregnancy, if the patient is, or has been, unable to stop smoking during pregnancy without pharmacotherapy, then the potential risks of pharmacotherapy to the pregnant woman or her fetus are very small. Leading, national clinical experts with experience treating tobacco-dependent patients and pregnant women would generally use at least one of the first-line medications cited earlier in this chapter.

Based on available published data, FDA pregnancy categories for these classes of medication were revised in 2007, in ways that can be confusing.

Varenicline has been FDA Pregnancy Category C since product launch in 2006 and remains so. Bupropion had been FDA Pregnancy Category B since at least 1997; however, in 2007, for reasons that were not specified, the FDA changed its rating to Pregnancy Category C. The FDA Physicians Prescribing Information did not contain new data to support that changes. Data published subsequently reaffirmed that bupropion—keeping in mind the severe paucity of data in pregnancy humans—is probably the safest medication to use initially in this setting. Other experts would recommend using nicotine medications initially, simply because we have so much experience with nicotine. Although most nicotine medications are now FDA Pregnancy Category D, using them is medically reasonable because the toxicity of nicotine to the fetus is known to follow dose-response patterns. Even using an individualized pharmacotherapy plan of multiple nicotine medications to completely suppress withdrawal symptoms, nicotine medication exposes both the mother and the fetus to only about one tenth to one twentieth of the nicotine dose from cigarette smoke and completely eliminates carbon monoxide (both dependent, known fetal teratogens and maternal toxins).

Based on the limited number of studies, the 2008 update of the Clinical Practice Guideline, Treating Tobacco Use and Dependence, states that the specific populations in which medication has not been shown to be effective include pregnant women, smokeless tobacco users, light smokers, and adolescents.[112]

Practice Concepts and Principles

33. Bupropion SR and varenicline are FDA Pregnancy Category C. Thus they would be first-line medications for pregnancy, tobacco-dependent smokers.
34. Bupropion nicotine medications and varenicline pose less risk to both the mother and the fetus than continued maternal smoking.
35. One or more medications should be used in pregnant smokers if their clinical history, including past experience in stopping smoking, FTND score, or nicotine withdrawal state, indicates that the pregnant patient will not likely be able to stop smoking without pharmacotherapy.
36. Because most nicotine medications are FDA Pregnancy Category D, they are probably best thought of as second-line medications for pregnant women.
37. Use of bupropion, varenicline, or nicotine medications will be safer for the fetus than continued maternal smoking.

DURATION OF TOBACCO-DEPENDENCE MEDICATION USE

All clinical trials show substantial relapse after medication use ends, even though relapse during treatment usually plateaus by about the twelfth week. Five randomized, double-blind, placebo-controlled trials have systematically evaluated various treatment durations, two for nicotine medications and one each for bupropion SR, nortriptyline, and varenicline. Treatment with transdermal nicotine for 6 months was no more effective than for 8 weeks.[99] In contrast, the four other long-term treatment trials show that longer treatment produces significantly and substantially better treatment outcome. Nicotine nasal spray used for 1 year was significantly more effective than placebo[88]; however, this study did not compare different medication treatment durations, as did the transdermal nicotine study.[99] One year of treatment with bupropion SR was significantly more effective than 7 weeks of treatment.[66] Twenty-four weeks of varenicline treatment was significantly more effective than 12 weeks.[61] The best-designed long-term treatment study showed that 1 year of treatment with nortriptyline was significantly and substantially (nearly three times) more effective than only 12 weeks.[20]

Manufacturers' recommendations for treatment duration with nicotine medications are not based on systematic research. Patients generally use nicotine medications for only 2 weeks[113]—not long enough to derive any clinical benefit. To obtain the best result, patients should receive at least a 3- to 6-month treatment course with nicotine medications.[2,3] The FDA specifically recommends a longer term (>3 to 6 months) maintenance treatment for bupropion SR, in part because of the strong supporting clinical trial data showing improved effectiveness with longer treatment.[66,114,115] The FDA recommends at least 6 months of treatment with varenicline and leaves the total treatment duration open-ended. Most clinical experts will treat for however long a patient needs; for as long as the patient lives, if necessary. (See also Practice Concepts and Principles #9 and #14 and their respective antecedent text regarding dosage.) In general, the dosage of nicotine medications should be gradually reduced at the end of treatment, but bupropion SR and varenicline can simply be discontinued.[3,12,61,66,114,115]

Practice Concepts and Principles

38. Because tobacco dependence is a chronic medical disease, most tobacco-dependent patients need to be treated for longer than 6 or 12 weeks. Many will need lifetime Controller Medication treatment to prevent or minimize relapse to cigarette or other tobacco use.

39. If patients experience significant nicotine withdrawal symptoms or start having occasional slips after tapering a dose or discontinuing a medication, the physician should increase the dose of that medication so that the patient is once again tobacco-use free and has no nicotine withdrawal symptoms. Then, attempt a slower rate of tapering.

Some patients are likely to benefit from more intensive and longer-duration treatment, including more frequent office visits, and combination pharmacotherapy rather than monotherapy. These patients include cigarette users who are highly nicotine dependent (as measured by the Fagerström Test for Nicotine Dependence [FTND]),[11,13,14,45,117-119] have a higher serum cotinine level while still smoking,[16,17] smoke more cigarettes per day,[99,120,121] are alcoholic,[122] are depressed,[123,124] are unmarried (divorced, separated, never married, or widowed), are female,[73,88,99,104,125-128] have another cigarette smoker in the household,[126,129] previously tried to quit smoking[126,129] and experienced nicotine withdrawal symptoms,[9,117,130] were younger than 17 years old when they started smoking,[17,129] or are younger at the start of treatment.[114,126,131]

Practice Concepts and Principles

40. Physicians should anticipate that tobacco users who are highly nicotine dependent, alcoholic, depressed, unmarried, female, have another cigarette user living in the same household, or began smoking when younger than 17 years of age are going to need more intensive medical treatment, including use of combination pharmacotherapy, more frequent follow-up visits, and a longer total duration of treatment.

Recommendations

4. Optimal tobacco cessation rates are achieved by individualizing all aspects of tobacco-dependence management, as is the current standard of care for asthma, COPD, and interstitial lung disease.

INEFFECTIVE MEDICATIONS FOR TREATING TOBACCO DEPENDENCE

Selective Serotonin Reuptake Inhibitors

Current scientific evidence shows that SSRIs, such as fluoxetine (Prozac), are not effective for treating tobacco dependence.[132] (*Note:* Any SSRI may be used conjointly with bupropion SR to optimize management of tobacco dependence, depression, or anxiety states, when two or more of these conditions are occurring in the same patient at the same time.)

Anxiolytics

Although initial studies suggested that buspirone (BuSpar) could be effective for tobacco dependence treatment,[133] a large-scale trial conducted by Bristol-Myers Squibb in the late 1990s failed to show any beneficial treatment effect of buspirone versus placebo.[134] There is no scientific evidence that any other anxiolytic is effective by itself for tobacco dependence treatment.

Practice Concepts and Principles

41. Underlying but clinically asymptomatic depression and anxiety are common comorbid conditions in tobacco-dependent patients. If depression, anxiety, or both emerge after the Target Quit Date, they need to be managed as separate conditions, with psychiatric referral, as indicated.

BEHAVIORAL INTERVENTION

Counseling

Although all of the first-line Controller and Rescue Medications discussed earlier in this chapter are effective when administered in a minimal intervention setting, their effectiveness is enhanced by even 3 minutes of physician counseling time.[3] Pharmacotherapy and physician counseling each *independently* improve treatment response, including smoking cessation rates.[3]

Also, physician counseling time and number of office visits are directly proportional to smoking cessation rates, independent of pharmacotherapy.[3,135] Six regular physician office visits over about 3 months provide a therapeutic benefit equivalent to six formal group-counseling sessions.

Residential Treatment Programs

There are only a few residential treatment programs available anywhere in the world, including well-established programs, such as the ones currently provided at the St. Helena Center for Health (St. Helena, Calif.) or the Mayo Clinic (Rochester, Minn.), and those that have been tested in pilot versions, such as at the Jerry L. Pettis Memorial Veterans Administration Medical Center (Loma Linda, Calif.) or the Durham Veterans Administration Medical Center (Durham, N.C.). These programs employ a comprehensive biobehavioral treatment model that includes group counseling, individual counseling, and educational seminars and lectures. They provide training in a range of skills, including stress management, relaxation, and relapse prevention, all accompanied by intensive, individualized pharmacotherapy with Controller and Rescue Medications.[91-93,136]

The St. Helena Center for Health established the first residential tobacco dependency program in 1969 and provided the behavioral treatment model for subsequently developed residential programs at the Mayo Clinic,[137] the Jerry L Pettis Veterans Administration Medical Center,[93,138] and the Durham Veterans Administration Medical Center.[92] The St. Helena Center for Health residential program provided comprehensive behavioral counseling without any pharmacotherapy until about 2001. Since 2005, it has consistently provided both comprehensive behavioral counseling and combination pharmacotherapy to most of its patients. Early data from the St. Helena program suggest that, in at least a subset of its program participants who agreed to have biofeedback from baseline pulmonary function testing along with monthly sputum cytology and comprehensive psychological counseling, 55% stopped smoking for 1 year.[139] Sixty-five percent of the participants in the St. Helena Center for Health Smoke-Free Life residential programs in 2006 reported that they were not smoking 1 year after completing the program (personal communication from John E. Hodgkin, MD, 2008).

The Mayo Clinic published data regarding intensive behavioral and pharmacologic residential treatment approach.[91] Between 1992 and 1996, patients self-selected to enter one of the following two programs: an 8-day residential program (n = 146) followed by regular counselor telephone contact, or an outpatient program (n = 292), also followed by regular, but less frequent, counselor telephone contact. One year after the initial intervention, 45% versus 23% (P <.001), respectively, had stopped smoking.[91] Both programs provided comprehensive behavioral and combination pharmacologic treatment. The residential program can provide much more thorough and intensive behavioral treatment as well as pharmacotherapy because it offers the patient 8 days of intensive, 8 hour/day professional staff interaction (with both physicians and trained counselors), whereas the outpatient program provides only a single, approximately 1-hour face-to-face session with a trained counselor.[91] For example, on the basis of objective rating of nicotine withdrawal symptom severity, the residential program could adjust Controller and Rescue Medication doses and combinations on a daily basis to bring nicotine withdrawal symptoms under optimal control.[91]

At the Jerry L. Pettis Memorial Veterans Administration Medical Center, an even more aggressive pilot behavioral and pharmacotherapeutic approach used a 7-day residential program with structured monthly outpatient face-to-face clinic visits for both refining behavioral and combination pharmacologic treatment, including bupropion. It showed 1-year nonsmoking rates of 75%.[92,93]

Finally, Green and colleagues[92] conducted a pilot 4-day residential study with 23 U.S. veterans who were severely nicotine dependent, had serious tobacco-caused medical diseases, had previously relapsed after a 6-week intensive behavioral and pharmacologic outpatient tobacco dependence treatment, and one-third of whom had significant psychiatric diagnoses (e.g., major depressive disorder, post-traumatic stress disorder). Pharmacotherapy provided up to 56 mg of nicotine per day via a Controller, transdermal nicotine, plus ad libitum Rescue Medication from a nicotine (oral) inhaler. While in the residential program, medication doses were adjusted to reduce nicotine withdrawal symptoms. Tobacco-dependence medications were tapered and discontinued rapidly, mostly within the first month postdischarge. Despite that approach, 26%

were not smoking at 1 year.[92] In this severely nicotine-dependent group (mean FTND score, 7.3/10), this finding is especially worth pursuing, because previous studies have shown re-treatment with standard-dose nicotine medications in an outpatient setting to be ineffective, with 100% relapsing by 6 months.[140]

MANAGING NICOTINE ADDICTION: PHARMACOTHERAPY TO ELIMINATE NICOTINE WITHDRAWAL

The greatest deficiency of most well-designed group counseling, behavior modification, and office practices is their failure to address the nicotine addiction side of the tobacco-dependency equation adequately. Providing effective pharmacotherapy to suppress all of the physiologically caused nicotine withdrawal symptoms significantly reduces the high relapse rates.[85,86,141-144]

The extent and severity of nicotine withdrawal symptoms directly predict relapse during the first 2 to 6 weeks of treatment after the Target Quit Date.[9,117,130] The more withdrawal symptoms the patient experiences and the greater their severity, the more likely the patient will resume smoking to eliminate those symptoms. The converse is also true: the fewer and less severe the nicotine withdrawal symptoms, the less likely the patient will slip, have occasional cigarettes, and then resume regular smoking. With more effective use of medications currently available to eliminate nicotine withdrawal symptoms, patients will experience less relapse.

MEDICAL RECORD: TOBACCO USE AND EXPOSURE HISTORY

In an earlier era, when the scientific community viewed cigarette smoking as a "lifestyle choice" or a "social habit," it was recorded under the heading of "Social History" in the initial outpatient or inpatient medical record. The scientific evidence no longer supports such categorization. Because tobacco smoke is the predominant pulmonary pathogen of the early 21st century, tobacco use should be recorded in a medically neutral, non-judgmental fashion.[2,5,131,145,146]

Recommendations

5. Printed and electronic medical history forms should include a value-neutral section heading such as "Tobacco Use and Exposure History." Information on secondhand tobacco smoke exposure, particularly the smoking history of the patient's immediate family members and coworkers, should also be included.

DIAGNOSIS CODING: ICD-9 AND CPT

An appropriate, chart-verifiable medical diagnosis should be established for patients. Examples would include bronchitis, bronchospasm, wheeze (especially on a forced expiratory maneuver), cough, emphysema, COPD, hypoxemia (using pulse oximetry), shortness of breath, asthma, chest pain, angina, or coronary artery disease. All these symptoms or diseases have standard, ICD-9 diagnostic codes. "Smoking cessation" is not an ICD-9

TABLE 16-7	Cost-Effectiveness Comparison of Tobacco-Dependence Treatment with Common Medical Tests and Interventions
Medical Screening Tests or Interventions	**Cost per Year of Life Saved[146,147]**
Tobacco-dependence pharmacotherapy and intensive physician involvement	$1,108
Pneumovax	$1,500
Tobacco dependence (minimal intervention)	$4,329
AIDS pharmacotherapy	$6,553
Renal transplantation	$9,756
Heart transplantation	$16,239
Hypertension screening	$23,335
Hyperlipidemia pharmacotherapy	$36,000
Postmyocardial infarction thrombolytic therapy	$55,000
Annual mammography	$61,744
Hypertension pharmacotherapy	$72,100

diagnosis code. The physician can provide more effective patient care and better treatment if tobacco-dependency treatment is part of the treatment plan for an appropriate medical diagnosis, as already noted. When used with appropriate ICD-9 diagnostic codes, insurance companies will reimburse at prevailing rates for corresponding standard CPT codes.

COST-EFFECTIVENESS

Treating tobacco dependence with pharmacotherapy and intensive physician involvement is exceptionally cost-effective: $3539 per year of life saved,[147] as opposed to most other common, accepted, and HMO-covered medical screening tests or interventions such as AIDS pharmacotherapy, renal transplantation, heart transplantation, hypertension screening, hyperlipidemia pharmacotherapy, post-myocardial infarction thrombolytic therapy, annual mammography, and hypertension pharmacotherapy[147,148] (Table 16-7). Many insurance companies view tobacco dependence pharmacotherapy from a return-on-investment model. Because, according to their model, it takes more than 1 year to recover the medical cost of treatment, such services and medications are not covered. Medi-Cal, the California Medicaid program, currently covers treatment for tobacco dependence at no cost to the patient, including nicotine patch, nicotine nasal spray, and bupropion SR, if prescribed by the treating physician.[149]

Practice Concepts and Principles

42. Medically managed tobacco-dependence treatment is cost-effective, more so than many usual treatments, such as moderate hypertension. In fact, more intensive tobacco-dependence treatment, involving extensive physician time and multiple Controller and Rescue Medications, is more cost-effective than less intensive tobacco-dependence treatment.

CONCLUSION

Smoking cessation paradigms dating from the 1960s are based on the incorrect assumption that tobacco dependence is a short-term, nonchronic, self-limited matter of willpower. Tobacco dependence, however, does have distinct, defined, neurogenetic and neuropathologic bases. Merely stopping smoking is an insufficient goal in tobacco-dependence treatment and sets the patient up for treatment failure and relapse. Rational pharmacotherapy is required, based on the "treat-to-effect" or "dose-to-effect" model used to treat many other complex chronic diseases, such as asthma, hypertension, or diabetes. This model includes providing adequate pharmacotherapy to suppress physiologically caused nicotine withdrawal symptoms (craving for cigarettes, increased anxiety, irritability, restlessness, dysphoria, depression, short-temperedness, increased appetite, or difficulty concentrating).

Treat-to-effect also means providing assistance, resources, and referral, if necessary, so that patients adequately attend to the psychological dependence side of tobacco dependence. Although medications suppress nicotine withdrawal symptoms, patients actively need to restructure their lives to reverse decades of conditioned responses that cause them to want a cigarette in certain "trigger" situations. For tobacco dependence to be effectively treated, both nicotine addiction and psychological dependence must be addressed.

Tobacco dependence is most effectively treated with combination pharmacotherapy or varenicline alone for at least 6 to 12 months, and even longer, if necessary. Throughout treatment and during medication tapering, the primary therapeutic goal is to enable the patient to lead a normal life. Nicotine withdrawal symptoms must be as completely suppressed as possible. This suppression is most effectively achieved with pharmacotherapy. If any withdrawal symptoms start to occur or recur as medications are tapered, then the dosage needs to be increased to restabilize the patient and then reduced more gradually.

Tobacco dependence is a chronic, relapsing, serious, life-threatening disease that physicians can effectively treat by long-term medical management. None of the medications currently available for tobacco-dependence treatment are known to reverse the underlying neuronal pathology of tobacco dependence. Consequently, as with asthma, some patients will need lifetime treatment in order to remain tobacco free.

ACKNOWLEDGMENTS

I appreciate the superb editorial and research assistance provided by Adina Kletter and the patience of the editors of this book.

References

1. Food and Drug Administration: Open Public Hearing on Improving the Prescription Labeling of Smoking Cessation Products. Paper presented at Drug Abuse Advisory Committee Meeting, with Representation from the Nonprescription Drugs Advisory Committee, June 9, 1997, Versailles Room, Holiday Inn, Bethesda, Md.

2. Fiore MC, Bailey WC, Cohen SJ et al: Treating tobacco use and dependence: clinical practice guideline, Rockville, Md, 2000, U.S. Department of Health and Human Services, Public Health Service.

3. Fiore MC: for the Tobacco Use and Dependence Clinical Practice Guideline Panel Staff and Consortium Representatives: A clinical practice guideline for treating tobacco use and dependence: a U.S. Public Health Service report, JAMA 283:3244-3254, 2000.

4. California Thoracic Society: Medical management for tobacco dependence: position paper, March 25, 2005. Available at www.thoracic.org/sections/chapters/thoracic-society-chapters/ca/publications/resources/tobacco-or-health/FINALTobaccoDependence Sum.pdf. Accessed July 21, 2008.

5. Sachs DPL: Tobacco dependence: pathophysiology and treatment. In Hodgkin JE, Celli BR, Connors GL, editors: Pulmonary rehabilitation: guidelines to success, ed 3, Philadelphia, 2000, Lippincott Williams & Williams, pp 261-301.

6. Food and Drug Administration: Regulations restricting the sale and distribution of cigarettes and smokeless tobacco to protect children and adolescents: final rule, Fed Regist 61:44396-45318, 1996. 21 CFR § 801, Washington DC, U.S. Department of Health and Human Services..

7. Garvey AJ, Bliss RE, Hitchcock JL et al: Predictors of smoking relapse among self-quitters: a report from the Normative Aging Study, Addictive Behaviors 17:367-377, 1992.

8. Hughes JR, Gulliver SB, Fenwick JW et al: Smoking cessation among self-quitters, Health Psychol 11:331-334, 1992.

9. West RJ, Hajek P, Belcher M: Severity of withdrawal symptoms as a predictor of outcome of an attempt to quit smoking, Psychol Med 19:981-985, 1989.

10. Transdermal Nicotine Study Group: Transdermal nicotine for smoking cessation: six-month results from two multicenter controlled clinical trials, JAMA 266:3133-3138, 1991.

11. Sachs DPL, Säwe U, Leischow SJ: Effectiveness of a 16-hour transdermal nicotine patch in a medical practice setting, without intensive group counseling, Arch Intern Med 153:1881-1890, 1993.

12. Hurt RD, Sachs DPL, Glover ED et al: A comparison of sustained-release bupropion and placebo for smoking cessation, N Engl J Med 337:1195-1202, 1997.

13. Tønnesen P, Fryd V, Hansen M et al: Effect of nicotine chewing gum in combination with group counseling on the cessation of smoking, N Engl J Med 318:15-18, 1988.

14. Sachs DPL: Effectiveness of the 4-mg dose of nicotine polacrilex for the initial treatment of high-dependent smokers, Arch Intern Med 155:1973-1980, 1995.

15. Tønnesen P, Nørregaard J, Mikkelsen K et al: A double-blind trial of a nicotine inhaler for smoking cessation, JAMA 269:1268-1271, 1993.

16. Paoletti P, Fornai E, Maggiorelli F et al: Importance of baseline cotinine plasma values in smoking cessation: results from a double-blind study with nicotine patch, Eur Respir J 9:643-651, 1996.

17. Sachs DPL, Benowitz NL: Individualizing medical treatment for tobacco dependence, Eur Respir J 9:629-631, 1996.

18. Jorenby DE, Hays JT, Rigotti NA et al: Efficacy of varenicline, an $\alpha_4\beta_2$ nicotinic acetylcholine receptor partial agonist, vs placebo or sustained-release bupropion for smoking cessation: a randomized controlled trial, JAMA 296:56-63, 2006.

19. Gonzales D, Rennard SI, Nides M et al: Varenicline, an $\alpha_4\beta_2$ nicotinic acetylcholine receptor partial agonist, vs sustained-release bupropion and placebo for smoking cessation: a randomized controlled trial, JAMA 296:47-55, 2006.

20. Hall SM, Humfleet GL, Reus VI et al: Extended nortriptyline and psychological treatment for cigarette smoking, Am J Psychiatry 161:2100-2107, 2004.

21. Kendler KS, Neale MC, MacLean CJ et al: Smoking and major depression: a causal analysis, Arch Gen Psychiatry 50:36-43, 1993.

22. Henningfield JE, Schuh LM, Jarvik MI: Pathophysiology of tobacco dependence. In Bloom FE, Kupfer DJ, editors: Psychopharmacology: the fourth generation of progress, New York, 1995, Raven Press, pp 1715-1730.

23. Hughes JR: Genetics of smoking: a brief review, Behav Ther 17:335-345, 1986.

24. Heath AC, Cates R, Martin NG et al: Genetic contribution to risk of smoking initiation: comparisons across birth cohorts and across cultures, J Subst Abuse 5:221-246, 1993.

25. Pomerleau OF: Individual differences in sensitivity to nicotine: implications for genetic research on nicotine dependence, Behav Genet 25:161-177, 1995.

26. Nakajima M, Yamamoto T, Nunoya K et al: Role of human cytochrome P4502A6 in C-oxidation of nicotine, Drug Metab Dispos 24:1212-1217, 1996.

27. Morgan JI, Curran TE: Proto-oncogenes: beyond second messengers. In Bloom FE, Kupfer DJ, editors: Psychopharmacology: the fourth generation of progress, New York, 1995, Raven Press, pp 631-642.

28. Chergui K, Nomikos GG, Mathé JM et al: Burst stimulation of the medial forebrain bundle selectively increases FOS-like immunoreactivity in the limbic forebrain of the rat, Neuroscience 72:141-156, 1996.

29. Svensson TH: Interview with Professor Torgny H. Svensson, MD, PhD, regarding the biology of nicotine addiction, conducted by David P.L. Sachs, MD, Palo Alto Center for Pulmonary Disease Prevention, 1997..

30. Lerman C, Caporaso N, Main D et al: Depression and self-medication with nicotine: the modifying influence of the dopamine D4 receptor gene, Health Psychol 17:56-62, 1998.

31. Lerman C, Caporaso NE, Audrain J et al: Evidence suggesting the role of specific genetic factors in cigarette smoking, Health Psychol 18:14-20, 1999.

32. Lerman C, Caporaso NE, Audrain J et al: Interacting effects of the serotonin transporter gene and neuroticism in smoking practices and nicotine dependence, Mol Psychiatry 5:189-192, 2000.

33. Lerman C, Caporaso NE, Bush A et al: Tryptophan hydroxylase gene variant and smoking behavior, Am J Med Genet 105:518-520, 2001.

34. Lerman C, Berrettini W: Elucidating the role of genetic factors in smoking behavior and nicotine dependence, Am J Med Genet B Neuropsychiatr Genet 118:48-54, 2003.

35. Miksys S, Lerman C, Shields PG et al: Smoking, alcoholism and genetic polymorphisms alter CYP2B6 levels in human brain, Neuropharmacology 45:122-132, 2003.

36. Kaufmann V, Lerman C: Genes, smoking, and treatment response, Am J Health Syst Pharm 60:1911, 2003.

37. Audrain-McGovern J, Lerman C, Wileyto EP et al: Interacting effects of genetic predisposition and depression on adolescent smoking progression, Am J Psychiatry 161:1224-1230, 2004.

38. Erblich J, Lerman C, Self DW et al: Effects of dopamine D2 receptor (DRD2) and transporter (SLC6A3) polymorphisms on smoking cue-induced cigarette craving among African-American smokers, Mol Psychiatry 10:407-414, 2005.

39. Lerman C, Patterson F, Berrettini W: Treating tobacco dependence: state of the science and new directions, J Clin Oncol 23:311-323, 2005.

40. Kellar KJ, Davila-Garcia MI, Xiao Y: Pharmacology of neuronal nicotinic acetylcholine receptors: effects of acute and chronic nicotine, Nicotine Tob Res 1(Supp. 2):S117-S120 discussion S139-S140, 1999.

41. Henningfield JE, Heishman SJ: The addictive role of nicotine in tobacco use, Psychopharmacology (Berl) 117:11-13, 1995.

42. Henningfield JE: Nicotine medications for smoking cessation, N Engl J Med 333:1196-1203, 1995.

43. Benowitz NL: Nicotine replacement therapy: what has been accomplished—can we do better?, Drugs 45:157-170, 1993.

44. Benowitz NL: Pharmacology of nicotine: addiction and therapeutics, Annu Rev Pharmacol Toxicol 36:597-613, 1996.

45. Heatherton TF, Kozlowski LT, Frecker RC et al: The Fagerström Test for Nicotine Dependence: a revision of the Fagerström Tolerance Questionnaire, Br J Addict 86:1119-1127, 1991.

46. Picciotto MR, Brunzell DH, Caldarone BJ: Effect of nicotine and nicotinic receptors on anxiety and depression, Neuroreport 13:1097-1106, 2002.

47. Balfour DJ: The neurobiology of tobacco dependence: a commentary, Respiration 69:7-11, 2002.

48. Hildebrand BE, Nomikos GG, Bondjers C et al: Behavioral manifestations of the nicotine abstinence syndrome in the rat: peripheral versus central mechanisms, Psychopharmacology (Berl) 129:348-356, 1997.

49. Hughes JR: Tobacco withdrawal in self-quitters, J Consult Clin Psychol 60:689-697, 1992.

50. Hughes JR, Hatsukami DK, Pickens RW et al: Consistency of the tobacco withdrawal syndrome, Addict Behav 9:409-412, 1984.

51. Shiffman SM, Jarvik ME: Smoking withdrawal symptoms in two weeks of abstinence, Psychopharmacology (Berl) 50:35-39, 1976.

52. Williamson DF, Madans J, Anda RF et al: Smoking cessation and severity of weight gain in a national cohort, N Engl J Med 324:739-745, 1991.

53. Rigotti NA: Clinical practice: treatment of tobacco use and dependence, N Engl J Med 346:506-512, 2002.

54. Buist AS, Rodriguez Roisin R, Anzneta A et al: GOLD Scientific Committee: Global strategy for the diagnosis, management, and prevention of chronic obstructive pulmonary disease. Update 2007. NHLBI/WHO Global Initiative for Chronic Obstructive Lung Disease (GOLD) workshop report. Available at www.goldcopd.com. Retrieved July 21, 2008.

55. U.S. Department of Health and Human Services: The health consequences of smoking: a report of the surgeon general. Atlanta, GA: U.S. Department of Health and Human Services. Centers for Disease Control and Prevention. National Center for Chronic Disease Prevention and Health Promotion. Office on Smoking and Health, 2004.

56. Varenicline (Chantix) for tobacco dependence, Med Lett Drugs Ther 48:66-68, 2006.

57. Drugs for tobacco dependence, Treat Guidel Med Lett 1:65-68, 2003.

58. Bupropion (Zyban) for smoking cessation, Med Lett Drugs Ther 39:77-78, 1997.

59. Coe JW, Brooks PR, Vetelino MG et al: Varenicline: an (4(2 nicotinic receptor partial agonist for smoking cessation, J Med Chem 48:3474-3477, 2005.

60. Obach RS, Reed-Hagen AE, Krueger SS et al: Metabolism and disposition of varenicline, a selective $\alpha_4\beta_2$ acetylcholine receptor partial agonist, in vivo and in vitro, Drug Metab Dispos 34:121-130, 2006.

61. Tonstad S, Tønnesen P, Hajek P et al: Effect of maintenance therapy with varenicline on smoking cessation: a randomized controlled trial, JAMA 296:64-71, 2006.

62. Klesges RC, Johnson KC, Somes G: Varenicline for smoking cessation: definite promise, but no panacea, JAMA 296:94-95, 2006.

63. Pfizer: Chantix™ (varenicline) tablets. Available at www.pfizer.com/files/products/uspi_chantix.pdf. Retrieved July 21, 2008.

64. Ascher JA, Cole JO, Colin JN et al: Bupropion: a review of its mechanism of antidepressant activity, J Clin Psychiatry 56:395-401, 1995.

65. Jorenby DE, Leischow SJ, Nides MA et al: A controlled trial of sustained-release bupropion, a nicotine patch, or both for smoking cessation, N Engl J Med 340:685-691, 1999.

66. Hays JT, Hurt RD, Rigotti NA et al: Sustained-release bupropion for pharmacologic relapse prevention after smoking cessation. a randomized, controlled trial, Ann Intern Med 135:423-433, 2001.

67. Ahluwalia JS, Harris KJ, Catley D et al: Sustained-release bupropion for smoking cessation in African Americans: a randomized controlled trial, JAMA 288:468-474, 2002.

68. Gonzales DH, Nides MA, Ferry LH et al: Bupropion SR as an aid to smoking cessation in smokers

treated previously with bupropion: a randomized placebo-controlled study, Clin Pharmacol Ther 69:438-444, 2001.

69. Zyban (bupropion hydrochloride sustained-release tablets), Physicians' Desk Reference, ed 61, Montvale, NJ, 2007, Medical Economics Data, pp 1644-1650.

70. Ferry LH, Robbins AS, Scariati PD et al: Enhancement of smoking cessation using the antidepressant bupropion hydrochloride, Circulation 86:1-167, 1992.

71. Ferry LH, Burchette RJ: Evaluation of bupropion versus placebo for treatment of nicotine dependence. Paper presented at the 147th Annual Meeting of the American Psychiatric Association, May 22-26, 1994, Philadelphia, Pa.

72. Ferry LH, Burchette RJ: Efficacy of bupropion for smoking cessation in non-depressed smokers, J Addict Dis 13:9A, 1994.

73. Fagerström KO, Sachs DPL: Medical management of tobacco dependence: a critical review of nicotine skin patches, Curr Pulmonol 16:223-238, 1995.

74. Glassman AH, Stetner F, Walsh BT et al: Heavy smokers, smoking cessation, and clonidine: results of a double-blind, randomized trial, JAMA 259:2863-2866, 1988.

75. Franks P, Harp J, Bell B: Randomized, controlled trial of clonidine for smoking cessation in a primary care setting, JAMA 262:3011-3013, 1989.

76. Hall SM, Reus VI, Munoz RF et al: Nortriptyline and cognitive–behavioral therapy in the treatment of cigarette smoking, Arch Gen Psychiatry 55:683-690, 1998.

77. Hall SM, Humfleet GL, Reus VI et al: Psychological intervention and antidepressant treatment in smoking cessation, Arch Gen Psychiatry 59:930-936, 2002.

78. Lunell E, Molander L, Ekberg K et al: Site of nicotine absorption from a vapour inhaler—comparison with cigarette smoking, Eur J Clin Pharmacol 55:737-741, 2000.

79. Schneider NG, Olmstead R, Nilsson F et al: Efficacy of a nicotine inhaler in smoking cessation: a double-blind, placebo-controlled trial, Addiction 91:1293-1306, 1996.

80. Schneider NG, Olmstead RE, Franzon MA et al: The nicotine inhaler: clinical pharmacokinetics and comparison with other nicotine treatments, Clin Pharmacokinet 40:661-684, 2001.

81. Gourlay SG, Benowitz NL: Arteriovenous differences in plasma concentration of nicotine and catecholamines and related cardiovascular effects after smoking, nicotine nasal spray, and intravenous nicotine, Clin Pharmacol Ther 62:453-463, 1997.

82. Schneider NG, Olmstead R, Mody FV et al: Efficacy of a nicotine nasal spray in smoking cessation: a placebo-controlled, double-blind trial, Addiction 90:1671-1682, 1995.

83. Schneider NG, Lunell E, Olmstead RE et al: Clinical pharmacokinetics of nasal nicotine delivery: a review and comparison to other nicotine systems, Clin Pharmacokinet 31:65-80, 1996.

84. Shiffman S, Dresler CM, Hajek P et al: Efficacy of a nicotine lozenge for smoking cessation, Arch Intern Med 162:1267-1276, 2002.

85. Bars MP, Banauch GI, Appel D et al: "Tobacco free with FDNY": the New York City Fire Department World Trade Center Tobacco Cessation Study, Chest 129:979-987, 2006.

86. Sachs DPL: Tobacco dependence treatment: time to change the paradigm, Chest 129:836-839, 2006.

87. Bohadana AB, Nilsson F, Rasmussen T et al: Nicotine inhaler and nicotine patch as a combination therapy for smoking cessation: a randomized, double-blind, placebo-controlled trial, Arch Intern Med 160:3128-3134, 2000.

88. Blöndal T, Gudmundsson LJ, Olafsdottir I et al: Nicotine nasal spray with nicotine patch for smoking cessation: randomised trial with six-year follow up, BMJ 318:285-288, 1999.

89. Kornitzer M, Boutsen M, Dramaix M et al: Combined use of nicotine patch and gum in smoking cessation: a placebo-controlled clinical trial, Prev Med 24:41-47, 1995.

90. Puska P, Korhonen HJ, Vartiainen E et al: Combined use of nicotine patch and gum compared with gum alone in smoking cessation: a clinical trial in north Karelia, Tobacco Control 4:231-235, 1995.

91. Hays JT, Wolter TD, Eberman KM et al: Residential (inpatient) treatment compared with outpatient treatment for nicotine dependence, Mayo Clin Proc 76:124-133, 2001.

92. Green A, Yancy WS, Braxton L et al: Residential smoking therapy, J Gen Intern Med 18:275-280, 2003.

93. Ferry LH (Loma Linda University, Loma Linda, CA): Personal communication: a pilot, 7-day, residential, tobacco-dependence treatment program at the Jerry L. Pettis Memorial Veterans Administration Medical Center using combination pharmacotherapy, group counseling, stress management, and relapse prevention training plus regular outpatient follow-up; as described in Green A, Yancy WS, Braxton L etal: Residential smoking therapy, J Gen Intern Med 18:275-280, 2003.

94. Young SJ: Panic associated with combining fluoxetine and bupropion, J Clin Psychiatry 57:177-178, 1996.

95. Gross J, Stitzer ML, Maldonado J: Nicotine replacement: effects of postcessation weight gain, J Consult Clin Psychol 57:87-92, 1989.

96. Jorenby D: Clinical efficacy of bupropion in the management of smoking cessation, Drugs 62(Supp. 2):25-35, 2002.

97. Johnston JA, Fiedler-Kelly J, Glover ED et al: Relationship between drug exposure and the efficacy and safety of bupropion sustained release for smoking cessation, Nicotine Tob Res 3:131-140, 2001.

98. Benowitz NL, Gourlay SG: Cardiovascular toxicity of nicotine: implications for nicotine replacement therapy, J Am Coll Cardiol 29:1422-1431, 1997.

99. Tønnesen P, Paoletti P, Gustavsson G et al: Higher dosage nicotine patches increase one-year smoking cessation rates: results from the European CEASE Trial. Collaborative European Anti-Smoking Evaluation, Eur Respir J 13:238-246, 1999.

100. Office on Smoking and Health, Centers for Disease Control and Prevention: The health

consequences of smoking: nicotine addiction—a report of the Surgeon General [DHHS publication No. (CDC) 88-8406], Rockville, Md, 1988, U.S. Department of Health and Human Services.

101. Benowitz NL, Fitzgerald GA, Wilson M et al: Nicotine effects on eicosanoid formation and hemostatic function: comparison of transdermal nicotine and cigarette smoking, J Am Coll Cardiol 22:1159-1167, 1993.

102. Benowitz NL, editor: Nicotine safety and toxicity, New York, 1998, Oxford University Press.

103. Sachs DPL, Säwe U: Transdermal nicotine patch and absence of myocardial infarction risk, Orlando, Fla, 1993, American College of Chest Physicians.

104. Sachs DPL, Benowitz NL, Bostrom AG et al: Percent serum replacement and success of nicotine patch therapy [abstract], Am J Respir Crit Care Med 151:A688, 1995.

105. Dale LC, Hurt RD, Offord KP et al: High-dose nicotine patch therapy: percentage of replacement and smoking cessation, JAMA 274:1353-1358, 1995.

106. Fredrickson PA, Hurt RD, Lee GM et al: High dose transdermal nicotine therapy for heavy smokers: safety, tolerability and measurement of nicotine and cotinine levels, Psychopharmacology (Berl) 122:215-222, 1995.

107. Zevin S, Jacob PIII, Benowitz NL: Dose-related cardiovascular and endocrine effects of transdermal nicotine, Clin Pharmacol Ther 64:87-95, 1998.

108. Murray RP, Bailey WC, Daniels K et al: Safety of nicotine polacrilex gum used by 3,094 participants in the Lung Health Study. Lung Health Study Research Group, Chest 109:438-445, 1996.

109. Working Group for the Study of Transdermal Nicotine in Patients with Coronary Artery Disease: Nicotine replacement therapy for patients with coronary artery disease, Arch Intern Med 154:989-995, 1994.

110. Mahmarian JJ, Moye LA, Nasser GA et al: Nicotine patch therapy in smoking cessation reduces the extent of exercise-induced myocardial ischemia, J Am Coll Cardiol 30:125-130, 1997.

111. Anthonisen NR, Skeans MA, Wise RA et al: The effects of a smoking cessation intervention on 14.5-year mortality: a randomized clinical trial, Ann Intern Med 142:233-239, 2005.

112. Fiore MC, Jaén CR, Baker TB et al: Treating tobacco use and dependence: 2008 update. Clinical Practice Guideline. Rockville, MD: U.S. Department of Health and Human Services. Public Health Service. May 2008.

113. Pierce JP, Gilpin EA: Impact of over-the-counter sales on effectiveness of pharmaceutical aids for smoking cessation, JAMA 288:1260-1264, 2002.

114. Hurt RD, Wolter TD, Rigotti N et al: Bupropion for pharmacologic relapse prevention to smoking: predictors of outcome, Addict Behav 27:493-507, 2002.

115. U.S. Food and Drug Administration: Zyban® (bupropion hydrochloride) sustained-release tablets: prescribing information (Publication No. NDA 20-711/S-027), Rockville, Md, 2007, U.S. Department of Health and Human Services.

116. U.S. Food and Drug Administration: Nicotrol: prescribing information, Rockville, Md, 1992, U.S. Department of Health and Human Services.

117. Nørregaard J, Tønnesen P, Petersen L: Predictors and reasons for relapse in smoking cessation with nicotine and placebo patches, Prev Med 22:261-271, 1993.

118. Glover ED, Sachs DPL, Stitzer ML et al: Smoking cessation in highly dependent smokers with 4-mg nicotine polacrilex, Am J Health Behav 20:319-332, 1996.

119. Sutherland G, Stapleton JA, Russell MAH et al: Randomised controlled trial of nasal nicotine spray in smoking cessation, Lancet 340:324-329, 1992.

120. Killen JD, Fortmann SP, Telch MJ et al: Are heavy smokers different from light smokers? A comparison after 48 hours without cigarettes, JAMA 260:1581-1585, 1988.

121. Hajek P, Jackson P, Belcher M: Long-term use of nicotine chewing gum: occurrence, determinants, and effect on weight gain, JAMA 260:1593-1596, 1988.

122. Hughes JR: Treatment of smoking cessation in smokers with past alcohol/drug problems, J Subst Abuse Treat 10:181-187, 1993.

123. Glassman AH, Helzer JE, Covey LS et al: Smoking, smoking cessation, and major depression, JAMA 264:1546-1549, 1990.

124. Covey LS, Glassman AH, Stetner F: Depression and depressive symptoms in smoking cessation, Compr Psychiatry 31:350-354, 1990.

125. Fiore MC, Bailey WC, Cohen SJ et al: Smoking cessation: clinical practice guideline no. 18 (AHCPR Publication No. 96-0692), Rockville, Md, 1996, U.S. Department of Health and Human Services.

126. Dale LC, Glover ED, Sachs DPL et al: Bupropion for smoking cessation: predictors of successful outcome, Chest 119:1357-1364, 2001.

127. Killen JD, Fortmann SP, Newman B et al: Evaluation of a treatment approach combining nicotine gum with self-guided behavioral treatments for smoking relapse prevention, J Consult Clin Psychol 58:85-92, 1990.

128. Sachs DPL, Leischow SJ: Differential gender treatment response: effectiveness of the 4 mg dose of nicotine polacrilex to treat low nicotine dependent male smokers but not women, paper presented at the Proceedings of the 54th Annual Scientific Meeting of the College on Problems of Drug Dependence, June 1992, Keystone, Col.

129. Sachs DPL, Bostrom AG, Hansen MD: Nicotine patch therapy: predictors of smoking cessation success [abstract], Am J Respir Crit Care Med 149:A326, 1994.

130. Killen JD, Fortmann SP: Craving is associated with smoking relapse: findings from three prospective studies, Exp Clin Psychopharmacol 5:137-142, 1997.

131. Lillington GA, Leonard CT, Sachs DPL: Smoking cessation: techniques and benefits, Clin Chest Med 21(xi):199-208, 2000.

Available at www.fda.gov/medwatch/safety/2007/Mar_PI/Zyban_PI.pdf. Retrieved July 21, 2008.

132. Hughes JR, Stead LF, Lancaster T: Antidepressants for smoking cessation, Cochrane Database Syst Rev 2:CD000031, 2003.

133. West R, Hajek P, McNeill A: Effect of buspirone on cigarette withdrawal symptoms and short-term abstinence rates in a smokers clinic, Psychopharmacology (Berl) 104:91-96, 1991.

134. Hughes JR, Stead LF, Lancaster T: Anxiolytics for smoking cessation, Cochrane Database Syst Rev 4:CD002849, 2000.

135. Wilson DM, Taylor DW, Gilbert JR et al: A randomized trial of a family physician intervention for smoking cessation, JAMA 260:1570-1574, 1988.

136. Sachs DPL, Hodgkin JE (The Center for a Smoke-Free Life, St. Helena Center for Health, St. Helena, Calif): Personal communication, 2008. *Note:* Drs. Sachs and Hodgkin served together as co-medical directors of the St. Helena Center for Health's residential smoke—free life program, January 2005—December 2006.

137. Hurt RD: Personal communication, 2001.

138. Ferry LH: Personal communication, 2003.

139. Swan GE, Hodgkin JE, Roby T et al: Reversibility of airways injury over a 12-month period following smoking cessation, Chest 101:607-612, 1992.

140. Tønnesen P, Nørregaard J, Säwe U et al: Recycling with nicotine patches in smoking cessation, Addiction 88:533-539, 1993.

141. Hurt RD: Personal communication, 2006.

142. Ferry LH: Personal communication, 2006.

143. Prezant DJ: Personal communication, 2006.

144. Sachs DPL: Personal communication, 2006.

145. Katz DA, Muehlenbruch DR, Brown RL et al: Effectiveness of implementing the Agency for Healthcare Research and Quality smoking cessation clinical practice guideline: a randomized, controlled trial, J Natl Cancer Inst 96:594-603, 2004.

146. Piper ME, Fox BJ, Welsch SK et al: Gender and racial/ethnic differences in tobacco-dependence treatment: a commentary and research recommendations, Nicotine Tob Res 3:291-297, 2001.

147. Cromwell J, Bartosch WJ, Fiore MC et al: Cost-effectiveness of the clinical practice recommendations in the AHCPR guideline for smoking cessation. Agency for Health Care Policy and Research, JAMA 278:1759-1766, 1997.

148. Croghan IT, Offord KP, Evans RW et al: Cost-effectiveness of treating nicotine dependence: the Mayo Clinic experience, Mayo Clin Proc 72:917-924, 1997.

149. Centers for Disease Control and Prevention (CDC): State Medicaid coverage for tobacco-dependence treatments—United States, 1994-2002, MMWR Morb Mortal Wkly Rep 53:54-57, 2004.

150. American Psychiatric Association: Nicotine-induced disorder, Diagnostic and statistical manual of mental disorders, ed 4, Washington DC, 1994, American Psychiatric Association, pp 244-245.

151. American Psychiatric Association: Nicotine-induced organic mental disorder, Diagnostic statistical manual of mental disorders, ed 3, Washington DC, 1987, American Psychiatric Association, pp 150-151 revised.

APPENDIX 1: RESOURCES

1. *Treating Tobacco Use and Dependence. Clinical Practice Guideline, 2008 Update. U.S. Department of Health and Human Services. Public Health Service. Available at www.surgeongeneral.gov/ tobacco/. Retrieved July 21, 2008.*

   • This document provides the interested physician with the most comprehensive meta-analysis of the scientific data, an evidence base for treating tobacco dependence.

2. *Helping Smokers Quit: A Guide for Clinicians.*

   • Available at www.ahrq.gov/clinic/tobacco/ clinhlpsmksqt.htm. Retrieved July 21, 2008.

3. *Consumer Guide: You Can Quit Smoking*

This document summarizes the findings of the complete *Clinical Practice Guideline* for patients. It is suitable for a medical office waiting room or examination room. It is available at *www.ahrq.gov/ consumer/tobacco/quits.pdf. Retrieved July 21,* 2008.

Any physician may obtain these documents free of charge by contacting:

   • Agency for Healthcare Research and Quality (AHRQ): www.ahrq.gov or 1-800-358-9295

   • Centers for Disease Control and Prevention (CDC): www.cdc.gov or 1-800-232-4636
   • National Cancer Institute (NCI): www.cancer.gov or 1-800-4-CANCER

4. *California Thoracic Society Position Paper: Medical Management for Tobacco Dependence, 2005.*

This evidence-based and consensus position paper is intended to provide the busy clinician with an update for the previously cited Public Health Service *Clinical Practice Guideline: Treating Tobacco Use and Dependence*, in exceptionally concise form.

   • The full text of the position paper is available at www.thoracic.org/sections/chapters/ thoracic-society-chapters/ca/publications/ resources/tobacco-or-health/FINALTobacco DependenceSum.pdf. Retieved July 21, 2008.

5. *American College of Chest Physicians Tobacco Cessation Tool Kit, 2004.*

Whereas the Public Health Service *Clinical Practice Guideline: Treating Tobacco Use and Dependence* provides the scientific base of data for rationally treating tobacco dependence, the American College of Chest Physicians (ACCP) *Tobacco Cessation Tool Kit* provides the practical "nuts-and-bolts" materials and procedures that the physician needs in order to readily implement effective tobacco-dependence treatment in the outpatient setting.

The *Tobacco Cessation Tool Kit*, provided as a CD-ROM in its 2004 second edition, is available for the nominal charge of $30.00. A completely revamped third edition will be available for purchase in the near future from the American College of Chest Physicians. Two patient education guides ("Thinking about Quitting Tobacco?" and "How to Quit Using Tobacco," in English or Spanish) are available in packages of 25 for $15. These may be ordered directly through the ACCP:

- American College of Chest Physicians (ACCP): www.chestnet.org or 800-343-ACCP (2227) or 847-498-1400
- Specific link for ordering Tool Kit: www.chestnet.org/education/guidelines/tctk.php

The *Tobacco Cessation Tool Kit* offers tremendous value to the practicing physician, because it literally provides a turnkey office setup. The ACCP *Tobacco Cessation Tool Kit*, 2004 includes:

- Complete, easy-to-use CD-ROM
- All necessary forms and chart flags
- Eight-minute training video (facilitating program implementation in medical office)
- Complete pharmacotherapeutic reference grid
- Guide for physician's nurse or cessation counselor in follow-up phone calls to:
  - Solicit progress
  - Document problems encountered
  - Address questions that the patient may want to ask
  - Verify compliance with the treatment regimen
- Two patient education brochures (available in English or Spanish):
  - To motivate the resistant patient to want to attempt quitting
  - To guide the patient who is ready to stop smoking
- Updated referral and resource list

The *Tobacco Cessation Tool Kit* also provides educational information about the biology of nicotine addiction, treating nicotine addiction as a chronic disease, multimodality treatment approaches, cost-benefits, motivating patients to quit, and relapse prevention, among other pertinent topics.

6. *Global Initiative for Chronic Obstructive Lung Disease (GOLD) Guidelines, 2004*

GOLD works with international experts to produce guidelines and other resources about the diagnosis, prevention, and management of COPD. The following documents are among those available for download from their Web site at www.goldcopd.com/GuidelinesResources.asp.

- *Global Strategy for Diagnosis, Management, and Prevention of COPD*, updated December 2007—Evidence-based guidelines for COPD diagnosis, management, and prevention, with citations from the scientific literature
- *GOLD Teaching Slide Set*, updated 2007—PowerPoint slide set summarizing the GOLD objectives, documents, and management recommendations, with background information about COPD and the burden of this disease

APPENDIX 2: CASE EXAMPLES: TREATMENT

CLINICAL CASE 1

Intense Craving for a Cigarette and Restlessness after Being Cigarette Deprived for 2 Hours

The patient was a 62-year-old male physician seeking definitive treatment for severe tobacco dependence and nicotine addiction. One year previously, he had been able to stop smoking for several months. After a left upper lobectomy for bronchogenic carcinoma, he had resumed smoking because of a severely stressful event in his life. Much to his frustration, he found that he simply could not stop smoking again. Craving for cigarettes was so severe that he could not effectively practice medicine. Thus, much to his frustration, despite several short-lived quitting attempts, he continued smoking.

On the day I first saw him, he had been in my office for about 2 hours and asked if he could go outside to smoke a cigarette because he noticed he was beginning to have severe cigarette cravings accompanied by marked restlessness. I asked him to wait a few minutes, until after one of my nurses had instructed him in the proper use of nicotine nasal spray and had him demonstrate proper use of the active device. He agreed. When I walked by him in our clinic waiting room about

15 minutes later, he mentioned that, much to his surprise, within 90 seconds after he had given himself the test dose from the active nicotine nasal spray (1 mg of nicotine delivered), he felt his cigarette craving and restlessness simply "melt away." He pointed out that in the past, only by smoking a cigarette had he been able to dissipate these symptoms so promptly. Not surprisingly, this experience gave him even greater confidence in the treatment plan I was about to outline and in his ability to stop smoking. It was also clinical "proof" to him of what he intellectually knew regarding the biology of nicotine addiction.

CLINICAL CASE 2

Difficulty Concentrating After Stopping Smoking Cold Turkey

The patient was a 54-year-old white male accountant presenting for tobacco dependence treatment. He had last tried to stop smoking about 3 years previously, stopping cold turkey on a Monday morning. Although he had been a practicing accountant for more than 20 years, he lacked the concentration skills to understand basic financial spreadsheets. When he tried to analyze the spreadsheet data, he "only saw a jumble of numbers." After 4 days of struggling unsuccessfully to practice accountancy, he smoked one cigarette and found that he could immediately think clearly again. His mind was functioning in its usual keen fashion, and he could analyze financial data with his usual skill and ability. As long as he continued to smoke, he could carry out his professional commitments. Because he really did want to stop smoking, he sought professional assistance to see if he could stop smoking without experiencing this horrendous and disruptive nicotine withdrawal symptom.

I reassured this patient at the initial visit, after he had told me about these concerns, that with current generation medications to treat tobacco dependence, he should be able to function normally, once he stopped smoking, without going through the ordeal he had several years earlier. (And he did.)

CLINICAL CASE 3

Increased Irritability and Anger After Stopping Smoking Cold Turkey

The patient was a 34-year-old white female management consultant presenting for treatment of severe nicotine withdrawal symptoms of 3 weeks' duration. The patient had successfully stopped smoking 3 weeks earlier, using a proprietary 1-week group-counseling program. Although she was pleased that she had been able to stop smoking on her own, she was concerned that she was about to lose all of her clients. She indicated that she had lost her usual tact and diplomacy when dealing with clients. Since stopping smoking, she noted that she had become hyperirritable, easily frustrated, and severely short-tempered. She had not been this way before stopping smoking. She had noticed no improvement in these symptoms since onset 3 weeks ago, when she stopped smoking. She decided she should seek treatment after the following episode occurred.

One of her clients was a large multinational hotel chain. She had just attended a daylong meeting with the board of directors to review their annual business development plan. When they made their presentation to her, she found their plan severely lacking. Rather than tactfully pointing out how it could be improved and strengthened, which she would have done before stopping smoking, she bluntly told them how poor it was. Moreover, she found herself shouting at them, telling them she was amazed at their stupidity and shortsightedness. She knew that if she continued in this hotheaded, short-tempered fashion, she would alienate and lose her clients, thus destroying her livelihood.

On the positive side, she noticed that even though she had been off cigarettes for only 3 weeks, her cough had nearly disappeared. Medically, she was feeling much improved, so she did not want to resume smoking. She knew, however, that if she could not regain her usual manner of dealing with her clients, she would have to resume smoking to avoid alienating them. Although the example she had just given me was unusually dramatic, she commented that since she had stopped smoking 3 weeks ago, she felt as if she were sitting on a keg of dynamite and that any little irritant would cause her to blow up and start screaming.

I congratulated her on stopping smoking and being cigarette-free for 3 weeks. I also explained to her that she was suffering from classic nicotine withdrawal symptoms: being more irritable, getting frustrated more easily, and becoming short-tempered. Moreover, these symptoms of nicotine withdrawal could be easily treated with a nicotine medication. I prescribed nicotine polacrilex, 4 mg, one piece to be chewed according to package instructions, every hour while awake, aiming for a minimum of 16 pieces per day.

Although the patient was skeptical this would do anything for her, she agreed to try it for a week. When she returned 1 week later, she reported that the day after she saw me, she began using the prescribed nicotine polacrilex daily dosage (approximately 64 mg of nicotine per day, from polacrilex medication). By that afternoon, she felt "95% back to normal." She reported that this level of mood and functioning had remained. Several days after she had started the medication, she had another major meeting with a different multinational client. At this meeting she felt she was functioning with her usual level of diplomacy, tact, skill, and creativity—all, of course, without needing a cigarette to restore her equanimity.

CLINICAL CASE 4

Effective Medical Management of Cigarette Slips Due to Acute Work-Related Stress During Tobacco-Dependence Treatment

cThe patient was a 54-year-old male Silicon Valley CEO presenting for tobacco-dependence treatment because his shortness of breath was interfering with all aspects of his life. He had only mild obstructive airway disease (mixed emphysematous and chronic bronchitic type) by pulmonary function testing but had hypoxemia (SpO$_2$ [oxygen saturation by pulse oximeter], 91%) on room air. He was smoking one and one-half packs per day and was highly nicotine dependent, on the basis of the Fagerström Tolerance Questionnaire scale, scoring 8 points (maximum, 11 points). He set his Target Quit Date (TQD) for September 13, 1993, using three standard-strength nicotine patches (delivering 45 mg of nicotine per 16 hr). The patient was delighted at how well he did initially. For the first 2 days, he had no nicotine withdrawal symptoms of any kind, including craving for cigarettes. (He also had no signs or symptoms of nicotine toxicity.) As the first week wore on, however, he noticed that he was becoming progressively more irritable. Also, he was becoming plagued by intermittent, incredibly intense, and frequent cigarette urges.

Late in the afternoon of the fourth day after his TQD, in response to severe stress at work, he had three cigarettes in rapid succession. He had no more cigarettes before returning to the clinic about 24 hours later. Because of those slips, however, as well as the increased cigarette craving and irritability, his nicotine patch dose was increased by 33% to four nicotine patches delivering 60 mg

of nicotine per 16 hours. Moreover, he was given a prescription for 4 mg of nicotine polacrilex as needed so that he could actively do something immediately to control intense cigarette urges.

Because of the medication changes and the patient's smoking in response to an acute stress situation, he was seen 10 days later, on September 27, 1993. He had used the four nicotine patches as prescribed and without difficulty. He was also using approximately four pieces of the 4-mg nicotine polacrilex daily, with no side effects whatsoever. The patient reported that after his previous visit on September 17, 1993, within 1 hour of putting on the fourth patch later that day he noted a marked decrease in irritability, anger, and cravings for cigarettes. During the following 10 days, however, he slipped on four separate days, having one cigarette on each of those days. The trigger was generally work-related stress, but one morning he rushed out of his house, forgetting his four nicotine patches. He continued to have intermittent slips, nearly all due to sudden work-related stress, for 6 weeks after his TQD. Finally, after he increased his daily use of 4-mg nicotine polacrilex, while continuing to wear four nicotine patches per day, he was able to stop smoking completely on September 27, 1993. Over the next 6 months, while not decreasing this nicotine patch dose, he slowly tapered off nicotine polacrilex. Then, during the next 4 months, he slowly tapered off his four nicotine patches. Throughout this time, he was seen about every 4 weeks. He knew to call immediately if he had any flare-ups in nicotine withdrawal symptoms, such as cigarette craving, irritability, or anger, as this nicotine dose reduction process was going on. (Of course, if he had a slip and smoked even part of a cigarette, that would be reason for a STAT phone call!)

Finally, 11 months after his quit date, he successfully tapered off all his nicotine medications. He had definitely needed the steady-state serum nicotine level that the four nicotine patches provided, but he also needed to be able to provide his CNS with periodic nicotine boosts, which the 4-mg dose of nicotine polacrilex provided. For approximately 2 months, from October to December 1993, his therapeutic nicotine dose, from both medications, was about 90 mg/day. He needed this dose to control his nicotine withdrawal symptoms and to enable him to stop smoking successfully (dose to therapeutic effect). He had no nicotine toxicity symptoms or adverse events of any kind.

APPENDIX 3

Pragmatic Method to Initiate Tobacco-Dependence Medications

If using varenicline:

Start varenicline, 0.5 mg once daily, 1.5 to 2 wk before the TQD.

Increase to 0.5 mg every 12 hr (total daily dose, 1 mg) for days 4 to 7.

Increase to the maintenance dose of 1 mg every 12 hr (total daily dose, 2 mg) for the next 4 days (treatment days 8 to 12) to allow medication to reach steady-state level before the TQD.*

If using bupropion sustained release:

Start bupropion at least 1 to 2 wk before the TQD.

Initial dose: 150 mg every morning for 3 to 7 days or longer if necessary or desired.

Increase to the therapeutic dose of 150 mg every 12 hr (total daily dose, 300 mg) at least 5 to 7 days before the TQD.

If using the nicotine patch determine initial dose:

Serum cotinine† ≥ 250 ng of cotinine per cubic milliliter: Start with two Step 1 nicotine patches delivering a total of 30 mg of nicotine every 16 hr.

Serum cotinine < 250 ng of cotinine per cubic milliliter: Start with one Step 1 nicotine patch delivering a total of 15 mg of nicotine every 16 hr.‡,§

Note: Realize that the preceding "simple" algorithm may underdose a large proportion of patients, so be prepared to increase the dose, even on the TQD.

Instruct the patient to start using the prescribed nicotine patch dose beginning the morning of the TQD.

Note: All nicotine patches should be removed after approximately 16 hr of use; otherwise the patient will be at high risk for severe insomnia or bizarre dreams.

See the patient back in the office 3 to 5 days after the TQD for evaluation:

Have the prescribed medication(s) produced the desired therapeutic effect?

Has the patient been able to stop smoking completely (and relatively easily)?

Are all nicotine withdrawal symptoms negligible or nonexistent?

Is the patient experiencing any medication side effects?

Adjust medication dose(s), as required.

Add Rescue Medications—nicotine nasal spray, inhaler, and/or polacrilex gum or lozenge (4-mg dose)—as necessary, if the patient is not taking varenicline.

Prescribe these as for a metered dose inhaler for asthma: Train the patient in the proper use technique and have the patient demonstrate the correct use technique before leaving the office.

If the patient is doing well, without any problems, then have him or her return in about 3 weeks.

If the patient is having difficult nicotine withdrawal symptoms, is smoking, or both, then have the patient come back in another 5 to 10 days, after dose adjustments. Use clinical judgment to determine the time interval between appointments; base visit frequency on the patient's response to revised treatment.

TQD, *Target Quit Date.*

This recommendation is different from the official prescribing instructions but is based on the 4-day period it takes to reach the steady-state level when the dose is changed.

†*Cotinine can be assayed in serum by most commercial laboratories (e.g., BioScience and SmithKline); cost varies, ranging from $35 to $75 per assay.*

‡*During the 16 hours that the patient is awake, it is desirable that nicotine delivery be approximately 0.9 mg of nicotine per hour per patch. All of the largest-size nicotine patches (30 cm²) currently on the market, including Habitrol (Nicotinell in Europe), NicoDerm, Nicotrol (Nicorette in Europe), and generics deliver 0.9 mg/hr per patch.[69] They all deliver 15 mg of nicotine during the first 16 hours of "wear" time. The major difference, in terms of nicotine delivery, occurs if the patch is worn for 24 hours. Then, each patch will deliver an additional 6 mg of nicotine during the 8 hours the patient is asleep (except for Nicotrol/Nicorette, which was designed to deliver nicotine for 16 hours only, so would only deliver 1 additional mg if left on all night). The more nicotine delivered to the CNS during the 8-hour sleep cycle, the greater the incidence of sleep disturbances and bizarre dreams.*

§*If serum cotinine levels are not available, the initial nicotine patch dose may be roughly approximated on the basis of the number of cigarettes smoked per day. This method will have only about one third the accuracy of a serum cotinine level. Measuring serum cotinine is far preferable. If, however, the physician elects not to order a serum cotinine assay, then the physician could initiate treatment with two Step 1 patches for a patient smoking more than 20 cigarettes per day and one Step 1 patch if the patient smokes fewer than 20 cigarettes per day.[105] The patients whose initial patch dose is determined on the basis of the number of cigarettes smoked per day will need to be monitored in the office even more closely than those whose initial patch dose is started on the basis of the serum cotinine level. Most patients will be underdosed, no matter what their starting patch dose is, using the method of Fredrickson and colleagues (see Frederickson PA, Hurt RD, Lee GM et al: High dose transdermal nicotine therapy for heavy smokers: safety, tolerability and measurement of nicotine and cotinine levels, Psychopharmacology 122:215–222, 1995). Be aware that the average number of Step 1 patches that a patient is going to need for the initial months of therapy will range widely, based on suppression of nicotine withdrawal symptoms, from only one Step 1 patch, or even less, to five or six Step 1 patches. In our clinical experience, a patient will need approximately 2.75 patches, on average. However, one cannot simply start a patient on 2.75 patches, because approximately half the patients being treated will be overdosed at that level. Thus, one should use a simple algorithm such as previously outlined in this appendix, using serum cotinine levels to set the starting patch dose and then adjusting the dose upward, if necessary, to suppress nicotine withdrawal symptoms, or downward for those few patients in whom the initial patch dose produces nausea or vomiting.*

Chapter 17

Behavioral Medicine in Pulmonary Rehabilitation: Psychological, Cognitive, and Social Factors

CHARLES F. EMERY • MICHELLE J. HUFFMAN • ANDREA K. BUSBY

CHAPTER OUTLINE

Psychological Functioning
  Depression
  Anxiety
  Personality
  Coping Skills and Self-Efficacy
  Assessment
  Treatment
Cognitive Functioning
  Assessment
  Treatment
Social and Marital Functioning

  Assessment
  Treatment
Behavioral Functioning
  Activities of Daily Living
  Smoking Cessation
  Dietary Factors
  Exercise
  Compliance/Adherence
  Education
Conclusion

PROFESSIONAL SKILLS

On completion of this chapter, the reader will be able to do
the following:
* Describe the psychological sequelae of pulmonary disease and the treatment strategies for improving psychological well-being
* Identify tools that assess levels of depression, anxiety, and psychological adjustment
* Describe the cognitive deficits that may be associated with pulmonary disease
* Describe the effects of pulmonary disease on social and marital relationships and identify tools for assessing social support
* Understand the physical and role limitations experienced by the patient with chronic obstructive pulmonary disease and understand how psychological and social factors can influence performance of daily activities

B ehavioral medicine research and clinical practice address the influence of behavioral, psychological, and social factors on physical functioning, and the way in which these factors interact to affect functioning among patients with pulmonary disease. The purpose of this chapter is to provide an overview of behavioral medicine research and clinical outcomes in patients with

TABLE 17-1   Common Symptoms Observed in Behavioral Medicine Evaluation of Patients in Pulmonary Rehabilitation

Psychological	Cognitive	Social	Behavioral
Depressed mood	Mild deficits	Reduced social activity	Impaired ADL
Anxiety	Impaired psychomotor speed	Change in family roles	Smoking
Anger	Impaired problem-solving	Reduced independence	Malnourishment
Guilt	Impaired attention		Decreased exercise capacity
Embarrassment			Medication noncompliance
Avoidance of expressing strong emotions			

ADL, *Activities of daily living.*

pulmonary disease, focusing on four primary areas of behavioral/psychological functioning: psychological well-being, cognitive performance, social functioning, and behavioral adaptation. Common symptoms associated with each area of functioning are summarized in Table 17-1. In addition to describing symptomatology in each of the four areas of functioning, this chapter (1) documents updated research literature supporting the relevance of each area of functioning for pulmonary disease and pulmonary rehabilitation, (2) summarizes the current relevant clinical data, (3) indicates common assessment procedures, and (4) provides treatment recommendations.

PSYCHOLOGICAL FUNCTIONING

Psychiatric symptoms and diminished psychological well-being frequently are observed among patients with pulmonary disease. Psychological sequelae of pulmonary disease may influence functional status and physical well-being, independent of disease severity.[1] Thus assessment and treatment of psychological factors are critical for effective treatment of the patient with pulmonary disease. Common psychological reactions among patients with pulmonary disease include anger, frustration, guilt, physical and emotional dependency, and embarrassment.[2,3] However, symptoms of depression and anxiety are the most frequently observed psychological symptoms among patients with pulmonary disease.

Depression

Although the prevalence of depression in patients with chronic obstructive pulmonary disease (COPD) is not greater than that found in other chronically ill groups, studies have found that 6% to 59% of patients with COPD have significant

symptoms of depression or clinical depression.[4-7] Depression in this population is typically characterized by hopelessness, pessimism, reduced sleep, decreased appetite, increased lethargy, difficulties in concentration, and increased social withdrawal.[3] In addition, depression in patients with COPD may have a negative effect on daily functioning. Studies consistently report that depressed mood predicts behavioral, social, and mental functioning and that greater depressive symptoms have been associated with increased impairment in activities of daily living[8-10] as well as significantly worse self-reported general and pulmonary health.[5] Depression also is associated with impaired self-management of disease exacerbations.[4] Although the correlation between depressed mood and disease severity is modest,[11] depression may have an influence on daily functioning that is independent of pulmonary functioning. In addition, subclinical depressive symptoms have been associated with poor health outcomes. In an observational study of 137 patients with COPD, subthreshold depressive symptoms predicted self-reported physical disability and quality of life.[7]

Anxiety

Anxiety is another common psychological consequence of COPD. Estimates indicate a prevalence of anxiety disorders and associated symptoms ranging from approximately 30% to 40%.[4,12] Symptoms of anxiety are manifested in a variety of ways, including accelerated speech, exaggerated body movements, and physiologic signs of arousal such as tachycardia, sweating, and dyspnea.[13] Up to 41% of patients with COPD may experience one or more panic attacks, as defined by bouts of intense anxiety, physiologic arousal, temporary cognitive impairment, and a desire to flee the situation.[4,14] Patients with panic report more catastrophic misinterpretations of their bodily symptoms, but do not differ from patients without panic on measures of physical functioning, disease severity, shortness of breath, or psychological distress. Thus, the experience of panic may reflect a cognitive interpretation of pulmonary symptoms rather than objective pulmonary status.[14]

Dyspnea itself, in conjunction with a fear of suffocation and death, is a source of significant anxiety.[3] The emotional arousal of anxiety increases ventilatory demands on the body, which may lead to hypoxia or hypercapnia. Increased physiologic arousal, in turn, exacerbates anxiety symptoms, which then produce greater physiologic insufficiency, resulting in a circular pattern that is difficult to break.[3] Although anxiety symptoms are commonly reported in patients with COPD, anxiety appears not to predict quality of life or directly influence functional status in this population.[10,15] Thus fluctuation of pulmonary symptoms associated with daily stressors does not appear to be influenced by anxiety symptoms per se.[16] However, symptoms of panic disorder may distract patients from self-management of severe disease exacerbations.[4] The small number of published studies in this area is confounded by variability in the measurement of anxiety.

Personality

Several studies have evaluated personality functioning among patients with COPD, but no specific personality disorder or profile for patients with COPD has been observed.[17] Strong emotional reactions such as anxiety, anger, and euphoria may exacerbate pulmonary symptoms by increasing energy expenditure and result in increased demands on ventilation and oxygenation. Emotions associated with decreases in arousal, such as feelings of depression and apathy, may decrease energy expenditure and result in decreased ventilatory demands and lower oxygen (O_2) consumption. Because either hyperarousal or hypoarousal may lead to exacerbations in pulmonary symptoms, it has been suggested that patients with COPD may tend to avoid expressing strong emotions in order to prevent physiologic changes that affect pulmonary symptoms.[18] However, there are no data to suggest that patients with COPD are more likely to avoid emotional expression than other groups with chronic illness. Thus no reliable pattern of personality functioning or personality disorder among patients with COPD has emerged.

Coping Skills and Self-Efficacy

Increasing attention has been devoted to examining coping styles among patients with pulmonary disease. In a 1-year longitudinal study of 40 patients with severe COPD, Parsons[19] observed stability of perceived well-being and a tendency to use more problem-focused coping strategies (e.g., problem solving and goal setting). However, women in the study tended to use more emotion-focused coping (e.g., minimization and avoidance) than did men, and emotion-focused coping was associated with lower levels of perceived well-being. Similarly, emotion-focused coping was independently associated with poorer health-related quality of life in a more recent study of 253 adults with COPD.[20] In a study of 64 outpatients with COPD, passive (avoidant) coping was associated with worse mental health.[21] Thus the data indicate that emotion-focused coping, especially avoidant coping, is associated with poorer quality of life and mental health.

In addition, there is evidence that religiosity and religious coping are common among patients with pulmonary disease. An exploratory, cross-sectional analysis of 90 presurgery patients with end-stage pulmonary disease revealed that religious coping strategies predicted 27% of the unique variance in depression and 14% of the unique variance in overall disability as measured with the Religious/Spiritual Coping Long Form (RCOPE).[22] Specifically, punishing reappraisal (e.g., "Decided that God was punishing me for my sins") and benevolent reappraisal (e.g., "Saw my situation as part of God's plan") accounted for the greatest variance in depression scores. Individuals with higher overall disability scores were more likely to seek spiritual support and a collaborative relationship with God. In addition, religious coping strategies accounted for 34% of the variance in psychosocial disability. Specifically, poorer psychosocial functioning was associated with perceiving lung disease as a punishment from God, as well as with seeking spiritual support and a collaborative relationship with God.[23] Thus, aspects of religious coping may be associated with poorer adjustment. Furthermore there are data suggesting that rational (problem-focused) coping is associated with poorer health-related quality of life.[20] Given these latter counterintuitive results, further research on coping styles is needed to clarify individual difference variables (such as illness severity, sex, and age) that may influence the degree to which coping strategies are effective among patients with COPD.

Self-efficacy also appears to play a role in physical well-being among patients with pulmonary disease. Self-efficacy is broadly defined as the expectation of one's own ability to complete a task. Self-efficacy expectations for walking were found to be a significant predictor of survival among patients with COPD.[24] Self-efficacy also may have an effect on functional status of patients with COPD. In an observational study of 208 patients with COPD, path analyses revealed that the association of pulmonary function with functional impairment was mediated by perceived self-efficacy for functional activities.[25] Relatedly, in a study of 97 patients with COPD, self-efficacy accounted for 36.5% of the variance in functional status among men (n = 52).[26] Self-efficacy expectations also are important for smoking cessation and exercise participation among patients with pulmonary disease.[27,28]

Assessment

Evaluation of psychological functioning often includes both general assessment tools and symptom-specific indicators. Two common tools used for evaluating psychological symptoms are the Brief Symptom Inventory (BSI)[29] and the Profile of Mood States-Short Form (POMS-SF).[30] The BSI is a 53-item multidimensional symptom inventory providing an overall index of symptoms as well as nine specific clinical subscales, including depression, anxiety, and hostility. The POMS-SF is a 30-item list of adjective ratings, providing an overall mood score as well as six mood subscores.

Symptom-specific indicators of psychological distress include measures of depression and anxiety. Common measures of depression include the Beck Depression Inventory (BDI)[31] and the Center for Epidemiological Studies-Depression Inventory (CES-D).[32] The BDI is a widely used, 21-item measure of depressive symptoms and the CES-D is a 20-item measure of depression validated in samples of community-residing older adults. Anxiety measures include the Beck Anxiety Inventory (BAI)[33] and the State-Trait Anxiety Inventory (STAI).[34] The BAI is a 21-item measure of symptoms of anxiety, and the STAI is a 40-item measure with 20 items assessing transient (state) anxiety and 20 items assessing long-standing (trait) symptoms of anxiety. All four of these measures are useful for evaluating change in symptoms of anxiety and depression. The CES-D and the state anxiety component of the STAI are research scales that could be used to measure changes in a clinical setting.

The COPE[35] is the most common measure of coping used in prior studies of COPD. The COPE is a 60-item, theoretically derived, self-report measure that identifies active and avoidant coping strategies across 15 different dimensions (planning, acceptance, denial, etc.). There are two versions of the COPE: the dispositional version and the situational version. For the dispositional version, respondents rate the degree to which they typically use each coping strategy when under stress. For the situational version, respondents rate the degree to which they use each coping strategy when confronted with a particular stressful event. The COPD Coping Questionnaire (CCQ), a disease-specific measure derived from the Asthma Coping Questionnaire,[36] has also been used in several studies as a measure of coping styles among patients with COPD.[20,37,38] The CCQ is a 34-item self-report measure that examines three specific coping styles: avoidant/passive coping, rational/problem-focused coping, and emotional coping. In addition, the RCOPE (Religious/Spiritual Coping Long Form)[22] has been used to assess religious coping among patients with COPD. The RCOPE is a 105-item self-report questionnaire that measures 5 religious functions (meaning, control, comfort/spirituality, intimacy/spirituality, and life transformation), and has 21 subscales (e.g., benevolent religious reappraisal, collaborative religious coping, seeking spiritual support, religious helping, and seeking religious direction).

The COPD Self-Efficacy Scale (CSES)[39] has shown use in measuring the degree of confidence patients with COPD have regarding their ability to avoid breathing difficulty while participating in specific activities. The CSES rates the strength of expectations of managing or avoiding breathing difficulty in 34 situations, and scores are obtained in the domains of negative affect, intense emotional arousal, physical exertion, weather/environment, and behavioral factors.

Treatment

Psychological distress among patients with COPD may be treated by means of group counseling, psychotherapy, medication, exercise rehabilitation, or a combination of modalities.

One prototype for treatment of pulmonary patients is the cognitive—behavioral group format, in which patients are taught relaxation skills combined with cognitive restructuring and identification of emotional changes.[40] Cognitive restructuring includes identification of stress-producing thought patterns (e.g., "I should have quit smoking 10 years ago") and replacing them with more adaptive thoughts (e.g., "I wish I had quit smoking 10 years ago, but I wasn't ready at that time"). Patients also are encouraged to identify emotions (e.g., depression, anxiety, anger, and guilt) and the stress-producing thoughts that contribute to the identified emotional state. This approach, in either a group or individual format, provides patients with a model for approaching psychological distress that can be used by the patient after pulmonary rehabilitation. An example of the stress-producing physical–cognitive–emotional cycle is shown in Figure 17-1.

Psychological treatments targeting catastrophic misinterpretations of bodily symptoms are thought to decrease experiences of panic in patients with COPD.[14] Although research in this area has not targeted symptoms of panic, one study suggests that cognitive restructuring may not significantly alter levels of overall anxiety or depression.[41] However, relaxation training, in which the patient is taught strategies for relaxing muscle groups throughout the body, may improve symptoms of anxiety, dyspnea, and airway obstruction in patients with COPD.[42]

Supportive coping skills interventions also may have a positive effect among patients with end-stage lung disease. In a randomized, controlled study of 328 patients with end-stage pulmonary disease awaiting lung transplantation, participants were randomized to either a 12-week telephone-based coping skills intervention or a usual care control condition.[43] Patients who received coping skills training experienced significant decreases in perceived stress, anxiety, and depression as well as increases in vitality, perceived social support, and perceived mental health.

In addition, there is evidence that standard pulmonary rehabilitation programs have positive psychological benefits. Studies have shown that rehabilitation programs consisting of pulmonary education and exercise conditioning may increase COPD self-efficacy,[44] 6-minute walk self-efficacy, overall quality of life, and emotional functioning.[40,45,46]

Psychotropic medications are sometimes included in the treatment of psychological distress among patients with pulmonary disease, and several studies have demonstrated benefits of

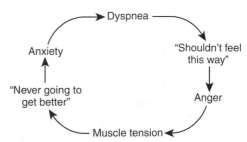

FIGURE 17-1 Model of interactive cycle of physical symptoms, cognitive distortions, and emotions, used in behavioral medicine treatment of patients in pulmonary rehabilitation.

psychotropic medication for reducing not only psychological symptoms, such as depression and anxiety, but also physical symptoms (e.g., feelings of suffocation and dizziness).[47,48] Medications may be used in conjunction with individual or group counseling, and behavioral approaches are often important in facilitating the patient's efforts to follow the treatment regimen or, alternatively, to work toward reducing the need for medication.

COGNITIVE FUNCTIONING

Mild cognitive deficits have been observed among patients with COPD. However, there is debate regarding the nature of the deficits and the extent to which they are related to hypoxemia. Studies have described impaired neuropsychological functioning among patients with COPD in problem-solving, psychomotor speed, attention, and verbal memory,[49-53] but verbal intelligence does not appear to be affected.[49] Other studies confirm that cognitive performance of patients with COPD reflects isolated deficits and does not resemble cognitive performance among patients with dementia.[51,54] Greater hypoxemia has been associated with more impairment in cognitive performance, but cognitive performance of severely hypoxemic subjects remains better than the performance of demented patients.

Data from the combined Nocturnal Oxygen Therapy Trial (NOTT) and the Intermittent Positive Pressure Breathing (IPPB) Trial have documented a positive correlation between neuropsychological impairment and hypoxemia.[49] Control subjects performed better than mildly hypoxemic patients, who in turn performed better than patients who were moderately or severely hypoxemic. However, data from these studies and others have indicated that neuropsychological functioning is not associated with standard pulmonary function variables (e.g., forced expiratory volume in 1 sec) and is only moderately associated with hypoxemia.[40] Age and education accounted for the greatest amount of variance in neuropsychological performance in the studies of Grant and colleagues.[49] Sleep disorders also are associated with hypoxemia and neuropsychological dysfunction.[55] Rourke and Adams[56] thus suggest that sleep-disordered breathing and sleep apnea may represent additional risk factors for neuropsychological impairment among patients with COPD.

Although past studies have evaluated self-perceptions of cognitive performance, studies have not evaluated the extent to which self-perceptions reflect objective cognitive performance. Mood or psychological functioning may be a confounding variable in the self-assessment of cognitive functioning, because previous studies have demonstrated an association of depression and anxiety with perceptions of poorer cognitive performance despite an absence of impairment on objective indicators.

Assessment

A number of neuropsychological measures have been used in studies evaluating cognitive performance among patients with COPD. Instruments include comprehensive indicators of intellectual functioning as well as measures tapping specific domains. The most common assessment battery, which provides measures of overall intellectual ability as well as subscale scores in verbal and performance domains, is the Wechsler Adult Intelligence Scale-III (WAIS-III).[57] Additional neuropsychological measures commonly used in evaluation of patients with COPD and patients with chronic illnesses include (1) the Trail Making Test, measuring sequencing ability and visual motor tracking,[58] (2) the Stroop Interference Test, designed to measure the patient's ability to shift perceptual set and meet changing demands of a task,[59] (3) the Wisconsin Card Sort,[60] a measure of abstract conceptual skills, cognitive flexibility, and ability to test hypotheses and use error feedback, (4) the Selective Reminding Task,[61] a measure of verbal learning and memory, and (5) the Wechsler Memory Scale-III,[62] which measures attention, concentration, visual memory, and verbal memory.

Treatment

Intervention studies have demonstrated that treatment with supplemental O_2 may reverse some of the deficits in neuropsychological functioning observed among patients with COPD.[63,64] However, improvements observed in neuropsychological performance are relatively mild and would not be considered clinically significant.[64,65] In addition, blood O_2 levels must be diminished to an extreme extent for metabolic alterations to occur in energy-producing pathways in the brain. Instead, the role of O_2 in neurotransmitter regulation has been outlined as the most probable cause of neuropsychological changes resulting from hypoxemia and from supplemental O_2 use.[56,66]

Exercise may have beneficial effects on aspects of cognitive functioning. Emery and colleagues[40] found improvements in verbal fluency among patients randomized to a 10-week exercise program compared with an education-only group and a wait-list control group. No changes were observed in other areas of cognitive functioning such as attention and motor speed. In a relatively brief 3-week exercise program, Kozora, Tran, and Make[67] found clinically significant improvements in sustained visual attention, verbal retention, and visuospatial ability among the most cognitively impaired patients, although improvements in the overall group did not differ significantly from those in a no-treatment comparison group. More recently, Kozora and colleagues[68] found significant improvement in delayed verbal memory and psychomotor speed among patients who had received lung volume reduction surgery in the National Emphysema Treatment Trial (NETT) versus no improvement among patients in a standard care control group.

SOCIAL AND MARITAL FUNCTIONING

Perceived social support contributes to enhanced well-being among patients with COPD[15] and may indirectly predict functional capacity.[8] In particular, marital support is an important predictor of patient well-being. In a prospective longitudinal study of 157 patients with severe COPD, living with a partner was associated with an additional 12 months of life.[69] However, the physical limitations experienced by patients with COPD may have profound effects on family relations and lifestyle. Five areas cited by Clough and colleagues[70] include diminished wage-earning ability, changes in family roles, reduced independence, reduced social activities, and effects of O_2 use in the home. Sexual functioning may be impaired[71] and spouses of patients with COPD may be prone to both depression and anxiety.[72] There may be important gender and individual differences that affect attitudes of the patient with COPD. For example, women with COPD report lower marital satisfaction than men with COPD.[73] In a study of 31 patients with COPD and their spouses, marital satisfaction among patients was associated with enhanced well-being and marital adjustment among spouses was related to the patient's level of physical functioning.[74] Thus physical functioning among patients with COPD is likely to have significant effects on both social functioning and marital functioning, and social/marital support is predictive of patient well-being. Further research is needed to investigate the influence of social support on health outcomes and the effect of social support interventions among patients with COPD.

Assessment

Social support has been broadly conceptualized in two domains: structural support and functional support.[75] *Structural support* refers to the number of social relationships and the connections between individuals in the network. *Functional support* refers to the support role (e.g., companionship, instrumental or material assistance, and information providing) of the social relationships. Therefore, measures of structural support typically evaluate the number of individuals in the support network, while measures of functional support assess the needs fulfilled by individuals in the social network. Both forms of assessment are subjective, relying on respondent perceptions, but structural measures may facilitate a somewhat more objective analysis.

Social support is typically assessed via self-report measures, sometimes within a larger multidimensional assessment of functional status or quality of life. For example, the Sickness Impact Profile (SIP)[76] and the Medical Outcomes Study 36-Item Short Form Health Survey (SF-36)[77] both assess social functioning as one area of overall patient functioning. In addition, specific measures of social support are also available and used widely. The Interpersonal Support Evaluation List-Short Form (ISEL-SF) is a 16-item measure of functional support assessing four different functions of the social support network: appraisal, self-esteem, belonging, and tangibility.[78] The Multidimensional Scale of Perceived Social Support (MSPSS) is a 12-item measure of structural support that assesses potential sources of social support, including family, friends, and significant others.[79] Social support has also been assessed using study-specific questions designed by individual investigators. Although the latter measures may provide useful data, they may have limited use in other clinical or research settings. Findings regarding social support among patients with COPD are based on a variety of social support measures, including measures targeting both the structure and function of the support network.

Treatment

Because of the importance of social support for health and psychological well-being of patients with pulmonary disease, pulmonary rehabilitation programs ideally would include spouses/caregivers in the educational components of the program. Inclusion of spouses/caregivers conveys to the patient the importance of the treatment (exercise) and contributes to the ability of the spouse/caregiver to facilitate exercise and proper medical care after the rehabilitation program has been completed. Psychological counseling may include spouses/caregivers as a way of providing a forum for discussion of spousal distress resulting from changes in the patient and the additional burdens of caregiving. For some patients, the spouse/caregiver may be attempting to provide more functional support than is required, which may undermine the patient's efforts at independent functioning. In such cases, the rehabilitation program may serve the important function of separating the patient from the spouse/caregiver for periods of time to allow the patient to engage in independent activities.

BEHAVIORAL FUNCTIONING

Activities of Daily Living

The lifestyle of individuals with COPD is often altered as a result of declining physical functioning associated with disease progression. Patients with COPD are typically confronted with difficulties in numerous areas of life functioning including bathing, grooming, dressing, eating, sleeping, and mobility.[11,80] In addition to difficulties in ambulation and home management, COPD also tends to hinder recreational activities and social interactions.[9,11,81]

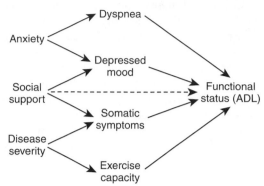

FIGURE 17-2 Model of psychological, social, and physical variables with direct and indirect influence on functional status among patients with pulmonary disease. ADL, activities of daily living.

Disease severity is often considered to be the primary factor contributing to functional impairments in this population, and a study of 56 patients with COPD revealed that disease severity predicted self-reported physical functioning.[82] No direct relationship between pulmonary function and functional status has been observed, but pulmonary function may indirectly affect functional status via its effect on exercise capacity.[10] Although studies have found significant associations between activities of daily living and exercise capacity, as measured by 6-Minute Walk Test, pulmonary function appears to be no more important in predicting exercise capacity than other, more subjective factors, including indicators of psychological well-being.[8-10,81]

Several psychological factors and behavioral symptoms appear to affect patient functioning, both directly and indirectly. Graydon and Ross[8] found that predictors of functional status varied according to whether or not patients used O_2. Among non–O_2-dependent subjects, the strongest predictor of exercise capacity was negative mood, not pulmonary function. Among O_2-dependent subjects, impaired functioning was found to be directly influenced by self-report ratings of somatic symptoms and indirectly influenced by pulmonary function.[8] Further, studies suggest that depressed mood may be a better predictor of functional status than other mood states.

In a sample of 104 patients with COPD, depressed mood, exercise capacity, and dyspnea were the only factors that directly influenced functional status, whereas anxiety had only an indirect impact through the pathways of depressed mood and dyspnea.[10] Additional findings suggest that depressed mood is a stronger predictor of exercise capacity than are anxiety and optimism.[15] Self-esteem has also been found to play a role in patient functioning, with at least two studies reporting direct effects on functional status[15,83] and at least one study reporting indirect effects through the pathway of depressed mood.[10] Although psychological factors may be less influential for patients receiving O_2 therapy, the data consistently suggest that subjective factors, especially depressed mood, are important when considering a patient's functional impairments. In a study of 334 patients with COPD, psychological distress was associated with difficulty in both self-care and performance of recreational activities.[84]

Perceived social support and satisfaction with social resources also appear to affect functional status, although data are inconsistent as to whether the influence is direct or indirect.[8,9,15,81] Studies indicate that social support may directly influence functional status or may indirectly influence functional status through the pathways of negative mood and somatic symptoms.[8,15]

Several models have been tested, resulting in support for the notion that functional status is best predicted by a combination of factors, rather than by any single factor in isolation.[10,15,81,83] Factors include pulmonary function, psychological well-being, and social support, as shown in Figure 17-2. Thus, numerous areas of functioning should be included in assessing functional status of patients and developing an optimal treatment plan. Enhancement of patient functioning may best be addressed by targeting factors that directly influence functional status, such as exercise capacity, depressed mood, self-esteem, exercise tolerance, dyspnea, and satisfaction with social support.

Assessment

Functional status can be assessed in several ways, most often using self-report instruments. Two commonly used general measures of quality of life are the Sickness Impact Profile (SIP)[76] and the Medical Outcomes Study 36-Item Short Form Health Survey (SF-36).[77] The SIP is a 136-item questionnaire evaluating 12 areas of daily functioning (ambulation, mobility, body care and movement, social interaction, communication, alertness behavior, emotional behavior, sleep and rest, eating, employment, home management, and recreation and pastimes) to reflect limitations in physical, psychological, and social functioning. More recently, a short form of the SIP has been developed, the SIP-68, with 68 items covering 6 dimensions of functioning (somatic autonomy, mobility control, psychic autonomy and communication, social behavior, emotional stability, and mobility range).[85] The SF-36 evaluates nine health-related dimensions: physical functioning, role functioning-physical, role functioning-emotional, social functioning, bodily pain, mental health, vitality, general health perceptions, and change in health. In addition, two common illness-specific measures of quality of life are the St. George's Respiratory Questionnaire (SGRQ)[86] and the Chronic Respiratory Disease Questionnaire (CRDQ).[87] The SGRQ is a 76-item self-administered questionnaire used to assess the impact of pulmonary disease on health and functioning. The SGRQ yields scores for three dimensions of functioning: symptom frequency, activities that either cause or are limited by breathing difficulties, and impact of disease on social and emotional functioning. The CRDQ is a 20-item measure of health-related quality of life in patients with chronic pulmonary disease yielding 4 scores: dyspnea, fatigue, emotional functioning, and mastery. Although the CRDQ is usually interviewer-administered, a study by Schünemann and colleagues[88] indicates reliability of a self-administered version of the questionnaire. All four of these measures could be used to evaluate change in quality of life among patients with COPD. The SF-36 would provide the most efficient assessment of generic quality of life, and the CRDQ would provide an illness-specific indicator of change with minimal burden to the patient.

Treatment

Exercise training is a critical factor in helping to increase activity levels, and improvements after exercise rehabilitation have been observed primarily in strenuous tasks such as cleaning, shopping, and personal care.[89] In addition, treatment strategies incorporate activity planning and pacing. Patients are encouraged to plan daily activities, list them on a daily planner, and mark off each activity as it is completed. Planning pleasurable activities is integral to this program to facilitate the patient's sense of control and to prevent depressive symptoms. Patients are encouraged to accept the pace at which they complete physical activities, and are helped to identify new aspects of their daily activities to enjoy.

Smoking Cessation

Smoking behavior is the primary risk factor for COPD. Although most patients have quit smoking before entering pulmonary rehabilitation, there are a number of important behavioral factors relevant for smoking cessation among patients who continue to smoke. Indeed, psychological factors, particularly self-efficacy and depressed mood, have been implicated in smoking cessation and relapse. In a study of smoking cessation among patients with COPD who have at least a 15-year smoking history, self-efficacy was the strongest predictor of cessation at 1 month and 3 months after baseline assessment. In addition, patient behaviors, motivation, and outcome expectancies were predictors, but only when they were combined with self-efficacy expectations.[27] Negative mood also may be associated with smoking cessation and abstinence. Depressed smokers may have more difficulty quitting than nondepressed smokers and may be more likely to relapse several months later.[90] In a sample of patients with COPD, depressed mood was significantly associated with reduced ability to quit smoking.[91]

Treatment

Behavioral medicine treatment of smoking often includes relaxation training, group support, nicotine fading via brand switching, and training in relapse prevention. Patients are encouraged to modify the home/work environment to minimize smoking temptations, and to enlist supportive allies in the home and work environments. Much of the initial work is devoted to establishing the patient's motivation and readiness for smoking cessation. Later sessions are devoted to preparing for becoming a nonsmoker and strategies for coping with smoking relapses.

The amount of support that a smoker receives while trying to quit is thought to be an important factor in predicting success. Therefore, patients should be encouraged to seek the support of a spouse or friend.[92] Smoking cessation treatment groups may be beneficial in this regard. Cognitive coping strategies also may influence success at maintaining abstinence. In a sample of 91 healthy adult ex-smokers, successful abstinence at 3-month follow-up was associated with the ability of subjects to use cognitive restructuring to modify an urge-to-smoke into an acknowledgment that smoking is not an optimal response. This cognitive process was associated with greater abstinence than was suppressing thoughts of smoking.[93]

Behavioral research suggests that comprehensive treatments targeting psychological functioning may increase the efficacy of smoking cessation. Specifically, empirical evidence suggests that multicomponent smoking cessation treatment may be more effective than treatment in a single modality. In addition, psychological variables seem to play a role in both the ability to quit smoking and the likelihood of relapse. In a Cochrane review of smoking cessation studies, most study therapists were clinical psychologists who used an array of psychological techniques, not a specific theoretical model.[94] The relative effectiveness of the various psychological approaches is unknown.

Several researchers have documented the beneficial effects of using a comprehensive treatment package for smoking cessation. Ockene and colleagues[95] randomly assigned 1200 healthy adult smokers to one of three conditions: (1) physician advice to stop smoking, (2) counseling in addition to advice, or (3) nicotine-containing gum in addition to counseling and advice. Rates of cessation were highest among subjects assigned to the most comprehensive treatment program. Additional studies have suggested that nicotine patches or nicotine nasal sprays may be ineffective unless combined with additional elements of a treatment plan, including a minimal addition such as a self-help booklet.[96,97] According to Kottke and colleagues,[98] no single strategy is more effective than another. Instead, the most important factor in smoking cessation is consistent repetition of the stop-smoking message. Thus, multimodal approaches and consistency of communications regarding smoking cessation appear to be critical to the success of smoking cessation interventions. Individual treatment and group treatment both increase the likelihood of quitting. Two trials comparing group and individual counseling for smoking cessation found no significant difference in outcomes.[99,100]

Motivational interviewing, a brief behavioral intervention that focuses on the patient's ambivalence to change, holds promise as a tool for smoking cessation. Motivational interviewing is a client-centered style of counseling in which motivation for change is explored without confrontation.[101] Motivational interviewing was developed for use with substance abuse patients[102] but is currently being used in a variety of domains. Although it has not been applied in a controlled study among patients with pulmonary disease, motivational interviewing to promote smoking cessation has shown promise in a variety of other populations including samples of college students[103] and hospitalized adolescents.[104]

Motivational interviewing appears to improve the likelihood of quitting smoking, but a combination of behavioral and drug therapies offers the greatest chance of successful smoking cessation.[105] Among patients who report they would like to quit smoking, 10.2% are successful in quitting following physician verbal advice alone.[106] However, the 12-month quit rate is increased to 35% when a combination of nicotine replacement, bupropion, and social or behavioral support is available.[107]

Dietary Factors

Studies indicate that a significant number of patients with COPD are malnourished, as indicated by lower than normal body weight, tricep muscle skinfold, arm muscle circumference, and caloric intake.[108,109] Behavioral research has indicated that malnourishment may be associated with psychological functioning and that dietary supplements may reverse the deterioration in psychological and physical functioning associated with depleted nutrition.[110]

Although few studies have investigated the degree to which nutrition is associated with psychological and behavioral factors, Efthimiou and colleagues[110] found that perceptions of general well-being were significantly greater in 7 well-nourished patients with COPD than in 14 malnourished patients. Similar degrees of breathlessness and physical capacity were observed in the two groups, but well-nourished patients demonstrated greater respiratory muscle strength and handgrip strength, as well as less muscle fatigue, which in turn may have contributed to greater feelings of well-being. Cochrane and Afolabi[111] assessed level of nourishment in 103 outpatients with COPD and found nutritional status to be related to fatigue, physical role limitation, energy/vitality, depression, and change in health. However, because their data are cross-sectional, the direction of the relationship between distress/depression and poor nutritional status is unknown.

Treatment

Dietary supplementation to increase caloric intake has been found to reverse some of the associated features of malnourishment. An 8-week course of dietary supplements has been associated with weight gain and increased caloric intake.[112,113] A 3-month course of supplements contributed to general well-being in addition to increases in percentage of ideal body weight, caloric intake, respiratory muscle functioning, handgrip strength, and physical capacity (as measured by the 6-Minute Walk Test), as well as decreases in level of breathlessness.[110] Thus, aspects of both psychological and physical health may be improved via nutritional manipulations.

Behavioral approaches to weight management include activity planning, meal planning, and helping the patient develop realistic goals for body weight. For patients who experience anxiety associated with eating, relaxation training may be useful. Stimulus control approaches (e.g., eating only while seated, and avoiding other activities while eating) are also important behavioral strategies for patients attempting weight loss.

Thus there is evidence supporting the idea that nutrition affects the functioning of pulmonary patients. Future research is needed to clarify the relationship of psychological well-being with nutritional intake in patients with pulmonary disease. No investigations to date have examined the effects of mood on nutritional and caloric intake, the effects of nutrition on cognitive functioning and mood, or psychological/cognitive factors that may predict nutritional status among pulmonary patients.

Exercise

Exercise is the core component of most pulmonary rehabilitation programs, and studies suggest that exercise is critical for achieving not only physical improvement in functioning, but also psychological improvement. One randomized study documented reductions in symptoms of anxiety and depression among patients with COPD participating in a 10-week exercise rehabilitation program.[40] Exercise also was associated with reductions in illness-related impairment (as measured by the Sickness Impact Profile) and improved cognitive performance on a task evaluating executive functioning. In a 1-year follow-up study of the same cohort, it was observed that patients who continued with the prescribed exercise routine maintained the gains that had been achieved during the 10-week exercise rehabilitation program, but patients who did not maintain the exercise routine experienced increased symptoms of depression and anxiety.[114]

Treatment

Exercise may be an important component of treatment to facilitate psychological gains. The study by Emery and colleagues[40] found no changes in psychological symptoms in a control group participating in education and social support without exercise, and similar negative results were observed in a 6-week nonexercise treatment of pulmonary patients.[115] These latter two studies suggest that psychological change in rehabilitation requires more than social support and knowledge. Increased physical activity seems to be an essential component.

Compliance/Adherence

Exercise compliance is at the heart of any rehabilitation program, and continued compliance (adherence) is essential for patients to maintain gains after the program has ended. The relapse prevention strategy appears to be useful with this patient group in that it prepares patients to acknowledge and cope with the inevitable occasions when they are reluctant or unable to exercise. In addition, because negative mood states may be associated with reduced energy and interest in activities such as exercise, strategies for improving mood also are likely to contribute to better exercise performance.

The medical regimen of individuals with COPD is often complex, with an average of 6.3 medications per patient.[116] Consequently, nonadherence is high, with about half of patients over- or underusing their medications.[116,117] Unfortunately, little is known about factors associated with noncompliance in patients with COPD or about ways in which compliance can be increased in this population. One study of medication compliance in the COPD population found that forgetting to use medication and declining to use medication were the two most frequent reasons for noncompliance, and that these reasons for noncompliance resulted from the patient feeling well enough without the medication.[116] Side effects, changes in daily routines, and running out of medication were also frequently reported as factors associated with noncompliance. In addition, impaired long-term memory has been associated with poor adherence among patients with COPD.[50] One study of medication adherence among patients with COPD revealed that demographic and medical history variables did not differ among compliant and noncompliant patients. Instead, adherence was associated with better understanding of the illness and greater confidence in the current medical management of the illness. Nonadherent patients reported greater difficulty or side effects with medications, greater confusion about medications, and a greater willingness to vary medications on the basis of their own perception of symptoms.[118] Among adult patients with asthma, stage of change (e.g., precontemplation, contemplation, and active) and readiness to change were predictors of adherence to medication regimens whereas self-efficacy was not associated with objective measures of adherence.[119]

No study to date has examined ways to increase medication compliance among patients with COPD. A review of studies among nonpulmonary patients suggests there are few solid quantitative data to support specific compliance recommendations.[120] This is due largely to inadequate methods of measuring drug compliance. Direct measurement of drug compliance is costly and inconvenient. Indirect methods such as self-report, interview, pill count, pharmacy records, and self-monitoring are less accurate and subject to other factors such as social desirability. Reinforcing patients for medical compliance or symptom reduction may be somewhat effective, but little evidence supports the use of self-monitoring techniques.[121]

Patients with pulmonary disease also may not comply with prescribed use of supplemental O_2. Earnest[122] completed a qualitative study of patterns of adherence and barriers to compliance among 27 patients with COPD using supplemental O_2. Use of supplemental O_2 was influenced by four domains of self-management: functional management, health management, social management, and symptom management. Functional management of adherence depended on whether or not O_2 was perceived as helpful or as cumbersome. The health management domain included the doctor's recommendation of O_2 use and the belief that it was supposed to be good for the patient's health. Patients also believed that O_2 could be harmful to their health, cause side effects such as nose bleeds and nasal dryness, and weaken the lungs. Patients who were less adherent to O_2 use believed that it compromised their social role. They cited embarrassment, self-consciousness, fear of burdening others, weak or sick appearance, and shame. For other patients, social pressure from family encouraged them to be compliant with O_2 use. Individuals who reported marked reduction of dyspnea when using O_2 were more likely to adhere to

doctor-recommended O_2 use than those who reported little change in dyspnea.

Treatment compliance is also critical to the success of pulmonary rehabilitation. Young and colleagues[123] conducted a cross-sectional study of 91 patients with COPD, comparing those who declined to participate or failed to complete a COPD rehabilitation program with those who completed the program. Members of the nonadherent group was more likely to be widowed or divorced, less likely to be currently married, more likely to live alone, and more likely to be current smokers. Inadequate social support was more common in the nonadherent group. No physiologic or psychological factors distinguished the two groups. Thus, these data emphasize the importance of a spouse or other source of social support for adherence to exercise rehabilitation.

Treatment

Treatment of noncompliance must address the source of the problem (e.g., lack of patient understanding, appropriateness of the intervention, absence of support at home for medication compliance, patient not trusting physician). When the source of noncompliance has been determined, then problem-solving can help the patient evaluate the extent to which medication compliance is feasible. Future investigations must address the role of behavioral and psychological factors in medical compliance among patients with COPD. Cognitive factors, mood, and social support should be examined further to determine their role in predicting or increasing medical compliance. Treatment efforts should then target modifiable factors associated with poor compliance.

Education

Education is a component in most pulmonary rehabilitation programs. The National Institute for Health and Clinical Excellence (NICE) guidelines[124] suggest topics to address in the education of patients, including smoking cessation, developing a plan for change, anxiety management, goal setting and rewards, relaxation, identifying and changing beliefs about exercise and health-related behaviors, and use of support groups. However, studies indicate that education alone does not lead to improvements in psychological functioning or quality of life[114] and that education in combination with exercise training is not as effective as activity-specific training (e.g., dyspnea management strategies) in combination with exercise training.[125]

Therefore education is viewed as a necessary component of pulmonary rehabilitation, but education alone is not sufficient to produce the behavioral and psychological changes commonly observed in association with exercise training.

CONCLUSION

Behavioral medicine components of pulmonary rehabilitation often incorporate evaluation and treatment of psychological functioning, cognitive performance, social functioning, and behavioral performance among patients with pulmonary disease. Data suggest the importance of addressing psychological factors, especially depression and anxiety, to help enhance functional abilities among patients. In addition, studies increasingly support the importance of examining the family and social context in which the patient functions and of helping the patient identify cognitive strategies that may be useful in coping with pulmonary disease. Behavioral factors also play a critical role in helping patients make changes in smoking, dietary intake, and exercise activity. Thus, behavioral and psychological factors are both directly and indirectly associated with health status among patients with pulmonary disease, and are important components of assessment and treatment in the context of a multidisciplinary pulmonary rehabilitation program.

References

1. Ashutosh K, Haldipur C, Boucher ML: Clinical and personality profiles and survival in patients with COPD, Chest 111:95, 1997.
2. Guyatt GH, Townsend M, Berman LB et al: Quality of life in patients with chronic airflow limitation, Br J Dis Chest 81:45, 1987.
3. Sandhu HS: Psychosocial issues in chronic obstructive pulmonary disease, Clin Chest Med 7:629, 1986.
4. Dowson CA, Town GI, Framptom C et al: Psychopathology and illness beliefs influence COPD self-management, J Psychosom Res 56:333, 2004.
5. Felker B, Katon W, Hedrick SC et al: The association between depressive symptoms and health status in patients with chronic pulmonary disease, Gen Hosp Psychiatry 23:56, 2001.
6. Mikkelsen RL, Middelboe T, Psinger C et al: Anxiety and depression in patients with chronic obstructive pulmonary disease (COPD): a review, Nord J Psychiatry 58:65, 2004.
7. Yohannes AM, Baldwin RC, Connolly MJ: Prevalence of sub-threshold depression in elderly patients with chronic obstructive pulmonary disease, Int J Geriatr Psychiatry 18:412, 2003.
8. Graydon JE, Ross E: Influence of symptoms, lung function, mood, and social support on level of functioning of patients with COPD, Res Nurs Health 18:525, 1995.
9. Leidy NK: Functional performance in people with chronic obstructive pulmonary disease, Image J Nurs Sch 27:23, 1995.
10. Weaver TE, Richmond TS, Narsavage GL: An explanatory model of functional status in chronic obstructive pulmonary disease, Nurs Res 46:26, 1997.
11. Engstrom C-P, Persson L-O, Larsson S et al: Functional status and well being in chronic obstructive pulmonary disease with regard to clinical parameters and smoking: a descriptive and comparative study, Thorax 51:825, 1996.
12. Kim HFS, Kunik ME, Molinari VA et al: Functional impairment in COPD patients: the impact of anxiety and depression, Psychosomatics 41:465, 2000.
13. Dudley DL, Glaser EM, Jorgenson BN et al: Psychosocial concomitants to rehabilitation in chronic obstructive pulmonary disease. 2. Psychosocial treatment, Chest 77:544, 1980.
14. Porzelius J, Vest M, Nochomovitz M: Respiratory function, cognitions, and panic in chronic obstructive pulmonary patients, Behav Res Ther 30:75, 1992.
15. Anderson KL: The effect of chronic obstructive pulmonary disease on quality of life, Res Nurs Health 18:547, 1995.
16. Goreczny AJ, Brantley PJ, Buss RR et al: Daily stress and anxiety and their relation to daily fluctuations of symptoms in asthma and chronic obstructive pulmonary disease (COPD) patients, J Psychopathol Behav Assess 10:259, 1988.
17. Bauer H, Duijsens IJ: Personality disorders in pulmonary patients, Br J Med Psychol 71:165, 1998.
18. Dudley DL, Wermuth C, Hague W: Psychosocial aspects of care in the chronic obstructive pulmonary disease patient, Heart Lung 2:289, 1973.
19. Parsons E: Coping and well-being strategies in individuals with COPD, Health Values 14:17, 1990.
20. Hesselink AE, Penninx BWJH, Schlosser MAG et al: The role of coping resources and coping style in quality of life of patients with asthma or COPD, Qual Life Res 13:509, 2004.
21. Scharloo M, Kaptein AA, Weinman JA et al: Physical and psychological correlates of functioning in patients with chronic obstructive pulmonary disease, J Asthma 37:17, 2000.
22. Pargament KI, Koenig HG, Perez LM: The many methods of religious coping: development and initial validation of the RCOPE, J Clin Psychol 56:519, 2000.
23. Burker EJ, Evon DM, Sedway JA et al: Religious coping, psychological distress and disability among patients with end-stage pulmonary disease, J Clin Psychol Med Settings 11:179, 2004.
24. Kaplan RM, Ries AL, Prewitt LM et al: Self-efficacy expectations predict survival for patients with chronic obstructive pulmonary disease, Health Psychol 13:366, 1994.
25. Kohler CL, Fish L, Greene PG: The relationship of perceived self-efficacy to quality of life in chronic obstructive pulmonary disease, Health Psychol 21:610, 2002.

26. Siela D: Use of self-efficacy and dyspnea perceptions to predict functional performance in people with COPD, Rehabil Nurs 28:197, 2003.

27. Devins GM, Edwards PJ: Self-efficacy and smoking reduction in chronic obstructive pulmonary disease, Behav Res Ther 26:127, 1988.

28. Ries AL, Kaplan RM, Limberg TM et al: Effects of pulmonary rehabilitation on physiologic and psychosocial outcomes in patients with chronic obstructive pulmonary disease, Ann Intern Med 122:823, 1995.

29. Derogatis LR, Spencer PM: Brief symptom inventory: administration, scoring, and procedures manual-I, Baltimore, 1982, Clinical Psychometric Research.

30. McNair DM, Lorr M, Droppelman LF: Profile of mood states, San Diego, Calif, 1981, Educational and Testing Service.

31. Beck AT: Depression inventory, Philadelphia, 1978, Center for Cognitive Therapy.

32. Radloff LS: The CES-D Scale: a self-report depression scale for research in the general population, Appl Psychol Meas 1:385, 1977.

33. Beck AT, Epstein N, Brown G et al: An inventory for measuring clinical anxiety: psychometric properties, J Consult Clin Psychol 56:893, 1988.

34. Spielberger CE, Gorsuch RL, Luschene RE: Manual for the State-Trait Anxiety Inventory, Palo Alto, Calif, 1970, Consulting Psychologist Press.

35. Carver CS, Scheier MF, Weintraub JK: Assessing coping strategies: a theoretically based approach, J Pers Soc Psychol 56:267, 1989.

36. Maes S, Schlosser MAG: The role of cognition and coping in health behaviour outcomes of asthmatic patients, Curr Psychol Res Rev 6:79, 1987.

37. Maes S, Schlosser MAG: Changing health behaviour outcomes in asthmatic patients: a pilot intervention study, Soc Sci Med 26:359, 1988.

38. Ketelaars CAJ, Abu-Saad HH, Halfens RJ et al: Long-term outcome of pulmonary rehabilitation in patients with COPD, Chest 112:363, 1997.

39. Wigal K, Creer TL, Kotses H: The COPD Self-efficacy Scale, Chest 99:1193, 1991.

40. Emery CF, Schein RL, Hauck ER et al: Psychological and cognitive outcomes of a randomized trial of exercise among patients with chronic obstructive pulmonary disease, Health Psychol 17:232, 1998.

41. Lisansky DP, Clough DH: A cognitive–behavioral self-help educational program for patients with COPD, Psychother Psychosom 65:97, 1996.

42. Gift AG, Moore T, Soeken K: Relaxation to reduce dyspnea and anxiety in COPD patients, Nurs Res 41:242, 1992.

43. Blumenthal JA, Babyak MA, Carney RM et al: Telephone-based coping skills training for patients awaiting lung transplantation, J Consult Clin Psychol 74:535, 2006.

44. Kara M, Asti T: Effect of education on self-efficacy of Turkish patients with chronic obstructive pulmonary disease, Patient Edu Counsel 55:114, 2004.

45. Lox CL, Freehill AJ: Impact of pulmonary rehabilitation on self-efficacy, quality of life, and exercise tolerance, Rehabil Psychol 44:208, 1999.

46. Guell R, Resqueti V, Sangenis M et al: Impact of pulmonary rehabilitation on psychosocial morbidity in patients with severe COPD, Chest 129:899, 2006.

47. Borson S, McDonald GJ, Gayle T et al: Improvement in mood, physical symptoms, and function with nortriptyline for depression in patients with chronic obstructive pulmonary disease, Psychosomatics 33:190, 1992.

48. Gordon GH, Michiels TM, Mahutte CK et al: Effect of desipramine on control of ventilation and depression scores in patients with severe chronic obstructive pulmonary disease, Psychiatry Res 15:25, 1985.

49. Grant I, Prigatano GP, Heaton RK et al: Progressive neuropsychologic impairment and hypoxemia, Arch Gen Psychiatry 44:999, 1987.

50. Incalzi RA, Gemma A, Marra C et al: Verbal memory impairment in COPD: its mechanisms and clinical relevance, Chest 112:1506, 1997.

51. Stuss DT, Peterkin I, Guzman DA et al: Chronic obstructive pulmonary disease: effects of hypoxia on neurological and neuropsychological measures, J Clin Exp Neuropsychol 19:515, 1997.

52. Vos PJE, Folgering HTM, van Herwaarden CLA: Visual attention in patients with chronic obstructive pulmonary disease, Biol Psychol 41:295, 1995.

53. Crews WD, Jefferson AL, Bolduc T et al: Neuropsychological dysfunction in patients suffering from end-stage chronic obstructive pulmonary disease, Arch Clin Neuropsychol 16:643, 2001.

54. Isoaho R, Puolijoki H, Huhti E et al: Chronic obstructive pulmonary disease and cognitive impairment in the elderly, Int Psychogeriatr 8:113, 1996.

55. Grant I, Heaton RK, McSweeny AJ et al: Neuropsychologic findings in hypoxemic chronic obstructive pulmonary disease, Arch Intern Med 142:1470, 1982.

56. Rourke SB, Adams KM: The neuropsychological correlates of acute and chronic hypoxemia. In Grant I, Adams KM, editors: Neuropsychological assessment of neuropsychiatric disorders, ed 2, New York, 1996, Oxford, pp 379-402.

57. Wechsler D: Wechsler Adult Intelligence Scale - third edition: administration and scoring manual, New York, 1997, The Psychological Corporation.

58. Reitan RM: Validity of the trail making test as an indicator of organic brain damage, Percept Mot Skills 8:271, 1958.

59. Stroop JR: Studies of interference in serial verbal reactions, J Exp Psychol 18:643, 1935.

60. Heaton RK, Chelune GJ, Talley JL et al: Wisconsin Card Sorting Test manual: revised and expanded, Odessa, Fla, 1993, Psychological Assessment Resources.

61. Buschke H, Fuld PA: Evaluating storage, retention, and retrieval in disordered memory and learning, Neurology 11:1019, 1974.

62. Wechsler D: WMS-III administration and scoring manual, San Antonio, Tex, 1997, The Psychological Corporation.

63. Krop H, Block AJ, Cohen E: Neuropsychologic effects of continuous oxygen therapy in chronic obstructive pulmonary disease, Chest 64:317, 1973.

64. Heaton RK, Grant I, McSweeny AJ et al: Psychologic effects of continuous and nocturnal oxygen therapy

in hypoxemic chronic obstructive pulmonary disease, Arch Intern Med 143:1941, 1983.

65. Hjalmarsen A, Waterloo K, Dahl A et al: Effect of long-term oxygen therapy on cognitive and neurological dysfunction in chronic obstructive pulmonary disease, Eur Neurol 42:27, 1999.

66. Dustman RE, Emmerson RY, Ruhling RO et al: Age and fitness effects on EEG, ERPs, visual sensitivity, and cognition, Neurobiol Aging 11:193, 1990.

67. Kozora E, Tran ZV, Make B: Neurobehavioral improvement after brief rehabilitation in patients with chronic obstructive pulmonary disease, J Cardiopulm Rehabil 22:426, 2002.

68. Kozora E, Emery CF, Ellison MC et al: Improved neurobehavioral functioning in emphysema patients following lung volume reduction surgery compared with medical therapy, Chest 128:2653, 2005.

69. Crockett AJ, Cranston JM, Moss JR et al: The impact of anxiety, depression, and living alone in chronic obstructive pulmonary disease, Qual Life Res 11:309, 2002.

70. Clough P, Harnisch L, Cebulski P et al: Method for individualizing patient care for obstructive pulmonary disease patients, Health Soc Work 12:127, 1987.

71. Rabinowitz B, Florian V: Chronic obstructive pulmonary disease: psycho-social issues and treatment goals, Soc Work Health Care 16:69, 1992.

72. Keele-Card G, Foxall MJ, Barron CR: Loneliness, depression, and social support of patients with COPD and their spouses, Public Health Nurs 10:245, 1993.

73. Isoaho R, Keistinen T, Laippala P et al: Chronic obstructive pulmonary disease and symptoms related to depression in elderly persons, Psychol Rep 76:287, 1995.

74. Ashmore JA, Emery CF, Hauck ER et al: Marital adjustment among patients with chronic obstructive pulmonary disease who are participating in pulmonary rehabilitation, Heart Lung 34:270, 2005.

75. Cohen S, Wills TA: Stress, social support, and the buffering hypothesis, Psychol Bull 98:310, 1985.

76. Bergner M, Bobbitt RA, Carter WB et al: The Sickness Impact Profile: development and final revision of a health status questionnaire, Med Care 19:787, 1981.

77. Ware JE, Sherbourne CD: The MOS 36-Item Short-Form Health Survey (SF-36). I. Conceptual framework and item selection, Med Care 30:473, 1992.

78. Cohen S, Mermelstein RL, Kamarck T et al: Measuring the functional components of social support. In Sarason IG, Sarason B, editors: Social support: theory, research, and applications, Dordrecht, The Netherlands, 1985, Martinus Nijhoff.

79. Zimet GD, Dahlem NW, Zimet SG et al: The Multidimensional Scale of Perceived Social Support, J Pers Assess 52:30, 1988.

80. Barstow RE: Coping with emphysema, Nurs Clin North Am 9:137, 1974.

81. Leidy NK, Traver GA: Psychophysiologic factors contributing to functional performance in people with COPD: are there gender differences? Res Nurs Health 18:535, 1995.

82. Arnold R, Ranchor AV, DeJongste MJL et al: The relationship between self-efficacy and self-reported physical functioning in chronic obstructive pulmonary disease and chronic heart failure, Behav Med 31:107, 2006.

83. Weaver TE, Narsavage GL: Physiological and psychological variables related to functional status in chronic obstructive pulmonary disease, Nurs Res 41:286, 1992.

84. Katz PP, Eisner MD, Yelin EH et al: Functioning and psychological status among individuals with COPD, Qual Life Res 14:1835, 2005.

85. De Bruin AF, Diederiks JPM, De Witte LP et al: The development of a short generic version of the Sickness Impact Profile, J Clin Epidemiol 47:407, 1994.

86. Jones PW, Quirk FH, Baveystock CM: The St. George's Respiratory Questionnaire, Respir Med 85:25, 1991.

87. Guyatt GH, Berman LB, Townsend M et al: A measure of quality of life for clinical trials in chronic lung disease, Thorax 42:773, 1987.

88. Schünemann HJ, Goldstein R, Mador MJ et al: A randomised trial to evaluate the self-administered standardised chronic respiratory questionnaire, Eur Respir J 25:31, 2005.

89. Bendstrup KE, Jensen JI, Holm S et al: Out-patient rehabilitation improves activities of daily living, quality of life and exercise tolerance in chronic obstructive pulmonary disease, Eur Respir J 10:2001, 1997.

90. Hall SM, Munoz RF, Reus VI et al: Nicotine, negative affect, and depression, J Consult Clin Psychol 61:761, 1993.

91. Daughton DM, Fix AJ, Kass I et al: Smoking cessation among patients with chronic obstructive pulmonary disease (COPD), Addict Behav 5:125, 1980.

92. Glynn TJ: Methods of smoking cessation: finally, some answers, JAMA 263:2795, 1990.

93. Haaga DA, Allison ML: Thought suppression and smoking relapse: a secondary analysis of Haaga (1989), Br J Clin Psychol 33:327, 1994.

94. Lancaster T, Stead L, Silagy C et al: Effectiveness of interventions to help people stop smoking: findings from the Cochrane Library, BMJ 321:355, 2000.

95. Ockene JK, Kristeller J, Goldberg R et al: Increasing the efficacy of physician-delivered smoking interventions: a randomized clinical trial J Gen Intern Med 6:1, 1991.

96. Fiore MC, Baker LJ, Deeren SM: Cigarette smoking: the leading preventable cause of pulmonary diseases. In Bone RC, Pulmonary and critical care medicine, vol 1, St. Louis, 1993, Mosby-Year Book.

97. Glover ED, Glover PN, Abrons HL et al: Smoking cessation among COPD and chronic bronchitis patients using the nicotine nasal spray, Am J Health Behav 21:310, 1997.

98. Kottke T, Battista RN, DeFriese GH et al: Attributes of successful smoking cessation interventions in medical practice: a meta-analysis of 39 controlled trials, JAMA 259:2883, 1988.

99. Stead LF, Lancaster T: Group behaviour therapy programmes for smoking cessation. In Cochrane Collaboration, Cochrane Library, 3, Oxford, 2000, Update Software.

100. Lancaster T, Stead LF: Individual behavioral counselling for smoking cessation. In Cochane Collaborations, Cochrane Library, 3, Oxford, 2000, Update Software.

101. Rollnick S, Miller WR: What is motivational interviewing? Behav Cogn Psychother 23:325, 1995.

102. Miller WR: Motivational interviewing with problem drinkers, Behav Psychother 11:147, 1983.

103. Herman KC, Fahnlander B: A motivational intervention to reduce cigarette smoking among college students: overview and exploratory investigation, J Coll Counsel 6:46, 2003.

104. Colby SM, Monti PM, Barnett NP et al: Brief motivational interviewing in a hospital setting for adolescent smoking: a preliminary study, J Consult Clin Psychol 65:531, 1998.

105. Mallin R: Smoking cessation: integration of behavioral and drug therapies, Am Fam Physician 65:1107, 2002.

106. Jorenby DE, Fiore MC: The Agency for Health Care Policy and Research smoking cessation clinical practice guidelines: basics and beyond, Prim Care 26:513, 1999.

107. Jorenby DE, Leischow SJ, Nides MA et al: A controlled trial of sustained-release bupropion, a nicotine patch, or both for smoking cessation, N Engl J Med 340:685, 1999.

108. McWhirter JP, Pennington CR: Incidence and recognition of malnutrition in hospital, BMJ 308:945, 1994.

109. Congleton J: The pulmonary cachexia syndrome: aspects of energy balance, Proc Nutr Soc 58:321, 1999.

110. Efthimiou J, Fleming J, Gomes C et al: The effect of supplementary oral nutrition in poorly nourished patients with chronic obstructive pulmonary disease, Am Rev Respir Dis 137:1075, 1988.

111. Cochrane WJ, Afolabi OA: Investigation into the nutritional status, dietary intake and smoking habits of patients with chronic obstructive pulmonary disease, J Hum Nutr Diet 17:3, 2004.

112. Lewis MI, Belman MJ, Dorr-Uyemura L: Nutritional supplementation in ambulatory patients with COPD, Am Rev Respir Dis 135:1062, 1987.

113. Knowles JB, Fairbarn MS, Wiggs BJ et al: Dietary supplementation and respiratory muscle performance in patients with COPD, Chest 93:977, 1988.

114. Emery CF, Shermer RL, Hauck ER et al: Cognitive and psychological outcomes of exercise in a 1-year follow-up study of patients with chronic obstructive pulmonary disease, Health Psychol 22:598, 2003.

115. Sassi-Dambron DE, Eakin EG, Ries AL et al: Treatment of dyspnea in COPD: a controlled clinical trial of dyspnea management strategies, Chest 107:724, 1995.

116. Dolce JJ, Crisp C, Manzella B et al: Medication adherence patterns in chronic obstructive pulmonary disease, Chest 99:837, 1991.

117. James PNE, Anderson JB, Prior JG et al: Patterns of drug taking in patients with chronic airflow obstruction, Postgrad Med J 61:7, 1985.

118. George J, Kong DCM, Thoman R et al: Factors associated with medication nonadherence in patients with COPD, Chest 128:3198, 2005.

119. Schmaling KB, Afari N, Blume AW: Assessment of psychological factors associated with adherence to medication regimens among adult patients with asthma, J Asthma 37:335, 2000.

120. Vermeire E, Hearnshaw H, Van Royen P et al: Patient adherence to treatment: three decades of research: a comprehensive review, J Clin Pharm Ther 26:331, 2001.

121. Epstein LH, Cluss PA: A behavioral medicine perspective on adherence to long-term medical regimens, J Consult Clin Psychol 50:950, 1982.

122. Earnest MA: Explaining adherence to supplemental oxygen therapy: the patient's perspective, J Gen Intern Med 17:749, 2002.

123. Young P, Dewse M, Fergusson W et al: Respiratory rehabilitation in chronic obstructive pulmonary disease: predictors of nonadherence, Eur Respir J 13:855, 1999.

124. National Collaborating Centre for Chronic Conditions: Chronic obstructive pulmonary disease: national clinical guideline on management of chronic obstructive pulmonary disease in adults in primary and secondary care, Thorax 59(Suppl 1):1, 2004.

125. Norweg AM, Whiteson J, Malgady R et al: The effectiveness of different combinations of pulmonary rehabilitation program components: a randomized controlled trial, Chest 128:663, 2005.

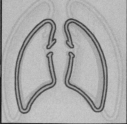

Chapter 18

Sexuality in the Patient with Pulmonary Disease

PAUL A. SELECKY

CHAPTER OUTLINE

Sex Versus Sexuality
Sexual Health Care
Sexuality Lasts a Lifetime
   Sexuality and the Aging Process
   Availability of a Sexual Partner
   Sexuality and Chronic Illness
What Can a Health Care Provider Do?
Sexual Counseling
   Permission Giving
   Limited Information

Specific Suggestions
Intensive Therapy
Sexuality and the Caregiver–Patient
   Relationship
Ethical Issues in Sexual Health Care
   Seductive Behavior
   Sexual Bias
   Sexual Abuse
   Sexual Interactions
Conclusion

PROFESSIONAL SKILLS

On completion of this chapter, the reader will be able to do
the following:
- Understand the integral role that sexuality plays in all human beings, both patients and caregivers
- Grasp the clinical responsibility of sexual health care
- Embrace the concept that sexuality lasts a lifetime
- Learn the role of a health care provider in sexual counseling
- Understand the potential positive and negative ways that sexuality can impact the caregiver–patient relationship

The primary basis for pulmonary rehabilitation is to help the patient understand and cope with his or her lung disease and to attempt to help the patient "…reduce symptoms, optimize functional status, increase participation…."[1] We therefore are interacting with the patient as a person, which includes his or her sexuality. Our patients are men and women of various ages who have differing sexual roles as husbands or wives or partners or single adults or youths who are involved in relationships in various ways. Caregivers also are sexual beings.

Our sexuality affects interpersonal relationships, including the interactions with our patients.

It is evident, therefore, that because sexuality is a far-reaching subject, addressing sexuality clearly comes within the scope of our responsibilities as members of a pulmonary rehabilitation team. It is our job to help our patients cope with the impact of the disease process on their lives in all its intricacies, including their lives as sexual beings. We should help them better understand this impact as a part of the rehabilitative process.

SEX VERSUS SEXUALITY

Jared Diamond, Pulitzer Prize–winning author and professor of physiology, in his book *Why Is Sex Fun? The Evolution of Human Sexuality*, wrote that "the subject of sex preoccupies us. It's the source of our most intense pleasure. Often it's also the cause of misery ... Understanding our sexuality is fascinating not only in its own right but also in order to understand our other distinctively human features."[2]

A discussion of sex within the context of a pulmonary rehabilitation program often begins with the focus on the physical aspects of sex, namely, sexual intercourse and other physical expressions of sexual functioning. This is understandably an area of great interest, but it is important that we paint a broader picture for ourselves and our patients. The word *sex* triggers many different images in each individual, depending on his or her experience and expectations as well as on the context in which the word is being used. *Sexuality* is a more complex term because it involves the total personality of an individual: how he or she thinks, how he or she acts and feels—in essence, who he or she is. It has been said that sex is something we do; sexuality is something we are.[3] Both are important and unique in each of us.

As described in Table 18-1, sex is a biologic term; sexuality addresses the total person. Our sex is our gender; it also establishes our role as male or female with a varying combination of masculine and feminine traits. Our sexuality colors our emotions, our understanding of ourselves, and our interactions with others. Together, sex and sexuality encompass the whole individual. Men and women respond differently to many situations in life because they are men or women. It is our responsibility as health care workers to better understand those differences if we are to be useful to our patients.

TABLE 18-1	Sex Versus Sexuality	
Sex as Biology	**Sexuality as Total Person**
Facts	Attitudes
Male/female	Maleness/femaleness
Genitality	Personality
Physical pleasure	Intimacy
Doing	Being
Self-oriented	Relational

BOX 18-1 | **World Health Organization Definitions of Sexuality**[4]

SEXUALITY

Sexuality is a central aspect of being human throughout life and encompasses sex, gender identities and roles, sexual orientation, eroticism, pleasure, intimacy, and reproduction. Sexuality is experienced and expressed in thoughts, fantasies, desires, beliefs, attitudes, values, behavior, practices, roles, and relationships. Although sexuality can include all of these dimensions, not all of them are always experienced or expressed. Sexuality is influenced by the interaction of biologic, psychological, social, economic, political, cultural, ethical, legal, historical, religious, and spiritual factors.

SEXUAL RIGHTS

Sexual rights embraces human rights that are already recognized in national laws, international human rights documents, and other consensus statements. They include the right of all persons, free of coercion, discrimination, and violence:

- To the highest attainable standard of sexual health, and to access to sexual health, and to access to sexual and reproductive health care services
- To seek, receive, and impart information related to sexuality
- To sexuality education
- To respect for bodily integrity
- To choose their partner
- To decide to be sexually active or not
- To consensual sexuality relations
- To consensual marriage
- To decide whether or not, and when, to have children
- To pursue a satisfying, safe, and pleasurable sexual life

SEXUAL HEALTH CARE

The World Health Organization defines sexual health in part as "a state of physical, emotional, mental, and social well-being in relation to sexuality."[4] It also defines sexuality and sexual rights in Box 18-1. Health care workers must attempt to achieve this objective through sexual health care, a concept that may seem a bit foreign to our roles as pulmonary rehabilitation team members. It requires us to focus on the impact of chronic lung disease and its attendant symptoms on the sexual health of the patient. It is not sufficient for us to inquire about physical sexual dysfunction alone, such as erectile dysfunction, decreased libido, painful intercourse, or ejaculatory problems. We must gain an understanding of the impact of chronic lung disease on the sexuality of our patient as a total person.

The delivery of sexual health care is a responsibility of the entire pulmonary rehabilitation team, which should integrate discussions of sexuality into the entire rehabilitative process. This is in contrast to assigning the team coordinator the responsibility to elicit responses to specific questions about sexual functioning and then to refer the patient as needed for specialty evaluation determined by any dysfunction that is uncovered. Schover and Jensen[5] describe this as a kind of "relay race" in which one health care worker "passes the baton" to the next. Instead, a more appropriate integrative approach should be applied that involves the entire rehabilitation team in a process that ideally includes the patient's sexual partner in the evaluation and treatment plan.

SEXUALITY LASTS A LIFETIME

The delivery of sexual health care is based on the thesis that sexuality lasts a lifetime, in contrast to the popular view expressed by the media that sexuality is relegated to the young. As Kaiser[6] has pointed out, "there is no age at which sexual activity, thoughts, or desire end." Sexual expression may change, but interest does not diminish. The significance of sexuality in later life is an extension of an individual's past life experiences, with the addition of (1) the normal expected aging process, (2) the availability of a sexual partner, and (3) one's general health. Alex Comfort, the noted gerontologist, and coauthor Lanyard Dial use a practical analogy, stating "most of our aged stop having sex for reasons similar to those why they stop riding a bicycle: general infirmity, fear that it would expose them to ridicule, and for most, lack of a bicycle."[7]

In simple analysis, a person who is sexually active during younger years is expected to become less active in later years, whereas the younger person who is sexually less active may likely become inactive. Comfort and Dial[7] point out that "as we age, the vast majority of us will notice little change in sexual function, except in the attitudes of other people. Sexuality will simply be transformed into a slightly different, probably quieter experience than it was in youth, but a no less sexual and no less worthwhile experience." Thienhaus[8] states that a reasonable attitude for caregivers to assume concerning sexual activity in later life is that "some do, some don't, and there's nothing wrong with either."

The patient with lung disease fits well into this concept of a lifetime of sexuality. He or she most often is an older individual who is facing the impact of aging on sexuality and sexual functioning, may be lacking a sexual partner, and is trying to cope with progressive breathing problems. It is important that the rehabilitation team be knowledgeable of these factors if it is to minister to the patient's concerns about sexuality.

Sexuality and the Aging Process

Aging is an ongoing process that affects all individuals and all bodily functions. Sexual health is not immune. Comfort and Dial[7] have pointed out, however, that "compared with the age changes in…the eyes' focusing ability or the lungs' vital capacity, sexual-organ changes are minimal." Nonetheless, despite the process of natural aging that one expects, changes in sexual functioning somehow seem to catch patients by surprise. This is more apparent in the aging male, largely because of the noticeable changes in his ability to achieve and maintain an erection. As a result, more studies and writings focus on the changes in the human sexual response during intercourse, as defined in the past by Masters and Johnson.[9] Details regarding both sexes are listed in Box 18-2. For the male, orgasm and sexual intercourse are of shorter duration, have fewer secretions, and the force and volume of ejaculation is less.[10,11] Andropause is multifactorial, and emcompasses sexual dysfunction, hypogonadism, and psychological changes.[11,12] A decrease in testosterone occurs although the aging male quickly forgets or ignores the fact that the peak of testosterone occurs around age 20 years, with a steady decline thereafter.[13] Conversely, testosterone replacement therapy for normal elderly men will not restore libido to the level of younger men, and according to the

BOX 18-2	Impact of Aging on Sexual Response

FEMALE
- Decrease in vaginal length and width
- Less vaginal elasticity
- Longer to achieve vaginal lubrication
- Less vaginal lubrication
- Decrease in frequency of orgasms

MALE
- Longer to achieve erection
- Less firm erection
- Longer to ejaculate
- Lower ejaculate volume
- Longer recovery time

American Urological Association in its 2005 guidelines, it will not aid the problem of impotence.[14]

The aging female continues to have the ability to have satisfying sexual relations despite a reduction in physiologic response, as described in Box 18-2. In fact, surprisingly little change occurs in sexual activity across the average woman's life span, except for the impact of social factors and general health.[15] Menopause, which occurs in most women at about age 50 years, is associated with substantial reductions in hormonal levels, leading to a variety of physical changes in genital anatomy and functioning, which can lead to dyspareunia, the most common sexual complaint among older women seeking gynecologic consultation.[13] This is less pronounced in women who continue to be sexually active, giving a biologic credence to the adage "use it or lose it."[16] The dyspareunia is often linked to delayed and/or reduced vaginal lubrication, which can be aided by topical lubricants or local or systemic estrogen replacement therapy. The latter remains a controversial subject since the 2002 report of the Women's Health Initiative Study that revealed increased health risks from use of combined estrogen plus progestin.[17]

Hysterectomy does not impair sexual function, although it can have a negative psychological effect on some women, who feel it has removed an essential part of their femininity.[18] Mastectomy can have even a greater impact on a woman's sense of her sexual attractiveness. Counseling by her physician and others can help the patient resolve these issues.

The expected physical changes associated with aging in both genders do not necessarily indicate that sexual desire and/or activity have ground to a halt, despite the myth and public perception that sexual functioning belongs to the younger set. Numerous studies have dispelled the myth of a declining sexual interest with advancing age.[6]

The 2004 results of a periodic survey of sexuality by the American Association of Retired Persons reveal that sexuality remains an essential element of the lives of U.S. adults ages 45 years and older. The details of the study can be found on their Web site at www.aarp.org. Data from the National Survey of Families and Households revealed that 53% of married persons 60 years and older, and 24% of those 76 years and older, have reported having sexual intercourse four times within the last month.[19] The study further found that these practices often were tied to the individual's sense of self-worth and competence and to his or her partner's health status. A study of sexual interest and behavior in healthy 80- to 102-year-olds revealed that the frequency of masturbation and sexual intercourse did not change greatly after age 80 years.[20] Both sexes who remain sexually active are likely to be more physically fit and to feel younger and are more likely to achieve sexual satisfaction.[21] Sexual dysfunction is more likely to be related to comorbid illnesses and/or psychosocial factors rather than aging alone.[22-25]

Ebersole and Hess[26] state that sexuality "is an affirmation that one's body functions well, maintains a strong sense of self-identity, and provides a means for self-assertion." It is a veritable measure of the quality of life.[7]

A survey of 27,500 men and women aged 40 to 80 years in 29 countries concluded that "sexual well-being was correlated with overall happiness in both men and women."[27] Sheryl Kingsberg,[28] in her article on the impact of aging on sexual function in women, writes that "regardless of the length or nature of the relationship, its quality is enhanced by emotional intimacy, autonomy without too much distance, an ability to manage stress, and to maintain a positive perception of self and the relationship." Moreover, a study in the *British Medical Journal* revealed that mortality risk was 50% lower in men who had a high frequency of sexual intercourse and orgasm.[29] An accompanying editorial compared this with the findings that suggest that alcohol might make one live longer. It stated "what we thought was bad for you may actually be good for you, but it may not be good to tell you in case you do it too much, and it is certainly not good to tell you it is good for you if you do too much of it already—assuming we could agree what was too much in the first place."[30] The study suggested tongue-in-cheek that public health intervention programs be considered, comparing them with the efforts at improving health by encouraging fruit and vegetable consumption with the phrase "at least 5 a day."

Andrew Greeley,[31] renowned sociologist and author who studied the sexual practices of aging Catholics, concluded that "one suspects that the older lovers for whom passion and play have not stopped after a long life together of cherishing one another will have the last laugh. They are entitled to that laugh and they can afford to have it."

Availability of a Sexual Partner

One of the greatest barriers to sexual activity in later life is the lack of a healthy sexual partner. It has long been known that women's life expectancy is much greater than men's, causing most married women to face a long period of widowhood. Data from the 1997 report of the Bureau of the Census reveal that there are eight women for every five men 75 years of age and older.[32] It is estimated that after age 80 years, there are about four women for every man.[33] Despite their diminishing numbers, approximately two-thirds of men 75 years and older are married. Two-thirds of women in the same age group are widowed. As a result, simple arithmetic indicates that older unmarried men have a greater likelihood of finding a female partner.

On the other hand, fate has dealt a cruel blow to many older women. Although they live longer, they are more likely to spend their later years alone because of the loss of their spouse. Some women may be open to choosing a second partner, but often this is thwarted by the progressively diminishing number of available male partners their age, particularly those men who remain healthy and active. They could seek the company of younger men, but their families and society in general seem to frown on such unions, whereas an older man is often applauded for being able to successfully win the heart of a younger woman.

These statistics are confirmed by a household survey in Michigan of individuals 60 years of age and older. Approximately 74% of married men responded as being sexually active compared with 31% of unmarried men. In contrast, 56% of married women were sexually active, whereas only 5% of unmarried women gave the same response.[34] Interestingly, the daily consumption of coffee correlated with sexual activity in women and potency in men.

Both genders may have the additional obstacle of lacking adequate privacy, either because of their living situation, such as rooming in their adult children's home, or concern about "what the neighbors might say." Health care institutions and staff may be another source of problems. For example, nursing home personnel generally frown on, if not prohibit, conjugal visits between residents, even though Medicaid-supported institutions are required to allow requesting married couples to be housed together.[26] Understandable concern exists that elderly residents not be abused by other residents, but a more liberal attitude would allow greater freedom of sexual interaction between consenting residents. Richardson and Lazur[35] describe several interventions that could lower the barriers.

Sexuality and Chronic Illness

Sexual functioning can be affected by chronic illness in a variety of ways.[36-38] Sometimes the effect is related to the specific disease, for example, impotence in diabetes, angina in coronary occlusive disease, or sometimes general frailty. Dyspnea is the major symptom of the patient with lung disease, but studies reveal that this does not seem to be a major obstacle to successful sexual intercourse, except perhaps for those with moderate to severe dyspnea.[39-41] Erectile dysfunction can occur, and is closely linked to the severity of the underlying lung disease.[42]

The impact of lung disease on sexual functioning is not to be measured by pulmonary function tests; rather, it is found in an understanding of the psychosocial impact of disease on the patient, as depicted in Box 18-3 (see also Chapter 17). Regardless of these factors, some patients have good coping skills and stand out as model patients because they are able to maintain an active lifestyle despite their chronic illness. This ability generally flows into their sexual functioning. A study of 49 male patients with chronic respiratory failure revealed sexual problems in 67%, but the importance of the problem was dependent on the degree of affection in the couple.[43]

Wise[44] organizes the obstacles to sexual functioning into three categories. The patient with lung disease must struggle with impersonal factors, such as limited exercise tolerance, chronic cough, sputum production, and the potential side effects of medications. He or she also often struggles with intrapersonal obstacles such as decreased self-esteem and an altered view of his

BOX 18-3	Psychosocial Composite of the Patient with Chronic Lung Disease

- Social, family, and sexual roles altered
- Limited activities of daily living
- Limited recreation
- Preoccupied with body functions
- Increased anxiety
- Decreased self-esteem
- Depressed
- Overdependent

or her masculine or feminine role with the accompanying anxiety. These then lead to interpersonal obstacles with a spouse or intimate other, including the fear of sexual failure and ultimately a suppression of sexual desire. It is important to realize, however, that this is not a universal finding linked only to chronic illness. Many healthy couples also complain of sexual problems. A survey of 987 women 20 to 65 years old revealed that 24% expressed distress about their sexual relationship and/or their own sexuality.[45] The best predictors of distress were markers of general emotional well-being and the emotional relationship with the partner during sexual activity. Physical aspects of sexual response were poor predictors of distress. Therefore, most patients continue to live full and satisfying sexual lives.

WHAT CAN A HEALTH CARE PROVIDER DO?

Our primary role as health care professionals is to attend to our patient's needs. In the field of sexual health care, this must begin with a self-examination of our knowledge and attitudes about sexuality. Any deficits in sexual information can be corrected by further study of a variety of published resources, but the facts we know are not nearly as important to our patients as are our attitudes concerning sex and sexuality. Ideally, we want our attitude to be "sex positive" and accepting of others' points of view and lifestyles, and we want to avoid making value judgments. Our lack of sexual knowledge can be an obstacle in communicating with our patients, but this obstacle is worsened by their perceiving negative nonverbal messages or hearing negative attitudes expressed concerning their sexual interests and behavior. Our patients plead for our help as health care providers,[33] as is revealed in the list of suggestions in Box 18-4 from a survey on this issue of almost 1500 persons 50 years of age and older.[46]

Before introducing the subject of sexuality in a rehabilitation program, it is important that the rehabilitation team conduct an introspective evaluation of their own sexual attitudes. This can be accomplished by conducting discussions of sexuality at team conferences. Team members might respond to probing questions such as "What are your attitudes about sexual activity in the elderly, masturbation, homosexuality, oral sex, and a wide variety of sexual subjects and practices?" and

BOX 18-4	**Older Adults' Suggestions for Health Care Providers Regarding Discussion About Sex**

- Spend time with older adults.
- Use clear and easy-to-understand words.
- Help older adults feel comfortable talking about sex.
- Be open-minded and talk openly.
- Listen closely.
- Treat older adults with a respectful and nonjudgmental attitude.
- Encourage discussion.
- Give advice or suggestions.
- Understand that sex is not just for the young.

"How comfortable are you talking about sex?"[47] Oregon State University[48] has developed a 30-minute board game to help caregivers examine their attitudes about aging and sexuality.

Ideally, training in the diagnosis and treatment of sexual dysfunctions should be sought. Schover and Jensen[49] describe a model for a 1-day training session. At the very least, we need to be good listeners. We must respond to our patients' needs and concerns and not shut them out or turn them away.

SEXUAL COUNSELING

Many health care workers feel unprepared to become involved in sexual counseling and feel more comfortable with discussion of almost every other subject in the field of pulmonary rehabilitation. Regardless of our hesitancy in discussing sexuality with our patients, we may have no choice other than to become involved when our patients ask questions. It is a subject for which the entire team should be prepared. The team should not relegate the responsibilities to just one member, such as the coordinator. Although the responsibility is often placed on the coordinator, the patient may feel more comfortable discussing questions concerning sexuality with some other members of the team. It is likely to be someone who appears to the patient to be most comfortable with the subject, someone who is approachable, or someone who appears able to discuss such intimate subjects in a relaxed and nonjudgmental manner. The coordinator may be the one to introduce the subject, but all members of the team should be open to continuing that discussion in their interactions with the patient.[50]

BOX 18-5	PLISSIT Model for Sexual Counseling

- P = Permission giving
- LI = Limited information
- SS = Specific suggestions
- IT = Intensive therapy

BOX 18-6	Giving Permission to Be Sexual

- Introduce the subjects of sex and sexuality.
- Communicate acceptance by your words and behavior.
- Use open-ended questions in the intake interview.
- Use terms comfortable to you and the patient.
- Be "sex positive."
- Be a good listener.
- Encourage and support the patient.
- Do not stereotype the patient's behavior.
- Provide educational materials.
- Consider using a structured survey tool.

Most questions can be addressed from the resource of our own life experiences without the need for specialized training. Francoeur[51] offers three cautions in this regard: (1) the health care worker should be aware of his or her limitations; (2) the health care worker should be sensitive to his or her position within the health care team so as not to interfere with the role of others, such as the primary care physician and (3) the health care worker should avoid making a detailed recommendation to a patient that may go beyond the team's limitations.

A model for sexual counseling that many have found useful has been described by Annon[52] as the PLISSIT model, a four-step process progressing from simple to complex counseling (P = permission-giving; LI = limited information; SS = specific suggestions; IT = intensive therapy). The caregiver proceeds through the four steps guided by the patient's needs and his or her own professional judgment and personal comfort. The steps are described in Box 18-5.

Permission Giving

The steps of this first level of counseling are listed in Box 18-6. They begin by merely introducing the subject to the pulmonary rehabilitation patient, and in doing so "give permission" to the patient to discuss his or her sexual concerns. It delivers a message from your team that says "It is OK to talk about sex here." This can be done by asking a few open-ended questions on the intake questionnaire and allowing time for the patient to elaborate on the responses during the intake interview. It is best to avoid questions that require a "yes" or "no" answer and instead to use probing and/or permission-giving questions, such as:

1. How has your breathing problem affected your view of yourself as a man or woman?
2. How does your breathing affect your sexual desire and activity?
3. You mentioned you were limited by your shortness of breath. How has it affected your sexual desire and functioning?
4. What do you find are the most troubling changes in your sexuality?
5. Many people have sexual concerns. What concerns you about your sexual functioning? What concerns your partner?

Ebersole and Hess[26] provide more detailed questions in their text *Toward Healthy Aging* that can be asked if the patient expresses greater interest.

It is important that the interviewer ask questions in a relaxed and comfortable manner, and then wait for the patient to respond. We must be cautious of our body language, which may be telling the patient that we really do not want to hear about his or her sexual problems because they embarrass us. The look on our faces is more important than the words we use. Structured survey tools are available to conduct a more formal inquiry.[53-55]

Ideally, such an interview should be conducted in privacy to maintain patient confidentiality. The interviewer should allow sufficient time for discussion, pointing out to the patient that additional opportunities will be available for addressing his or her concerns during the rehabilitation program. The patient's sexual partner should be involved in these discussions at some point, although initially it may be more comfortable for the patient to address the subject alone with the interviewer.

Schover and Jensen[56] point out that couple therapy is more productive than addressing the patient alone. The interviewer often is able to assess the potential benefit of involving the patient's sexual partner in the discussion by assessing the role that the partner is already playing in the patient's illness. These authors point out that "general coping skills and sexual function are linked in the chronically ill" and advise the clinician that the best way to treat any sexual concerns is by fostering the strengths of the couple's relationship. They identify a strong relationship as one in which the couple has developed four important skills: (1) they are comfortable and flexible in allocating their individual roles; (2) they respect each other's boundaries and allow these boundaries to change over time; (3) they have achieved good communication; and (4) they have reached agreement on the rules of their relationship that govern its daily functioning. The same four skills apply to their sexual relationship as well.

The first step of permission giving may generate no response from the patient. It should be remembered that "some do, some don't, and there is nothing wrong with either."[8] Nonetheless, sexual concerns are common. Giving permission to discuss them is likely to bring results. A study in a general practice of adults of all ages, both sexes, different marital statuses, and different education levels revealed that more than 50% reported sexual problems or concerns, for example, frequency of intercourse, lack of sexual desire, marital or relationship problems, painful intercourse, and difficulties achieving an erection.[57] We should be prepared to address these concerns.

The solution to many patients' sexual concerns lies in education. Various institutions have produced printed materials that can be offered to patients or placed in the packet of education materials that they receive as part of the rehabilitation program.[58-61] Information for patients is also available on the Internet, for example, on the Web site of the National Institute on Aging at www.nih.gov/nia; other Internet resources are listed in Box 18-7. [62] Such educational efforts introduce the subject of sexuality but are of only limited usefulness unless the patient is given an opportunity to discuss individual concerns. Some programs introduce the topic of sexuality for discussion in patient support groups; this requires the presence of an experienced facilitator to make the discussion productive.

Limited Information

Introducing the topic of sexuality may open the door to further discussion. If such is the case, the clinician should be prepared to offer at least limited information of a general nature, such as listed in Box 18-8. The first step is to broaden the patient's focus from genital functioning to the impact of sexuality on their total being, explaining that sexuality also includes how a person thinks and feels, not just what he or she does. This is

---

BOX 18-7	**Internet Resources for Patient Education on Sexuality**

- National Institute on Aging: Sexuality in later life: www.niapublications.org/agepages/sexuality.asp
- American Heart Association: www.americanheart.org/presenter.jhtml?identifier=1200000
- American Cancer Society: www.cancer.org/docroot/home/index.asp
- National Library of Medicine: Medline Plus: www.nlm.nih.gov/medlineplus/medlineplus.html
- National Jewish Center: www.nationaljewish.org/
- Mayo Clinic: Sexual Health: www.mayoclinic.com/health/sexual-health/HA00035
- Cystic Fibrosis Worldwide: www.cfww.org
- National Center on Elder Abuse: http://www.ncea.aoa.gov

Box 18-8	**Provide Limited Information**

- Sexuality involves the total person
- Aging has predictable effects on sexual function
- Fears and myths about sex are to be dispelled
- Physiologic stress of lovemaking is limited
- Some medication can impair or aid sexual function
- Sexual dysfunction can be treated
- Discuss sexual concerns with your partner
- Address and resolve impact of any comorbid conditions

---

particularly important for the patient with lung disease who has often developed a negative self-image and who chooses to focus on his or her own frailties and limitations. This negative attitude often springs from society's image of the sexually active person as being young and attractive. Many patients unfortunately succumb to these myths, feeling that they are too old, too unattractive, or too sickly to have sexual feelings, let alone to consider being sexually active.

It is important that patients understand the impact of normal aging on sexual functioning, as described in Box 18-2. Although this knowledge does not resolve patients' concerns entirely, it often alleviates their fear that they are not normal. Patient education materials are available on this subject as well in Box 18-7.

Although there are no true aphrodisiacs, some medications can improve sexual desire and/or functioning by having a beneficial effect on an underlying medical disorder. Certain drugs used

TABLE 18-2	Some Medications That Can Affect Sexual Functioning
Erectile Dysfunction	**Decreased Libido**
Diuretics	Antihypertensive drugs
Antihypertensive drugs	Antihistamines
Anticholinergic drugs	Psychiatric drugs
Antihistamines	Sedatives
Antidepressants	Alcohol
Anorectic drugs	Anxiolytics
Alcohol	
Anxiolytics	

BOX 18-9	Specific Suggestions for Lovemaking

- Be physically and emotionally rested
- Ensure your privacy
- Start and progress slowly
- Choose the "best breathing" time
- Avoid a "touchdown" mentality
- Concentrate on mutual touch
- Avoid after alcohol consumption and heavy meals
- Use O_2 and/or medications to your advantage
- Choose less stressful positions
- Be creative and romantic

O_2, Oxygen.

to treat Parkinson's disease, for example, have resulted in improved sexual functioning. Some antidepressants have improved libido in the absence of any antidepressant effect.[63]

More likely, medications can be the source or an aggravating factor for sexual dysfunction, particularly contributing to impotence in the male. Antihypertensive medications are commonly the culprit, but not all are known to cause this problem. Patients should be made aware of the potential for this side effect and advised to discuss it with their prescribing physician or a clinical pharmacist to see if an alternative medication can be substituted. Other medications may result in decreased libido in both sexes, as noted in Table 18-2.[64,65] Fortunately, few of the pulmonary medications suppress sexual functioning, and they in fact may enhance it by decreasing exertional dyspnea. On the other hand, decreased testosterone levels in men with chronic lung disease have been correlated with glucocorticoid therapy and with hypoxemia.[66]

Patients and their sexual partners may limit sexual activity because they fear that the physical exertion and associated increase in breathing may trigger an attack of coughing or dyspnea. They need to be reassured that although the breathing rate increases, the physical stress of sexual intercourse is limited and often lasts only a few minutes in most circumstances.[67,68] Individual styles of lovemaking, however, are varied.

A significant proportion of patients with chronic obstructive pulmonary disease have coexisting coronary heart disease, not surprising because of the link between cigarette smoking and those two diseases. These patients may fear that sexual activity will put them at cardiac risk. Cheitlin and coworkers[68] point out that sexual intercourse increases oxygen (O_2) consumption to only a modest extent (3 to 5 metabolic equivalents), and lasts only a brief period. The metabolic cost is equivalent to walking at 3 mph on level ground or walking up two flights of stairs. Moreover, the duration is only a few minutes. The absolute risk of myocardial infarction with sexual activity is therefore extremely low.[69]

Specific Suggestions

As we move through this model of progressive counseling in sexual health, patients may ask for specific suggestions to address their problems or concerns. These also may be presented in a general way as one of the lectures given to patients in the pulmonary rehabilitation program or to patient support groups or at general patient education forums, such as the Better Breathers Clubs of the American Lung Association. A list of suggestions that focus on ways to enhance sexual performances is found in Box 18-9. Many of these suggestions are based on common sense, but are worth reiterating for the patient and his or her sexual partner. Making these suggestions often reassures both partners and may encourage their discussing the subject further in private.

The rehabilitation team can advise patients to schedule lovemaking for the "best breathing" time. This usually is in the late morning or early afternoon after their daily morning bronchial hygiene has been completed and before late afternoon fatigue has begun to set in. In addition, older men often are better able to achieve an erection in the morning.[26] Regardless of the time of day chosen, patients should be sure they have taken their bronchodilator treatments before the lovemaking, and to use O_2 therapy if prescribed by their physician. Advise patients to be creative and romantic in their sexual encounters, and urge them to avoid the "touchdown" mentality that often has been the driving force for many patients, that is, attempting to achieve orgasm or "score" on every sexual encounter. They need to be reminded of the sexual benefits of touch, for example, cuddling, caressing, and just spending some sexual time together.[26] They should be encouraged to explore a wide range of sexual behaviors "from smiling to orgasm."[70]

Specific variations on body position can be offered as an alternative to their usual habits of lovemaking.[61,71,72] For the male patient, the female-on-top position has been shown to have a lower metabolic expenditure.[67,68] Such a suggestion is less important if the change in position appears too unnatural to the couple. The male patient using the male-on-top position with someone other than his spouse expends the greatest amount of energy. For the male or female patient with coexisting symptomatic coronary occlusive disease, obtaining guidance from his or her physician on a safe level of physical activity would be an appropriate suggestion. Our role is simply to offer the suggestions in an attempt to give them permission to change their habits if they so desire and to point out the wide variety of ways in which couples conduct their lovemaking.

The team can remind patients to avoid lovemaking after a heavy meal or the use of alcohol because of the tendency to generate fatigue. Alcohol also can be a risk factor for male impotence, as Shakespeare pointed out in *Macbeth*, stating that "drink... provokes the desire, but it takes away the performance." Cigarette smoking also is a risk factor for male impotence because the vasoconstrictive effects of nicotine alter the complex vascular mechanism associated with erection of the penis. More often than not, physicians have convinced their male patients to stop smoking because of its impact on their lung disease.

Intensive Therapy

If our suggestions have not resolved the patient's concerns up to this point, or if we detect problems that need specialty care, appropriate referrals should be made. Care options are described in Box 18-10. Referral requires our having knowledge of appropriate resources that are available in the community. Types of sexual dysfunction are listed in Box 18-11.

Erectile dysfunction, that is, impotence, can be a problem for the aging male. Estimates indicate

---

BOX 18-10	Intensive Therapy for Sexual Problems

- Training in communication techniques
- Marriage counseling
- Urologic/gynecologic consultation
- Psychological counseling
- Psychiatric counseling
- Sex therapy

BOX 18-11	Sexual Dysfunctions

- Erectile dysfunction/impotence
- Premature ejaculation
- Dyspareunia
- Vaginismus
- Inhibited sexual desire
- Inhibited sexual arousal
- Inhibited orgasm

---

that as many as 55% of men report problems with impotence by age 75 years.[13] It is not an all-or-nothing symptom. Impotence is defined as "the inability to attain and/or maintain penile erection sufficient for satisfactory sexual performance."[73] Regardless of the expected increase in incidence with age, impotence in elderly men should not be accepted as a normal course of events. Many patients can be successfully treated.

An erection is the result of a complex physiologic process that can go awry in a variety of ways.[26] This emphasizes the importance of appropriate diagnosis and treatment, which usually begins with the primary care physician.[74] The patient can be referred for further evaluation as needed to such specialists as an endocrinologist, urologist, vascular surgeon, or perhaps sex therapist. The population being studied influences the results of studies that identify the various causes, but most indicate that most patients with impotence have an organic cause. Possible organic causes include medication effects, endocrine abnormalities, neurologic diseases, and vascular dysfunction. The effects of alcohol and nicotine have already been mentioned.

The complex nature of impotence requires the physician to perform a physical examination and compile a thorough history that includes a detailed discussion of the sexual dysfunction.[14] This often is supplemented by appropriate laboratory studies as needed. A variety of treatment modalities are available, guided by evaluation.

It includes such therapies as testosterone supplementation for the rare patient with hypogonadism, oral drug therapy, intracavernous injections of vasoactive medications, vacuum constriction devices, and penile prosthesis implantation.[14,75] Particular to our patients, a study of a small number of male patients with chronic obstructive pulmonary disease placed on long-term O_2 therapy to treat hypoxemia revealed an improvement in oxygenation followed by a reversal of sexual impotence in 42% after 1 month of O_2 use.[76] Regardless of the modality, sexual counseling is often an important part of each of these varied therapies.[77]

Oral medications for the treatment of erectile dysfunction did not show reliable results until the introduction of a phosphodiesterase-5 (PDE5) inhibitor, sildenafil, in the United States, which dramatically revolutionized the awareness and treatment of this sexual dysfunction.[78] Originally introduced as a vasodilator for the treatment of coronary artery disease, sildenafil quickly gained greater use for the treatment of impotence. The new drug became the topic of discussion in newspapers, magazines, and talk shows. Its popularity soared, with pharmaceutical sales increasing dramatically in just the first few months of use.

Subsequent clinical experience has revealed that sildenafil improves erections in 63% to 82%, depending on the dose.[79] Its pharmacologic effect is to increase blood flow to the penis in response to sexual stimulation, not causing penile erections directly, and it has been shown to be effective in many causes of erectile dysfunction, including diabetes.[80] Its principal side effects relate to the vasodilatation and include headache, flushing, and small decreases in blood pressure. Although generally well tolerated by healthy individuals, serious cardiovascular events can occur in patients who are concurrently taking organic nitrates because the drug can cause potentially life-threatening hypotension. Deaths that have been reported to the U.S. Food and Drug Administration were related to probable cardiac events in patients who already were at risk because of their underlying cardiovascular disease. As a result, it has been difficult to discern whether the drug or the associated increase in physical sexual activity played the major role in these incidents.

Three PDE5 inhibitors (sildenafil, tadalafil, and vardenafil) are now available. Sildenafil has a short half-life (4 hours), making it the drug of choice in patients with more severe cardiovascular disease. Vardenafil has a similar chemical structure to sildenafil, and thus a similar clinical profile. Tadalafil has a longer half-life (17.5 hours), and has a similar safety and efficacy profile to sildenafil.[81,82]

Many consider erectile dysfunction as a marker for vascular disease, urging a thorough evaluation for asymptomatic coronary artery disease.[81] In the patient with known cardiac disease, the Second Princeton Consensus Conference has published guidelines on the treatment of erectile dysfunction.[83] Patients with congestive heart failure are often treated with medications that can aggravate erectile dysfunction, and thus require special attention.[84]

The same caution applies to the use of sildenafil when used in postmenopausal women with sexual dysfunction.[85] The effect of the drug in this population in limited studies revealed that although overall sexual function did not improve significantly, vaginal lubrication and clitoral sensitivity changed. The role of this medication in this population thus remains to be determined. On the other hand, women's sexual function has been shown to improve when their partner's erectile dysfunction was treated with a PDE5 inhibitor.[86,87]

Attention is often paid to the treatment of erectile dysfunction in men, but women can have disorders of sexual desire and arousal that deserve attention. As many or 10% to 51% of women surveyed in various countries complain of too little sexual desire. This requires an overall evaluation of their sexual difficulties, as well as those of their partners, and includes an assessment of "her mental health, feelings, medical history, and her thoughts and emotions during sexual activity."[88] Recommendations for the evaluation and treatment of sexual disorders in women have been presented by various organizations, including the issues of the impact of menopause and the use of testosterone therapy in women.[89-91]

Review of Box 18-12 indicates that there are also many nonorganic causes of sexual problems

BOX 18-12	Nonorganic Causes of Sexual Problems

- Lack of a partner
- Monotonous sexual interactions
- Marital disharmony
- Unreasonable sexual expectations
- Fear of failure in sexual performance

that can occur at any age and that can be corrected or alleviated by ongoing counseling.[26] The patient and his or her sexual partner should focus on the problems they are having in their sexual interactions, but these problems may be a symptom of a more general problem with their relationship.[92]

Couples need to be reminded that their lovemaking at night is an extension of their daytime interactions. They may be suffering from monotony and boredom in their daily life together, which can flow over into their love life. Both partners need to be reminded that each needs to continue to work on their relationship on an ongoing basis and to continue to romance each other. Patients with lung disease are often so involved in the management of their illness that they neglect their personal relationships.[38] They may need to be reminded that they must work at being feminine or masculine and focus on expressing their sexuality in the way they dress, their general attitude, and how they interact with others. Most individuals enjoy being attractive and gaining the attention of others. We may need to remind patients how they pursued those goals in the past.

SEXUALITY AND THE CAREGIVER–PATIENT RELATIONSHIP

To a certain extent, our own sexuality has an effect on all the relationships we have with our patients. Sometimes this effect is brief and passing, such as when a caregiver administers a nebulizer treatment to a patient during a hospital stay. On the other hand, it can be ongoing over a period of time, such as in a pulmonary rehabilitation program or when delivering home care on a recurring basis to a patient. As discussed previously, we are sexual beings as males or females and thus cannot divorce sexuality from our interpersonal relationships. Male and female caregivers may act differently with male patients than with female patients. The difference in these interactions is not necessarily good or bad, but it is important that the caregiver be aware of how sexuality might have a negative impact on these relationships.

It is natural that a caregiver might be sexually attracted to a patient, more commonly male caregiver and female patient.[93] Many people in the world are beautiful in mind, body, and soul, and it is understandable that we might be sexually attracted to them. These feelings are neither right nor wrong; they simply exist. However, we must recognize our sexual feelings and deal with them if they interfere with the professional nature of our relationship.

We are told to be loving and caring individuals, and at the same time we are expected to be scientifically objective. This combination can be difficult. We must compromise each of these goals in some way. If we are to be successful caregivers, we must be loving and caring, but we must also be aware of our own sexual feelings, needs, and desires to guard against their interfering with our roles as loving and caring health care professionals.

The relationship with our patients is unique. Farber, Novack, and O'Brien[94] point out that it is based on a bond characterized by an agape or brotherly love that can be beneficial to the caregiver–patient relationship. It also has been described as a fiduciary relationship, that is, the patient has the trust and confidence that the caregiver will act in his or her best interest.[95] It is not unique to health care, as other professions (e.g., clergy, lawyers, teachers, and coaches), to have similar relationships.[93] By its very nature, this relationship is asymmetric, with the patient being in a dependent and vulnerable role. The patient entrusts us with many personal and sometimes intimate aspects of his or her life, and we are obliged to preserve the patient's dignity and privacy. This ranges from how we address the patient to how we physically touch the patient and maintain an ongoing relationship.

As professionals, we have developed a sensitivity of calling the patient by his or her proper name and to avoid using familiar and potentially insulting labels. We have also learned about respecting the patient's "personal space" and about assessing when and how it is appropriate to touch the patient, either in the process of physical examination or in social touching. Touch can be an important part of healing, but limits and boundaries to touching exist and may vary from patient to patient.[26] It may seem appropriate at times to hold the hand of a depressed patient to offer comfort and support. Other patients may consider this gesture an intrusion. Our actions are generally guided by our own common sense and by the awareness of our own personal level of comfort. Regardless, the asymmetric and fiduciary nature of the relationship must be kept in mind, particularly when we may sense sexual feelings rising to the surface, either in ourselves or in our patients.

ETHICAL ISSUES IN SEXUAL HEALTH CARE

Acknowledging the impact of sexuality on our professional relationships brings the realization that sexual feelings sensed or expressed by either the caregiver or the patient can disrupt and alter the goals of the professional relationship. This leads to a variety of concerns regarding medical ethics. The caregiver may inadvertently or sometimes consciously become involved in circumstances with a patient that might be termed "boundary violations," which implies that the professional nature of the relationship has been breached. Farber, Novack, and O'Brien[94] define boundaries in patient care as "mutually understood, unspoken, physical and emotional limits of the relationship between the trusting patient and the caring physician or provider." Violations, even just the giving of gifts, can disrupt the efforts to establish and maintain a trusting provider–patient relationship.[96]

The "violations" by either the caregiver or the patient may at times be seemingly innocent and perhaps trivial—such as an inappropriate word or action, or unwelcome familiarity—and simply be excused as a brief intrusion into the privacy of either the caregiver or the patient. On the other hand, the slippery slope of this behavior can lead to more significant violations, which if not corrected can lead to complete disruption of the relationship and sometimes become associated with charges of impropriety or ethical misconduct. Examples potentially leading to boundary violations are listed in Box 18-13.[97]

Most health care professionals have had little or no training on how to identify and avoid or correct sexually oriented disruptions in the professional relationship. Those in the field of psychiatry and related professions who become involved in long-term counseling have been the most vocal in addressing these issues.[98] We can learn from their experiences as they apply to the field of pulmonary rehabilitation.

Seductive Behavior

The caregiver may sometimes find that a patient exhibits behavior that is sexually seductive, and he or she may be at a loss as to how to respond, except for the instinctual urge to turn and run. Such seductive behavior may be subtle and actually may be innocent, such as a wink of an eye, a touch, a comment, or other behavior by the patient that makes the caregiver feel uncomfortable. On the other hand, the behavior may be blatant, such as the male patient exposing his genitals to the female caregiver when she enters his hospital room, or the female patient whose manner of dress or draping is seductive with a male caregiver. Regardless of the intent of the behavior, its sexual content is disruptive to the relationship and needs to be recognized and perhaps addressed.

At times, the caregiver may sense a sexual attraction to the patient, which by itself is neither right nor wrong but clearly must be recognized by the caregiver and suppressed. Sexual feelings are natural and spontaneous in each of us and should be recognized for what they are, that is, simply feelings. Acting on those feelings, on the other hand, is inappropriate and unethical. Seductive behavior by a patient to a vulnerable caregiver is understandably a formula for disaster for both individuals.

The caregiver should try to analyze and interpret the motivation for the patient's behavior. Is it expressing a truly sexual need or physical urge, or is the patient lonely and depressed and craving personal attention? Is the patient using this inappropriate behavior in an attempt to fulfill those needs? Perhaps the behavior is merely representative of the patient's personality, that is, he or she might be flirtatious or a sexual tease by nature. Conversely, the behavior may represent the patient's attempt to control the relationship by manipulating the caregiver's feelings by making inappropriate sexual comments. Under these circumstances, the caregiver should suppress the urge to "play along," however tantalizing it might appear. It is important to realize that the patient is responding to the relationship with the caregiver, not to the caregiver as an individual. It is at this point that the caregiver should identify

---

> **BOX 18-13** **Examples of Potential Boundary Blurring**[97]
>
> - Gift giving from/to the patient
> - Patient or provider having or wanting access to provider's or patient's home phone number, or other personal information
> - Patient or provider expectations that the provider will provide care or socialize outside of clinical care settings
> - Provider or patient providing excessive personal information with patient or provider

---

BOX 18-14	Self-reflection on Potential Professional–Patient Boundaries[94]

- Am I treating this patient differently than I do my other patients?
- What emotions of my own does this trigger, and are the emotions impacting my clinical decision making?
- Are any actions truly therapeutic for the patient, or am I acting in a manner to meet my personal needs?
- Would I be comfortable if this gift/action was known to the public or my colleagues?

BOX 18-15	Responses to a Seductive Patient

- Do not play along.
- Identify the patient's motive.
- Indicate discomfort.
- Reaffirm the professional relationship.
- Preserve the patient's self-esteem.
- Acknowledge the patient's sexuality.
- Address the patient's emotional needs.
- Transfer care to a different caregiver if necessary.

---

what it is in his or her own behavior that may be generating sexual attraction by the patient. Ideas for self-reflection are described in Box 18-14.[97]

If possible, the caregiver should try to preserve the relationship unless the behavior is totally disruptive. Suggestions for this are listed in Box 18-15.[95] It is important to reaffirm the professional nature of the relationship. Words or touches by the patient that are blatantly sexual must be addressed, and it must be pointed out to the patient that such liberties are not acceptable. The male patient who exposes his genitals during the female caregiver's visit to his hospital room should be told to cover up and that such actions are not welcomed and that they make the caregiver uncomfortable. More subtle behavior by the patient may be more difficult to address. The situation may be resolved simply by refocusing the relationship, pointing out to the patient that the behavior suggests that his or her feelings for the caregiver may be other than professional and thus are not appropriate.

It is important to preserve the patient's self-esteem by acknowledging and affirming his or her sexuality. The patient may feel sickly and unattractive and fear that the caregiver looks on him or her with pity or disgust. A negative response by the caregiver would then confirm the patient's low

self-worth. The caregiver should try not to focus on the actual behavior but rather on the reason for the behavior. At times, unfortunately, the professional nature of the relationship is beyond repair, and this relationship must be severed. In such cases, the caregiver should transfer the patient to the care of another if possible. It is wise that the caregiver discuss this problem with the rehabilitation team or an appropriate supervisor.

Sexual Bias

Another sexual issue that may impact negatively on the caregiver–patient relationship is a preexisting sexual bias. As discussions concerning sexuality ensue in a pulmonary rehabilitation program, the caregiver may learn of sexual behavior or preferences of the patient that the caregiver finds personally unacceptable. Learning about a patient's homosexual preference, for example, may activate a sexual bias in the caregiver if he or she feels that homosexual behavior is morally wrong or somehow abnormal. As has been stated many times, feelings about sexuality are an integral part of our personality. The rightness or wrongness of a sexual bias is not the subject of this discussion. Rather, it is important that the caregiver recognize a personally sexual bias and take precautions that it does not interfere with the professional relationship.

Gender conflicts can disrupt the caregiver–patient relationship. The male patient may feel that he has to remain strong and fearless concerning the impact of the disease on his masculinity, and thus not be able to reveal his concerns to a female caregiver. One might think that he would be more open with a male caregiver, but the same macho attitude may prevail. This seems to be less of an obstacle in female caregiver/female patient interactions. Gender conflicts also can occur out of a sense of control, the male patient feeling that he has to be in charge all the time.

This re-emphasizes the importance of preparing for patient encounters by examining one's feelings and attitudes about sexuality and sexual behavior and by coming to grips with one's own sexual values and levels of comfort. It is not our place to make value judgments about the sexual preferences or behavior of our patients, unless they think that the behavior is harmful to the patient or to others. Although we may avoid making any comments to the patient, we must guard against sending nonverbal messages and disapproval, such as the look on our faces or our body language or how we choose to continue the discussion. We may not agree with the patient's choices, but we must accept them and work to accept the patient unconditionally as a person.

Sexual Abuse

Our interactions with patients may reveal evidence or generate suspicion of sexual abuse of the patient. It most commonly involves individuals who depend on others for their care and support, such as children and the elderly. All health care professionals are legally required in most states to report suspected incidents of abuse and neglect, and legal immunity is provided for those making such reports. Victims of such abuse would seem to be unlikely participants in a pulmonary rehabilitation program, but this depends on the age and nature of the population that the program is serving.

The sexual abuse of children is a major problem in the United States, and we must be knowledgeable of the behavioral and physical signs that indicate that such abuse may be taking place. This is particularly important for caregivers who serve children and young adults.[99,100] The 2005 American Academy of Pediatrics Clinical Report on the evaluation of sexual abuse in children reviews those signs.[101]

Although sexual abuse is often thought of as occurring mainly in children, the caregiver must also consider whether elderly patients have been abused sexually. Most commonly, the patient who has been abused is an elderly woman who has lost her spouse and is physically or mentally dependent on another person for care. Often the abused person will be unwilling to talk about the abusive incidents because he or she is afraid that the abuser will find out and that the abuse will worsen. The caregiver is obliged to protect the patient from injury and thus should be familiar with the necessary steps to obtain protection or to seek appropriate professional resources.[102-105] The reader is referred to The National Center on Elder Abuse, which can be accessed at www.ncea.aoa.gov/.

Sexual Interactions

It is difficult for a caregiver to know how to respond when the patient expresses attraction or "makes a pass" at him or her. The initial reaction may be one of flattery, the caregiver feeling pleased that the patient has found him or her to be attractive. However, it is important to focus on the nature of the relationship. The patient's response may seem genuine, but it is more commonly an expression of transference.[95] This is a behavioral phenomenon first identified by Freud, who noted that patients displace previous experiences, behavior, and emotions onto the caregiver, viewing him/her as parent, spouse, lover, adversary, or friend.[93] This can be a source of confusion for both the patient and the caregiver. Transference is not necessarily pathologic or sexual, but it can be either or both. Regardless of its nature, it must be recognized and understood by the caregiver and be addressed when their behavior oversteps the boundary limitations of the relationship.

It is understandable that patients may confuse their feelings toward the caregiver with feelings that may have been expressed to others in intimate relationships in their past. The patient may feel lonely and unloved and sense that the caregiver is beginning to fill those needs. After all, our professional behavior is to focus on the patient as a person, giving him or her our attention and addressing his or her needs and desires. Our actions tell the patient that we think he or she is a special person and worthy of our attention. The patient may feel the desire to respond to that attention, even though that desire is misguided.

Countertransference is a caregiver's return response to the patient. Again, such interaction is not necessarily bad and can sometimes act to cement the relationship, such as talking about things that both have in common, for example, a certain hobby, travel experiences, or interest in sports. Such discussions make the patient and caregiver feel more familiar and thus more comfortable with each other. Conversely, sexual transference and countertransference are generally disruptive. In these circumstances, the caregiver must be reminded of the asymmetric nature of the relationship and the fact that the patient is vulnerable and at risk for exploitation. Most would say that mutual consent is thus not possible. Any encouragement that the caregiver gives to the patient's expression of sexual interest is a violation of the trust that the patient has placed in the relationship, with the patient suffering the consequences of the breach of that trust. Even if the patient continues to pursue the caregiver and seems to consent to an ongoing sexual relationship, many would argue that the initial fiduciary basis for the relationship prevents any true consent from occurring.[106] As a result, the AMA

Council on Ethical and Judicial Affairs and other professional organizations have determined that sexual interactions between caregiver and patient, particularly sexual intercourse, are unethical.[93,107,108]

CONCLUSION

Sexuality is an integral part of the human experience and thus is an integral part of the rehabilitative process of an individual disabled by a chronic illness, often complicated by the natural aging process. We as health caregivers have a responsibility to understand this aspect of our patients' lives and to be prepared to minister to their needs. As our country ages, we must strive to meet this challenge and, as Comfort and Dial[7] state, strive "to make them welcome—now, because they include our parents, and in the future, because they will include ourselves."

References

1. Nici L, Donner C, Wouters E et al: American Thoracic Society/European Respiratory Society Statement on pulmonary rehabilitation, Am J Respir Crit Care Med 173:1390-1413, 2006.
2. Diamond JM: Why is sex fun? The evolution of human sexuality, New York, 1998, Basic Books.
3. Selecky PA: Sexuality and the patient with lung disease. In Casaburi R, Petty TL, editors: Principles and practice of pulmonary rehabilitation, Philadelphia, 1993, WB Saunders, p 382.
4. World Health Organization: Report of a technical consultation on Sexual health: defining sexual health, Geneva, 2005, World Health Organization.
5. Schover LR, Jensen SB: Sexuality and chronic illness: a comprehensive approach, New York, 1988, Guilford Press, p 3.
6. Kaiser FE: Sexuality in the elderly, Urol Clin North Am 23:99-109, 1996.
7. Comfort A, Dial LK: Sexuality and aging, Clin Geriatr Med 7:1, 1991.
8. Thienhaus OJ: Practical overview of sexual function and advancing age, Geriatrics 43:63-67, 1988.
9. Masters WH, Johnson VE: Human sexual response, New York, 1981, Bantam Books.
10. Bellastella A, Esposit D, Conte M et al: Sexuality in aging male, J Endocrinol Invest 28:55-60, 2005.
11. Schow DA, Redmon B, Pryor JL: Male menopause: how to define it, how to treat it, Postgrad Med 101:62-64, 67-68, 71-74, 1997.
12. Araujo AB, Mohr BA, McKinlay JB: Changes in sexual function in middle-aged and older men: longitudinal data from the Massachusetts Male Aging Study, J Am Geriatr Soc 52:1502-1509, 2004.
13. Meston CM: Aging and sexuality, West J Med 167:285-290, 1997.
14. Montague DK, Jarow JP, Broderick GA et al: Chapter 1: the management of erectile dysfunction: an AUA update, J Urol 174:230-239, 2005.
15. Barber HR: Sexuality and the art of arousal in the geriatric woman, Clin Obstet Gynecol 39:970-973, 1996.
16. Gentili A, Mulligan T: Sexual dysfunction in older adults, Clin Geriatr Med 14:383-393, 1998.
17. Women's Health Initiative: Risks and benefits of estrogen plus progestin in healthy postmenopausal women, JAMA 288:321-333, 2002.
18. Goldstein MK, Teng NN: Gynecologic factors in sexual dysfunction of the older woman, Clin Geriatr Med 7:41-61, 1991.
19. Marsiglio W, Donnelly D: Sexual relations in later life: a national study of married persons, J Gerontol 46:s338-s344, 1991.
20. Bretschneider JG, McCoy NL: Sexual interest and behavior in healthy 80- to 102-year-olds, Arch Sex Behav 17:109-129, 1988.
21. Bortz WM II, Wallace DH: Physical fitness, aging, and sexuality, West J Med 170:167-169, 1999.
22. Mulligan T, Retchin SM, Chinchilli VM et al: The role of aging and chronic disease in sexual dysfunction, J Am Geriatr Soc 36:520-524, 1988.
23. Mooradian AD: Geriatric sexuality and chronic diseases, Clin Geriatr Med 7:113-131, 1991.
24. Zeiss RA, Delmonico RL, Zeiss AM et al: Psychologic disorder and sexual dysfunction in elders, Clin Geriatr Med 7:133-151, 1991.
25. Chiechi LM, Granieri M, Lobascio A et al: Sexuality in the climacterium, Clin Exp Obstet Gynecol 24:158-159, 1997.
26. Ebersole P, Hess P: Intimacy, sexuality, and aging. In Ebersole P, Hess P, editors: Toward healthy aging, ed 6, St. Louis, 2004, Mosby.
27. Laumann EO, Paik A, Glassen DB et al: A cross-national study of subjective sexual well-being among older women and men: findings from the Global Study of Sexual Attitudes and Behaviors, Arch Sex Behav 35:145-161, 2006.
28. Kingsberg SA: The impact of aging on sexual function in women and their partners, Arch Sexual Behav 31:431-437, 2002.
29. Davey Smith G, Frankel S et al: Sex and death: are they related? Findings from the Caerphilly Cohort Study, BMJ 315:1641-1644, 1997.
30. Cleare AJ, Wessely SC: Just what the doctor ordered—more alcohol and sex, BMJ 315:1637-1638, 1997.
31. Greeley A: Sex: the Catholic experience, Allen, Tex, 1994, Tabor, p 149.
32. U.S. Bureau of the Census: Statistical abstract of the United States: 1998, ed 118, Washington, DC, 1998, U.S. Bureau of the Census.
33. Holzapfel S: Aging and sexuality, Can Fam Physician 40:748-750, 753-754, 757-758, 1994.
34. Diokno AC, Brown MB, Herzog AR: Sexual function in the elderly, Arch Intern Med 150:197-200, 1990.
35. Richardson JP, Lazur A: Sexuality in the nursing home patient, Am Fam Physician 51:121-124, 1995.
36. McInnes RA: Chronic illness and sexuality, Med J Aust 179:263-266, 2003.

37. Kuyper MB, Wester F: In the shadow: the impact of chronic illness on the patient's partner, Qual Health Res 18:237-253, 1998.

38. Kralik D, Koch T, Telford K: Constructions of sexuality for midlife women living with chronic illness, J Adv Nurs 35:180-187, 2001.

39. Fletcher EC, Martin RJ: Sexual dysfunction and erectile impotence in chronic obstructive pulmonary disease, Chest 81:413-421, 1982.

40. Meyer IH, Sternfels P, Fagan JK et al: Asthma-related limitations in sexual functioning: an important but neglected area of quality of life, Am J Pub Health 92:770-772, 2002.

41. Schonhofer B, von Sydow K, Bucher T et al: Sexuality in patients with noninvasive mechanical ventilation due to chronic respiratory failure, Am J Respir Crit Care Med 164:1612-1617, 2001.

42. Koseoglu N, Koseoglu H, Ceylan E et al: Erectile dysfunction prevalence and sexual function status in patients with chronic obstructive pulmonary disease, J Urol 174:249-252, 2005.

43. Ibanez M, Aguilar JJ, Maderal MA et al: Sexuality in chronic respiratory failure: coincidences and divergences between patient and primary caregiver, Respir Med 95:975-979, 2001.

44. Wise TN: Sexual dysfunction in the medically ill, Psychosomatics 24:787-801, 805, 1983.

45. Bancroft J, Loftus J, Long JS: Distress about sex: a national survey of women in heterosexual relationships, Arch Sex Behav 32:209-211, 2003.

46. Johnson B: Older adults' suggestions for health care providers regarding discussions of sex, Geriatr Nurs 18:65-66, 1997.

47. Drench ME, Losee RH: Sexuality and sexual capacities of elderly people, Rehabil Nurs 21:118-123, 1996.

48. Oregon State University Extension Service: Sex and aging: a game of awareness and interaction [board game], Corvallis, Ore, 1980, Oregon State University. (http://extension.oregonstate.edu/catalog).

49. Schover LR, Jensen SB: Sexuality and chronic illness: a comprehensive approach, New York, 1988, Guilford Press, p 293.

50. Spica MM: Educating the client on the effects of COPD on sexuality: the role of the nurse, Sex Disabil 10:91-101, 1992.

51. Francoeur RT: Sexual components in respiratory care, Respir Manage 18:35-39, 1988.

52. Annon JS: Brief therapy. In Annon JS, editor: The behavioral treatment of sexual problems, Honolulu, Hawaii, 1974, Enabling Systems, p 1.

53. Taylor JF, Rosen RC, Leiblum SR: Self-report assessment of female sexual function: psychometric evaluation of the Brief Index of Sexual Functioning for Women, Arch Sex Behav 23:627-643, 1994.

54. Clayton AH, McGarvey EL, Clavet GJ: The Changes in Sexual Functioning Questionnaire (CSFQ): development, reliability, and validity, Psychopharmacol Bull 33:731-745, 1997.

55. Derogatis LR: The Derogatis Interview for Sexual Functioning (DISF/DISF-SR): an introductory report, J Sex Marital Ther 23:291-304, 1997.

56. Schover LR, Jensen SB: Sexuality and chronic illness: a comprehensive approach, New York, 1988, Guilford Press, p 14.

57. Ende J, Rockwell S, Glasgow M: The sexual history in general medicine practice, Arch Intern Med 144:558-561, 1984.

58. Selecky PA: Sexuality and chronic breathing problems [brochure], Santa Ana, Calif, 1989, American Lung Association of Orange Country.

59. Eckert RC, Bartsch K, Dowell D et al: Being close, Denver, 1984, National Jewish Hospital. Available at www.nationaljewish.org. Retrieved June 10, 2008.

60. Butler RN, Lewis MI: The new love and sex after 60, revised edition, New York, 2002, Ballantine Books.

61. Good JT, Petty TL: Frontline advice for the COPD patient, Denver, 2005, Snowdrift Pulmonary Foundation.

62. National Institute on Aging Information Center: AgePage: sexuality in later life, Bethesda, Md, 2005, National Institute on Aging, National Institutes of Health. Available at www.niapublications.org/engagepages/sexuality.asp. Retrieved June 10, 2008.

63. Yates A, Wolman W: Aphrodisiacs: myth and reality, Med Aspects Hum Sexuality 67:58, 1991.

64. Deamer RL, Thompson JF: The role of medications in geriatric sexual function, Clin Geriatr Med 7:95-111, 1991.

65. Schwarz ER, Rastogi S, Kapar V et al: Erectile dysfunction in heart failure patients, J Am Coll Cardiol 48:1111-1119, 2006.

66. Kamischke A, Kemper DE, Castel MA et al: Testosterone levels in men with chronic obstructive pulmonary disease with or without glucocorticoid therapy, Eur Respir J 11:41-45, 1998.

67. Cheitlin MD, Hutter AM Jr, Brindis RG et al: Use of sildenafil (Viagra) in patients with cardiovascular disease: Technology and Practice Executive Committee, Circulation 99:168-177, 1999.

68. Cheitlin MD: Sexual activity and cardiac risk, Am J Cardiol 96(suppl):24M-28M, 2005.

69. Cheitlin MD: Sexual activity and cardiovascular disease, Am J Cardiol 92(suppl):3M-8M, 2003.

70. Romano MD: Sexuality and the disabled female, Accent Living 18:28, 1973.

71. Sipski ML: Sexuality and individuals with respiratory impairment. In Bach JR, editor: Pulmonary rehabilitation, Philadelphia, 1996, Hanley & Belfus, p 203.

72. Cole SS, Hossler CJ: Intimacy and chronic lung disease. In Fishman AP, editor: Pulmonary rehabilitation, New York, 1996, Marcel Dekker, p 251.

73. NIH Consensus Development Panel on Impotence: NIH consensus conference: impotence, JAMA 270:83-90, 1993.

74. Sadovsky R, Nusbaum M: Sexual health inquiry and support is a primary care priority, J Sex Med 3:3-11, 2006.

75. Montague DK, Barada JH, Belker AM et al: Clinical guidelines panel on erectile dysfunction: summary report on the treatment of organic erectile dysfunction: the American Urological Association, J Urol 156:2007-2011, 1996.

76. Aasebo U, Gyltnes A, Bremnes RM et al: Reversal of sexual impotence in male patients with chronic

obstructive pulmonary disease and hypoxemia with long-term oxygen therapy, J Steroid Biochem Mol Biol 46:799-803, 1993.

77. Althof SE, Leiblum SR, Chevret-Measson M et al: Psychological and interpersonal dimensions of sexual function and dysfunction, J Sex Med 2:793-800, 2005.

78. Goldstein I, Lue TF, Padma-Nathan H et al: Oral sildenafil in the treatment of erectile dysfunction: Sildenafil Study Group, N Engl J Med 338:1397-1404; 1998. [Erratum appears in N Engl J Med 1998;339:59.]

79. Sildenafil: an oral drug for impotence. Med Lett Drugs Ther. 1998, 40:51-52.

80. Rendell MS, Rajfer J, Wicker PA et al: Sildenafil for treatment of erectile dysfunction in men with diabetes: a randomized controlled trial: Sildenafil Diabetes Study Group, JAMA 281:421-426, 1999.

81. Jackson G, Rose RC, Kloner RA et al: The second Princeton consensus on sexual dysfunction and cardiac risk: new guidelines for sexual medicine, J Sex Med 3:28-36, 2006.

82. Kloner RA: Cardiovascular effects of the 3 phosphodiesterase-5 inhibitors approved for the treatment of erectile dysfunction, Circulation 110:3149-3155, 2004.

83. Kostis JB, Jackson G, Rosen R et al: Sexual dysfunction and cardiac risk (the Second Princeton Consensus Conference), Am J Cardiol 96:313-321, 2005.

84. Schwarz ER, Rastogi S, Kapur V et al: Erectile dysfunction in heart failure patients, J Am Coll Cardiol 48:1111-1119, 2006.

85. Kaplan SA, Reis RB, Kohn IJ et al: Safety and efficacy of sildenafil in postmenopausal women with sexual dysfunction, Urology 53:481-486, 1999.

86. Fisher WA, Rosen RC, Earley I et al: Sexual experience of female partners of men with erectile dysfunction: the Female Experience of Men's Attitudes to Life Events and Sexuality (FEMALES) Study, J Sex Med 2:675-684, 2005.

87. Goldstein I, Fisher WA, Sand M et al: Women's sexual function improves when partners are administered vardafenil for erectile dysfunction: a prospective, randomized, double-blind, placebo-controlled trial, J Sex Med 2:819-832, 2005.

88. Basson R: Sexual desire and arousal disorders in women, N Engl J Med 354:1497-1506, 2006.

89. Basson R: Clinical updates in women's health care monograph, vol 2, no 2: sexuality and sexual disorders in women, Washington DC, 2003, American College of Obstetricians and Gynecologists, pp 1-94.

90. Blake J, Belisle S, Basson R et al: SOGC clinical practice guideline: Canadian Consensus Conference on Menopause, 2006 update [No. 171], J Obstet Gynecol Can February, S7-S10, 2006. Available at www.sogc.org/jogc/abstracts/200602_SOGCClinical PracticeGuidelines_1.pdf. Retrieved June 17, 2008.

91. North American Menopause Society: The role of testosterone therapy in postmenopausal women: position statement of the North American Menopause Society, Menopause 12:497-511, 2005.

92. Plaud JJ, Dubbert PM, Holm J et al: Erectile dysfunction in men with chronic medical illness, J Behav Ther Exp Psychiatry 27:11-19, 1996.

93. Gabbard GO, Nadelson CN: Professional boundaries in the physician–patient relationship, JAMA 273-1445-1449, 1995.

94. Farber NJ, Novack DH, O'Brien MK: Love, boundaries, and the patient–physician relationship, Arch Intern Med 157:2291-2294, 1997.

95. Selecky PA: Sexuality in respiratory care. In Pierson DJ, Kacmarek R, editors: Foundations of respiratory care, New York, 1992, Churchill Livingstone, p 1237.

96. Spence S: Patients bearing gifts: are there strings attached? BMJ 331:1527-1529, 2005.

97. Barbour LT: Professional–patient boundaries in palliative care. Fast Fact and Concept #172. End-of-Life/Palliative Education Resource Center. Available at www.eperc.mcw.edu/fastFact/ff_172.htm. Retrieved June 17, 2008.

98. Schafer P: When a client develops an attraction: successful resolution versus boundary violation, J Psych Mental Health Nursing 4:203-211, 1997.

99. AMA issues diagnostic and treatment guidelines on child sexual abuse, Am Fam Physician 47:1519-1520, 1993.

100. Vandeven AM, Newton AW: Update on child physical abuse, sexual abuse, and prevention, Curr Opin Pediatr 18:201-205, 2006.

101. Kellogg N: American Academy of Pediatrics Committee on Child Abuse and Neglect: The evaluation of sexual abuse in children, Pediatrics 116:506-512, 2005.

102. Geroff AJ, Olshaker JS: Elder abuse, Emerg Med Clin N Am 24:491-505, 2006.

103. Schneider DC, Li X: Sexual abuse of vulnerable adults: the medical director's response. J Am Med Dir Assoc 7:442-445, 2006.

104. Aravanis SC, Adelman RD, Breckman R et al: Diagnostic and treatment guidelines on elder abuse and neglect, Arch Fam Med 2:371-388, 1993.

105. Council on Scientific Affairs: Elder abuse and neglect, JAMA 257:966-971, 1987.

106. Kennedy E: Sexual counseling: a practical guide for those who help others, New York, 1989, Continuum, p 63.

107. Sexual misconduct in the practice of medicine. Council on Ethical and Judicial Affairs, American Medical Association, JAMA 266:2741-2745, 1991.

108. American Psychiatric Association: The principles of medical ethics with annotations especially applicable to psychiatry, Washington DC, 1998, American Psychiatric Association.

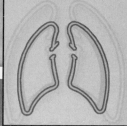

Chapter 19

Preventive Strategies for the Patient with Chronic Lung Disease

BRIAN W. CARLIN • VIJAY SUBRAMANIAM

CHAPTER OUTLINE

Primary Prevention
Secondary Prevention
Tertiary Preventionc

Other Preventive Measures
Conclusion

PROFESSIONAL SKILLS

Upon completion of this chapter, the reader will be able to
do the following:
* Identify the various types of preventive measures (e.g., primary, secondary, and tertiary measures)
  available in the management of a patient with lung disease
* Identify measures used to detect abnormalities in lung function before the development of signs and
  symptoms associated with chronic obstructive pulmonary disease
* Describe measures used to reduce the complications resulting from chronic lung disease (e.g., smoking
  cessation, pulmonary rehabilitation, supplemental oxygen (O_2) use, vaccination, and treatment of
  exacerbations).

Chronic obstructive pulmonary disease (COPD), including emphysema, chronic bronchitis, and asthma, is a considerable cause of morbidity and is currently the fourth leading cause of death in the United States.[1] An estimated 3.6 million people have emphysema, 9 million people have chronic bronchitis, and at least another 20 million people have asthma. Of all the leading causes of death in the United States, COPD is the only one that has shown a relative increase (by 47%) during the past 20 years.

There is often a long disease-free interval between the onset of the disease and the actual development of symptoms. Patients with mild and some with moderate disease often have minimal, if any, symptoms and thus do not seek medical attention. It is only with the development of symptoms that interfere with a person's lifestyle that a person seeks medical attention. In many instances this long disease-free interval adds to the morbidity and mortality associated with the disease. Strategies designed to diagnose the disease earlier in its course and to alter the progression of the disease are of great importance when attempting to decrease morbidity and mortality.

Opportunities for the prevention of chronic lung disease exist, including both health promotion and disease management. Health promotion requires the active participation of the patient in the treatment plan. Disease management requires the input of the patient and health care providers. The combination of health promotion and disease management can provide the person with

BOX 19-1	Strategies for Preventing Chronic Lung Disease

PRIMARY STRATEGIES
- Smoking/nicotine abstinence, cessation
- Health education
- Components of comprehensive pulmonary rehabilitation

SECONDARY STRATEGIES
- Smoking cessation
- Spirometric measurement of expiratory flow rates in high-risk patients (e.g., smokers)
- α1-Antitrypsin replacement therapy (for patients with the genetic deficiency syndrome)
- Components of comprehensive pulmonary rehabilitation
- Nutritional support
- Pulmonary hygiene

TERTIARY STRATEGIES
- Smoking cessation
- Vaccination (pneumococcal, influenza)
- Pulmonary rehabilitation
- O_2 supplementation (for patients with hypoxemia)
- Nutritional support
- Pulmonary hygiene
- Treatment of exacerbations (e.g., antibiotic therapy)

O_2, *Oxygen.*

chronic lung disease the necessary strategies to allow optimal functionality.

Preventive strategies can occur at a variety of levels (primary, secondary, and tertiary). Primary strategies focus on prevention of development of the disease, secondary strategies focus on early detection and prevention of symptomatic disease, and tertiary strategies focus on reduction of complications associated with symptomatic disease (Box 19-1). Comprehensive pulmonary rehabilitation often includes only tertiary prevention strategies; however, incorporation of primary and secondary prevention strategies into a comprehensive pulmonary rehabilitation program should be afforded.

PRIMARY PREVENTION

The greatest risk factor for the development of chronic lung disease is cigarette smoking, with up to 90% of cases of COPD in the United States being caused by exposure to cigarette smoke.[2] Smoking rates are currently declining; however, the incidence of lung disease continues to increase because of the long latency period from the initiation of cigarette smoking to the development of symptomatic disease. A primary preventive strategy is to avoid cigarette smoke altogether. With avoidance of cigarette smoking, the overall development of chronic lung disease can be reduced.

The greatest potential for prevention occurs through efforts to encourage children and teenagers to abstain from smoking. Twenty-two percent of high school students report smoking cigarettes. Although most teenagers who begin to smoke will stop smoking by early adulthood, ongoing strategies to encourage abstinence must be promoted. Health care professionals are important role models in community antismoking campaigns. Educational efforts beginning with grade school children may be the most effective method to prevent the development of chronic lung disease.

How important is it to encourage smoking cessation in patients who are elderly or who already have chronic lung disease? Most of the changes in the lung that are related to smoking are irreversible. Although overall lung function may not improve significantly after cessation of cigarette smoking, the rate of decline of lung function will be reduced and may eventually approach the usual age-related rate of decline.[3] Smoking cessation is of great importance (regardless of the age of the patient) in an attempt to reduce the morbidity and mortality associated with chronic lung disease.[4]

SECONDARY PREVENTION

Secondary prevention includes the early detection of disease and the prevention of symptomatic disease. Early detection of obstructive lung disease is problematic. Every person has a significant amount of "reserve" lung function and it is not until relatively late in the disease course that a patient will exhibit symptoms. Up to 50% of "lung function" (as measured by lung volumes and/or flow rates) can be lost with little or no change in the patient's symptoms or functional capacity. Early detection efforts cannot be based solely on the presence and/or development of symptoms.

Early detection efforts should therefore be based on a simple reproducible means to assess airway function. The clinical examination may be helpful in the evaluation of a patient suspected of having airway obstruction. The presence of wheezing or a prolongation of a forced exhalation time to longer than 6 seconds suggests significant airway obstruction. Spirometry should then be used to confirm the presence of airway obstruction.

Simple spirometry offers the most advantageous way to assess airway function. Spirometry is recommended as part of the routine management of patients at high risk for the development of lung disease (e.g., smokers). The National Lung Health Education Program recommends that anyone who currently smokes or is routinely exposed to environmental tobacco smoke or work place irritants and who has symptoms of chronic cough, wheezing, persistent mucus, or shortness of breath should have simple spirometry performed. Serial determination of the flow rates over time can then be used to determine whether a greater than usual decline in flow rates is occurring.[5] Population screening through the measurement of flow rates might appear to be beneficial, but no data exist to support its use for this purpose. Intervention, provided in the form of intensive smoking cessation programs, could then be afforded in an attempt to minimize ongoing decline of lung function and to improve functional status.

One of the difficulties encountered with the performance of spirometry involves the quality of performance of this testing in primary care environments. As most patients with symptoms of cough, dyspnea, and sputum production will be initially seen by a primary care physician or primary caregiver, the importance of being able to perform spirometry accurately in the primary care setting is necessary.[6] In a study involving 30 primary care practices, acceptable results from spirometry were obtained in only a few patients evaluated (3.4% of patients in practices that received no training in the performance of spirometry and 13.5% of patients in practices that received minimal training), despite the use of quality assurance devices that were built into the equipment being used for the testing.[7] Another study has shown that spirometry in the primary care setting influences the physician's diagnosis of airflow obstruction and management plans, particularly for patients with moderate to severe obstructive lung disease.[8] The availability and reliability of screening under these circumstances needs to be more completely evaluated to ensure that accurate testing is performed. Close cooperation between primary care providers and pulmonary medicine specialists will be necessary in these endeavors.[9]

Another tool that can be used to help assess the effects of smoking-related lung disease on the individual's spirometry test results is the "lung age."[10] Lung age equations have been developed from reference linear regression equations and nomograms, allowing lung age estimation in

---

BOX 19-2	Equations for Estimation of Lung Age

WOMEN

FEV_1 (L)
Lung age = $3.560H - 40.000(\text{Obs } FEV_1) - 77.280$

$FEF_{25\%-75\%}$ (L/sec)
Lung age = $2.000H - 33.333(\text{Obs } FEF_{25\%-75\%}) + 18.367$

MEN

FEV_1 (L)
Lung age = $2.870H - 31.250(\text{Obs } FEV_1) - 39.375$

$FEF_{25\%-75\%}$ (L/sec)
Lung age = $1.044H - 22.222(\text{Obs } FEF_{25\%-75\%}) + 55.844$

$FEF_{25-75\%}$, Forced expiratory flow during the middle half of the forced vital capacity; FEV_1, forced expiratory volume in 1 second; H, height (inches); L, liters; Obs, observed. Lung age is given in years.

---

terms of ventilatory function (Box 19-2). Lung age can then be compared with the person's chronologic lung age and can then be used during patient counseling and may be particularly useful for people who continue to smoke to help encourage discontinuation of smoking.

The early detection of lung function abnormalities may be useful in the individual patient to encourage smoking cessation (if the patient remains a smoker), to enable other risk reduction interventions (e.g., annual influenza vaccination), and to promote entry into a comprehensive pulmonary rehabilitation program. Although definitive studies showing the benefits of such strategies have yet to be performed, this approach for the person at high risk for the development of chronic lung disease should ultimately result in a reduction of the morbidity and mortality associated with the disease.

TERTIARY PREVENTION

The focus of tertiary prevention is to reduce complications resulting from a disease process. Smoking cessation, comprehensive pulmonary rehabilitation, supplemental O_2 administration (when significant hypoxemia is present), pneumococcal and influenza immunization, and exacerbation prevention are tertiary preventive strategies useful in the management of a patient with chronic lung disease.

Although many people who smoke try to quit each year, only about 6% are successful in the long term.[11] Most smokers have visited their primary care provider within the past year and a significant proportion say they would quit smoking had they been advised to do so by their physician, yet many say that they have not been advised by their physician. Physicians may not feel comfortable in the process of assisting a patient to quit smoking[12] but need to remember that physician counseling, even if limited, can result in a doubling of the annual rate of smoking cessation.

The "5 A's" can be an effective means to inquire about the patient's smoking habits and can assist the patient with smoking cessation: *ask* (the patient about tobacco use at every office visit), *advise* (the patient of the dangers associated with smoking in a compassionate way), *assess* (the patient's readiness to quit smoking), *assist* (the patient who is ready to quit), and *arrange* (follow up during the treatment period). In patients who are not ready to quit, it is important to promote motivation to quit, using the "5 R's": *relevance* (to encourage contemplation on personal relevance), *risks* (to discuss personal negative consequences), *rewards* (to show the benefits of smoking cessation), *roadblocks* (to determine barriers to the smoking cessation process), and *repetition* (to repeat these messages during every patient encounter).[13]

Smoking cessation can result in a reduction of the decline in lung function in patients with established disease, as noted in the Lung Health Study.[3] A significant reduction in the rate of decline of forced expiratory volume in 1 second (FEV_1) was noted in those patients who quit smoking and continued as nonsmokers during the 5 years of the trial. This group underwent a comprehensive management program, including the use of nicotine replacement, psychosocial counseling, and frequent follow-up visits to assess the patient's adherence to the regimen.

The addiction associated with cigarette smoking arises from the effects of the nicotine that is delivered to the bloodstream. Physiologic withdrawal symptoms occurring with the decrease in the blood level of nicotine cause a patient to want to continue smoking. Several formulations of nicotine replacement therapy (e.g., patch, gum, nasal spray, lozenge, or inhaler form) are currently available. Each effectively delivers nicotine to the bloodstream and assists with nicotine abstinence. In some instances doubling of the abstinence rates has been noted.[14] Physician counseling

during this process is extremely important during the process of nicotine abstinence. Adjustment of the dose and delivery route of the medication(s), side effect development, assessment for side effects, and provision of ongoing patient support are of importance in this process. Several follow-up office visits during the 2 months following initiation of the medication are advisable.

Varenicline, a partial agonist/antagonist of the $\alpha_4\beta_2$ nicotinic acetylcholine receptor, has been approved for smoking cessation. Varenicline is an oral medication started 1 week before the quit date and titrated to a dose of 1 mg twice per day and continued for 12 weeks. In comparison with other medications and placebo, varenicline has been shown to result in a significant improvement with both short-term and long-term abstinence from smoking[15-18] (Table 19-1). The most common adverse event (and reason for stopping treatment) was nausea, which occurred in 30% of the patients treated with varenicline.

Several other medications are available to assist in the smoking cessation process. Bupropion hydrochloride and nortriptyline have been shown to increase the abstinence rates from 13% to 23% at a 1-year follow-up.[19] Nortriptyline has also been shown to result in a 13% abstinence rate at 26 weeks.[20] Combination therapy has been shown to result in a further increase in the abstinence rate. Treatment with sustained-release bupropion hydrochloride in combination with a nicotine patch resulted in significantly higher long-term rates of smoking cessation than did use of either the nicotine patch alone or placebo (35.5% rate in the group receiving bupropion hydrochloride and nicotine patch, 30.3% in the group receiving bupropion, 16.4% in the group receiving the nicotine patch, and 15.6% in the group receiving placebo). Varenicline has not yet been studied for combination therapy. Several other medications

TABLE 19-1	Smoking Cessation Rates Associated with Varenicline and Bupropion		
	Varenicline (%)	Placebo (%)	Bupropion (SR) (%)
Short-term abstinence	44	17.7	29.5
Long-term abstinence	21.9	8.4	16.1

SR, *Sustained release.*

(e.g., caffeine, buspirone, cytisine, and mecamylamine)[21] have also been used in the treatment of smoking cessation, although few data exist regarding their overall effectiveness.

Formal smoking cessation programs are available in most communities. The most successful programs include those that are at least 2 weeks in duration with a minimum of four to seven sessions, those that offer a variety of interventions from a variety of professionals, and those that offer social support. Knowledge of the psychological effects that are associated with tobacco use and with tobacco cessation are essential components of these programs.[22] A smoking cessation program can be a component of the pulmonary rehabilitation program or can be a part of another community-based program (e.g., a local lung association or a hospital).

Smoking cessation is probably the most important factor responsible for a reduction in the number of complications in patients with symptomatic disease.[23] The comprehensive management of smoking cessation (including education, psychological counseling, medication administration, and social support) has been shown to result in 1-year abstinence rates of up to 44%. Practice guidelines for smoking cessation have been developed and are the core components of successful programs (Table 19-2). One concern of many patients regards the potential weight gain associated with smoking cessation. A mean weight gain of only 2.1 kg has been noted however.[24] In addition, strategies to educate the patient about potential side effects (or lack thereof) should be developed.

Comprehensive pulmonary rehabilitation has been shown to effectively reduce dyspnea, improve exercise tolerance, improve health-related quality of life, and reduce hospitalizations necessary for COPD-related causes. Pulmonary rehabilitation includes patient assessment and evaluation, education regarding lung disease, psychosocial intervention, methods to minimize dyspnea, upper and lower extremity exercise in a monitored setting, measurement of various patient and program outcomes, and long-term adherence of the patient to the regimen. Initially performed in an outpatient setting during an 8- to 12-week period, pulmonary rehabilitation provides effective therapy for patients with established, symptomatic lung disease. Current guidelines, including both evidence- and practice-based, show the essential components of a pulmonary rehabilitation program

and the associated benefits.[25-28] Benefits following continuation of pulmonary rehabilitation after the initial outpatient program have also been shown.[29,30] Many physicians are unaware of the benefits associated with pulmonary rehabilitation or have failed to accept pulmonary rehabilitation as an important and effective modality of therapy and thus have not offered pulmonary rehabilitation to their patients with symptomatic lung disease.

Administration of supplemental O_2 to patients with COPD and resting hypoxemia has been shown to reduce morbidity and improve survival as documented by two landmark studies (the British Medical Research Council and the Nocturnal Oxygen Therapy Trial) performed in the early 1980s.[31,32] A reduction in mortality in addition to a decrease in pulmonary artery pressure, an improvement in exercise tolerance, and an improvement in cognitive function have also been shown. Patients who have COPD and arterial hypoxemia should thus be offered long-term O_2 therapy (Box 19-3). The beneficial effects of the administration of O_2 for patients who exhibit oxyhemoglobin desaturation only during exercise or during sleep are less well documented; however, most physicians offer supplemental O_2 to those patients as well.

O_2 can be administered in various forms (gas, concentrator, or liquid) and modalities (nasal cannula, conserving device, pulse demand device, mask, or transtracheal device). The ambulatory status of each patient is important in the determination of the type of O_2 supply/device that will be of most benefit. The system that allows for maximal ambulation should be afforded. It is important to test each patient in the use of the prescribed O_2 system (including a conserving device) to guarantee appropriate levels of O_2 administration. Combinations of O_2 delivery modalities can be administered depending upon the patient's clinical status (e.g., the use of an O_2 concentrator during sleep and a liquid system during ambulation for the patient who is ambulatory). A strategy for the choice of delivery system for patients who require supplemental O_2 is presented in Figure 19-1.

Exacerbations of COPD (including exacerbations of chronic bronchitis or pneumonia) account for more than 600,000 hospitalizations each year, with a high associated mortality. Various types of disruption in the host defenses can allow the development of lower respiratory

TABLE 19-2	Key Clinical Practice Guideline Recommendations for Smoking Cessation[23]
Recommendation No.	**Description**
1	Tobacco dependence is a chronic condition that often requires repeated interventions; however, effective treatments exist that can produce long-term or even permanent abstinence
2	Because effective tobacco-dependence treatments are available, every patient who uses tobacco should be offered at least one of these treatments: • Patients willing to try to quit tobacco should be provided with treatments that are identified as effective in the guideline • Patients unwilling to try to quit tobacco use should be provided with a brief intervention that is designed to increase their motivation to quit
3	It is essential that clinicians and health-care delivery systems (including administrators, insurers, and purchasers) institutionalize the consistent identification, documentation, and treatment of every tobacco user who is seen in a health-care setting
4	Brief tobacco-dependence treatment is effective, and every patient who uses tobacco should be offered at least brief treatment
5	There is a strong dose-response relationship between the intensity of tobacco-dependence counseling and its effectiveness; treatments involving person-to-person contact (via individual, group, or proactive telephone counseling) are consistently effective, and their effectiveness increases with treatment intensity (e.g., minutes of contact)
6	Three types of counseling and behavioral therapies were found to be especially effective and should be used with all patients who are attempting tobacco use cessation: • Provision of practical counseling (problem solving/skills training) • Provision of social support as part of treatment (intratreatment social support); and • Help in securing social support outside of treatment (extratreatment social support)
7	Numerous effective pharmacotherapies for smoking cessation now exist; except in the presence of contraindication, these should be used with all patients who are attempting to quit smoking • Five first-line pharmacotherapies were identified that reliably increase long-term smoking abstinence rates: Bupropion SR Nicotine patch Nicotine gum Nicotine inhaler Nicotine nasal spray
8	Tobacco-dependence treatments are both clinically effective and cost-effective relative to other medical and disease prevention interventions; as such, insurers and purchasers should ensure the following: • All insurance plans include, as a reimbursed benefit, the counseling and pharmacotherapeutic treatments that are identified as being effective in this guideline • Clinicians are reimbursed for providing tobacco-dependence treatment just as they are reimbursed for treating other chronic conditions

SR, Sustained release.

tract illness. Disruption of the epithelial surface of the airways promotes microbial colonization and, in some instances, invasive infection. Other abnormal host defenses (including the loss of normal mucociliary function, production of abnormal mucus and immunoglobulins, susceptibility for aspiration of oropharyngeal and stomach secretions, and reduced cough effectiveness) may play a role in the retention of microbial organisms within the tracheobronchial tree.

Viral infections (e.g., influenza viruses A and B, rhinovirus, respiratory syncytial virus, and adenovirus) have been associated with the development of COPD exacerbations. Viral infections usually occur during the winter months and prevention of influenza can be successfully accomplished through vaccination. The vaccine is commercially prepared from purified egg-grown viruses that contain inactivated antigens from the influenza A and influenza B viruses. Protective antibodies can be expected to rise in the individual patient within several weeks of vaccination but depend on the individual's general health and immune status. Because the antibody response decreases with time and the

BOX 19-3	Indications for the Prescription of Long-term Oxygen Therapy

- Clinical stability of the patient
- Demonstration of arterial hypoxemia or oxyhemoglobin desaturation:
  - Pa_{O_2} < 55 mm Hg
  or
  - Pa_{O_2} 56–59 mm Hg and one of the following:
    - P pulmonale noted on electrocardiogram
    - Presence of edema
    - Cor pulmonale

This demonstration can be made with the patient during rest, exercise, or under sleep conditions.

Pa_{O_2}, *Arterial partial pressure of oxygen.*
Note: Sa_{O_2} (arterial oxygen saturation) of 88% or less can be used in place of the Pa_{O_2} value.

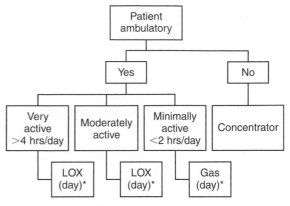

LOX-liquid oxygen system
Gas-gaseous oxygen system

FIGURE 19-1 Oxygen (O_2) delivery device selection. An asterisk (*) indicates that continuous flow or use of an O_2-conserving device with a nasal cannula should be used if applicable. Continuous flow O_2 via a concentrator can be used during sleep. The actual amount of O_2 liter flow to be administered should be determined through performance of an O_2 titration study under rest and exercise conditions. Such studies should be performed with the actual O_2 therapy equipment (e.g., gaseous or liquid system, O_2-conserving device) that the patient will be using in the ambulatory setting.

influenza virus exhibits antigenic drift from one year to the next, annual vaccination is recommended. The vaccine is usually administered as an intramuscular injection although a trivalent, live attenuated virus vaccine is now available and is administered as an intranasal spray.[33]

Vaccination of patients at increased risk for infection is the single most important method to reduce the morbidity associated with influenza, with an efficacy rate varying from 30% to 85%.[34,35] In a systematic review, it was found that administration of the inactivated vaccine reduces the exacerbation rate (3 or more weeks after vaccination) in patients with COPD. A mild increase in local adverse effects with vaccination was noted.[36] Despite the efficacy and low adverse effect rates, few people at risk for influenza infection are actually vaccinated each year.

Vaccination for influenza is recommended for adults and children who have chronic lung and/or cardiac disease, are immunosuppressed, diabetic, or have renal disease. It is also recommended for people who are older than 65 years, residents of chronic care facilities (including personal care homes and nursing homes), and persons who live with or care for persons at high risk (including household contacts who have frequent contact with persons at high risk and who can transmit influenza to those persons at high risk) and health care workers.[37] Vaccination should occur in the fall on a yearly basis. Side effects are usually of minimal consequence (e.g., soreness around the injection site, fever, malaise, and myalgias) and the only absolute contraindication to vaccination is an egg allergy. Certain patients should not be vaccinated with the live attenuated vaccine, including those who are younger than 5 years or older than

50 years; those who have asthma, reactive airway disease, or other chronic disorders of the pulmonary or cardiovascular systems; and those with known or suspected immunodeficiency diseases, or other underlying medical conditions. In most instances, the inactivated vaccine should be the type of vaccination used.

For those patients who have influenza infection, antiviral medications (e.g., amantadine and rimantidine) have been shown to reduce the signs and symptoms associated with influenza A infection by up to 50%, if given within 48 hours of the onset of clinical symptoms. More recent data, however, indicate widespread resistance of influenza virus to these medications and thus neither should be used for the treatment or chemoprophylaxis of influenza A in the United States.[38] Zanamavir and oseltamivir are approved for use in the treatment of influenza infection and for use as chemoprophylaxis. Their use has been shown to reduce the rate of viral shedding and the duration of clinical symptoms associated with influenza in healthy adults.[39,40] Zanamavir is administered via an inhaler and its use is discouraged in patients with airway disease (e.g., asthma) because of its potential for airway irritation. Oseltamivir is delivered in pill form.

Pneumococcal vaccine is the other vaccination generally recommended for patients with chronic lung disease. The 23-valent vaccine contains serotypes that are responsible for more than 85% of invasive pneumococcal infections. A significant effect of reducing invasive pneumococcal disease in adults after vaccination has been shown.[41] Although some debate exists as to the efficacy of the vaccine and duration of protection in patients with COPD, efficacy for such patients approached 65%.[42,43] In addition, colonization of the airway with pneumococci has been shown to increase the exacerbation risk in patients with COPD. In those patients, pneumococcal antibody titers were lower than in healthy vaccinated adults. Thus, it can be postulated that vaccination may benefit patients with COPD as an increase in the antibody titer rate for those colonized with pneumococci may ultimately reduce the exacerbation rate.[44]

Pneumococcal vaccination is recommended for all patients older than 65 years and revaccination is recommended after 6 years for those at high risk of fatal complications from pneumococcal infection (e.g., patients with asplenia or chronic lung disease).[45] Whether revaccination should be given routinely in other patient groups has not yet been answered. The side effects associated with revaccination are minimal, usually pain and induration at the injection site. More serious local effects (e.g., skin necrosis) have rarely been noted.[46]

The overall administration rate of both the influenza and pneumococcal vaccinations is low across the population at risk for the development of either type of infection. Vaccination rates as low as 20% of the potential at-risk population have been reported. A well-designed vaccination administration protocol is necessary and should be available in physician offices and hospitals to ensure that patients and health care workers who might benefit from the vaccination actually receive it.

Awareness of the signs and symptoms associated with a lower respiratory tract infection (e.g., bronchitis and pneumonia) is an important component of the disease management strategy for patients with chronic lung disease. An increase in shortness of breath, increase in sputum production, or change in the character of the sputum should prompt immediate consultation with the primary care provider. In patients who have at least two of these three symptoms antibiotic therapy has been shown to result in an improvement in the patient's clinical condition.[47,48] Symptoms such as

chest pain, fever, sore throat, and myalgias should also prompt concern. Other causes for these symptoms should be considered (e.g., heart failure, myocardial infarction, arrhythmias, and pulmonary embolism) because many patients with COPD have comorbid illnesses. Guidelines for the treatment of patients with exacerbations of chronic bronchitis and community-acquired pneumonia can be helpful in the management strategy for these patients.[49,50]

Prevention of exacerbations is an important part of the overall management of patients with chronic lung disease. By reducing the exacerbation rate, a reduction in overall morbidity and mortality should occur. Both pharmacologic and nonpharmacologic interventions are used in such preventive efforts. Pharmacologic therapy (including anticholinergics, β_2-agonists, and inhaled corticosteroids) has been shown to reduce the exacerbation rate.[51-56] Nonpharmacologic therapy (e.g., pulmonary rehabilitation) has been shown to reduce hospitalizations due to exacerbations of COPD.[57-59]

Other types of pharmacologic interventions are being investigated regarding a reduction in the exacerbation rate for patients with COPD. One intervention involves the use of medication therapy to augment the patient's innate defense mechanisms. Viewed by some with skepticism, a recent meta-analysis (albeit of poor quality) suggests these drugs may have a positive effect on exacerbations.[60] Phosphodiesterase inhibitors (e.g., theophylline, cilomilast, and roflumilast) may also help to reduce exacerbation rates but again conclusive data are lacking.[61,62]

The presence of gastroesophageal reflux should be suspected in patients who have COPD. Several studies have shown that patients with COPD have an increase in gastrointestinal symptoms (e.g., heartburn, regurgitation, chronic cough, and dysphagia) compared with control subjects.[63] Work has shown an increase in gastroesophageal reflux disease in patients with severe COPD.[64] Although the impact of reflux on respiratory symptoms is unknown, suspicion for the presence of reflux should prompt investigation and appropriate therapeutic intervention.

General health measures for patients with chronic lung disease should be discussed with each patient. Avoidance of people who might potentially have any respiratory illnesses (e.g., people who are in health care facilities or children) is an important component of these preventive efforts. Routine hand washing is the most important method that can be used to prevent the transmission of infection, especially when one is caring for children. Handshakes are a potential source for transmission of infection and although it is not possible to perform hand washing after each handshake, appropriate precautions should be taken. These measures should be discussed during the educational component associated with a pulmonary rehabilitation program.

One the most significant difficulties encountered in the management of a person with chronic illness is the issue of adherence with the recommended medical regimen. Even the most complete medical assessment and treatment plan can be effective only if the patient adheres to the recommendations made by the health care provider. The health care provider must be aware that most patients do not satisfactorily comply with a suggested medical regimen. To gain such adherence to a treatment plan, the patient must become an active participant in the evaluation and treatment plan. Adherence to a medical regimen (both the daily regimen and the regimen associated with an acute illness [e.g., use of antibiotics for an acute exacerbation in a patient with underlying chronic lung disease, smoking cessation, and exercise]) needs to be assessed continually. The most effective adherence-enhancing interventions are designed to improve patient self-management capabilities.[65]

OTHER PREVENTIVE MEASURES

The American Cancer Society estimates that more than 213,000 Americans are diagnosed yearly with lung cancer and that more Americans will die of lung cancer than of colon, breast, and prostate cancer combined.[66] The Lung Health Study showed that among middle-aged men and women with even mild degrees of airflow obstruction, deaths from lung cancer outnumbered deaths from COPD, coronary artery disease, or stroke.[3] Treatment of early-stage lung cancer (stage 1) by surgical resection is often effective, with a 5-year survival of about 70%. Unfortunately, by the time most lung cancers are detected, only 25% are resectable. The 5-year survival in this group is only 14%. Because of its significant association with the development of lung cancer, cessation from cigarette smoking must be addressed with each smoker.[67]

Identification of lung cancer during the earlier stages should result in reduced morbidity and mortality. Screening for lung cancer is feasible if there is a detectable presymptomatic phase of the disease and an established means of intervention (i.e., surgical resection) during this presymptomatic phase. Patients at risk for the development of lung cancer include those with a family history of lung cancer, preexisting COPD, a history of previous smoking-associated cancer (of the lung or head and neck), occupational exposures (e.g., silica, heavy metals, radon, and asbestos), or preexisting pulmonary fibrosis.[68] In one study, 51 consecutive patients with either clinical symptoms of or occupational exposures to uranium or asbestos were identified by sputum cytology to have lung carcinoma and 46 of these patients had early-stage disease. Twenty-seven were deemed to be surgical candidates with a 5-year actuarial survival, including deaths from all causes of 55%.[69] In another study of 632 patients who had a greater than 40–pack-year smoking history and an FEV_1 less than 70% predicted, screening sputum cytology revealed 9 carcinomas (in situ or invasive).[70]

Sputum and bronchoalveolar lavage cytology studies are a primary means to detect lung cancer. Other modalities are also being used in the early identification of the disease in those patients who are at risk but without significant symptomatology (e.g., spiral computed tomography [CT] scanning). In one group of male smokers older than 50 years, 14 of the 15 cancers detected by spiral CT were stage 1, and only 4 of these were visible by chest radiograph.[71] In another study, the use of CT scanning of the chest helped to detect a significant number of patients with lung cancer who would not have been otherwise diagnosed as they were asymptomatic.[72]

Autofluorescence bronchoscopy offers yet another technique for early detection. An 89% improvement in the sensitivity for identification of moderate to severe endobronchial dysplasia has been shown using this technique.[73] Newer biochemical and immunologic methods (e.g., the use of monoclonal antibodies for small-cell and non–small-cell carcinoma on sputum cytologic specimens) may allow lung cancer to be detected months to years earlier than would be possible compared with routine sputum cytology.[74] Eventually, hematologic gene markers for cancer will be used to detect lung cancer. Further investigations must be performed to determine the exact role for each of these techniques in the early detection process. At present, an annual chest radiograph coupled with sputum cytology for people at high risk for lung cancer is recommended by some.[75] Studies are underway to more completely evaluate the value of a yearly spiral CT scan combined with sputum cytology for patients in high-risk groups.[76]

An intriguing potential approach to the prevention of chronic lung disease involves the identification of lung disease at the genetic level. Symptomatic lung disease develops in only 15% to 20% of white individuals who are heavy cigarette smokers. Differences have been noted in the development of lung disease in different ethnic groups (e.g., the low prevalence of COPD noted in China).[77] The prevalence of airflow obstruction and pulmonary disease symptoms in Japanese Americans who reside in Hawaii is significantly lower than in white Americans who reside there.[78] An increased prevalence of airflow obstruction within families not accounted for by smoking has also been suggested.[79] The Framingham Study provided the ability to analyze a subset of more than 5000 subjects from more than 1000 families, suggesting that after correction for smoking, polygenic gene effects and other environmental factors determine FEV_1.[80] It has been suggested for more than 30 years that some patients have airflow obstruction at an earlier age than others, suggesting that genetic factors may be playing a role in the development of symptomatic disease.[81] Finally, because the mortality rate from COPD has increased in women, such genetic differences also need to be considered when evaluating and managing patients.

Genetics may play a role in both the development of the disease and in a patient's response to therapy. Women appear to benefit less from nicotine replacement therapy and experience less physiologic addiction and greater behavioral dependence. Thus, women may benefit more than men from a smoking cessation program that includes the use of bupropion and intensive counseling. Women also appear to derive greater benefits (e.g., greater initial rise and a slower age-related decline in FEV_1) from a sustained quit attempt.[82,83]

Another consideration for preventive therapy centers on the potential for the development of osteoporosis. Women are at higher risk than men for the development of osteoporosis.[84] People with COPD have several risk factors that predispose to accelerated bone loss and osteoporosis, including the direct effects of smoking on bone metabolism, premature menopause, vitamin D deficiency, immobility, and long-term corticosteroid use.[85] Baseline and follow-up bone mineral density scans should be performed in women who have COPD. For those without evidence of osteoporosis or osteopenia, exercise and calcium and vitamin D supplements should be considered in most women. Postmenopausal women with established osteoporosis or osteopenia are candidates for bisphosphonates, estrogen, calcitonin, or a selective estrogen receptor modulator. Smoking cessation is mandatory and the use of systemic corticosteroids should be avoided as much as possible.[86]

The overall effects of the various factors involved in the development of chronic lung disease (whether it is related to the inflammatory response, the protease–antiprotease imbalance, or various immunoglobulin abnormalities) have yet to be fully defined from a genetic perspective. Through the use of positional cloning, candidate genes, or whole genome screens, identification of various genetic defects can potentially be found early and appropriate intervention(s) can then be administered.[87]

Newer therapies in addition to those already discussed are being investigated and may be beneficial in this prevention of the progression of COPD. The use of inhaled corticosteroids has been shown in the TORCH (*To*wards a *R*evolution in *C*OPD *H*ealth) Study to result in a 17% relative reduction in mortality over a 3-year period as well as a reduction in the COPD exacerbation rate and improvement in quality of life in the treatment group.[88,89] Such therapies in combination with other types of therapy (e.g., pulmonary rehabilitation and smoking cessation) should prove to result in a further decline in the morbidity and mortality associated with COPD.

CONCLUSION

Preventive strategies for patients with chronic lung disease can be afforded through a variety of interventions (Box 19-4). Primary strategies (e.g., health promotion), secondary strategies (e.g., spirometry in high-risk patients, smoking cessation and components of pulmonary rehabilitation), and tertiary strategies (e.g., comprehensive pulmonary rehabilitation, supplemental O_2 use, influenza and pneumococcal vaccinations, and prevention of exacerbations) can be used to help reduce the morbidity and mortality associated with chronic lung disease.[90]

BOX 19-4	Preventive Measures to Be Included as Part of a Pulmonary Rehabilitation Program

- Smoking cessation, nicotine intervention (knowledge of addictive properties of nicotine)
- Controls of environment (crowds, humidity)
- Proper hand-washing technique
- Vaccination (influenza, pneumococcal)
- Nutrition
- Exercise
- Mental wellness
- Knowledge of course of lung disease
- Knowledge of warning signs of an infection, prevention of exacerbations
- Knowledge of warning signs of lung cancer
- Knowledge of osteoporosis risk factors
- Adherence to medication program, smoking cessation, and exercise program

References

1. Mannino DM, Homa DM, Akinbami LJ et al: Chronic obstructive disease surveillance—United States, 1971-2000, MMWR Surveill Summ 51:1-16, 2002.
2. U.S. Department of Health and Human Services: Chronic obstructive lung disease: the health consequences of smoking: a report of the Surgeon General (DHHS Publication 84, 2677), Washington DC, 1984, U.S. Office of the Assistant Secretary for Health. Office of Smoking and Health.
3. Anthonisen NR, Connett JE, Kiley JP et al: Effects of smoking intervention and the use of an inhaled anticholinergic bronchodilator on the rate of decline of FEV_1: the Lung Health Study, JAMA 272:1497-1505, 1994.
4. Fletcher C, Peto R: The natural history of chronic airflow obstruction, BMJ 1:1645-1648, 1977.
5. National Lung Health Education Program Executive Committee: Strategies in preserving lung health and preventing COPD and associated diseases: the National Lung Health Education Program (NLHEP), Chest 113(suppl):123S-155S, 1998.
6. Hankinson JL: Office spirometry: does poor quality render it impractical? Chest 116:276-277, 1999.
7. Eaton T, Withy S, Garrett JE et al: Spirometry in primary care practice, Chest 116:416-423, 1999.
8. Dales RE, Vandenheen KL, Clinch J et al: Spirometry in the primary care setting, Chest 128:2443-2447, 2005.
9. Lusuardi M, De Benedetto F, Paggiaro P et al: A randomized controlled trial on office spirometry in asthma and COPD in standard general practice, Chest 129:844-852, 2006.
10. Morris JF, Temple W: Spirometric "lung age" estimates for motivating smoking cessation, Prev Med 14:655-662, 1985.
11. Centers for Disease Control and Prevention (CDC): Smoking cessation during previous year among adults—United States 1990 and 1991, MMWR Morb Mortal Wkly Rep 42:504-507, 1993.
12. Russell MAH, Wilson C, Taylor C et al: Effects of general practitioner's advice against smoking, BMJ 2:231-235, 1989.
13. Anderson JE, Jorenby DE, Scott WJ et al: Treating tobacco use and dependence: an evidence-based clinical practice guideline for tobacco cessation, Chest 121:932-941, 2002.
14. Henningfield JE: Nicotine medications for smoking cessation, N Engl J Med 333:1196-1203, 1995.
15. Gonzales D, Rennard SI, Nides M et al: Varenicline Phase 3 Study Group: Varenicline, and $\alpha_4\beta_2$ nicotinic acetylcholine receptor partial agonist vs. sustained-release bupropion and placebo for smoking cessation: a randomized controlled trial, JAMA 296:47-55, 2006.
16. Jorenby DE, Hays JT, Rigotti NA et al: Varenicline Phase 3 Study Group: Efficacy of varenicline, an $\alpha_4\beta_2$ nicotinic acetylcholine receptor partial agonist vs. placebo or sustained-release bupropion for smoking cessation: a randomized controlled trial, JAMA 296:56-63, 2006.
17. Nides M, Oncken C, Gonzales D et al: Smoking cessation with varenicline, a selective $\alpha_4\beta_2$ nicotinic receptor partial agonist, Arch Intern Med 166:1561-1568, 2006.
18. Oncken C, Gonzales D, Nides M et al: Efficacy and safety of the novel selective nicotinic acetylcholine receptor partial agonist, varenicline, for smoking cessation, JAMA 166:1571-1577, 2006.
19. Hurt RD, Sachs DPL, Glover ED et al: A comparison of sustained release bupropion and placebo for smoking cessation, N Engl J Med 337:1195-1202, 1997.
20. Wagena EJ, Knipschild PG, Huibers MJ et al: Efficacy of bupropion and nortriptyline for smoking cessation among people at risk for or with chronic obstructive pulmonary disease, Arch Intern Med 165:2286-2292, 2005.
21. Etter JF: Cytisine for smoking cessation: a literature review and a meta-analysis, Arch Intern Med 166:1553-1559, 2006.
22. Williams JM, Ziedonis D: Addressing tobacco among individuals with a mental illness or addiction, Addict Behav 29:1067-1083, 2004.
23. Fiore MC, Bailey WC, Cohen SC et al: Smoking cessation: clinical practice guideline No. 18 (AHCPR publication 90-0692), Rockville, Md, 1996, Agency for Health Care Policy and Research.
24. Jorenby DE, Leischow SJ, Nides MA et al: A controlled trial of sustained release bupropion, a nicotine patch, or both for smoking cessation, N Engl J Med 340:685-691, 1999.
25. Ries AL, Bauldoff GS, Carlin BW et al: Pulmonary rehabilitation: joint ACCP-AACVPR evidenced based clinical practice guidelines, Chest 131:1S-42S, 2007.
26. Hill NS: Pulmonary rehabilitation, Proc Am Thorac Soc 3:66-74, 2006.
27. Troosters T, Casaburi R, Gosselink R et al: Pulmonary rehabilitation in chronic obstructive pulmonary disease, Am J Respir Crit Care Med 172:19-38, 2005.
28. Nici L, Donner C, Wouters E et al: on behalf of the ATS/ERS Pulmonary Rehabilitation Writing

Committee: American Thoracic Society/European Respiratory Society statement on pulmonary rehabilitation, Am J Respir Crit Care Med 1390-1413, 2006.

29. Ries AL, Kaplan RM, Myers R et al: Maintenance after pulmonary rehabilitation in chronic lung disease: a randomized trial, Am J Respir Crit Care Med 167:880-888, 2003.

30. Guell R, Casan P, Belda J et al: Long-term effects of outpatient rehabilitation of COPD: a randomized trial, Chest 117:976-983, 2000.

31. Medical Research Council Working Party: Long-term domiciliary oxygen therapy in chronic hypoxic cor pulmonale complicating chronic bronchitis and emphysema, Lancet 1:1681-1686, 1981.

32. Nocturnal Oxygen Therapy Trial Group: Continuous or nocturnal oxygen therapy in hypoxemic chronic obstructive lung disease: a clinical trial, Ann Intern Med 93:391-398, 1980.

33. Nichol KL, Mendelmann PM, Mallon KP et al: Effectiveness of live, attenuated intranasal influenza virus vaccine in healthy, working adults, JAMA 282:137-144, 1999.

34. Govaert TME, Thijs CTMCN, Masurel N et al: The efficacy of influenza vaccination in elderly individuals: a randomized double-blind placebo-controlled trial, JAMA 272:1661-1665, 1994.

35. Gross PA, Hermogenes AW, Sacks HS et al: The efficacy of influenza vaccine in elderly persons: a meta-analysis and review of the literature, Ann Intern Med 123:518-527, 1995.

36. Poole PJ, Chacko E, Wood-Baker RWB et al: Influenza vaccine for patients with chronic obstructive pulmonary disease, Cochrane Database Syst Rev 1: CD002733, 2006.

37. Smith NA, Bresee JS, Shay DK et al: Advisory Committee on Immunization Practices: Prevention and control of influenza: recommendations of the Advisory Committee on Immunization Practices (ACIP), MMWR Recomm Rep 55(RR-10):1-42, 2006. [Erratum in MMWR Morb Mortal Wkly Rep 2006;55(29):800.]

38. Atkinson WL, Arden NH, Patriarca PA et al: Amantadine prophylaxis during an institutional outbreak of type A influenza, Arch Intern Med 146:1751-1756, 1986.

39. Monto AS, Fleming DM, Henry D et al: Efficacy and safety of the neuraminidase inhibitor zanamavir in the treatment of influenza A and B virus infections, J Infect Dis 180:254-261, 1999.

40. Monto AS, Robinson DP, Herlacher ML et al: Zanamavir in the prevention of influenza among healthy adults, JAMA 282:31-35, 1999.

41. Dear KBG, Andrews RR, Holden J et al: Vaccines for preventing pneumococcal infections in adults [review], Cochrane Database Syst Rev 4: CD000422, 2003.

42. Shapiro ED, Berg AT, Austrian R et al: The protective efficacy of polyvalent pneumococcal polysaccharide vaccine, N Engl J Med 325:1453-1460, 1991.

43. Butler JC, Breiman RF, Campbell JF et al: Pneumococcal polysaccharide vaccine efficacy: an evaluation of current recommendations, JAMA 270:1826-1831, 1993.

44. Bogaert D, van der Valk P, Ramdin R et al: Host—pathogen interaction during pneumococcal infection in patients with chronic obstructive pulmonary disease, Infect Immun 72:818-823, 2004.

45. Harper SA, Fukuda K, Uyeki TM et al: Centers for Disease Control and Prevention (CDC) Advisory Committee on Immunization Practices (ACIP): Prevention and control of influenza: recommendations of the Advisory Committee on Immunization Practices (ACIP), MMWR Recomm Rep 53(RR-6):1-40, 2004. [Erratum in MMWR Recomm Rep 2004;53(32):743; update in MMWR Recomm Rep 2005;54(RR-8):1-40.]

46. Artz AS, Eishler WB, Longo DL: Pneumococcal vaccination and revaccination of older adults, Clin Microbiol Rev 16:303-318, 2003.

47. Anthonisen NR, Manfreda J, Warren CPW et al: Antibiotic therapy in exacerbations of chronic obstructive pulmonary disease, Ann Intern Med 106:196-204, 1987.

48. Saint S, Bent S, Vittinghoff E et al: Antibiotics in chronic obstructive pulmonary disease exacerbations: a meta-analysis, JAMA 273:957-960, 1995.

49. Balter MS, La Forge J, Low DE et al: Chronic Bronchitis Working Group; Canadian Thoracic Society; Canadian Infectious Disease Society: Canadian guidelines for the management of acute exacerbations of chronic bronchitis: executive summary, Can Respir J 10:248-258, 2003.

50. Pauwels PA, Buist AS, Calverley PM et al; GOLD Scientific Committee: Global strategy for the diagnosis, management, and prevention of chronic obstructive pulmonary disease. NHLBI/WHO Global Initiative for Chronic Obstructive Lung Disease (GOLD) workshop summary, Am J Respir Crit Care Med 163:1256-1276.

51. Szafranski W, Cukier A, Ramirez A et al: Efficacy and safety of budesonide/formoterol in the management of chronic obstructive pulmonary disease, Eur Respir J 21:74-81, 2003.

52. Calverley PMA, Pauwels R, Vestbo J et al: TRISTAN Study Group: Combined salmeterol and fluticasone in the treatment of chronic obstructive pulmonary disease: a randomized controlled trial, Lancet 361:449-456, 2003.

53. Casaburi RA, Mahler DA, Jones PW et al: A long-term evaluation of once daily inhaled tiotropium in chronic obstructive pulmonary disease, Eur Respir J 19:217-224, 2002.

54. Burge PS, Calverley PMA, Jones PW et al: Randomised, double blind, placebo controlled study of fluticasone propionate in patients with moderate to severe chronic obstructive pulmonary disease: the ISOLDE Trial, BMJ 320:1297-1303, 2000.

55. Pauwels PA, Lofdahl C, Laitinen LA et al: European Respiratory Society Study on Chronic Obstructive Pulmonary Disease: Long-term management with inhaled budesonide in persons with mild chronic obstructive pulmonary disease who continue smoking, N Engl J Med 340:1948-1953, 1999.

56. Vestbo J, Sorensen T, Lange P et al: Long-term effects of inhaled budesonide in mild and

moderate chronic obstructive pulmonary disease: a randomized controlled trial, Lancet 353:1819-1823, 1999.

57. California Pulmonary Rehabilitation Collaborative Group: Effects of pulmonary rehabilitation on dyspnea, quality of life, and health care costs in California, J Cardiopulmonary Rehabil 24:52062, 2004.

58. Griffiths TL, Phillips CJ, Davies S et al: Cost effectiveness of an outpatient multidisciplinary rehabilitation programme, Thorax 56:779-784, 2001.

59. Bourbeau J, Julien M, Maltais F et al: Reduction of hospital utilization in patients with chronic obstructive pulmonary disease: a disease specific self-management intervention, Arch Intern Med 163:585-591, 2003.

60. Stuerer-Stey C, Bachmann LM, Steurer J et al: Oral purified bacterial extracts in chronic bronchitis and COPD: systematic review, Chest 126:1645-55, 2004.

61. Gamble E, Grootendorst DC, Brightling CE et al: Antiinflammatory effects of the phosphodiesterase-4 inhibitor cilomilast in chronic obstructive pulmonary disease, Am J Respir Crit Care Med 168:976-982, 2003.

62. Rabe KF, Bateman ED, O'Donnell D et al: Roflumilast: an oral anti-inflammatory treatment for chronic obstructive pulmonary disease, Lancet 366:563-571, 2005.

63. Casanova C, Baudet JS, del Valle Velasco M et al: Increased gastroesophageal reflux disease in patients with severe COPD, Eur Respir J 841-845, 2004.

64. Mohklesi B, Morris AL, Huang CF et al: Increased prevalence of gastroesophageal reflux symptoms in patients with COPD, Chest 119:1043-1048, 2005.

65. World Health Organization: Adherence to long-term therapies: evidence for action, Annex 1: Behavioral mechanisms explaining adherence. Geneva, 2003, WHO Press, p 143.

66. American Cancer Society: Cancer facts and figures 2007. Atlanta, Ga, 2007, American Cancer Society.

67. Tockman MS, Anthonisen NR, Wright EC et al: Airways obstruction and the risk for lung cancer, Ann Intern Med 106:512, 1987.

68. Saraceno J, Spivack SD: Strategies for early detection of lung cancer, Clin Pulm Med 6:66-72, 1999.

69. Bechtel JJ, Kelley WR, Petty TL et al: Outcome of 51 patients with roentgenographically occult lung cancer detected by sputum cytology testing: a community hospital program, Arch Intern Med 154:975-980, 1994.

70. Kennedy TC, Proudfoot SP, Franklin WA et al: Cytopathological analysis of sputum in patients with airflow obstruction and significant smoking histories, Cancer Res 56:4673-4678, 1996.

71. Kaneko M, Eguchi K, Ohmatsua H et al: Peripheral lung cancer: screening and detection with low-dose spiral CT versus radiography, Radiology 201:798-802, 1996.

72. Herschke CI, McCauley DI, Yankelevitz DF et al: Early Lung Cancer Action Project: overall design and findings from baseline screening, Lancet 354:99-105, 1999.

73. Lam S, Kennedy T, Under M et al: Localization of bronchial intraepithelial neoplastic lesions by fluorescence bronchoscopy, Chest 113:696-702, 1999.

74. Tockman MS, Gupta PK, Myers JD et al: Sensitive and specific monoclonal antibody recognition of human lung cancer antigen on preserved sputum cells: a new approach to early lung cancer detection, J Clin Oncol 6:1685-1693, 1988.

75. Midthun DE, Jett JR: Early detection of lung cancer: today's approach, J Respir Dis 19:59-70, 1998.

76. Saraceno J, Spivack SD: Strategies for early detection of lung cancer, Clin Pulm Med 6:66-72, 1999.

77. Buist AS, Vollmer WM, Wu Y et al: Effects of cigarette smoking on lung function in four population samples in the People's Republic of China: the PRC-US Cardiovascular and Cardiopulmonary Research Group, Am J Respir Crit Care Med 151:1393-1400, 1995.

78. Marcus EB, Buist AS, Curb AJ et al: Correlates of FEV1 and prevalence of pulmonary conditions in Japanese-American men, Am Rev Respir Dis 138:1398-1404, 1988.

79. Higgins M, Keller J: Familial occurrence of chronic respiratory disease and familial resemblance in ventilatory capacity, J Chronic Dis 28:239-251, 1975.

80. Givelber RJ, Couropmitree NN, Gottlieb DJ et al: Segregation analysis of pulmonary function among families in the Framingham Study, Am J Respir Crit Care Med 157:1445-1451, 1998.

81. Burrows B, Knudson RJ, Cline MG et al: Quantitative relationships between cigarette smoking and ventilatory function, Am Rev Respir Dis 115:195-205, 1977.

82. Bohadana A, Nilsson F, Rasmussen T et al: Gender differences in quit rates following smoking cessation with combination nicotine therapy: influence of baseline smoking behavior, Nicotine Tob Res 5:111-116, 2003.

83. Connett JE, Murray RP, Buist AS et al: Changes in smoking status affect women more than men: results of the Lung Health Study, Am J Epidemiol 157:973-979, 2003.

84. NIH Consensus Development Panel on Osteoporosis Prevention, Diagnosis, and Therapy: Osteoporosis prevention, diagnosis, and therapy, JAMA 285:785-795, 2001.

85. Biskobing DM: COPD and osteoporosis, Chest 121:609-20, 2002.

86. Ionescu AA, Schoon E: Osteoporosis in chronic obstructive pulmonary disease, Eur Respir J 22:s46,64s-75s, 2003.

87. Barnes PJ: Molecular genetics of chronic obstructive pulmonary disease, Thorax 54:245-252, 1999.

88. Vestbo J TORCH Study Group: The TORCH (Towards a Revolution in COPD Health) survival study protocol, Eur Respir J 24:206-210, 2004.

89. Calverley PM, Celli B, Anderson JA et al: TORCH Investigators: Salmeterol and fluticasone propionate and survival in chronic obstructive pulmonary disease, N Engl J Med 356:775-789, 2007.

90. Connors GL, Hilling L: Prevention, not just treatment, Respir Care Clin N Am 4:1-12, 1998.

Chapter 20

Adherence in the Patient with Pulmonary Disease

ROBERT M. KAPLAN • ANDREW L. RIES

CHAPTER OUTLINE

Extent of the Problem
Physician Awareness of the Problem
Adherence in Chronic Obstructive
   Pulmonary Disease
Adherence to Pharmacologic
   Interventions
   Overadherence
   Rational Nonadherence
   Practical Suggestions on Medication
      Adherence

Adherence to Exercise
   Exercise as a Component
      of Rehabilitation
   Practical Suggestions on Exercise
      Promotion
Adherence to Smoking Cessation
   Programs
Conclusion

PROFESSIONAL SKILLS

On completion of this chapter, the reader will be able to do
the following:

* Recognize the extent of nonadherence among patients with chronic obstructive pulmonary disease
  (COPD)
* Be able to differentiate different adherence behaviors
* Summarize unique medicine adherence problems for patients with COPD
* Define overadherence and rational nonadherence
* Describe steps to improve adherence to exercise for patients with COPD
* Discuss behavioral interventions to improve adherence
* Recognize problems of relapse among smokers
* Identify Internet resources to help patients stop smoking

Medical encounters typically end with advice and recommendations. Patients are advised to fill a prescription, take a medication, stay on a prescribed diet, or give up cigarettes.[1] Often medical advice is provided by nonphysician health care professionals or nonprofit agencies such as the American Lung Association. Chronic disease management modules provide instructions for self-care and physician records are used as evidence that certain services have been completed by the patient.[2]

Several groups offer guidelines. For example, the American Lung Association recommends that people with chronic bronchitis be vaccinated against influenza and pneumococcal pneumonia (see www.lungusa.org). Patients are asked to adhere to many different instructions. *Nonadherence* is defined as the failure to follow such advice. This same phenomenon is also called *noncompliance*. Although we prefer the term *nonadherence*, we use it interchangeably with noncompliance.

EXTENT OF THE PROBLEM

A large amount of literature suggests that failure to comply with medical advice is a major problem that results in adverse consequences for consumers of health care. Published figures suggest that nonadherence rates vary between 15% and 93%, depending on the patient population and the definition of adherence.[3] A summary review suggested that approximately 50% of all patients fail to adhere to treatment recommendations.[4] However, another systematic review of 569 studies over a 50-year period suggested that the average nonadherence rate was 24.8%. Among a variety of chronic conditions, adherence rates tended to be lowest for patients with pulmonary diseases, diabetes, or sleep disorders.[1]

PHYSICIAN AWARENESS OF THE PROBLEM

Although evidence consistently demonstrates that patient nonadherence is common, many physicians do not appear to appreciate the problem. DiMatteo and DiNiccola[5] reviewed a variety of studies on practitioner awareness. They found that physicians most often overestimated the extent to which their patients cooperated with recommendations. Several studies have suggested that physicians typically are inaccurate in their estimates of patient adherence and that they generally overestimate correspondence between their orders and patient behavior.[6] These problems raise serious doubts about the validity of physicians predictions of future patient adherence.[4,5,7-9]

ADHERENCE IN CHRONIC OBSTRUCTIVE PULMONARY DISEASE

Despite major advances in diagnosis and medical therapeutics, many patients do not receive optimal benefit from standard medical care. Although some aspects of chronic obstructive pulmonary disease (COPD) are treatable, the medical regimen is extremely complex. Medical management of COPD requires multiple medications. George and colleagues,[10] using self-report measures, noted that only 37% of patients with chronic lung diseases fully adhere to their medical treatments. However, treatment may also include respiratory chest physiotherapy techniques, exercise, and advice to quit smoking. Most patients are confronted with complex combinations of antibiotics, bronchodilators, anti-inflammatory drugs, and, in some cases, supplemental oxygen (O_2). In the following sections, we consider adherence to various components of the regimen for patients with COPD.

ADHERENCE TO PHARMACOLOGIC INTERVENTIONS

In previous editions of this book, we identified all papers on adherence to the COPD regimen back to 1980. In addition, we examined literature reviews published before 1980. Overall the search revealed few studies that have directly addressed adherence, especially regarding traditional medical regimens. The studies considered different treatments in diverse samples and employed various definitions of, and measurements for, adherence. Unfortunately, few conclusions, if any, can be drawn from the current literature. A few of the most recent studies are summaries in Table 20-1.

Published studies have considered adherence regarding a variety of different regimens. Adherence to O_2 therapy in Scotland was reported by Morrison, Skwarski, and MacNee.[11] Among patients with COPD prescribed 24-hour O_2, only 14% were in full adherence. The average use was 14.9 hours/day and 44% used their O_2 less than 15 hours/day. These patients also had poor adherence to other aspects of the regimen. Although all patients were requested to undergo acute arterial blood gas measurements within 12 months, only about half obtained the tests. In another study from the United Kingdom, it was shown that patients who are prescribed O_2 for less than 24 hours, in this case 15 hours/day, obtained high levels of adherence to the prescription.[12] In Denmark, about 66% of patients appear to have appropriate follow-up when receiving O_2 therapy.[13] However, compliance with therapy is often low.

TABLE 20-1   Summary of Selected Studies on Adherence Published Since 2005

Citation	Regimen	Sample	Measure	Definition	Adherence
Arnold, Bruton, and Ellis-Hill (2006)[42]	Pulmonary rehabilitation	20 patients with COPD; age, 45-85 yr	Qualitative semistructured interview	Not defined	Patients were more adherent when physician was enthusiastic about treatment. Social support was also an important predictor of adherence
Lin, Kuna, and Bogen (2006)[22]	Long-term O$_2$ therapy	10 patients with COPD	Percentage of time on O$_2$ therapy	Not defined	Measures of O$_2$ inhalation may be more accurate than measures of O$_2$ expenditure for measuring adherence
Cochram, Cecins, and Jenkins (2006)[48]	Exercise in COPD rehabilitation	172 Australian patients with COPD, participating in rehabilitation	Self-reported exercise	Exercise three to five times per week	67% of those attending a weekly community-based class adhered to the exercise program
George et al (2005)[10]	Medication use	276 patients with chronic lung disease; mean age, 71 yr	Self-report Medication Adherence Report Scale (MARS)	Perfect self-reported adherence on the MARS	37% self-reported perfect adherence. One third used complementary or alternative medicines (not prescribed)
Neri et al (2005)[14]	Long-term O$_2$ therapy	1504 Italian patients with COPD, using O$_2$ therapy for at least 6 mo	Self-reported O$_2$ use	Not defined	84% had a mobile O$_2$ device, but only 40% used the device daily
Ringbaek (2005)[13]	Long-term O$_2$ therapy	8487 Danish patients with COPD	Correct prescription of O$_2$ therapy	Patient received appropriate follow-up	65% of patients had appropriate follow-up

COPD, *Chronic obstructive pulmonary disease; O$_2$, oxygen.*

Neri and colleagues[14] studied more than 1500 patients in Italy. They found that 84% of their sample had a mobile O_2 delivery device, but that only 40% of these patients used the device daily.

Long-term adherence to inhaled medications was evaluated in the Lung Health Study.[15] This was one of the first trials to evaluate inhaled bronchodilator medication used regularly over a long period of time. The Lung Health Study was a large clinical trial (N = 3923) of smoking intervention and bronchodilator therapy for the early stages of COPD. Early in the trial, self-report data suggested that nearly 70% of the patients adhered to the regimen. This rate dropped off only slightly over the next 18 months. In addition to self-reports, the investigators weighed the canisters containing the medications. Self-reports confirmed by canister weights showed that 48% of the patients had good adherence at 1 year. Some nonadherence involved overuse of medication. Further analysis demonstrated that those who overuse medication are also likely to incorrectly report their true smoking status.

Personality measures tend not to be good predictors of adherence. A scale designed to assess medication adherence in COPD has been developed and reported by Powell,[16] but it is not clear that it will be of great clinical value because it does a poor job of predicting adherence. A variety of studies have investigated demographic characteristics associated with COPD self-care behaviors. For example, the Lung Health Study suggested that adherence was associated with being married, older, white, and having more severe disease. More adherent patients also had less shortness of breath and were hospitalized or confined to bed less often.[16] Studies of adherence to nebulizer therapy from the Intermittent Positive Pressure Breathing (IPPB) Study showed that about half of the patients were adherent and half were nonadherent. Predictors of adherence included white race, married, abstinence from alcohol and cigarette use, and more severe shortness of breath. Further, those patients with more severe disease were also more likely to adhere to the therapy.[17] Few trials have evaluated interventions to improve adherence. Solomon and colleagues[18] failed to demonstrate that instructions by clinical pharmacy residents significantly improved adherence over usual care.

Some variables thought to predict adherence often fail to do so. For example, it is commonly assumed that heavy drinkers will be less likely to follow a recommended health care regimen than those who drink less. In the Lung Health Study alcohol consumption was used as a predictor of the ability to quit smoking. The results revealed that heavy alcohol use greater than 25 drinks per week was not a significant predictor of relapse in smoking cessation. However, binge drinking defined as eight or more drinks per occasion once a month or more was associated with greater relapse.[19]

Estimated or measured adherence values do not appear to converge on a specific rate or even a specific pattern. James and colleagues[20] reported that only half of their patients took their medicine regularly. Corden and colleagues[21] also found that about half (56%) of their patients failed to comply with home nebulized therapy. The IPPB clinical trial, which used objective assessments of actual time on IPPB therapy, found that only half of the patients used the nebulizer at least 25 minutes/day. Interventions by clinical pharmacists appear to have relatively small effects on adherence.[18] Adherence does appear to be related to health quality of life. Patients with higher scores on the St. George's Respiratory Questionnaire have been shown more likely to comply with nebulized therapy.[21]

Electronic medication monitors may be valuable methods for improving adherence among patients with COPD. Evidence suggests that measures of O_2 expenditure may not be the most accurate estimates of adherence. New methods that allow direct assessment of O_2 inhalation may be more reliable.[22] One study evaluated 251 patients with COPD participating in a multisite clinical trial of nebulizer therapy with inhalers. The patients were allocated to intervention and control groups. Using an electronic medication monitor known as the nebulizer chronolog, the intervention group received feedback on the accuracy of their medication use. Patients receiving feedback were significantly more likely to adhere to the regimen and to use medications correctly than those in the control group.[23]

The traditional view of adherence/nonadherence, in which the patient either strictly follows or fails to follow a treatment recommendation, may no longer be the optimal direction of adherence research. The degree of adherence required for the desired outcome, be it adherence to a prescribed regimen or maximizing quality of life, varies from treatment to treatment, and should be considered. To date, few studies have systematically evaluated adherence regarding the COPD regimen, and in these few cases, the focus has been on drug and O_2 therapy. Further, only a few studies evaluating interventions to improve the ability of patients with COPD to manage their disease have been reported. Several commentaries have offered strategies for enhancing adherence; however, none have been systematically studied. Some individuals with asthma mistakenly stop steroid inhalers, but continue bronchodilator inhalers, because they do not notice any acute effect from the steroid inhaler.

Overadherence

Most of the literature on adherence behaviors focuses on the extent to which patients underuse medications. A less common, but perhaps equally important, problem involves the overuse of medication. Overadherence is a more common problem when medications provide prompt symptomatic relief. Chryssidis and colleagues,[24] for example, reported that the use of high doses of aerosol therapy often exceeded prescription rates. The mean percentage of prescribed dose actually used was 98.5% at 1 month follow-up and 110.8% at 2 months follow-up. Because there was variability for each of these estimates, it appears that some portion of the patients took considerably more medication than was prescribed.[24] It is not surprising that patients with COPD, a highly symptomatic disorder, would overuse a medication that provides rapid symptomatic relief.

Some of the evidence for patient overadherence comes from innovative studies on the assessment of adherence. For example, in one clinical trial on antihypertensive medications, patients were asked to bring their medications with them for follow-up visits. Adherence rates were remarkably high—sometimes approaching 100%. However, there was considerable variability among subjects, with those at higher adherence levels obtaining better clinical results. Using innovative methods to attach microprocessors to pill blister packs or to the caps of standard pill bottles, it was possible to estimate not only how many of the pills were removed from the packages, but also specifically when they were removed. Studies using these methods suggest that patients often have lapses in adherence in periods between visits or that medicine taking is erratic. Also, they may overuse medication or engage in "pill dumping" just before a clinic visit.[15,25] These findings imply that medications may not be used as prescribed.

Often, patients overuse medication before a clinic visit. Erratic medication use may substantially bias estimates of dose response in clinical trials as well as providing an inaccurate measure of treatment side effects.[15,25]

Rational Nonadherence

There are several competing theories about why patients fail to comply with medical regimens. Explanations for why patients fail to adhere might be divided into three categories: those that focus on the patient, those that focus on the patient's environment, and those that focus on the interaction between the patient and the provider. Patient-oriented explanations suggest that certain personalities fail to adhere to medical treatments or that patients intentionally reject therapy because of some flaw in their personality.[4,20,23,26,27] These explanations have failed to gain empirical support. There is some evidence that patients misunderstand instructions,[20] but relatively little evidence that patients intentionally try to harm themselves by ignoring advice.

Environmental explanations suggest that elements in the patient's environment, such as family influences, reminders, or other environmental stimuli, influence adherence behavior. Evidence for this view of adherence is suggested by studies demonstrating that telephone reminders and simple environmental cues increase adherence.[28] These simple reminders might be notes attached to a refrigerator or electronic devices that beep when a dose of medication is indicated.

The third view of adherence emphasizes the role of the patient–provider relationship. Although the evidence cannot be reviewed in detail here, substantial literature demonstrates that information exchanged between patients and providers is often poor.[5,7] This view of adherence suggests that the remedy to the problem is to improve communication between patients and their health care providers.

In considering the three views of noncompliant behavior, we find little evidence that patient personality variables explain much of the variability in nonadherence.[2,8,27] The environmental view is valuable in identifying simple manipulations that may enhance adherence behavior in some settings.[29-31] However, the environmental view is not a comprehensive explanation that considers the patient's role in the choice to use or not use medications. The patient–provider interaction view comes closest to dealing with the realities of the problem.[32] Substantial evidence suggests that patients often do not comprehend instructions offered to them by their providers.[5] Conversely, providers often have an inadequate picture of the responses their patients have to treatment recommendations. In the following sections, we explore this issue in more detail.

Liang[33] offered reasons why his chronically ill patients failed to take their medications. Common explanations were, "I forgot," "too expensive," "felt dopey," "felt constipated," and "didn't work." Patients often have poor responses to medications, find that the medications are not providing the expected benefit, or cannot afford to purchase the medications. These patients are taking several factors into consideration in their decision to use or not use a product. Whereas the provider may condemn the patient as irrational, the patient may be making what he or she considers to be an informed choice. Kaplan and Simon[34] suggested that patients are more likely to comply with treatment when they perceive a net health benefit. Nonadherence occurs when the perceived negative consequences outweigh expected benefits. In this decision process, patients may discount future benefits because of current side effects. A corollary of the theory is that treatments that produce a short-term benefit may evoke better adherence than those that produce a delayed benefit. For example, treatments that provide immediate symptomatic relief, such as inhalers, may be associated with higher adherence than those such as antihypertensive therapies that exchange current inconvenience for future benefit.

One major reason for nonadherence is that patients experience treatment side effects and, therefore, increased medicine use results in increased discomfort.[35] The Institute of Medicine estimated that 98,000 people in the United States die each year as a result of medical errors.[36] A meta-analysis of 39 studies in U.S. hospitals suggested that adverse drug reactions occur in 6.7% of hospitalized patients and fatal adverse drug reactions occur in 0.32% of the cases. In the United States, this amounts to more than 2 million cases per year.[37]

Several authors have argued that nonadherence can be rational.[38] Patients may adhere to a regimen but fail to obtain the desired benefit. If the probability of an expected benefit is low and there are undesirable side effects, nonadherence may enhance health outcome. For example, a patient with streptococcal pharyngitis who discontinues an antibiotic on the eighth day of a 10-day course might be regarded as a noncomplier. However, if the patient decides that the inconvenience and side effects associated with the medication are a greater concern than the low probability of developing rheumatic fever the decision may be regarded as rational. Nonadherence might also be regarded as rational when the patient achieves the desired result despite nonadherence. Although results are mixed, many studies in many areas do not show a systematic relationship between adherence and health outcome.[25] Many studies in the adherence literature fail to take health outcomes into consideration.

Practical Suggestions on Medication Adherence

Several practical suggestions emerge from the review of research on adherence to medical regimens. These suggestions parallel discussions on the locus of the problem. First, alterations in the patient's environment may increase adherence behavior. Simple techniques, such as using mailed reminders, placing reminder magnets on refrigerators, or phone call reminders, have been successful in several studies. Some new products provide auditory cues as reminders. Patients might also purchase digital watches that beep according to their medical regimen schedule.

Behavioral contracts have also been used with some success. These contracts specify precise regimens and often require the patient to make some desired event or activity contingent upon medicine use. For example, the contract might make some highly probable behavior, such as watching television, contingent upon medicine use.

A second approach to increasing medicine-taking adherence requires enhanced physician–patient communication. A major focus of pulmonary rehabilitation programs is in educating patients and family members about their disease and treatments and in enhancing their ability to communicate with their physicians. Several studies have shown that patients often have misconceptions about their illness and about the expected effects of medications.[39-41] Furthermore, patients often experience side effects of medication. Rarely is this information fully communicated to the provider. Physicians should ask about all reactions to medication and barriers to taking medication in the patient's environment, and should clarify the patient's view of why the medications may or may not be effective. Some evidence indicates that adherence is better when physicians are enthusiastic about the treatment.[42]

Finally, evidence suggests that interventions designed to increase a patient's involvement might increase adherence and ultimately affect patient outcome. In one experiment, patients were coached on which questions to ask their provider before their encounter. In comparison with a group that received traditional patient education, those in the coaching group had actually achieved better health outcomes. Analysis of audio tapes of these physician—patient interactions demonstrated that those in the experimental group were twice as effective as those in the control group in obtaining appropriate information from their physician.[43] The patient-counseling sessions involved the use of a disease-specific algorithm and a set of diagnostic and therapeutic guidelines presented in the branching logic format. The purpose of the session was to identify important components of medical decisions and to increase the patient involvement at each decision point. Other algorithms have now been developed for several chronic disease conditions.[44,45]

ADHERENCE TO EXERCISE

An important component of most pulmonary rehabilitation programs has been the establishment of a regular exercise regimen. Specific physical conditioning exercises, such as walking, can be undertaken by the patient to help maintain lung function and to improve the remainder of the O_2 delivery system.[46] Specifically, appropriate physical conditioning exercises can improve maximal O_2 consumption and endurance, reduce heart rate, improve ventilatory efficiency, and increase tolerance for exercise. Lacasse and colleagues[47] reviewed 23 randomized controlled trials on pulmonary rehabilitation and found significant improvements on all measured aspects of quality of life, including functional or maximal exercise capacity and dyspnea. Some evidence suggests that community-based programs can significantly improve adherence to exercise in patients with COPD.[48]

Few studies have evaluated factors associated with long-term exercise maintenance among patients with COPD. However, a rich literature in cardiac rehabilitation may provide useful suggestions. One literature review analyzed 24 studies that had reported 12 or more months of follow-up.[49] Long-term maintenance of exercise was associated with supervision of the exercise, availability of equipment, more frequent contact with program staff, the inclusion of a behavioral component, maintaining moderate as opposed to high-intensity activity, and specific interventions to maintain the behavior. Some success has been shown for difficult-to-reach patients. For example, Friedman, Williams, and Levine[50] offered a rehabilitation program to the medically indigent. By individualizing instructions and providing guidance for specific community activities such as mall walking, stair climbing, and use of neighborhood facilities, they were able to obtain a self-reported adherence rate of 90%.

Exercise as a Component of Rehabilitation

A few controlled trials documented the benefits of exercise programs for patients with COPD.[51] Cockcroft, Saunders, and Berry[52] randomly assigned 39 patients to a 6-week exercise program or to a no-treatment control group. In comparison with the control group, patients in the exercise group experienced subjective benefits and increased the amount of distance they could walk in 12 minutes. However, the length of follow-up was only 2 months. McGavin and colleagues[53] randomly allocated 24 patients with COPD to a 3-month unsupervised stair-climbing home exercise program or to a nonexercise control group. The 12 patients in the exercise group noted subjective improvements and an increased sense of well-being and decreased breathlessness. They also reported an objective increase in the 12-minute walk distance and maximal level of exercise on a cycle ergometer. These changes did not occur in the control group. However, the length of follow-up was limited to 3 months. Ambrosino and colleagues[54] randomly assigned 23 patients to a 1-month medical and rehabilitative therapy group and 28 patients to medical therapy alone without exercise training. The experimental group improved in exercise tolerance and respiratory pattern as evidenced by a decrease in respiratory rate and increase in tidal volume. Again, these changes were not present in the control group.

One argument for the importance of exercise is that programs that do not have an exercise component are less effective. Sassi-Dambron and colleagues[55] conducted a randomized clinical trial to evaluate a modified pulmonary rehabilitation program focused on coping strategies for shortness of breath, but without exercise training. Eighty-nine patients with COPD were randomly assigned to the 6-week treatment or to a 6-week general health education control group.

The treatment consisted of instruction and practice in techniques of progressive muscle relaxation, breathing retraining, pacing, self-talk, and panic control. Outcomes included the 6-Minute Walk Test, quality of well-being, depression and anxiety scales, and six commonly used dyspnea shortness of breath measures. There were no significant differences between the treatment and control groups at the end of treatment or 6-month follow-ups. The authors conclude that although dyspnea management strategies are an important component of COPD management, they should be taught in combination with other aspects of comprehensive pulmonary rehabilitation, namely structured exercise training.

We have conducted several studies designed to improve adherence to exercise for patients with COPD. One of these experiments randomly assigned 119 patients with COPD to either comprehensive rehabilitation or to an education control group. Pulmonary rehabilitation consisted of 12 four-hour sessions distributed over an 8-week period. The content of the sessions was education, physical and respiratory care, psychosocial support, and supervised exercise. The education control group attended four 2-hour sessions that were scheduled twice per month. These education sessions did not include any individual instruction or exercise training. Topics included medical aspects of COPD, pharmacy use, breathing techniques, and a variety of interviews about smoking, life events, and social support. Lectures covered pulmonary medicine, pharmacology, respiratory therapy, and nutrition. Outcome measures included lung function, maximal exercise tolerance and endurance, symptoms of perceived breathlessness and perceived fatigue, self-efficacy for walking, depression (measured by Centers for Epidemiologic Studies Depression Scale), and sense of well-being (measured by Quality of Well-being Scale). The patients were evaluated at baseline and then again after 2, 6, 12, 24, 36, 48, and 60 months.

Figure 20-1 shows the differences between those in pulmonary rehabilitation and the education control groups over the first year of the study. The top portion of Figure 20-1 shows changes in exercise endurance. Those randomly assigned to rehabilitation had significantly higher endurance at 2, 6, and 12 months. This was complemented

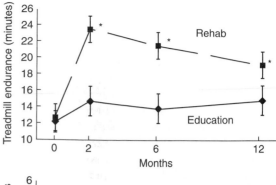

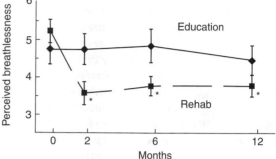

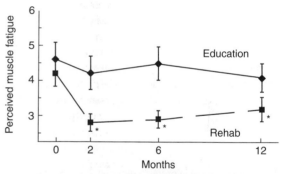

FIGURE 20-1 Results of treadmill endurance exercise tests for patients in rehabilitation (Rehab) and education groups at baseline and for 12 months of follow-up. **Top,** Exercise endurance time. **Middle,** Perceived breathlessness rating at the end of exercise. **Bottom,** Perceived muscle fatigue rating at the end of exercise. *$P < .05$ for within-group change from baseline; values and error bars represent the mean ± SE.

by differences in breathlessness: those in the rehabilitation program were less breathless at the end of the treadmill exercise after 2, 6, and 12 months. Similarly, patients in the rehabilitation group experienced significantly lower perceived muscle fatigue at each follow-up period (see Figure 20-1, *bottom*).[56] There were no differences between groups for measures of lung function, depression, or quality of life. However, both groups experienced reductions in quality of life. For exercise variables, benefits tended to relapse toward baseline after 18 months of follow-up.

We have reason to believe that there is a systematic relationship between compliance with physical activity and a variety of outcomes. In an earlier study we demonstrated a linear relationship between quartile of compliance with physical activity and exercise endurance measured in minutes. The study involved 57 patients with moderate to severe COPD who were participating in a rehabilitation program. Each patient kept a log of physical activity, making it possible to determine self-reported compliance with the exercise component of the program. Each 3 minutes of compliance per day translated into an estimated 1 minute of improvement on treadmill exercise endurance (Figure 20-2).[57]

In a more recent study, 160 patients with chronic lung disease participated in a comprehensive rehabilitation program. At the end of the program the patients were randomly assigned to a program designed to improve compliance and maintenance of the rehabilitation lessons or to routine follow-up. Outcome measures included quality of life, symptoms, health care use, measures of pulmonary function, measures of psychological function, and survival. All patients were evaluated before the pulmonary rehabilitation and then again after the 8-week program had been completed. After the second evaluation, patients were evaluated at 6, 12, and 24 months.[58] The patients were further divided into those who were regular walkers and those who walked irregularly. Regular walking was defined as walking most days or every single day, whereas irregular walking was defined as walking some days, rarely, or never. The core psychosocial measures included the Quality of Well-being (QWB) Scale, the UCSD Shortness of Breath Questionnaire, and a measure of self-efficacy for walking. Quality of life results are summarized in Figure 20-3. Regular walkers maintained better quality of life scores than irregular walkers. Similarly, those who walked on an irregular basis had more shortness of breath than those who walked on a regular basis.[59]

Our group has produced other evidence that walking compliance is related to better health outcomes. In one of our earlier studies, patients with COPD were randomly assigned to one of five groups. One group was designed to increase compliance with physical activity by using cognitive–behavior modification. Cognitive–behavior modification combines traditional behavior modification with cognitive therapy. Cognitive–behavior modification is believed to be superior to either the cognitive component alone (the second group) or behavior modification alone (the third group). The fourth group got attention while the fifth group received no treatment. All patients were evaluated at baseline and monitored over the course of 12 weeks. Cumulative time spent walking was measured on the basis of patient reports in a diary. Those in the cognitive–behavior modification group accumulated significantly more walking time than did those in the control groups. Compliance with physical

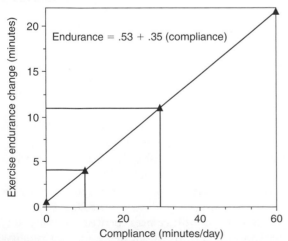

Expected increase in exercise endurance by exercise/day

$Endurance = .53 + .35 (compliance)$

FIGURE 20-2 Dose–response relationship between compliance quartile and exercise endurance. A linear regression equation suggests that each 3 minutes of compliance per day translates into 1 minute of improved endurance.

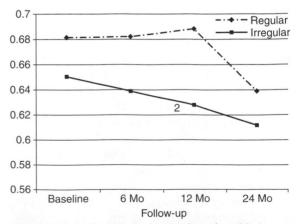

FIGURE 20-3 Changes in the Quality of Well-being Scale, excluding deaths for regular and irregular walkers, at postrehabilitation and 6-, 12-, and 24-month follow-ups. Higher scores indicate better overall health-related quality of life.

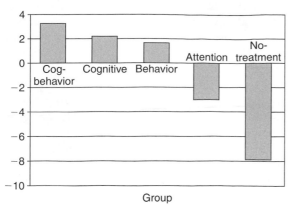

FIGURE 20-4 Mean change in Quality of Well-being Scale (multiplied by 100) by group. Cog-Behavior, group undergoing cognitive–behavior modification.

activity was associated with changes in endurance as evaluated on a treadmill after 12 weeks. Further, these changes in endurance were associated with changes on the QWB Scale (Figure 20-4). All three groups experiencing a cognitive or behavioral intervention showed imp-rovements on the QWB Scale, whereas those in the two control groups declined on the QWB Scale.[60]

There are several potential explanations for the failure to demonstrate long-term benefits from comprehensive pulmonary rehabilitation. One explanation is that behavioral interventions, without long-term follow-up or maintenance sessions, such as rehabilitation, are inadequate to produce long-term change. Long-term maintenance of behavior change has also been difficult to demonstrate in research on smoking cessation,[58] weight loss,[59] and exercise adherence.[60] The finding that patients experience behavior change during treatment that is not maintained after treatment is consistent across a variety of different behavioral interventions.[3] Discovering ways to maintain behavior change over extended periods of time remains a high priority for research.

Practical Suggestions on Exercise Promotion

In summary, patient adherence to exercise is perhaps the most difficult and least studied component of pulmonary rehabilitation. Exercise requires alteration in lifestyle, coping with uncomfortable sensations, and changes in daily schedules. To improve adherence to an exercise program, we recommend the following:

Set realistic goals: Patients who set goals too high become discouraged.

Perform a functional analysis: This involves identifying highly probable enjoyable behaviors such as watching television, reading a novel, or having a cup of coffee. These activities will differ from patient to patient. Once identified, the highly probable behaviors can be used as reinforcers for the exercise activity. The patient might be asked to sign a contract in which he or she agrees to make enjoyable activities contingent upon completion of an exercise session.

Use cognitive techniques: Identify negative things a patient may say to himself or herself during an exercise session. Then teach the patient to use realistic, but positive, self-talk. For example, for a person who says to him- or herself, "This is painful, I can't stand this," the positive coping self-statements of, "Although this is painful, I know it will be good for me in the end" might be substituted. These statements must be rehearsed and practiced. Techniques for developing these statements have been described elsewhere.[60]

ADHERENCE TO SMOKING CESSATION PROGRAMS

Because of the well-documented association between smoking and COPD, successful smoking prevention programs are expected to reduce the incidence of these diseases. Smoking cessation programs are also valuable. There is considerable interest in the effects of smoking cessation for smokers with mild airway obstruction who may be at risk for COPD. In addition to the role of smoking as a cause of COPD, active cigarette smoking also affects the course of the illness. For example, cigarette smoking is associated with mucous hypersecretion, acute respiratory illnesses, altered airway reactivity, and increased risk of mortality from other causes, including coronary heart disease. Some of the relations between smoking and problems in the airways have been reviewed elsewhere.[61] A variety of studies have suggested that loss in lung function is associated with total duration of cigarette use.[62] Longitudinal studies indicate that there is a progressive loss of pulmonary function with continued cigarette smoking. However, there is at least some evidence that there is partial recovery of lung function for those who cease cigarette smoking, particularly for those who do so early in life.[63]

Because of the potential benefits of smoking cessation, efforts to improve adherence to smoking cessation programs are of great importance.

Evidence has accumulated suggesting that the physician may play a critical role in helping patients to stop smoking and to maintain this behavioral change.[64] Several experimental trials have trained physicians to deliver a smoking cessation intervention. The components of the intervention include approaches for taking a smoking history, personalizing the health risks, setting a quit date, prescribing nicotine chewing gum, and counseling techniques for follow-up. In one study, Ockene and colleagues[65] assigned physicians to receive training in behaviorally oriented counseling techniques or to a control group in which patients were provided with only brief advice to stop smoking. Some of the interventions involved the use of nicotine gum, whereas others did not. The results suggested that the behavioral intervention, with or without the use of nicotine gum, resulted in greater reductions in cigarette use among patients. Further, differences between these groups remained at 6-month follow-up.

The Agency for Health Care Policy and Research (AHCPR) offered guidelines for smoking cessation in primary care medicine.[66] Despite the well-established health consequences of tobacco use, less than one half of physicians commonly advise their patients to give up cigarettes.[67] Among those who discuss smoking with their patients, few go much further. For example, only about one in four physicians make any effort beyond simply stating that the patient should quit smoking.[67] One of the biggest challenges in getting patients to quit smoking is the recognition that relapse is common. Most smokers who stop will begin using cigarettes again within 3 months. Among smokers who have abstained for 48 hours, nearly 20% relapse within the first week and an additional 13% relapse during the second week.[68] About 23% remain smoke free for 6 months. Relapse rates among those who participate in formal programs are somewhat better than they are for self-quitters.[69] Studies suggest that those smokers who slip are most likely to relapse. For example, a smoker who takes an occasional cigarette is significantly more likely to relapse than one who does not slip.[69,70] Readiness to change should also be assessed. Many smokers may be in a "precontemplation" phase in which they are nonreceptive to messages about quitting. Those who are already contemplating quitting might be better targets for a stop-smoking message.[71,72]

Perhaps the best predictor of relapse is low personal expectations for remaining smoke free.[68,72] Using electronic daily diaries, Shiffman and colleagues[73,74] have been able to determine what factors precipitate relapse. These studies suggest that lapses associated with self-reported stress or good mood were more likely to progress to relapses than those associated with eating or drinking.

Considerable literature on smoking cessation techniques has developed and is best summarized in the AHCPR Smoking Guideline.[66] Overall, self-help groups tend not to achieve better outcomes than control groups.[75] We urge the use of self-help materials in combination with some counseling intervention. Telephone counseling appears to offer significant benefits. In addition, several toll-free 800 numbers are now available. Many of these are summarized at www.helpguide.org/mental/quit_smoking_cessation.htm. Evidence does suggest that physicians and other health care providers can offer brief smoking cessation counseling in combination with pharmacologic intervention[75] and that these simple interventions enhance abstinence rates at 6 and 12 months.[76] The addition of nicotine replacement therapy has also been shown to increase long-term maintenance. Pharmacotherapy may be more effective for men than for women, particularly when it is used with combination with smoking cessation counseling.[77]

In an analysis of the potential for smoking cessation programs, the AHCPR considered the impact of applying their *Smoking Cessation Clinical Practice Guideline* for the U.S. population. The *Clinical Practice Guideline* identifies 15 different smoking cessation guidelines, ranging from minimal counseling to intensive counseling. Each intervention is considered with or without concomitant use of nicotine replacement in the form of gum or nicotine patches. The analysis assumed that the interventions would be available to 75% of adult smokers, which corresponds to the proportion that made a previous quit attempt. The model assumes that the program would yield 1.7 million new quitters, of whom 40% would have quit on their own and 60% may have been influenced in some way by the program to quit. Further, the model assumed that 8.8% of smokers would quit with no intervention, 10.7% would quit with minimal counseling, 12.1% would quit with brief counseling, and 18.7% would quit with counseling lasting more

TABLE 20-2	The 5-A Behavioral Counseling Framework for Helping Patients to Quit Smoking

Step	A	Task
1	Ask	*Ask* about tobacco use
2	Advise	*Advise* to quit through clear personalized messages
3	Assess	*Assess* willingness to quit
4	Assist	*Assist* to quit
5	Arrange	*Arrange* follow-up and support

Adapted from 2006 United States Preventive Services Taskforce, p 121.

than 10 minutes. Use of nicotine replacement would boost these effects further. The program would cost an estimated $6.3 billion, or about $32 per smoker. Cost per quality-adjusted life year (QALY) was estimated at $1915, placing it well below that of most programs that have been analyzed.[78]

A variety of excellent materials are available to help the patient through the cessation process. Some excellent self-help Web sites include the following:

- www.cancer.org/docroot/PED/content/ PED_10_13X_Guide_for_Quitting_ Smoking.asp
- www.lungusa.org/site/pp.asp? c=dvLUK9O0E&b=22931
- www.helpguide.org/mental/quit_smoking_ cessation.htm

However, a recent systematic review of randomized clinical trials and observational studies raised some questions about self-help strategies. When used alone, self-help appears to be ineffective. Person-to-person contact is an important aspect of intervention. Quit attempts are higher for tobacco counseling and pharmacotherapy, either used independently or in combination. Among pharmacotherapies, some of the best results have been obtained with buproprion.[79]

The United States Preventive Services Taskforce recommends a five-step approach for clinicians to guide tobacco-dependent patients toward smoking cessation. The five steps are described as the "5-A" behavioral framework. The 5 As are summarized in Table 20-2.

CONCLUSION

The typical regimen for patients with COPD requires many different behaviors. These might include the use of several different medications, exercise, O_2, respiratory and physiotherapy techniques, and other aspects of self-care. Adherence to this regimen can be challenging. In contrast to nearly every other medical condition, there are relatively few published studies evaluating the benefits of interventions to improve adherence among patients with COPD. Further, we do not know the extent to which overuse of medication is associated with poor outcomes for patients with COPD. Behavioral intervention may enhance adherence with medicine taking, smoking cessation, and exercise. However, considerably more research is necessary to evaluate the long-term benefits of these interventions.

References

1. DiMatteo MR: Variations in patients' adherence to medical recommendations: a quantitative review of 50 years of research, Med Care 42:200-209, 2004.
2. Dunbar-Jacob J: Chronic disease: a patient-focused view, J Prof Nurs 21:3-4, 2005.
3. Haynes RB, Taylor DW, Sackett DL: Compliance in health care, Baltimore, 1979, Johns Hopkins University Press.
4. Schlenk EA, Dunbar-Jacob J, Engberg S: Medication non-adherence among older adults: a review of strategies and interventions for improvement, J Gerontol Nurs 30:33-43, 2004.
5. DiMatteo MR, DiNicola DD: Achieving patient compliance: the psychology of the medical practitioner's role, New York, 1982, Pergamon Press.
6. Norell SE: Accuracy of patient interviews and estimates by clinical staff in determining medication compliance, Soc Sci Med [E] 15:57-61, 1981.
7. DiMatteo MR: Evidence-based strategies to foster adherence and improve patient outcomes, JAAPA 17:18-21, 2004.
8. DiMatteo MR, Giordani PJ, Lepper HS et al: Patient adherence and medical treatment outcomes: a meta-analysis, Med Care 40:794-811, 2002.
9. Norell SE: Memory and medication compliance, J Clin Hosp Pharm 10:107-109, 1985.
10. George J, Kong DC, Thoman R et al: Factors associated with medication nonadherence in patients with COPD, Chest 128:3198-3204, 2005.
11. Morrison D, Skwarski K, MacNee W: Review of the prescription of domiciliary long term oxygen therapy in Scotland, Thorax 50:1103-1105, 1995.
12. Restrick LJ, Paul EA, Braid GM et al: Assessment and follow up of patients prescribed long term oxygen treatment, Thorax 48:708-713, 1993.
13. Ringbaek TJ: Continuous oxygen therapy for hypoxic pulmonary disease: guidelines, compliance and effects, Treat Respir Med 4:397-408, 2005.
14. Neri M, Melani AS, Miorelli AM et al: Long-term oxygen therapy in chronic respiratory failure: a

Multicenter Italian Study on Oxygen Therapy Adherence (MISOTA), Respir Med 100:795-806, 2006.

15. Rand CS, Nides M, Cowles MK et al: Long-term metered-dose inhaler adherence in a clinical trial: the Lung Health Study Research Group, Am J Respir Crit Care Med 152:580-588, 1995.

16. Powell SG: Medication compliance of patients with COPD, Home Healthcare Nurse 12:44-50, 1994.

17. Turner J, Wright E, Mendella L et al; Predictors of patient adherence to long-term home nebulizer therapy for COPD. The IPPB Study Group: Intermittent Positive Pressure Breathing, Chest 108:394-400, 1995.

18. Solomon DK, Portner TS, Bass GE et al: Clinical and economic outcomes in the hypertension and COPD arms of a multicenter outcomes study, J Am Pharm Assoc (Wash) 38:574-585, 1998.

19. Nides MA, Rakos RF, Gonzales D et al: Predictors of initial smoking cessation and relapse through the first 2 years of the Lung Health Study, J Consult Clin Psychol 63:60-69, 1995.

20. James PN, Anderson JB, Prior JG et al: Patterns of drug taking in patients with chronic airflow obstruction, Postgrad Med J 61:7-10, 1985.

21. Corden ZM, Bosley CM, Rees PJ et al: Home nebulized therapy for patients with COPD: patient compliance with treatment and its relation to quality of life, Chest 112:1278-1282, 1997.

22. Lin SK, Kuna ST, Bogen DK: A novel device for measuring long-term oxygen therapy adherence: a preliminary validation, Respir Care 51:266-271, 2006.

23. Nides MA, Tashkin DP, Simmons MS et al: Improving inhaler adherence in a clinical trial through the use of the nebulizer chronolog, Chest 104:501-507, 1993.

24. Chryssidis E, Frewin DB, Frith PA et al: Compliance with aerosol therapy in chronic obstructive lung disease, N Z Med J 94:375-377, 1981.

25. DiMatteo MR, Haskard KB: Further challenges in adherence research: measurements, methodologies, and mental health care, Med Care 44:297-299, 2006.

26. Chia LR, Schlenk EA, Dunbar-Jacob J: Effect of personal and cultural beliefs on medication adherence in the elderly, Drugs Aging 23:191-202, 2006.

27. Stilley CS, Sereika S, Muldoon MF et al: Psychological and cognitive function: predictors of adherence with cholesterol lowering treatment, Ann Behav Med 27:117-124, 2004.

28. Rigsby MO, Rosen MI, Beauvais JE et al: Cue-dose training with monetary reinforcement: pilot study of an antiretroviral adherence intervention, J Gen Intern Med 15:841-847, 2000.

29. Adherence strategies. Telephone follow-ups improve virologic outcomes. Program could be worked into regular budget, AIDS Alert 21:113-114, 2006.

30. Downer SR, Meara JG, Da Costa AC et al: SMS text messaging improves outpatient attendance, Aust Health Rev 30:389-396, 2006.

31. Wu JY, Leung WY, Chang S et al: Effectiveness of telephone counselling by a pharmacist in reducing mortality in patients receiving polypharmacy: randomised controlled trial, BMJ 333:522, 2006.

32. Johnson MO, Chesney MA, Goldstein RB et al: Positive provider interactions, adherence self-efficacy, and adherence to antiretroviral medications among HIV-infected adults: a mediation model, AIDS Patient Care STDs 20:258-268, 2006.

33. Liang MH: Compliance and quality of life: confessions of a difficult patient, Arthritis Care Res 2:S71-S74, 1989.

34. Kaplan RM, Simon H: Compliance in medical care: reconsideration of self-predictions, Ann Behav Med 12:66-71, 1990.

35. Rains JC, Lipchik GL, Penzien DB: Behavioral facilitation of medical treatment for headache. I. Review of headache treatment compliance, Headache 46:1387-1394, 2006.

36. Richardson WC, Berwick DM, Bisgard JC et al The Institute of Medicine report on medical errors: misunderstanding can do harm. Quality of Health Care in America Committee, MedGenMed 2:E42, 2000.

37. Lazarou J, Pomeranz BH, Corey PN: Incidence of adverse drug reactions in hospitalized patients: a meta-analysis of prospective studies, JAMA 279:1200-1205, 1998.

38. Becker MH: Patient adherence to prescribed therapies, Med Care 23:539-555, 1985.

39. Halm EA, Mora P, Leventhal H: No symptoms, no asthma: the acute episodic disease belief is associated with poor self-management among inner-city adults with persistent asthma, Chest 129:573-580, 2006.

40. Idler E, Leventhal H, McLaughlin J et al: In sickness but not in health: self-ratings, identity, and mortality, J Health Soc Behav 45:336-356, 2004.

41. Kelly K, Leventhal H, Andrykowski M et al: Using the common sense model to understand perceived cancer risk in individuals testing for BRCA1/2 mutations, Psychooncology 14:34-48, 2005.

42. Arnold E, Bruton A, Ellis-Hill C: Adherence to pulmonary rehabilitation: a qualitative study, Respir Med 100:1716-1723, 2006.

43. Greenfield S, Kaplan S, Ware JE Jr: Expanding patient involvement in care: effects on patient outcomes, Ann Intern Med 102:520-528, 1985.

44. Schneider J, Kaplan SH, Greenfield S et al: Better physician–patient relationships are associated with higher reported adherence to antiretroviral therapy in patients with HIV infection, J Gen Intern Med 19:1096-1103, 2004.

45. Belfiglio M, De Berardis G, Franciosi M et al: The relationship between physicians' self-reported target fasting blood glucose levels and metabolic control in type 2 diabetes: the QuED Study Group—quality of care and outcomes in type 2 diabetes, Diabetes Care 24:423-429, 2001.

46. Ries AL: The importance of exercise in pulmonary rehabilitation, Clin Chest Med 15:327-337, 1994.

47. Lacasse Y, Goldstein R, Lasserson TJ et al: Pulmonary rehabilitation for chronic obstructive pulmonary disease, Cochrane Database Syst Rev 4:CD003793, 2006.

48. Cockram J, Cecins N, Jenkins S: Maintaining exercise capacity and quality of life following pulmonary rehabilitation, Respirology 11:98-104, 2006.

49. Simons-Morton DG, Calfas KJ, Oldenburg B et al: Effects of interventions in health care settings on physical activity or cardiorespiratory fitness, Am J Prev Med 15:413-430, 1998.

50. Friedman DB, Williams AN, Levine BD: Compliance and efficacy of cardiac rehabilitation and risk factor modification in the medically indigent, Am J Cardiol 79:281-285, 1997.

51. Resnikoff PM, Ries AL: Maximizing functional capacity: pulmonary rehabilitation and adjunctive measures, Respir Care Clin N Am 4:475-492, 1998.

52. Cockcroft AE, Saunders MJ, Berry G: Randomised controlled trial of rehabilitation in chronic respiratory disability, Thorax 36:200-203, 1981.

53. McGavin CR, Gupta SP, Lloyd EL et al: Physical rehabilitation for the chronic bronchitic: results of a controlled trial of exercises in the home, Thorax 32:307-311, 1977.

54. Ambrosino N, Paggiaro PL, Macchi M et al: A study of short-term effect of rehabilitative therapy in chronic obstructive pulmonary disease, Respiration 41:40-44, 1981.

55. Sassi-Dambron DE, Eakin EG, Ries AL et al: Treatment of dyspnea in COPD: a controlled clinical trial of dyspnea management strategies, Chest 107:724-729, 1995.

56. Ries AL, Kaplan RM, Limberg TM et al: Effects of pulmonary rehabilitation on physiologic and psychosocial outcomes in patients with chronic obstructive pulmonary disease, Ann Intern Med 122:823-832, 1995.

57. Eakin EG, Kaplan RM, Ries AL: Measurement of dyspnoea in chronic obstructive pulmonary disease, Qual Life Res 2:181-191, 1993.

58. Ries AL, Kaplan RM, Myers R et al: Maintenance after pulmonary rehabilitation in chronic lung disease: a randomized trial, Am J Respir Crit Care Med 167:880-888, 2003.

59. Heppner PS, Morgan C, Kaplan RM et al: Regular walking and long-term maintenance of outcomes after pulmonary rehabilitation, J Cardiopulm Rehabil 26:44-53, 2006.

60. Atkins CJ, Kaplan RM, Timms RM et al: Behavioral exercise programs in the management of chronic obstructive pulmonary disease, J Consult Clin Psychol 52:591-603, 1984.

61. Redline S, Tager IB, Speizer FE et al: Longitudinal variability in airway responsiveness in a population-based sample of children and young adults: intrinsic and extrinsic contributing factors, Am Rev Respir Dis 140:172-178, 1989.

62. Dockery DW, Speizer FE, Ferris BG Jr et al: Cumulative and reversible effects of lifetime smoking on simple tests of lung function in adults, Am Rev Respir Dis 137:286-292, 1988.

63. Camilli AE, Burrows B, Knudson RJ et al: Longitudinal changes in forced expiratory volume in one second in adults. Effects of smoking and smoking cessation, Am Rev Respir Dis 135:794-799, 1987.

64. Ockene JK, Zapka JG: Physician-based smoking intervention: a rededication to a five-step strategy to smoking research, Addict Behav 22:835-848, 1997.

65. Ockene JK, Adams A, Pbert L et al: The Physician-Delivered Smoking Intervention Project: factors that determine how much the physician intervenes with smokers, J Gen Intern Med 9:379-384, 1994.

66. Fiore MC: Overview of the Agency for Health Care Policy and Research guideline, Tob Control 7(suppl):S14-S16[discussion S24-S15], 1998.

67. Ockene JK, Aney J, Goldberg RJ et al: A survey of Massachusetts physicians' smoking intervention practices, Am J Prev Med 4:14-20, 1988.

68. Gulliver SB, Hughes JR, Solomon LJ et al: An investigation of self-efficacy, partner support and daily stresses as predictors of relapse to smoking in self-quitters, Addiction 90:767-772, 1995.

69. Brandon TH, Tiffany ST, Obremski KM et al: Postcessation cigarette use: the process of relapse, Addict Behav 15:105-114, 1990.

70. Baer JS, Kamarck T, Lichtenstein E et al: Prediction of smoking relapse: analyses of temptations and transgressions after initial cessation, J Consult Clin Psychol 57:623-627, 1989.

71. Boudreaux E, Carmack CL, Searinci IC et al: Predicting smoking stage of change among a sample of low socioeconomic status, primary care outpatients: replication and extension using decisional balance and self-efficacy theories, Int J Behav Med 5:148-165, 1998.

72. Boudreaux ED, Hunter GC, Bos K et al: Predicting smoking stage of change among emergency department patients and visitors, Acad Emerg Med 13:39-47, 2006.

73. Shiffman S: Reflections on smoking relapse research, Drug Alcohol Rev 25:15-20, 2006.

74. Shiffman S, Scharf DM, Shadel WG et al: Analyzing milestones in smoking cessation: illustration in a nicotine patch trial in adult smokers, J Consult Clin Psychol 74:276-285, 2006.

75. Ranney LM, Melvin CL, Rohweder CL: From guidelines to practice: a process evaluation of the National Partnership to Help Pregnant Smokers Quit, AHIP Cover 46:50-52, 2005.

76. Morgan GD, Noll EL, Orleans CT et al: Reaching midlife and older smokers: tailored interventions for routine medical care, Prev Med 25:346-354, 1996.

77. Perkins KA, Grobe JE, Caggiula A et al: Acute reinforcing effects of low-dose nicotine nasal spray in humans, Pharmacol Biochem Behav 56:235-241, 1997.

78. Cromwell J, Bartosch WJ, Fiore MC et al: Cost-effectiveness of the clinical practice recommendations in the AHCPR guideline for smoking cessation: Agency for Health Care Policy and Research, JAMA 278:1759-1766, 1997.

79. Ranney L, Melvin C, Lux L et al: Systematic review: smoking cessation intervention strategies for adults and adults in special populations, Ann Intern Med 145(11):845-856, 2006.

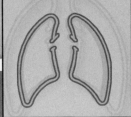

Chapter 21

Outcome Assessment

RICHARD ZuWALLACK

CHAPTER OUTLINE

Rationale for Outcome Assessment
Tests of Exercise Performance
  Incremental Exercise Testing
  Endurance Exercise Testing
  Walk Tests
Dyspnea Assessment
  Exertional Breathlessness
  Breathlessness Associated
    with Activities
Health-Related Quality of Life
  The CRQ
  The SGRQ
  The SF-36

Questionnaire-Measured Functional
    Status
  EADL Scale
  The PFSS
  The PFSDQ
Direct Measurements of Physical
    Activity
Nutritional Status
Multidimensional Staging of Chronic
    Obstructive Pulmonary Disease
    and Pulmonary Rehabilitation
Survival
Health Care Use
Which Outcome Measure(s) to Choose

PROFESSIONAL SKILLS

On completion of this chapter, the reader will be able to do
the following:
* Explain the importance and rationale of outcome assessment in pulmonary rehabilitation
* Describe the availability of outcome assessment in several areas, including exercise ability, dyspnea,
  health-related quality of life (HRQL), functional status, and nutritional status
* List the advantages and disadvantages of various forms of exercise testing for chronic lung disease,
  such as incremental exercise testing, endurance testing at a constant workload, the timed walk test,
  and the incremental shuttle walking test
* Specify the two major forms of dyspnea assessment in chronic lung disease: the rating of exertional
  dyspnea during exercise testing and questionnaire-measured dyspnea, usually in association with daily
  activities
* Describe the concept and rationale of HRQL measurement in respiratory assessment and appreciate
  the differences between generic and respiratory-specific instruments
* Explain the differences between functional status and quality of life instruments and the importance of
  evaluating the effect of severe lung disease on activities of daily living
* Indicate the importance of nutritional and body composition abnormalities in advanced chronic lung
  disease

RATIONALE FOR OUTCOME ASSESSMENT

The American Thoracic Society/European Respiratory Society Statement on Pulmonary Rehabilitation indicates that its goals include reduced symptoms, optimized functional status, increased participation, and reduced health care costs.[1] In general, outcome assessment is used to quantify the improvement in these and other outcome areas. This can be in the form of documenting individual patient gains or assessing the overall effectiveness of the program.

Although the pulmonary physiologic abnormalities associated with advanced chronic lung disease are usually irreversible, pulmonary rehabilitation often leads to measurable and clinically meaningful benefits.[2] The reason is that a substantial portion of the morbidity from chronic respiratory disease is not directly related to the respiratory disease. For instance, although pulmonary rehabilitation does not increase the forced expiratory volume in 1 second (FEV_1) in chronic obstructive pulmonary disease (COPD), it improves peripheral muscle and cardiovascular conditioning, alleviates dyspnea through better pacing and breathing strategies, and reduces anxiety associated with dyspnea-producing activities. The role of outcome assessment in pulmonary rehabilitation is to capture these and other favorable changes.

Box 21-1 lists some of the rationale for outcome assessment in pulmonary rehabilitation. In view of its complexity, no single outcome assessment can capture the degree and breadth of improvement from the pulmonary rehabilitation intervention. Therefore, assessment in multiple areas is often advisable. Some areas of outcome assessment are listed in Box 21-2.

Outcome assessment can also be viewed from three perspectives: the individual patient's, the pulmonary rehabilitation program's, and the third-party payer's. Monitoring progression toward specific patient-centered goals may help provide positive feedback to the patient and enhance motivation and outcome. Evaluation of outcome across several areas allows the program to provide a quality assessment and may help direct changes toward improving the intervention. The objective demonstration of improvement in outcomes, especially in areas of health care use, may provide support among third-party payers to increase necessary funding for pulmonary rehabilitation.

BOX 21-1	Rationale for Outcome Measurement in Pulmonary Rehabilitation

- Outcomes such as decreased dyspnea and improved quality of life are of paramount importance to the patient yet correlate poorly with physiologic abnormalities. These outcomes are easily measured before and after rehabilitation.
- Baseline impairment in symptoms, exercise performance, functional status, and quality of life varies widely among patients entering pulmonary rehabilitation. Knowledge of baseline status might allow the rehabilitation staff to focus intervention on those areas most affected.
- Although the individual program's pulmonary rehabilitation intervention is usually roughly the same for each patient, the degree of improvement among patients often varies widely.
- Patients allowed to see objective evidence of their improvement might be better motivated to continue with long-term rehabilitation efforts.
- Feedback on outcomes can be useful for rehabilitation staff in maintaining morale and in adjusting rehabilitation therapy components to provide optimal results.
- Prerehabilitation to postrehabilitation outcome assessment provides objective evidence for third-party payers on the effectiveness of the individual pulmonary rehabilitation program.
- Clinical research on the effectiveness of pulmonary rehabilitation or its components requires accurate outcome measurement.

For scientific studies of pulmonary rehabilitation outcome, randomization of patients to a treatment or control group is usually necessary. However, the inclusion of an untreated or partially treated control group is not feasible for typical clinically oriented pulmonary rehabilitation programs. For these, simple assessment of prerehabilitation to postrehabilitation changes in a few outcome areas without a control group is usually sufficient to document individual patient gains and the overall effectiveness of the program.

Even in randomized, controlled clinical trials, the patient obviously cannot be blinded to the pulmonary rehabilitation intervention. Therefore effort-dependent outcome measures, such as the timed walk test, are potentially influenced by motivation or encouragement.[3] Other outcome areas, such as questionnaire-measured health-related quality of life (HRQL), are subjective and potentially affected by the patient's desire to please the rehabilitation staff.

BOX 21-2	Examples of Outcome Assessment in Pulmonary Rehabilitation

Laboratory tests of exercise performance
- Incremental exercise test to peak workload
- Steady state endurance test

Field tests of exercise performance
- Self-paced: the 6-minute timed walk test
- Externally paced: the incremental and steady state shuttle walking tests

Dyspnea
- Exertional dyspnea: the Visual Analog Scale and Borg category scale
- Overall dyspnea: the Baseline and Transitional Dyspnea Indexes and the Medical Research Council Dyspnea Scale

Questionnaire measures of health-related quality of life
- Generic: the Medical Outcomes Study Short-Form 36
- Respiratory specific: the Chronic Respiratory Disease Questionnaire and the St. George's Respiratory Questionnaire

Questionnaire measure of functional status
- Generic: the Extended Activities of Daily Living Scale
- Respiratory specific: the Pulmonary Functional Status Scale and the Pulmonary Functional Status and Dyspnea Questionnaire

Nutritional status
Activity measurement
Survival
Health care use

The mere demonstration that a change resulting from pulmonary rehabilitation is statistically significant is not sufficient for clinical purposes—ideally, the favorable effect should also be demonstrated to be clinically relevant and meaningful.[4] Established or suggested clinically meaningful changes for the 6-Minute Walk Test (approximately 50 m)[5]; two HRQL measures, including the Chronic Respiratory Disease Questionnaire (CRQ)[6] (0.5 unit per question) and the St. George's Respiratory Questionnaire (SGRQ)[7] (4 units); and the Transition Dyspnea Index (TDI) (1 unit)[8] are available at this time.

Although outcome assessments before and shortly after rehabilitation treatment are easiest to perform, the documentation of long-term benefit is also important. It has become clear that some of the gains made from pulmonary rehabilitation wane over the ensuing year.[9,10] Therefore consideration should be given to assessment at intervals of months or years after completion of the formal program.

TESTS OF EXERCISE PERFORMANCE

Incremental Exercise Testing

Incremental exercise testing on a bicycle ergometer or treadmill to maximal tolerance or to a heart rate of about 85% of predicted provides an objective and reproducible measurement of exercise performance. Measurements of heart rate, respiratory rate, blood pressure, electrocardiographic tracings, and oxygen saturation are routinely monitored. With analysis of expired gases, the determination or calculation of minute ventilation, oxygen consumption, carbon dioxide production, anaerobic threshold, and respiratory dead space is possible. Additional information can be obtained by having the patient rate the level of exertional dyspnea or leg fatigue at intervals during the testing. In patients with COPD, dyspnea or leg fatigue may be the predominant exercise-limiting symptom in this testing.

A listing of some randomized, controlled trials of pulmonary rehabilitation or exercise training demonstrating the usefulness of incremental exercise testing is given in Table 21-1. In general, these studies have shown relatively small increases in peak oxygen consumption but more impressive increases in peak exercise workload after the period of exercise training. For example, in a study by Ries and colleagues[10] comparing comprehensive outpatient pulmonary rehabilitation with education alone, the rehabilitation group did not significantly increase their peak oxygen consumption at 2 months after therapy (+0.11 L/min; $P = .10$) but did increase their maximal treadmill workload by 1.5 metabolic equivalents—a 33% improvement over baseline. Similarly, a randomized, controlled study of 6 weeks of supervised exercise training in COPD[11] showed no significant change in peak oxygen consumption after exercise training (0.92 vs. 0.97 L/min) but did show a 33% increase in peak cycle work rate, from 36 to 48 W. Finally, in an 18-month study comparing hospital-based outpatient pulmonary rehabilitation with a home-based setting, the hospital-based program resulted in a 20% increase in peak workload at 3 months, with a gradual decrease in effectiveness at 12 and 18 months. In contrast, the home-based program resulted in a gradual increase in maximal workload during this time period, peaking at 21% over baseline at 18 months.[12]

In addition to quantifying improvement in peak exercise performance, incremental exercise testing is useful in demonstrating changes in

TABLE 21-1	Examples of Incremental Exercise Testing in Pulmonary Rehabilitation Outcome Assessment		
Investigator	**Intervention**	**Incremental Test**	**Results**
Casaburi et al (1991)[13]	8 wk of inpatient rehabilitation; low (n = 8) vs. high (n = 11) work rate exercise training groups	Cycle ergometer	Both groups had a low lactate threshold; the higher work rate group had more training effect demonstrated by greater decreases in heart rate, lactate, $\dot{V}_E$, $\dot{V}CO_2$, and $\dot{V}_E/\dot{V}O_2$ at identical postexercise work rates
Reardon et al (1994)[38]	6 wk of comprehensive outpatient rehabilitation (n = 10) vs. untreated control group (n = 10)	Treadmill	No significant improvement occurred in maximal exercise performance after pulmonary rehabilitation; the treatment group, however, did have significant decreases in VAS-rated dyspnea measured during incremental testing
Ries et al (1995)[10]	8 wk of outpatient rehabilitation (n = 57) vs. education alone (n = 62)	Treadmill	The rehabilitation group had greater increases in maximal exercise work load and $\dot{V}O_2$ and greater decreases in perceived dyspnea and fatigue at maximal workload than did the education control group
O'Donnell et al (1995)[11]	Outpatient exercise training (n = 30) vs. an untreated, matched control group	Cycle ergometer	The treatment group showed preintervention to postintervention improvement in peak work rate and significant reductions in dyspnea and leg effort
Strijbos et al (1996)[12]	Hospital-based outpatient (n = 15) vs. home care–based outpatient rehabilitation (n = 15) vs. an untreated control group (n = 15)	Cycle ergometer	The hospital-based outpatient group showed a 19.8% increase in Wmax at 3 mo, and then a gradual decrease in this improvement over time; the home-based group showed a more gradual increase in Wmax over time, with a 20.7% increase over baseline by 18 mo
Wijkstra et al (1996)[52]	12 wk of comprehensive home rehabilitation (n = 23) vs. no rehabilitation (n = 15)	Cycle ergometer	Thirty-nine of 43 patients had a ventilatory limitation to their exercise; the rehabilitation group had a greater increase in Wmax and peak $\dot{V}O_2$ and a greater decrease in dyspnea at Wmax than the control group

VAS, *Visual Analog Scale*; $\dot{V}CO_2$, *peak carbon dioxide uptake*; $\dot{V}_E$, *minute ventilation*; $\dot{V}O_2$, *peak oxygen uptake*; Wmax, *maximal work level.*

physiology resulting from exercise training. This is usually accomplished by measuring variables at *identical* workloads before and after therapy. This utility is demonstrated in a study by Casaburi and colleagues,[13] who compared high- and moderate-intensity stationary bicycle exercise training in individuals with moderately severe COPD. Eleven patients were randomized to the high-intensity exercise and nine to the moderate-intensity exercise protocol. Lactate production and resultant increased ventilatory demand was present in both groups at low exercise workloads. After the course of exercise training, only the group given high-intensity exercise training showed a true physiologic training effect, with decreases in blood lactate and minute ventilation at identical levels of exercise at follow-up testing (Figure 21-1). In addition, their reduction in minute ventilation was proportional to their decrease in lactate production.

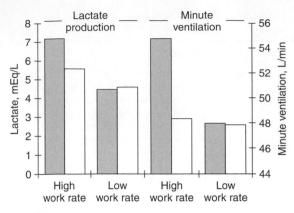

FIGURE 21-1 A comparison of high and low levels of exercise training on the physiologic adaptation to exercise. Eleven patients with chronic obstructive pulmonary disease were given high-intensity exercise training and 9 were given low-intensity exercise training for 8 weeks. Baseline values are represented by the *shaded columns*, postexercise training values by the *open columns*. Post-training responses were measured at the same work rate as in the pretraining study. The group given the high-intensity training had greater reductions in lactate and minute ventilation, indicating a greater physiologic training effect.

As the previously described study illustrates, incremental exercise testing can uncover the physiologic basis for favorable effects of exercise training in pulmonary rehabilitation. Despite this advantage, this type of exercise testing is limited by the expertise it requires, its expense, and some inconvenience to the patient.

Endurance Exercise Testing

Endurance testing on a stationary bicycle or treadmill usually involves exercising at a constant work rate for as long as tolerated. The work rate is usually set at a constant fraction of a peak work rate (such as 85%) determined at a previous incremental exercise test. The duration for which the patient can perform at this constant, high work rate is the outcome measure. Because the exercise level is set by the investigator, self-pacing is not a potential confounding variable as with self-paced tests, such as the timed walk test. Exercise endurance measured in this fashion often shows considerable improvement after pulmonary rehabilitation,[10,14,15] probably reflecting the latter's emphasis on lower extremity exercise training.

The usefulness of endurance exercise testing in demonstrating improvement is illustrated in the randomized, controlled study of pulmonary rehabilitation by Ries and associates.[10] A total of 119 patients with COPD were randomized to either

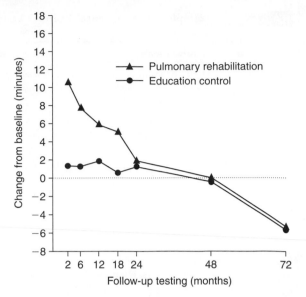

FIGURE 21-2 The effect of comprehensive pulmonary rehabilitation on treadmill exercise endurance time.

comprehensive outpatient rehabilitation (n = 57) or education only (n = 62) groups. Treadmill exercise endurance testing was performed at approximately 95% of the patient's maximal exercise tolerance. The initial exercise endurance times in the rehabilitation and control groups (12.4 ± 8.4 and 11.8 ± 8.0 minutes, respectively) were similar. Figure 21-2 shows changes in this outcome measure over the study period. Treadmill endurance time was essentially unchanged in the control group, but did increase significantly in the rehabilitation group in the months immediately after pulmonary rehabilitation. For the latter group, the 10.5-minute increase in endurance time at 2 months represented an 85% increase over baseline. The favorable effects of rehabilitation remained statistically significant at 6 months and tended to be greater up to 18 months later. After this, any beneficial effect was lost.

More recently, endurance exercise testing has also been useful in demonstrating underlying physiologic mechanisms responsible for decreases in dyspnea and increases in exercise performance. For instance, in COPD static and dynamic hyperinflation of the lungs contribute to the sensation of dyspnea and limit exercise performance.[16] Spirometry during exercise testing done before and after a treatment (such as bronchodilators or exercise training) *at identical work rates* (isowork or isotime) can detect differences in lung volumes such as the inspiratory capacity. Assuming there is no change in total lung capacity, a decrease in inspiratory capacity at isowork or isotime indicates the end-expiratory lung volume (and degree of hyperinflation) has increased. Lung hyperinflation in patients with COPD is decreased after pulmonary rehabilitation when lung volumes are assessed at isowork endurance testing. This probably reflects less ventilatory demand from the prolonged exercise training stimulus, allowing for a lower respiratory rate at isowork, thereby allowing more time for expiration and emptying of the lungs.[17]

Walk Tests

Timed Walk Test

The timed walk test has probably become the most widely used measure of exercise performance in pulmonary rehabilitation. For this test, the patient is given instructions to walk as far as possible in a corridor or large room during an allotted period of time, usually 6 or 12 minutes.[18,19] More recently a 2-Minute Walk Test has been demonstrated to be reliable and valid,[20] although, by far, most clinical and research experience is with the 6-minute test. The distance covered is recorded as the outcome measure.

The popularity of the timed walk test in pulmonary rehabilitation probably results from several features: (1) it is easy to administer, requires no special equipment, and is well tolerated by the patient; (2) the type and intensity of the exercise are relevant to many common daily activities; (3) it is responsive to pulmonary rehabilitation intervention; and (4) reasonable estimates exist of what represents a clinically meaningful change in the 6-minute walk distance.[5] The importance of the walk test is underscored by its incorporation as the major outcome variable in the National Emphysema Therapy Trial, a multicenter investigation to evaluate the effectiveness of lung volume reduction surgery for emphysema.[21]

Despite its advantages, the walk test is potentially biased by practice or learning effect and the positive effect of encouragement from rehabilitation personnel. For instance, in a study by Larson and colleagues[22] evaluating weekly 12-Minute Walk Test performance in stable patients, a 7% increase in distance was present at the second walk, a 4% further increase was found at the third walk, and a 2% improvement at the fourth walk. This 7% increase from the first to the second walk was also seen in the National Emphysema Therapy Trial study.[23] Therefore a minimum of two timed walks (with rests of approximately 15 minutes between them) is needed to reduce practice effect to a reasonably low level. Encouragement, supplied by the staff member administering the test, has been shown to increase the 6-minute walk distance by approximately 30 m[24]—a change not too different from that attributed to the rehabilitation intervention in some studies. For this reason, standardization of encouragement is also a necessary component of the timed walk test. The American Thoracic Society has published guidelines on how to perform a 6-Minute Walk Test.[25] A protocol giving specific directions for 6-minute walk testing[26] is outlined in Box 21-3.

The timed walk test is usually responsive to pulmonary rehabilitation intervention, probably reflecting the emphasis most programs give to lower extremity training. This is illustrated in Figure 21-3, which shows a meta-analysis of the effects of pulmonary rehabilitation on walk test performance from 11 randomized, controlled clinical trials. The favorable effect of treatment, which was +55.7 m, was not only statistically significant but exceeded the estimated minimal clinically important difference for the 6-minute walk distance of 54 m.[5]

Shuttle Walking Test

The progressive 10-m shuttle walking test[27] is an externally paced measure of exercise capacity for individuals with chronic lung disease. For this test the patient must walk up and down a 10-m distance defined by marker cones 0.5 m from either end. Walking pace is set by repetitive beeping signals from an audiocassette player. Instructions are given to walk at a steady pace with a goal of reaching the opposite marker cone at the next beeping signal. Initially, the time interval between the beeping signals is such that the patient must walk at 0.5 m/second to get to the opposite end in time. This speed is increased at 1-minute intervals by shortening the time between beeping signals. The test end point is determined when the patient becomes too breathless to keep up with the pace or is unable to complete the shuttle in the time allowed. The total distance (number of completed shuttles times 10 m) is calculated as the outcome.

Although the timed walk test and the shuttle walking tests are "field" measures of distance walked, they differ in certain areas, as outlined in Table 21-2. Being incremental in nature, the shuttle walking test is more a measure of exercise capacity. In contrast, the timed walk test is probably more a measure of exercise endurance.

BOX 21-3   **Recommended Protocol for the Timed Walk Test**

EQUIPMENT

Rolling distance marker and stopwatch; spirometer; pulse oximeter

EXCLUSION CRITERIA

Patients with musculoskeletal problems that significantly limit walking such as paralysis, pain, and psychiatric problems that would contribute to suboptimal walking performance; uncontrolled angina or hypertension, hypoxia, recent history of cardiac dysrhythmia or myocardial infarction; and other significant medical conditions that might be exacerbated by physical exertion

PROCEDURE

1. Before the first walk, dyspnea (10-point Borg Scale), blood pressure, pulse, and respiratory rate are measured and recorded for all patients. In addition, any medications, such as an inhaled β-agonist or nitroglycerine, that might ordinarily be taken before activity should be self-administered. For patients with COPD and asthma, postbronchodilator spirometry and baseline oximetry should be carried out 15 minutes after taking their β-agonist.

2. Walks will take place at approximately the same time of day, at least 2 hours after a meal.

3. Patients will be asked to walk from end to end of the walking track, covering as much ground as possible in 6 minutes.

4. The walks should be carried out in an area with minimal traffic that is at least 100 ft in length. Ambient temperature at that location should be recorded.

5. Two walks will be carried out with at least 15 minutes of rest between each walk. Consider carrying out the tests with more time between each walk or over two consecutive days for more disabled individuals.

6. The following instructions will be given to subjects: "The purpose of this test is to find out how far you can walk in 6 minutes. You will start from this point [indicate marker at one end of the course] and follow the hallway to the marker at the end, then turn around and walk back. When you arrive back at the starting

point, you will go back and forth again. You will go back and forth as many times as you can in the 6-minute period. If you need to, you may stop and rest. Just remain where you are until you can go on again. However, the most important thing about the test is that you cover as much ground as you possibly can during the 6 minutes. I will tell you the time, and I will let you know when the 6 minutes are up. When I say 'stop,' please stand right where you are." Subjects are then asked to repeat the gist of the instructions to validate understanding.

7. During the first walk, pulse oximetry will be carried out during the test on everyone. Patients receiving supplemental oxygen will use their oxygen at the prescribed flow rate for exercise. Patients who desaturate to levels below 85% will be asked to stop walking and the walk test will be discontinued. Oxygen therapy may be considered, and if instituted, these patients may then be restudied.

8. During the walks, the following words of encouragement will be provided at 30-second intervals: "You're doing well," "keep up the good work," "good job," "you're doing fine."

9. With the exception of the first walk, during which pulse oximetry will be performed, staff will walk behind the patient so as not to influence his or her pace and will attempt to face the patient only when offering encouragement.

10. Patients are told when 2, 4, and 6 minutes (Stop) have elapsed.

11. The longest distance walked of the three trials will be noted, although all distances will be documented. Duration of time spent resting will also be recorded.

12. Immediately after completion of each walking test, patients will be asked to rate their level of breathing effort on the Borg Scale and to indicate which symptom limited walking (shortness of breath, leg pain, etc.)

From Steele B: Timed walking tests of exercise capacity in chronic cardiopulmonary disease, J Cardiopulm Rehab 16:25-33, 1996.

In addition, unlike the timed walk test, the shuttle test is not affected by self-pacing because pace is externally set.

As might be expected, the shuttle walking distance correlates well with peak oxygen consumption ($r = 0.88$) from incremental treadmill exercise.[28] The Incremental Shuttle Walk Test is responsive to therapy. In a randomized, controlled trial of pulmonary rehabilitation of patients with COPD, those given hospital-based rehabilitation had an 88-m increase in shuttle distance, representing a 46% increase over baseline.[29]

The Endurance Shuttle Walk Test is a constant rate, field-based, endurance test developed to complement the Incremental Shuttle Walk Test. For this, patients are instructed to walk around the 10-m shuttle course at an externally paced speed of approximately 80% of their maximum, which was determined from an earlier incremental test.[30] This type of testing is similar to constant

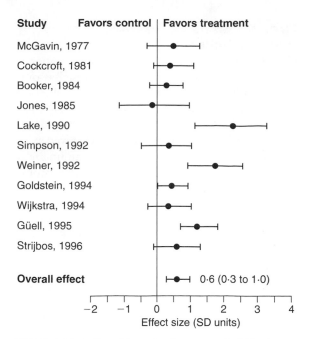

FIGURE 21-3 The effect of pulmonary rehabilitation on walking distance.

TABLE 21-2	Comparison of the Timed Walk Test and Incremental Shuttle Walking Test

Timed Walk Test	Incremental Shuttle Walking Test
Testing is done in the "field"	Testing is done in the "field"
Walking distance is the outcome measured	Walking distance is the outcome measured
More of a steady state measure of exercise endurance	An incremental measure of exercise capacity
Self-pacing is potentially important in influencing performance	Speed is set externally, reducing or eliminating self-pacing effects

work rate treadmill or bicycle endurance testing. After pulmonary rehabilitation the endurance shuttle walk distance increased by 24%, demonstrating its responsiveness to this intervention.[30]

DYSPNEA ASSESSMENT

Dyspnea, or breathlessness, is usually the principal symptom limiting exercise in patients with advanced pulmonary disease and is probably the most important factor influencing their health-related quality of life.[31,32] In patients with

COPD, breathlessness is often most pronounced during tasks requiring unsupported arm exercise, probably because this type of activity places both ventilatory and nonventilatory burdens on the accessory respiratory muscles.[33] Dyspnea is correlated with respiratory physiologic abnormalities such as airway obstruction or lung hyperinflation.[16] It is also modulated by other factors, such as anxiety, depression, hysteria, social support, grief, fear, and past life experiences.[34] In addition, the effort component of dyspnea can be distinguished from its anxiety and distress components,[35] although the clinical importance of this distinction has yet to be determined.

In pulmonary rehabilitation outcome assessment, two forms of dyspnea measurement are generally used: (1) the level of exertional breathlessness during a specific task, such as exercise testing or a timed walk, and (2) overall breathlessness during daily activities.

Exertional Breathlessness

In moderately advanced respiratory disease, either dyspnea or leg discomfort (or both) usually limits exercise, whereas in severe disease dyspnea is usually the limiting symptom.[36] Exertional dyspnea can be measured with a 10- or 20-point category scale, such as the Borg Scale,[37] or it can be rated with a Visual Analog Scale. For the latter, the patient rates the intensity of dyspnea by pointing along a 100- or 200-mm vertical line. The vertical distance from the bottom of the line to this point is the level of dyspnea. The line is often anchored at either end with descriptors such as "greatest breathlessness" and "no breathlessness."

Pulmonary rehabilitation is an effective treatment for exertional dyspnea in patients with COPD. An example of its effectiveness is demonstrated in a study by Reardon and colleagues,[38] who randomized patients referred for pulmonary rehabilitation into either a treatment group (6 weeks of outpatient rehabilitation, n = 10) or a control group (6-week waiting period, n = 10). Incremental treadmill exercise testing was performed before and after the rehabilitation intervention or the waiting period. At 1-minute intervals during the testing, the patient rated his or her level of exertional dyspnea, using a linear Visual Analog Scale. Exertional dyspnea was unchanged in the control group but significantly reduced in the rehabilitation group. For the latter, the reduction in dyspnea was detectable early in the exercise and was maintained until peak workload

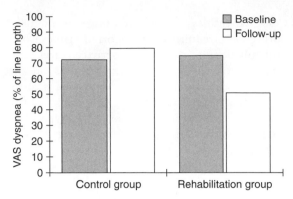

FIGURE 21-4 Changes in exertional dyspnea with pulmonary rehabilitation. Patients referred for outpatient pulmonary rehabilitation were randomized into a treatment group (n = 10) given 6 weeks of pulmonary rehabilitation or into a control group (n = 10) that waited 6 weeks to begin rehabilitation. Dyspnea was measured with a Visual Analog Scale (VAS) at regular intervals during incremental treadmill exercise. The *columns* represent VAS values at peak workload at baseline and after either the waiting period or the rehabilitation period. Maximal exercise capacity did not change significantly in either group. Pulmonary rehabilitation patients, however, had significant decreases in VAS-measured exertional dyspnea.

was reached. The ratio of dyspnea to minute ventilation was also decreased in this study, suggesting that the improvement in dyspnea was not just owing to a decreased ventilatory demand resulting from exercise training. The changes in dyspnea at peak workload are depicted in Figure 21-4.

Another example of exertional dyspnea as an outcome measurement for pulmonary rehabilitation is given in a study by O'Donnell and colleagues,[11] who studied the impact of 6 weeks of exercise conditioning on dyspnea and leg fatigue of individuals with COPD. Results were compared with a control group that did not receive exercise training. Exercise was limited primarily by dyspnea and secondarily by leg fatigue, both before and after intervention. Despite an increase in exercise performance on cycle ergometer testing after the exercise training period, exertional dyspnea in the treatment group decreased, dropping from 5.3 to 3.8 ($P < .001$) on a 10-point Borg Scale at peak exercise.

The exercise training group also had a significant reduction in minute ventilation (due primarily to a decrease in respiratory frequency) at a standardized work rate. In multiple regression analysis, the reduction in dyspnea was predicted best by the reduction in ventilatory demand.

Breathlessness Associated with Activities

Overall dyspnea associated with daily activities is measured by questionnaire. Examples used as outcome measures for pulmonary rehabilitation include the Medical Research Council Dyspnea Scale; the Baseline Dyspnea Index and Transitional Dyspnea Index (BDI and TDI)[39-41]; the University of California, San Diego, Dyspnea Questionnaire[10]; and the dyspnea domain of the Chronic Respiratory Disease Questionnaire (CRQ).[42]

For the modified Medical Research Council Dyspnea Scale, the patient rates his or her level of dyspnea by choosing, from a scale of 0 to 4, that descriptor which best gives the degree of breathlessness:

MMRC 0: Not troubled with breathlessness except with strenuous exercise

MMRC 1: Short of breath when hurrying or walking up a slight hill

MMRC 2: Walks slower than people of same age due to breathlessness or has to stop when walking at own pace on the level

MMRC 3: Stops for breath after walking about 100 meters or after a few minutes on the level

MMRC 4: Too breathless to leave the house or breathless when dressing or undressing

Originally the MRC was developed on a scale of 1 to 5, with the same descriptors, so the reader should be sure what scale range is being used.

The BDI and TDI are interviewer-administered questionnaires that assess dyspnea through its effect on daily activities. The instrument takes about 3 to 4 minutes to complete.[39] The BDI has three scales: functional impairment, magnitude of task, and magnitude of effort. Each is scored on a 0 (severe) to 4 (no impairment) scale. The focal score, which sums the three, can therefore range from zero (most limitation from dyspnea) to 12 (no limitation from dyspnea). Changes in limitation in the areas of functional impairment, magnitude of task, and magnitude of effort are rated with the TDI. Each is scored on a −3 (major deterioration) to 0 (no change) to +3 (major improvement) scale. The focal TDI score, which sums the three, therefore, can range from −9 (greatest increase in limitation owing to dyspnea) to +9 (greatest reduction in limitation owing to dyspnea).

Some pulmonary rehabilitation studies using the BDI and TDI in outcome measurement are listed in Table 21-3. These studies indicate that

TABLE 21-3 Examples of Randomized Controlled Studies of Pulmonary Rehabilitation with Dyspnea Measured by Questionnaire

Study	Treatment Intervention	Dyspnea Measure	Outcome
Reardon et al (1994)[38]	6 wk of OPR	BDI/TDI	TDI increased significantly in the treatment group (+2.3 units) compared with control subjects (0.2) (P = .006)
Goldstein et al (1994)[14]	8 wk of IPR and 16 wk of supervised outpatient training	BDI/TDI, CRQ dyspnea	TDI increased by 2.7 units (P = .005); CRQ dyspnea increased by a clinically meaningful 3.0 units (P = .006)
Ries et al (1995)[10]	8 wk of OPR	UCSD Shortness of Breath Questionnaire	Improvement in questionnaire score by 7.0 units at 2-mo measurement after OPR (P < .01); beneficial effect gradually waned over ensuing months
O'Donnell et al (1995)[11]	6 wk of a multimodality exercise endurance program	BDI/TDI	TDI increased by 2.8 units (P < .001)
Cambach et al (1997)[15]	3 mo of home-based pulmonary rehabilitation	CRQ dyspnea	Significant and clinically meaningful improvement in CRQ dyspnea at 3 mo (+6 units) and 6 mo (+5 units) after pulmonary rehabilitation

BDI, *Baseline Dyspnea Index*; CRQ, *Chronic Respiratory Disease Questionnaire*; IPR, *inpatient pulmonary rehabilitation*; OPR, *outpatient pulmonary rehabilitation*; TDI, *Transitional Dyspnea Index*; UCSD, *University of California, San Diego*.

the mean improvement in overall dyspnea during daily activities as reflected in the focal TDI score is between 2 and 3 units. In contrast, a clinical trial comparing the bronchodilators ipratropium and salmeterol in COPD demonstrated 1.18 and 1.07 units, respectively, in TDI dyspnea resulting from these drugs.[43]

The University of California, San Diego Shortness of Breath Questionnaire is a 24-item instrument developed by the pulmonary rehabilitation program at that institution. It assesses dyspnea associated with 21 activities of daily living (ADLs) by having the patient rate each on a six-point scale. The questionnaire also has three additional questions that assess limitations caused by shortness of breath, fear of overexertion, and fear of shortness of breath. The usefulness of this questionnaire as an outcome measure was demonstrated by the controlled trial of pulmonary rehabilitation by Ries and colleagues.[10] Although the education-treated control group had no significant change in dyspnea by this measure, the rehabilitation group had a significant, 7.0-unit decrease in dyspnea by 2 months. This represents a 19.6% improvement over baseline.

The CRQ is a 20-item instrument that measures HRQL for patients with COPD. (This is discussed in more detail later in this chapter.) The dyspnea domain of this questionnaire consists of five questions that require the patient to rate five dyspnea-producing activities, each on a 1-to-7 scale. The activities must be dyspnea producing, performed regularly, and of importance to the patient. Thus, the dyspnea assessment is unique to the individual.

HEALTH-RELATED QUALITY OF LIFE

Quality of life is a somewhat nebulous concept that refers to the individual's satisfaction or happiness with life in domains that he or she considers important. In this general sense, quality of life is affected by factors not necessarily related to health, such as job satisfaction, quality of housing, financial security, family and social interaction, and spiritual fulfillment.[44] HRQL, on the other hand, focuses only on those areas of life satisfaction affected by alterations in health and its treatments.[45] Instruments measuring this, therefore, must quantify the impact of disease and its treatment on important daily life activities and the sense of well-being.[46]

Because a cure for COPD is not possible and standard medical therapy is often only partially effective in relieving symptoms, improvement in HRQL is important to consider in evaluating the effectiveness of its therapy. HRQL measurement provides useful complementary information to physiologic measurements such as the FEV_1. HRQL is, by nature, specific to the individual patient. Therefore, the questions are answered by the patient, never by a spouse or a member of the pulmonary rehabilitation staff. Questionnaires can be generic and applicable to most disease states or respiratory specific, focusing on aspects of health influenced by lung disease. Areas of respiratory-specific HRQL measurement may include the effects of respiratory symptoms (especially dyspnea or fatigue), social or role function, emotional function, limitation of activity, the impact of the disease on the individual, and the patient's sense of mastery over the disease.

HRQL is usually informally assessed by the health care provider in the clinical setting, using unstructured questions aimed at assessing the patient's symptoms, functional limitations, participation in social activities, and sense of well-being. The clinician probably does not consider this routine activity as HRQL assessment, but it is. Validated questionnaires provide a more formalized assessment of HRQL. These were designed to assess groups of patients such those in a clinical trial or those completing pulmonary rehabilitation, and results are usually expressed in the aggregate. Whether results from an HRQL questionnaire prove useful in assessing the status or response to therapy of an *individual* patient is not clear.

The ideal HRQL questionnaire for pulmonary rehabilitation should be short and easy to understand and should be self-administered or easy for staff to administer. In addition, it should have both discriminative and evaluative properties. The former refers to its ability to distinguish individuals with better HRQL from those with worse HRQL, whereas the latter refers to its ability to detect small changes after therapy or over time.

The following discussion touches on three HRQL questionnaires commonly used in pulmonary rehabilitation assessment: the respiratory-specific Chronic Respiratory Disease Questionnaire (CRQ), the St. George's Respiratory Questionnaire (SGRQ), and the generic Medical Outcomes Study Short-Form 36 (SF-36).

The CRQ

The CRQ[41] is perhaps the most widely used HRQL questionnaire in pulmonary rehabilitation assessment. This 20-item interviewer-administered questionnaire, which takes about 20 minutes to

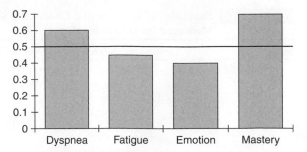

FIGURE 21-5 The effect of pulmonary rehabilitation on HRQL. The *columns* represent treatment effects: change in the CRQ domain scores for rehabilitation patients minus corresponding changes in the domain scores for the untreated control group. Results are expressed as mean per-question changes. Each question can range from 1 (lowest score) to 7 (highest score). The *horizontal line* indicates a clinically meaningful 0.5-unit change per question.

complete, has a total score and four domain scores: dyspnea, fatigue, emotion, and mastery—the sense of control over the disease. The dyspnea domain consists of five questions unique to the individual. For these, the patient must identify five important activities done in the preceding 2 weeks that were associated with breathlessness. A list of 26 activities is provided for suggestions. The dyspnea associated with each of the five chosen activities is then scored with a seven-point scale ranging from 1, extremely short of breath, to 7, not at all short of breath. The 15 questions used to assess the three remaining domains are also scored with a seven-point scoring system, with higher scores indicating less impairment in HRQL. A 0.5-unit per question change resulting from therapy is considered clinically meaningful (Figure 21-5).[47]

The tailoring of the dyspnea questions to the individual patient enhances the ability of the questionnaire to detect changes in HRQL, making this a desirable tool for outcome assessment in pulmonary rehabilitation. Its responsiveness is probably further enhanced by allowing patients to see their previous responses.[48] The five individual-specific questions rating dyspnea, however, diminish the discriminative abilities of this questionnaire. For example, one patient with mild respiratory disease might choose a dyspnea-producing activity such as jogging and another with severe disease might choose walking. The usefulness of the CRQ in the outcome assessment of pulmonary rehabilitation is shown in Figure 21-5.

The original CRQ is interviewer administered. However, two validated, self-administered versions

TABLE 21-4 Examples of Randomized, Controlled Studies of Pulmonary Rehabilitation Using the Chronic Respiratory Disease Questionnaire to Measure Health-related Quality of Life

Study	Type of Rehabilitation	Change in CRQ* in Treatment Group
Goldstein et al (1994)[14]	Inpatient pulmonary rehabilitation for 8 wk followed by supervised outpatient training for 16 wk	Improvements in dyspnea (0.6 units, $P = .006$), emotion (0.4 units, $P = .015$), and mastery (0.7 units, $P = .0002$) domains; the change in fatigue approached statistical significance (0.45, $P = .051$)[†]
Wijkstra et al (1994)[52]	Home-based comprehensive pulmonary rehabilitation for 12 wk	Improvements in dyspnea (0.9 units), emotion (0.6 units), fatigue (0.9 units), and mastery (0.6 units) domains (all, $P < .001$)
Cambach et al (1997)[15]	3 mo of home-based pulmonary rehabilitation	Improvements in dyspnea (1.2 units), fatigue (1.0 units), emotion (0.9 units), and mastery (0.75 units) domains at 3 mo[‡]
Bendstrup et al (1997)[54]	Comprehensive outpatient pulmonary rehabilitation for 12 wk	Improvement in the total CRQ score by 0.3 units at 6 wk, 0.4 units at 12 wk, and 0.6 units at 24 wk; the improvement in the 24-wk measurement was statistically significant
Wedzicha et al (1998)[29]	8 wk of comprehensive outpatient pulmonary rehabilitation; hospital based for those with moderate dyspnea, home based for those with severe dyspnea	For patients with moderate dyspnea given hospital-based intervention, the total CRQ score increased by 0.7 units ($P < .0001$); for those given home pulmonary rehabilitation, total CRQ score increased by 0.2 units, which was significantly greater than its baseline ($P < .05$), not different from the change in an education control group

*CRQ domain scores are expressed as mean change per question. Each question is scored on a scale of 1 to 7. A 0.5-unit change per question is considered clinically significant.
†Treatment effects (change in rehabilitation group CRQ minus change in control group CRQ).
‡Patients with asthma and COPD were studied. These results are from the subgroup (RC) with COPD.
CRQ, Chronic Respiratory Disease Questionnaire.

of this instrument have been developed.[49,50] These should greatly facilitate HRQL assessment in the clinical setting. Controlled clinical trials of pulmonary rehabilitation using the interviewer-administered CRQ in outcome assessment are listed in Table 21-4.[51-54]

The SGRQ

The SGRQ[7] is a 76-item respiratory-specific self-administered questionnaire requiring about 15 minutes to complete. Unlike the CRQ, the instrument can also be used for asthma as well as COPD. It measures HRQL in three domains: symptoms (distress owing to respiratory symptoms), activity (the effects owing to impairment of mobility or physical activity), and impacts (the psychosocial impact of the disease). A summary score can also be calculated. Another feature of the SGRQ is that the scoring of individual questions is weighted on the basis of empirically derived weights. Each of the three domains and the total score can range from 0 (no reduction in HRQL) to 100 (maximal reduction in HRQL). Questions specifically related to anxiety or

depression were intentionally excluded from the SGRQ, and thus a separate questionnaire would have to be given to capture this outcome area.

Because HRQL is a multidimensional concept, it should be understandable that it is influenced by several aspects of the individual's morbidity. For example, a multiple regression analysis evaluating factors related to the SGRQ[55] identified dyspnea, depression, wheeze, and the 6-minute walk distance as predictors of the total SGRQ score. Interestingly, the FEV_1 was not significantly predictive in this model. These varied factors, however, explained less than 50% of the variance in HRQL. Dyspnea is a strong predictor of SGRQ-measured HRQL,[31] as illustrated in Figure 21-6.

A decrease in an SGRQ domain or total score by 4 units or more (i.e., 4% of its range) is considered a clinically meaningful improvement. The questionnaire has adequate reliability and validity and has been shown to be able to detect clinically meaningful changes in HRQL in patients with COPD given the long-acting bronchodilator salmeterol (Figure 21-7).[56] The SGRQ has also been able to detect favorable change resulting from the use of nasal intermittent positive-pressure ventilation in hypoxemic, hypercapnic COPD.[57] The SGRQ has not been shown, however, to be particularly responsive to detecting favorable changes resulting from pulmonary rehabilitation. For instance, in a randomized, controlled study of pulmonary rehabilitation by Wedzicha and colleagues[29] that used both the CRQ and the SGRQ as outcome measures, the investigators were able to show improvement in the treatment group with the CRQ but not the SGRQ. The SGRQ, however, has been used successfully to discriminate

between groups of patients with varying levels of disease severity. For example, in a study evaluating the effects of long-term oxygen therapy,[58] patients with hypoxemic COPD had much higher SGRQ scores (i.e., worse quality of life) than their nonhypoxemic counterparts.

The SF-36

The SF-36 is a 36-item self-complete questionnaire that measures general HRQL in eight areas.[59] Five of its scales (physical functioning, role-physical, bodily pain, social functioning, and role-emotional) define HRQL as the absence of limitation or disability. For these, a score of 100 indicates no limitations or disabilities. Three scales (general health, vitality, and mental health) are bipolar and measure negative and positive states. For these, a score of 50 indicates no limitations or disability and scores between 50 and 100 indicate positive health states. Two SF-36 summary scores, the physical component summary and the mental component summary, have been introduced.[60] These summary scores are standardized to have a mean of 50 and a standard deviation of 10 in normal populations. The SF-36 questionnaire takes just a few minutes to complete, but its scoring requires a considerable amount of hand calculation or computer assistance.

A general HRQL measure such as the SF-36 might be expected to be less able to detect changes

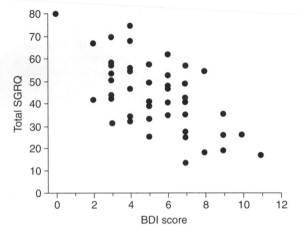

FIGURE 21-6 The relationship between dyspnea and health-related quality of life. BDI, Baseline Dyspnea Index; SGRQ, St. George's Respiratory Questionnaire.

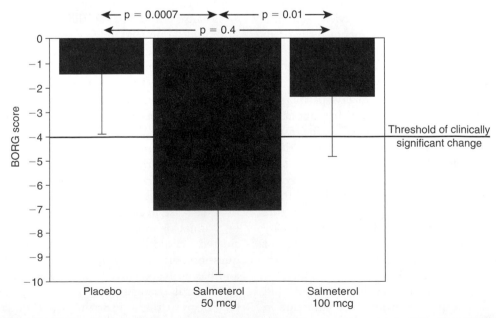

FIGURE 21-7 The effect of long-acting bronchodilator therapy on the health-related quality of life of patients with COPD. SGRQ, St. George's Respiratory Questionnaire.

resulting from pulmonary rehabilitation than respiratory-specific measures such as the CRQ. However, the SF-36 is indeed sensitive enough to demonstrate improvement in HRQL resulting from pulmonary rehabilitation.[61,62] Furthermore, its wider scope might allow for better detection of comorbidity, which is so common and important in individuals referred to pulmonary rehabilitation. One shortcoming is that a threshold for clinically meaningful change with this instrument has not been clearly defined. Changes in the SF-36, however, have been shown to correlate with changes in patient-perceived health over time.[63] Several questionnaire scales, especially physical functioning, social functioning, role-physical, pain, vitality, and general health, have been found to correlate well with measures of COPD disease severity.[64] In patients with COPD, dyspnea is, by far, the strongest predictor of SF-36 scores.[64]

QUESTIONNAIRE-MEASURED FUNCTIONAL STATUS

Functional status refers to the extent individuals perform their usual behaviors and activities without limitation from health problems.[65] For individuals with advanced lung disease, functional status relates predominantly to the individual's ability to perform ADLs.[66] ADLs serve to meet basic physical, psychological, social, or spiritual needs; fulfill usual roles; and maintain health and well-being.[67] In a model by Leidy,[68] functional status can be considered as having four dimensions: capacity, performance, reserve, and capacity utilization (Figure 21-8). *Functional capacity* refers to the maximal potential to perform daily activities, analogous to the peak oxygen consumption in incremental exercise testing. *Functional performance* refers to the daily activities

actually done, which for most individuals is considerably less than functional capacity. *Functional reserve* reflects the difference between performance and capacity, and *functional capacity utilization* indicates how close functional performance approaches functional capacity.

ADLs, which are physical components of functional performance, can be divided into basic and instrumental activities.[69] Basic ADLs include tasks concerned with daily self-care, such as feeding, dressing, personal hygiene, bowel function, and physical mobility. Many patients with chronic lung disease have dyspnea with these activities but remain able to perform them. Instrumental ADLs include higher level tasks necessary to adapt independently to the environment,[70] such as cooking, shopping, home chores, walking outdoors, housework, doing laundry, driving a car, and gardening. Because they are more complex and require more energy expenditure than basic ADLs, they are more likely to be affected by respiratory disease. Limitation or elimination of instrumental ADLs, usually from associated dyspnea or fatigue, is a major component of the handicap from advanced chronic lung disease.

The concepts, functional status and HRQL, are not interchangeable. HRQL represents the gap between what is desired and what is achievable within the confines of the disease process.[71] In essence, it reflects in large part the impact of symptoms and limitation in ADLs on the individual patient. Therefore functional status is an important *component* of HRQL.

Patients with chronic respiratory disease that is severe enough to warrant referral for pulmonary rehabilitation often have significant impairments in ADLs. Milder disease usually is associated with unpleasant symptoms such as dyspnea or fatigue attached to that activity, but the activity is still performed as usual. With more severe disease and activities that require higher energy expenditure, physical activities may have to be decreased in frequency or intensity because of symptom limitation. Finally, in advanced disease, more and more physical activities are given up altogether. In this sense, the decreased physical activity becomes adaptive through keeping distressing symptoms at a minimum.

Although HRQL instruments have items pertaining to functional status, questionnaires that focus on ADLs explore this area of morbidity in more depth. The generic Extended Activities of Daily Living (EADL) Scale[72] and two respiratory-specific

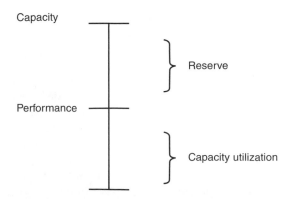

FIGURE 21-8 Functional status components.

questionnaires, the Pulmonary Functional Status Scale (PFSS)[73] and the Pulmonary Functional Status and Dyspnea Questionnaire (PFSDQ),[74] which have been used in pulmonary rehabilitation assessment, are discussed.

EADL Scale

The EADL Scale, a 22-item generic questionnaire, rates the performance (yes–no) in 22 extended (i.e., instrumental) ADLs in four domains: (1) *mobility* (walking outside, climbing stairs, getting in and out of a car, walking over uneven ground, crossing the street, using public transport), (2) *kitchen activities* (eating, making a hot drink, carrying hot drinks from room to room, washing, preparing a snack), (3) *domestic tasks* (managing money, washing small clothing items, housework, shopping, full laundry), and (4) *leisure activities* (reading newspaper or book, telephoning, writing letters, going out socially, gardening, driving a car).

The EADL Scale was able to discriminate between 23 patients with COPD who were oxygen dependent and 19 patients with slightly less severe airflow obstruction but no oxygen dependency.[75] In contrast, the HRQL measure, the SGRQ, was not significantly different for the two groups. EADL Scale scores were related to the degree of airflow obstruction, HRQL, and mood state.

The PFSS

The PFSS is a 56-item, self-administered questionnaire that gives a total score and subscores of daily activities/social functioning, dyspnea, and psychological status. Completion time is about 15 minutes. The daily activities/social functioning subscore, which measures functional performance, has components of self-care, daily activities, household tasks, grocery shopping and meal preparation, transportation (mobility), and relationships. PFSS functional activities correlates strongly ($r = 0.76$) with the timed walk distance.[76] Although this questionnaire to date has not been used much as an evaluative instrument, an uncontrolled study showed its ability to detect a positive response to rehabilitative intervention.[76,77] The responsiveness of the individual daily activities/social functioning component scores to inpatient pulmonary rehabilitation is depicted in Figure 21-9.

The PFSDQ

The PFSDQ is a 164-item, self-administered questionnaire that requires about 15 to 20 minutes

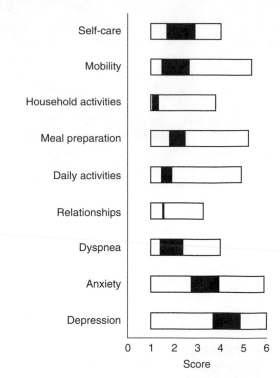

FIGURE 21-9 The effect of inpatient pulmonary rehabilitation on functional activities. The *left* and *right margins* of the *solid bars* indicate the preinpatient and postinpatient pulmonary rehabilitation mean scores, respectively; the *left* and *right margins* of the *open bars* indicate minimal and maximal attainable scores, respectively.

to complete. The limitation in performance and the level of dyspnea are rated separately for each activity. The questionnaire has component scores of self-care, mobility, eating, home management, social activities, and recreational activities. Its activity total score correlates weakly with the percent-predicted FEV_1 and moderately with maximal oxygen consumption on exercise testing.[78] The PFSDQ can discriminate varying degrees of airway obstruction in COPD[79] and can detect change resulting from pharmacologic intervention.[80]

A much-shortened, modified version of the PFSDQ, the PFSDQ-M, has been developed. Ten common activities are rated separately for activity (whether it is still done), associated dyspnea, and associated fatigue. These categories include brushing or combing hair, putting on a shirt, washing hair, showering, raising arms over head, preparing a snack, walking 3.5 m, walking on inclines, walking on bumpy terrain, and climbing three stairs.

Both the PFSDQ and the PFSDQ-M hold promise as measures of activity limitation and associated dyspnea for individuals with advanced lung disease. However, their ability to detect changes resulting from pulmonary rehabilitation has not been fully explored.

DIRECT MEASUREMENTS OF PHYSICAL ACTIVITY

One of the goals of pulmonary rehabilitation is to increase physical activity. This has become even more important because lower activity levels are now known to be associated with increased health care use and mortality in COPD.[81] Furthermore, patients with COPD have been found to be quite inactive physically when sophisticated activity monitors are used to measure this activity.[82] This activity is especially decreased for prolonged periods of time after an exacerbation of COPD.[83] It is unclear at the present time whether the increases in exercise performance that follow pulmonary rehabilitation are necessarily translated into increased physical activity in the home setting. In this vein, direct measurement of activity might become a useful outcome measure for pulmonary rehabilitation. This will require the development and testing of a sensitive motion detector (pedometers may be too insensitive to detect some of the slow-motion activity of people with advanced lung disease) that would be relatively inexpensive and reliable. Furthermore, there would have to be the development of an understanding of what actually represents a clinically meaningful change in activity counts from direct measurements.

NUTRITIONAL STATUS

Abnormalities in nutritional status in individuals with chronic lung disease include increases or decreases in body weight and abnormalities in body composition. Body weight can be assessed as a percentage of ideal body weight or as the body mass index (expressed as kilograms per meter squared). In patients with COPD, decreased weight is associated with increased mortality independent of lung function.[84] Low body weight is also associated with decreased exercise performance on timed walk testing[85] and reduced muscle aerobic capacity during incremental stationary bicycle exercise.[86]

Body composition can be evaluated by anthropometry or bioelectrical impedance analysis, which estimate fat-free mass, or dual-energy X-ray absorptiometry, which estimates lean mass.

Reductions in fat-free or lean body mass, which reflect the impact of advanced pulmonary disease on the peripheral musculature, may even be present in patients with normal weight.[87] Alterations in body composition are correlated with impaired performance on timed walk testing and poorer HRQL independent of body weight. An example of the effect of body weight and composition on HRQL is given in Figure 21-10.

In view of its prevalence and its relationship to the morbidity and mortality of patients with advanced chronic lung disease, the measurement of nutritional status should be considered as an

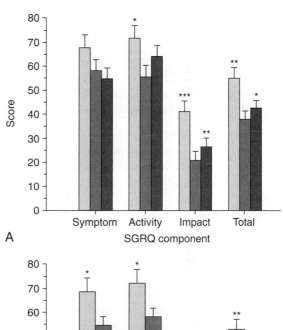

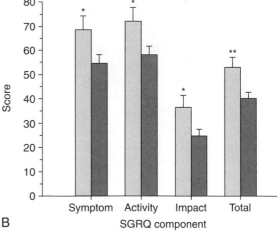

FIGURE 21-10 The relationship between **A,** body weight (*open columns,* underweight patients; *hatched columns,* normal-weight patients; *cross-hatched columns,* overweight patients) and **B,** body composition, (*open columns,* patients with low lean mass; *hatched columns,* patients with normal lean mass) and SGRQ-measured HRQL. *$P < .05$, **$P < .01$, and ***$P < .001$ versus patients with normal weight and normal composition. SGRQ, St. George's Respiratory Questionnaire.

outcome measure for pulmonary rehabilitation. However, to date, nutritional intervention has met with questionable success in patients with COPD,[88] and more recent studies have focused on hormonal supplementation to increase lean mass.[89] Six months of therapy with oral anabolic steroids in nutritionally depleted patients with COPD did increase the body mass index, lean body mass, and arm and leg circumference, but it did not affect endurance exercise capacity.[90] More recently, the combination of testosterone and resistance weight training in hypogonadal men with COPD did increase lean body mass and strength more than either component alone.[91] The role of hormonal therapy remains to be determined.

MULTIDIMENSIONAL STAGING OF CHRONIC OBSTRUCTIVE PULMONARY DISEASE AND PULMONARY REHABILITATION

Although the objective diagnosis of chronic obstructive pulmonary disease rests on the demonstration of airflow limitation (i.e., FEV_1/FVC [forced vital capacity] <0.70 on spirometry), patients with this disease often have important systemic manifestations not captured by the FEV_1. For instance, dyspnea, exercise performance on a cycle ergometer, the 6-Minute Walk Test, and mean leg or arm circumference are all more robust predictors of survival than the FEV_1. The reason is that COPD is, in reality, a systemic disease. This knowledge has led to the development of a multi-component scoring system to better characterize the severity of the disease. In 2004 Celli and colleagues[92] reported on the BODE scoring, which included four variables: *b*ody mass index, airflow *o*bstruction (FEV_1 percent predicted), *d*yspnea level (modified MRC dyspnea score), and *e*xercise capacity (6-Minute Walk Test distance). Scores in each of these four areas were combined to give a composite BODE score, which can range from 0 (best health) to 10 (worst health). The BODE score proved to be a better predictor of risk of death from COPD than the FEV_1. In a subsequent study testing patients with COPD in a veterans hospital,[93] the BODE score significantly improved (a 19% increase over baseline) after pulmonary rehabilitation. This improvement is shown in Figure 21-11. This study demonstrates the potential usefulness of the BODE Index as an outcome measure for pulmonary rehabilitation.

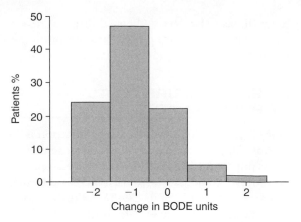

FIGURE 21-11 The effect of pulmonary rehabilitation on the BODE score. The BODE Index is a multidimensional index incorporating the following four variables: *b*ody mass index, airway *o*bstruction (the FEV_1), *d*yspnea, and *e*xercise capacity (the 6-Minute Walk Test). The score can range from 0 (worst) to 10 (best).

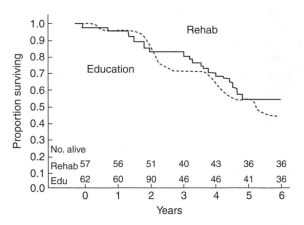

FIGURE 21-12 The effect of outpatient pulmonary rehabilitation on survival.

SURVIVAL

To date, only one randomized, controlled study of pulmonary rehabilitation has evaluated the effect of pulmonary rehabilitation on long-term survival. Ries and colleagues[10] randomly assigned patients with COPD to either an 8-week comprehensive outpatient pulmonary rehabilitation program (57 patients) or to a control group given educational sessions (62 patients). Although 67% of the rehabilitation group versus 56% of the education control group were still alive at 6 years, this difference was not statistically significant ($P = .3$). The survival graph from this study is given in Figure 21-12.

HEALTH CARE USE

Uncontrolled studies of health care use in pulmonary rehabilitation generally compare the number of hospital days or emergency department visits during a period of time before rehabilitation with a period of time after rehabilitation. These studies are subject to a regression to the mean bias because patients are often referred to pulmonary rehabilitation after a deterioration in condition that resulted in medical resource consumption.

One controlled study of outpatient pulmonary rehabilitation by Ries and colleagues[10] included an analysis of health care use, which consisted of self-reports of hospitalizations at each annual follow-up visit during a 6-year period. The mean number of hospital days in the year before randomization was not significantly different for the two groups: 6.4 days for the rehabilitation group and 3.6 days for the control group. At 12 months, the mean number of days for the rehabilitation group decreased by 2.4 days, whereas it increased by 1.3 days for the control group. This difference, however, was not statistically significant ($P = .2$).

A study by Bourbeau and colleagues[94] evaluated the effectiveness of a COPD-specific self-management intervention in patients with COPD who had at least one hospitalization for exacerbation. The intervention consisted of a comprehensive patient education program administered through weekly visits by trained health professionals over a 2-month period, followed up by monthly telephone calls. Hospitalizations for exacerbations of COPD decreased by 39.8% with this intervention compared with a group that received usual care. These positive results suggest that self-management education is complementary to exercise training in pulmonary rehabilitation. More outcome research is needed in this area. Two collaborative studies that used a before-after design without a control group have demonstrated health care use reductions in California[95] and the northeastern United States.[96]

WHICH OUTCOME MEASURE(S) TO CHOOSE

Measurement of outcomes should be incorporated into every comprehensive pulmonary rehabilitation program. The extent of assessment will logically depend on the purpose of the measurement, the goals of the program, and the level of clinician expertise in the evaluation of outcomes. Most clinical programs are not equipped to do a survival or

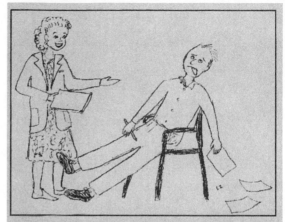

"Well, Mr. Smith, you've completed your PFTs, your exercise test, two practice and one real six-minute walk, the SF-36, the CRDQ and the SGRQ - now it's time to begin your exercise training!"

FIGURE 21-13 The potential effect of including too many outcome measures in pulmonary rehabilitation. CRDQ, Chronic Respiratory Disease Questionnaire; PFTs, pulmonary function tests; SF-36, Medical Outcomes Study Short-Form 36; SGRQ, St. George's Respiratory Questionnaire.

cost-effectiveness analysis of their patients—that is best reserved for multicenter, controlled trials. The BODE score, which incorporates body mass index, airway obstruction, dyspnea, and exercise capacity, might prove to be a useful outcome tool in patients with COPD but will not be applicable to patients with other diseases.

For clinical purposes, assessment of exercise ability, dyspnea, and HRQL is reasonable and probably not too burdensome to the staff. The 6-Minute Walk Test has proved to be an excellent field measure of functional exercise performance for pulmonary rehabilitation. The BDI and TDI, likewise, are valid and able to detect changes resulting from pulmonary rehabilitation. The CRQ has the best track record as a responsive instrument for evaluating pulmonary rehabilitation, and the newer, self-administered versions will greatly facilitate its administration.

Whichever measures are chosen for outcome assessment, certainly the situation portrayed in Figure 21-13[97] is to be avoided.

References

1. Nici L, Donner C, Wouters E et al: American Thoracic Society/European Respiratory Society Statement on Pulmonary Rehabilitation, Am J Respir Crit Care Med 173:1390-1413, 2006.

2. Ries AL, Bauldoff GS, Carlin BW et al: Pulmonary rehabilitation: joint ACCP/AACVPR evidence-based clinical practice guidelines, Chest 131(5 suppl):4S-42S, 2007.

3. Guyatt GH, Pugsley O, Sullivan MJ et al: Effect of encouragement on walking test performance, Thorax 39:818-822, 1984.

4. Juniper EF: Quality of life questionnaires: does statistically significant = clinically important? J Allergy Clin Immunol 102:16-17, 1998.

5. Redelmeier DA, Bayoumi AM, Goldstein RS et al: Interpreting small differences in functional status: the Six Minute Walk Test in chronic lung disease patients, Am J Respir Crit Care Med 155:1278-1282, 1997.

6. Guyatt GH, Townsend M, Pugsley SO et al: Bronchodilators in chronic air-flow limitation, Am Rev Respir Dis 135:1069-1074, 1987.

7. Jones PW, Quirk FH, Baveystock CM et al: A self-complete measure for chronic airflow limitation: the St. George's Respiratory Questionnaire, Am Rev Respir Dis 145:1321-1327, 1992.

8. Witek TJ, Mahler DA: Minimal important difference of the transition dyspnoea index in a multinational clinical trial, Eur Respir J 21:267-272, 2003.

9. Vale F, Reardon JZ, ZuWallack RL: The long-term benefits of outpatient pulmonary rehabilitation on exercise endurance and quality of life, Chest 103:42-45, 1993.

10. Ries AL, Kaplan RM, Limberg TM et al: Effects of pulmonary rehabilitation on physiologic and psychosocial outcomes in patients with chronic obstructive pulmonary disease, Ann Intern Med 122:823-832, 1995.

11. O'Donnell DE, McGuire M, Samis L et al: The impact of exercise reconditioning on breathlessness in severe chronic airflow limitation, Am J Respir Crit Care Med 152:2005-2013, 1995.

12. Strijbos JH, Postma DS, van Altena R et al: A comparison between an outpatient hospital-based pulmonary rehabilitation program and a home-care pulmonary rehabilitation program in patients with COPD, Chest 109:366-372, 1996.

13. Casaburi R, Patessio A, Loli F et al: Reductions in exercise lactic acidosis and ventilation as a result of exercise training in patients with obstructive lung disease, Am Rev Respir Dis 143:9-18, 1991.

14. Normandin EA, McCusker C, Connors M et al: An evaluation of two approaches to exercise conditioning in pulmonary rehabilitaion, Chest 121:1085-1091, 2002.

15. Casaburi R, Kufafka D, Cooper CB et al: Improvement in exercise tolerance with the combination of tiotropium and pulmonary rehabilitaion in patients with COPD, Chest 127:809-817, 2005.

16. O'Donnell DE, Revill SM, Webb KA: Dynamic hyperinflation and exercise intolerance in chronic obstructive pulmonary disease, Am J Respir Crit Care Med 164:770-777, 2001.

17. Porszasz J, Emtner M, Goto S et al: Exercise training decreases ventilatory requirements and exercise-induced hyperinflation at submaximal intensities in patients with COPD, Chest 128:2025-2034, 2005.

18. McGavin CR, Gupta SP, McHardy GJR: Twelve-minute walking test for assessing disability in chronic bronchitis, Br Med J 1:822-823, 1976.

19. Mungall IPF, Hainsworth R: Assessment of respiratory function in patients with chronic obstructive airways disease, Thorax 34:254-258, 1979.

20. Leung ASY, Chan KK, Sykes K et al: Reliability, validity, and responsiveness of a 2-min walk test to assess exercise capacity of COPD patients, Chest 130:119-125, 2006.

21. National Emphysema Treatment Trial Research Group: A randomized trial comparing lung-volume-reduction surgery with medical therapy for severe emphysema, N Engl J Med 348:2059-2073, 2003.

22. Larson JL, Covey MK, Vitalo CA et al: Reliability and validity of the 12-minute distance walk in patients with chronic obstructive pulmonary disease, Nurs Res 45:203-210, 1996.

23. Sciurba F, Criner GJ, Lee SM et al: Six-minute walk distance in chronic obstructive pulmonary disease. reproducibility and effect of walking course layout and length, Am J Respir Crit Care Med 167:1522-1527, 2003.

24. Guyatt GH, Pugsley O, Sullivan MJ et al: Effect of encouragement on walking test performance, Thorax 39:818-822, 1984.

25. American Thoracic Society: Guidelines for the Six-Minute Walk Test, Am J Respir Crit Care Med 166:111-117, 2002.

26. Steele B: Timed walking tests of exercise capacity in chronic cardiopulmonary disease, J Cardiopulm Rehab 16:25-33, 1996.

27. Singh SJ, Morgan MDL, Scott S et al: Development of a shuttle walking test of disability in patients with chronic airways obstruction, Thorax 47:1019-1024, 1992.

28. Singh SJ, Morgan MDL, Hardman AE et al: Comparison of oxygen uptake during a conventional treadmill test and the shuttle walking test in chronic airflow limitation, Eur Respir J 7:2016-2020, 1994.

29. Wedzicha JA, Bestall JC, Garrod R et al: Randomized controlled trial of pulmonary rehabilitation in severe chronic obstructive pulmonary disease patients, stratified with the MRC Dyspnoea Scale, Eur Respir J 12:363-369, 1998.

30. Revill SM, Morgan MDL, Singh SJ et al: The Endurance Shuttle Walk: a new field test for the assessment of endurance capacity in chronic obstructive pulmonary disease, Thorax 54:213-222, 1999.

31. Shoup R, Dalsky G, Warner S et al: Body composition and health-related quality of life in patients with chronic obstructive airways disease, Eur Respir J 10:1576-1580, 1997.

32. Siafakas NM, Schiza S, Xirouhaki N et al: Is dyspnoea the main determinant of quality of life in the failing lung? A review, Eur Respir Rev 7:53-56, 1997.

33. Celli B, Rassulo J, Make B: Dyssynchronous breathing during arm but not leg exercise in patients with chronic airflow obstruction, N Engl J Med 314:1485-1490, 1986.

34. Sweer L, Zwillich CW: Dyspnea in the patient with chronic obstructive pulmonary disease: etiology and management, Clin Chest Med 11:417-439, 1990.

35. Carrieri-Kohlman V, Gormley JM, Douglas MK et al: Differentiation between dyspnea and its affective components, West J Nurs Res 18:626-642, 1996.

36. Simoni P, Foglio K, Zanoni C et al: Symptom limited exercise in COPD: do dyspnea and leg discomfort identify different groups of patients?, Eur Respir J 10:373s, 1997.

37. Borg GAV: Psychophysical bases of perceived exertion, Med Sci Sports Exerc 14:377-381, 1982.

38. Reardon J, Awad E, Normandin E et al: The effect of comprehensive outpatient pulmonary rehabilitation on dyspnea, Chest 105:1046-1052, 1994.

39. Mahler DA, Weinberg DH, Wells CK et al: The measurement of dyspnea: contents, interobserver agreement, and physiologic correlations of two new clinical indexes, Chest 85:751-758, 1984.

40. Mahler DA, Wells CK: Evaluation of clinical methods for rating dyspnea, Chest 93:580-586, 1988.

41. Mahler DA, Tomlinson D, Olmstead EM et al: Changes in dyspnea, health status, and lung function in chronic airway disease, Am J Respir Crit Care Med 151:61-65, 1995.

42. Guyatt GH, Berman LB, Townsend M et al: A measure of quality of life for clinical trials in chronic lung disease, Thorax 42:773-778, 1987.

43. Mahler D, ZuWallack R, Rickard K et al: Effects of salmeterol and ipratropium on dyspnea as measured by the Six Minute Walk and Baseline Dyspnea Index/Transitional Dyspnea Index (BDI/TDI), Am J Respir Crit Care Med 155:A278, 1997.

44. Gill TM, Feinstein AR: A critical appraisal of the quality of quality-of-life measurements, JAMA 272:619-626, 1994.

45. Guyatt GH, Feeny DH, Patrick DL: Measuring health-related quality of life, Ann Intern Med 118:622-629, 1993.

46. Jones PW: Health status: what does it mean for payers and patients? Proc Amer Thor Soc 3:222-226, 2006.

47. Jaeschke R, Singer J, Guyatt GH: Measurement of health status: ascertaining the minimal clinically important difference, Control Clin Trials 10:407-415, 1989.

48. Guyatt GH, Berman LB, Townsend M et al: Should study subjects see their previous responses? J Chronic Dis 38:1003-1007, 1985.

49. Williams JE, Singh SJ, Sewell L et al: Health status measurement: sensitivity of the self-reported Chronic Respiratory Questionnaire (CRQ-SR) in pulmonary rehabilitation, Thorax 58:515-518, 2003.

50. Schunemann HJ, Goldstein R, Mador MJ et al: A randomised trial to evaluate the self-administered standardised chronic respiratory questionnaire, Eur Respir J 25:31-40, 2005.

51. Goldstein RS, Gort EH, Stubbing D et al: Randomised controlled trial of respiratory rehabilitation, Lancet 344:1394-1397, 1994.

52. Wijkstra PJ, Van Altena R, Krann J et al: Quality of life in patients with chronic obstructive pulmonary disease improves after rehabilitation at home, Eur Respir J 7:269-273, 1994.

53. Cambach W, Chadwick-Straver RVM, Wagenaar RC et al: The effects of a community-based pulmonary rehabilitation programme on exercise tolerance and quality of life: a randomized controlled trial, Eur Respir J 10:104-113, 1997.

54. Bendstrup KE, Ingemann Jensen J, Holm S et al: Out-patient rehabilitation improves activities of daily living, quality of life and exercise tolerance in chronic obstructive pulmonary disease, Eur Respir J 10:2801-2806, 1997.

55. Jones PW: Issues concerning health-related quality of life in COPD, Chest 107:187s-192s, 1995.

56. Jones PW, Bosh TK: In association with an international study group: quality of life changes in COPD treated with salmeterol, Am J Respir Crit Care Med 155:1283-1289, 1997.

57. Meecham Jones DJ, Paul EA, Jones PW et al: Nasal pressure support ventilation plus oxygen compared to oxygen therapy alone in hypercapneic COPD, Am J Respir Crit Care Med 152:538-544, 1995.

58. Okubadejo AA, Paul EA, Jones PW et al: Does long-term oxygen therapy affect quality of life in patients with chronic obstructive pulmonary disease and severe hypoxaemia? Eur Respir J 9:2335-2339, 1996.

59. Ware JE: SF-36 health survey manual and interpretation guide, The Health Institute, Boston, 1993, New England Medical Center.

60. Ware JE, Kosinski M, Keller SD: SF-36 Physical & Mental Health Summary Scales: a user's manual, The Health Institute, Boston, 1994, New England Medical Center.

61. Benzo R, Flume PA, Turner D et al: Effect of pulmonary rehabilitation on quality of life in patients with COPD: the use of SF-36 summary scores as outcomes measures, J Cardiopulm Rehab 20:231-234, 2000.

62. Boueri FMV, Bucher-Bartelson BL, Glenn KA et al: Quality of life measured with a generic instrument (Short Form-36) improves following pulmonary rehabilitation in patients with COPD, Chest 119:77-84, 2001.

63. Harper R, Brazier JE, Waterhouse JC et al: Comparison of outcome measures for patients with chronic obstructive pulmonary disease (COPD) in an outpatient setting, Thorax 52:879-887, 1997.

64. Mahler DA, Mackowiak JI: Evaluation of the short-form 36-item questionnaire to measure health-related quality of life in patients with COPD, Chest 107:1585-1589, 1995.

65. Ware JE: SF-36 health survey manual and interpretation guide (Glossary:3). Boston, 1993. The Health Institute, New England Medical Center.

66. Lareau SC, Breslin EH, Meek PM: Functional status instruments: outcome measure in the evaluation of patients with chronic obstructive pulmonary disease, Heart Lung 25:212-224, 1996.

67. Leidy NK: Functional status and the forward progress of merry-go-rounds: toward a coherent analytical framework, Nurs Res 43:196-202, 1994.

68. Leidy NK: Using functional status to assess treatment outcomes, Chest 106:1645-1646, 1994.

69. Guccione AA: Functional assessment. Physical medicine and rehabilitation: assessment and treatment, Philadelphia, 1994, FA Davis, pp 193-208.

70. Spector WD, Katz S, Murphy JB et al: The hierarchical relationship between activities of daily living and instrumental activities of daily living, J Chronic Dis 40:481-489, 1987.

71. Jones PW: Issues concerning health-related quality of life in COPD, Chest 107:187s-193s, 1995.

72. Lincoln NB, Gladman JRF: The extended Activities of Daily Living Scale: a further validation, Disabil Rehabil 14:41-43, 1992.

73. Weaver TE, Narsavage GL: Physiological and psychological variables related to functional status in chronic obstructive pulmonary disease, Nurs Res 41:286-291, 1992.

74. Lareau S, Carrieri-Kohlman V, Janson-Bjerklie Roos P: Development and testing of the Pulmonary Functional Status and Dyspnea Questionnaire (PFSDQ), Heart Lung 23:242-250, 1994.

75. Okubadejo AA, O'shea L, Jones PW et al: Home assessment of activities of daily living in patients with severe chronic obstructive pulmonary disease on long-term oxygen therapy, Eur Respir J 10:1572-1575, 1997.

76. Haggerty MC, Stockdale-Wolley R, ZuWallack R: Functional status in pulmonary rehabilitation participants, J Cardiopulm Rehabil 19:35-42, 1999.

77. Votto J, Bowen J, Scalise P et al: Short-stay comprehensive inpatient pulmonary rehabilitation for advanced chronic obstructive pulmonary disease, Arch Phys Med Rehabil 77:1115-1118, 1996.

78. Lareau SC, Breslin EH, Meek PM: Functional status instruments: outcome measure in the evaluation of patients with chronic obstructive pulmonary disease, Heart Lung 25:212-224, 1996.

79. Lareau SC, Breslin EH, Anholm JD et al: Reduction in arm activities in patients with severe obstructive pulmonary disease, Am Rev Respir Dis 145:A476, 1990.

80. Borson S, McDonald GJ, Gayle T et al: Improvement in mood, physical symptoms, and function with nortriptyline for depression in patients with chronic obstructive pulmonary disease, Psychosomatics 33:190-201, 1992.

81. Garcia-Aymerich J, Lange P, Benet M et al: Regular physical activity reduces hospital admission and mortality in chronic obstructive pulmonary disease: a population based cohort study, Thorax 61:772-778, 2006.

82. Pitta F, Troosters T, Probst VS et al: Characteristics of physical activities in daily life in COPD, Am J Respir Crit Care Med 171:972-977, 2005.

83. Pitta F, Troosters T, Probst VS et al: Physical activity and hospitalization for exacerbation of COPD, Chest 129:536-544, 2006.

84. Gray-Donald K, Gibbons L, Shapiro SH et al: Nutritional status and mortality in chronic obstructive pulmonary disease, Am J Respir Crit Care Med 153:961-966, 1996.

85. Schols AMWJ, Mostert R, Soeters PB et al: Body composition and exercise performance in patients with chronic obstructive pulmonary disease, Thorax 46:695-699, 1991.

86. Palange P, Forte S, Onorati P et al: Effect of reduced body weight on muscle aerobic capacity in patients with COPD, Chest 114:12-18, 1998.

87. Schols AMWJ, Soeters PB, Dingemans AMC et al: Prevalence and characteristics of nutritional depletion in patients with stable COPD eligible for pulmonary rehabilitation, Am Rev Respir Dis 147:1151-1156, 1993.

88. Fitting JW: Nutritional support in chronic obstructive lung disease, Thorax 47:141-143, 1992.

89. Casaburi R, Carithers E, Tosolini J et al: Randomized controlled trial of growth hormone in severe COPD patients undergoing endurance training, Am J Respir Crit Care Med 155:A498, 1997.

90. Ferreira IM, Verreschi IT, Nery LE et al: The influence of 6 months of oral anabolic steroids on body mass and respiratory muscles in undernourished COPD patients, Chest 114:19-28, 1998.

91. Casaburi R, Bhasin S, Cosentino L et al: Effects of testosterone and resistance training in men with chronic obstructive pulmonary disease, Am J Respir Crit Care Med 170:870-878, 2004.

92. Celli BR, Cote CG, Marin JM et al: The body-mass index, airflow obstruction, dyspnea, and exercise capacity index in chronic obstructive pulmonary disease, N Engl J Med 350:1005-1012, 2004.

93. Cote CG, Celli BR: Pulmonary rehabilitation and the BODE Index in COPD. Eur Respir J 26:630-636, 2005.

94. Bourbeau J, Julien M, Maltais F et al: Reduction of hospital utilization in patients with chronic obstructive pulmonary disease: a disease-specific self-management intervention, Arch Intern Med 163:585-591, 2003.

95. California Pulmonary Rehabilitation Collaborative Group: Effects of pulmonary rehabilitation on dyspnea, quality of life, and healthcare costs in California, J Cardiopulm Rehabil 24:52-62, 2004.

96. Raskin J, Spiegler P, McCusker C et al: The effect of pulmonary rehabilitation on healthcare utilization in chronic obstructive pulmonary disease: the Northeast Pulmonary Rehabilitation Consortium, J Cardiopulm Rehabil 26:231-236, 2006.

97. ZuWallack RL: Selection criteria and outcome assessment in pulmonary rehabilitation, Monaldi Arch Chest Dis 53:429-437, 1998.

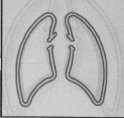

Chapter 22

Home Mechanical Ventilation

JOSHUA O. BENDITT • LOUIS BOITANO

CHAPTER OUTLINE

Demographics of Home Ventilation
Methods of Mechanical Ventilation
   Invasive Positive-Pressure Ventilation
   Noninvasive Mechanical Ventilation
Secretion Management
Selection of Patients for Home
   Mechanical Ventilation

Selection Factors Common
   to NPPV and TPPV
Selection Factors for NPPV
Selection Factors for TPPV
Costs of Home Mechanical Ventilation
Evidence Regarding Home Mechanical
   Ventilation
Conclusion

PROFESSIONAL SKILLS

On completion of this chapter, the reader will be able to do
the following:
* Gain knowledge of the various methods of home ventilation that are available for the individual with
  chronic respiratory failure
* Be able to select appropriate individuals for home mechanical ventilation
* Understand the similarities and differences between invasive (tracheostomy) and noninvasive ventilation
  and be able to select appropriate candidates for each

Home mechanical ventilation as a treatment for chronic respiratory failure has been the subject of increased interest for several reasons, including the following: improved survival after episodes of respiratory failure, development of compact portable ventilators as well as noninvasive modes of ventilation, and financial incentives for moving care for chronically ill individuals from the hospital to the home.[1,2] A wide variety of causes of chronic respiratory failure have been treated at home with mechanical ventilation (Box 22-1). These disease processes fall into four major categories and include the following:

1. Impaired ventilatory control (e.g., central alveolar hypoventilation)

2. Restrictive neuromuscular diseases (e.g., muscular dystrophies, spinal cord injury)
3. Chest wall diseases (e.g., kyphoscoliosis)
4. Primary pulmonary disease (e.g., chronic obstructive pulmonary disease)

DEMOGRAPHICS OF HOME VENTILATION

The frequency of ventilation in the home has increased over the past several decades. The two main reasons for this appear to be an increase in the number of patients who are discharged from intensive care and are left with residual chronic respiratory failure and a dramatic upsurge in the

351

use of noninvasive positive-pressure ventilation (NPPV). Survey studies estimated that between 1983 and 1990 there was a doubling in the number of patients on long-term ventilation (>3 weeks) in the United States, from approximately 3 per 100,000[3] to 6 per 100,000.[4] This increase in patients surviving on ventilation in the intensive care unit has resulted in the development of long-term acute care facilities to try to reduce the high costs of therapy in that setting.[5] In turn, some patients who are discharged from long-term facilities to home may do so on either partial or full-time ventilation. However, it appears that a major reason for the growth in home ventilation is the greater use of NPPV. Adams, Shapiro, and Marini[6] reported that 47% of the increase in home ventilation in Minnesota between 1992 and 1997 was due to an increase in the use of noninvasive ventilation and that 34% of patients were using ventilation less than 24 hours/day. In France, where a national database of home ventilation is in place, exponential growth in the use of NPPV has occurred: 500 individuals received NPPV in 1988, rising to 4500 in 1998.[7] In contrast, individuals using tracheostomy positive-pressure ventilation (TPPV) ventilation remained at approximately 2000.

METHODS OF HOME MECHANICAL VENTILATION

The methods of delivering home mechanical ventilation can be divided into two major categories: invasive positive-pressure ventilation or TPPV, and noninvasive ventilation, of which in turn there are several varieties (Box 22-2). Full-time or part-time ventilation can be accomplished by either method of ventilation. Although equipment varies somewhat between the two methods, the characteristics of the patient, family, and caregivers that lead to successful home ventilation are similar.

Invasive Positive-Pressure Ventilation

Invasive positive-pressure ventilation at home, using tracheostomy or TPPV, has been used successfully in several large series of patients.[8-10] Benefits of this type of ventilatory support include complete control of the machine-delivered tidal gas volume and ease of access to the central airways for suctioning of secretions. In addition, treatment during episodes of acute respiratory failure requires no change in the method of ventilation.

Unfortunately, a number of serious complications of TPPV have been cited. Damage to the trachea from the indwelling tracheostomy tube including necrosis, stenosis, and hemorrhage, as well as tracheo-esophageal fistulas, have been reported.[11-13] Food aspiration and swallowing problems can also occur because of interference with the normal swallowing mechanism. An increased risk of airway colonization with bacteria and lower respiratory tract infection has also been noted.[14-16] The use of a tracheostomy tube requires supplemental humidification, an additional daily respiratory care task. Finally, social interactions and patient psychological well-being may be impaired by the fact that the tracheostomy tube prevents the patient from speaking. A number of devices and techniques have been designed to allow speech and communication while being ventilated; however, these cannot be used by all individuals.[17]

There are a number of instances, however, in which TPPV will be required over NPPV: (1) when the patient lacks the bulbar function to be able to tolerate the noninvasive interfaces, (2) if local health care providers are not familiar with noninvasive techniques, or (3) if the patient prefers this form of ventilation.[18,19]

Noninvasive Mechanical Ventilation

NPPV was first used during the polio epidemics of the 1950s to allow patients time out of the iron lung.[20] More recently, there has been significant renewed interest in this technique. There are currently three ways in which NPPV may be delivered (Figure 22-1): (1) via mouthpiece with or without a lip seal, (2) via full facemask, or (3) via a nasal mask. Nasal interfaces are by far the most popular. There are relatively few serious side effects and, in general, leakage around the mask is not a major problem limiting effective ventilation[21]; however, in those patients for whom leakage around the mask is a problem, use of an oral–facial mask interface or chinstrap may be appropriate.[22,23]

The ventilators used for NPPV are generally pressure-preset devices that are often equipped with a back-up rate and thus supply pressure support breaths without a preset tidal volume. These devices have the advantage that they can compensate for mask leakage. However, it is also possible to use volume ventilators with a mask interface.[24,25]

Mask-type noninvasive ventilation is most often used at night, when the mask will not interfere with activities such as speaking and eating. However, during the daytime, when speech and eating are needed and when wearing a bulky mask would be socially uncomfortable, mouth ventilation can be used for patients for whom a daytime noninvasive device is needed.[26,27] The mouthpiece device can be used on an as-needed basis and allows the patient complete control over ventilation (Figure 22-2). In addition, the mouthpiece allows the patient to take in multiple breaths, increasing the volume of the lungs as far as possible (maximal insufflation capacity maneuver), which have been shown to improve

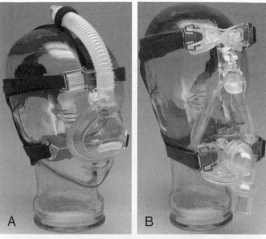

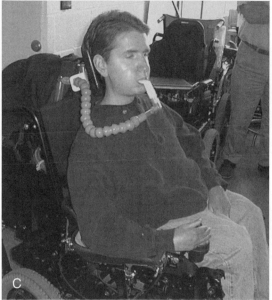

FIGURE 22-1 Noninvasive positive-pressure ventilation interfaces. **A,** Nasal mask; **B,** full facemask; **C,** patient using mouthpiece ventilation device.

compliance of the lung[28] as well as allowing independent cough function.[29,30]

Other forms of noninvasive ventilation, called "body ventilators," are available but rarely used today. Negative-pressure ventilation with devices such as the iron lung[31] or cuirasse ventilator[32] is not popular because of their bulkiness as well as because obstructive apnea, often present in these patients at night, can be worsened by patient-ventilator dyssynchrony.[33-35] Another device, called the pneumobelt,[36,37] can be used to assist ventilation in the upright individual. On activation, an air-filled bladder strapped to the anterior abdominal wall inflates, displacing the diaphragm upward and causing exhalation. When the device

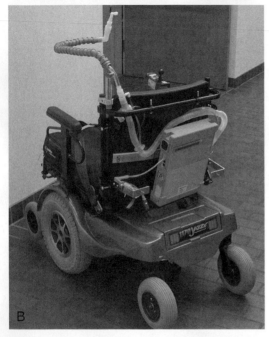

BOX 22-3 | **Methods of Secretion Management**

COUGH AUGMENTATION
- Manually assisted cough ("quad" cough)
- Breath-stacking
  - Resuscitator bag
  - Glossopharyngeal breathing
  - With mouthpiece ventilator
  - Mechanical insufflation–exsufflation

SECRETION MOBILIZATION
- Chest wall oscillation therapy
- Intrapulmonary percussive ventilation
- Tracheal suction with catheter

FIGURE 22-2 Mouthpiece ventilation (MPV) device. **A,** Schematic of MPV setup; **B,** MPV setup on motorized wheelchair.

shuts off the diaphragm descends under the force of gravity, causing inflation of the lungs. This device, popular after the polio epidemic, is rarely used today.

Electric stimulation of the diaphragm by pacing with implanted electrodes is a technique that is available to those patients with intact phrenic nerves and diaphragm muscle adequate to sustain ventilation when stimulated.[38,39] It is, in essence, a form of invasive ventilation as it requires surgery and oftentimes continued use of a tracheostomy to avoid upper airway obstruction due to patient–ventilator dyssynchrony. It is most often used in patients with central alveolar hypoventilation and patients with paralysis of the respiratory muscles secondary to high (C1–C2)

cervical cord injuries.[19,40] The procedure requires operative implantation of the electrodes and receiver and is relatively expensive, with costs sometimes exceeding $200,000, although a newer and potentially less expensive method for implanting the pacing wires has been described more recently.[41]

SECRETION MANAGEMENT

Secretion management is an important issue for patients receiving home ventilation via TPPV or noninvasive ventilation, especially for those with cough impairment due to neuromuscular disease. Various methodologies are available to assist cough and secretion removal (Box 22-3). These include catheter suction for those with a tracheostomy, manually assisted cough, breath-stacking, the mechanical insufflator–exsufflator, and a variety of chest wall oscillatory devices.

Manually assisted cough is a method of applying positive pressure to the abdomen, pleural space, and airway leading to adequate cough expiratory flow rates. A number of techniques are available for an attendant to apply rapid abdominal thrusts resulting in effective clearance of secretions.[42] Increasing the volume of air in the respiratory system before the assisted breath increases the volume of gas in the lungs for exhalation and also increases the inward elastic recoil pressure of the lung and chest wall, which can increase the exhalatory pressures and cough effectiveness.[30]

An effective secretion management device, available for more than 50 years but only more recently used to any great extent, is the mechanical insufflator–exsufflator or CoughAssist (Respironics, Murrysville, Pa.)[43,44] (Figure 22-3). This device consists of an electric motor that can generate positive

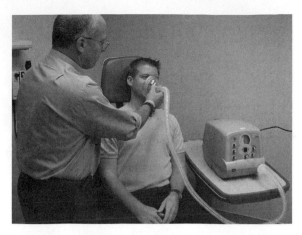

FIGURE 22-3 Mechanical insufflator—exsufflator in use.

and negative pressures of up to 50 cm H_2O to the airways of patients who are unable to cough. The device can be used with a tracheostomy[45] or via a facemask for those ventilated noninvasively. The device removes secretions from the airway by mimicking the native cough and essentially "vacuuming" secretions from the airway.

Other noninvasive mechanical aids include devices that oscillate the chest wall or airway directly.[46] Although effective for patients with bronchiectasis and cystic fibrosis,[47] their role in support of home ventilation is unclear.

SELECTION OF PATIENTS FOR HOME MECHANICAL VENTILATION

Patients who are candidates for home mechanical ventilation will generally follow one of two pathways. They may come from an inpatient setting where they received mechanical ventilation for an acute or progressive chronic condition and were unable to wean from the mechanical ventilator. These patients are often, although not always, receiving invasive TPPV. Other patients, often with chronic progressive neuromuscular diseases, will have home mechanical ventilation started as an outpatient or may be admitted for short hospital stays for adjustment and titration of ventilation. These patients are most often treated by noninvasive methodologies. The selection of patient candidates for home mechanical ventilation involves careful analysis not only of the type of disease the patient has, and his or her equipment and support service requirements, but also but also other factors that will have a significant impact on the successful outcome of the endeavor. It is imperative that the patient's directives be

discussed as part of the process as many of these patients may develop significant complications that are life threatening. The participation of the patient in setting the directives will go a long way in facilitating the overall management of the patient over time.

Selection Factors Common to NPPV and TPPV

Patients who require either invasive or noninvasive ventilation are experiencing ventilatory failure. This may require either full-time or part-time ventilator support, the latter most often occurring at night. Although mild hypoxemia may be a part of the presentation of respiratory failure, the major problem for patients undergoing home ventilation is hypercarbic respiratory failure because they are unable to maintain ventilation and gas exchange without at least part-time ventilation.

There are patient personality characteristics that lend themselves to successful implementation of home mechanical ventilation. The most successful candidates for successful home ventilation are highly motivated individuals with interested family members who can help care for the patient at home.[2] Considerable stress and frustration can be involved in the preparation for movement to the home environment, so that flexibility and patience are also important characteristics.

Patients who may be considered successful candidates for long-term home mechanical ventilation may have other associated medical illnesses. These illnesses do not necessarily disqualify them from receiving home mechanical ventilation if the problems can be dealt with in the home and do not necessitate frequent admission to a medical facility for evaluation or treatment. In general, the patient should be clinically and physiologically stable enough to remain out of an acute care setting for at least 1 month.[1,2] In particular, if associated lung disease is present there may be increased need for airway hygiene in the form of frequent airway suctioning. To be candidates for home treatment programs, these patients must be able to clear their secretions either by assisted cough techniques or by airway suctioning via tracheostomy.

Some characteristics of the families of individuals who decide to attempt home mechanical ventilation have been recognized.[48,49] The requirements of a home ventilation program as well as the potential pitfalls and drawbacks must be well understood by the patient and family.

Frequently one or more members of the family will assume part or all of the responsibility for daily care of the patient. This can create significant psychological stress within the family. An assessment of the ability of the family to accept the ventilator-dependent patient into the home before discharge from the acute care facility or in the outpatient setting must be made.

Although home mechanical ventilation is frequently less expensive than in-hospital care, many third-party carriers cover only 80% of the costs of prescribed durable medical equipment, so that the patient and family may end up taking on a substantial financial burden. A careful analysis of resources for supporting the ventilator-dependent individual must be undertaken before discharge.

Selection Factors for NPPV

A consensus statement by the American College of Chest Physicians has defined the major criteria for NPPV for chronic respiratory failure applicable to home mechanical ventilation needed because of restrictive lung disease, COPD, and other conditions as shown in Table 22-1.[50] Patients should have symptoms related to hypoventilation, such as dyspnea or those of sleep-disordered breathing, but should also meet objective criteria such as reduced muscle strength or elevated pulmonary arterial carbon dioxide pressure (Pa_{CO_2}). In addition to the criteria listed patients should also have adequate bulbar function to protect their airway during noninvasive

ventilation, as pressure delivered to the nose and mouth can force secretions into the airway, potentially increasing the risk of pneumonia.[51] Patients must also be able to manage secretions effectively either on their own or with devices that can assist them to do so.[43,52,53]

Selection Factors for TPPV

Unlike NPPV, precise selection criteria have not been established for TPPV, although similar considerations apply. Practically speaking, many patients requiring TPPV will have been shown the need for ventilation following repeated attempts either in the hospital or an intermediate care facility.[5,54] On occasion, transition from NPPV to TPPV will be required if patients develop bulbar dysfunction and cannot protect their airway and adequately handle secretions. In this case, TPPV provides some protection against aspiration and allows direct access to the airway for secretion management. Finally, some patients may require oxygen (O_2) or positive end-expiratory pressure continuously, factors that TPPV can more reliably deliver. Even so, a fraction of inspired O_2 requirement less than 40 or a positive end-expiratory pressure less than 10 cm H_2O makes home ventilation more feasible.[1]

COSTS OF HOME MECHANICAL VENTILATION

The cost of caring for patients who require prolonged mechanical ventilation can be high.

TABLE 22-1	Criteria for Candidate Selection for NPPV	
Restrictive Thoracic/Neuromuscular Disease	**Obstructive Lung Disease**
APPROPRIATE DIAGNOSIS	
ALS, muscular dystrophy, postpolio, etc.	COPD, bronchiectasis, cystic fibrosis, etc.
SYMPTOMS	
Dyspnea	Dyspnea
Symptoms of sleep-disordered breathing	Symptoms of sleep-disordered breathing
Snoring	Snoring
Morning headache	Morning headache
Frequent nocturnal awakenings	Frequent nocturnal awakenings
Etc.	
PHYSIOLOGIC CRITERIA (ONE OF THE FOLLOWING)	
$Pa_{CO_2} \geq 45$ mm Hg	$Pa_{CO_2} \geq 55$ mm Hg
Nocturnal O_2 saturation $\leq 88\%$ for 5 consecutive minutes	$Pa_{CO_2} \geq 54$ mm Hg and nocturnal O_2 saturation $\leq 88\%$ for 5 consecutive minutes during sleep
Maximal inspiratory pressure < 60 cm H_2O	Pa_{CO_2} between 50 and 54 mm Hg and ≥ 2 hospitalizations in 1 year due to hypercarbia
Forced vital capacity $< 50\%$ predicted	

ALS, *Amyotrophic lateral sclerosis*; COPD, *chronic obstructive pulmonary disease*; NPPV, *noninvasive positive-pressure ventilation*; O_2, *oxygen*; Pa_{CO_2}, *Pulmonary arterial carbon dioxide pressure*.

Bach and colleagues studied the hospital costs of patients requiring mechanical ventilation for more than 48 hours.[55] In their study, the mean charge for these patients per hospitalization was approximately eight times that for all other hospitalized patients. In patients who are unable to wean from the ventilatory and require chronic care, costs can range up to $66,000/month.[55] It is clear that substantial cost savings can be obtained by moving chronic care into the home. Lafond, Make, and Gilmartin have estimated the average monthly costs at approximately $3000 for their series of patients.[56] In a careful estimate of costs for home ventilation versus in-hospital care in London, Creese and Fielden[57] indicated that savings of approximately 32% could be expected by moving the patient from the hospital to home with 24-hour attendants. The American Association for Respiratory Care conducted a 20-state hospital survey in 1980, estimating hospital cost of $22,569 versus home care cost of $1766 for chronically ventilated patients.[58]

A significant financial disincentive to care of ventilated patients in the home is the fact that most insurers will reimburse only 80% of home care costs.[56] This places a significant financial burden on even the most affluent families and serves to prevent consideration of moving patients into the home. Few insurers will cover the costs of full-time nursing care ("custodial care") for those who are paralyzed or disabled to the point of being unable to perform the activities of daily living. One solution to this problem may be provided by some European experiences. England and France have used small chronic care facilities focused on ventilator-assisted individuals.[59] The organization of regional centers for overseeing the care of home ventilator patients has had a significant positive effect in maintaining appropriate resource use. A number of states have established programs for dealing with these issues.[55] Given the current need for controlling ever-increasing medical costs it is likely that organization and guidelines at the national level in the United States will become stronger.

EVIDENCE REGARDING HOME MECHANICAL VENTILATION

Neuromuscular diseases were some of the first maladies for which home mechanical ventilation was employed. This was in large part because of the polio epidemics that occurred during the 1940s and 1950s. Noninvasive ventilation in the form of the iron lung, rocking bed, and even mouthpiece positive pressure was used first in the hospital and later at home as patients convalesced. A 46-year experience of noninvasive ventilation at one such center has been published.[60] This case series presents data on 560 patients with sequelae of polio as well as other neuromuscular diseases such as Duchenne muscular dystrophy, amyotrophic lateral sclerosis, and chest wall deformities. Although not a randomized trial, the study showed that noninvasive home ventilation could be carried out for long periods of time (years to decades) with good self-reported quality of life in patients with neuromuscular disease. Of note, patients receiving NPPV (mask or mouthpiece) as opposed to negative-pressure ventilation such as the iron lung or cuirasse went on to tracheostomy less frequently and had fewer problems with discomfort and self-discontinuation of ventilation. It is clear that home ventilation with TPPV or NPPV leads to improved survival.[7,61,62] A number of studies have shown that morbidities such as hospitalization as well as quality of life are improved with noninvasive home mechanical ventilation. Leger and colleagues[63] showed that the number of days spent in hospital decreased for two or more years after initiation of noninvasive ventilation at home. Noninvasive home ventilation has been shown to improve survival, quality of life, and cognitive function in amyotrophic lateral sclerosis.[64-68]

At this time for neuromuscular disease, NPPV is preferred over TPPV unless bulbar involvement prevents the patient from protecting the airway during ventilation or hypercarbia persists despite adequate noninvasive ventilation because of the risks and side effects of TPPV.[7,69,70]

Both TPPV and noninvasive ventilation have been tried extensively in patients with COPD. In a retrospective cohort study in which TPPV was compared with long-term O_2 therapy benefit initially appeared to favor TPPV although long-term survival was no different.[71] NPPV has become the preferred modality, again because of the potential negative side effects of TPPV. Few randomized trials of noninvasive ventilation in COPD have been performed. A large multicenter trial from Italy showed improvements in $Paco_2$ and dyspnea scores, and improved quality of life scores among patients receiving NPPV compared with those who received long-term O_2 therapy.[72,73] Hospital admissions did not differ between the groups; mortality was not studied as an end point. Quality of life for individuals using noninvasive ventilation was examined in a study by Meecham-Jones and colleagues.[74] Quality of life was improved among patients with COPD using noninvasive ventilation compared with long-term O_2 therapy. Interestingly, patients with COPD receiving noninvasive ventilation had poorer quality of life than patients with neuromuscular disorders such as Duchenne muscular dystrophy. Other studies have shown that patients with COPD are much less likely to tolerate NPPV and may discontinue use on their own.[63] Overall it appears that patients with COPD do not fare as well with noninvasive ventilation as patients with neuromuscular diseases. The reasons for this are not clear but may relate to the fact that hypercarbic respiratory failure for which NPPV is designed is less frequently found in patients with COPD.

CONCLUSION

Economic pressures within the medical system make it likely that chronic ventilation of patients with neuromuscular disease respiratory failure will occur more and more frequently outside of the hospital setting. This may occur either in the home or in a long-term acute care facility or nursing home. Some authors have suggested that home care for ventilator-dependent patients be regionalized to standardize therapy and reduce costs as has been adopted in some European countries.[59,75] Also, licensing of less highly trained individuals to care for the ventilator-dependent patient in the home is likely to become an important issue as this has been shown to be a safe and cost-saving measure.

It is clear that home mechanical ventilation in the United States and across the world is increasing significantly in large part because of the growing use of NPPV. For those patients who are appropriate candidates for noninvasive ventilation, wide arrays of options are available. In particular, NPPV has showed a strong upsurge in use and will likely continue to do so compared with TPPV. Noninvasive methods tend to be less costly and may be considered a better option by patients.[76,77]

References

1. Make BJ, Gilmanton ME: Mechanical ventilation in the home, Crit Care Clin N Am 6:785-796, 1990.
2. O'Donohue WJ Jr, Giovannoni RM, Goldberg AI et al: Long-term mechanical ventilation. Guidelines for management in the home and at alternate community sites. Report of the Ad Hoc Committee, Respiratory Care Section, American College of Chest Physicians, Chest 90(1 suppl):1S-37S, 1986.
3. Make B, Gilmartin M: Care of the ventilator-assisted individual in the home and alternative and community sites. In Hodgkin JE, Connors GL, Bell CW, editors: Pulmonary rehabilitation: guidelines to success, Philadelphia, 1993, JB Lippincott, pp 359-391.
4. Milligan S: AARC and Gallup estimate numbers and costs of caring for chronic ventilator patients, AARC Times 15:30-36, 1991.
5. Scheinhorn DJ, Chao DC, Stearn-Hassenpflug M: Liberation from prolonged mechanical ventilation, Crit Care Clin 18:569-595, 2002.
6. Adams AB, Shapiro R, Marini JJ: Changing prevalence of chronically ventilator-assisted individuals in Minnesota: increases, characteristics, and the use of noninvasive ventilation, Respir Care 43:635-636, 1998.
7. Simonds AK: Home ventilation, Eur Respir J Suppl 47:38s-46s, 2003.
8. Burr BH, Guyer B, Todres ID et al: Home care for children on respirators, N Engl J Med 309:1319-1323, 1983.
9. Make BJ: Long-term management of ventilator-assisted individuals: The Boston University experience, Respir Care 31:303-310, 1986.
10. Splaingard ML, Frates RC Jr, Harrison GM et al: Home positive-pressure ventilation: twenty years' experience, Chest 84:376-382, 1983.
11. Epstein SK: Late complications of tracheostomy, Respir Care 50:542-549, 2005.
12. Durbin CG Jr: Early complications of tracheostomy, Respir Care 50:511-515, 2005.
13. Sue RD, Susanto I: Long-term complications of artificial airways, Clin Chest Med 24:457-471, 2003.
14. Brook I: Role of anaerobic bacteria in infections following tracheostomy, intubation, or the use of ventilatory tubes in children, Ann Otol Rhinol Laryngol 113:830-834, 2004.
15. Jarrett WA, Ribes J, Manaligod JM: Biofilm formation on tracheostomy tubes, Ear Nose Throat J 81:659-661, 2002.
16. Harlid R, Andersson G, Frostell CG et al: Respiratory tract colonization and infection in patients with chronic tracheostomy: a one-year study in patients living at home, Am J Respir Crit Care Med 154:124-129, 1996.
17. Manzano JL, Lubillo S, Henr'iquez D et al: Verbal communication of ventilator-dependent patients [see comments], Crit Care Med 21:512-517, 1993.
18. Finder JD, Birnkrant D, Carl J et al: Respiratory care of the patient with Duchenne muscular dystrophy: ATS consensus statement, Am J Respir Crit Care Med 170:456-465, 2004.
19. Garrido-Garcia H, Mazaira Alvarez J, Martin Escribano P et al: Treatment of chronic ventilatory failure using a diaphragmatic pacemaker, Spinal Cord 36:310-314, 1998.
20. Hill NS: Clinical applications of body ventilators, Chest 90:897-905, 1986.
21. Meyer TJ, Pressman MR, Benditt J et al: Air leaking through the mouth during nocturnal nasal ventilation: effect on sleep quality, Sleep 20:561-569, 1997.

22. McDermott I, Bach JR, Parker C et al: Custom-fabricated interfaces for intermittent positive pressure ventilation, Int J Prosthodont 2:224-233, 1989.

23. Bach JR, Alba AS: Sleep and nocturnal mouthpiece IPPV efficiency in postpoliomyelitis ventilator users, Chest 106:1705-1710, 1994.

24. Bach JR, Alba AS: Management of chronic alveolar hypoventilation by nasal ventilation, Chest 97:52-57, 1990.

25. Bach JR, Alba A, Mosher R et al: Intermittent positive pressure ventilation via nasal access in the management of respiratory insufficiency, Chest 92:168-170, 1987.

26. Bach JR, Alba AS, Saporito LR: Intermittent positive pressure ventilation via the mouth as an alternative to tracheostomy for 257 ventilator users, Chest 103:174-182, 1993.

27. Boitano LJ, Benditt JO: An evaluation of home volume ventilators that support open-circuit mouthpiece ventilation, Respir Care 50:1457-1461, 2005.

28. Lechtzin N, Shade D, Clawson L et al: Supramaximal inflation improves lung compliance in subjects with amyotrophic lateral sclerosis, Chest 129:1322-1329, 2006.

29. Bach JR: Mechanical insufflation—exsufflation: comparison of peak expiratory flows with manually assisted and unassisted coughing techniques, Chest 104:1553-1562, 1993.

30. Kang SW, Bach JR: Maximum insufflation capacity: vital capacity and cough flows in neuromuscular disease, Am J Phys Med Rehabil 79:222-227, 2000.

31. Drinker P, Shaw LA: An apparatus for the prolonged administration of artificial respiration, J Clin Invest 7:229-247, 1929.

32. Gilmartin ME: Body ventilators: equipment and techniques, Respir Care Clin N Am 2:195-222, 1996.

33. Levy RD, Bradley TD, Newman SL et al: Negative pressure ventilation: effects on ventilation during sleep in normal subjects, Chest 95:95-99, 1989.

34. Corrado A, Gorini M: Long-term negative pressure ventilation, Respir Care Clin N Am 8:545-557, v-vi, 2002.

35. Bach JR, Penek J: Obstructive sleep apnea complicating negative-pressure ventilatory support in patients with chronic paralytic/restrictive ventilatory dysfunction, Chest 99:1386-1393, 1991.

36. Dettenmeier PA, Jackson NC: Chronic hypoventilation syndrome: treatment with non-invasive mechanical ventilation, AACN Clin Issues Crit Care Nurs 2:415-431, 1991.

37. Miller HJ, Thomas E, Wilmot CB: Pneumobelt use among high quadriplegic population, Arch Phys Med Rehabil 69:369-372, 1988.

38. Glenn WWL, Hogan JF, Loke JS et al: Ventilatory support by pacing of the conditioned diaphragm in quadriplegia, N Engl J Med 310:1150-1155, 1984.

39. Elefteriades JA, Quin JA, Hogan JF et al: Long-term follow-up of pacing of the conditioned diaphragm in quadriplegia, Pacing Clin Electrophysiol 25:897-906, 2002.

40. Chen ML, Tablizo MA, Kun S et al: Diaphragm pacers as a treatment for congenital central hypoventilation syndrome, Expert Rev Med Devices 2:577-585, 2005.

41. DiMarco AF, Onders RP, Ignagni A et al: Phrenic nerve pacing via intramuscular diaphragm electrodes in tetraplegic subjects, Chest 127:671-678, 2005.

42. Bach JR: Pulmonary rehabilitation: the obstructive and paralytic conditions, Philadelphia, 1995, Hanley and Belfus.

43. Hardy KA, Anderson BD: Noninvasive clearance of airway secretions, Respir Care Clin N Am 2:323-345, 1996.

44. Bach JR: Mechanical insufflation/exsufflation: has it come of age? A commentary, Eur Respir J 21:385-386, 2003.

45. Sancho J, Servera E, Vergara P et al: Mechanical insufflation—exsufflation vs. tracheal suctioning via tracheostomy tubes for patients with amyotrophic lateral sclerosis: a pilot study, Am J Phys Med Rehabil 82:750-753, 2003.

46. Chang HK, Farf A: High-frequency ventilation: a review, Respir Physiol 57:135-152, 1984.

47. Arens R, Gozal D, Omlin KJ et al: Comparison of high frequency chest compression and conventional chest physiotherapy in hospitalized patients with cystic fibrosis, Am J Respir Crit Care Med 150:1154-1157, 1994.

48. Gilgoff I, Prentice W, Baydur A: Patient and family participation in the management of respiratory failure in Duchenne's muscular dystrophy, Chest 95:519-524, 1989.

49. Sivak ED, Gibson WT, Hanson MR: Long-term management of respiratory failure in amyotrophic lateral sclerosis, Ann Neurol 12:18-23, 1982.

50. National Association for Medical Direction of Respiratory Care: Clinical indications for noninvasive positive pressure ventilation in chronic respiratory failure due to restrictive lung disease, COPD, and nocturnal hypoventilation: a consensus conference report, Chest 116:521-534, 1999.

51. Bach JR: Amyotrophic lateral sclerosis: prolongation of life by noninvasive respiratory AIDS, Chest 122:92-98, 2002.

52. Bach JR, Smith WH, Michaels J et al: Airway secretion clearance by mechanical exsufflation for postpoliomyelitis ventilator-assisted individuals, Arch Phys Med Rehabil 74:170-177, 1993.

53. Lahrmann H, Wild M, Zdrahal F et al: Expiratory muscle weakness and assisted cough in ALS, Amyotroph Lateral Scler Other Motor Neuron Disord 4:49-51, 2003.

54. Nevins ML, Epstein SK: Weaning from prolonged mechanical ventilation, Clin Chest Med 22:13-33, 2001.

55. Bach JR, Intinola BA, Alba AS et al: The ventilator-assisted individual: cost analysis of institutionalization vs rehabilitation and in-home management, Chest 101:26-29, 1992.

56. Lafond L, Make BJ, Gilmartin ME: Home care costs for ventilator-assisted individuals, Am Rev Respir Dis 137:62, 1988.

57. Creese AL, Fielden R: Hospital or home care for the severely disabled: a cost comparison, Br J Prev Soc Med 31:116-121, 1977.

58. Times A: Association holds press conference on ventilator survey, AAR Times 8:28-31, 1984.

59. Goldberg A: Home care for life-supported persons: is a national approach the answer?, Chest 90:744-748, 1986.

60. Baydur A, Layne E, Aral H et al: Long term non-invasive ventilation in the community for patients with musculoskeletal disorders: 46 year experience and review, Thorax 55:4-11, 2000.

61. Mehta S, Hill NS: Noninvasive ventilation, Am J Respir Crit Care Med 163:540-577, 2001.

62. Simonds AK, Muntoni F, Heather S et al: Impact of nasal ventilation on survival in hypercapnic Duchenne muscular dystrophy, Thorax 53:949-952, 1998.

63. Leger P, Bedicam JM, Cornette A et al: Nasal inter-mittent positive pressure ventilation: long-term follow-up in patients with severe chronic respira-tory insufficiency, Chest 105:100-105, 1994.

64. Aboussouan LS, Khan SU, Meeker DP et al: Effect of noninvasive positive-pressure ventilation on sur-vival in amyotrophic lateral sclerosis [see com-ments], Ann Intern Med 127(6):450-453, 1997.

65. Bourke SC, Bullock RE, Williams TL et al: Noninvasive ventilation in ALS: indications and effect on quality of life, Neurology 61:171-177, 2003.

66. Kleopa KA, Sherman M, Neal B et al: Bipap improves survival and rate of pulmonary function decline in patients with ALS, J Neurol Sci 164:82-88, 1999.

67. Lyall RA, Donaldson N, Fleming T et al: A prospective study of quality of life in ALS patients treated with noninvasive ventilation, Neurology 57:153-156, 2001.

68. Pinto AC, Evangelista T, Carvalho M et al: Respiratory assistance with a non-invasive ventilator (Bipap) in MND/ALS patients: survival rates in a controlled trial, J Neurol Sci 129(suppl):19-26, 1995.

69. Bach JR: Noninvasive mechanical ventilation, ed 1, Philadelphia, 2002, Hanley and Belfus.

70. Benditt JO, Boitano L: Respiratory support of indi-viduals with Duchenne muscular dystrophy: toward a standard of care, Phys Med Rehabil Clin N Am 16:1125-1139, xii, 2005.

71. Muir JF: Multicentre study of 259 severe COPD patients with tracheostomy and home mechanical ventilation. In Proceedings of the World Congress on Oxygen Therapy and Pulmonary Rehabilitation, 1987; Denver.

72. Clini E, Sturani C, Rossi A et al: The Italian multi-centre study on noninvasive ventilation in chronic obstructive pulmonary disease patients, Eur Respir J 20:529-538, 2002.

73. Vitacca M, Clini E, Pagani M et al: Physiologic effects of early administered mask proportional assist ventilation in patients with chronic obstruc-tive pulmonary disease and acute respiratory fail-ure, Crit Care Med 28:1791-1797, 2000.

74. Meecham Jones DJ, Paul EA, Jones PW et al: Nasal pressure support ventilation plus oxygen compared with oxygen therapy alone in hypercapnic COPD, Am J Respir Crit Care Med 152:538-544, 1995.

75. Gajdos P: The French organisation of mechanical ventilation at home for neuromuscular diseases, Paraplegia 31:147-149, 1993.

76. Bach JR, Campagnolo DI, Hoeman S: Life satisfac-tion of individuals with Duchenne muscular dys-trophy using long-term mechanical ventilatory support, Am J Phys Med Rehabil 70:129-135, 1991.

77. Bach JR, Alba AS: Noninvasive options for ventila-tory support of the traumatic high level quadriple-gic patient, Chest 98:613-619, 1990.

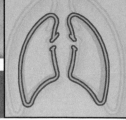

Chapter 23

Pulmonary Rehabilitation and Lung Transplantation

STEVEN D. NATHAN • OKSANA A. SHLOBIN

CHAPTER OUTLINE

Lung Allocation Score
General Inclusion Criteria
Contraindications to Lung
    Transplantation
    Absolute Contraindications
    Relative Contraindications
Candidate Selection
Chronic Obstructive Pulmonary Disease
Idiopathic Pulmonary Fibrosis
Nonspecific Interstitial Pneumonia
Cystic Fibrosis
Idiopathic Pulmonary Arterial
    Hypertension (Primary Pulmonary
    Hypertension)
Eisenmenger Syndrome
Sarcoidosis
Organ Donor
Rehabilitation and Lung Transplantation
    Pretransplantation Rehabilitation
    Post-transplantation Rehabilitation

Medications
    Cyclosporine A (Neoral, Gengraf,
        Sandimmune)
    Tacrolimus (FK506, Prograf)
    Azathioprine (Imuran)
    Mycophenolate mofetil (CellCept)
    Sirolimus (Rapamycin, Rapamune)
    Corticosteroids (Prednisone,
        Prednisolone, Deltasone)
Effects of Medications on Pulmonary
    Rehabilitation
Complications
    Primary Graft Dysfunction
    Airway Complications
    Acute Rejection
    Chronic Rejection
    Infection
Lung Transplantation Outcomes
Conclusion

PROFESSIONAL SKILLS

On completion of this chapter, the reader will be able to do
the following:

- Understand the general inclusion criteria for lung transplantation and absolute contraindications
- Know the candidate selection process for lung transplantation for various lung diseases, including guidelines for referral and listing for lung transplantation
- Explain the differences in pulmonary rehabilitation treatment of patients before and after lung transplantation
- Know the most common maintenance immunosuppression drug regimen for post–lung transplantation patients and how the medications affect pulmonary rehabilitation
- Recognize the complications that can occur after lung transplantation
- State the outcomes of lung transplantation including projected survival and functional and health related quality of life

The first human transplantation is credited to Dr. James Hardy and colleagues, who performed the procedure at the University of Mississippi in 1963.[1,2] Until 1974, 36 transplants were performed around the world but because of rejection-related graft failure only 2 patients survived.[3] It was not until cyclosporine was introduced in the early 1980s that solid-organ transplantation was reattempted. The 1990s witnessed the resurgence of the field of lung transplantation and today it is an established option for patients with various forms of advanced lung disease.[4-7]

LUNG ALLOCATION SCORE

The aim of transplantation is to improve longevity and the quality of life of the recipient. This requires an intimate knowledge of the course and prognosis of the primary disease as well as post-transplantation outcomes. Despite this, a significant number of patients succumb to their disease while on the waiting list. In deference of this, the United Network for Organ Sharing (UNOS), the organization that oversees organ allocation in the United States, implemented a new lung allocation system in the spring of 2005 based on need and outcomes to maximize the impact of this scarce resource. The new system calls for patients to be allocated into one of four groups based on their underlying primary disease. Models incorporating numerous factors have been developed for each of these groups to determine the prognosis during the ensuing year with and without transplantation. Patients are allocated a score based on a combination of these considerations. According to the new lung allocation system, transplantation benefits for each patient are computed on the basis of the difference between these projected outcomes. This is then balanced against wait list urgency based on the patient listing characteristics to determine organ allocation.[8]

Conditions for which lung transplantation may be considered as a potential therapeutic option and the type of transplant for which patients may be considered are summarized in Box 23-1.[1,8,9]

GENERAL INCLUSION CRITERIA

Patients may be considered for lung transplantation if they present with end-stage lung disease from any of the aforementioned conditions and meet the following criteria:

BOX 23-1	Conditions for Which Lung Transplantation May Be Considered

INDICATIONS FOR SINGLE LUNG TRANSPLANTATION
- COPD
- α_1-Antitrypsin deficiency-induced emphysema
- Pulmonary fibrosis of any etiology
- Sarcoidosis
- Eosinophilic granuloma
- Lymphangiolyomyomatosis
- Bronchiolitis obliterans
- Idiopathic pulmonary arterial hypertension (primary pulmonary hypertension)/Eisenmenger syndrome

INDICATIONS FOR BILATERAL LUNG TRANSPLANTATION
- Select patients with COPD (e.g., young age)
- Bronchiectasis
- Cystic fibrosis
- Bilateral pulmonary sepsis
- Idiopathic pulmonary arterial hypertension (primary pulmonary hypertension)/Eisenmenger syndrome with repairable cardiac defects

INDICATIONS FOR HEART–LUNG TRANSPLANTATION
- Eisenmenger syndrome with irreparable cardiac defect(s) or irreversible cardiac failure
- Pulmonary sarcoidosis with significant cardiac involvement

COPD, *Chronic obstructive pulmonary disease.*

---

1. Age:
   - Younger than 65 to 70 years for single lung transplants
   - Younger than 60 years for bilateral lung transplants
   - Younger than 55 years for heart–lung transplants
2. Failure to respond to conventional treatment
3. Limited life expectancy (less than 2 to 3 yr)
4. Patients cannot be too sick as to limit their likelihood of a successful outcome and therefore they need to at least be ambulatory with oxygen (O_2)
5. Patients should be judged to have the social and psychological profile to be able to adhere to a disciplined medical regimen

CONTRAINDICATIONS TO LUNG TRANSPLANTATION

Absolute Contraindications

1. Smoking: Patients should have abstained from smoking for at least 6 months before being considered for transplantation

2. Psychiatric disorders and psychosocial problems that cannot be resolved and that have a high likelihood of impacting negatively on the patient's outcome
3. Recent drug/alcohol abuse problems
4. Noncompliance with medical care or treatment plans even in the absence of documented psychiatric problem
5. Active malignancy within the past 2 years (except basal cell and squamous cell cancer of the skin) with a 5-year disease-free interval for extracapsular renal cell tumors, breast cancer stage 2 or higher, colon cancer staged higher than Dukes A, and melanoma, level III or higher
6. A history of primary or metastatic lung malignancy
7. Morbid obesity
8. Systemic disease
   - Renal (creatinine clearance < 50 ml/min)
   - Liver disease (cirrhosis, chronic active or chronic persistent hepatitis, hepatitis B, hepatitis C with evidence of liver disease)
   - Insulin-dependent diabetes mellitus, which is not well controlled or has resulted in significant end-organ dysfunction
   - Chronic pancreatitis
   - Active connective tissue disorder
9. Human immunodeficiency virus (HIV) positivity or other active chronic infection
10. Disabling arthritis or other limitation to exercise
11. Progressive neuromuscular disorders

Relative Contraindications

1. Coronary artery or other cardiac disease
2. Systemic hypertension that requires more than two drugs for adequate control
3. Severe right-sided heart failure
4. Multidrug-resistant/pan-resistant organism(s)
5. Insulin-dependent diabetes mellitus
6. Symptomatic osteoporosis
7. Severe musculoskeletal disease affecting the thorax
8. Poor nutritional status (body mass index <17 or >32)
9. Seizure disorder that is not well controlled
10. Steroid dependency (>20 mg/day)
11. Significant pleural disease/prior chest surgery

12. Colonization with fungi or atypical mycobacteria

CANDIDATE SELECTION

Timing of referral for prospective transplantation in appropriate lung candidates remains a decision that is dependent on a number of dynamic variables. Careful consideration of the natural history and prognosis of the underlying primary disease needs to be weighed against the projected survival after transplantation. Not only does survival need to be factored into the decision regarding transplant listing, but quality of life also needs to be taken into consideration. There are a number of quality of life instruments available that have been validated for the various primary diseases as well as for lung transplant recipients.[10-14] When survival benefits appear marginal, for example, for patients with chronic obstructive pulmonary disease (COPD), changes in quality-adjusted life years may be sufficient to justify transplantation. Last, the anticipated wait time on the transplant list also needs to be accounted for. The ultimate goals remain the obtaining of "maximal mileage" from the patient's native lung(s), conferring a greater chance of survival with a new lung; and the avoidance of death while on the transplant list.

The International Society for Heart and Lung Transplantation (ISHLT) published an updated consensus statement in 2006, which provided guidelines for referral and listing for lung transplantation.[15] Changes in the recommendations have been predicated by new knowledge of the natural history of the various diseases as well as more recently described prognostic factors.[16] How these recommendations will perform in the context of the new allocation system in effect in the United States remains uncertain. It is noteworthy, however, that the statement provides recommendations both for when to refer and when to list for transplantation.

CHRONIC OBSTRUCTIVE PULMONARY DISEASE

COPD is the one condition for which the survival benefit of transplantation has been challenged.[17] This is likely due to prior imprecise candidate selection, when this was based on the forced expiratory volume in 1 second (FEV_1) alone.[18] There is a growing appreciation that the FEV_1 should not be viewed in isolation, but in the context of other pulmonary function tests and other parameters.

Other indices that have been shown to correlate strongly with mortality include subjective breathlessness, weight loss, exercise tolerance, hospitalizations, and lung morphology.[19,20] In one study, categorization of the level of dyspnea, using a simple scale of questions, has been shown to be a better predictor of mortality than the FEV_1.[21] Patients were categorized as having grade IV dyspnea if they acknowledged having to stop for breath after walking about 100 yards on the level. With this level of dyspnea, patients were shown to have a median survival of about 3 years, which is comparable to the 3-year post-transplantation survival (61%). In contrast, those patients with the most severe disease based on FEV_1 (<35%) had a median survival in excess of 5 years.

A number of studies have shown weight loss to be a significant independent risk factor for mortality in patients with COPD.[22-24] This is thought to be due to the elevated energy metabolism related to an increased work of breathing and a catabolic state related to inflammatory cytokines.[25,26] Patients with severe COPD are often capable only of small meals and therefore this energy consumption is unmatched by an adequate dietary intake. Those patients with the lowest body mass indices, especially less than 20 kg/m^2, are at greatest risk of death.[27,28]

Hospital admissions for acute exacerbations appear to have a significant impact on subsequent mortality. Interestingly, a minority of this mortality is during the hospitalization itself, with rates of 8% to 11% being reported in two large studies.[29,30] In one of these studies, the 1-year mortality after admission was 23%; however, if patients had been admitted to an intensive care unit, the 1-year mortality then increased to 35%. For those patients whose partial pressure of carbon dioxide (CO_2) was greater then 50 mm Hg on admission, the 1-year mortality was 43%. All of the preceding mortality rates exceed the current 1-year mortality for patients with COPD who become lung recipients (21%). Therefore any patient with COPD requiring hospitalization for an exacerbation should be considered for transplantation, if they are otherwise appropriate candidates.

With improving computerized axial tomography (CAT) techniques, determination of lung morphology may ultimately provide the best index of outcomes. In patients with α_1-antitrypsin deficiency, it has been shown that CAT-based morphology, specifically in the upper lobes, correlates best with survival when compared with subjective symptoms, FEV_1, or diffusing capacity of the lung for carbon monoxide (D_{LCO}). Although patients with emphysema due to α_1-antitrypsin deficiency may have a different course compared with those with smoking-induced emphysema, these patients do represent a younger group of emphysema patients with less comorbidity; any mortality is more likely related to their underlying lung disease, and therefore they represent a more desirable group to study prognostic factors directly attributable to COPD.

Because many different factors appear to play a role, a model incorporating a number of these parameters might correlate best with survival in patients with COPD. The BODE score, incorporating *b*ody weight, *o*bstruction, level of *d*yspnea, and *e*xercise tolerance, has been proposed and validated.[31,32] On the basis of these four parameters, patients are scored on a 10-point scale. Those patients in the highest quartile (BODE score of 7 to 10) have 80% mortality at 52 months, which is clearly worse than the expected mortality with transplantation. Patients with BODE scores of less than 7 have 5-year survivals of greater than 50%, which is more than can be expected from transplantation. Therefore these patients with less severe disease should not be considered for transplantation. The degree of obstruction in this study was based on the American Thoracic Society criteria of disease severity.[33] Therefore patients with FEV_1 less than 35% were all given the same score for obstruction. The factors proposed as indicating the need for lung transplantation in the 2006 consensus guidelines include the following[15]:

- BODE (body mass, obstruction, dyspnea, and exercise) score of 7 to 10 or at least one of the following[31]:
- FEV1 less than 25% of predicted and either D_{LCO} less than 20% or homogeneous distribution of emphysema, and/or
- History of hospitalization associated with acute hypercapnea (arterial partial pressure of CO2 $\geq$ 55 mm Hg), and/or
- Pulmonary hypertension or cor pulmonale, or both, despite O2 therapy

Another issue that needs to be addressed when assessing patients with end-stage COPD is whether the patient might be an appropriate lung volume reduction surgery (LVRS) candidate.[34,35]

BOX 23-2	LVRS Physiologic and Morphologic Inclusion/Exclusion Criteria

INCLUSION

- FEV_1 15% to 45% of predicted
- TLC > 100% predicted
- Residual volume > 150% predicted
- P_{CO_2} < 60 mm Hg
- P_{O_2} > 45 mm Hg (at rest on room air)
- 6-Minute Walk Test distance > 459 ft

EXCLUSION

- FEV_1 15% to 20% of predicted with homogeneous disease on chest CAT scan or with D_{LCO} < 20% predicted
- FEV_1 < 15% or > 45% predicted
- Homogeneous disease and exercise capacity > 40% predicted

CAT, Computerized axial tomography; D_{LCO}, diffusing capacity of the lung for CO; FEV_1, forced expiratory volume in 1 second; LVRS, lung volume reduction surgery; P_{CO_2}, carbon dioxide pressure; P_{O_2}, oxygen pressure; TLC, total lung capacity.

After undergoing LVRS, patients still may be candidates for transplantation in the future. How does one then place these two procedures in context? It is important to be aware of the National Emphysema Treatment Trial (NETT) inclusion criteria before considering LVRS (Box 23-2). On the basis of these criteria, five groups of patients were identified.[35] The first of these was identified in an earlier analysis and constituted those patients with an FEV_1 less than 20% of predicted accompanied by either homogeneous disease on chest CAT scan and/or a diffusing capacity of less than 20% of predicted. These patients were shown to have a higher mortality with LVRS and therefore their characteristics represent a contraindication to this form of surgery. From the remaining patients, four groups were identified on the basis of exercise capacity and CAT scan appearance. Patients with homogeneous disease and a high exercise capacity constituted a second high-risk group whose mortality was increased by LVRS. Two groups, constituted by those patients with homogeneous disease and a low exercise capacity and those with a high exercise capacity and upper lobe—predominant disease, did not have a survival advantage, but enjoyed quality of life improvements with LVRS. The last group of patients was defined by having predominantly upper lobe disease and a low exercise capacity. This was the only group in which a survival advantage was demonstrated. Figure 23-1 shows a suggested algorithm for patients who are both

LVRS as well as potential lung transplantation candidates. Long-term follow-up shows that the salutary effects of LVRS may last up to 5 years.[36] For those patients who have a prior history of LVRS with an inadequate or unsustained response, it does appear that lung transplantation remains a viable option without compromise of results provided they remain appropriate candidates.[37]

IDIOPATHIC PULMONARY FIBROSIS

Idiopathic pulmonary fibrosis (IPF), a disease characterized pathologically by usual interstitial pneumonitis (UIP), is associated with a median survival time of approximately 3 years from the time of diagnosis.[38-40] It is therefore not surprising that patients with IPF have previously had the highest attrition rate on the transplantation wait list, with mortality rates in excess of 30%. In the 2005 ISHLT consensus statement, it was acknowledged that even patients with minimal symptoms should be referred for transplantation evaluation.[15] The poor prognosis for this condition and the high mortality on the transplant list were the impetus for this recommendation as well as the reason these patients were given 3 months of credit on the transplant list under the old allocation system. Survival does appear to be age dependent, and therefore the prognosis in the subgroup of patients who are transplantation candidates is superior, with median survivals of 63 months for patients between ages 50 and 60 years and 116 months for those younger than 50 years.

If all patients with IPF are referred at the time of diagnosis, the issue then evolves to identifying the minority group of patients with a better prognosis, who might live 5 to 10 years beyond their diagnosis without transplantation. Traditionally, the forced vital capacity (FVC) and D_{LCO} have the parameters used to indicate the need for transplantation referral. Breakpoints of 60% to 70% for the FVC and 50% to 60% for the D_{LCO} have been regarded as indicative of a poor outcome.[41] The data attesting to the utility of the FVC, or any other pulmonary function parameter, as a prognosticator for IPF have been inconsistent and imperfect at best.[42]

Many different factors have been linked to prognosis including age; gender; smoking status; presence of clubbing; serial change in the FVC,

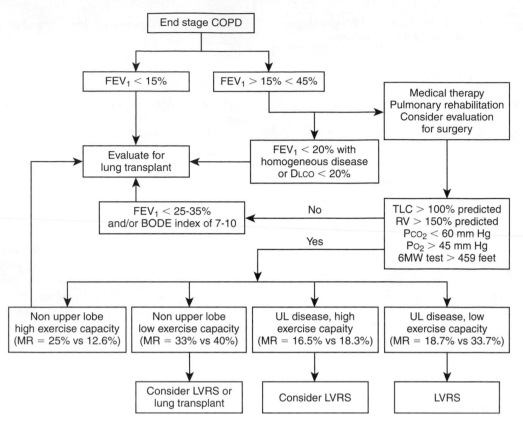

FIGURE 23-1 Suggested algorithm of surgical options for patients with chronic obstructive pulmonary disease (COPD). Shown are comparisons of lung volume reduction surgery (LVRS) versus medical therapy in each of the four United Network for Organ Sharing–defined groups, with a median follow-up of 29 months. 6MW test, 6-Minute Walk Test; BODE, body weight, obstruction, level of dyspnea, and exercise tolerance score; DLCO, diffusing capacity of the lung for carbon monoxide; FEV₁, forced expiratory capacity in 1 second; MR, mortality rates; Non upper lobe, non–upper lobe disease distribution; PCO₂, partial pressure of carbon dioxide; PO₂, partial pressure of oxygen; RV, residual volume; TLC, total lung capacity; UL disease, upper lobe–predominant disease.

DLCO, FEV_1/FVC ratio, and various biomarkers; presence of pulmonary hypertension; exercise desaturation; fibroblastic foci on surgical lung biopsy; and CAT characteristics.[43-45] Some of these factors have been incorporated into models in order to discern prognosis with greater accuracy. One of these models was specifically derived from a group of lung transplantation candidates. Of the data collected at the time of evaluation, it was found that a DLCO less than 39% of predicted together with a high-resolution computed tomography (HRCT) fibrosis score of 2.25 yielded a sensitivity and specificity for death within the next 2 years of 82% and 84%, respectively. Use of this or other models requires further prospective validation, especially for potential lung transplantation candidates.[46-48]

Clinical or physiologic parameters apart, HRCT morphologic characteristics have been shown to be important in predicting outcomes. In addition

to the extent of fibrosis, it appears that categorization of patients with histologic UIP into those with HRCT features typical of UIP and those with atypical HRCT appearance might have important prognostic implications. Patients with histologic UIP and an HRCT consistent with definite or probable UIP have a median survival of about 2 years, whereas those patients with histologic UIP and an HRCT that is indeterminate for UIP or suggestive of nonspecific interstitial pneumonia (NSIP) have a median survival of 5.76 years.[49] Serial pulmonary function tests, resting arterial partial pressure of oxygen (PaO₂), and desaturation on the 6-Minute Walk Test (6MWT) might also help discern those patients with a better prognosis. Regarding the latter test, it has been shown that patients who desaturate below 89% on a 6-minute walk study had a 4-year survival of 34.5% versus 69% for those who did not.[50] This latter 4-year survival far surpasses the 42% survival for the same period in IPF transplant recipients. Therefore, it would appear that as long as patients maintain this level of saturation on serial 6-minute walk studies, the need for transplantation might be deferred.

Two studies described groups of patients whose FVCs improved over the course of 6 months and of whom approximately two thirds survived beyond 5 years.[51,52] These patients constituted only 11 and 19% of the patients with IPF in these respective studies. These low percentages underscore the risk of monitoring patients expectantly to assess for improvement before referring them for transplantation. Patients should, rather, be monitored simultaneously while undergoing an evaluation or while listed for transplantation. If they do show improvement, then they can be delisted or made inactive on the transplant list.

Approximately 30% of patients with IPF will manifest serial deterioration in their spirometric indices at 6 months after their initial presentation. This portends the worst prognosis with median survivals of less than 2 years. What has previously been underappreciated is that even those patients who maintain their FVC within 10% of their baseline are at risk of succumbing to their disease. Data from the study of interferon γ-1b, in which spirometry was performed every 3 months, attest to patients succumbing before manifesting a significant reduction in FVC.[53] Therefore stability of spirometry should not be regarded as stability of disease and these patients might still be best served with transplantation.

On the basis of the information presented, the ISHLT recommends that patients with IPF be transplanted when they demonstrate any of the following: (1) a D_{LCO} less than 39% of predicted, (2) a 10% of greater decrement in FVC during the 6 months of follow-up, (3) a decrease in pulse oximetry below 88% during the 6MWT, or (4) the presence of honeycombing on HRCT with a fibrosis score greater than 2.[15]

NONSPECIFIC INTERSTITIAL PNEUMONIA

The pathologic pattern of nonspecific interstitial pneumonia (NSIP) was first described in 1994 as a separate entity with a more benign course than IPF.[53] Until 2005, there had been no transplant listing recommendations for this relatively newly described condition. There is no separate designation for NSIP when patients are listed for transplantation and such patients are listed as "IPF" with UNOS. The initial report of NSIP described a mortality of only 11% and subsequent reports have attested to median survivals anywhere from more than 5 to greater than 10 years.[54] Although this overall survival is better than what can be expected with transplantation, there does appear to be a group of patients whose prognosis is worse and who might best be served by transplantation. The salient issue then becomes trying to identify those patients who are at highest risk for disease progression and mortality.

Although pathologic temporal homogeneity is what binds these cases, it is apparent that NSIP can be seen in conjunction with a heterogeneous group of conditions. This pathologic injury pattern can be seen in association with collagen vascular diseases, various inhalational exposures, resolving diffuse alveolar damage, and UIP.[55] Thus it is likely that there is a spectrum of outcomes among such cases, including some whose prognosis warrants consideration for transplantation. NSIP-like changes can be seen in conjunction with UIP in anywhere from 12.5% to 25% of cases.[56,57] If the two coexist, then UIP becomes the default diagnosis, because such cases have a prognosis that most closely approximates that of UIP.

The one group of patients with NSIP whose prognosis is excellent includes those with the cellular variant, in whom 5- and 10-year survivals of 100% have been reported. Unfortunately, this variant is three times less common than the fibrotic form and likely represents a different disease with a course that more closely parallels that of desquamative interstitial pneumonia. Patients with NSIP with a D_{LCO} less than 35% or a decrease in D_{LCO} greater than 15% of predicted have been shown to have an outcome that approximates that of patients with UIP, with a median survival of about 2 years. The current ISHLT recommendations for transplantation for NSIP include (1) a D_{LCO} less than 35% predicted and/or (2) a 10% or greater decrement in FVC or 15% decrement in D_{LCO} during 6 months of follow-up.[15]

CYSTIC FIBROSIS

The criteria proposed in the consensus statement from 2006 for patients with cystic fibrosis to be referred for lung transplantation included

(1) an FEV₁ not exceeding 30% predicted, or a rapid decline in FEV_1, especially in young female patients; (2) exacerbation of pulmonary disease requiring a stay in the intensive care unit; (3) increasing frequency of exacerbations requiring antibiotic therapy; (4) refractory or recurrent pneumothoraces; and/or (5) recurrent hemoptysis not controlled by embolization.[15]

The largest series of outcomes reported has been based on analyses from the Cystic Fibrosis Foundation National Patient Registry.[58-62] The utility of the FEV_1 as a predictor of outcomes at 2 years has been examined with data derived from this registry. On the basis of this, an FEV_1 less than 30% was shown to have a sensitivity for predicting death within the next 2 years of 42% with a specificity of 95%. The associated negative predictive value was 97%, indicating that transplantation could be deferred if a patient's FEV_1 remained above this level. This FEV_1 cutoff performed as accurately as a multiple logistic regression model comprising six different factors.[63] However, a study assessing 5-year survival has shown that a model comprising nine factors was most predictive of outcomes. These factors include age, FEV_1, gender, weight-for-age z score, pancreatic insufficiency, diabetes mellitus, infection with *Staphylococcus aureus*, infection with *Burkholderia cepacia*, and the number of acute exacerbations per year. The effect of each of these variables on 5-year survival in FEV_1 equivalency is shown in Table 23-1.[64] With the new transplant allocation system in place in the United States, no patient should wait as long as 5 years for a transplant. This appears to be especially true in the case of patients with cystic fibrosis, whom the allocation system appears to favor.

The 2006 guidelines for transplantation, interestingly, do not include the FEV_1 criteria, and are composed of the following: (1) O_2-dependent respiratory failure, (2) hypercapnea, and/or (3) pulmonary hypertension.[15]

IDIOPATHIC PULMONARY ARTERIAL HYPERTENSION (PRIMARY PULMONARY HYPERTENSION)

Of all the conditions for which lung transplantation is performed, idiopathic pulmonary arterial hypertension (IPAH) (formerly known as primary pulmonary hypertension) is the only one for which there have been significant strides made in medical

TABLE 23-1	Covariate Influence on 5-Year Survival Expressed as FEV₁ Equivalent
Covariate	FEV₁ Equivalence*
Age (per year)	−0.7
Sex (male = 0, female = 1)	−6
FEV₁ (per %)	1
Weight-for-age z score†	10
Pancreatic insufficiency (0 or 1)	12
Diabetes mellitus (0 or 1)	−13
Staphylococcus aureus infection (0 or 1)	6
Burkholderia cepacia infection (0 or 1)	−48
No. of acute exacerbations (0-5)	−12

*The FEV₁ equivalence column shows the survival effect of each variable expressed as the effective equivalent change in FEV_1 expressed as a percentage of the predicted value (FEV_1%). For example, a diagnosis of diabetes mellitus has the same survival effect as subtracting 13% from the actual measured FEV_1%.
†Measure of bone density adjusted for age.
From Liou TG, Adler FR, FitzSimmons SC et al: Predictive 5-year survivorship model of cystic fibrosis, Am J Epidemiol 153:345-352, 2001.

management. An attestation to this is the ever-decreasing number of patients with IPAH who ultimately receive lung transplants. In 1990, approximately 10.5% of all lung transplants were for patients with primary pulmonary hypertension, whereas in 2001 only 3.6% of lung transplantations performed were for patients with this condition. There are now five U.S. Food and Drug Administration (FDA)–approved medical therapies for IPAH (epoprostenol, bosentan, sildenafil, inhaled iloprost, and treprostinil). Epoprostenol was the first of these agents to become available, having received FDA approval in 1995. Although initially touted as a bridge to transplantation, it has since been realized that the need for transplantation can be averted in some cases.[65-68] There is indirect evidence that the other agents might also confer a survival advantage.[69] There are also a number of new agents in various stages of development, as well as studies of combination therapy, which may further diminish the need for lung transplantation.

Before the advent of these effective therapies, the decision to list patients with IPAH was relatively easy, because the median survival was only about 2.8 years.[70] In the current era, patients who have New York Heart Association (NYHA) class III or IV symptoms, and hemodynamics that are compromised to the point that they are considered transplantation candidates, should be given the gold standard of therapy, which remains continuous intravenous prostanoid therapy. Whether other agents should be added initially or in combination is open to debate and requires further study. It is tempting to treat patients with multiple agents acting on different pathways up front, especially when one considers that the alternative to treatment failure is transplantation. Depending on the characteristics of the local median waiting time, consideration should be given to listing at the same time that therapy is initiated.

Response to therapy can be assessed as early as 3 months after the initiation of therapy. Patients who remain NYHA class III or IV after 3 months of intravenous epoprostenol or treprostinil have a 2-year survival of 46% and therefore warrant ongoing listing for transplantation. On the other hand, those who have been converted to NYHA class I or II have a 2-year survival of 93% and therefore can be made inactive or delisted.

The 2006 ISHLT guidelines for listing include (1) persistent NYHA class III or IV status despite maximal medical therapy, (2) low (<350 m) or declining 6MWT, (3) failing therapy with intravenous epoprostenol, or equivalent, (4) cardiac index of less than 2 L/min/m^2, and/or (5) right atrial pressure exceeding 15 mm Hg.[15]

EISENMENGER SYNDROME

It is difficult to decide the appropriateness and timing of transplantation for patients with Eisenmenger syndrome. These patients tend to have a better prognosis than patients with IPAH despite similar pulmonary arterial pressures.[71] They also constitute a group of patients concerning whom doubt has been cast as to the risk/benefit of lung transplantation. These patients can also now be successfully managed with continuous intravenous epoprostenol, and in some cases therapy may render previously inoperable patients operable.[72] It is hoped that this will further lessen the need for transplantation consideration in this difficult group. Historically, the procedure of choice for these patients has evolved from heart—lung transplantation to lung transplantation alone with repair of the cardiac defect. However, there are now data suggesting that heart—lung transplantation might be the procedure that confers the greatest survival advantage, especially for those patients with Eisenmenger syndrome due to ventricular

septal defects.[73] The 2006 ISHLT consensus statement did not offer transplantation guidelines for Eisenmenger syndrome.[15]

SARCOIDOSIS

After COPD, sarcoidosis is the second most common condition for which lung transplantation may be an option. However, because most patients run a benign course and only about 10% to 20% sustains permanent sequelae, sarcoidosis contributes only 2.5% of all lung transplant recipients. The 2006 ISHLT guidelines statement was the first time that specific referral and transplant guidelines were recommended for sarcoidosis.[15]

There is the possibility of spontaneous reversal in the earlier stages, and therefore only those patients with stage IV sarcoidosis should be considered for transplantation. This stage is radiographically characterized by advanced fibrotic changes, honeycombing, hilar retraction, bullae, cysts, and emphysema.[74] Listed patients with sarcoidosis have a high risk of dying while awaiting transplantation, with 28% of them succumbing before transplantation. This approximates the wait list mortality of patients with IPF. Because patients with sarcoidosis are generally diagnosed and in the medical system earlier than patients with IPF, this high attrition rate on the list likely reflects late consideration and referral for transplantation. Predictors of mortality on the transplant list include the presence of underlying pulmonary hypertension, amount of supplemental O_2 needed, and African American race.[75,76] There is a paucity of data looking at pulmonary function test predictors of mortality in patients with sarcoidosis. One such study has shown that those patients with an FVC less than 1.5 L are at greatest risk of death. For those patients whose highest FVC falls below this threshold, the positive predictive value for death is 46% with a negative predictive value of 98%.[75] Characteristics of listed patients with sarcoidosis include a mean FVC of 42.6% of predicted and a mean FEV_1 of 36% of predicted. Therefore consideration for transplantation when the FVC is less than 50% predicted or the FEV_1 is less than 40% predicted seems reasonable.[77]

The 2006 ISHLT guidelines recommend referral for transplantation when patients remain in NYHA functional class III or IV despite therapy. Transplantation is recommended when the preceding functional status is accompanied by (1) hypoxemia at rest, (2) pulmonary hypertension, and/or (3) elevated right atrial pressure exceeding 15 mm Hg.[15]

ORGAN DONOR

Most solid organs for transplantation are obtained from heart-beating, brain-dead donors. After brain death criteria have been fulfilled and family permission has been granted, lungs and other organs can be procured. In the United States, this process is coordinated by local organ procurement organizations (OPOs). Local OPO representatives manage the donor process based on the UNOS guidelines published in 1993.[78]

On the recipient end, the pulmonary and surgical teams make decisions about donor acceptability and potential donor–recipient matching. General guidelines for donor selection include (1) age younger than 65 years; (2) absence of significant lung disease, including asthma; (3) limited cumulative cigarette-smoking history (less than 30 pack-years); (4) satisfactory bronchoscopic appearance without evidence of aspiration; (5) clear lung fields on chest radiograph; (6) adequate oxygenation ($PaO_2 > 300$ on a fraction of inspired oxygen [FIO_2] of 100%); and (7) acceptable lung compliance.[1]

General exclusionary criteria include viral infections such as HIV, encephalitis, and hepatitis, untreated septicemia or primary lung infection, malignancy other than primary unmetastasized brain tumor, and current intravenous drug use.[79]

Donor and recipient should match by blood type and thoracic size dimensions, although some programs use donors with a modest size discrepancy. Size is gauged mostly by donor and recipient height because this is the factor that is the strongest determinant of lung volumes.

REHABILITATION AND LUNG TRANSPLANTATION

Pretransplantation Rehabilitation

Most centers require that potential candidates for lung transplantation undergo a comprehensive pulmonary rehabilitation (PR) program before transplantation.[80] PR is useful in patients undergoing lung transplantation, although the goals are different before and after surgery. The primary goal of pretransplantation rehabilitation is to optimize and maintain the patient's functional status while continuing close monitoring of the underlying disease and to provide psychosocial support.[81] The secondary goal is to thereby improve post-transplantation compliance, morbidity, hospital length of stay, and possibly even mortality. Some patients who present for transplantation evaluation may be too limited and deconditioned to be regarded as appropriate candidates. A further goal for such patients would be to improve their functional status to the point that they can be regarded as appropriate candidates. At the other end of the "window for transplantation," some patients might have sufficient improvement to delay their listing. Even patients with severe respiratory impairment may experience a reduction in dyspnea and an improvement in functional status with PR.[82,83] One of the goals in the immediate post-transplantation period is to mobilize the patient and implement post-transplantation PR as soon as possible. The more mobile the patient going into the surgery, the greater the likelihood that PR can be resumed expeditiously after transplantation.

Several small studies have shown that pretransplantation PR maintains or increases exercise capacity as measured by the 6MWT.[81-86] In addition, a study of patients with severe pulmonary hypertension undergoing an intensive inpatient PR program showed that significant improvement in the 6MWT distance, quality of life scores, World Health Organization functional class, peak O_2 consumption, O_2 consumption at the anaerobic threshold, and maximal workload was achieved.[86] Interestingly, the improvement in the 6MWT distance with PR was greater than that achieved in studies of pulmonary hypertension medications. Because no significant differences were documented in hemodynamic data of the patients before and after the program, the authors postulated that the physiologic improvements were due to improved efficacy of muscular gas exchange and metabolism and reversal of skeletal muscle atrophy. At the molecular level, exercise-induced attenuation of endothelial dysfunction and inflammatory mediators may also play a role.

Patients awaiting lung transplantation carry a variety of diagnoses, and the rehabilitation center should be prepared to tailor goals to the various patient groups and individual patients. The initial assessment of all patients should include an evaluation of the musculoskeletal system, the degree of endurance and strength, the severity of desaturation (assessed with a 6MWT), and mobility limitations.[80]

Exercise training is a cornerstone of any PR program and usually involves three sessions per week that concentrate on flexibility exercises, stretching, muscle strengthening, and endurance training.[80] The most important goals of exercise conditioning are the effects on skeletal muscle strength and endurance, including the diaphragm fibers.[87] Data suggest that survival after lung transplantation is significantly related to ventilatory muscle strength.[84] Secondary goals include the assessment and reinforcement of patient compliance and motivation.

Pre–lung transplantation patients typically have the most severe underlying pulmonary disease, and therefore the intensity of exercise training may need to be reduced. In patients with chronic lung disease, use of target heart rate might not be appropriate because these patients frequently reach a ventilatory limitation before achieving target heart rates.[80] Patients should exercise close to the highest workload that can be tolerated as gauged by their symptoms, which might include dyspnea, generalized fatigue, leg fatigue, or dizziness.[88] Patients usually train to a level of dyspnea that can be sustained with reasonable comfort for several minutes. Gradual increases are then made in the duration or intensity of training. Interval training, including alternating brief periods of high and low intensity exercise, may be beneficial. Finally, exercise should be supervised to ensure that the prescribed workload can be safely tolerated but is intense enough to have a beneficial effect.

Ambulation performed with or without a rolling walker or on a treadmill is a valuable mode of conditioning while promoting improved functional status. Ambulation-based exercises are considered superior to other methods of conditioning training.[89] However, they are also associated with increased work of breathing and metabolic cost in comparison with less intense modes of exercises. Using a walker or handlebars on a treadmill reduces work of breathing and allows for increased exercise duration.[90]

Stationary bicycle ergometry is the mode of exercise used for most debilitated patients. It eliminates the adverse effects of body weight and thoracic instability encountered during most other forms of aerobic exercise while optimizing the accessory muscles to assist with respiration. Proper use of the handle bars appears to elevate and stabilize the thorax, which may facilitate diaphragmatic descent, thereby enabling a decrease in the work of breathing and metabolic cost of exercise.[87] The most debilitated patients can benefit from using the restorator bicycle, which is a pedal-system bicycle that allows patients to sit comfortably in the chair while stabilizing the back, thorax, and arms. This system allows the overcoming of isometric arm contractions that occur with use of treadmill and stationary bicycles.[87]

Upper extremity work is accompanied by a higher ventilatory demand than lower extremity exercises, with consequent development of symptoms of severe dyspnea. Upper extremity training is included in most comprehensive PR programs, as it has been shown to decrease metabolic and ventilatory requirements for arm exercises.[80]

It is important that the patient maintain the intensity of exercise achieved up to the time of surgery, preferably by undertaking exercise in a PR center complemented by home-based exercise. Ongoing attendance in a rehabilitation maintenance exercise program and periodic review of the home exercise prescription allow frequent reassessment by the PR team. This allows for the ongoing serial assessment of the patient in terms of his or her compliance, change in medical condition, and other potential issues that might impact transplantation status. PR provides an ideal setting for education about the transplantation process and the management of expectations after the procedure. It also can provide psychosocial support for patients and family members who are coping with end-stage lung disease[91] and help prepare them for the psychological and physiologic stress of surgery.[80] PR also provides the opportunity to impart information about nutrition, stress management, and relaxation techniques. One of the prerequisites for successful transplantation is patient compliance. Ongoing PR is an ideal forum for monitoring the desire and ability of patients to follow and understand instruction. Previously unappreciated social, financial, or logistic issues might also be uncovered during the course of a PR program. As such, members of the PR team are integral members of the transplantation team. Transplantation team members might only have a few select opportunities to interact with patients before the transplantation procedure. Therefore such issues might escape detection without feedback and input from the PR team members. In the context of PR programs directly associated with transplantation centers, pretransplantation patients frequently interact with transplant recipients, enabling an informal support network and mentorship opportunities.

Post-transplantation Rehabilitation

Successful postoperative rehabilitation depends largely on successful participation in and completion of a preoperative PR program. Any propensity for noncompliance with PR or resistance to mobilization is apt to manifest further in the postoperative period. This may be compounded or precipitated by postanesthetic effects, pain, and narcotic medications. In addition to precipitating or perpetuating any deconditioning, immobilization can have profound effects on the allograft with incomplete alveolar expansion.

Inadequate lung expansion, alone or in combination with prolonged bed rest, can result in atelectasis, secretion pooling, and predisposition to pulmonary infection. Lung transplantation patients are particularly at risk for the latter complication. The nature of the lung donors is such that recipients frequently "inherit" an aspiration or ventilator-associated pneumonia from their lung donors. Patients are routinely administered broad-spectrum antibiotics for this reason. A contributory factor to the predisposition for pulmonary infections includes denervation of the newly implanted allograft with the resultant loss of the cough reflex distal to the anastomosis. For this reason pulmonary toilet is critical and should include devices that facilitate the mobilization of secretions. Deliberate coughing is encouraged to mobilize any distal secretions. Once secretions are mobilized proximal to the anastomosis, the patient's own intrinsic cough reflex should be stimulated. Other contributory factors for infection include impairment of mucociliary clearance, loss of the pulmonary lymphatics, and early post-transplantation changes in the composition of surfactant, which affects its antimicrobial properties.[80,92] In addition, patients can develop sterile (noninfectious) secretions and mucous plugs, which can predispose to infections and atelectasis. The reason for this is related to bronchial airway ischemia, which results from the bronchial circulation being sacrificed as part of the transplantation procedure. In extreme cases, self-limiting sloughing of the airways might ensue.

In addition to infection, there are multiple potential complications that can result from transplantation. These include primary graft dysfunction, rejection, and bleeding. Frequently other organ complications can also ensue, such as cardiovascular instability or renal failure. Patients who remain immobile as a result of serious post-transplantation complications are at risk of entering the cascade of deconditioning. Medications including high-dose steroids and calcineurin inhibitors (cyclosporine and tacrolimus) are unavoidable, but can contribute to weakness and further compound the problem. In more complicated cases, the use of paralytic agents and aminoglycosides might become necessary, which themselves can lead to profound, protracted weakness. Patients who have such a "rocky" course often require long-term physical therapy and PR after transplantation.

The main goal of early post-transplantation rehabilitation is to minimize atelectasis and aid in the clearance of airway secretions.[80] Positive end-expiratory pressure and postural drainage by manual or bed chest percussion are applied with the patient still intubated to enable these goals.[93] Early positioning in a chair also helps decrease atelectasis and improves chest tube drainage. Once extubated, incentive spirometry and flutter devices can further aid in the prevention of atelectasis and strengthening of the diaphragm.[94]

Rehabilitation in the early postoperative period also should include range of motion, basic transfer activities (e.g., sitting to standing), breathing pattern efficiency, upper and lower extremity strengthening, and functional mobility. An exercise program based on a restorator bicycle and early ambulation is employed once a patient is determined to be stable. Special walkers can be used to facilitate walking while chest tubes are still in place. Resistive exercise of the upper and lower extremities can be performed in addition to simple ambulation. Analgesia to control incisional and chest tube—related pain needs to be titrated appropriately to enable the prescribed exercise.[95]

Before discharge, it is important to check that the patient's gait is stable and that lower extremity strength is adequate for the independent performance of tasks such as transferring into and out of bed and stair climbing.[96] At discharge, patients are instructed on how to record their daily spirometry to monitor for the early detection of pulmonary events such as episodes of acute rejection and infection.[80]

After discharge, patients are expected to continue with PR to maximize their strength and endurance. Most programs use exercise regimens similar to those initiated in the pretransplantation period. Transplant recipients are at high risk of osteoporosis due to the prolonged use of immunosuppressive medications.[96] Therefore maintenance of good posture and back protection measures, avoiding rotation and flexion, needs to be addressed to prevent spinal compression fractures. A modified upper extremity training program is designed for each patient individually postoperatively because of healing and pain issues related to the chest wall surgery.[80] PR is an ideal setting for continuing patient education with a focus on health maintenance, nutrition counseling, as well as the early detection of infection and rejection, and recognizing other signs of long-term posttransplantation complications including medication side effects.

Despite significant improvements in pulmonary function and gas exchange, cardiopulmonary exercise test responses remain abnormally low, with O_2 consumptions of only 40% to 60% of predicted.[97] There may be an important contributory role of immunosuppressive medications in this regard, specifically calcineurin inhibitors, which have been reported to affect oxidative metabolism at the mitochondrial level.[98,99] Nevertheless, multiple studies demonstrate overall improvement in exercise tolerance and quality of life after transplantation.[100]

In summary, although there are a few studies examining the impact of PR in lung transplantation candidates, PR is commonly accepted as an integral bridge between the pre— to post—lung transplantation periods. PR can have a significant influence on multiple domains of the patients' pretransplantation status as well as important enduring post-transplantation benefits.

MEDICATIONS

Maintenance immunosuppression for most transplantation patients includes a three-drug regimen including a calcineurin inhibitor (cyclosporine A [CSA] or tacrolimus [FK506]), a purine synthesis inhibitor (mycophenolate mofetil [MMF] or azathioprine [AZA]), and corticosteroids (Table 23-2).[101]

Cyclosporine A (Neoral, Gengraf, Sandimmune)

Cyclosporine A (CSA) binds to an intracellular protein, cyclophilin, and the formed complex binds to calcineurin, an enzyme vital to the transcription of several T-cell cytokines, including interleukin-2. The final result is a specific and reversible inhibition of immunocompetent T-cell activation, mainly $CD4^+$ T cells.

The major CSA side effects are listed in Table 23-2. Nephrotoxicity occurs in one third of patients as a result of renal vasoconstriction of afferent arterioles. Clinically, fluid retention, hyperkalemia, and hyperchloremia may accompany elevated creatinine levels. It is often associated with high trough levels, and is mostly reversible, upon dose reduction. Chronic CSA renal toxicity is due to irreversible glomerular fibrosis. Hypertension, both systolic and diastolic, occurs in 50% of patients and usually develops within few days to a few months after CSA administration. Neurotoxicity, including headaches and fine hand tremors, occur in 30% of patients and may improve without halting therapy. Peripheral neuropathy with symptoms of numbness, tingling, and burning may also occur, as can mild alterations in mental status. Seizures, especially when CSA is used with high-dose steroids, have also been reported. Severe neurotoxicity, with characteristic white matter changes on magnetic resonance imaging, is rare. Mild hirsutism on the face, arms, eyebrows, and back occurs in 30% of patients. Gingival hyperplasia occurs in 10% of patients and may improve with vigorous oral hygiene. Hepatotoxicity occurs in less than 5% and is characterized by cholestatic jaundice.

Tacrolimus (FK506, Prograf)

Tacrolimus is pharmacologically related to CSA. Like CSA, it inhibits T-cell activation by binding to the FK-binding protein, and inhibits activity of calcineurin. A side effect profile not unlike that of CSA is seen with similar rates of nephrotoxicity, neurotoxicity, and hypertension. Unlike CSA, it can also cause diabetes mellitus. Tacrolimus is cleared by the liver, and the levels rise rapidly in patients with severe liver dysfunction.

There are some data that a tacrolimus-based regimen (versus a cyclosporine regimen) results in fewer acute rejections and a lower incidence of bronchiolitis obliterans syndrome.[102]

Azathioprine (Imuran)

Azathioprine (AZA) inhibits lymphocyte replication and function. It is metabolized by the liver to 6-mercaptopurine, which in turn is converted to the active metabolite, thioinosinic acid. The latter inhibits

TABLE 23-2	Immunosuppressive Medications	
	Mechanism of Action	Side Effects
CSA	Blocks calcineurin (inhibits T-cell activation)	Nephrotoxicity, hypertension, neurotoxicity, hirsutism, gingival hyperplasia, hepatotoxicity
Tacrolimus	Blocks calcineurin (inhibits T-cell activation)	Nephrotoxicity, hypertension, neurotoxicity, diabetes mellitus
MMF	Purine synthesis inhibitor (inhibits lymphocyte replication)	Leukopenia, thrombocytopenia, gastrointestinal symptoms
AZA	Purine synthesis inhibitor (inhibits lymphocyte replication)	Hematotoxicity, alopecia, hepatotoxicity, pancreatitis, rash, gastrointestinal symptoms, teratogenicity
Prednisone	Alteration of T-cell proliferation, inhibition of cytokine production, suppression of macrophage function	Cushing's syndrome, hypertension, hyperglycemia, infections, osteoporosis, cataracts, mood alterations
Sirolimus	Suppression of cytokine-driven T-cell differentiation	Hypertriglyceridemia, hypercholesterolemia, rash, hypokalemia, leukopenia, thrombocytopenia, gastrointestinal symptoms

AZA, *Azathioprine*; CSA, *cyclosporine A*; MMF, *mycophenolate mofetil.*

DNA synthesis with the resultant effect of inhibition of cell division by activated lymphocytes.

Major side effects include hematologic toxicity, temporary hair loss, hepatotoxicity, pancreatitis, rash, and gastrointestinal (GI) side effects. Hematologic toxicity manifests as dose-dependent leukopenia, although all bone marrow lines may be suppressed. The dose should be adjusted to maintain a white blood cell count of 4000 to 6000/mm^3. Liver function abnormalities may require dosage decreases or discontinuation of the medication. Pancreatitis mandates discontinuation of the medication, although it may persist despite this. Rash is infrequent and likely represents an allergic reaction. GI side effects are also usually infrequent and include mostly nausea and vomiting.

AZA should never be given with allopurinol, as the combination can cause severe bone marrow suppression. AZA is removed by dialysis and the dose should therefore be administered thereafter.

Mycophenolate Mofetil (CellCept)

Mycophenolate mofetil (MMF) inhibits late-stage T-cell activation by interfering with purine synthesis, antibody formation, and cytotoxic T-cell generation. Potential toxicities include leukopenia, thrombocytopenia, and GI side effects, such as nausea, vomiting, and diarrhea. GI side effects may be reduced by splitting the daily dose into three or four smaller doses. A microemulsion formulation is also available that may ameliorate

GI symptoms. MMF is considered to be teratogenic, with birth defects having been reported in animal studies. MMF is not dialyzable.

Sirolimus (Rapamycin, Rapamune)

Sirolimus binds to the FK-binding protein 12 (FKBP12), and the complex then binds to a regulatory protein mammalian target of rapamycin (mTOR), thereby inhibiting its activation. This in turn results in suppression of cytokine-driven T-cell differentiation. Despite binding to the same protein, sirolimus and tacrolimus can be successfully used together.

Sirolimus can cause hypertriglyceridemia and hypercholesterolemia in a dose-dependent fashion. It can also result in bone marrow suppression with leukopenia and thrombocytopenia, especially when used with MMF. Hypokalemia, rash, nausea, and vomiting have been reported. Although not thought to be nephrotoxic, increases in serum creatinine, especially in combination with CSA, can be seen. It is nonetheless often used as a renal preserving agent in patients with nephrotoxicity. There have also been anecdotal reports of sirolimus-related interstitial pneumonitis in all forms of solid-organ transplantation.

Corticosteroids (Prednisone, Prednisolone, Deltasone)

Corticosteroids have multiple immunosuppressive mechanisms, including alteration of T-cell proliferation, inhibition of cytokine production (interleukin-2 and interleukin-6), suppression of macrophage function, reduction of adhesion molecule expression, and induction of lymphocyte apoptosis.

Toxicities are multiple and include Cushing's syndrome, hyperglycemia and increased appetite, fluid retention, hypertension, cataracts, mood alterations, candidiasis, GI ulcers, increased risk of infections, leukocytosis, musculoskeletal symptoms, and osteoporosis. Efforts are usually made to reduce the steroid dose expeditiously because of its broad side effect profile.

EFFECTS OF MEDICATIONS ON PULMONARY REHABILITATION

The development of any myopathy after transplantation can have a profound effect on the ability of patients to engage in PR. This is especially true for patients who have had a protracted course in an intensive care unit, where they might have received multiple agents that could precipitate or predispose to a myopathy. These agents include but are not limited to high-dose steroids, paralytic agents, and aminoglycoside antibiotics. The calcineurin inhibitors may also affect oxidation at the cellular mitochondrial level.[98,99] This is thought to be responsible for patients attaining maximal O_2 consumption only in the 40% to 60% range. This level of function is fully compatible with a normal lifestyle and does not affect the ability of patients to participate in PR.

COMPLICATIONS

Primary Graft Dysfunction

Primary graft dysfunction (PGD) is a devastating form of acute lung injury that afflicts about 10% to 25% of patients in the first hours to days —after lung transplantation.[103-105] This term, previously known as reperfusion injury or pulmonary reimplantation response, refers to a clinical scenario of hypoxemia and diffuse allograft infiltrates. Histologically, early graft dysfunction is characterized by diffuse alveolar damage.[106] It results from acute lung injury with increased vascular permeability that is presumably secondary to preservation and ischemia—reperfusion injury. A variety of factors have been linked to a higher incidence of PGD, including greater donor age, lower donor oxygenation, and greater need for inotropic support.[107]

The incidence of PGD depends on how it is defined. This was not standardized until a consensus panel under the auspices of the ISHLT proposed a grading system for PGD. The classification scheme contains a grading for severity of PGD based on the ratio of O_2 delivered to the lung to the partial pressure of O_2 measured by arterial blood gas determination (P/F ratio) at different time points: grade 0, Pao_2/Fio_2 greater than 300 with absent radiographic changes of pulmonary edema; grade 1, Pao_2/Fio_2 greater than 300 with radiographic findings consistent with pulmonary edema; grade 2, Pao_2/Fio_2 between 200 and 300 with radiographic findings consistent with pulmonary edema; and grade 3, Pao_2/Fio_2 less than 200 with radiographic findings consistent with pulmonary edema.[103] The presence of PGD is assessed at the following time points: immediately postoperatively (T0) and 24 hours (T24), 48 hours (T48), and 72 hours (T72) postoperatively. Other entities that should be excluded before the diagnosis include hyperacute rejection, venous anastomotic obstruction, pneumonia, and cardiogenic pulmonary edema.[103]

In a review of the UNOS database with more than 5500 patients, the incidence of PGD was reported to be approximately 10.2%. When present, it greatly influences short-term mortality, with an all-cause 30-day mortality of 42.1% in patients with early graft dysfunction versus 6.1% in unaffected patients.[108] PGD can result in protracted periods of intubation, increased length of stay in an intensive care unit, hospital length of stay, and prolonged disability.[109] Among the patients who survived to 1 year after transplantation, mortality was also much higher in the former group, with a hazard ratio of 1.35.[108] Treatment includes supportive principles of acute lung injury including the limitation of intravenous fluids and appropriate diuresis.[110]

Airway Complications

Dehiscence of the airway anastomosis was the surgical Achilles' heel of lung transplantation in the early days of transplantation.[111] In contemporary series, the prevalence of airway complications, including dehiscence, stenosis, and bronchomalacia, has been between 10% and 20%, but the associated mortality is low.[112-117] Stenosis is considered to be significant if airway obstruction by bronchoscopic evaluation is more than 50%. Bronchomalacia causes dynamic, expiratory collapse best observed bronchoscopically when patients breathe spontaneously. Treatment options for stenosis include laser resection and dilatation; however, stent placement is often required, especially if bronchomalacia is present.[118]

Acute Rejection

Acute rejection remains one of the most common complications after lung transplantation. It is a T-cell—mediated response directed against "nonself" antigens that include both HLA and non-HLA proteins.

Acute rejection is usually not seen before day 6 after transplantation, but only 24% to 40% of patients remain rejection free at 1 year after transplantation.[119] The greatest risk for development of acute rejection is in the first several months after transplantation.[119,120] The reason for such an exceedingly high rate of rejection is multifocal, including the constant exposure of the lung to the environment and its large vascular and lymphatic network.

The presentation of acute rejection is usually nonspecific and can range in severity from asymptomatic to acute respiratory failure. Patients may have increased shortness of breath, desaturation, fever, leukocytosis, or reduced spirometry. Infiltrates on chest radiograph or CAT scan are uncommon but are more likely to be seen with early rejection.[121,122]

The management of acute rejection is usually in the form of high-dose bolused methylprednisolone sodium succinate (Solu-Medrol). Early episodes of acute rejection typically respond rapidly to treatment with resolution of clinical symptoms and improvement in spirometric and radiographic findings. However, a significant portion of patients with later episodes of rejection will stabilize with lower post-treatment spirometric values.[123] A small subset of patients has rejection that is refractory to repeated treatment courses of corticosteroids. In such cases, other therapies including cytolytics and total lymphoid irradiation; photophoresis may be useful.[124-126] The use of high-dose steroids can predispose to myopathy especially in patients who are receiving concomitant aminoglycosides or paralytic agents. This may impact on the need and duration of PR in the post-transplantation period. Recurrent episodes of acute rejection have been consistently implicated in the later development of bronchiolitis obliterans syndrome (BOS), which is the physiologic correlate of chronic allograft rejection.[127-133]

Chronic Rejection

Increasing success early after transplantation has been tempered by the long-term development of chronic allograft dysfunction, which is histologically characterized by obliterative bronchiolitis. Pathologically, obliterative bronchiolitis is characterized by the presence of dense mononuclear inflammation in the walls of the airways with partial or total obliteration of airway lumens.[134] Because the yield of pathologic diagnosis on transbronchial biopsy is relatively low, the physiologic entity of bronchiolitis obliterans syndrome (BOS) has been created. BOS is characterized by progressive airflow obstruction with a permanent decrement in FEV_1. It is defined as a drop in the FEV_1 greater than 20% from the best previous baseline in the absence of acute rejection, infection, bronchial stricture, or any other abnormality that could potentially cause impairment in pulmonary function.[135] BOS is staged by degree of FEV_1 decrease from baseline. The following staging system has been defined[136]:

Stage 0-p (potential): FEV_1 80% to 89% of baseline

Stage I: FEV_1 65% to 79% of baseline

Stage II: FEV_1 50% to 64% of baseline

Stage III: FEV_1 less than 50% of baseline

The development of BOS is the primary determinant of long-term outcome for lung transplantation. It can occur any time after the first few months after transplantation. The cumulative probability of developing chronic rejection is 35% to 60% 5 years after transplantation.[137]

Probable risk factors for the development of BOS include acute rejection and infection. Potential risk factors include gastroesophageal reflux disease; the presence of donor-specific anti-HLA antibodies; infection, especially community-acquired respiratory viruses; older donor age; and prolonged ischemic time.[136,138-140] There are no proven treatments, although a variety of reports attest to the potential utility of macrolides, statin therapy, and the treatment of gastroesophageal reflux disease, including the use of surgical modalities. Changes in immunosuppressive regimens, including implementation of sirolimus and inhaled cyclosporine therapy, have been reported to slow the progression of disease.[141-147]

Infection

Infection is one of the greatest threats to both short-term and long-term survival after lung transplantation. Bacterial pneumonias, viral infections (especially cytomegalovirus [CMV]), and fungal infections, especially *Candida* and *Aspergillus* species, are common in lung transplant recipients. There are a number of factors that place the allograft at higher risk compared with recipients of other solid organs, including the following[148]:

- Direct communication with the outside environment
- Blunted cough reflex
- Impaired mucociliary clearance
- Early alterations in surfactant
- Lack of pulmonary lymphatics
- Greater levels of immunosuppression
- Native lung infection/prior colonization

The high predisposition for infection is most evident in the early post-transplantation period. Therefore aggressive efforts should be made to mobilize patients early. Pulmonary toilet should be emphasized in the early postextubation period. Devices such as incentive spirometers and flutter valves can be helpful in clearing secretions and stimulating cough. Patients can be instructed to cough volitionally in lieu of the loss of their cough reflex distal to the anastomosis. Early bronchoscopy is often performed to facilitate the removal of secretions, which can result not only from infection but also from airway ischemia, which in its most extreme form can result in sloughing of the bronchial epithelium.

Measures to prevent infectious complications after transplantation center on antimicrobial prophylaxis. Antibacterial prophylaxis in lung transplant recipients is typically more aggressive than in other solid-organ recipients.[149] Aside from the factors described previously, it is often prudent to assume that the donor may have aspirated at some stage of their terminal course and/or developed ventilator-associated pneumonia. Therefore, antibacterial prophylaxis in the recipient should be implemented with these risks in mind and should include broad-spectrum coverage.

CMV is a common infection in lung transplant recipients.[150] CMV prophylaxis is usually administered to recipients who are at risk, anywhere from a few weeks to 1 year after transplantation. Various centers have different protocols for CMV prophylaxis.[151,152] In our institution, we use valganciclovir at high doses for the first month and in decreased doses up to the first year after transplantation.

Candida initially and *Aspergillus* and *Pneumocystis* further out, are the fungal pathogens of concern. Antifungal prophylaxis may take the form of mono- or combination therapy with an azole (voriconazole, itraconazole, or fluconazole), clotrimazole troches/nystatin swish and swallow, and inhaled amphotericin B (usually 15 to 25 mg daily or twice per day).[153,154]

LUNG TRANSPLANTATION OUTCOMES

Outcomes for lung transplantation demonstrate survivals of 87% at 3 months, 78% at 1 year, 61% at 3 years, 49% at 5 years, and 25% at 10 years after transplantation. The mortality rate is highest in the first year, and there is slow attrition thereafter.[155] At 10 years after transplantation, patients with primary pulmonary hypertension (IPAH), cystic fibrosis, and α_1-antitrypsin deficiency have the best survival statistics, whereas patients with COPD and IPF fare the worst. Patients in the former groups tend to be younger in comparison with the latter groups. Five years after transplantation, younger patients (18 to 49 years) did better overall than older patients (50 years of age and older), most likely due to age-related comorbidities and the deleterious effect of the post-transplantation regimen on some of these age-related conditions.[155]

In the first 30 days, graft failure, non-CMV infections, and cardiovascular and technical complications were the principal fatal complications. In the first year acute rejection and CMV infections commonly occur, although neither has a large impact on mortality. BOS remained the leading cause of morbidity and mortality after the first year after transplantation. By 5 years after transplantation, 43% of recipients who survived at least 90 days developed BOS. Moreover, malignancy (lymphoid neoplasms in the first year, and skin cancers in 5- and 7-year survivors) and non-CMV infections were increasingly important contributors to mortality in recipients dying more than 1 year after transplantation.[155]

After lung transplantation, patients have a number of comorbidities, many caused or potentiated by immunosuppressive medications. Data from the ISHLT Official Adult Lung and Heart-Lung Transplantation Report[155] attest to hypertension and renal dysfunction as the most common complications, with prevalences of 51.3% and 25.7% at 1 year, and 85.9% and 39.4% (with 3.2% requiring chronic dialysis) at 5 years, respectively. Hyperlipidemia and diabetes mellitus were also reported with prevalences of 49.3 and 31.5% at

5 years, respectively. From the same data source, BOS developed in 33.5% of patients within 5 years of transplantation and in 44% of patients 5 years after transplantation.

Functional outcomes were first analyzed in a 1998 ISHLT report representing data through March 1998.[156] At 3 years after transplantation, 89.6% of recipients reported no activity limitations, 9.3% were able to perform activity with some assistance, and 1% required total assistance. In that report, despite the functional improvements achieved with transplantation, only a minority of patients (29.1%) were employed full-time 3 years after transplantation. A majority of patients (54.8%) required repeat hospitalization during the first year of follow-up, but by the third year the rehospitalization rate fell to 38.2%. The most common reason for repeat hospitalization was infection and rejection.[156] The 2006 ISHLT report[155] had limited statistics about functional outcomes, with more than 80% of 1-, 3-, 5-, and 8-year survivors reporting no activity limitation at follow-up, and approximately 40% working full or part-time.

Although data are limited, studies have assessed specific measurements of lung function and exercise tolerance after transplantation. With single-lung transplantation, because the native lung contributes to the overall pulmonary function, pulmonary function outcomes depend on the underlying primary disease.[157] With obstructive lung disease, a component of airflow obstruction may persist after transplantation, whereas with restrictive lung disease, a degree of restriction may be observed. The FEV_1 is expected to rise to 50% to 75% of predicted for patients with COPD, whereas the FVC usually rises to 65% to 69% of predicted in patients with pulmonary fibrosis.[158,159] Perfusion and ventilation have also been assessed after single-lung transplantation. In patients with pulmonary fibrosis, the transplanted lung has been shown to receive 69% to 82% of ventilation and 79% to 85% of perfusion; whereas in patients with pulmonary hypertension, the transplanted lung receives 44% to 65% of ventilation and 95% to 99% of perfusion 12 weeks postoperatively.[160]

Several studies have assessed cardiopulmonary function at maximal tolerable constant work rate exercise after lung transplantation. In patients transplanted for IPAH with a heart–lung procedure, gas exchange and ventilation were essentially normal.[161] Although improved, circulatory limitations to maximal exercise still persisted. After both single- and double-lung transplantation, a reduction in exercise tolerance, maximal O_2 uptake, and anaerobic threshold has been reported.[162] Exercise limitation was often attributed to chronic muscle deconditioning, possibly due to chronic steroid[163,164] and cyclosporine use,[165,166] as well as residual muscle weakness.[167] No significant difference in work capacity, O_2 pulse, tidal volume, or peak minute ventilation has been observed in patients with single-lung, double-lung, or heart-lung transplants.[168]

There has been increased interest in research on health-related quality of life after transplantation. The overall consensus is that the health-related quality of life benefit conferred from lung transplantation renders it a worthwhile option for patients with end-stage lung disease who have significant physical limitations.[169-173] Successful lung transplantation largely reverses the energy and mobility deficits reported by pre-transplantation patients. The type and amount of quality of life benefit can also differ depending on the underlying primary lung disorder.[170] Health-related quality of life is also dependent on the incidence of infections, rejection episodes, and the development of BOS. Many patients experience frequent symptoms associated with immunosuppression that may limit the full benefit of transplantation, and these may worsen over time.[172] Overall, although lung transplant recipients must cope with the side effects of immunosuppression, they report a highly satisfying quality of life regarding physical and emotional well-being and social and sexual function.[173]

CONCLUSION

This chapter serves as an overview of lung transplantation and disease-specific indications for transplantation referral and work-up. It further concentrates on the role of PR during all phases of the process, including before transplantation, the immediate perioperative period, and after transplantation.

References

1. Trulock EP: Lung transplantation, Am J Respir Crit Care Med 155:789-818, 1997.
2. Blumenstock DA, Lewis C: The first transplantation of the lung in a human revisited, Ann Thorac Surg 56:1423-1425, 1993.

3. Veith FJ, Koerner SK: Problems in the management of human lung transplant patients, Vasc Surg 8:273-282, 1974.

4. Reitz BA, Wallwork JL, Hunt SA et al: Heart—lung transplantation: successful therapies for patients with pulmonary vascular disease, N Engl J Med 306:557-564, 1982.

5. Toronto Lung Transplant Group: Unilateral lung transplant for pulmonary fibrosis, N Engl J Med 314:1140-1145, 1986.

6. Cooper JD, Patterson GA, Grossman A et al: Toronto Lung Transplant Group: Double-lung transplant for advanced chronic obstructive lung disease, Am Rev Respir Dis 139:303-307, 1989.

7. Theodore J, Lweiston N: Lung transplant comes of age, N Engl J Med 322:772-774, 1990.

8. Nathan S: Lung transplant candidate selection and clinical outcomes: strategies for improvement in prioritization, Curr Opin Organ Transplant 10:216-220, 2005.

9. International guidelines for the selection of lung transplant candidates. Joint statement of the American Society for Transplant Physicians (ASTP)/ American Thoracic Society (ATS)/, European Respiratory Society (ERS)/International Society for Heart and Lung Transplantation(ISHLT), Am J Respir Crit Care Med 158:335-339, 1998.

10. Ramsey SD, Patrick DL, Lewis S et al: Improvement in quality of life after lung transplantation: a preliminary study, J Heart Lung Transplant 14:870-877, 1995.

11. Limbos MM, Joyce DP, Chan CK et al: Psychological functioning and quality of life in lung transplant candidates and recipients, Chest 118:408-416, 2000.

12. Stavem K, Bjortuft O, Lund MB et al: Health-related quality of life in lung transplant candidates and recipients, Respiration 67:159-165, 2000.

13. Lanuza DM, Lefaiver C, McCabe M et al: Prospective study of functional status and quality of life before and after lung transplantation, Chest 118:115-122, 2000.

14. TenVergert VM, Essink-Bot ML, Geertsma A et al: The effect of lung transplantation on health-related quality of life: a longitudinal study, Chest 113:358-364, 1998.

15. Orens JB, Estenne M, Arcasoy S et al: International guidelines for the selection of lung transplant candidates: 2006 update—a consensus report from the Pulmonary Scientific Council of the International Society for Heart and Lung Transplant. J Heart Lung Transplant 25:745-755, 2006.

16. International Society for Heart and Lung Transplantation: ISHLT International Registry for Heart and Lung Transplantation. Available at http://www.ishlt.org/registries/slides.asp. Retrieved January 11, 2007.

17. Hosenpud JD, Bennett LE, Keck BM et al: Effect of diagnosis on survival benefit of lung transplantation for end-stage lung disease, Lancet 351:24-27, 1998.

18. Liou TG, Adler FR, Cahill BC et al: Survival effect of lung transplantation among patients with cystic cibrosis, JAMA 286:2683-2689, 2001.

19. Dawkins PA, Dowson LJ, Guest PJ et al: Predictors of mortality in α_1-antitrypsin deficiency, Thorax 58:1020-1026, 2003.

20. Oga T, Nishimura K, Tsukino M et al: Analysis of the factors related to mortality in chronic obstructive pulmonary disease, Am J Respir Crit Care Med 167:544-549, 2003.

21. Nishimura K, Izumi T, Tsukino M et al: Dyspnea is a better predictor of 5-year survival than airway obstruction in patients with COPD, Chest 121:1434-1440, 2002.

22. Schols AM, Slangen J, Volovics L et al: Weight loss is a reversible factor in the prognosis of chronic obstructive pulmonary disease, Am J Respir Crit Care Med 157:1791-1797, 1998.

23. Wilson DO, Rogers RM, Wright E et al: Body weight in chronic obstructive pulmonary disease, Am J Respir Crit Care Med 139:1435-1438, 1989.

24. Gray-Donald K, Gibbons L, Shapiro SH et al: Nutritional status and mortality in chronic obstructive pulmonary disease, Am J Respir Crit Care Med 153:961-966, 1996.

25. Schols AM, Buurman AJ, Staal van den Brekel AJ et al: Evidence for a relation between metabolic derangements and elevated inflammatory mediators in a subset of patients with chronic obstructive pulmonary disease, Thorax 51:819-824, 1996.

26. Di Francia M, Barbier D, Mege JL et al: Tumor necrosis factor α levels and weight loss in chronic obstructive pulmonary disease, Am J Respir Crit Care Med 150:1453-1455, 1994.

27. Schols AM, Slangen J, Volovics L et al: Weight loss is a reversible factor in the prognosis of chronic obstructive pulmonary disease, Am J Respir Crit Care Med 157:1791-1797, 1998.

28. Landbo C, Prescott E, Lange P et al: Prognostic value of nutritional status in chronic obstructive pulmonary disease, Am J Respir Crit Care Med 160:1856-1861, 1999.

29. Connors AF, Dawson NV, Thomas C et al: Outcomes following acute exacerbation of severe chronic obstructive lung disease, Am J Respir Crit Care Med 154:959-967, 1996.

30. Groenewegen KH, Schols AM, Wouters EF: Mortality and mortality-related factors after hospitalization for acute exacerbation of COPD, Chest 124:459-467, 2003.

31. Celli BR, Cote CG, Marin JM et al: The body-mass index, airflow obstruction, dyspnea, and exercise capacity index in chronic obstructive pulmonary disease, N Engl J Med 350:1005-1012, 2004.

32. Cote CG, Gomez NA, Celli BR: Effects of pulmonary rehabilitation on a multivariate disease severity score (BODE) in patients with COPD, Am J Respir Crit Care Med 167:A432, 2003.

33. American Thoracic Society: Lung function testing: selection of reference values and interpretative strategies [American Thoracic Society statement], Am Rev Respir Dis 144:1202-1218, 1991.

34. National Emphysema Treatment Trial Research Group: A randomized trial comparing lung volume reduction surgery with medical therapy for severe emphysema, N Engl J Med 348:2059-2073, 2003.

35. National Emphysema Treatment Trial Research Group: Patients at high risk of death after lung-volume-reduction surgery, N Engl J Med 345:1075-1083, 2001.

36. Nathan SD, Edwards LB, Barnett SD et al: Outcomes of COPD lung transplant recipients after lung volume reduction surgery, Chest 126:1569-1574, 2004.

37. Tutic M, Lardinois D, Imfeld S et al: Lung volume redusction surgery as an alternative or bridging procedure to lung transplantation, Ann Thorac Surg 82:208-213, 2006.

38. Daniil ZD, Gilchrit FC, Nicholson AG et al: A histologic pattern of nonspecific interstitial pneumonia is associated with a better prognosis then usual interstitial pneumonia in patients with cryptogenic fibrosing alveolitis, Am J Respir Crit Care Med 160:899-905, 1999.

39. Bjoraker JA, Ryu JH, Edwin MK et al: Prognostic significance of histopathologic subsets in idiopathic pulmonary fibrosis, Am J Respir Crit Care Med 157:199-203, 1998.

40. Latsi PI, du Bois RM, Nicholson AG et al: Fibrotic idiopathic interstitial pneumonia: the prognostic value of longitudinal functional trends, Am J Respir Crit Care Med 168:531-537, 2003.

41. Noon RA, Garrity ER: Lung transplantation for fibrotic diseases, Am J Med Sci 315:146-154, 1998.

42. Mogulkoc N, Brutsche MH, Bishop PW et al: Pulmonary function in idiopathic pulmonary fibrosis and referral for lung transplantation, Am J Respir Crit Care Med 164:103-108, 2001.

43. Gay SE, Kazerooni EA, Toews GB et al: Idiopathic pulmonary fibrosis: predicting response to therapy and survival, Am J Respir Crit Care Med 157:1063-1072, 1998.

44. Greene KE, King TE, Kuroki Y et al: Serum surfactant proteins-A and -D as biomarkers in idiopathic pulmonary fibrosis, Eur Respir J 19:439-446, 2002.

45. Schwartz DA, Helmers RA, Galvin JR et al: Determinants of survival in idiopathic pulmonary fibrosis, Am J Respir Crit Care Med 149:450-454, 1994.

46. Perez A, Rogers RM, Dauber JH: The prognosis of idiopathic pulmonary fibrosis, Am J Respir Cell Mol Biol 29:S19-S26, 2003.

47. Wells AU, Desai SR, Rubens MB et al: Idiopathic pulmonary fibrosis: a composite index derived from disease extent observed by computed tomography, Am J Respir Crit Care Med 167:962-969, 2003.

48. King TE, Tooze JA, Schwarz MI et al: Predicting survival in idiopathic pulmonary fibrosis, Am J Respir Crit Care Med 164:1171-1181, 2001.

49. Flaherty KR, Thwaite EL, Kazerooni EA et al: Radiological versus histological diagnosis in UIP and NSIP: survival implications, Thorax 58:143-148, 2003.

50. Lama VN, Flaherty KR, Toews GB et al: Prognostic value of desaturation during a 6-Minute Walk Test in idiopathic interstitial pneumonia, Am J Respir Crit Care Med 168:1084-1090, 2003.

51. Collard HR, King TE, Bartelson BB et al: Changes in clinical and physiologic variables predict survival in idiopathic pulmonary fibrosis, Am J Respir Crit Care Med 168:538-542, 2003.

52. Martinez FI, Bradford WZ, Safrin S: Rates and characteristics of death in patients with IPF, Chest 124:117S, 2003.

53. Katzenstein AL, Myers JL: Nonspecific interstitial pneumonia/fibrosis: histologic features and clinical significance, Am J Surg Pathol 18:136-147, 1994.

54. Travis WD, Matsui K, Moss J et al: Idiopathic nonspecific interstitial pneumonia: prognostic significance of cellular and fibrosing patterns, Am J Surg Pathol 24:19-33, 2000.

55. Flaherty KR, Travis WD, Colby TV et al: Histopathologic variability in usual and nonspecific interstitial pneumonias, Am J Respir Crit Care Med 164:1722-1727, 2001.

56. Monaghan H, Wells AU, Colby TV et al: Prognostic implications of histologic patterns in multiple surgical lung biopsies from patients with idiopathic interstitial pneumonias, Chest 125:522-526, 2004.

57. Katzenstein AL, Zisman DA, Litzky LA et al: Usual interstitial pneumonia: histologic study of biopsy and explant specimens, Am J Surg Pathol 26:1567-1577, 2002.

58. Kerem E, Reisman J, Corey M et al: Prediction of mortality in patient with cystic fibrosis, N Engl J Med 326:1187-1191, 1992.

59. Vizza CD, Yusen RD, Lynch JP et al: Outcome of patients with cystic fibrosis awaiting lung transplantation, Am J Respir Crit Care Med 162:819-825, 2000.

60. Tantisira KG, Systrom DM, Ginns LC: An elevated breathing reserve index at the lactate threshold is a predictor of mortality in patients with cystic fibrosis awaiting lung transplantation, Am J Respir Crit Care Med 165:1629-1633, 2002.

61. Sharma R, Florea VG, Bolger AP et al: Wasting as an independent predictor of mortality in patients with cystic fibrosis, Thorax 56:746-750, 2001.

62. Stanchina ML, Tantisira KG, Aquino SL et al: Association of lung perfusion disparity and mortality in patients with cystic fibrosis awaiting lung transplantation J Heart Lung Transplant 21 217-225, 2003.

63. Mayer-Hamblett N, Rosenfeld M, Emerson J et al: Developing cystic fibrosis lung transplant referral criteria using predictors of 2-year mortality, Am J Respir Crit Care Med 166:1550-1555, 2002.

64. Liou TG, Adler FR, FitzSimmons SC et al: Predictive 5-year survivorship model of cystic fibrosis, Am J Epidemiol 153:345-352, 2001.

65. Sitbon O, Humbert M, Nunes H et al: Long-term intravenous epoprostenol infusion in primary pulmonary hypertension, J Am Coll Cardiol 40:780-788, 2002.

66. Kuhn KP, Byrne DW, Arbogast PG et al: Outcome in 91 consecutive patients with pulmonary arterial hypertension receiving epoprostenol, Am J Respir Crit Care Med 167:580-586, 2003.

67. McLaughlin VV, Shillington A, Rich S: Survival in primary pulmonary hypertension, Circulation 106:1477-1482, 2002.

68. Conte JV, Gaine SP, Orens JB et al: The influence of continuous intravenous prostacyclin therapy for primary pulmonary hypertension on the timing

and outcome of transplantation, J Heart Lung Transplant 17:679-685, 1998.

69. McLaughlin V, Sitbon O, Rubin LJ et al: The effect of first-line bosentan on survival of patients with primary pulmonary hypertension, Am J Respir Crit Care Med 167:A442, 2003.

70. D'Alonzo GE, Barst RJ, Ayres SM et al: Survival in patients with primary pulmonary hypertension, Ann Intern Med 115:343-349, 1991.

71. Hopkins WE, Ochoa LL, Richardson GW et al: Comparison of the hemodynamics and survival of adults with severe primary pulmonary hypertension or Eisenmenger syndrome, J Heart Lung Transplant 15:100-105, 1996.

72. Rosenzweig EB, Kerstein D, Barst RJ: Lon-term prostacyclin for pulmonary hypertension with associated congenital heart defects, Circulation 99:1858-1865, 1999.

73. Waddell TK, Bennett L, Kennedy R et al: Heart–lung or lung transplantation for Eisenmengers syndrome, J Heart Lung Transplant 21:731-737, 2002.

74. Statement on sarcoidosis. Joint Statement of the American Thoracic Society (ATS): the European Respiratory Society (ERS) and the World Association of Sarcoidosis and Other Granulomatous Disorders (WASOG) adopted by the ATS Board of Directors and by the ERS Executive Committee, February 1999, Am J Respir Crit Care Med 160:736-755, 1999.

75. Baughman RP, Winget DB, Bowen EH et al: Predicting respiratory failure in sarcoidosis patients, Sarcoidosis Vasc Diffuse Lung Dis 14:154-158, 1997.

76. Shorr AF, Davies DB, Nathan SD: Predicting mortality in patients with sarcoidosis awaiting lung transplantation, Chest 124:922-928, 2003.

77. Shorr AF, Davies DB, Nathan SD: Outcomes for patients with sarcoidosis awaiting lung transplantation, Chest 122:233-238, 2002.

78. United Network for Organ Sharing: Guidelines for multiorgan organ management and procurement. UNOS Update 9:14-15, 1993.

79. Darby JM, Stein K, Grenvik A et al: Approach to management of the heartbeating "brain dead" donor, JAMA 261:2222-2228, 1989.

80. Palmer SM, Tapson VF: Pulmonary rehabilitation in the surgical patient, Respir Care Clin N Am 4:71-83, 1998.

81. Sheldon JB, Carroll BA, Ries AL et al: Pulmonary rehabilitation before lung transplantation, Am Rev Respir Dis 47:A597, 1993.

82. Niederman MS, Clemente PH, Fein AM et al: Benefits of a pulmonary rehabilitation program: improvements are independent of lung function, Chest 99:798-804, 1991.

83. Biggar D: Medium term results of pulmonary rehabilitation before lung transplantation, Am Rev Respir Dis 47:A33, 1993.

84. Nomori H, Kobayashi R, Fuyuno G et al: Preoperative respiratory muscle training: an assessment in thoracic surgery patients with special reference to postoperative pulmonary complications, Chest 105:1782-1788, 1994.

85. Saltin B, Bromqvist G, Mitchell JH et al: Response to exercise after bed rest and after training: a longitudinal study of adoptive changes in oxygen transport and body composition, Circulation 38:1, 1968.

86. Mereles D, Ehlken N, Kreuscher S et al: Exercise and respiratory training improve exercise capacity of life in patients with severe chronic pulmonary hypertension, Circulation 114:1482-1489, 2006.

87. Cahalin LP: Preoperative and postoperative conditioning for lung transplantation and volume-reduction surgery, Crit Care Nurs Clin N Am 8:305-322, 1996.

88. Surgit O, Ersoz G, Gursel Y et al: Effects of exercise training on specific immune parameters in transplant recipients, Transplant Proc 33:3298, 2001.

89. Cooper JD, Trulock EP, Triantafillou AN et al: Bilateral pneumonectomy (volume reduction) for chronic obstructive pulmonary disease, J Thorac Cardiovasc Surg 109:106-116, 1995.

90. Delgado HR, Braun SR, Scatrud JB et al: Chest wall and abdominal motion during exercise in patients with chronic lung disease, Am Rev of Respir Dis 126:200-205, 1982.

91. Resinkoff PM, Ries A: Pulmonary rehabilitation for chronic lung disease, J Heart Lung Transplant 17:643-650, 1998.

92. Downs AM: Physical therapy in lung transplantation, Phys Ther 76:626-642, 1996.

93. Forshag MS, Cooper AD: Postoperative care of the thoracotomy patient, Clin Chest Med 13:33-45, 1992.

94. Barlett RH, Brennon ML, Bazzaniga AB et al: Studies on the pathogenesis and prevention of post-operative pulmonary complications, Surg Gynecol Obstet 137:925-933, 1973.

95. Biggar DG, Mallen J, Trulock EP: Pulmonary rehabilitation before and after transplantation. In Casaburi R, Petty T, editors: Principles and practice of pulmonary rehabilitation, Philadelphia, 1993, WB Saunders, pp 459-469.

96. American Association of Cardiovascular and Pulmonary Rehabilitation: Disease-specific approaches in pulmonary rehabilitation. In Guidelines for pulmonary rehabilitation programs, ed 3, Champaign, Ill, 2004, Human Kinetics, pp 67-92.

97. Howard DK, Iademarco EI, Trulock EP: The role of cardiopulmonary exercise testing in lung and heart–lung transplantation, Clin Chest Med 15:405-420, 1994.

98. Hokanson JF, Mercier JG, Brooks GA: Cyclosporine A decreases rat skeletal muscle mitochondrial respiration in vitro, Am J Respir Crit Care Med 151:1848-1851, 1995.

99. Mercier JG, Hokanson JF, Brooks G: Effects of cyclosporine A on skeletal muscle mitochondrial respiration and endurance time in rats, Am J Respir Crit Care Med 151:1532-1536, 1995.

100. Craven JL, Bright J, Dear CL: Psychiatric, psychosocial and rehabilitative aspects of lung transplantation, Clin Chest Med 11:247-257, 1990.

101. Hertz MI, editor: Manual of lung transplant medical care, ed 2, Minneapolis, Minn, 2001, Fairview Press, pp 22-41.

102. Keenan RJ, Konishi H, Kawai A et al: Clinical trials of tacrolimus versus cyclosporine in lung transplantation, Ann Thorac Surg 60:580-584, 1995.

103. Christie JD, Bavaria JE, Palevsky HI et al: Primary graft failure following lung transplantation, Chest 114:51-60, 1998.

104. Christie JD, Kotloff RM, Pochettino A et al: Clinical risk factors for primary graft failure following lung transplantation, Chest 124:1232-1241, 2003.

105. Christie JD, Sager JS, Kimmel SE et al: Impact of primary graft failure on outcomes following lung transplantation, Chest 127:161-165, 2005.

106. Yousem SA, Duncan SR, Kormos RL et al: Interstitial and airspace granulation tissue reactions in lung transplant recipients, Am J Surg Pathol 16:877-884, 1992.

107. Pilcher DV, Snell GI, Scheinkestel CD et al: High donor age, low donor oxygenation, and high recipient inotrope requirements predict early graft dysfunction in lung transplant recipients, J Heart Lung Transplant 24:1814-1820, 2005.

108. Christie JD, Carby M, Bag R et al: Report of the ISHLT Working Group on Primary Lung Graft Dysfunction. II. Definition [a consensus statement of the International Society for Heart and Lung Transplantation], J Heart Lung Transplant 24(10):1454-1459, 2005.

109. Christie JD, Kotloff RM, Ahya VN et al: The effect of primary graft dysfunction on survival after lung transplantation, Am J Respir Crit Care Med 171:1312-1316, 2005.

110. Date H, Triantafillou AN, Trulock EP et al: Inhaled nitric oxide reduces human allograft dysfunction, J Thorac Cardiovascular Surg 111:913-919, 1996.

111. Veith FJ, Koerner SK: Problems in the management of human lung transplant patients, Vasc Surg 8:273-282, 1974.

112. Shennib H, Massard G: Airway complications in lung transplantation, Ann Thorac Surg 57:506-511, 1994.

113. Griffith BP, Magee MJ, Gonzalez IF et al: Anastomotic pitfalls in lung transplantation, J Thorac Cardiovasc Surg 107:743-754, 1994.

114. Schafers HJ, Haydock DA, Cooper JD: The prevalence and management of bronchial anastomotic complications in lung transplantation, J Thorac Cardiovasc Surg 101:1044-1052, 1991.

115. Patterson GA: Airways complications, Chest Surg Clin N Am 3:157-173, 1993.

116. Cooper JD, Patterson GA, Trulock EP et al: Results of single and bilateral lung transplantation in 131 consecutive recipients, J Thorac Cardiovasc Surg 107:460-471, 1994.

117. Higgins RK, McNeil K, Dennis A et al: Airway stenoses after lung transplantation: management with expanding stents, J Heart Lung Transplant 13:774-778, 1994.

118. Colt H, Janssen JP, Dumon JF et al: Endoscopic management of bronchial stenosis after double lung transplantation, Chest 102:10-16, 1992.

119. Hopkins, PM, Aboyoun CL, Chhajed PN et al: Prospective analysis of 1,235 transbronchial biopsies in lung transplant patients, J Heart Lung Transplant 21:1062-1067, 2002.

120. Baz MA, Layish DT, Govert JA et al: Diagnostic yield of bronchoscopies after isolated lung transplantation, Chest 110:84-88, 1996.

121. Millet B, Higenbottam TW, Flower CD et al: The radiographic appearance of infection and acute rejection of the lung after heart—lung transplantation, Am Rev Respir Dis 140:62-67, 1989.

122. Kundu S, Herman SJ, Larhs A et al: Correlation of chest radiographic findings with biopsy-proven rejection, J Thorac Imaging 14:178-184, 1999.

123. Kesten S, Maidenberg A, Winton T et al: Treatment of presumptive and proven acute rejection following six months of lung transplant survival, Am J Respir Crit Care Med 152:1321-1324, 1995.

124. Valentine VG, Robbins RC, Wehner JH et al: Total lymphoid irradiation for refractory acute rejection in heart—lung and lung allografts, Chest 109:1184-1189, 1996.

125. Andreu G, Achkar A, Couetil JP et al: Extracorporeal photochemotherapy treatment for acute lung rejection episode, J Heart Lung Transplant 14:793-796, 1995.

126. Villanueva J, Bhorade SM, Robinson JA et al: Extracorporeal photophoresis for the treatment of lung allograft rejection, Ann Transplant 5:44-47, 2000.

127. Bando K, Paradis IL, Similo S et al: Obliterative bronchiolitis after lung and heart—lung transplantation: an analysis of risk factors and management, J Thorac Cardiovasc Surg 110:4-13, 1995.

128. Whitehead B, Rees P, Sorensen K et al: Incidence of obliterative bronchiolitis after heart—lung transplant in children, J Heart Lung Transplant 12:903-908, 1993.

129. Girgis RE, Tu I, Berry GJ et al: Risk factors for the development of obliterative bronchiolitis after lung transplantation, J Heart Lung Transplant 15:1200-1208, 1996.

130. Scott JP, Higenbottam TW, Sharples L et al: Risk factors for obliterative bronchiolitis in heart-lung transplant, Transplantation 51:813-817, 1991.

131. Sharples LD, Tamm M, McNeill K et al: Development of bronchiolitis obliterans syndrome in recipients of heart—lung transplantation: early risk factors, Transplantation 61:560-566, 1996.

132. Husain AN, Siddiqui MT, Holmes EW et al: Analysis of risk factors for development of bronchiolitis obliterans syndrome, Am J Respir Crit Care Med 159:829-833, 1999.

133. Kroshus TJ, Kshettry VR, Savik K et al: Risk factors for the development of bronchiolitis obliterans syndrome after lung transplantation, J Thorac Cardiovasc Surg 114:195-202, 1997.

134. Yousem SA, Berry GJ, Cagle PT et al: Revision of the 1990 working formulation for the classification of pulmonary allograft rejection: Lung

Rejection Study Group, J Heart Lung Transplant 15:1-15, 1996.

135. Cooper JD, Billingham M, Egan T et al: A working formulation for the standardization of nomenclature and for clinical staging of chronic dysfunction of the lung allografts, J Heart Lung Transplant 12:713-716, 1993.

136. Estenne M, Maurer JR, Boehler A et al: Bronchiolitis obliterans syndrome 2001: an update of the disgnostic criteria, J Heart Lung Transplant 21:297-310, 2002.

137. Valentine VG, Robbins RC, Berry GJ et al: Actuarial survival of heart–lung and bilateral sequential lung transplant recipients with obliterative bronchiolitis, J Heart Lung Transplant 15:371-383, 1996.

138. Khalifah AP, Hachem RR, Chakinala MM et al: Minimal acute rejection after lung transplantation: a risk of bronchiolitis obliterans syndrome, Am J Transplant 5:2022-2030, 2005.

139. Kumar D, Erdman D, Keshavjee S et al: Clinical impact of community-acquired respiratory viruses on bronchiolitis obliterans after lung transplant, Am J Transplant 5:2031-2036, 2005.

140. Girnita AL, Duquesnoy R, Yousem SA et al: HLA-specific antibodies are risk factors for lymphocytic bronchiolitis and chronic lung allograft dysfunction, Am J Transplant 5:131-138, 2005.

141. Iacono AT, Corcoran TE, Griffith BP et al: Aerosol cyclosporin therapy in lung transplant recipients with bronchiolitis obliterans, Eur Respir J 23:384-390, 2004.

142. Johnson BA, Iacono AT, Zeevi A et al: Statin use is associated with improved function and survival of lung allografts, Am J Respir Crit Care Med 167:1271-1278, 2003.

143. Gerhardt SG, McDyer JF, Girgis RE et al: Maintenance azithromycin therapy for bronchiolitis obliterans syndrome: results of a pilot study, Am J Respir Crit Care Med 168:121-125, 2003.

144. Shitrit D, Bendayan D, Gidon S et al: Long-term azithromycin use for treatment of bronchiolitis obliterans syndrome in lung transplant recipients, J Heart Lung Transplant 24:1440-1443, 2005.

145. Yates B, Murphy DM, Forrest IA et al: Azithromycin reverses airflow obstruction in established bronchiolitis obliterans syndrome, Am J Respir Crit Care Med 172:772-775, 2005.

146. Azzola A, Havryk A, Chhajed P et al: Everolimus and mycophenolate mofetil are potent inhibitors of fibroblast proliferation after lung transplantation. Transplantation 77:275-280, 2004.

147. Dosanjh A, Pirfenidone: Anti-fibrotic agent with a potential therapeutic role in the management of transplantation patients, Eur J Pharmacol 536:219-222, 2006.

148. Dauber JH, Paradis IL, Dummer JS: Infectious complications in pulmonary allograft recipients, Clinics Chest Med 11:291-308, 1990.

149. Maurer JR, Tullis DE, Grossman RF et al: Infectious complications following isolated lung transplantation, Chest 101:1057-1059, 1992.

150. Zamora MR, Davis RD, Leonard C; CMV Advisory Board Expert Committee: Management of cytomegalovirus infection in lung transplant recipients: evidence-based recommendations, Transplantation 80:157-163, 2005.

151. Ruttmann E, Geltner C, Bucher B et al: Combined CMV prophylaxis improves outcome and reduces the risk for bronchiolitis obliterans syndrome (BOS) after lung transplantation, Transplantation 81:1415-1420, 2006.

152. Zamora MR, Nicolls MR, Hodges TN et al: Following universal prophylaxis with intravenous ganciclovir and cytomegalovirus immune globulin, valganciclovir is safe and effective for prevention of CMV infection following lung transplantation, Am J Transplant 4:1635-1642, 2004.

153. Shitrit D, Ollech JE, Ollech A et al: Itraconazole prophylaxis in lung transplant recipients receiving tacrolimus (FK 506): efficacy and drug interaction, J Heart Lung Transplant 24:2148-2152, 2005.

154. Capitano B, Potoski BA, Husain S et al: Intrapulmonary penetration of voriconazole in patients receiving an oral prophylactic regimen, Antimicrob Agents Chemother 50:1878-1880, 2006.

155. Trulock EP, Edwards LB, Taylor DO et al: Registry of the International Society for Heart and Lung Transplantation: Twenty-second official adult lung and heart–lung transplant report—2005, J Heart Lung Transplant 24:956-967, 2005.

156. Hosenpud JD, Bennett LE, Keck BM et al: Registry of the International Society for Heart and Lung Transplantation: fifteenth official report—1998, J Heart Lung Transplant 17:656-668, 1998.

157. Orens J, Martinez F, Becker F et al: Cardiopulmonary exercise testing following lung transplantation for different underlying diseases, Chest 107:144-149, 1995.

158. Mal H, Sleiman C, Jebrak G et al: Functional results of single-lung transplantation for chronic obstructive lung disease, Am J Respir Crit Care Med 149:1476-1481, 1994.

159. Grossman R, Frost A, Zamel N et al: Results of single lung transplantation for bilateral pulmonary fibrosis, N Engl J Med 322:727-733, 1990.

160. Kramer MR, Marshall SE, McDougall IR et al: The distribution of ventilation and perfusion after single-lung transplantation in patients with pulmonary fibrosis and pulmonary hypertension, Transplant Proc 23:1215-1216, 1991.

161. Theodore J, Morris A, Burke C et al: Cardiopulmonary function at maximum tolerable constant work rate exercise following human heart–lung transplant, Chest 93:433-439, 1987.

162. Miyoshi S, Trulock E, Schaefers H et al: Cardiopulmonary exercise testing after single and double lung transplantation, Chest 97:1130-1136, 1990.

163. Williams T, Patterson A, McClean P et al: Maximal exercise testing in single and double lung transplant recipients, Am Rev Respir Dis 145:101-105, 1992.

164. Ross D, Waters P, Mohsenifar Z et al: Hemodynamic responses to exercise after lung transplantation, Chest 103:46-53, 1993.

165. Gibbons W, Levine S, Bryan C et al: Cardiopulmonary exercise responses after single lung

transplant for severe obstructive lung disease, Chest 100:106-111, 1991.

166. Horber FF, Hoppeler H, Scheidegger JR et al: Impact of physical training on the ultrastructure of mid-thigh muscle in normal subjects and in patients treated with glucocorticoids, J Clin Invest 79:1181-1190, 1987.

167. Reinsma GD, ten Hacken NH, Grevink RG et al: Limiting factors of exercise performance 1 year after lung transplant, J Heart Lung Transplant 25:1310-1316, 2006.

168. Schwaiblmair S, Reichenspruner H, Muller C et al: Cardiopulmonary exercise testing before and after lung and heart–lung transplantation, Am J Respir Crit Care Med 159:1277-1283, 1999.

169. Vasiliadis HM, Collet JP, Poirier C: Health-related quality-of-life determinants in lung transplantation, J Heart Lung Transplant 25:226-233, 2006.

170. Gross CR, Raghu G: The cost of lung transplantation and the quality of life post-transplant, Clin Chest Med 18:391-403, 1997.

171. Kugler C, Fischer S, Gottlieb J et al: Health-related quality of life in two hundred-eighty lung transplant recipients, J Heart Lung Transplant 24:2262-2268, 2005.

172. Rodrigue JR, Baz MA, Kanasky WF et al: Does lung transplantation improve health-related quality of life? The University of Florida experience, J Heart Lung Transplant 24:755-763, 2005.

173. Smeritsching B, Jaksch P, Kocher A et al: Quality of life after lung transplantation: a cross-sectional study, J Heart Lung Transplant 24:474-480, 2005.

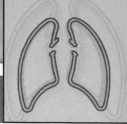

Chapter 24

Pulmonary Rehabilitation and Lung Volume Reduction Surgery

MeiLan K. Han • Steven E. Gay • Fernando J. Martinez

CHAPTER OUTLINE

**Functional Changes After Lung Volume
Reduction Surgery**
  Pulmonary Function and Exercise
  Health Status
Patient Selection
  Clinical Features

Physiologic Features
Imaging
**Rehabilitation Needs and Results
in the LVRS Population**
Conclusion

PROFESSIONAL SKILLS

On completion of this chapter, the reader will be able to do
the following:

- Discuss the short- and long-term benefits of lung volume reduction surgery (LVRS) in terms of
  pulmonary function, exercise, and overall health
- Evaluate and apply patient selection criteria for LVRS
- Explain the role of imaging in patient evaluation
- Appraise the use of preoperative and postoperative pulmonary rehabilitation in combination with LVRS

The current era of surgical lung volume reduction was ushered in by Cooper and colleagues,[1] who reported dramatic improvement after bilateral lung volume reduction surgery (LVRS) performed via median sternotomy. Subsequently multiple investigators reported more limited improvement.[2-4] The results of the National Emphysema Treatment Trial (NETT)[5,6] and other randomized trials[7-9] provided more definitive insight into the role of LVRS in patients with advanced emphysema. In this chapter, results of LVRS in case series and randomized trials are discussed, while providing insight into the role of pulmonary rehabilitation in the preoperative evaluation of patients considered for LVRS.

FUNCTIONAL CHANGES AFTER LUNG VOLUME REDUCTION SURGERY

Pulmonary Function and Exercise

Although the initial report by Cooper and colleagues[1] documented an 82% improvement in forced expiratory volume in 1 second (FEV_1) approximately 6 months after bilateral LVRS via median sternotomy, subsequent studies confirmed significant mean improvements in spirometry although to a lesser extent than initially suggested.[3] Reported changes in pulmonary function clearly indicated a short-term improvement in spirometry, favoring surgery over medical therapy. This has been confirmed by the results of randomized trials.[5,10] In general, bilateral LVRS resulted in greater short-term improvement, although there were few direct comparisons between unilateral and bilateral procedures. One multicenter prospective study comparing unilateral video-assisted thoracic surgery (VATS) LVRS with bilateral VATS LVRS noted that pulmonary function improvement favored the bilateral approach.[11] The results of laser procedures appeared to be worse than stapling techniques.[12] Several groups have compared the short-term physiologic results of bilateral LVRS performed by VATS or median sternotomy.[13] Data from the NETT have confirmed similar functional benefits between bilateral LVRS performed by median sternotomy or VATS.[6]

A significant heterogeneous spirometric response has been reported.[14] The NETT has confirmed this finding.[5,13] A significant proportion of patients experienced little improvement in FEV_1, even in the short term. Interestingly, many of the patients experiencing limited spirometric improvement demonstrate significant improvement in breathlessness, highlighting the limitation of FEV_1 as a sole measure of improvement.[15]

Data regarding long-term functional follow-up are limited. Brenner and colleagues[16] reported the rate of FEV_1 change greater than 6 months after LVRS. They noted a greater decrease in rate of change in FEV_1 (0.255 ± 0.057 L/year) in those patients experiencing the greatest improvement in the initial 6 months after surgery. The lowest rate of drop in FEV_1 appeared in those with the least initial improvement. Flaherty and colleagues[17] documented a gradual decrement in FEV_1 over the course of 3 years after bilateral LVRS, whereas another group presented a median of 4 years of follow-up in 200 patients treated with bilateral LVRS.[18] Although data collection was not complete, a majority of patients still exhibited spirometric improvement 3 and 5 years after surgery.

Most available data on exercise response have described simple measures of exercise capacity such as timed measures of walk distance. Consistent improvements in walk distance have been reported.[3] The NETT investigators[5] confirmed a modest improvement in 6-minute walk distance for surgically treated patients, with a consistent decrease in medically treated patients. Several groups have reported consistent, short-term increases in maximal work load, oxygen (O_2) consumption, and minute ventilation.[3] The improved maximal ventilation was achieved through increased tidal volume, with a modest change in respiratory rate.[19] Benditt and

colleagues[20] reported improved exercise capacity but decreased heart rate at similar work loads after bilateral LVRS. Martinez and colleagues[15] reported that improved dyspnea at isowork correlated best with decreased dynamic hyperinflation. In addition, Tschernko and colleagues[21] noted a significant decrease in the work of breathing during exercise after LVRS. Ferguson and colleagues[22] reported an improved tidal volume at submaximal work loads during steady state testing while physiologic dead space improved. The NETT investigators[5] confirmed an increase in maximal achieved wattage during O_2-supplemented cycle ergometry in surgically patients; lesser improvement was noted in patients who continued aggressive medical management. Dolmage and colleagues[23] reported improved peak O_2 consumption and power with greater minute ventilation and tidal volume. Importantly, this study confirmed an improvement in operational lung volumes among patients undergoing operation. NETT investigators[24] noted that surgical patients, in contrast to medically treated patients, were more likely to maintain improved maximal wattage during O_2-supplemented cardiopulmonary exercise testing during long-term follow-up.

Health Status

Numerous investigative groups have confirmed short-term improvement in breathlessness either with the Medical Research Council dyspnea scores and/or the Transitional Dyspnea Index.[25] The NETT investigators[5] have presented a detailed assessment of breathlessness demonstrating improvement with the University of California, San Diego Shortness of Breath Questionnaire. A heterogeneous response was noted, although a clear benefit was noted in the surgically treated group compared with medically managed patients. Results of formal health status measurement have been reviewed by others.[26] Improvement has been reported with general instruments including the Medical Outcomes Survey-Short Form 36 and the Nottingham Health Profile.[1,27] The improvement reported after LVRS included measures of vitality, social functioning, physical functioning, and general health, and an increased ability to perform various roles.

Improvement after LVRS has also been reported with disease-specific instruments, including the Chronic Respiratory Questionnaire[28] and the St. George's Respiratory Questionnaire.[29] The Canadian controlled trial focused on health status, documenting improvement with the Chronic

Respiratory Questionnaire.[8] Similarly, the NETT investigators[5] reported significant improvement in the St. George's Respiratory Questionnaire of surgically treated patients compared with medically treated patients. Long-term improvement in St. George's Respiratory Questionnaire among surgically treated patients have been reported by NETT investigators.[24]

PATIENT SELECTION

Clinical Features

The clinical evaluation should identify patients with predominant emphysema.[25] The presence of frequent respiratory infections and/or chronic, copious sputum production may be useful in identifying patients with primarily airway disease.[30] In addition, clinical assessment should attempt to identify patient features predicting a higher mortality or likelihood of poor functional result, such as unstable cardiac disease or severe pulmonary hypertension. On the other hand, coronary artery disease should not be considered an absolute contraindication to surgery, as LVRS successfully combined with cardiac surgery has been well documented.[31,32] Less favorable outcomes have been reported in the presence of α_1-antitrypsin deficiency,[27,33-36] although this has not been a totally consistent finding.[37] An impaired nutritional status, such as a low body mass index or a decreased percentage of ideal body weight or fat-free mass index, has been associated with increased perioperative complications.[38,39]

Physiologic Features

Pulmonary function testing has proven instrumental in identifying optimal candidates for surgery.[25] Although a lower limit of FEV_1 that identifies individuals at prohibitive risk has not been agreed upon, the NETT investigators[40] noted that a lower FEV_1 was independently predictive of greater postoperative pulmonary morbidity. Some investigators have reported acceptable outcomes in patients with severely decreased FEV_1 (<500 ml).[41-44] Several groups have suggested that a low diffusing capacity of the lung for carbon monoxide (D_{LCO}) increases risk,[45-47] whereas others did not confirm these findings.[48] The most definitive data come from the NETT, which identified two subgroups of patients at particularly high risk of surgical mortality after bilateral LVRS.[5,24] Patients with a postbronchodilator

FEV_1 not exceeding 20% predicted and a D_{LCO} not more than 20% predicted exhibited much higher mortality with LVRS than with medical management (odds ratio, 2.98; 95% confidence interval, 1.3 to 7.7). This same group has confirmed that a lower D_{LCO} was independently associated with postoperative pulmonary morbidity.[40] Although arterial blood gas abnormalities have been suggested as predictive of a bad outcome, the NETT did not identify baseline arterial partial pressure of carbon dioxide as suggestive of impaired outcome despite more than 30% of randomized patients exhibiting baseline hypercapnia.[5]

The most compelling data supporting the role of preoperative exercise capacity comes from the NETT, one of the primary end points of which was maximal achieved work load achieved on a cycle ergometer while breathing 30% supplemental O_2.[5] A threshold of 40% of the baseline workload (corresponding to a work load of 25 W for females and 40 W for male patients) was a clear threshold for mortality for the overall study group.[5] These thresholds, in conjunction with computed tomography data, allowed a clear separation of non–high-risk patients into four distinct categories.

Imaging

Thoracic imaging is crucially important for the evaluation of patients for LVRS.[49] Computed tomography has proven particularly valuable.[50-52] The importance of emphysema heterogeneity has been highlighted by NETT investigators.[5] Radiologists at 17 participating clinical centers classified high-resolution computed tomography (HRCT) scans as exhibiting predominantly upper lobe or non–upper lobe emphysema, based on visual scoring of disproportionate disease between nonanatomic thirds divided equally from apex to the base.[53] Using this methodology, in conjunction with the maximal achieved workload during O_2-supplemented maximal cycle ergometry, NETT investigators clarified the role of CT imaging in the evaluation of patients for LVRS. Early work identified an increased risk of surgical mortality among patients with severe obstruction ($FEV_1 \leq 20\%$ predicted) and either diffuse emphysema on HRCT or a D_{LCO} not more than 20% predicted (relative risk, 3.9; 95% confidence interval, 1.9 to 9.0).[5] Patients with upper lobe–predominant emphysema and low postrehabilitation exercise tolerance exhibited a decreased risk of mortality during long-term follow-up (relative risk, 0.57; $P = .01$) after LVRS.[24]

Patients with non–upper lobe–predominant emphysema and a high postrehabilitation exercise capacity exhibited an increased risk of death during follow-up after LVRS that did not achieve statistical significance. Patients with upper lobe–predominant emphysema and a high postrehabilitation exercise capacity or patients with non–upper lobe–predominant emphysema and a low postrehabilitation exercise capacity did not have a survival advantage or disadvantage.[5,24] Importantly, homogeneous emphysema alone was found to confer increased odds of 90-day mortality, regardless of postrehabilitation exercise capacity (odds ratio, 2.99; P = .009).[40]

Unfortunately, the definition of emphysema heterogeneity has varied widely in the published literature.[53] As such, many investigators have used quantitative CT methodology to define disease heterogeneity. Several groups have confirmed moderately strong correlations between quantitative CT values and outcomes.[17,54] This includes measures of emphysema severity and peripheral distribution[55] and quantitation of the number and size of emphysematous lesions.[56]

REHABILITATION NEEDS AND RESULTS IN THE LVRS POPULATION

It is evident that pulmonary rehabilitation has played an important role in the evaluation and preparation of patients for LVRS. Before controlled trials, these concepts evolved from noncontrolled studies. Most of the case series have required pulmonary rehabilitation before LVRS, including the earliest reports in the new era[57] (Table 24-1). The value of such an approach was highlighted by Moy and colleagues,[58] who reported Medical Outcomes Survey-Short Form 36 values before and after comprehensive pulmonary rehabilitation and again after bilateral LVRS via VATS in 19 patients. These investigators noted no significant change in any of the domains after pulmonary rehabilitation although significant improvement was noted in vitality after LVRS. When compared with the baseline scoring, the combination of rehabilitation and bilateral LVRS resulted in significant improvement in four of the eight domains. Importantly, pulmonary rehabilitation accounted for most of the

---

TABLE 24-1 **Pulmonary Rehabilitation in Representative Case Series and Randomized Trials of Lung Volume Reduction Surgery**

Reference	Rehabilitation Requirement	Rehabilitation Format
CASE SERIES		
Ojo et al[63]	Required	Not specified
Criner et al[64]	Required	8-wk outpatient program
Moy et al[58]	Required	At least 6- to 8-wk outpatient program
Nezu et al[65]	Not required; encouraged	Minimum of 1 mo
Cassart et al[66]	Not required	NA
Flaherty et al[67]	Required	Not specified
Fujimoto et al[68]	Required	3 to 4 wk of inpatient rehabilitation
Hamacher et al[69]	Not required	NA
Ciccone et al[70]	Required	Not specified; median, 97 days of participation
Ingenito et al[71]	Required	6-wk outpatient program; multidisciplinary
CONTROLLED TRIALS		
Criner et al[59]	Required	8-wk outpatient program followed by either 3 mo of additional rehabilitation or LVRS
National Emphysema Treatment Trial Research Group[5,72]	Required	Three phases: (1) prerandomization (16 to 20 sessions over 6 to 10 wk); (2) postrandomization (10 sessions over 8 to 9 wk); (3) long-term maintenance (duration of trial). Regimented, multicomponent, closely monitored
Mineo et al[61]	Not required in LVRS group	None
	Comparator rehabilitation group	3 hr/5 days per week/6 wk; multidisciplinary including interval training
Dolmadge et al[23]; Goldstein et al[8]	Required	6-wk outpatient program; multidisciplinary
Hillerdal et al[73]	Required	6-wk multidisciplinary program
Miller et al[10,74]	Required	8 wk

LVRS, *Lung volume reduction surgery*; NA, *not applicable*.

improvement in role limitations whereas LVRS accounted for most of the improvement in physical functioning, vitality, and social functioning.

The onset of controlled trials shed additional light on the role of pulmonary rehabilitation in LVRS evaluation. Criner and colleagues[59] compared functional results after an initial 8 weeks of pulmonary rehabilitation followed by an additional 3 months of rehabilitation or bilateral LVRS. Patients receiving pulmonary rehabilitation exhibited modest improvement in exercise capacity and health status but little change in spirometry. LVRS was associated with more impressive physiologic and functional improvements. The NETT formalized and highlighted the importance of pulmonary rehabilitation before LVRS. A rigorous protocol was used at central centers or local satellites and included three phases: prerandomization, postrandomization, and long-term maintenance.[60] The prerandomization phase included a total of 16 to 20 supervised sessions completed over a period of 6 to 10 weeks. The comprehensive nature of the program was exemplified by components of exercise training, education, psychosocial assessment and treatment, and nutritional assessment and management. Despite the severe nature of disease in the participants, improvement was noted in exercise capacity, dyspnea, and health status; this was particularly evident among those subjects who had not undergone previous rehabilitation (Figure 24-1). Interestingly, it has also been estimated that approximately 10% of patients in

the NETT trial who participated in prerandomization pulmonary rehabilitation experienced such significant improvement that they were unwilling to proceed with randomization and accept the risks associated with surgery.[60] This emphasizes the tangible improvements experienced by many patients who undergo pulmonary rehabilitation.

Not all randomized trials have included a preoperative period of pulmonary rehabilitation (see Table 24-1). Mineo and colleagues[61] specifically tested results of LVRS only versus pulmonary rehabilitation in 60 patients with emphysema. For the 17 patients who underwent bilateral LVRS and the 13 who underwent unilateral LVRS, there was no difference in 6-month mortality or late morbidity (>30 days) compared with patients treated solely by pulmonary rehabilitation. Early morbidity was higher in surgically treated patients although overall functional and physiologic results favored surgical therapy. Interestingly, there was little change in the domains of vitality or physical role, which the authors thought could reflect the lack of preoperative pulmonary rehabilitation.

It is evident that clear recommendations regarding the role of pulmonary rehabilitation in LVRS require additional well-designed studies. Unfortunately, it is unlikely that these will be forthcoming in the near future. As such, recommendations can be made only on the basis of the existing data set. Importantly, in the United States Centers for Medicare & Medicaid Services coverage for the procedure is contingent on the completion of a

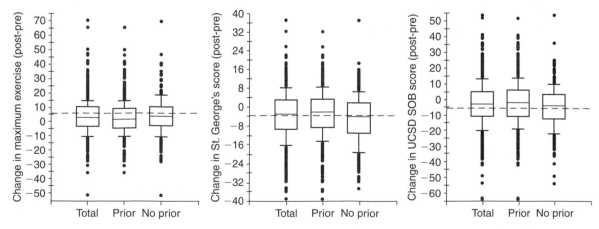

FIGURE 24-1 Box plots of changes from prerandomization pulmonary rehabilitation program in exercise capacity (maximal workload), health-related quality of life (St. George's Respiratory Questionnaire total score), and dyspnea (UCSD Shortness of Breath [SOB] Questionnaire score) for all 1218 patients in the National Emphysema Treatment Trial, as well as for subgroups with and without prior pulmonary rehabilitation experience. *Dashed lines* represent the following estimated minimal clinically important differences: 5-W increase for maximal workload; 4-unit decrease for the St. George's Respiratory Questionnaire total score; and 5- unit decrease for the UCSD Shortness of Breath Questionnaire score.

TABLE 24-2   Suggested Pulmonary Rehabilitation Approach to Patients Being Evaluated for and Who Have Undergone Lung Volume Reduction Surgery

Phase	Approach	
Presurgical	Comprehensive evaluation	
	Exercise	
	Lower extremity	
	Upper extremity	
	Flexibility	18 to 24 sessions over 6 to 10 wk
	Strength training	
	Education	
	Psychosocial counseling	
	Nutritional counseling	
Perioperative	Rapid mobilization	
	Two sessions per day, 7 days/wk	
	Chest physical therapy	
	Pulmonary toileting	
Postoperative	Inpatient rehabilitation (if needed)	
	Outpatient similar to presurgical	

Adapted from references 60 and 62.

comprehensive pulmonary rehabilitation program (http://www.cms.hhs.gov/transmittals/downloads/R3NCD.pdf). The format for pulmonary rehabilitation in the available case series and randomized trials is highly variable, as noted in Table 24-1. An excellent review has provided insight into the optimal delivery of rehabilitation in this setting.[62] Table 24-2 enumerates an approach to patients being evaluated for LVRS, management in the immediate postsurgical period, and management in the later postoperative period.

CONCLUSION

Exercise limitation is severe before LVRS and pulmonary rehabilitation is likely an important adjunctive therapy among these patients. The majority of published case series and randomized trials have required aggressive preoperative and postoperative pulmonary rehabilitation. Although data are not conclusive, a comprehensive approach to rehabilitation in patients evaluated for LVRS and for those undergoing LVRS seems appropriate.

References

1. Cooper JD, Trulock EP, Triantafillou AN et al: Bilateral pneumectomy (volume reduction) for chronic obstructive pulmonary disease, J Thorac Cardiovasc Surg 109:106-116, 1995.
2. Utz J, Hubmayr R, Deschamps C: Lung volume reduction surgery for emphysema: out on a limb without a NETT, Mayo Clin Proc 73:552-556, 1998.
3. Flaherty KR, Martinez FJ: Lung volume reduction surgery for emphysema, Clin Chest Med 21:819-848, 2000.
4. Benditt J: Surgical therapies for chronic obstructive pulmonary disease, Respir Care 49:53-61, 2004.
5. National Emphysema Treatment Trial Research Group: A randomized trial comparing lung-volume-reduction surgery with medical therapy for severe emphysema, N Engl J Med 348:2059-2073, 2003.
6. National Emphysema Treatment Trial Research Group: Safety and efficacy of median sternotomy versus video-assisted thoracic surgery for lung volume reduction surgery, J Thorac Cardiovasc Surg 127:1350-1360, 2004.
7. Pompeo E, Marino M, Nofroni I et al: Pulmonary Emphysema Research Group: Reduction pneumoplasty versus respiratory rehabilitation in severe emphysema: a randomized study, Ann Thorac Surg 70:948-953[discussion 954], 2000.
8. Goldstein R, Todd T, Guyatt G et al: Influence of lung volume reduction surgery (LVRS) on health related quality of life in patients with chronic obstructive pulmonary disease, Thorax 58:405-410, 2003.
9. Geddes D, Davies M, Koyama H et al: Effect of lung-volume-reduction surgery in patients with severe emphysema, N Engl J Med 343:239-245, 2000.
10. Miller J, Malthaner R, Goldsmith C et al: for the Canadian Lung Volume Reduction Surgery Study: A randomized clinical trial of lung volume reduction surgery versus best medical care for patients with advanced emphysema: a two-year study from Canada, Ann Thorac Surg 81:314-321, 2006.
11. Lowdermilk GA, Keenan RJ, Landreneau RJ et al: Comparison of clinical results for unilateral and bilateral thoracoscopic lung volume reduction, Ann Thorac Surg 69:1670-1674, 2000.
12. McKenna R, Brenner M, Gelb A et al: A randomized, prospective trial of stapled lung reduction

versus laser bullectomy for diffuse emphysema, J Thorac Cardiovasc Surg 111:317-322, 1996.

13. Chang A, Chan K, Martinez F: Lessons from the National Emphysema Treatment Trial, Semin Thorac Cardiovasc Surg 19:172-180, 2007.

14. Kotloff R, Tino G, Bavaria J et al: Bilateral lung volume reduction surgery for advanced emphysema: a comparison of median sternotomy and thoracoscopic approaches, Chest 110:1399-1406, 1996.

15. Martinez F, Montes de Oca M, Whyte R et al: Lung volume reduction improves dyspnea, dynamic hyperinflation and respiratory muscle function, Am J Respir Crit Care Med 155:1984-1990, 1997.

16. Brenner M, McKenna R Jr, Gelb A et al: Rate of FEV1 change following lung volume reduction surgery, Chest 113:652-659, 1998.

17. Flaherty KR, Kazerooni EA, Curtis JL et al: Short-term and long-term outcomes after bilateral lung volume reduction surgery: prediction by quantitative CT, Chest 119:1337-1346, 2001.

18. Yusen R, Lefrak S, Gierada D et al: A prospective evaluation of lung volume reduction surgery in 200 consecutive patients, Chest 123:1026-1037, 2003.

19. Keller C, Ruppel G, Hibbett A et al: Thoracoscopic lung volume reduction surgery reduces dyspnea and improves exercise capacity in patients with emphysema, Am J Respir Crit Care Med 156:60-67, 1997.

20. Benditt JO, Lewis S, Wood DE et al: Lung volume reduction surgery improves maximal O2 consumption, maximal minute ventilation, O2 pulse, and dead space-to-tidal volume ratio during leg cycle ergometry, Am J Respir Crit Care Med 156:561-566, 1997.

21. Tschernko E, Gruber E, Jaksch P et al: Ventilatory mechanics and gas exchange during exercise before and after lung volume reduction surgery, Am J Respir Crit Care Med 158:1424-1431, 1998.

22. Ferguson G, Fernandez E, Zamora M et al: Improved exercise performance following lung volume reduction surgery for emphysema, Am J Respir Crit Care Med 157:1195-1203, 1998.

23. Dolmage T, Waddell T, Maltais F et al: The influence of lung volume reduction surgery on exercise in patients with COPD, Eur Respir J 23:269-274, 2004.

24. Naunheim K, Wood D, Mohsenifar Z et al: Long-term follow-up of patients receiving lung-volume reduction surgery versus medical therapy for severe emphysema by the National Emphysema Treatment Trial Research Group, Ann Thorac Surg 82:431-443, 2006.

25. Martinez F, Chang A: Surgical therapy for chronic obstructive pulmonary disease, Semin Respir Crit Care Med 26:167-191, 2005.

26. Yusen R, Morrow L, Brown K: Health-related quality of life after lung volume reduction surgery, Semin Thorac Cardiovasc Surg 14:403-412, 2002.

27. Cooper JD, Patterson GA, Sundaresan RS et al: Results of 150 consecutive bilateral lung volume reduction procedures in patients with severe emphysema, J Thorac Cardiovasc Surg 112:1319-1329[discussion 1329-1330], 1996.

28. Bagley P, Davis S, O'Shea M et al: Lung volume reduction surgery at a community hospital: program development and outcomes, Chest 111:1552-1559, 1997.

29. Norman M, Hillerdal G, Orre L et al: Improved lung function and quality of life following increased elastic recoil after lung volume reduction surgery in emphysema, Respir Med 92:653-658, 1998.

30. Flaherty K, Kazerooni E, Martinez F: Differential diagnosis of chronic airflow obstruction, J Asthma 37:201-223, 2000.

31. Whyte R, Bria W, Martinez F et al: Combined lung volume reduction surgery and mitral valve reconstruction, Ann Thorac Surg 66:1414-1416, 1998.

32. Schmid R, Stammberger U, Hillinger S et al: Lung volume reduction surgery combined with cardiac interventions, Eur J Cardiothorac Surg 15:585-591, 1999.

33. Teschler H, Thompson A, Stamatis G: Short- and long-term functional results after lung volume reduction surgery for severe emphysema, Eur Respir J 13:919-925, 1999.

34. Stoller J, Gildea T, Ries A et al: for the National Emphysema Treatment Trial Research Group: Lung volume reduction surgery in patients with emphysema and α-1 antitrypsin deficiency, Ann Thorac Surg 83:241-251, 2007.

35. Cassina P, Teschler H, Konietzko N et al: Two-year results after lung volume reduction surgery in α-1 antitrypsin deficiency versus smoker's emphysema, Eur Respir J 12:1028-1032, 1998.

36. Gelb A, McKenna R, Brenner M et al: Lung function after bilateral lower lobe lung volume reduction surgery for α1-antitrypsin emphysema, Eur Respir J 14:928-933, 1999.

37. Tutic M, Bloch K, Lardinois D et al: Long-term results after lung volume reduction surgery in patients with α-1 antitrypsin deficiency, J Thorac Cardiovasc Surg 128:408-413, 2004.

38. Mazolewski P, Turner J, Baker M et al: The impact of nutritional status on the outcome of lung volume reduction surgery: a prospective study, Chest 116:693-696, 1999.

39. Nezu K, Yoshikawa M, Yoneda T et al: The effect of nutritional status on morbidity in COPD patients undergoing bilateral lung reduction surgery, Thorac Cardiovasc Surg 49:216-220, 2001.

40. Naunheim K, Wood D, Krasna M et al: for the National Emphysema Treatment Trial Research Group: Predictors of operative mortality and cardiopulmonary morbidity in the National Emphysema Treatment Trial, J Thorac Cardiovasc Surg 131:43-53, 2006.

41. Eugene J, Dajee A, Kayaleh R et al: Reduction pneumoplasty for patients with a forced expiratory volume in 1 second of 500 milliliters or less, Ann Thorac Surg 63:186-192, 1997.

42. Argenziano M, Moazami N, Thomashow B et al: Extended indications for lung volume reduction surgery in advanced emphysema, Ann Thorac Surg 62:1588-1597, 1996.

43. McKenna RJ Jr, Brenner M, Fischel RJ et al: Patient selection criteria for lung volume reduction surgery, J Thorac Cardiovasc Surg 114:957-964[discussion 964-967], 1997.

44. Naunheim K, Hazelrigg S, Kaiser L et al: Risk analysis for thoracoscopic lung volume reduction: a

multi-institutional experience, Eur J Cardiothorac Surg 17:673-679, 2000.

45. Brenner M, Kayaleh R, Milne E et al: Thoracoscopic laser ablation of pulmonary bullae: radiographic selection and treatment response, J Thorac Cardiovasc Surg 107:883-890, 1994.

46. Keenan R, Landrenau R, Sciurba F et al: Unilateral thoracoscopic surgical approach for diffuse emphysema, J Thorac Cardiovasc Surg 111:308-316, 1996.

47. Hazelrigg S, Boley T, Henkle J et al: Thoracoscopic laser bullectomy: a prospective study with three-month results, J Thorac Cardiovasc Surg 112:319-327, 1996.

48. McKenna R Jr, Brenner M, Fischel R et al: Patient selection criteria for lung volume reduction surgery, J Thorac Cardiovasc Surg 114:957-967, 1997.

49. Gierada D: Radiologic assessment of emphysema for lung volume reduction surgery, Semin Thorac Cardiovasc Surg 14:381-390, 2002.

50. Kazerooni E: Radiologic evaluation of emphysema for lung volume reduction surgery, Clin Chest Med 20:845-861, 1999.

51. Goldin J: Quantitative CT of the lung, Radiol Clin North Am 40:45-58, 2002.

52. Madani A, Keyzer C, Gevenois PA: Quantitative computed tomography assessment of lung structure and function in pulmonary emphysema, Eur Respir J 18:720-730, 2001.

53. Sciurba F: Preoperative predictors of outcome following lung volume reduction surgery, Thorax 57(suppl II):ii47-ii52, 2002.

54. Gierada DS, Slone RM, Bae KT et al: Pulmonary emphysema: comparison of preoperative quantitative CT and physiologic index values with clinical outcome after lung-volume reduction surgery, Radiology 205:235-242, 1997.

55. Nakano Y, Coxson HO, Bosan S et al: Core to rind distribution of severe emphysema predicts outcome of lung volume reduction surgery, Am J Respir Crit Care Med 164:2195-2199, 2001.

56. Coxson H, Whittall K, Nakano Y et al: Selection of patients for lung volume reduction surgery using a power law analysis of the computed tomographic scan, Thorax 58:510-514, 2003.

57. Cooper J, Trulock E, Triantafillou A et al: Bilateral pneumectomy (volume reduction) for chronic obstructive pulmonary disease, J Thorac Cardiovasc Surg 109:106-116, 1995.

58. Moy M, Ingenito E, Mentzer S et al: Health-related quality of life improves following pulmonary rehabilitation and lung volume reduction surgery, Chest 115:383-389, 1999.

59. Criner G, Cordova F, Furukawa S et al: Prospective randomized trial comparing bilateral lung volume reduction surgery to pulmonary rehabilitation in severe chronic obstructive pulmonary disease, Am J Respir Crit Care Med 160:2018-2027, 1999.

60. Ries A, Make B, Lee S et al. for the National Emphysema Treatment Trial Research Group: The effects of pulmonary rehabilitation in the National Emphysema Treatment Trial, Chest 128:3799-3809, 2005.

61. Mineo T, Ambrogi V, Pompeo E et al: Impact of lung volume reduction surgery versus rehabilitation on quality of life, Eur Respir J 23:275-280, 2004.

62. Bartels M, Kim H, Whiteson J et al: Pulmonary rehabilitation in patients undergoing lung-volume reduction surgery, Arch Phys Med Rehabil 87(supp. 1):S84-S88, 2006.

63. Ojo T, Martinez F, Paine RIII et al: Lung volume reduction surgery alters management of pulmonary nodules in patients with severe COPD, Chest 112:1494-1500, 1997.

64. Criner G, Cordova F, Leyenson V et al: Effect of lung volume reduction surgery on diaphragm strength, Am J Respir Crit Care Med 157:1578-1585, 1998.

65. Nezu K, Yoshikawa M, Yoneda T et al: The change in body composition after bilateral lung volume reduction surgery for underweight patients with severe emphysema, Lung 178:381-389, 2000.

66. Cassart M, Hamacher J, Verbandt Y et al: Effects of lung volume reduction surgery for emphysema on diaphragm dimensions and configuration, Am J Respir Crit Care 163:1171-1175, 2001.

67. Flaherty K, Kazerooni E, Curtis J et al: Short-term and long-term outcomes after bilateral lung volume reduction surgery: prediction by quantitative CT, Chest 119:1337-1346, 2001.

68. Fujimoto T, Teschler H, Hillejan L et al: Long-term results of lung volume reduction surgery, Eur J Cardiothorac Surg 21:483-488, 2002.

69. Hamacher J, Buchi S, Georgescu C et al: Improved quality of life after lung volume reduction surgery, Eur Respir J 19:54-60, 2002.

70. Ciccone A, Meyers B, Guthrie T et al: Long-term outcome of bilateral lung volume reduction in 250 consecutive patients with emphysema, J Thorac Cardiovasc Surg 125:513-525, 2003.

71. Ingenito E, Loring S, Moy M et al: Physiological characterization of variability in response to lung volume reduction surgery, J Appl Physiol 94:20-30, 2003.

72. National Emphysema Treatment Trial Research Group: Rationale and design of the National Emphysema Treatment Trial: a prospective randomized trial of lung volume reduction surgery, Chest 116:1750-1761, 1999.

73. Hillerdal G, Lofdahl C, Strom K et al. Swedish VOLREM Group: Comparison of lung volume reduction surgery and physical training on health status and physiologic outcomes: a randomized controlled clinical trial, Chest 128:3489-3499, 2005.

74. Miller J, Berger R, Malthaner R et al: Lung volume reduction surgery vs medical treatment: for patients with advanced emphysema, Chest 127:1166-1177, 2005.

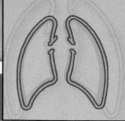

Chapter 25

Ethical and End-of-Life Issues for the Care of Patients with Advanced Lung Disease

JOHN E. HEFFNER • J. RANDALL CURTIS

CHAPTER OUTLINE

Rationale for Advance Care Planning
Barriers to Advance Care Planning
Potential Role for Pulmonary
    Rehabilitation in Initiating Advance
    Care Planning
Advance Planning Curricula Within
    Pulmonary Rehabilitation
      Selecting Patients for Advance Care
        Planning

Helping Patients Make Valid End-
    of-Life Decisions
Toward an Expanded Definition
    of Advance Care Planning
Supporting the End-of-Life Needs of
    Patients Beyond Advance Directives
Conclusion

PROFESSIONAL SKILLS

On completion of this chapter, the reader will be able to do
the following:
* Understand the difficulties that exist with predicting which patients with advanced lung disease will
  benefit from intubation and mechanical ventilation for respiratory failure
* Recognize the role of advance care planning to assist patients in making their end-of-life decisions
* Identify the shortcomings of present efforts to promote the adoption of advance directives
* Denote the interests of patients with severe lung disease for advance care planning
* Select patients for advance care education
* Provide patients with chronic lung disease a framework for discussing advance directives with their
  families and physicians

Patients with advanced lung disease frequently present difficult ethical dilemmas during the course of their care. Regardless of the nature of the underlying pulmonary condition, most patients with chronic respiratory disorders experience a slowly progressive course punctuated by episodes of acute worsening of their lung function. Each episode of pulmonary decompensation poses questions regarding the appropriateness of life-sustaining interventions, such as intubation and mechanical ventilation. For some patients, life-supportive care may promote survival and allow recovery to a baseline level of function. For others, intubation and mechanical ventilation may leave patients with a restricted level of activity or simply prolong the dying process when respiratory failure occurs at the terminal stage of disease. In an effort to assist patients with their decision regarding the acceptability of life-sustaining care, clinicians are often called on to estimate both the likelihood of survival for their patients and the anticipated quality of their postrecovery lives.

Unfortunately, clinicians have a limited ability to predict the outcome of acute respiratory failure for individual patients with chronic lung disease.[1] Multiple studies indicate that patients with chronic obstructive lung disease (COPD) admitted for an acute exacerbation of airway disease have an overall survival to hospital discharge that ranges from 66% to 94%.[2-4] Survival to hospital discharge of patients with COPD who require assisted ventilation is lower, ranging from 60% to 74%.[5-8] Although overall short-term survival is good, the median survival of patients hospitalized with an acute exacerbation of COPD is only 2 years, and 50% of patients are readmitted to the hospital within 6 months.[9]

Unfortunately, no clinical factors, including the severity of blood gas abnormalities or the presence of comorbid factors at the time of hospital admission, accurately identify the subset of patients who will fail to survive hospitalization[1] or will survive but with a decreased functional level and diminished quality of life. Even fewer data exist to describe the probability of survival or postrecovery function of patients who require hospitalization for advanced lung diseases other than COPD.[10]

In the ambulatory setting, patients with advanced emphysema can be categorized on the basis of age, oxygen use, physiologic measures, exercise capacity, and emphysema distribution to identify those at increased risk of death.[11] The BODE (body mass, obstruction, dyspnea, and exercise) Index, a simple grading system, and measures of quality of life[12] have improved our ability to identify groups of patients with COPD at increased risk of all-cause and respiratory-related death.[13] However, the ability to identify patients who will most likely die in the next 6 months remains limited. It is therefore problematic to select patients for advance care planning by the results of prediction rules. Consequently, for advance care planning to be effective, it must be provided to a broader group of patients with moderate to severe lung disease.

In the absence of accurate prognosticating tools, the care of patients with advanced lung disease presents ethical dilemmas and challenging patient care considerations. The ethical dilemmas often focus on decisions regarding the withholding or withdrawal of life-supportive care, such as cardiopulmonary resuscitation, artificial airways, and mechanical ventilators. The patient care considerations encompass effective use of palliative care measures and social support for patients who are experiencing severe discomfort at the terminal stages of their disease. Considering that COPD is the fourth leading cause of death,[14] it is remarkable that few empiric studies have examined clinical approaches to these ethical dilemmas and unique management needs presented by patients with chronic lung disease at the end of life. Consequently, expert panel clinical practice guidelines on COPD have either no content related to end-of-life care[15] or limited information based on a small body of investigative data.[16] The importance of this neglect is profound considering the evidence that end-of-life care is commonly worse for patients with COPD compared with those with other respiratory diseases, such as lung cancer.[17,18] This chapter reviews important ethical considerations in the care of these patients and provides recommendations for using opportunities provided by pulmonary rehabilitation, as well as other outpatient programs for chronic lung disease, to help patients as they prepare for and pass through the terminal stages of their disease.

RATIONALE FOR ADVANCE CARE PLANNING

Considerable ethical, social, and legal support exists for allowing patients to refuse life-sustaining medical care even when such refusal would result in their death.[19,20] In most jurisdictions, living wills and durable powers of attorney for health care are recognized instruments for conveying patients' health care wishes when they become incapacitated. These documents address the observation that most patients with advanced lung disease wish to direct their own end-of-life decisions even after they lose decision-making capacity. A questionnaire study of patients enrolled in pulmonary rehabilitation indicates that more than 80% of patients prefer to direct decisions regarding intubation and mechanical ventilation by either communicating with their physicians directly, through a written advance directive, or through their appointed surrogate decision makers.[21]

Patients' interests to direct their end-of-life decisions mandates that caregivers assist patients with advanced lung disease in making end-of-life decisions that reflect their unique clinical circumstances, life values, and goals. Unfortunately, most studies indicate that less than 15% of elderly care planning discussions.[21,23-25,39,40] In groups of patients with advanced lung disease, information is desired on advance directives by 89% and explicit explanations of the nature and value of life-supportive care by 69%.[21] When these discussions do occur, patients rate the quality of the discussions high.[38]

It has been suggested that several barriers exist for physicians to initiate these discussions, including time constraints,[27,41] their concerns that patients are "not sick enough yet,"[27] and their perceptions that they already understand the end-of-life preferences of their patients.[42-44] This latter barrier is a risky assumption, because multiple studies indicate that physicians consistently underestimate patients' interests in advanced life support because physicians make assumptions based on their perceptions of the quality of their patients' lives, which physicians also consistently underestimate.[45,46] Furthermore, patients' assessments of their own quality of life are not associated with their treatment preferences for life-sustaining treatments.[37] It is important, therefore, that physicians examine their own assumptions and obtain treatment preferences directly from patients.[47] An additional barrier is the discomfort some physicians experience with discussing end-of-life issues.[48] Studies indicate that pulmonary physicians who feel personal discomfort in discussing end-of-life decisions are more likely to postpone these discussions with their patients with COPD.[48] Other barriers include little available time, fears that discussions with extinguish patient hope, and concern that the patient is not ready for a talk.[27]

POTENTIAL ROLE FOR PULMONARY REHABILITATION IN INITIATING ADVANCE CARE PLANNING

Programs directed toward physicians to promote more patient–physician discussions on advance care planning have produced mixed results. The SUPPORT (Study to Understand Prognoses and Preferences for Outcomes and Risks of Treatments) investigators[44] observed negligible effects of an inpatient program to notify physicians of patients who would benefit from end-of-life discussions. In contrast, a comprehensive effort to change the culture within a medical center regarding the importance of advance directives promoted a greater patient–physician dialogue.[49] This latter study, however, was limited

to inpatient care and did not examine the effect of physician education on patient-physician discussions about advance care planning in the ambulatory setting. Other studies in general patient populations indicate that policy interventions, computer prompts to electronic medical records, and physician education have only marginal success in promoting these discussions and the proportion of patients with completed advance directives.[24,49-65]

Promoting discussions on advance planning in the ambulatory setting is important because most patients with advanced lung disease indicate a preference for such discussions to occur during periods of stable health.[21] Only 19% of patients with chronic lung disease would choose to defer advance care planning to an acute hospitalization, when the need for life-supportive care seems imminent.[21]

Unfortunately, observational studies indicate that most advance planning occurs during critical illnesses when patients have already lost their decision-making capacity.[49,66,67] Only 20% of patients who have a do-not-resuscitate order placed in their medical record have had an opportunity to participate in the decision-making process.[68]

The reluctance of physicians to initiate end-of-life discussions has produced interest in promoting advance care planning by encouraging patients with chronic lung disease to initiate these discussions with their physicians. Physician behavioral studies indicate that patient expectations and requests for specific components of care are potent influences for altering physician practice patterns.[69]

Success in initiating end-of-life discussions can be achieved by developing a team-based approach with incorporation of nonphysician clinicians.[36,70] Rabow and colleagues[70] demonstrated that an outpatient consultative team that provided educational and supportive services was well accepted by patients with serious illnesses and their families.

Pulmonary rehabilitation offers patients with advanced lung disease a multidisciplinary team that provides broad education and support for problems related to the underlying condition. It would seem, therefore, that enrollment in pulmonary rehabilitation would be an opportunity to inform patients regarding the importance of advance care planning and of discussing end-of-life issues with their physicians. The success of such a program would depend on the willingness patients under the long-term care of physicians and patients with chronic health conditions have had discussions with their physicians about end-of-life care.[21-26] Similarly, only 19% to 32% of patients with advanced lung disease have discussions with their physicians about the appropriateness of life support in various clinical circumstances,[21,27] and 15% have participated in discussions regarding the nature of life-supportive care.[21] Although most patients with chronic lung disease have formulated opinions regarding the acceptability of intubation and mechanical ventilation, less than 15% of these patients feel confident that their physicians understand their wishes.[21]

The importance of this patient-physician dialogue is underscored by the observation that patients need medical information from their caregivers to formulate their advance care decisions. Patients often have an inflated estimation of the value of life-sustaining care.[28]

When geriatric patients are presented with realistic estimations of the likelihood of survival after cardiopulmonary resuscitation, they often alter their willingness to undergo life-sustaining care.[29,30] Patients with chronic lung disease similarly demonstrate a lower interest in accepting intubation and mechanical ventilation as the probability of survival decreases and when baseline or postrecovery respiratory function diminishes.[21] Unfortunately, patients with advanced lung disease are more likely than patients with cancer to indicate that they lack education about their disease, treatment, prognosis, and advance care planning.[31] Box 25-1 shows some of the specific aspects of education that many patients with COPD report they want.

Patients with advanced lung disease, therefore, have a greater opportunity to make end-of-life decisions that result in the outcomes they desire if they gain an accurate knowledge of the nature of life-sustaining interventions and their probabilities of success in different clinical circumstances. Because this information needs to be tailored to the unique health circumstances of each patient, physicians and other caregivers with an awareness of the patient's condition are in the best position to inform their patients regarding these issues. Helping patients prepare for decisions that may entail the withholding or withdrawing of life-sustaining care should emulate the approach care providers use to inform patients about the nature of surgical procedures before requesting consent for an operative procedure.

BOX 25-1	Components of Communication about End-of-Life Care That Patients with COPD Report They Would Like to Discuss with Their Physician

- Details about their diagnosis and nature of their disease process
- The role and limitations of the available treatments in improving symptoms, quality of life and duration of life
- Their prognosis both for survival and for quality life
- What the dying process might be like and how symptoms can be controlled at the end of life
- Advance care planning for future medical care exacerbations of COPD

COPD, *Chronic obstructive pulmonary disease.*
Adapted from Curtis and colleagues.[31]

BARRIERS TO ADVANCE CARE PLANNING

It remains uncertain why few patients chronic health conditions discuss end-of issues with their physicians. Physicians seem wait for patients to request information advance directives because they interpret s initiatives as evidence that patients are emoti ally ready to discuss these topics.[21] Most patie do not demonstrate initiative and instead wait their physicians to introduce advance care pla ning.[21] The resulting communication "standof leaves patients uninformed regarding the value life-supportive care in their unique circumstances

The barriers to communication are not entirely defined. We currently have only a limited understanding of the perspective of patients with severe COPD regarding the problems they face in attaining advance-care planning.[17,18,27,32] Patients state, however, issues of preferring to "concentrate on staying alive than talking about death," lack of certainty as to "what physician will be providing care during a severe illness," and fears of "abandonment" if they adopt advance directives.[33-36] Other factors, such as depression, also impede communication.[37,38] The relative roles of these factors for an individual patient and physician are highly variable and require conversations with a specific patient to identify the importance of each.[27]

Although barriers exist, multiple studies indicate that most patients are receptive to advance of patients to participate in advance care planning educational programs within pulmonary rehabilitation and their opinions regarding the suitability of receiving this information from nonphysician educators.

To address these issues, a study examined the attitudes of patients with advanced lung disease enrolled in pulmonary rehabilitation programs.[21] The authors found that patients identified pulmonary rehabilitation educators and lawyers in addition to physicians as the most important sources of information on advance directives (Table 25-1). Pulmonary rehabilitation educators and physicians were identified as the preferred sources of information on life-supportive care. This receptiveness to information from a variety of sources provides an opportunity to develop curricula within pulmonary rehabilitation that prepare patients to initiate discussions with their physicians and approach advance care planning in an informed manner.

The effectiveness of advance care planning curricula in pulmonary rehabilitation, however, has received little investigational attention. One study examined a brief educational intervention about advance directives directed toward patients with chronic lung disease enrolled in pulmonary rehabilitation. The study determined that education increased the proportion of patients who had completed written advance directives from 34% to 86% but had a smaller effect on increasing the number of patients who had discussed these issues with their physicians (22% to 58%). Moreover, only 44% of patients had confidence at the end of the study that their end-of-life wishes were understood by their physicians. These results support the utility of end-of-life education within pulmonary rehabilitation, especially considering that the educational intervention was brief and did not provide follow-up monitoring of patients for completion of advance planning. However, it highlights the need for involving the primary physicians involved in the patient's care. The advantages of different approaches to advance care planning education within pulmonary rehabilitation warrant further evaluation.

Although pulmonary rehabilitation seems to be a potentially valuable site for advance planning information for patients with advanced lung disease, most programs do not offer end-of-life educational opportunities. In a survey study, fewer than 10% of pulmonary rehabilitation programs in the United States provide information on end-of-life issues.[71] More than 70% of nonphysician directors of rehabilitation programs, however, state a willingness to include such education into their curricula.[71] Some program directors responding to this survey, however, stated a reluctance to present sessions on advance care planning, voicing a concern that education on end-of-life issues might be unsettling or depressing to their patients.

The psychological impact of advance care planning has been examined in several studies.

TABLE 25-1 Subject Preferences* for Sources of Information on Advance Directives and the Life Support Interventions of Intubation and Mechanical Ventilation

	PREFERENCE RATING	
Source	**Advance Directives**	**Life Support**
Pulmonary rehabilitation	1.75 ± 0.74[†]	1.63 ± 0.67[‡]
Lawyer	1.77 ± 0.91[§]	2.48 ± 0.92
Physician	1.80 ± 0.77[§]	1.34 ± 0.50[‖]
Family	2.02 ± 1.01[¶]	1.74 ± 0.84[‡]
Reading	2.10 ± 0.74[¶]	NA
Community class	2.31 ± 0.81	2.38 ± 0.81[¶]
Clergy	2.58 ± 0.85	2.70 ± 0.80

*Preference ratings calculated from the mean ± SD of a four-level Likert scale, with "1" corresponding to highly preferred and "4" corresponding to very undesirable.
[†]$P < .05$ compared with clergy, community class, and reading.
[‡]$P < .05$ compared with clergy, lawyer, and community class.
[§]$P < .05$ compared with clergy and community class.
[‖]$P < .05$ compared with clergy, lawyer, community class, and family.
[¶]$P < .05$ compared with clergy.
NA, Not assessed.
Reprinted with permission from Heffner JE, Fahy B, Hilling L et al: Attitudes regarding advance directives among patients in pulmonary rehabilitation, Am J Respir Crit Care Med 154:1735, 1996.

These studies indicate that discussions on end-of-life issues do not cause the patient depression or provoke excessive anxiety or a sense of hopelessness.[68,72-75] Geriatric patients participating in end-of-life discussions with their physicians have demonstrated a decrease in measured anxiety and depression scores.[75] Elderly patients and patients with chronic health conditions identify loss of control over their lives and fears of becoming a burden to their families as their greatest concerns. Advance care planning may decrease anxiety and depression by providing patients with approaches to retaining control over their health care and avoiding prolonged illnesses before their deaths.[76]

The psychological impact of advance care planning for patients with advanced lung disease has not been extensively investigated. Existing data, however, indicate that more than 88% of patients with advanced lung disease enrolled in pulmonary rehabilitation state an interest in learning more about advance care planning.[22] Nearly all (>99%) of these patients indicate that end-of-life discussions would not provoke unacceptable levels of concern or anxiety.[21]

ADVANCE PLANNING CURRICULA WITHIN PULMONARY REHABILITATION

The foregoing discussion indicates that patients with advanced lung disease wish to learn more about advance care planning so as to participate effectively in their end-of-life decisions. At present, however, patients do not often participate in discussions on advance care planning with their physicians and have limited resources to learn about end-of-life issues tailored to their unique respiratory conditions. Previous studies suggest that curricula on advance care planning within pulmonary rehabilitation would assist patients in making valid end-of-life decisions. Also, pulmonary rehabilitation could provide patients with advanced lung disease the continuity they seek in their end-of-life care.[36,77]

Unfortunately, formal curricula for educating patients on advance care planning have not been developed and validated to date. If such a curriculum were to be designed, it would need to contain elements that would assist rehabilitation directors to select patients for advance care planning and provide information that would allow patients to participate in a meaningful way in their end-of-life decisions.

Selecting Patients for Advance Care Planning

Although most patients want their caregivers to initiate discussions regarding end-of-life care, it should be noted that a proportion do not.[21,78-80] In a survey of patients with advanced lung disease, 4% of patients indicated that they would prefer their caregivers to make all of their end-of-life decisions without being included in the decision-making process.[21] Similarly, although most patients do not think that end-of-life discussions would promote undue anxiety, 1% indicate that such discussion would be too anxiety provoking to pursue.[21] Also, some members of certain ethnic groups are reluctant to engage in discussions about end-of-life issues. Mexican Americans, Korean Americans, and Navajos are less receptive to making their own life support decisions.[78,81] Receptiveness to participating in advance planning increases as members of ethnic groups begin to assimilate into the dominant culture.[81] An educational program within pulmonary rehabilitation on advance care planning, therefore, would need to respect the reluctance of some patients to participate.

One acceptable approach for selecting patients for discussing end-of-life care entails presenting patients with an invitation to participate in educational sessions without exposing them to the contents of the program. End-of-life topics can be introduced while discussing other components of health care planning, such as vaccinations, health screening, and disease prevention activities. An appropriate invitation would come in the form of a statement of rationale and a question: "Patients with chronic lung conditions can develop respiratory complications that might require life-supportive care, such as mechanical ventilation. It is important for your physician to understand your attitudes and beliefs about life-prolonging care in different circumstances. Would you be willing to participate in an educational program intended to assist you with making decisions about your care if you developed a severe illness?" It may also be helpful to frame discussions of advance care planning within the context of "hoping for the best while preparing for the worst."[33]

Patients who voice a reluctance to participate may respond more favorably as they learn more about the nature of their lung conditions in pulmonary rehabilitation and the possibility for progressive deterioration. Periodic invitations to participate as patients demonstrate increasing trust and comfort within the rehabilitation program may allow patients to become more receptive to advance care planning. Also, some patients with anxiety about discussing life-sustaining treatment still want to have these discussions take place after receiving reading material on advance planning and additional opportunities and encouragement.[21,25] As an alternative approach, patients may be administered a questionnaire that could select patients for further discussions.[38]

Pulmonary rehabilitation programs can also develop profiles of patients with COPD who are at increased risk of hospitalization and who would especially benefit from end-of-life discussions.[82] Reasonable criteria would assess patients for an FEV_1 (forced expiratory volume in 1 second) less than 30% of predicted, one or more hospital admissions in the last year for COPD exacerbations, comorbidities such as heart failure or lung cancer, older age, living alone, depression, and increasing dependence on home caregivers.[82] Use of the BODE Index[13] or measures of quality of life,[12] which are predictors of hospitalization and all-cause mortality, may also help patient selection.

Helping Patients Make Valid End-of-Life Decisions

An important component of advance care planning involves the completion of a written document that is intended to direct patients' care when they have lost their decision-making capacity or can no longer communicate their wishes. A living will provides caregivers a statement regarding a patient's wishes for life-supportive care in various clinical circumstances, often limited in some jurisdictions to the existence of a terminal disease. A durable power of attorney for health care provides an opportunity to appoint a health care proxy who can represent the patient's wishes through surrogate decision making.

Unfortunately, written advance directives have been only marginally successful in allowing patients to direct their end-of-life care.[83] As previously stated, only a small proportion of patients with chronic health conditions[23-25,39] and patients with advanced lung disease have completed these documents.[21] Also, physicians often are unaware of the existence of formal advance directives and do not adhere to the written

directives when critical illnesses arise.[44,84,85] Moreover, patients with written advance directives frequently fail to understand the contents and implications of their complete documents,[86] and surrogate decision makers usually have a poor understanding of the end-of-life wishes of patients.[87] These shortcomings have created concern that written advance directives have little utility for supporting patient autonomy at the end of life.[88,89]

Although advance directives have been promoted as instruments that direct end-of-life care for patients, most patients intend that their surrogates and physicians overrule their advance directives in some clinical situations as circumstances dictate.[90,91] Advance directives, therefore, should be considered for many patients to represent general statements regarding treatment preferences. Patients need to be asked how specifically their advance directives should be respected. Without an ongoing dialogue, physicians generally demonstrate a poor understanding of the preferences of their patients for overruling advance directives, which is associated with more interventional end-of-life care.[92]

Despite these efforts to assist patients to formulate valid written advance directives, it seems that written instruments will always fall short in providing accurate and comprehensive descriptions of patients' wishes in all conceivable clinical circumstances. Discussions on end-of-life planning have recommended a conceptual shift in our thinking about advance care planning.[93] This shift directs us to understand how patients rather than caregivers perceive advance care planning and to participate in an expanding definition of advance care planning.

TOWARD AN EXPANDED DEFINITION OF ADVANCE CARE PLANNING

Caregivers tend to perceive written advance directives as operational tools that direct the selection of life-sustaining interventions when patients can no longer participate in health care decision making. From the patients' perspectives, advance directives are only one of the many resources available to patients for achieving their end-of-life goals. These goals extend beyond the usual choices between specific life-supportive interventions presented to patients during episodes of respiratory failure. The more comprehensive goals of patients at the end of life center on preparing for death, achieving a sense of control over their lives, and fortifying personal relationships with friends and families.[93]

The goals of advance care planning from patients' perspectives, therefore, are more psychosocial and less operational or oriented toward accepting or rejecting specific interventions. The goals of advance care planning may consequently shift from patient-physician communication focused on the withholding or withdrawing of various life-sustaining interventions toward communication between family members about goals and values. This communication within a patient's family has a purpose of strengthening family relationships and offering mutual support as patients anticipate the end of their lives.

Educators in pulmonary rehabilitation and other ambulatory health care settings who care for patients with advanced lung disease nearing the end of life can facilitate this strengthening of family relationships. Appropriate efforts would involve families in advance care planning and promote a dialogue between patients and their families regarding the prognosis of the patient's lung disease and the decisions regarding care that they will eventually face. Educators can identify patient and family needs for resources to enrich these discussions and provide specific respiratory-related information tailored to a specific patient's unique health circumstances and stage of disease. Educators can also make themselves available to respond to patients' questions and concerns or direct patients to appropriate palliative care resources. During enrollment in pulmonary rehabilitation, educators can monitor their patients' advance care planning and obtain copies of written directives to be certain that they accurately reflect their patients' stated preferences, life values, and goals.[93]

In this model, an ongoing dialogue about end-of-life decisions—rather than a written advance directive itself—becomes the purpose of advance care planning. This purpose fulfills the needs of patients to know their prognosis, to understand what it is like to die from advanced lung disease, to prepare for death, to enhance family relationships, and to receive the end-of-life care that best conforms to their wishes and preferences.[31,47] Enrollment in pulmonary rehabilitation may provide the suitable environment to assist patients with initiating and maintaining this family-oriented dialogue.

SUPPORTING THE END-OF-LIFE NEEDS OF PATIENTS BEYOND ADVANCE DIRECTIVES

Many patients with advanced lung disease will experience progression of their respiratory condition. Eventually, coping mechanisms that previously alleviated the discomforts of chronic dyspnea will fail and patients will experience ongoing respiratory distress. If such patients choose to forego life-supportive care with ventilatory support, they require reassurance that effective palliative measures will limit suffering as they approach the end of life and that they will not be abandoned by their care providers.[94] For example, most pulmonary rehabilitation programs educate patients regarding the progressive nature of their disease.[71] Most programs, however, have not included education on the availability and effectiveness of palliative care and community resources for managing the difficulties that progressive respiratory diseases present at the end of life. This omission may be unfortunate because patients with lung disease commonly harbor an unspoken fear of experiencing the distress of suffocating as they die. This fear seems reasonable considering that severe dyspnea is a common experience of patients dying from any cause.[95] Also, almost all of the patients with COPD monitored in the SUPPORT study experienced dyspnea during the last few days of their life.[96] Patients with advanced lung disease have an all too familiar understanding of the discomforts produced by unremitting dyspnea.

To address these and other issues, physicians, nurses, and pulmonary rehabilitation educators will need to acquire new skills in communicating to patients topics related to end-of-life care and advance planning. No research addresses the components of these skills within pulmonary rehabilitation. Curtis and coworkers, however, have examined the important components of physicians' skills in providing excellent end-of-life care from the perspective of patients and their families (Box 25-2).[35,47] Among the identified 12 domains, communication, emotional support, and accessibility proved to be the most highly valued content areas. The domains may also be applicable to pulmonary educator skills. Providers can learn such communication skills as demonstrated by a randomized controlled trial wherein oncologists participated in a 3-day communications skills workshop and improved their abilities to communicate effectively with patients.[97] Similar skills workshops

---

BOX 25-2	Physician Skills in Providing End-of-Life Care Most Valued by Patients

- Accessibility and continuity
- Team coordination and communication
- Communication with patients
- Patient education
- Inclusion and recognition of the family
- Competence
- Pain and symptom management
- Emotional support
- Personalization
- Attention to patient values
- Respect and humility
- Support of patient decision making

BOX 25-3	Parameters for Identifying Patients Who Qualify for Hospice Services

I. Severity of chronic lung disease documented by
  A. Disabling dyspnea at rest; poorly or unresponsive to bronchodilators, resulting in decreased functional activity, for example, bed-to-chair existence, often exacerbated by other debilitating symptoms such as fatigue and cough. FEV_1 greater than 30% predicted, after bronchodilator use, is helpful supplemental objective evidence but should not be required if not already available
  B. Progressive pulmonary disease
    1. Increasing visits to the emergency department or hospitalizations for pulmonary infections and/or respiratory failure
    2. Decrease in FEV_1 on serial testing of more than 40 ml/year is helpful supplemental objective evidence but should not be required if not already available
II. Presence of cor pulmonale or right heart failure
  A. These should be caused by advanced pulmonary disease, not primary or secondary to left heart disease or valvulopathy
  B. Cor pulmonale may be documented by:
    1. Echocardiography
    2. Electrocardiogram
    3. Chest radiograph
    4. Physical signs of right heart failure
III. Hypoxemia at rest on supplemental oxygen:
  A. $Po_2 \leq 55$ mm Hg on supplemental oxygen
  B. Oxygen saturation $\leq 88\%$ on supplemental oxygen
IV. Hypercapnia:
  A. $Pco_2 \geq 50$ mm Hg
V. Unintentional progressive weight loss exceeding 10% of body weight over the preceding 6 months
VI. Resting tachycardia greater than 100/minute in a patient with known severe chronic obstructive pulmonary disease

FEV_1, *Forced expiratory volume in 1 second;* Pco_2, *partial pressure of carbon dioxide.* Po_2; *partial pressure of oxygen. Data from Stuart B, Alexander C, Arenella C et al: Medical guidelines for determining prognosis in selected non-cancer diseases, Arlington, Va, 1996, National Hospice Organization.*

---

could be provided for pulmonary rehabilitation educators in the domain of advance care planning.

Community resources have not matured for patients with advanced lung disease as they have for patients with terminal malignancies. Palliative care teams, however, do exist within some health care systems and are rapidly increasing in numbers and capacity.[98] The goal of palliative care is to prevent and relieve suffering and to support the best possible quality of life for patients and their families, regardless of the stage of disease or the need for other therapies.[99] As such, palliative care expands traditional disease-model medical treatment to include the goals of enhancing quality of life, optimizing function, helping with decision making, and providing opportunities for personal growth.[99] Physicians, nurses, and pulmonary rehabilitation programs should help identify patients who could benefit from palliative care services and design education to include information on available palliative resources in the community.

Alternatives to hospitalization for terminal patients with advanced lung disease, however, do exist. The National Hospice Organization revised their guidelines for selecting patients with noncancer diseases for access to hospice services.[100] These guidelines discuss the difficulties in accurately predicting the prognosis of patients with advanced COPD but recognize the appropriateness of providing hospice services for subsets of these patients (Box 25-3).[100] Educational programs within pulmonary rehabilitation can serve as contact resources to advise patients and their families regarding these community resources. Such guidance from pulmonary rehabilitation directors could address observations that patients with COPD are now more likely to die in the intensive care unit on a ventilator as compared with patients with lung cancer and less likely to have received palliative care services.[17,101]

Perhaps one of the most important roles of nurses, social workers, and pulmonary rehabilitation educators is to bridge patients with their physicians to help facilitate the advance care planning discussions that patients desire but now do not have with their doctors. Because multiple patient-related and physician-related barriers exist for these discussions, patient advocates should target both patients and physicians to facilitate this important dialogue.[47] Guidance from informed pulmonary rehabilitation directors can prime patients to expect these discussions and alert physicians for when their patients are ready, willing, and in need for these discussions to occur.

CONCLUSION

End-of-life care of patients with advanced lung disease can be enhanced with the adoption of well-conceived advance directives that reflect the end-of-life preferences of patients. Advance directives by themselves, however, cannot communicate the full spectrum of patient preferences in all conceivable health care circumstances. They should serve as a component of an ongoing dialogue between patients, families, and care providers that promotes an understanding of the patient's life values and goals. With this understanding, patients have the greatest opportunity to approach the end of their life with confidence that their wishes will be honored, their dying experience will strengthen their family relationships, and they will gain support from the family relationships that advance care planning engendered. Education on life-supportive interventions and end-of-life issues within the pulmonary clinical practice and the pulmonary rehabilitation program can foster this expanded role of advance care planning for patients with advanced lung disease and guide patients toward palliative care services.

References

1. Heffner JE: Chronic obstructive pulmonary disease: ethical considerations of care, Clin Pulm Med 3:1-8, 1996.
2. Warren PM, Flenley DC, Millar JS et al: Respiratory failure revisited: acute exacerbations of chronic bronchitis between 1961-68 and 1970-76, Lancet 1:467-470, 1980.
3. Bone RC, Pierce AK, Johnson RL: Controlled oxygen administration in acute respiratory failure in chronic obstructive pulmonary disease: a reappraisal, Am Rev Respir Dis 65:896-902, 1978.
4. Martin TR, Lewis SW, Albert RK: The prognosis of patients with chronic obstructive pulmonary disease after hospitalization for acute respiratory failure, Chest 82:310-314, 1982.
5. Portier F, Defouilloy C, Muir JF: Determinants of immediate survival among chronic respiratory insufficiency patients admitted to an intensive care unit for acute respiratory failure, Chest 101:204-210, 1992.
6. Rieves RD, Bass D, Carter RR et al: Severe COPD and acute respiratory failure: correlates for survival at the time of tracheal intubation, Chest 104:854-860, 1993.
7. Menzies R, Gibbons W, Goldberg P: Determinants of weaning and survival among patients with COPD who require mechanical ventilation for acute respiratory failure, Chest 95:398-405, 1989.
8. Gillepsie DJ, Marsh MM, Divertie MB et al: Clinical outcome of respiratory failure in patients requiring prolonged (>24 hours) mechanical ventilation, Chest 90:364-369, 1986.
9. Connors AF, Dawson NV, Thomas C et al: Outcomes following acute exacerbations of severe chronic obstructive lung disease: the SUPPORT investigators, Am J Respir Crit Care Med 154:959-967, 1996.
10. Noble PW: Idiopathic pulmonary fibrosis: natural history and prognosis, Clin Chest Med 27(1 supp 1):S11-S16 v, 2006.
11. Martinez FJ, Foster G, Curtis JL et al: Predictors of mortality in patients with emphysema and severe airflow obstruction, Am J Respir Crit Care Med 173:1326-1334, 2006.
12. Fan VS, Curtis JR, Tu SP et al: Using quality of life to predict hospitalization and mortality in patients with obstructive lung diseases, Chest 122:429-436, 2002.
13. Celli BR, Cote CG, Marin JM et al: The body-mass index, airflow obstruction, dyspnea, and exercise capacity index in chronic obstructive pulmonary disease, N Engl J Med 350:1005-1012, 2004.
14. Mannino DM: COPD: epidemiology, prevalence, morbidity and mortality, and disease heterogeneity, Chest 121(5 suppl):121S-126S, 2002.
15. Pauwels RA, Buist AS, Calverley PM et al: GOLD Scientific Committee: Global strategy for the diagnosis, management, and prevention of chronic obstructive pulmonary disease: NHLBI/WHO Global Initiative for Chronic Obstructive Lung Disease (GOLD) workshop summary, Am J Respir Crit Care Med 163:1256-1276, 2001.
16. American Thoracic Society/European Respiratory Society Task Force: Standards for the diagnosis and management of patients with COPD [Internet], version 1.2. New York, 2004, American Thoracic Society. Available at http://www.thoracic.org/sections/copd. Retrieved October 11, 2006.
17. Claessens MT, Lynn J, Zhong Z et al: Dying with lung cancer or chronic obstructive pulmonary disease: insights from SUPPORT. Study to Understand Prognoses and Preferences for Outcomes and Risks of Treatments. J Am Geriatr Soc 48(5 suppl):S146-S153, 2000.
18. Gore JM, Brophy CJ, Greenstone MA: How well do we care for patients with end stage chronic obstructive pulmonary disease (COPD)? A comparison of palliative care and quality of life in COPD and lung cancer, Thorax 55:1000-1006, 2000.
19. President's Commission for the Study of Ethical Problems in Medicine and Biomedical and Behavioral Research: Deciding to forgo life-sustaining treatment: a report on the ethical, medical, and legal issues in treatment decisions, Washington DC, 1983, U.S. Government Printing Office.
20. Lanken PN, Ahlheit BD, Crawford S et al: Withholding and withdrawing life-sustaining therapy, Am Rev Respir Dis 144:726-731, 1991.

21. Heffner JE, Fahy B, Hilling L et al: Attitudes regarding advance directives among patients in pulmonary rehabilitation, Am J Respir Crit Care Med 154:1735-1740, 1996.

22. Emanuel LL, Emanuel EJ, Stoeckle JD et al: Advance directives: stability of patients' treatment choices, Arch Intern Med 154:209-217, 1994.

23. La Puma J, Orentlicher D, Moss R: Advance directives on admission: clinical implications and analysis of the Patient Self-determination Act of 1990, JAMA 266:402-405, 1991.

24. Rubin SM, Strull WM, Fialkow MF et al: Increasing the completion of the durable power of attorney for health care: a randomized, controlled trial, JAMA 271:209-212, 1994.

25. Virmani J, Schneiderman LJ, Kaplan RM: Relationship of advance directives to physician-patient communication, Arch Intern Med 142:909-913, 1994.

26. Lo B, McLeod GA, Saika G: Patient attitudes to discussing life-sustaining treatment, Am J Med 146:1613-1615, 1986.

27. Knauft E, Nielsen EL, Engelberg RA et al: Barriers and facilitators to end-of-life care communication for patients with COPD, Chest 127:2188-2196, 2005.

28. Miller DL, Jahnigen DW, Gorbien MJ et al: Cardiopulmonary resuscitation: how useful? Attitudes and knowledge of an elderly population, Arch Intern Med 152:578-582, 1992.

29. Murphy DJ, Burrows D, Santilli S et al: The influence of the probability of survival on patients' preferences regarding cardiopulmonary resuscitation, N Engl J Med 330:545-549, 1994.

30. Frankl D, Oye RK, Bellamy PE: Attitudes of hospitalized patients toward life support: a survey of 200 hospitalized medical patients, Am J Med 86:645-648, 1989.

31. Curtis JR, Wenrich MD, Carline JD et al: Patients' perspectives on physician skill in end-of-life care: differences between patients with COPD, cancer, and AIDS, Chest 122:356-362, 2002.

32. Edmonds P, Karlsen S, Khan S et al: A comparison of the palliative care needs of patients dying from chronic respiratory diseases and lung cancer, Palliat Med 15:287-295, 2001.

33. Back AL, Arnold RM, Quill TE: Hope for the best, and prepare for the worst, Ann Intern Med 138:439-443, 2003.

34. Hofmann JC, Wenger NS, Davis RB et al: Patient preferences for communication with physicians about end-of-life decisions. SUPPORT Investigators. Study to Understand Prognoses and Preference for Outcomes and Risks of Treatment, Ann Intern Med 127:1-12, 1997.

35. Curtis JR, Wenrich MD, Carline JD et al: Understanding physicians' skills at providing end-of-life care perspectives of patients, families, and health care workers, J Gen Intern Med 16:41-49, 2001.

36. Carline JD, Curtis JR, Wenrich MD et al: Physicians' interactions with health care teams and systems in the care of dying patients: perspectives of dying patients, family members, and health care professionals, J Pain Symptom Manage 25:19-28, 2003.

37. Stapleton RD, Nielsen EL, Engelberg RA et al: Association of depression and life-sustaining treatment preferences in patients with COPD, Chest 127:328-334, 2005.

38. Curtis JR, Engelberg RA, Nielsen EL et al: Patient—physician communication about end-of-life care for patients with severe COPD, Eur Respir J 24:200-205, 2004.

39. Emanuel LL, Barry MJ, Stoekle JD et al: Advance directives for medical care: a case for greater use, N Engl J Med 324:889-895, 1991.

40. Guthrie SJ, Hill KM, Muers ME: Living with severe COPD: a qualitative exploration of the experience of patients in Leeds, Respir Med 95:196-204, 2001.

41. Wolf SM, Boyle P, Callahan D et al: Sources of concern about the Patient Self-determination Act, N Engl J Med 325:1666-1671, 1991.

42. Lo B: "Do not resuscitate" decisions: a prospective study at three teaching hospitals, Arch Intern Med 145:1115, 1985.

43. Uhlmann RF, Pearlman RA, Cain KC: Physicians' and spouses' predictions of elderly patients' resuscitation preferences, J Gerontol 43:115-121, 1988.

44. A controlled trial to improve care for seriously ill hospitalized patients: the Study to Understand Prognoses and Preferences for Outcomes and Risks of Treatments (SUPPORT). The SUPPORT Principal Investigators, JAMA 274:1591-1598, 1995.

45. Sprangers MA, Aaronson NK: The role of health care providers and significant others in evaluating the quality of life of patients with chronic disease: a review, J Clin Epidemiol 45:743-760, 1992.

46. Wilson KA, Dowling AJ, Abdolell M et al: Perception of quality of life by patients, partners and treating physicians, Qual Life Res 9:1041-1052, 2000.

47. Curtis JR, Engelberg RA, Wenrich MD et al: Communication about palliative care for patients with chronic obstructive pulmonary disease, J Palliat Care 21:157-164, 2005.

48. Sullivan KE, Hébert PC, Logan J et al: What do physicians tell patients with end-stage COPD about intubation and mechanical ventilation? Chest 109:258-264, 1996.

49. Reilly BM, Wagner M, Magnussen R et al: Promoting inpatient directives about life-sustaining treatments in a community hospital: results of a 3-year time-series intervention trial, Arch Intern Med 155:2317-2323, 1995.

50. Hanson LC, Tulsky JA, Danis M: Can clinical interventions change care at the end of life? Ann Intern Med 126:381-388, 1997.

51. Cohen-Mansfield J, Rabinovich BA, Lipson S et al: The decision to execute a durable power of attorney for health care and preferences regarding the utilization of life-sustaining treatments in nursing home residents, Arch Intern Med 151:289-294, 1991.

52. Hare J, Nelson C: Will outpatients complete living wills? A comparison of two interventions, J Gen Intern Med 6:41-46, 1991.

53. Sachs G, Stocking C, Miles S: Empowerment of the older patient? A randomized, controlled trial to increase discussion and use of advance directives, J Am Geriatr Soc 40:269-273, 1992.

54. High D: Advance directives and the elderly: a study of interventional strategies to increase their use, Gerontologist 33:342-349, 1993.

55. Holley JL, Nespor S, Rault R: The effects of providing chronic hemodialysis patients written material on advance directives, Am J Kidney Dis 22:413-418, 1993.

56. Luptak MK, Boult C: A method for increasing elders use of advance directives, Gerontologist 34:409-412, 1994.

57. Markson LJ, Fanale J, Steel K et al: Implementing advance directives in the primary care setting, Arch Intern Med 154:2321-2327, 1994.

58. Cuglian AM, Miller T, Sobal J: Factors promoting completion of advance directives in the hospital, Arch Intern Med 155:1893-1898, 1995.

59. Silverman HJ, Tuma P, Schaeffer MH et al: Implementation of the Patient Self-determination Act in a hospital setting, Arch Intern Med 155:502-510, 1995.

60. Duffield P, Podzamsky JE: The completion of advance directives in primary care, J Fam Pract 42:378-384, 1996.

61. Meier DE, Fuss BR, O'Rourke D et al: Marked improvement in recognition and completion of health care proxies: a randomized controlled trial of counseling by hospital patient representatives, Arch Intern Med 156:1227-1232, 1996.

62. Meier DE, Gold G, Mertz K et al: Enhancement of proxy appointment for older persons: physician counseling in the ambulatory setting, J Am Geriatr Soc 44:37-43, 1996.

63. Sulmasy DP, Song KY, Marx ES et al: Strategies to promote the use of advance directives in a residency outpatient practice, J Gen Intern Med 11:657-663, 1996.

64. Landry FJ, Kroenke K, Lucas C et al: Increasing the use of advance directives in medical outpatients, J Gen Intern Med 12:412-415, 1997.

65. Richter KP, Langel S, Fawcett SB et al: Promoting the use of advance directives: an empirical study, Arch Fam Med 64:609-615, 1995.

66. Quill TE, Bennett NM: The effects of a hospital policy and state legislation on resuscitation orders for geriatric patients, Arch Intern Med 15:569-572, 1992.

67. Cohen-Mansfield J, Droge JA, Billig N: The utilization of the durable power of attorney for health care among hospitalized elderly patients, J Am Geriatr Soc 39:1174-1178, 1991.

68. Stolman CJ, Gregory JJ, Dunn D et al: Evaluation of the do not resuscitate orders at a community hospital, Arch Intern Med 149:1851-1856, 1989.

69. Maly RC, Abrahamse AF, Hirsch SH et al: What influences physician practice behavior? An interview study of physicians who received consultative geriatric assessment recommendations, Arch Fam Med 5:448-454, 1996.

70. Rabow MW, Petersen J, Schanche K et al: The comprehensive care team: a description of a controlled trial of care at the beginning of the end of life, J Palliat Med 6:489-499, 2003.

71. Heffner JE, Fahy B, Barbieri C: Advance directive education during pulmonary rehabilitation, Chest 109:373-379, 1996.

72. Bedell SE, Delbanco TL: Choices about cardiopulmonary resuscitation in the hospital: when do physicians talk with patients? N Engl J Med 310:1089-1093, 1984.

73. Reilly BM, Magnussen CR, Ross J et al: Can we talk? Inpatient discussions about advance directives in a community hospital, Arch Intern Med 154:2299-2308, 1994.

74. Pfeifer MP, Sidorov JE, Smith AC et al: Discussion of end of life medical care by primary care physicians and patients: a multicenter study using qualitative interviews, J Gen Intern Med 9:82-88, 1994.

75. Kellogg FR, Crain M, Corwin J et al: Life-sustaining interventions in frail elderly persons: talking about choices, Arch Intern Med 152:2317-2320, 1992.

76. Reid DW, Ziegler M: Validity and stability of a new desired control measure pertaining to psychological adjustment of the elderly, J Gerontol 35:395-402, 1980.

77. Steinhauser KE, Christakis NA, Clipp EC et al: Factors considered important at the end of life by patients, family, physicians, and other care providers, JAMA 284:2476-2482, 2000.

78. Carrese JA, Rhodes LA: Western bioethics on the Navajo reservation, JAMA 274:826-829, 1995.

79. Jones I, Kirby A, Ormiston P et al: The needs of patients dying of chronic obstructive pulmonary disease in the community, Fam Pract 21:310-313, 2004.

80. Fried TR, Bradley EH, O'Leary J: Prognosis communication in serious illness: perceptions of older patients, caregivers, and clinicians, J Am Geriatr Soc 51:1398-403, 2003.

81. Blackhall LJ, Murphy ST, Frank G et al: Ethnicity and attitudes toward patient autonomy, JAMA 274:820-825, 1995.

82. Hansen-Flaschen J: Chronic obstructive pulmonary disease: the last year of life, Respir Care 49:90-97, 2004.

83. Miles SH, Koepp R, Weber EP: Advance end-of-life treatment planning: a research review, Arch Intern Med 156:1062-1068, 1996.

84. Teno J, Lynn J, Wenger N et al: Advance directives for seriously ill hospitalized patients: effectiveness with the Patient Self-determination Act and the SUPPORT intervention, J Am Geriatr Soc 45:500-507, 1997.

85. Phillips RS, Wenger NS, Teno J et al: Choices of seriously ill patients about cardiopulmonary resuscitation: correlates and outcomes, Am J Med 100:128-137, 1996.

86. Jacobson JA, White BE, Battin MP et al: Patients' understanding and use of advance directives, West J Med 160:232-236, 1994.

87. Hare J, Pratt C, Nelson C: Agreement between patients and their self-selected surrogates on difficult medical decisions, Arch Intern Med 152:1049-1054, 1992.

88. Tonelli MR: Pulling the plug on living wills: a critical analysis of advance directives, Chest 110:816-822, 1996.

89. Heffner JE: End-of-life ethical decisions, Semin Respir Crit Care Med 19:271-282, 1998.

90. Seghal A, Galbraith A, Chesney M et al: How strictly do dialysis patients want their advance directives followed? JAMA 267:59-63, 1992.

91. Mazur DJ, Hickman DH: Patients' preferences for risk disclosure and role in decision making for invasive medical procedures, J Gen Intern Med 12:114-117, 1997.

92. Teno JM, Hakim RB, Knaus WA et al: Preferences for cardiopulmonary resuscitation: physician–patient agreement and hospital resource use, J Gen Intern Med 10:179-186, 1995.

93. Martin DK, Thiel EC, Singer PA: A new model of advance care planning, Arch Intern Med 159:86-92, 1999.

94. Youngner SJ, Lewandowsky W, McClish DK et al: "Do not resuscitate" orders: incidence and implications in a medical intensive care unit, JAMA 253:54-57, 1985.

95. Rousseau P: Nonpain symptom management in terminal care, Clin Geriatr Med 12:313-327, 1996.

96. Lynn J, Teno JM, Phillips RS et al: Perceptions by family members of the dying experience of older and seriously ill patients. SUPPORT Investigators. Study to Understand Prognoses and Preferences for Outcomes and Risks of Treatments [see comments], Ann Intern Med 126:97-106, 1997.

97. Fallowfield L, Jenkins V, Farewell V et al: Efficacy of a cancer research UK communication skills training model for oncologists: a randomised controlled trial, Lancet 359:650-656, 2002.

98. Morrison RS, Maroney-Galin C, Kralovec PD et al: The growth of palliative care programs in United States hospitals, J Palliat Med 8:1127-1134, 2005.

99. National Consensus Project for Quality Palliative Care: Clinical practice guidelines for quality palliative care: executive summary, J Palliat Med 7:611-627, 2004.

100. Stuart B, Alexander C, Arenella C et al: Medical guidelines for determining prognosis in selected non-cancer diseases, ed 2, Arlington, Va, 1996, National Hospice and Palliative Care Organization.

101. Au DH, Udris EM, Fihn SD et al: Differences in health care utilization at the end of life among patients with chronic obstructive pulmonary disease and patients with lung cancer, Arch Intern Med 166:326-331, 2006.

Chapter 26

Social and Recreational Support of the Patient with Pulmonary Disease

JAMES J. BARNETT • MARY BURNS

CHAPTER OUTLINE

Establishment of a Patient Support
  Group
  Location
  Time of Meetings
  First Meeting
  Telephone Committee
  Patient Board of Directors
  Offices in the Board of Directors
  Organization Name
  Funding
Social Activities
Holidays
  Picnics

General Guidelines for Other Events
  Refund Policy
  Longer Group Trips
  Hospital Policy
  Oxygen Needs
  Transportation
Encouraging Patient Involvement
Encouraging Physical Activity While
  Socializing
Respiratory Rally
  Rally, or Special Event, Timetable
Conclusion

PROFESSIONAL SKILLS

On completion of this chapter, the reader will be able to do the following:
* Understand how to establish a Better Breathers Club
* Know how to encourage patient participation
* Be able to plan patient social activities
* Know how to increase physical involvement
* Be able to plan a rally or other large event
* Know how to plan recreational trips for groups of patients

Pulmonary rehabilitation (PR) is now accepted as the standard of care for patients with respiratory disability.[1-4] Many studies have shown important benefits, including increased exercise tolerance, decreased symptoms, and improved quality of life, after PR.[3-5] Unfortunately, of the few studies looking at long-range benefits of this improvement, most show that 1 year after PR many of these benefits begin to diminish.[5]

To prevent this, we need to understand that social support and recreation will significantly decrease the loneliness, anxiety, and poor self-image so often seen in respiratory patients before PR. Therefore offering a social and recreational support system not only becomes an integral part of the continuum of care, but it will in most cases extend their benefits well beyond 1 year after PR.

ESTABLISHMENT OF A PATIENT SUPPORT GROUP

Once the need for a social and recreational support system for the respiratory patient population is agreed on, holding a monthly group meeting is usually the first step in implementing this. It is helpful to enlist the aid of the hospital respiratory committee, a supportive physician,[6] or a PR department manager to obtain the necessary cooperation of hospital administration usually needed to establish this group. The American Lung Association may also have suggestions for establishing a support group, often called a Better Breathers Club (BBC).

Location

The next challenge is to find a suitable room or auditorium in which to hold BBC meetings. If the hospital does not have space, other areas to investigate are the local American Lung Association, YMCA or YWCA, church halls, community centers, VFW halls, Elks Lodge, local restaurants with a banquet room, or senior centers. For the small group just getting started, a physician may offer his waiting room. However, this will be only a temporary solution because the goal should be eventually to have a much larger group than can fit into the limited space of an office.

It is important to make sure that the meeting area is easy to reach, bearing in mind the physical limitations of this population. If it is held in an auditorium that has theater-style seating with a down slope it may be hard for the patients to exit because they will have to walk up a ramp. Parking access is important but difficult to obtain in some large facilities. Solutions include blocking off close parking spots for BBC members on the day of the meeting, valet parking, parking lot shuttle service, or arranging for transportation, or door-to-door dial-a-ride service. The hospital social services department or City Hall might have other suggestions for assisting with transportation to the meetings.

If the group is small, try to get the local American Lung Association to put an ad in the local newspaper about upcoming meetings. If this is not possible the local home care companies could get involved to tell their patients about the BBC.

If it is decided that a cruise or a bus trip may be unrealistic for the group, try to plan an activity at a location where everyone can drive. This may be a restaurant, dinner theater, a local garden, or anywhere they can get away to enjoy the day.

Time of Meetings

The day of the week and time of day on which to meet are the next two items for consideration. Most BBCs meet once a month, although a few meet weekly. Depending on the weather, some BBCs may wish to skip a few meetings during the summer or worst months of winter. Once the program becomes established, however, the group may not wish any break in the schedule. For the most part, it is better to avoid Monday and Friday for meetings. Monday is sometimes a universal holiday and meetings on either of these two days may interfere with long weekends for staff, speakers, and attendees.

Patients with respiratory disorders often have trouble getting started in the morning and are reluctant to drive at night; therefore, midday meetings work best. Making a lecture part of the meeting provides a focal point. Scheduling the lecture to conclude before 2 PM makes it feasible for a busy physician to speak to the group and yet get back to the office in time for afternoon appointments. It is important to allow time before and after the lecture for socializing. If the meeting is held in a hospital, perhaps a buffet luncheon can be arranged. Bringing a box lunch, or sandwiches from home, is another option. Many groups serve beverages only, with members bringing snacks. Meals can then be reserved for special occasions once or twice a year.

First Meeting

Plan the first BBC meeting far enough in advance to arrange for adequate publicity. If a PR program is already in operation, graduates, of course, are the first to be sent a printed invitation. Active members can be asked to assist with planning and hosting the event. Make sure the announcement makes it clear that a spouse or friend is equally welcome. The hospital newsletter, local newspaper, and local chapter of the American Lung Association may assist with publicizing the event. Often, local radio and TV stations deliver free public service announcements that can help publicize the event. Flyers can also be posted in offices of physicians. It is usually wise to enlist the help of the hospital public relations department for assistance, permission, and additional ideas. This is a good time to establish cordial relations with a department that can be of great assistance in the future.

Make this first meeting as special as circumstances allow. A few balloons, colorful napkins, and a little extra effort on the refreshments go a long way. Have several chairs at the entrance, along with a table equipped with pens, nametags, and markers. Use PR graduates, or a nucleus of individuals interested in a support group, from the start. Two can sit at the sign-in table to ensure that everyone entering signs a sheet with their name, address, and telephone number before filling in a name tag to wear. Others can act as official hosts and hostesses to warmly welcome guests and help them find a seat. Make sure volunteers have a name tag or an official badge.

Introduce new guests to the person they are seated next to, even if it is necessary to read their name tag to do so. Do everything possible to provide a warm, welcoming atmosphere for this and all future meetings.

If a BBC has not been developed and a PR program is being established, have the first BBC meeting after the first graduating class. This provides something for the patients to look forward to. Because they have something to look forward to, their attitude will be more positive and they will want to keep active and learn more about their breathing problem. The participants will feel that they are part of something new, if they help make plans for future meetings.

The first speaker should be someone who will give a talk that will stimulate the interest and enthusiasm of the group. A topic that includes the word "new" usually will guarantee a large audience. Asthma, medications, and discussions on how to handle stress are high on the interest list of patients with respiratory disorders.

Have an audiocassette recorder or video camera ready to record the guest speaker. Consider asking a patient to be responsible for tending to the recording process. This can be the first item in the group library. The video recording can be used for future attendees who have missed a meeting, for those who are homebound, or for those who wish to hear the topic again. It also is useful for reviewing the lecture to summarize it for a patient newsletter. Be sure to have a camera and take a few pictures to document this special occasion. At least one of the patients is likely to have an interest in photography and may be willing to help in this area.

Guest speakers donating their time appreciate a thank-you. Ask one or two patients to write short notes of appreciation.

Although a monthly patient meeting is an important part of the continuum of care for a PR program, it can also be of value if the PR program has not yet been established. The patient with respiratory disease is usually hungry for knowledge, help, and empathy from others with a similar disability. Although a BBC cannot take the place of PR, it does help to fulfill a need until the PR program can be established. At that time it will also become a referral source as well as being of key importance in maintaining social and recreational support while updating knowledge.

Telephone Committee

At the first BBC meeting, or even before, solicit several patients to do the telephoning for the group. Even the most physically limited are able to assist in this way. It is a good way to establish group cohesiveness, which is so important, and to start involvement of even the homebound patient in the group process.

If the initial first meeting is from the first graduating class of a newly established PR program, ask for a volunteer from that group to be the phone caller for that group. As the group grows, a chairperson can be appointed to whom the phone callers report. Limit each caller's responsibility to 10 names, if possible. As the group grows, appoint team leaders to whom callers report, and then the team leaders can report to the chairperson.

Calls should be made several days before each monthly luncheon, and before other activities, to encourage people to come as well as to get an attendance count. Most people like being called, reinforcing that someone cares. Friendships develop, and some people on the calling list may like to be called more often, especially if they become homebound.

Callers should notify the chairperson of the telephone committee about attendance, illness in a family, or any special information that would be helpful to the PR staff. After all the information for the month is collected, the chairperson telephones a member of the staff to report. This means that only one telephone call each month to the staff will keep them informed about the entire patient population. This committee is of major importance. It helps the busy staff keep in close contact with support group members with a minimal expenditure of time.

Patient Board of Directors

A patient Board of Directors (BOD) designed to oversee BBC operations can be established in several ways. If the group is small, consider inviting everyone to join the initial planning sessions, where responsibilities are discussed and divided.

If the group is large and better established, a slate of names can be submitted and voted on. Another way to appoint a BOD is to ask for volunteers. Many people will be so appreciative they will ask if there is anything they can do to help.

Often potential officers are concerned about not having enough energy or health to fulfill the job requirements. It helps to reassure them that the workload will be modest and that they can always resign. This is one reason why primary offices may have two people in each position, with the spouse automatically included if the patient is elected. This lessens the workload and allays concerns about being able to fulfill the office. It also encourages involvement of the (usually) healthier spouse. A healthy spouse can be a vital member of the organization and should also be allowed to run for office. This process strengthens spousal relationships, as well as making the core working group larger. The members of the BOD will become the strongest advocates for the BBC and PR program, even after their term of office is completed.

Offices in the Board of Directors

Patients who have moderate disease and are not yet severely limited by their breathing problem, and who have recently retired, may want to help. These people would be effective in the role of administrative assistant, especially if they are computer literate. They could start a database of all the necessary information such as birthdays, graduation date, address, and phone numbers and any other information that may be appropriate.

If the main offices for the BOD include two people for each position, there will be two cochairpersons, co–vice chairpersons, cosecretaries, and cotreasurers. The telephone chairperson, whose duties have already been discussed, should definitely be a member of the BOD. Another important member is someone who will keep track of birthdays and also send get-well cards to group members. This member, or another, should be responsible for a short thank-you note to the monthly guest speaker. A librarian can help start, and then keep track of, the lending library of medical books, compact disks (CDs), and videocassettes the group may wish to provide members.

A historian can be responsible for scrapbooks and pictures to document the history of the group. If this task is left to the busy PR staff, the group is apt to be left with boxes of unidentified slides and pictures.

Someone who enjoys decorating for holidays and special events should hold an arts and crafts office. If the group decides to hold an annual holiday boutique, this is the person who would help organize it.

If the group is fortunate, someone will be willing to accept the office of editor and send out a monthly flyer or newsletter about BBC activities to all members. A social chairperson can help plan and organize group events.

All of these chairpersons can enlist the assistance of as many others on their committees as they wish. If people are left over and eager to participate, think of a title for them such as "at large." The more people actively participating, the more fun they have and the more active the organization. A health care professional, or PR staff member, should attend BOD meetings as an advisor.

Organization Name

Encourage the group to pick a name that has special meaning for them. BBC leaves a bit to be desired as a name that inspires feelings of group loyalty. Rather than having a name chosen by one person, or the BOD, get a slate of suggestions and vote on the choice. The winner should get some sort of prize, such as dinner for two donated by a local restaurant. Examples of a few names others have chosen for support groups include the PEP Pioneers, The Inspirations, The Breathsavers, The Senior Puffers, The PREP Airwaves, The Breathing Buddies, and the Wheezenpuffs.

Funding

Discourage dues for the BBC because the object is to include everyone as a member, regardless of income. A raffle at the monthly BBC meeting can be fun and also raise a little money. Raffle tickets should be inexpensive, such as a dollar each. Raffle prizes can include home-baked goods, or home-grown fruits and vegetables. A home care company should be happy to donate a nice prize such as a dinner at a restaurant or a gift card.

Encourage group involvement. Have one or two patients sell tickets, another pick the winning tickets out of a hat, and yet another read off the winner. This activity may not raise much money, but valuable group interaction will result.

An annual holiday boutique can be a fundraiser. Depending on the group, a baked goods table, white elephant table, and other crafts can be considered. A raffle with three or four special prizes may be even more successful. These special prizes

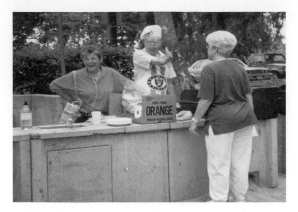

FIGURE 26-1 The staff helps, but patients do more and more as they gain confidence. They learn it is fun. Here they barbecue hot dogs and hamburgers even though on oxygen.

can be something handmade and donated by members of the group or gift certificates for dinners solicited from local restaurants. Local stores will sometimes donate gift baskets or gift certificates, or a free trip on the next outing.

SOCIAL ACTIVITIES

The BOD can also plan other activities and social events during the year. The social events chairperson is in charge of generating ideas and organizing events. This is too large a task for one person, however, and needs the involvement of many in the group.

HOLIDAYS

An annual holiday party is a must. If the group has a large enough treasury, the lunch or refreshments can be free. It is advisable to get a vote from the group as to whether a fee should be charged. The holiday party can be held at the same place as the meetings. If the group is large, try one of the local hotel banquet rooms. Be sure to decorate so as to make this a special function. Arrange early in the year for a local high school chorus to come and sing holiday carols for, and with, the group. Bring a CD player to play songs, and consider having a person who can play a violin go from table to table and play requests. Have special guest speakers. This would also be a good time for the PR coordinator or medical director to recognize the patient BOD and the committees for their hard work and to give them a small token of appreciation. Help them

feel special, because they are. Try to get a spouse to dress up as Santa Claus and pass out candy canes. Although fun-loving patients may attempt this, the beard can cause feelings of suffocation. Have a big decorated box where toys and gifts for the needy can be collected. Be sure to take pictures for the group's albums.

Picnics

A summer picnic is another popular event and is easy to organize. Hot dogs and hamburgers can be barbecued, and, yes, patients receiving oxygen can do the barbecuing if they wish (Figure 26-1). Find a local park with easy access to parking and bathrooms. Get a head count of the number of people wishing to come, families included. Purchase paper plates, napkins, condiments, soft drinks, and other supplies at a discount store. Charge a minimal amount to cover expenses for the barbecue of hamburgers, hot dogs, and other purchased food. Have the patients bring a side dish or a dessert. A local home care company could also be asked to provide the main dish with the condiments. This makes for a fun day for everyone. Mingle and have the patients get to know each other better. Bring a CD player for music, consider playing bingo with silly prizes. A camera is a must, to make a record of a great day.

General Guidelines for Other Events

If patients wish to attempt other events, start with something easy to organize and for which to arrange transportation. An example would be a group meeting for lunch and then attending a matinee movie. Later, this can be expanded to something like an afternoon at a local dinner theater, a play, or even the circus. Tickets are purchased in advance, but everyone is responsible for their own transportation. For all activities:

- Plan ahead. This cannot be stressed often enough.
- Get suggestions from the patient group.
- Look for activities that will be low in physical stress.
- Aim for lighthearted fun, for example, a musical matinee with lunch rather than a museum tour with a lot of walking.
- Have a sign-up sheet. Get commitments on patient interest in the specific activity before proceeding with plans.
- Arrange end seats for those using oxygen or canes.

- Make sure that stairs are limited and that bathroom access is easy.
- Book early to get the best seats.
- Group tickets, especially for the handicapped or seniors, are often discounted, especially if purchased in advance.
- Request a block of seats so that everyone can sit together.
- Request early seating to avoid standing in lines and to ensure a leisurely entrance.
- A reminder call to participants before the trip is helpful. A volunteer can assist with this.

Refund Policy

Refunds can be a problem with a group that tends to get sick, but it is important to discourage the attendance of anyone who does not feel well. The group needs to feel safe in joining these excursions. Try to have a standby or waiting list. If refunds are not possible, the individual canceling needs to find his or her own replacements or pay for the already purchased tickets. If all else fails, suggest donating the tickets for use by someone who cannot afford the price or is hesitant to attempt something new.

Longer Group Trips

When ready to attempt longer group trips, the possibilities are numerous. Important considerations for longer group trips include hospital policy and oxygen needs.

Hospital Policy

- Get permission from the medical director and the hospital administrator.
- The legal department may request written signed consents and physician approval.
- Clarify hospital policy for staff liability coverage.

Oxygen Needs

- Know the patients' oxygen needs.
- Note the type of oxygen unit used by each patient.
- Make sure each patient has an adequate oxygen supply to last the trip, including transportation time to and from home.
- Allow for delays and half-filled containers.
- Consider whether the trip will be to an elevation that will require extra oxygen.
- Make friends with the local oxygen suppliers. They may be willing to donate oxygen, or extra containers, for these trips.

- For longer trips, make sure to have oxygen waiting in patient rooms on arrival. Payment should be worked out in advance. The local supplier may be of help with this.
- Make sure to have extra oxygen tubing, connectors, a wrench, and an oximeter.

The technology for delivering portable oxygen has improved. The Inogen One (Inogen, Goleta, Calif) and the AirSep LifeStyle and AirSep FreeStyle (the latter weighing only 4.4 lb; AirSep, Buffalo, NY) have pulse–dose technology. These concentrators have been approved for airline travel. Another portable oxygen concentrator, the Advantage: Eclipse (SeQual Technologies, San Diego, Calif), has both continuous flow (up to 3 L/minute) and pulse–dose technology. It weighs approximately 17.5 lb but is mounted on wheels and easy to maneuver. This concentrator has also been approved by the airlines. When making arrangements to fly, ask the medical desk at the airlines which portable oxygen concentrators they have approved.

Transportation
Buses

- Shop around. Deal with the manager. Don't be afraid to discuss specific needs, such as a non-smoking driver willing to help with patients and carry-ons; a bus with a restroom; a step stool for getting off and on the bus; and promptness.
- Have a checklist with the names of all patients to make sure everyone is on board before departure and on the return trip!
- Keep the patients' welfare in mind at all times. Let those receiving oxygen, or the most handicapped, board first.
- Provide beverages and snacks on a long trip. Include this in the cost of the ticket.
- Travel during daylight hours.
- Everyone should make arrangements for their own transportation to and from the bus.
- Have cost include the tip for the driver.
- Make friends with senior bus drivers. They are a good source of valuable information.
- Find a tour company that can make most of the arrangements such as booking the hotel, arranging a stop for lunch at the halfway point so the patients can get off and stretch their legs and get something to eat. Larger tour companies usually maintain their buses in excellent condition, which is extremely important.

• Find a tour company that will ensure that the bus is well maintained; check on the maintenance schedules of their buses. Also, a tour company may have other trips that might be of interest to the patients. If the same company is used more than once, they will get to know the group and understand their needs, which helps to ensure an enjoyable trip.

Boats

Boats can be fun for short river cruises or harbor cruises.

- Ensure ease of access to the boat.
- Be aware that the boarding ramp is sometimes long or steep.
- Reserve seating on the main deck, if possible. Avoid climbing the steep stairs to upper decks.

Ships

Many travel agencies can now handle longer group cruises.[7] See Figure 26-2 and Figure 26-3. However, keep in mind the following:

- PR staff is responsible for patients' remains.
- Verify oxygen acceptance by the cruise line well in advance,
- Verify oxygen delivery to the ship by the vendor well in advance.
- Start plans 1 year in advance, taking the weather into consideration.Use this time as an incentive to get patients into a regular exercise program to increase fitness.
- Refer to Chapter 29 travel for other specifics.

Be a good customer. Appreciate the kindness and generosities of those who go the extra mile to make the trip a success. They always welcome a brief thank-you note and often remember it the next time a trip is booked with them.

After PR graduation, many patients will be eager to attempt a long-delayed trip. Although the PR program usually conducts a class on travel, the PR staff remains a good resource for patients about to embark on their own.

ENCOURAGING PATIENT INVOLVEMENT

Although this chapter deals with the social and recreational support of the patient, it is important to remember why this is considered to be so important. The goal is to help patients remain actively involved and to maintain maximal fitness. With that in mind, remember that opportunities for patients to assume social responsibility should be considered along with offering them social support. Patients thrive on being able to help others rather than always being on the receiving end of assistance. Use volunteer assistance from patients as much as possible. This really is part of their therapy.

Ask several graduates to greet and welcome each new group on the first day of the PR class. Encourage them to tell the new class how much PR helped enrich their lives. Encourage them also to occasionally drop by during later classes to say hello and offer support to the current class. On the last day of class, they may enjoy being asked to welcome the new graduates to the BBC, with the presentation of a name tag along with a special invitation to the next BBC meeting.

On the day of graduation present them with a certificate of achievement and take a class picture. Give them their exercise prescriptions and

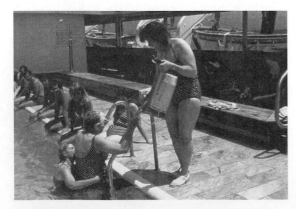

FIGURE 26-2 In the ship's pool with oxygen, swimming for the first time in 20 years.

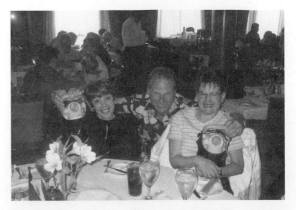

FIGURE 26-3 Enjoying the cruise ship's fine dining, with the convenience of portable oxygen.

encourage them to join a maintenance program. Be available for them if they have questions, but encourage independence. On the day of graduation have a potluck or have everyone contribute their favorite snack. Provide a cake that says "Congratulations, Graduates," and be approachable so that the patients will feel comfortable and want to be a part of the group.

Other suggestions have been presented earlier on ways that patients can help at BBC meetings, such as acting as hosts or hostesses, recording the guest speaker's lecture, taking pictures, helping with the raffle, and writing thank-you notes to the guest speaker.

Some patients enjoy taking part in research and feeling that they contribute to science, helping others with respiratory disease as they have been helped. Research participation may only mean taking part in a small study done by a local university. If a nearby teaching hospital has a pulmonary division, check to see if they are doing anything that might be of interest to the BBC. The physicians there will be delighted to have potential access to a pool of volunteer patients and will reciprocate by providing speakers for the BBC meetings.

ENCOURAGING PHYSICAL ACTIVITY WHILE SOCIALIZING

One of the reasons to work so hard at the social support system of our patients is to keep them active and to help them maintain the physical fitness gains they have made during PR. Maintenance of these physical gains is essential. Social and physical support is often interrelated. Many health care practitioners will testify that part of the success of a maintenance program is the group socialization that takes place at these sessions.

There is a lot to offer patients in addition to the very important maintenance exercise classes. This is especially important to remember if room for a maintenance exercise program is not available.

Check with the local YMCA or YWCA. Ask them to set aside the outside lane of the pool so patients with oxygen can swim without getting tangled in their 50-ft oxygen tubing. Low-level exercise classes for patients with arthritis are also suitable for pulmonary patients. Community colleges are beginning to offer classes for pulmonary patients, such as water aerobics, and the local high school might be convinced to offer a slow dance class suitable for the respiratory impaired. And yes, patients receiving oxygen can dance.

At all of these classes, it is much easier for patients to participate in a group rather than struggling alone. Walking clubs can be formed in which the group meets once a week to walk together followed by lunch or a snack. Local parks, malls, and walking areas can be mapped out, complete with distance. Meeting with the mall manager might result in a formal arrangement between the mall and the walking group. It can be good publicity for both. Sometimes the mall can be opened an hour before the stores are opened. Perhaps they will agree to a measured walking route. The group may wish to make up cards that patients can fill out, on the honor system, and turn in as they complete set distances. Recognition can be given in various ways, such as a "wall of fame" with names and pictures on the wall of the PR gym.

Another idea that has had great success is a planned group walk to a destination across the country or to a special location. This is a simulated walk, of course, in which each 15 or 30 minutes of walking or bike riding can equal a mile. Mileage can be collected monthly from individual group members. The accumulated distances are plotted on a large map. This has the potential of becoming an elaborate project that generates much enthusiasm as well as the desired effect of an increase in the activity level of the group.

RESPIRATORY RALLY

A respiratory rally is the ultimate BBC meeting. The PEP Pioneers, of Torrance, California, have been holding an annual rally for the past 20 years. See Figure 26-4. Patients, family members, and the medical staff of hospitals and PR

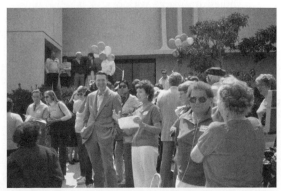

FIGURE 26-4 Dr. Tom Petty and Mary Burns participate in a PEP Pioneers Respiratory Rally, along with patients and friends.

programs from the southern part of the state gather for a day of fun, fellowship, and education. Variations on this event now take place in other areas of the world with equal success. One example is Dr. Freddy Smeets of Belgium, who held his rally in a local castle!

Highlights of the day may include a well-known pulmonary physician as a speaker or a panel of speakers. A suggested requirement is that each speaker include some jokes in his or her presentation. The rally should be fun, with everyone going home at the end of the day in high spirits.

Some form of physical activity is usually also part of a rally. In Torrance, it is the Pace Race, whereas other areas may have a 1-km or 1-mile walk. What is a Pace Race? It is a walk covering a measured distance short enough for anyone to cover without difficulty, such as a hospital parking lot or lawn. Each participant estimates the amount of time it will take to complete the course comfortably, without marked shortness of breath. The three who guess their time most accurately are the winners. Because distances are very short, these guesses are narrowed down to hundredths of a second, with an official race stopwatch marking the time. Anyone has the potential to come in first, including the most handicapped of patients. Everyone gets a certificate for participation in the race.

An annual rally can have 200 or 300 people attending, Plan carefully in advance for any large event to ensure that everything will run smoothly.

Rally, or Special Event, Timetable
Nine Months to One Year in Advance
- Notify the medical director and hospital public relations department of the rally plans.
- Get their input and support.

Date. When setting the date, avoid days that coincide with other events, such as the annual meeting of respiratory associations and national holidays.
- Remember to allow for the vagaries of the weather.
- Decide on the day of the week, taking into consideration the physicians who will attend.

Location
- Find an area with easy access that is large enough to hold the number of people anticipated to attend.
- Ensure adequate bathrooms, kitchen facilities, sound system, and parking.

- Consider cost. A hospital auditorium will often work well as long as it provides the ability to have tables where the people can sit and socialize. A cultural arts center or civic auditorium can sometimes be reserved at no cost, or minimal cost, for nonprofit organizations. Just remember to try to stay away from theater seating.

You are on your own on how to find a castle!

Theme
- Pick a catchy phrase, such as "Humor for the Health of It," "Pioneer Days," "Breath of Spring."
- Assign someone to be in charge of decorations, using the theme as a guide.
- Ask speakers to have topics appropriate to the theme.

Speakers. The medical director of PR should be on the panel, introduce the panel, or be master of ceremonies.
- Although telephoning potential speakers is acceptable, always follow up with a written letter repeating the date, time, topic, and length of time desirable for them to speak.
- Most local physicians are happy to volunteer their time.
- If the desired speaker is nationally known, or from out of the area, he or she will need to be reimbursed for expenses.

Vendors and Funding. Industry support is vital in helping with expenses and honorariums.
- Some of the larger companies may provide an educational grant.
- Contact all the drug representatives of companies producing the medications that patients use.
- Call all the local home care companies as well as the oxygen suppliers. Ask them if they can provide oxygen, so the patients will be comfortable knowing that oxygen will be available.
- Check with respiratory departments for the names of companies from which they make large purchases.
- The amount of money that can be requested from each company will depend on the size of the group that is expected to attend the event.
- Some vendors will explain what their budget limit is for an event or suggest a reasonable amount. Because they have an annual budget it is important to get their commitment as early as possible.
- It will often be necessary to follow through with a formal letter explaining the event and providing a tax ID number.

Six Months in Advance
Food
- If the event is to be held in a hospital, find out the policy of the dietary department. Do they want to provide the food or do they have a caterer whom they recommend?
- Find out what the charge is.
- If the hospital requires an outside caterer, box lunches are usually the easiest way to go.
- Have several vegetarian lunches available.
- Remember that many of these patients are on salt-restricted diets.
- Sometimes costs can be kept down by buying soft drinks and bottled water at a large discount store.
- Remember to provide snacks for volunteers arriving early.

Cost
- Add up the cost of the meeting area and speaker expenses, plus the cost of food and beverages for the projected number of participants.
- Remember that volunteers will have free lunches.
- Add on another dollar or two for decorating expenses and entertainment.
- Deduct the amount of money pledged from participating vendors.
- The final cost for the day for each individual can range from as high as $8 or $9 to being cost free for all participants.

Letters
- Send an initial letter to all PR programs in the area explaining the plan, along with specifics including the date, guest speakers, and an estimate of cost per ticket.
- Suggest that they contact local home care companies or drug representatives to see if their program can obtain sponsorship to help defray the costs of their bus or lunch.
- Send this letter to the hospital public relations department and to anyone else it is hoped will attend.
- Send a copy to all the physicians in the area.

Entertainment
- Contact the local hospital volunteer department for ideas.
- Request clowns or other forms of entertainment that they may be able to provide.
- Check other local agencies for volunteer talent.
- Have clowns greet the arriving buses and cars to create a festive mood.
- Piano players for background music or even patient groups with musical or comedic talents also can be of value.

- Remember that the object is to provide a fun-filled day.

Volunteer Help
- Put in an early request with the volunteer department of the local hospital.
- Telephone the respiratory therapy or nursing school departments of the local college. They may wish to make attendance part of their curriculum and it may also lead to further interaction with them in the future.
- Do not forget to involve the patients and their families. The more involved they are the more they will enjoy themselves and the more creative they will become at turning this into an extravaganza.

Door Prizes
- Try to arrange to offer dinners for two from chain restaurants rather than from a local eatery if some participants are from outside the area.
- Send letters requesting donations of gift certificates to all the large chain restaurants.
- Gift baskets make excellent door prizes.
- Vendors will often provide a prize in addition to financial support.

Equipment
- Make a detailed checklist of everything that will be needed.
- Write down the date each item was ordered and the date that each item is received.
- Now is the time to reserve such things as helium for balloons, race timers from the local high school, linens, and a piano.

One or Two Months in Advance
- Step up the publicity.
- Send letters to all participating hospitals.
- Request estimates of numbers planning to attend from each participating program. Don't forget to add in vendors and volunteers.
- Have each group keep track of their own patients.
- After payment has been received, promptly send admission raffle tickets along with name tags to save time and confusion on the day of the rally.
- Note the number of display tables needed for sponsoring vendors.
- Remind the oxygen companies about providing oxygen.

Two or Three Days in Advance
- Confirm the participating number attending from any group that has not responded.
- Provide a final count to the caterer.

- Go over the checklist.
- Assign duties to various individuals to avoid last-minute confusion.
- Make a detailed timed schedule of the final day's events.

This schedule may sound like overkill, but it is essential for a smoothly running event of this size. Also, by spreading the work out over a long time, it is possible to continue the day-to-day activities of the PR program.

CONCLUSION

It is important to provide social and recreational support for pulmonary patients. We have seen the impact on our patients first-hand. The support group enables patients to improve their exercise maintenance, self-sufficiency, and increased community involvement. By talking to other patients they will learn more about different types of portable oxygen systems, along with other therapies, which will enable them to be more mobile and to have a better quality of life. As patients communicate with each other they learn special strategies in problem solving and about the various opportunities available to them. Social and recreational support of the pulmonary patient should no longer be considered a luxury but an integral part of the continuum of care.

Many patient groups have been formed, dedicated to promoting wellness and increased awareness of COPD. Such groups are the National Emphysema/COPD Association (NECA), Emphysema Foundation for Our Right To Survive (EFFORTS), the National Home Oxygen Patients Association (NHOPA), the Pulmonary Education and Research Foundation (PERF), and the U.S. COPD Coalition, which was responsible for planning the first-ever National COPD Conference in November 2003 outside Washington, DC. This conference brought together leaders in COPD management, education, research, patient advocacy, and public policy. From this conference the COPD Caucus was officially launched in March 2003. The Congressional COPD Caucus gives the COPD community a public platform in Congress to bring attention to critical issues that have been identified by the U.S. COPD Coalition.

Today, patients are better informed, live more productive lives, and have more resources than ever before. Over the past few decades PR has transitioned from a therapy that very few accepted to the standard of care for patients with chronic lung disease.

References

1. California Thoracic Society: Position paper: the principles of pulmonary rehabilitation, Tustin, Calif, 1998, California Thoracic Society.
2. Nici L, Donner C, Wouters E et al: ATS/ERS Pulmonary Rehabilitation Writing Committee: ATS/ERS statement on pulmonary rehabilitation, Am J Respir Crit Care Med 173:1390-1413, 2006.
3. Ries AL: Position paper of the American Association of Cardiovascular and Pulmonary rehabilitation: scientific basis of pulmonary rehabilitation, J Cardiopulm Rehabil 10:418, 1990.
4. Ries AL, Bauldoff GS, Carlin BW et al: Pulmonary rehabilitation: joint ACCP/AACVPR evidence-based clinical practice guidelines, Chest 131(5 suppl):4S-42S, 2007.
5. Ries AL, Kaplan RM, Limberg TM et al: Effects of pulmonary rehabilitation on physiologic and psychosocial outcomes in patients with chronic obstructive pulmonary disease, Ann Intern Med 122:823-834, 1995.
6. Burns MR: Travel with oxygen. In Tiep BL, editor: Portable oxygen including oxygen conserving devices, Spring Valley, NY, 1991, Futura Press, pp 421-436.
7. Burns M: Cruising with COPD, Am J Nurs 87:479-482, 1987.

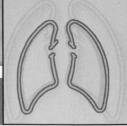

Chapter 27

Sleep Disorders in Patients with Pulmonary Disease

DANIEL O. RODENSTEIN

CHAPTER OUTLINE

Sleep
  Basic Facts
  Mechanisms of Sleep
  Physiologic Consequences of Sleep
  Respiratory Consequences of Sleep
  Sleep Failure
Sleep in Patients with Respiratory Disease
  Chronic Obstructive Pulmonary
    Disease
  Restrictive Ventilatory Defects

Specific Sleep-Related Disorders That May Affect Patients with Pulmonary Disease
  Nocturnal Myoclonus and Periodic
    Limb Movements
  Obstructive Sleep Apnea Syndrome
  Other Types of Sleep Apnea
  Obesity–Hypoventilation Syndrome
Diagnostic Approach to Sleep Disorders in Patients with Pulmonary Disease
Therapeutic Considerations in Patients with Pulmonary Disease
Conclusion

PROFESSIONAL SKILLS

On completion of this chapter, the reader will be able to do
the following:
* Understand the sleep process in healthy subjects
* Have a solid knowledge of the physiologic consequences of sleep on the various systems of the
  organism, especially on the respiratory system
* Understand the special problems that sleep poses to the patient with pulmonary disorders
* Recognize some sleep-related diseases that may affect patients with pulmonary diseases

Like any other people, patients with pulmonary diseases go to sleep at least once a day. Although at first this seems an obvious fact, sleeping is not always trivial. Indeed, sleep by itself represents a serious physiologic challenge for patients with chronic respiratory disease, a challenge that many fail to manage well.

The patient with pulmonary disease may experience serious problems during sleep on two accounts. First, sleep may have a primary deleterious effect on the pulmonary disease. Second, sleep may add the effect of specific sleep-related disorders to the basic underlying pulmonary disease. This chapter reviews some basic notions about sleep, points out the influence of sleep physiology on the respiratory system in healthy subjects and especially in patients with respiratory disease, and describes some sleep-related disease in patients with respiratory illness. The combined effect of these two types of disorders in an individual may result in severe complications and even death.

SLEEP

Basic Facts

Although nobody knows the exact vital function of sleep, it is nonetheless true that after a number of hours of active wakefulness, people have a feeling of tiredness and sleepiness. Keeping awake becomes more difficult, and finally the body enters a physiologic state different from wakefulness, known as sleep. The most obvious difference between wakefulness and sleep is that in the latter state the subject becomes "disconnected" from the external world. External stimuli (auditory, visual, and tactile) are ignored by the sleeping person, but this state of unresponsiveness is partial (i.e., stronger stimuli will induce an interruption of sleep) and spontaneously reversible: after several hours of sleep, the subject wakes up refreshed, and sleepiness has vanished.

This cycle of events repeats itself with striking regularity about every 24 hours. In human beings, sleepiness generally peaks in the late evening, and sleep occurs generally during the night. A second, less potent peak in sleepiness normally occurs after midday. Many people in the world respond to this weak sleepiness sensation in the form of a short period of sleep, known as siesta, whereas it is ignored by most people in the "developed" world.

Sleep may be viewed as a physiologic state that depends on a particular functional organization of the central nervous system. If the electrical activity of the cerebral cortex is examined by recording the electroencephalogram with surface electrodes, sleep is characterized (with respect to wakefulness) both by a slowing down of the frequency of the waves of the recordings and by an increase in the voltage amplitude of these electrical waves. As amplitude increases and frequency decreases progressively, sleep is defined as deeper (meaning, among other things, that the subject is less and less responsive to external and proprioceptive stimuli). In addition to the slowing frequency and increasing amplitude in the electroencephalogram, the eyeballs move slowly behind the closed eyelids, and the tonic activity of all skeletal muscles decreases progressively as sleep deepens. After a variable period of time in these stages, a new sleep state emerges: the electroencephalographic pattern has a higher frequency and lower voltage, like the one during wakefulness; the eyes show fast, coordinated movements; and the muscular tone is practically abolished, as if the subject were paralyzed. This sleep stage has been termed rapid eye movement (REM) sleep, whereas the other type of sleep is accordingly known as non-REM sleep. The latter is usually divided into stages 1 to 4, depending on the particular frequency and voltage of the electrical waves.[1] Dreams are thought to occur almost exclusively in REM sleep.

The architecture of normal sleep varies with age. In the healthy adult, sleep progresses from stage 1 to stage 4 non-REM sleep, and this is followed by a period of REM sleep. This succession is known as a sleep cycle and lasts for about 60 to 90 minutes. Four to seven cycles occur during a night. Stages 3 and 4 predominate in the first part of the night, whereas REM sleep predominates in the last half of the night (Figure 27-1). REM sleep is more prevalent in babies than later in life, whereas after age 50 to 60 years, it is common for stages 3 and 4 to nearly completely disappear.

Mechanisms of Sleep

Contrary to what may be believed, sleep is an active, not a passive, energy-dependent process. Sleep depends on active inhibition of neuronal activity in the brain. This active inhibition is initiated by neurons located in the preoptic area and around the lower brain stem reticular formation. Their action is to inhibit the excitatory waking neurons located in the reticular formation and other areas of the brain stem that are essential for the maintenance of the wake state. REM sleep seems to have a specific neuronal control, different from that of non-REM sleep. It is supposed that as wakefulness continues, sleep-promoting substances accumulate, increasing sleepiness until the sleep state becomes evident. Sleep-promoting neurochemicals and cytokines have already been described. For instance, acetylcholine seems to promote wakefulness and REM sleep, whereas norepinephrine, histamine, and serotonin levels are very high during wakefulness. Orexin may act as a wakefulness organizer, and its deficiency appears to be strongly linked to an REM sleep disorder called narcolepsy. Non-REM sleep seems to be promoted by γ-aminobutyric acid and by galanine-containing neurons from the ventrolateral preoptic area of the brain. Several non-neural substances may also have sleep-promoting characteristics, such as adenosine, interleukin-1β, tumor necrosis factor-α, prostaglandin D_2, and growth hormone–releasing hormone.[2]

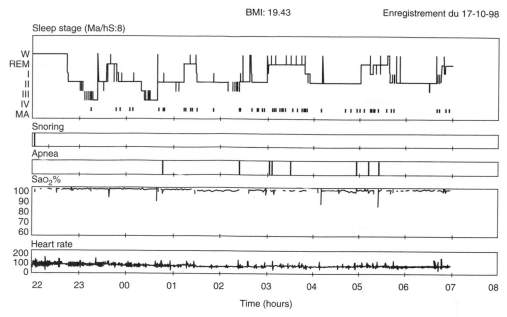

FIGURE 27-1 Schematic representation of a sleep recording in a healthy individual. The *horizontal axis* represents time in hours. The graph starts at 22:00 hours and ends at 08:00 hours. The resolution of the graph is 30 seconds. Above the boxes are depicted the date of the recording (to the right), the body mass index (BMI) of the individual (center, in kilograms per square meter), and the index of movement arousals per hour of sleep (Ma/hS). From top to bottom, the first box represents the hypnogram (schematic representation of the vigilance states). Each bar indicates that during that period of 30 seconds, a movement arousal has occurred. The second box represents snoring. The heights of the bars indicate the total noise recorded during that 30 seconds. The third box depicts apneas; each bar indicates that during that 30 seconds at least one apnea occurred. The fourth box represents arterial oxygen saturation (Sao_2%) measured transcutaneously with an oximeter. Each bar represents the mean ± 2 standard deviations of all measures recorded during that 30 seconds. The scale ranges from 100% to 60% saturation. The last box represents heart rate, with the scale ranging from 200 to 0 beats/min. Again, each bar is the mean ± 2 standard deviations of all measurements performed during that 30 seconds. Note that in this normal young female, sleep latency (the period from the start of the recording to the first sleep period) lasts for about 45 minutes. Five sleep cycles (a sleep cycle is the combination of stages of non-REM sleep followed by a period of REM sleep) occur during the night. Note that from time to time brief awakenings (return to wakefulness) and some movement arousals occur. Also note that stages 3 and 4 non-REM sleep predominate in the first half of the night, whereas REM sleep predominates in the second half of the night. No snoring and only a few apneas occur. Oxygen saturation remains high during the whole night. Note that both heart rate and heart rate variability decrease during sleep. I, II, III, and IV, the stages of non-REM or slow wave sleep; MA, movement arousal; REM, rapid eye movement sleep; W, wakefulness.

Physiologic Consequences of Sleep

As the responsiveness to external stimuli changes, so does the responsiveness to "internal" (proprioceptive) stimuli. In addition, sleep affects every physiologic system in the body. For instance, the heart rate decreases by about 5 to 10 beats/minute with respect to the resting, supine, awake heart rate. This decrease is sleep specific and goes beyond the effects of posture and rest in wakefulness. Similarly, blood pressure decreases by about 10 mm Hg.[3] Kidney function also changes during sleep: glomerular filtration decreases, as do urine production and sodium excretion, whereas sodium and water resorption increases.[4]

Salivary secretion stops at sleep onset, and the swallowing reflex is abolished during sleep. Peristaltic waves in the gastrointestinal system seem to slow down during sleep, although discrepancies are present between different gastrointestinal segments. Motor activity seems to be reduced much more consistently in the colon than in the esophagus. The endocrine system has tight connections with sleep and with the circadian rhythm. For instance, the secretion of growth hormone peaks during the first half of the sleeping time, synchronous with a period of stage 3 to 4 slow wave sleep.[5] About 80% of the daily secretion of growth hormone takes place during this sleep-related period. Cortisol secretion also peaks during the night, in fact during the early morning hours, and usually coincides with sleep. However, cortisol secretion seems to be independent of sleep per se; even if a subject sleeps during the day and stays awake during the night, cortisol secretion will still peak in the early morning hours.[5] Prolactin secretion significantly increases during sleep, whereas thyroid-stimulating hormone levels are depressed during sleep.

Respiratory Consequences of Sleep

Minute ventilation decreases during sleep, by about 10% to 15% beyond the supine awake basal volumes.[6] The decrease is caused mainly by a reduction in tidal volume, whereas average respiratory frequency remains similar in wakefulness and sleep.[7] However, frequency variability is strikingly reduced during non-REM sleep, during which breathing becomes regular, especially during stages 3 and 4 non-REM sleep. In contrast, frequency is irregular during REM sleep, and the tidal volume variability also increases in this stage, perhaps in relation to the content of dreams (this has been frequently postulated but not demonstrated).

Blood gases also change during sleep. Arterial partial pressure of carbon dioxide ($Paco_2$) increases by about 3 to 8 mm Hg, and arterial partial pressure of oxygen (Pao_2) decreases by about 2 to 5 mm Hg.[8] The various mechanisms causing these changes are complex and are briefly described here. Ventilation depends schematically on two different control systems: the metabolic controller and the volitional controller. The former adjusts ventilation so that the $Paco_2$ value remains almost constant whatever the activity of the body. Thus $Paco_2$ is allowed to fluctuate minimally around a given value (the so-called set point, usually 39 mm Hg) by modifying ventilation as a function of the carbon dioxide (CO_2) production of the body so that CO_2 excretion matches CO_2 production. The volitional system attributes a higher hierarchy to the nonmetabolic roles of the respiratory system, overriding the metabolic controller. For instance, during speech or singing, it may be necessary to allow for enough expiratory time (i.e., time useful for speech) to reduce respiratory frequency to less than 4 to 5 breaths/minute. This will result in CO_2 accumulation and increases in $Paco_2$, but the metabolic controller will not react by increasing ventilation until the volitional task is finished. During sleep, ventilation is governed by the metabolic controller because the volitional

controller is inhibited. As a consequence, the drive to breathe is reduced. Indeed, the set point of CO_2 is determined at least partly by a stimulation that depends on the wakefulness state, probably mediated by the volitional controller. Therefore the "retreat" of this wakefulness drive to breathe will result in an increase in the set point of CO_2 and hence in a decrease in ventilation. The sleep CO_2 set point is about 42 to 45 mm Hg.[9]

Together with the sleep-related disappearance of volitional control and of the wakefulness drive to breathe, the sensitivity of the metabolic respiratory controller to hypercapnia and probably also to hypoxia decreases.[10,11] The ventilatory responses to a resistive load are also decreased compared with wakefulness, a change with important physiologic consequences (see the section on obstructive sleep apnea). This means that during sleep, if the $Paco_2$ increases, or if the Pao_2 decreases, the respiratory controller will react less briskly than in wakefulness so that the increase in ventilation in response to these stimuli will be less, and the correction of hypoxia or hypercapnia will be incomplete. Similarly, if the resistance to airflow increases, the response in terms of augmented efforts to breathe will be less than during wakefulness, meaning that ventilation will be less well defended, and thus will decrease during sleep. During wakefulness, however, it would be maintained by the increased efforts of the respiratory pump.

Ventilation depends on the contraction of a series of skeletal muscles, usually referred to collectively as the respiratory pump. The muscle pump includes the diaphragm (the main respiratory muscle) and the intercostals and scaleni (accessory respiratory muscles), but also a series of muscles distributed along the upper airways, from the nose to the glottis. These muscles are activated with each inspiration in descending order so that the dilators of the nares are activated first and the diaphragm and intercostals last. As for all skeletal muscles, the tonic activity of these upper airway muscles decreases during sleep. In the nose, a reduction in muscular activity of the alae nasi dilator muscles (the muscles that dilate the nares when inspiratory airflow has to increase to slightly decrease nasal airflow resistance) has no important consequences. However, a reduction in muscular activity of the muscles that constitute the walls of the pharynx results in a significant increase in total airway resistance to flow.[12] Indeed, the pharynx is the only portion of the upper airway that lacks rigid or semirigid structural support. The nose has bony walls, whereas the larynx has cartilaginous support, but the pharyngeal walls are formed just by muscles. Sleep decreases muscle tone, with two important consequences. First, the pharyngeal walls lose some rigidity, that is, the pharyngeal compliance increases. In other words, the walls become more floppy. Second, the cross-sectional area of the pharynx decreases, that is, anteroposterior and especially lateral diameters become narrower and the pharyngeal surface decreases. When a fluid flows through a tube, the resistance to flow depends on a series of parameters, the most important of which is the cross-sectional area of the tube. The reason is that the resistance is inversely proportional to the fourth power of the radius of the tube, whereas it is directly proportional to the simple length of the tube. This means, for instance, that if the tube doubles its length, resistance doubles. But if the tube radius is halved, the resistance increases 16 times. Thus the decrease in pharyngeal cross-sectional area secondary to the sleep-related decrease in the muscle tone of its walls results in a 300% to 400% increase in total airflow resistance.[13]

This increase in resistance should immediately lead to a decrease in ventilation. Even during sleep, the metabolic controller will react to this impedance by increasing as much as possible (which is, however, less than during wakefulness) the efforts to breathe via the respiratory pump muscles. This will in turn result in an increase in negative pressure inside the thorax, transmitted through the airways to the airway opening (the nose or mouth). Indeed, the negative inspiratory pressure is the motor force causing inspiratory airflow. However, this enhanced negative inspiratory pressure will find a floppy tubing at the pharyngeal level, and instead of sucking air from the ambient inside the lungs, it will suck the pharyngeal walls inward, provoking a further reduction in pharyngeal surface and a further increase in pharyngeal resistance. In healthy people this leads to a new equilibrium, contributing to the sleep-related decrease in ventilation and to the increase in Pa_{CO_2} and decrease in Pa_{O_2}.

The sleep-related generalized decrease in muscle tone also affects the respiratory pump muscles, sparing only the diaphragm (the diaphragm is a vital muscle that cannot be shut down even during sleep, a characteristic shared with the cardiac muscle). Hence, the activity of the intercostal muscles, the scaleni, and the pectoral muscles will decrease during sleep.[14] Again, this will have important ventilatory consequences. The contraction of the main respiratory muscle, the diaphragm, leads to an increase in the three diameters of the lower thoracic cage. The descent of the dome of the diaphragm increases the vertical dimension of the thorax. The upward lift given by the vertical costal fibers of the diaphragm to the lower ribs will result, because of the particular geometric form of the ribs, in an increase in the lateral and anteroposterior dimensions of the thorax. This latter effect is enhanced by the increased abdominal pressure (a result of the descent of the diaphragmatic dome) pushing the lower ribs outward (the content of the thoracic segment covered by the lower ribs is the abdomen, not the lungs). The increase in the dimensions of the thorax creates the negative inspiratory pressure inside the thorax.[15] Curiously enough, this negative intrathoracic pressure will tend to draw the upper ribs inward, thus reducing the anteroposterior and lateral dimensions of the upper thorax and wasting the effects of the contraction of the diaphragm in distorting the rib cage rather than in inspiring ambient air into the lungs. This is usually avoided by the simultaneous contraction of the upper thorax accessory respiratory muscles, essentially the scaleni and upper ribs intercostals.

When the accessory respiratory muscles lose their activity during REM sleep, the diaphragm is almost left alone as the only contracting respiratory muscle, with a consequent decrease in the overall mechanical efficiency of the ventilatory pump. However, in a healthy individual, tidal volume is still maintained because of the tight coupling between the upper and lower rib cage. In patients, alterations in this coupling have important detrimental implications, as is discussed later.

Normally, when secretions accumulate in the bronchial tree because of hypersecretion, reduction in clearing efficiency, or a combination of both factors, airway sensory receptors are stimulated. This results in the series of events characteristic of the cough reflex: rapid contraction of expiratory muscles against a closed glottis, followed by fast opening of the glottis and the production of high expiratory flows. The cough reflex is abolished during sleep, when secretions can accumulate in the bronchial tree. Only when the level of secretions is exceedingly high will cough occur. However, cough must be preceded by sleep

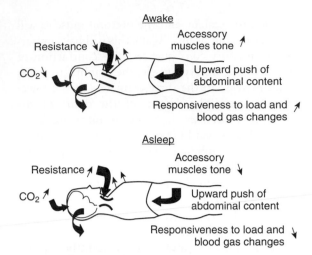

FIGURE 27-2 Schematic representation of the main respiratory consequences of sleep. For details, see the section on respiratory consequences of sleep. CO_2, carbon dioxide.

interruption because cough is impossible during sleep. Therefore for cough to proceed, first an awakening from sleep occurs, resulting in sleep disruption.

Figure 27-2 summarizes the main respiratory consequences of sleep.

Sleep Failure

Abnormal sleep generates a series of changes during wakefulness. In other words, sleep abnormalities are perceived mainly through their consequences during wakefulness. The consequences may range from minimal alterations in the quality of life to situations of severe lifestyle compromise for some persons. Sleep may be abnormal for different reasons, which can be schematically divided into three domains: abnormalities in sleep duration, sleep continuity, and sleep architecture.

Normal sleep duration varies among individuals, with an average daily duration of about 8 hours. Some healthy people function well with only 3 to 4 hours of sleep per day, whereas others need close to 10 hours. Whatever the normal sleep duration needed by an individual, if this value is not achieved (sleep deprivation), the usual consequence is an increase in sleepiness during the following 24-hour cycle. This mild level of enhanced sleepiness can usually be easily tolerated. However, when sleep duration is significantly reduced for more than a couple of days, sleepiness begins to pose more serious problems and is less easily managed, especially during sedentary and routine activities.

Even if sleep duration is sufficient for a given individual, sleep function may be lost owing to sleep discontinuity (sleep fragmentation). This means that sleep is frequently interrupted, either by complete awakenings or by arousal reactions. An arousal reaction is defined as a short-duration (2 to 15 seconds) return to an electroencephalographic pattern characteristic of wakefulness, interspersed in a sleep period (i.e., preceded and followed by a sleep pattern). Normally, 10 or so such episodes of arousals occur per hour of sleep.[16] Some think that they are important in allowing frequent changes in position and in this way avoiding pressure sores. When sleep is abnormally fragmented, usually in excess of 20 to 25 arousals per hour, the daytime consequences are important.[17]

The last form of abnormal sleep is the loss of normal sleep architecture. This means decreased or absent deep (stages 3 and 4) non-REM sleep, decreased or absent REM sleep, or, on the other hand, excessive amounts of REM sleep that may alter the usual pattern in which REM sleep follows a more or less lengthy period of non-REM sleep. This kind of abnormality may have few consequences or may be manifested by severe daytime sleepiness.

The main chronic consequences of sleepiness are psychosocial and are characterized by a decrease in the capability for sustained attention, decreases in short-term memory, aggressiveness or its opposite, depression and disinterest, and cognitive dysfunction.[18] When these consequences are very serious, they may be mistaken for early dementia. When sleep deprivation or sleep fragmentation with a concomitant loss of normal sleep architecture is severe and long-standing, the degree of sleepiness may be so intense that short periods (2 to 5 seconds in duration) of electroencephalographic patterns typical of sleep, called microsleep periods, may intersperse during wakefulness so that during every minute of wakefulness some seconds of sleep always occur; the individual is never fully alert and awake.

So far problems that make people feel sleepy, or unable to remain fully awake, have been referred to. Many other subjects have trouble with falling asleep, or with remaining asleep once they have succeeded in falling asleep. This is usually called insomnia, of which two essential types have been described: subjective insomnia (people think that they have not slept at all, whereas in fact sleep time is normal) and objective insomnia (people sleep few hours during the night and remain awake for hours during their sleep time). Insomnia may be normal in periods of emotional crisis, mourning, before passing examinations, moving, and so on. But many persons have insomnia for months or years, longing for some sleep without being able to get enough. In general, these people do not feel daytime sleepiness; they do not get enough sleep either at day or night. Some think that insomnia is a disorder of "excessive wakefulness." Insomnia is prevalent, especially in the elderly, among whom it coexists with an abnormal sleep distribution; elderly people frequently nap during the daytime, consuming their sleep time and finding themselves unable to have a full-night sleep period. This is of course not insomnia, because the 24-hour total sleep time is normal. However, this may be taken for insomnia, with some possible untoward consequences that are reviewed at the end of this chapter.

SLEEP IN PATIENTS WITH RESPIRATORY DISEASE

Chronic Obstructive Pulmonary Disease

Patients with chronic bronchitis and emphysema may be seriously challenged during sleep. It is not at all infrequent to see deep falls in oxygen (O_2) saturation during sleep in patients with borderline normal awake O_2 saturation owing to a variety of factors that have already been described. Patients decrease their ventilation during sleep for the same reasons that healthy people do: decrease in tidal volume resulting from the "dampened" wakefulness drive, with an increase in upper airway resistance; a decrease in the respiratory center reactivity to hypercapnia, hypoxia, and resistive loading; and a decrease in the activity of the respiratory pump muscles. However, patients with chronic obstructive pulmonary disease (COPD) manifest some specific features that add complexity to these factors.[19]

O_2 is mainly transported in the blood attached to the hemoglobin, enclosed in the red blood cells. Depending on the PaO_2 dissolved in the blood in gaseous form, the hemoglobin molecule will incorporate more or less O_2. When the hemoglobin carries all the O_2 it can incorporate, the hemoglobin is said to be fully saturated with O_2, or 100% saturated. Lower levels of PaO_2 will result in the hemoglobin being less saturated. However, this relationship is not linear. When O_2 saturation is high (usually above 90%), the relationship is horizontal; large increases in PaO_2 result in small increases in

O_2 saturation. Similarly, PaO_2 can significantly decrease without resulting in significant decreases in O_2 saturation. At about the level of 90% saturation (which corresponds roughly to a PaO_2 of 60 mm Hg), the relationship has an inflection point and becomes much more steep. Below this point, minimal changes in O_2 partial pressure result in larger changes in O_2 saturation. This has striking consequences for the O_2 saturation of patients with advanced COPD during sleep, who already during wakefulness have a PaO_2 close to 60 mm Hg. When these patients sleep, the resulting "normal" decrease in ventilation leads to a normal decrease in PaO_2 of about 5 mm Hg. However, because they are on the elbow of the hemoglobin dissociation curve, this small normal decline in PaO_2 will result in a 5% to 10% loss in hemoglobin O_2 saturation, leading them to a nocturnal saturation level near 80%.

If patients with COPD have a significant degree of airflow obstruction, they usually have an increase in the physiologic dead space. Because during sleep the tidal volume decreases and dead space does not significantly change, the proportion of the tidal volume that is wasted increases, leaving less effective tidal air for gas exchange. This may lead to a decrease in PaO_2 that is in excess of that of a healthy individual, which, coupled with the fact that the patient is already on the steep part of the hemoglobin O_2 dissociation curve, results in large falls in O_2 saturation during sleep.

When COPD includes a significant component of emphysema, hyperinflation is common. Hyperinflation, characterized by an increase in total lung capacity, is accompanied by some noteworthy changes in the mechanics of the chest wall. The diaphragm is flattened and the ribs adopt an inspiratory, horizontal position. Thus the vertical disposition of the costal fibers of the diaphragm is lost, and this impairs the ability of the diaphragm to exert an inspiratory action. As a consequence, the patient has to rely increasingly on his or her accessory respiratory muscles to maintain adequate ventilation during wakefulness. However, during sleep the activity of these accessory muscles is, normally, inhibited so that the patient is left, especially during REM sleep, with a lone and inefficient diaphragm. This leads to a striking reduction in ventilation during REM sleep periods, which, added to the previously mentioned factors, results in the typical deep falls in O_2 saturation (down to levels of 60% or less) during REM sleep. At the same time, hypercapnia develops or increases to levels above those of wakefulness.

The aggravation of hypoxemia and hypercapnia related to sleep is facilitated by the sleep-related decrease in the central ventilatory response to hypoxia and hypercapnia. Moreover, hypoxia is not a potent stimulus for awakening, and sleep may continue uninterrupted despite severe levels of hypoxemia. Of course, hypoxia will lead to increases in heart rate (to try to maintain O_2 delivery to the peripheral tissues), increases in pulmonary artery pressure, and a variety of other deleterious cardiovascular consequences, which by and large go unnoticed by the patient until late in the natural course of the disease, when the patient may have signs and symptoms of cor pulmonale.

Obesity in these patients adds a particular problem that merits some comments. When an obese patient (in particular, a patient with abdominal obesity) lies down, the abdominal contents displace cephalad, which pushes the diaphragm toward the rib cage. The craniocaudal diameter of the thorax is therefore reduced, and the functional residual capacity and the expiratory reserve volume decrease. This has two consequences: a decrease in the functional residual capacity and the closure of small airways in the more dependent parts of the lung, where blood perfusion is usually greater. Thus a loss of functional alveolar units in the areas of good perfusion enhances the ventilation–perfusion mismatch already present in the lungs of these patients. This is perhaps the most important mechanism responsible for the decrease in Pao_2.[19]

In addition to these features, which are strictly related to sleeping per se, sleep continuity and duration may be impaired in patients with COPD. Chronic bronchitis is characterized by increased bronchial mucus secretion and an impaired bronchial clearance mechanism. Thus, these patients frequently awaken during the night to cough up the accumulated mucus (which may well take 30 to 60 minutes) and may have trouble returning to sleep. Indeed, cough represents an effort that worsens shortness of breath so that patients may need an aerosol with medication in the middle of the night. If all this happens after 4 hours of sleep, for instance, sleepiness will be decreased by the preceding sleep period, and falling back asleep may take longer. Hence, nocturnal total sleep time may be reduced even if the patients spend a normal amount of time in bed. Figure 27-3 shows data from a representative polysomnogram of a patient with COPD.

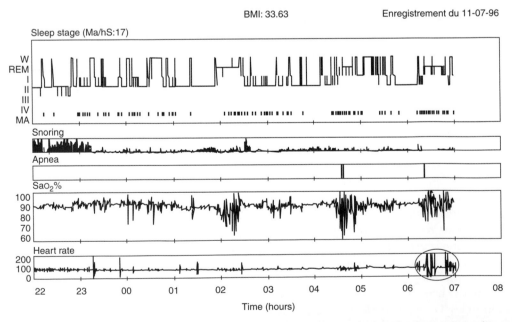

FIGURE 27-3 Schematic representation of a polysomnogram in a patient with chronic obstructive pulmonary disease and moderate obesity. For abbreviations and symbols, see the legend to Figure 27-1. Note first that sleep is not excessively fragmented (arousal index, 17 per hour), that only a few minutes of stage 3 non-REM sleep occur, and that stage 4 non-REM sleep is absent. Two periods of wakefulness (at 00:30 hours and 05:15 hours) occur because of the need to cough and expectorate, in addition to several other short periods of wakefulness. The patient snores mildly but consistently throughout the night. Note that oxygen saturation is about 90% in wakefulness as well as in non-REM sleep but that during REM sleep it falls to 70% or less. The extreme variations in heart rate at the end of the night are a recording artifact.

Finally, some of the medications these patients use may have deleterious effects on sleep. The β_2-agonists may provoke tachycardia and premature heart beats that can disturb sleep initiation if taken just before going to bed. Theophylline derivatives can also impair sleep by increasing sleep latency (the time from lights off to the first minutes of sleep) and decreasing sleep efficiency (the ratio of total sleep time to the time in bed period).

Thus patients with advanced COPD share with all other human beings the ventilatory challenges of sleep. However, because of their specific disease, they may fail to maintain adequate levels of ventilation during the night, whereas at the same time their disease will lead to inadequate sleep time, with the consequent daytime sleepiness and other symptoms owing to insufficient and unrefreshing sleep.

Restrictive Ventilatory Defects
Extrapulmonary Disorders

Extrapulmonary disorders are those that lead to respiratory failure in patients whose lungs are, basically, normal. These patients do not have airflow obstruction, or parenchymal abnormalities, yet are unable to breathe normally. The problem may arise in the skeleton (the best example is kyphoscoliosis); in the skeletal muscles, including the respiratory muscles (e.g., all the myopathies, such as Duchenne muscular dystrophy); in the central neural system (as in spinal muscular atrophy or poliomyelitis); in the peripheral nerves (as in idiopathic diaphragmatic paralysis); in the neuromuscular junction (as in myasthenia gravis); or in the pleura (as in extended pleural fibrosis secondary to pleural tuberculosis).

The most important mechanism leading to sleep-related respiratory failure in these types of disorders is weakness or inefficient contractile properties of the respiratory muscles.[20] In kyphoscoliosis, for instance, the diaphragm may be normal, but deformation of the thoracic cage distorts its insertion points so that the net result is a loss in the inspiratory action of diaphragmatic contraction. In Duchenne muscular dystrophy, the primary defect is weakness of the muscles so that the contraction force is decreased. Whatever the reason, the final result is hypoventilation, which is aggravated by sleep because of the additional loss of muscular activity linked to the sleep process. These patients hypoventilate during sleep, and their hypoventilation is even further aggravated during REM sleep, when they

lose the activity of the accessory muscles that have become "essential" muscles of respiration. As a consequence, the high levels of hypercapnia at the end of the night result in morning headaches. Hypoxia may be severe, with saturation levels below 60% for extended periods of the night. Nocturnal saturation abnormalities can be the first manifestation of progression of the disease and are worth monitoring while these patients are monitored over time.

It is not unusual that REM sleep decreases first in these patients while the disease progresses. As they enter REM sleep, ventilation falls dramatically, and after 1 to 2 minutes an arousal occurs, and patients go into non-REM sleep. Stages 3 and 4 of non-REM sleep are less affected initially but may also decrease or even disappear totally afterward. Sleep is then limited to stages 1 and 2 of non-REM sleep, with a few minutes of REM sleep.

Patients generally complain of sleepiness, morning headaches, difficulties in concentrating, and even of severe dyspnea during the night awakenings. However, they do not usually volunteer these complaints unless specific questions are asked. Children may become aggressive, or school performances may deteriorate. The need for naps during the day may be the first symptom of severe sleep-related respiratory failure, itself heralding a progression of the disease that will lead to overt daytime respiratory failure. Figure 27-4 shows a typical example of a sleep recording from a patient with severe kyphoscoliosis.

Restrictive Pulmonary Disorders

Patients with pulmonary fibrosis and other restrictive pulmonary disorders behave like other individuals during sleep, until the progression of their disease leads to the development of daytime hypoxemia in the range of a Pao_2 of 60 mm Hg. At this point, as in patients with obstructive conditions and because of the particular characteristics of the hemoglobin O_2 dissociation curve, further sleep-related decreases in ventilation will lead to impressive falls in nocturnal O_2 saturation. However, these patients will usually maintain the $Paco_2$ at normal or below-normal levels.[20]

Asthma

The existence of a specific entity labeled nocturnal asthma has been debated. Nocturnal asthma is characterized by episodes of shortness of breath and wheezing in the early morning hours, usually

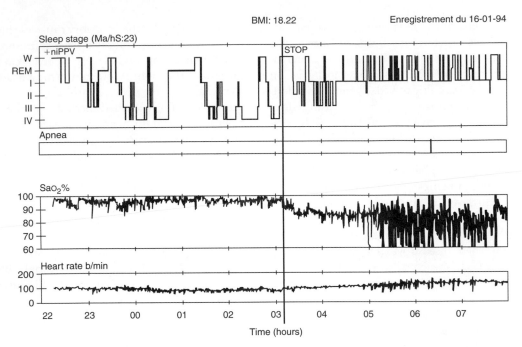

FIGURE 27-4 Schematic representation of a polysomnogram in a patient with severe kyphoscoliosis and respiratory failure. For abbreviations and symbols, see the legend to Figure 27-1 (MAs are not shown on this record). During the first part of the night the patient is under noninvasive mechanical ventilation with a volumetric ventilator in the controlled mode, using a nasal mask. At 03:00 hours the treatment is interrupted, and the patient is allowed to go back to sleep, breathing spontaneously. Note that during noninvasive ventilation, all sleep stages are present, sleep is stable, oxygen saturation stays above 95%, and heart rate decreases during sleep. After treatment interruption, sleep becomes fragmented, stage 4 non-REM sleep disappears, only a few minutes of REM sleep occur, oxygen saturation is almost constantly below 85% (with frequent falls below 60%), and heart rate increases well beyond 100 beats/minute.

causing awakening, and subsiding after several minutes, sometimes after the expectoration of a variable quantity of thick phlegm. When the attacks become frequent, they may impair total sleep duration (i.e., result in sleep deprivation) and lead to daytime sleepiness, to a decrease in the ability to stay fully alert and to concentrate, and to a deterioration in cognitive functioning. Much research has been conducted on this particular topic. The conclusion seems to be that nocturnal asthma is nothing else than the nocturnal manifestations of poorly controlled bronchial asthma. Nevertheless, it is crucial to be aware of the existence of these nocturnal asthma attacks because they may be the initial sign that asthma is being poorly controlled and that a medication adjustment is needed. Nocturnal asthma symptoms may also indicate that compliance with medication is less than optimal, which is a common occurrence in chronic diseases such as asthma. Again, specific questions should be asked or the information about nocturnal attacks may go unnoticed.[21]

SPECIFIC SLEEP-RELATED DISORDERS THAT MAY AFFECT PATIENTS WITH PULMONARY DISEASE

Sleep disorders are too numerous and varied to be considered here at any length. However, some are worth mentioning as examples of the interaction between sleep disorders and pulmonary diseases, which sometimes may have deleterious consequences in particular patients.

Nocturnal Myoclonus and Periodic Limb Movements

Nocturnal myoclonus or nocturnal restless legs syndrome is a common condition present in middle-aged and elderly individuals. It consists of repetitive—every 20 to 30 seconds—contractions of lower limb muscles with a resulting leg jerk. These repetitive contractions occur in clusters of 30 minutes to 1 hour or more in duration, and two or three such episodes may be seen during a single night. They are generally present only during sleep,

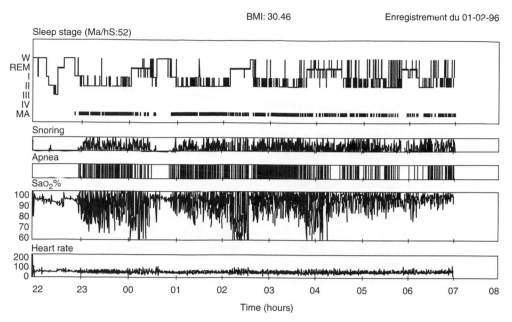

FIGURE 27-5 Schematic representation of a sleep recording in a patient with obstructive sleep apnea syndrome. For abbreviations and symbols, see the legend to Figure 27-1. Note that sleep is abnormally fragmented (52 arousals per hour of sleep, nearly 1 arousal per minute) and that stages 3 and 4 non-REM sleep are almost absent. Snoring is of high intensity and constant throughout the night. Apneas are numerous, but their frequency decreases in the last quarter of the night. Apneas result in deep falls in oxygen saturation and in increases and decreases in heart rate. Note that in this moderately obese patient (BMI, 30.46 kg/m^2), REM sleep has a deleterious effect on oxygen saturation.

although some patients experience them during wakefulness. Patients may complain of leg "tiredness" at awakening, of nocturnal cramps, but they may also refer to disturbing excessive daytime sleepiness. The reason is that each contraction of the lower limb muscles may (but not necessarily) lead to a short arousal from sleep. This produces sleep fragmentation, with the consequent excessive daytime sleepiness, sensation of unrefreshing nocturnal sleep, and other psychosocial consequences of chronic sleep failure. If nocturnal myoclonus is present in a patient with pulmonary disease of enough severity to produce in itself an impairment in sleep quality or duration, the resulting daytime symptoms will aggravate an already stressful situation.

Some patients may feel an imperious need to move, stand up, and walk during wakefulness, especially during the evening hours, with or without concomitant nocturnal complaints. This is called restless legs syndrome, or periodic limb movement disorder. Symptoms may be just annoying, with an explanation being enough to comfort patients, or may disturb social life to the point that a pharmacologic treatment is justified.

Obstructive Sleep Apnea Syndrome

Obstructive sleep apnea is characterized by the occurrence of multiple episodes of complete or almost complete upper airway occlusion during sleep. The floppy pharyngeal walls collapse inward, favored by the high negative inspiratory pressure. It follows a series of ineffective inspiratory efforts, of increasing intensity, as hypoxemia and hypercapnia develop. After 10 to 60 seconds under these asphyxic conditions, a reaction is elicited: an arousal from sleep, allowing for the opening of the pharynx, the resumption of breathing, and the correction of hypoxemia and hypercapnia. Whereas one such isolated episode is of no consequence, the occurrence of 20 to 70 episodes per hour of sleep for months or years results in a well-defined clinical entity known as obstructive sleep apnea syndrome.[22] Figure 27-5 shows a sleep recording from a patient with this syndrome.

A series of other phenomena take place in conjunction with the basic apnea—arousal mechanism. During apneas, partly owing to the decrease in the amplitude of lung expansion, a decrease in heart frequency occurs. After the arousal reaction, a surge in sympathetic activity (both neural and hormonal) occurs, with an acceleration in heart frequency. In some patients, a typical bradycardia—tachycardia pattern emerges that can be recognized on a Holter monitoring tracing. Simultaneously, alveolar hypoxia leads to pulmonary vasoconstriction and increases in pulmonary artery pressure. On the other hand, systemic arterial pressure decreases during apneas but increases after arousals because of the sympathetic surge.[23] For reasons not fully understood, kidney function is altered, with an inversion of the normal biphasic urinary output; patients with obstructive sleep apnea increase nocturnal diuresis and decrease diurnal diuresis. As a consequence, nocturia is common and may be mistaken for early prostatic troubles.[24] Snoring, loud and disturbing for the bed partner, is almost constant in this disorder. Indeed, with each arousal, breathing resumes with high-frequency oscillations of the pharyngeal walls, producing the typical harsh sound known as snoring.

Patients with obstructive sleep apnea experience the full-blown array of clinical manifestations of sleep failure: excessive daytime sleepiness, unrefreshing sleep, morning headaches, morning sleep drunkenness (they need some time to get out of sleep and feel alert), intellectual deterioration, personality changes, and memory impairment. Impotence is frequently reported by males. The prevalence of this disorder is about 1% to 5% of the adult population, and it seems to be severe enough to require treatment in about 1%. Obstructive sleep apnea is favored by maleness, obesity, and a short mandibular bone. The typical patient is a rather overweight male in his fifth decade with a long-standing history of loud snoring. However, lean patients and women are not at all infrequent. Obstructive sleep apnea seems to be a result of a reduction in pharyngeal cross-sectional surface, perhaps because of fat apposition on the lateral pharyngeal walls, which is counterbalanced successfully during wakefulness by the increased activity of pharyngeal dilator muscles, mainly the genioglossus. The sleep-related decrease in the activity of these dilators "reveals" the structural pharyngeal narrowing, resulting in high pharyngeal airflow resistance that leads to increased respiratory muscle pump efforts and to increases in the negative inspiratory pressures that favor the collapse of the floppy pharyngeal walls, finally resulting in complete or near complete pharyngeal

occlusion and apnea.[25] Studies have pointed to obstructive sleep apnea as a serious risk factor for arterial hypertension, stroke, and increased mortality.[26-28] In addition, patients with obstructive sleep apnea have a threefold increase in the risk of motor vehicle accidents.

The main treatment of obstructive sleep apnea is the application of continuous positive airway pressure during sleep, generally through a mask covering the nose (nCPAP). CPAP reverses all aspects of the disease and seems even to "normalize" survival in these patients.

A different pattern may be seen in children, where enlarged tonsils (common in this age group) lead to pharyngeal obstruction during sleep. The extension of the disease is less well known than in adults, but recent data seem to show that it is quite prevalent. In children, the main symptoms are daytime restlessness and agitation (this may be taken for a hyperactivity disorder), nocturnal snoring, a decrease in school performances, and a decrease in height increase leading to a short stature. In children, the main treatment is tonsillectomy.

A subset of patients have a severe form of obstructive sleep apnea that is accompanied by signs of right heart failure, ankle edema, and pulmonary hypertension. In general, these patients have at the same time obstructive sleep apnea syndrome and a coexisting lung disorder, most usually COPD, which is an especially dreadful combination. In a patient with a low awake level of Pao_2 owing to his or her lung disorder, sleep-related apneas will lead to extreme falls in Pao_2 (with the consequent rise in pulmonary artery pressure owing to pulmonary vasoconstriction) and arterial O_2 saturation. Hypercapnia at the end of apneas will not be easily corrected during the few seconds of free breathing during the arousal reaction in a patient with impaired lung function, all the more so if the patient already has chronic daytime hypercapnia with a reduced ventilatory response. This will finally lead to the development of right heart failure and respiratory insufficiency.[29]

Other Types of Sleep Apnea

Some sleep studies show episodes of apneas without obstruction of the upper airway, which are less frequent than obstructive sleep apnea syndrome. Patients just stop breathing for some time (usually 10 to 60 seconds), and then breathing resumes, generally without snoring. This syndrome may lead to respiratory failure, needing noninvasive assisted ventilation as a treatment. An example of central apneas is seen in the so-called Ondine's curse, a rare genetic disorder in children that can also be seen as an acquired disorder in adults. A much more frequent type of central apneas is seen in patients with severe cardiac failure, in whom breathing progressively becomes less ample until it finally stops for 10 to 20 seconds and then resumes with a progressive increase in amplitude until a maximum is reached and a new decrease proceeds. This is called Cheyne-Stokes breathing and can also accompany some neurologic disorders, such as after a stroke.

In some patients, central and obstructive apneas coexist, and it is not impossible to see central apneas appearing in a patient with previously observed obstructive apneas when the latter are treated with positive pressure during sleep.

Obesity–Hypoventilation Syndrome

Obesity–hypoventilation syndrome is defined as the presence of severe obesity (body mass index, $>30 \text{ kg} \cdot \text{m}^{-2}$) accompanied by chronic hypoventilation characterized by the presence of daytime hypercapnia unexplained by pulmonary disease. With the increase in obesity in industrialized countries, the incidence of obesity–hypoventilation syndrome is expected to increase. Many patients seem to experience a severe form of sleep apnea syndrome with right-side heart failure, which can be treated with assisted mechanical ventilation for a short period of time, and reverts to simple obstructive sleep apnea in obese individuals. However, in many other patients chronic hypoventilation remains present, probably indicating a low response of the respiratory center to CO_2. This represents perhaps the lowest normal ventilatory response to CO_2 or perhaps an abnormal absence of response. Obesity–hypoventilation syndrome seems to respond well to noninvasive nocturnal assisted mechanical ventilation, either with a volumetric or barometric ventilator.[30]

DIAGNOSTIC APPROACH TO SLEEP DISORDERS IN PATIENTS WITH PULMONARY DISEASE

Patients with pulmonary disease should be asked periodically about sleep quality and symptoms of sleep failure, especially when an obvious change occurs in their status that is not easily explainable by other factors. When poor sleep quality is suspected or a rapid unexplained deterioration in the condition of the patient occurs, a nocturnal oximetric recording is a useful initial screening test. If the oximetry result is strictly normal, either no special sleep-related disorder of respiration is present or the patient has not slept at all during that night (this is not an unusual occurrence). The next step is to repeat the oximetric recording (it is easily available, with little if any cost, and the devices are reliable). When the recording is abnormal and typical of the sleep-related oximetric consequences of the disease of the patient, it may be confidently concluded that the patient has a sleep disorder. When doubts persist or an atypical oximetric pattern is seen, obtain a full-night polysomnogram at a sleep center experienced in the management of patients with pulmonary disease and sleep-related breathing disorders. This is usually not necessary for patients with COPD but may be worthwhile for patients with restrictive disorders of extrapulmonary origin.

THERAPEUTIC CONSIDERATIONS IN PATIENTS WITH PULMONARY DISEASE

As we have seen, sleep represents a formidable challenge for patients with severe respiratory disorders. Sleep worsens the consequences of respiratory diseases, unraveling the fragility of the adaptive mechanisms developed to try to maintain normal blood gas levels. Is this enough to consider specific treatments to help these patients sleep? The answer is clearly *yes* for some patients, clearly *no* for others, and *perhaps* for still others.

Patients with restrictive extrapulmonary disorders and sleep-related hypoventilation benefit when they receive ventilatory assistance during sleep (see Figure 27-4). This assistance may be in the form of noninvasive positive-pressure ventilation or invasive (usually via tracheostomy) mechanical ventilation. This allows for normal sleep, normalization of breathing during sleep, correction or nearly complete normalization of nocturnal and daytime blood gases, decreases in the need for hospital admissions, enhanced quality of life, and increased survival.[31]

In contrast, patients with stable COPD and sleep-related falls in O_2 saturation do not seem to benefit from ventilatory assistance. Of course, when long-term O_2 therapy (>15 hour/day) is needed, night use of supplemental O_2 is mandatory, not only because this is practical (the sleep period already represents a sizable part of the minimal 15-hour daily period) but also because sleep represents that portion of the day during which gas exchange is least effective. Sleep duration may be normalized in these patients, and thus daytime symptoms of sleep failure may be decreased by paying special attention to such issues as timing of administration of sleep-disturbing drugs, management of nocturnal secretions, and management of nocturnal shortness of breath with long-acting bronchodilators. In patients with asthma, sleep may be improved by better control of the overall disease, with close follow-up of nocturnal attacks as a useful indication of suboptimal treatment.

In patients with a combination of diseases, it is important to adequately treat all conditions because a potentiating treatment effect seems to be present, because there is a potentiating effect in patients with coexisting sleep disorders and respiratory disease.

Finally, a word of caution is needed concerning the use of sleeping pills. Hypnotic and sedative drugs are among the most popular medications. Patients frequently overuse them. For patients with respiratory disease, sleeping pills have several undesirable effects that may in fact jeopardize the ability of these patients to breathe during sleep. Hypnotics and sedatives decrease minute ventilation, the tone of upper airway muscles, the arousal threshold of the brain, and the cough reflex threshold. These effects will worsen the sleep-related consequences of respiratory diseases. It is not uncommon that a borderline patient is precipitated into respiratory failure after the administration of hypnotics. A good example is the patient with COPD who has excessive mucous secretion that awakens him or her during the night. Frequently, patients will complain of awakening in the middle of the night, with subsequent difficulty in going back to sleep. This may be interpreted as insomnia and inadequately treated with hypnotics. The use of hypnotics and sedatives should be avoided in patients with severe respiratory disease. The same holds true for alcohol, which has similar effects and should also be avoided in these patients.

CONCLUSION

Sleep, unavoidable as it is, represents a stressful period for patients with respiratory disease. When the fragile equilibrium between the need to sleep and the need to breathe is altered, both abnormal breathing and abnormal sleep will occur. This will lead to the appearance of daytime symptoms that may greatly impair the ability of patients to enjoy life, an ability already hampered by respiratory symptoms. It is crucial to take due notice of these facts not only to avoid harming the patient but especially to realize that the disease has progressed to a stage in which the sleep challenge can no longer be adequately met by the failing respiratory system. Treatment optimization is then necessary, and the improvement of sleep-related symptoms may constitute the best indication of a successful intervention.

References

1. Rechtschaffen A, Kales A: A manual of standardised terminology, techniques, and scoring system for sleep stages of human subjects (publication No. 204), Washington DC, 1968, National Institutes of Health.
2. Kapsimalis F, Richardson G, Opp MR et al: Cytokines and normal sleep, Curr Opin Pulm Med 5:11-16, 2005.
3. Khatri IM, Fries ED: Haemodynamic changes during sleep, J Appl Physiol 22:867-873, 1967.
4. Koopman MG, Koomen GCM, Krediet RT et al: Circadian rhythm of glomerular filtration rate in normal individuals, Clin Sci 77:105-111, 1989.
5. Van Cauter E, Plat L, Copinschi G: Interrelations between sleep and the somatotropic axis, Sleep 21:553-556, 1998.
6. Krieger J: Breathing during sleep in normal subjects. In Kryger MH, Roth T, Dement WC, editors: Principles and practice of sleep medicine, Philadelphia, 1994, WB Saunders, p 217.
7. Stradling JR, Chadwick GA, Frew AJ: Changes in ventilation and its components in normal subjects during sleep, Thorax 40:364-370, 1985.
8. Bulow K: Respiration and wakefulness in man, Acta Physiol Scand 59(Suppl 209):1-110, 1963.
9. Colrain IM, Trinder J, Fraser G: Ventilation during sleep onset in young adult females, Sleep 13:491-501, 1990.
10. Gleeson K, Zwillich CW, White DP: Chemosensitivity and the ventilatory response to airflow obstruction during sleep, J Appl Physiol 67:1630-1637, 1989.
11. Douglas NJ, White DP, Weil JV: Hypoxic ventilatory response decreases during sleep in normal men, Am Rev Respir Dis 125:286-289, 1982.
12. Remmers JE, Sauerland WJ, Anch AM: Pathogenesis of upper airway occlusion during sleep, J Appl Physiol 44:931-938, 1978.
13. Hudgel DW, Hendrickx C, Hamilton HB: Characteristics of the upper airway pressure–flow relationship during sleep, J Appl Physiol 64:1930-1935, 1988.
14. Smith PE, Edwards RH, Calverley PM: Ventilation and breathing pattern during sleep in Duchenne muscular dystrophy, Chest 96:1346-1351, 1989.

15. De Troyer A, Estenne M: Coordination between rib cage muscles and diaphragm during quiet breathing in humans, J Appl Physiol 57:899-906, 1984.

16. Collard P, Dury M, Delguste P et al: Movement arousals and sleep-related disordered breathing in adults, Am J Respir Crit Care Med 154:454-459, 1996.

17. Roehrs T, Merlotti L, Petrucelli N et al: Experimental sleep fragmentation, Sleep 17:438-443, 1994.

18. Engelman H, Joffe D: Neuropsychological function in obstructive sleep apnoea, Sleep Med Rev 31:59-78, 1999.

19. Folgering H, Vos P: Sleep and breathing in chronic obstructive pulmonary disease, Eur Respir Monograph 10:303-323, 1998.

20. Shneerson J: Sleep in neuromuscular and thoracic cage disorders, Eur Respir Monograph 10:324-344, 1998.

21. Fitzpatrick MF, Jokic R: Nocturnal asthma, Eur Respir Monograph 10:285-302, 1998.

22. Krieger J: Clinical presentations of sleep apnoea, Eur Respir Monograph 10:75-105, 1998.

23. Hedner J, Grote L: Cardiovascular consequences of obstructive sleep apnoea, Eur Respir Monograph 10:227-265, 1998.

24. Rodenstein DO, d'Odemont JP, Pieters T et al: Diurnal and nocturnal diuresis and natriuresis in obstructive sleep apnea: effects of nasal continuous positive airway pressure therapy, Am Rev Respir Dis 145:1367-1371, 1992.

25. Deegan PC, McNicholas WT: Pathophysiology of obstructive sleep apnoea, Eur Respir Monograph 10:28-62, 1998.

26. Yaggi HK, Concato J, Kernan WN et al: Obstructive sleep apnea as a risk factor for stroke and death, N Engl J Med 353:2034-2041, 2005.

27. Becker HF, Jerrentrup A, Ploch T et al: Effect of nasal continuous positive pressure treatment on blood pressure in patients with obstructive sleep apnea, Circulation 107:68-73, 2003.

28. Marin JM, Carrizo SJ, Vicente E et al: Long-term cardiovascular outcomes in men with obstructive sleep apnoea-hypopnoea with or without treatment with continuous positive airway pressure: an observational study, Lancet 365:1046-1053, 2005.

29. Chaouat A, Weitzenblum E, Krieger J et al: Association of chronic obstructive pulmonary disease and obstructive sleep apnea syndrome, Am J Respir Crit Care Med 151:82-86, 1995.

30. Olson AL, Zwillich C: The obesity hypoventilation syndrome, Am J Med 118:948-956, 2005.

31. Hill NS: Noninvasive positive pressure ventilation in neuromuscular disease: enough is enough! Chest 105:337-338, 1994.

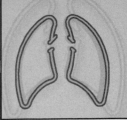

Chapter 28

Role of Respiratory Home Care

SUSAN L. McINTURFF

CHAPTER OUTLINE

**Respiratory Home Care: Now
   and Looking Ahead**
   Benefits of Home Care
   Candidates for Home Care
Delivery of Home Care Services
   Home Care Team
   Home Medical Equipment Provider
   Role of the Home Care Respiratory
      Therapist
   Home Visit
   Home Care Plan
Respiratory Home Medical Equipment
   Oxygen Therapy Devices

Aerosol Therapy Devices
Airway Clearance Devices
Ventilatory Assist Devices
Diagnostic and Monitoring Devices
Reimbursement Issues
   Medicare
   Medicaid
   Private Commercial Insurance
   Managed Care
   Documentation of Medical Necessity
   Reimbursement for Respiratory
      Therapy Services
Conclusion

PROFESSIONAL SKILLS

On completion of this chapter, the reader will be able to do
the following:
* Understand the reasons behind the shift of health care from the institutional setting to the home
* Identify patients who would benefit from and are candidates for respiratory home care
* Describe the role of the respiratory therapist in the patient's home care program
* Understand the types of respiratory home medical equipment commonly used
* Recognize the importance of proper equipment selection for patients needing home oxygen (O_2)
* Know the guidelines Medicare has for reimbursement of home O_2 therapy
* Understand the home respiratory care program from acuitization, follow-up care to determining when
  the patient is ready for discharge from the program

An important aspect of a patient's comprehensive medical management takes place away from the physician's office, the acute care hospital, and the pulmonary rehabilitation program. It involves a multidisciplinary team that can provide continuity to the services of a comprehensive pulmonary rehabilitation program, the physician's plan of care, or the hospital discharge plan. Respiratory home care is considered an essential component of the short- and long-term treatment of the patient with pulmonary disease. This chapter focuses on the respiratory home care needs of pulmonary patients, provided by home medical equipment (HME) companies, and does not expand into the home health agency role (e.g., nurse, physical therapist, and occupational therapist).

RESPIRATORY HOME CARE: NOW AND LOOKING AHEAD

Chronic obstructive pulmonary disease (COPD) is the fourth most common cause of death in the United States and although its overall mortality has been slowly decreasing since 1999, the death rate for females has been steadily increasing.[1] It is estimated that more than 12 million Americans received a diagnosis of COPD in 2003.[2] Pneumonia and influenza ranked as the seventh most common cause of death in 2003.[1] Pair these statistics with the fact that within the next 25 years, that population of Americans aged 65 years and older is expected to double in size and that life expectancy is increasing. People 85 years of age and older are now the fastest growing segment of the population.[3] This is a staggering number of people who will be consuming health care. Indeed, health care expenditures for our aging population continue to outpace overall inflation at a nearly doubled ratio.[4,5]

With the advent of managed care and continual changes in Medicare reimbursement to reflect fixed payments for services based on diagnosis-related groups, health care providers are looking for ways to limit the costs of providing that care. Hospitals are discharging patients much earlier in their course of care, often referred to as "quicker and sicker." These patients often have continued medical needs that were formerly met by an extended length of stay in the hospital, and in the case of patients requiring high technology such as assisted invasive ventilation, several additional months or longer. Extended survival of chronic lung disease and catastrophic illnesses such as acute respiratory failure is now common.[6]

What happens to patients who have continuing or ongoing medical needs or are being discharged from the acute care setting before they have all the information and skills they need to care for themselves? Respiratory home care is the answer to this question. Indeed, studies have revealed promising data that suggest that home care is a safe and suitable substitute for hospital care of select patients; that is, in the traditional model a patient would be admitted to an acute care facility, but in this model the admission is bypassed and hospital care is provided at home.[7,8]

Employment in home health care services continues to outpace growth in nearly all other health service sites.[4]

A well-structured home care program will allow the continued treatment of the patient with nearly any type of health problem and with most of the therapeutic modalities available in the acute or long-term care setting. Intravenous therapy, wound care, oxygen (O_2) and aerosol therapy, and invasive and noninvasive mechanical ventilation are all commonly performed in the patient's home. Home care also allows for ongoing assessment, education, and training of the patient. Home care can reinforce what a patient has been taught in a pulmonary rehabilitation program. For many patients, a good home care program is vital to their quality of life and long-term survival.

This chapter describes how to develop a comprehensive program for the respiratory home care patient and discusses the roles of the members of the home care team. It reviews the common types of home medical equipment (HME), also referred to as durable medical equipment, that are used as well as reimbursement issues that are important to home care providers. The home visit, the plan of care, and determining when the patient is ready for discharge from the home care program are also discussed.

Benefits of Home Care

The goal of any outpatient treatment program is to perform a medical service outside the acute care facility. Home care permits these medical services to be rendered in the comfort and convenience of the patient's own home, which is also the least expensive site of care.[7-9] Home care allows for ongoing evaluation and treatment, which can identify urgent problems and often prevent a hospitalization, an emergency department or urgent care clinic visit, or a visit to the physician's office. For example, a nurse or respiratory therapist (RT) performing a home visit may assess a patient and find that he or she has an increased cough, is now producing purulent sputum, and has abnormal breath sounds and a fever. The nurse or RT can relay these symptoms to the patient's physician, who may then decide to treat the patient with antibiotic therapy without bringing him or her into the office. The nurse or RT performs a follow-up visit to evaluate the patient's response to therapy and compliance with the medication program.

BOX 28-1	Benefits of Home Care

Improves quality of life
Is cost-effective
Encourages self-management and independence
Allows for ongoing monitoring of patient response
  to treatment
Reduces the need for clinic visits, emergency
  department visits, and hospital admissions
Reduces risk of nosocomial infections
Improves mental health and social independence

From McInturff SL, O'Donohue WJ: Respiratory care in the home and alternate sites. In Burton GC, Hodgkin JE, Ward JJ, editors: Respiratory care: a guide to clinical practice, ed 4, Philadelphia, 1997, Lippincott.

BOX 28-2	Candidates for Home Care

Patients who are newly diagnosed with a disease
  and require education and training for that
  disease
Patients with the desire to be treated at home,
  particularly those with terminal illnesses
Patients who have had repeated hospitalizations
Patients with adequate family, caregivers, and
  financial resources
Patients with physical limitations
  • Dyspnea that limits ADLs
  • Ambulatory difficulties
  • Difficulties with vision, speech, or hearing
Patients with functional impairments
  • Cognitive disabilities
  • Inability to perform ADLs
  • Inability to monitor and administer medications
    and other treatments
Patients requiring medical devices that necessitate
  monitoring and maintenance

ADLs, Activities of daily living.
Adapted from McInturff SL, O'Donohue WJ: Respiratory care in the home and alternate sites. In Burton GC, Hodgkin JE, Ward JJ, editors: Respiratory care: a guide to clinical practice, ed 4, Philadelphia, 1997, Lippincott.

The patient's home environment can enhance learning and provides a sense of control that is often lost in the acute care setting. Patients are happier at home and are more willing to cooperate with their medical program when they feel they have some control and input.[10] Box 28-1 reviews some of the benefits of home care.

Candidates for Home Care

A large and varied population of patients exists who could be considered candidates for home care; most of them are elderly and many of them have pulmonary disease. By 1999, 6.8 million Americans had chronic disabilities and used assistive services.[5] It has been estimated that 44% of all patients discharged from the hospital require posthospital medical or nursing care that cannot be provided by the family.[9] More than one-third of people aged 65 years and older and living in the community reported limitations in activity, and it is estimated that 20% of patients older than 65 years have functional and physical problems that impair their ability to perform the essential activities of daily living.[9] Approximately 1.4 million Medicare beneficiaries received assisted home health care services in 2000.[6]

Data from 2000 show that pneumonia and COPD were among the top 10 diagnoses of patients discharged to home care.[11] Asthma affects 20.7 million Americans and is increasing in prevalence and mortality.[2] It is estimated that up to 5% of adults have obstructive sleep apnea;[12] more than 40 million Americans may be chronically ill with sleep-related disorders.[10] Many of these people have concomitant or comorbid health conditions. These patient populations often require short- or long-term home care; however, diagnosis alone does not make a patient a candidate for home

care. Box 28-2 reviews the types of patients who are considered potential candidates for home care.

DELIVERY OF HOME CARE SERVICES

The delivery of home care services has many elements, and many personnel are involved in providing these services.

Home Care Team

It has been shown that the use of multidisciplinary teams in patient care can improve quality of care and enhance patient satisfaction.[9,10,13] The team provides continuity of care when transitioning from acute and skilled care to the home care setting. This team would include the following, as appropriate:

• The patient
• The patient's family
• Other caregivers
• The patient's physician(s)
• The hospital's discharge planner
• The home health agency, including nursing; physical, occupational, and speech therapy; and social services
• The hospital-based RT
• The home care RT
• The HME provider

- The insurance company's case manager or other liaison
- The pulmonary rehabilitation staff

Each member of the team has an integral function and purpose. For example, the discharge planner coordinates the predischarge activities of the other team members. The insurance case manager provides guidance as to the patient's health care benefits relative to the services required. The pulmonary rehabilitation staff provides recommendations as to the types of ongoing rehabilitation services the patient needs as well as a discharge plan. The HME company provides the equipment and related services the patient will need at home. The team members act cooperatively to help the patient achieve the goals established in the discharge plan.

Once the patient is discharged to a home care program, this team continues to evolve to reflect the patient's changing needs. The hospital staff would not remain on the team, but new members would most certainly be added. For example, a patient undergoing outpatient dialysis might now have a dialysis nurse on the team. A patient dying of lung cancer would have a hospice nurse and perhaps a hospice volunteer coordinator join the team. This team continues to customize its care to suit the patient's needs for the duration of the home care program.

Home Medical Equipment Provider

Once the physician has determined that the patient needs HME, the referral source (e.g., the discharge planner or pulmonary rehabilitation staff) will contact an HME provider to arrange for delivery of the equipment. The referral source must be prepared to provide specific information to the HME provider; Table 28-1 reviews the information the referral source should have in hand when making the referral.

Several factors must be considered when selecting an HME provider for the patient (if the patient has not already chosen one):[14]

- Does the company provide service to the area in which the patient resides?
- Does the company have the equipment the patient needs?
- Does the company also carry any supplies or soft goods the patient needs?
- Will the company bill the patient's insurance for the equipment?
- Does the company provide 24-hour emergency service?
- Will the company deliver on weekends?
- Does the company charge for deliveries? For off-schedule or after-hour deliveries?
- Does the company have RTs or nurses on staff?

The HME provider may assist in determining what type of equipment the patient needs, based on the information given by the referral source. For example, the referral source may request an aspirator for a child of school age. The provider, understanding that the patient attends school, might supply the child with a small, battery-powered

TABLE 28-1 Information Required When Ordering Home Medical Equipment

Personal Information	Billing Information	Equipment Information
Name	Primary health insurance carrier	Type of equipment needed, including portability if home O_2 is being ordered
Physical address	Primary policy number	
Mailing address	Primary group number	
Telephone number	Billing address	Frequency of use
Date of birth	Billing telephone number, contact person	Hours of use
Social security number		Medications necessary
Height	Secondary health insurance carrier	Allergy status
Weight		Qualifying medical data (e.g., room air blood gas or oximetry results)
Next of kin	Secondary policy number	
Ordering physician	Secondary group number	
Primary physician	Billing address	Delivery location
Primary diagnosis	Billing telephone number, contact person	Delivery date, approximate time as appropriate
Secondary diagnosis		

O_2, *Oxygen.*

machine in a carry bag instead of a heavy-duty stationary unit. If the physician desires a specific piece of equipment, such as a liquid oxygen system (LOX) instead of a concentrator, the provider cannot substitute any other type of O_2 equipment to reduce costs.

The HME provider has certain responsibilities to the patient. The provider is responsible for delivering the equipment in a timely manner, for example, O_2 equipment that has been ordered for a patient being discharged from the hospital should be delivered within a stated number of hours, not the next day. In fact, the O_2 equipment may need to be set up in the home before the patient arrives, and a portable system might need to be delivered to the patient's hospital room for use during transport home. The provider will also need to make arrangements with the patient to refill the O_2 as necessary.

The HME provider is responsible for the routine and ongoing maintenance of all equipment placed on rental to the patient. Such maintenance is performed at the time intervals recommended by the manufacturer or more frequently as needed. This service is performed at no charge to the patient if the equipment is rented. In the event that the equipment has been purchased, either privately by the patient or by the health insurance company, the patient must be informed of the required maintenance, the existence of any warranties, and whether a service contract is necessary. Many health insurance companies pay for service contracts as well as repairs on purchased equipment.

Depending on the type of respiratory equipment that is ordered, the HME provider will use a specially trained driver/technician to deliver and set up the equipment.[11,15] This practice varies by provider, but it is common for a technician to set up and teach patients to use O_2 equipment and compressor nebulizers. Some companies use technicians to set up equipment such as continuous positive airway pressure (CPAP) or apnea monitors, but this is not as common.

Role of the Home Care Respiratory Therapist

The primary duty of the home care RT is patient education and training.[9,16] Most home care RTs are employed by HME providers to teach patients how to correctly and safely use respiratory care equipment that has been prescribed by their physician. The education and training provided to the patient is not always a "one-time" service but rather continues as changes occur in the status of the patient. For example, a patient using home O_2 equipment might be instructed in its use during the initial setup, but it is discovered later that he or she does not remember how to clean the filter on the concentrator. The RT would then retrain the patient and encourage him or her to refer to the written instructions whenever uncertainty arises concerning any care instructions. Perhaps a couple of months later the patient is changed to an LOX; the RT would then instruct the patient in the use of this equipment.

The home care RT also provides education and training to the other members of the home care team. A patient using invasive mechanical ventilation may have a new caregiver who needs instruction on ventilator care. A home health nurse may need instruction about how to properly titrate a patient's O_2 flow, using pulse oximetry. A patient's spouse may need training on proper technique for filling a portable liquid tank.

The RT also trains the patient and caregivers to perform many types of respiratory care procedures. Many of these care procedures are done similarly to how they are done in the acute care facility. The major differences are the using of clean technique instead of sterile technique when performing those procedures and the reusing of items that are normally considered "disposable," such as medication nebulizers and suction catheters.[17] Box 28-3 lists some of the respiratory care procedures that are done in the home care setting.

The secondary responsibility of the RT" is assessment.[16] The RT evaluates many different

---

BOX 28-3	Respiratory Care Procedures Commonly Taught by the Home Care Respiratory Therapist

Tracheostomy tube and stoma care
Oral and endotracheal suctioning
Ventilator management
O_2 administration
Nebulized medication administration
Peak flow monitoring
Infection control practices
Basic assessment (heart rate, blood pressure, chest auscultation in some instances, color)
Airway clearance techniques, postural drainage, and percussion
Breathing retraining, energy conservation

O_2, Oxygen.

elements of the patient's care. For example, the RT assesses the patient for retention of instructions on using the prescribed medical equipment or performing a respiratory care procedure. The RT would physically assess a patient with a new, congested cough. The RT evaluates a patient's compliance with his or her O_2 therapy prescription. Good assessment skills are essential to the home care RT.

Home Visit

After receiving the referral, the home care RT will either set up the prescribed equipment or contact the patient, usually within the first 48 hours after the equipment has been set up by the driver/technician. This initial contact is usually done by telephone to assess the patient's understanding of the use of the equipment, and a home visit is scheduled.

The initial home visit accomplishes several things. It is used to evaluate the appropriateness of the equipment and to determine whether it meets the patient's needs. It is used to evaluate the patient's knowledge of and ability to safely operate the prescribed equipment. It is used to train or evaluate the patient's ability to perform any related care procedures, that is, oral or tracheal suctioning or taking a nebulizer treatment. It also establishes the patient's medical status. Elements of the initial visit should include the following:

- Patient evaluation, including relevant medical history, symptom profile, and barriers to learning
- Physical assessment, including identification of functional abilities and disabilities
- Evaluation of the patient's physical environment
- Evaluation of psychosocial issues
- Caregiver involvement
- Need for ancillary services (e.g., home health agency)
- Equipment needs
- Financial resources

Patient Evaluation

The patient's current medical condition(s), diagnosis, chief complaint, and previous medical history should be obtained through direct interview or by interview with appropriate family members. This information can also be obtained from medical records when available. Smoking status and other pulmonary risk factors should be identified.[9,10,18,19] The patient should be questioned about his or her immunizations for influenza and pneumococcal pneumonia.[20] Symptom profile; prescribed, over-the-counter, and herbal medications and dietary supplements; and alcohol and tobacco use should also be identified.[16,17]

The patient's nutritional status should be evaluated because lung disease frequently contributes to undernutrition and dehydration.[21] Patients should be questioned as to their current diet and eating habits as well as any problems they have in preparing meals. Patients receiving O_2 by nasal cannula often report a reduced sense of smell and taste, and elderly patients are known to have a decreased sense of smell, which can decrease appetite and contribute to malnutrition.[22]

Physical Assessment

Physical assessment includes routine vital signs, such as the following:

- Blood pressure
- Heart rate
- Respiratory rate
- Breath sounds
- Height and weight
- Temperature
- Inspection for cyanosis and clubbing
- Inspection for peripheral edema
- General appearance
- Blood O_2 levels by blood gas or pulse oximetry (when ordered by the physician)

The physical assessment of the patient should also identify any physical or functional limitations. Elderly patients frequently have sensory impairments that can inhibit their ability to care for themselves.[22] Decreased color discrimination can make it difficult for the patient to tell one colored pill from another. Nearly half of men and one third of women age 65 years or older undergo hearing loss,[5] which reduces speech perception and comprehension; this can impair their ability to understand instructions. Overall sensory loss in the elderly contributes to impaired balance and coordination, decreased tactile sensation, and decreased response to pain.

Assessment of the Physical Environment

One of the first things that must be determined when evaluating the patient's home environment is whether the patient is willing to allow home health care providers into the home. Some patients do not think that they need home care services or do not like admitting outsiders into their home. Ultimately, the patient has the right to refuse these services.

The home must also be appropriate and conducive to care. For example, the home needs to have adequate electrical wiring to power any HME that uses electricity. The home must present no fire, safety, or health risks to the patient; it may be necessary to make adaptations to improve the home's safety and accessibility.[23,24] Is the home one or two story? What are the patient's mobility needs in that space? What is the equipment range of use?

Patients with an asthmatic component to their health problems need to have their homes evaluated for allergens and irritants that can trigger an asthma flare-up. Dust mites, mold, cigarette smoke, pet dander, the presence of household cleaners, and many other factors can contribute to asthma symptoms.

Space must be adequate to place all the necessary equipment and supplies, and appropriate facilities must be available to clean the equipment as required. The kitchen or laundry room might be used to clean equipment. The pantry might be used to store not only food items but also O_2 tubing and suction catheters as well.

The home's geographic location must also be considered. Patients needing HME may live in an area not serviced by an HME company or home health agency. They may live in a remote area where medical care is not easily accessed. In these situations, special arrangements need to be made for temporary placement in another home or care facility until the patient no longer requires home health care services.

Although it is ideal to evaluate the home for these potential problems before discharge from the hospital or pulmonary rehabilitation program, this does not always occur. Instead, personnel from the home health agency or HME provider may identify problems during the initial home visit. In that event, the home care personnel will work with the patient and his or her physician to facilitate the prescribed program within the confines of those problems.

Psychosocial Issues

Another important element is the psychosocial evaluation. Many issues can greatly enhance the success or failure of the home care program.[9,10,13,25,26] Box 28-4 reviews psychosocial issues that should be evaluated.

Caregiver Involvement

Patients who are unable to perform their own medical care will need the assistance of caregivers.

BOX 28-4	Psychosocial Issues That Are Important to Evaluate

Patient's perception and acceptance of disease
Depression
Family dynamics, roles
Work history
Cultural issues, language barriers
Religious beliefs
Substance abuse by patient or family
Support system availability, ability and willingness to participate in plan of care
Financial resources
Domestic violence, child abuse

In fact, *family caregivers* provide 80% to 90% of all long-term home care services to family members.[2] Their work, if added to the market economy, would equal about 20% of all health care expenditures.[27] Examples of other caregivers include the following:

- Immediate and extended family
- Friends
- Home health nurses
- Home health aides or chore workers
- Privately funded lay caregivers
- Volunteers (e.g., hospice)

Depending on the type and amount of care the patient requires, the patient must have an adequate number of people to provide that care. For example, a quadriplegic patient whose lungs are being mechanically ventilated would require around-the-clock assistance and a "backup" list of caregivers in the event someone is unable to work his or her allotted shift. A patient who only needs assistance with bathing may only need the assistance of a home health aide three times a week. Family and friends are frequently used for patients with only basic needs such as assistance with cooking and cleaning. Family and friends are also frequently used to provide care for high-tech patients.

Regardless of the type of assistance needed, every caregiver must be evaluated to determine his or her appropriateness to provide that care. They must be evaluated for physical and functional disabilities just as the patient is evaluated. A caregiver, be it the patient's wife or the home health nurse, will not be adequate if he or she has a bad back and the patient needs assistance turning in bed. A caregiver with arthritic hands may not be capable of turning on or changing a regulator on an O_2 cylinder. A person with poor vision might not be able to read prescription labels or distinguish different medications.

Need for Ancillary Services

Once the need for home care has been identified, referrals are made to the appropriate members of the home care team. One of the most beneficial aspects of home care is the opportunity for visits from a variety of specialty practitioners employed by the home health agency that receives the referral. During the discharge planning process or during the initial home visit by the home care RT or nurse, it may be determined that the patient needs the services of a physical or occupational therapist, for example. This therapist might be needed to assess the effectiveness of the prescribed exercise program or to train the patient in energy conservation techniques. They may work with the patient on performing activities of daily living or using a wheeled walker.

It may be determined that the patient needs not only nursing visits but also visits by a home health aide to assist the patient with bathing, or a chore worker to help with cooking and cleaning. The psychosocial evaluation might reveal that the patient and family are having coping problems and would benefit from a visit by the home health agency's social worker. Box 28-5 lists the medical specialists typically available from a home health agency.

Equipment Needs

Patients with acute and chronic lung disease represent one of the largest population groups using HME, often also referred to as durable medical equipment. Depending on his or her medical condition and needs, a patient's physician may prescribe one or more pieces of equipment, ranging from walking aids, bathroom safety equipment, or nutritional support devices to O_2 equipment, aerosol administration devices, or invasive mechanical ventilation. Table 28-2 lists some common types of HME.

It is important to consider the HME provider when a patient needs equipment. All HME companies are not the same. Many specialize in respiratory care equipment, whereas others focus mainly on durable medical equipment. Some companies have RTs on staff, whereas others use specially trained driver/technicians to set up respiratory therapy equipment.

Financial Issues

A common misconception among health care professionals and lay people alike is that if a physician orders home care equipment or services, it must be covered by the patient's medical insurance. That is unfortunately not the case. It is essential to determine whether the patient's medical insurance includes that service or equipment as a benefit in the patient's particular plan. For example, Medicare, the federally funded insurance for

---

BOX 28-5   Medical Specialists Employed by Home Health Agencies

Registered nurses
Physical therapists
Licensed vocational and practical nurses
Occupational therapists
Respiratory therapists*
Speech therapists
Nursing aides
Social workers

Respiratory therapists (RTs) are not commonly employed by home health agencies because there is no direct payment for services rendered by RTs under many health insurance plans, particularly Medicare. Home health agencies may include the RT's wages in their overhead. Services rendered by RTs are often included in a home health agency's contract as negotiated with managed care organizations.

TABLE 28-2   Common Types of Home Medical Equipment

Respiratory Care Equipment	Durable Medical Equipment
O_2 therapy devices: stationary, portable, and ambulatory systems	Walking aids: crutches, walkers, canes
Aerosol therapy devices: medication and large-volume nebulizers, humidifiers	Wheelchairs: standard, lightweight, reclining, customized
Ventilatory assist devices: invasive and noninvasive mechanical ventilators, CPAP and BiPAP devices, IPPB	Hospital beds and related aids: traction devices, trapezes, air flotation devices for decubitus prevention
Home diagnostic and monitoring equipment: oximeters, sleep-recording devices, basic spirometry devices	Bathroom safety aids: commodes, bath or shower chairs, bath transfer benches, grab bars, hand-held shower attachments

BiPAP, *Bilevel positive airway pressure;* CPAP, *continuous positive airway pressure;* IPPB, *intermittent positive-pressure breathing;* O_2, *oxygen.*

people older than 65 years, has specific criteria the patient must meet to qualify for such things as O_2 therapy equipment. Some equipment is not covered at all by Medicare, such as bathroom safety equipment. Medicare and many other health insurance plans will cover equipment to treat obstructive sleep apnea if the patient meets specific criteria. Some plans have a lifetime "cap" for specific services or equipment. The area of reimbursement is constantly changing and patients needs to know what their insurance plans cover and the HME company needs to be aware of the latest reimbursement regulations.

It should never be assumed that the patient is willing or able to pay for medical equipment or services in the event that they are not covered by their health insurance. Consider also how large a patient's copayment is; copayment amounts can be up to as much as 50% of the total monthly charge. Many health insurance plans, including Medicare, require a copayment of 20% of the allowed charges. Depending on the type and amounts of equipment or services needed, a patient's total copayment may be cost prohibitive.

Home Care Plan

The purpose of all the assessments done during the initial visit is to use it to develop the home care plan. This plan is the comprehensive blueprint that identifies the patient's home care needs. It also identifies the services that are needed to meet those needs, as well as expected outcomes of those services. The plan incorporates both clinical and equipment monitoring. This information is communicated to the referring physician.

A tool to aid the development of the home care plan is *acuity scoring*.[28] It uses weighted criteria against which the patient is compared and categorized. The patient's "score" dictates the type of follow-up care; for example, using one acuity scoring model, a higher score would indicate that the patient is poorly compliant, is medically unstable, and possesses a less than satisfactory understanding of how to use the home care equipment. This patient would need more monitoring and follow-up than would a patient who had a low score. Table 28-3 illustrates a type of acuity scoring.

Follow-up Care

On the basis of the home care plan and the patient's acuity score, the patient will be seen on a periodic basis by members of the home care team. The home care RT, in particular, will check on the patient to monitor the goals of care and adjust those goals as necessary. For example, the RT may need to do

---

TABLE 28-3   Example of Acuity Scoring*

Assessment Parameter Point Value (Score 1-5)	Best Case, Needs Little or No Monitoring, Modification = 1	Satisfactory but Needs Monitoring, Modification = 3	Worst Case, Needs Close Monitoring, Extensive Modification = 5
Patient's medical status	Medically stable	Recent exacerbation, hospital discharge	Medically complex, unstable
Physical abilities	No or mild physical impairments	Moderate physical impairments, needs some assistance	Severe physical impairments, needs assistance for all activities
Caregiver needs	Independent	Needs intermittent caregiver assistance	Needs caregivers around-the-clock
Physical environment	Safe, clean, suitable	Safe, needs minor modifications	Unsatisfactory, needs major modifications
Equipment needs	Low-tech, single piece (e.g., nebulizer, O_2)	Low-tech, multiple pieces (e.g., nebulizer + O_2, CPAP + O_2)	High-tech (e.g., high-flow O_2, apnea monitor, ventilator)
Knowledge base	Good comprehension, performs skills as instructed	Fair comprehension, performs most skills as instructed, needs some review	Poor comprehension, cannot perform skills as instructed, needs assistance

*Scoring key: 6 to 13 points: follow-up in 1 month to reassess, then quarterly; 14 to 24 points: follow-up in 2 to 4 weeks to reassess, then monthly or quarterly as necessary; 25 to 30 points: follow-up in 1 week (or sooner if necessary) to reassess, then in 2 to 4 weeks as needed, then monthly.
CPAP, Continuous positive airway pressure; O_2, oxygen.

follow-up visits daily with a new O_2 client to titrate the O_2 flow rate during different activities. Once the titration is complete, the follow-up visit may be reduced to monthly to monitor the patient's progress with exercise tolerance. Acuity scoring is done during each follow-up visit to evaluate the patient's progress. The home care plan is then revised as indicated by changes in the patient's condition, psychosocial status, prognosis, and equipment needs and goals that are not achieved.[10,29,30]

A fairly recent development in technology is now making it possible for follow-up care to be done by telemonitoring.[31] Special computers and videophones allow the patient to measure vitals signs and transmit this information to the care provider. It is also possible for home O_2 providers to monitor O_2 equipment via computer link. The provider can check for contents, use time, and other equipment parameters at any time; the rationale for this type of telemonitoring is that it improves patient care through tighter equipment maintenance. It also potentially reduces the provider's service calls for complaints of equipment malfunction and empty tanks.

Discharging the Patient from Home Care Services

Most patients receiving clinical respiratory home care services will at some point likely be discharged from those services. Several areas need to be considered:

- Diagnosis and any change in condition from baseline or start of care
- The patient's ability to manage his or her own care
- The family's ability to manage the patient's care
- The patient's ability to independently manage activities of daily living
- The patient's acuity score
- The patient's ongoing equipment needs

The home care plan was used to establish specific goals related to the patient's care. Once those goals are met, the patient may no longer need the services of the RT. Regardless of this, patients will continue to need equipment services as long as they continue to use any respiratory HME.

RESPIRATORY HOME MEDICAL EQUIPMENT

As previously discussed, one of the major components of a home care program is the provision of medical equipment. Technology of HME has expanded greatly in the past 20 years to include many of the same technologies seen in acute care. It is not uncommon to see home care patients who need invasive and noninvasive ventilatory support, intravenous pumps, enteral or parenteral nutrition therapy, or diagnostic testing. The challenge is in determining the most appropriate device to meet the patient's medical needs within the boundaries of the third-party payer's guidelines.

Oxygen Therapy Devices

O_2 therapy has been proven to reduce mortality, reduce dyspnea, increase performance of activities of daily living, and improve quality of sleep and cognitive function in patients for whom it is medically indicated.[18,32] Patients with chronic lung disease and resultant chronic hypoxemia represent one of the largest population groups using home medical equipment.

Three distinct types of stationary O_2 systems are used in home care:

- High-pressure cylinders
- O_2 concentrators
- LOXs

Two distinct types of portable or ambulatory O_2 systems are used in home care:

- Small high-pressure cylinders
- Small LOXs

High-pressure Cylinders

The use of seamless steel or aluminum to contain gaseous O_2 under high pressure is the oldest and most reliable method of storing O_2 for subsequent administration. O_2 is compressed to pressures of 2200 to 2400 psi (15,169 to 16,548 kPa) in cylinders of various sizes. The larger the cylinder, the more cubic feet (liters) of O_2 can be contained at the filling pressure of 2200 psi (15,169 kPa). The most common sizes seen in the home are H or K tanks, containing 244 cu ft (6910 L); E tanks, containing 22 cu ft; and D tanks, with 13 cu ft.

The high-pressure stationary O_2 system has several advantages: no external power supply is required for operation; O_2 is not lost when the system is not in use; and it can also be used to power other pieces of respiratory equipment such as nebulizers, blenders, or ventilators. However, this type of stationary system has several disadvantages: each cylinder has a fixed capacity, necessitating frequent changes and refills; cylinders are heavy and are not easily moved; high-pressure O_2 cylinders pose a safety risk and must be properly secured; and moderate hand strength is required to open valves and change regulators.

Stationary compressed O_2 tanks are rarely used as a patient's primary source of O_2 because of the limited amount of use time the tank has; for example, a patient receiving O_2 at 2 liters per minute (lpm) with continuous use would empty an H or K tank in less than 3 days. These tanks are instead used as a backup source of O_2 in the event that the primary source has failed in some way.

Oxygen Concentrators

An O_2 concentrator is an electrically powered device capable of separating O_2 from room air. A concentrator is boxlike and is about the size of an end table (Figure 28-1). O_2 concentrators use a molecular sieve of zeolite to absorb nitrogen from room air gas that is drawn into a compressor, pressurized to a relatively low level of 4 to 10 psi (27.6 to 69.0 kPa), and directed through the sieve bed. As the gas passes through the sieve bed, nitrogen is absorbed by the zeolite and the remaining O_2 is collected, concentrated, and passed through a flowmeter, where it is then delivered to the patient. O_2 concentrators are capable of providing flow rates up to 6 lpm at concentrations of 85% or more. In general, the lower the flow rate, the higher the O_2 concentration. Many concentrators have an O_2 concentration indicator that alerts the user should the concentration drop below an acceptable level.

O_2 concentrators offer many advantages when used as a stationary O_2 system. The concentrator has the ability to provide O_2 without the need to be refilled. Concentrators are designed to run continuously, when properly maintained, and do so with minimal interruption. The console itself has an aesthetically pleasing appearance, and the patient or caregiver can easily operate the device. Concentrators have casters and weigh approximately 50 lb (22.5 kg), facilitating relocation throughout the home.

The use of O_2 concentrators has several disadvantages. A concentrator requires a source of electrical power (115 VAC) and, depending on the model, can consume up to 450 W per hour. Any interruption in electrical power obviously renders the unit inoperable, which can be a problem if the patient lives in an area that experiences frequent power outages. The additional power usage will increase the patient's utility bill, and for some patients this is cost prohibitive. Some utility companies offer special consideration and reduced rates for patients using electrically powered life support devices such as concentrators. Concentrators produce extraneous noise in the range of 50 to 60 dB, which some patients find bothersome, particularly at night. Concentrators also produce a moderate amount of heat that is exhausted into the room.

Because concentrators are low-pressure systems, they cannot be used to power other equipment such as nebulizers or blenders. A concentrator is also a sophisticated piece of equipment and requires routine and periodic maintenance to ensure optimal performance. Patients are responsible for cleaning the foam intake filter on a weekly basis and for cleaning and disinfecting the humidifier if one is being used. They must also change the O_2 tubing and cannula as recommended by the provider. The HME provider is responsible for performing the preventive maintenance as recommended by the manufacturer.

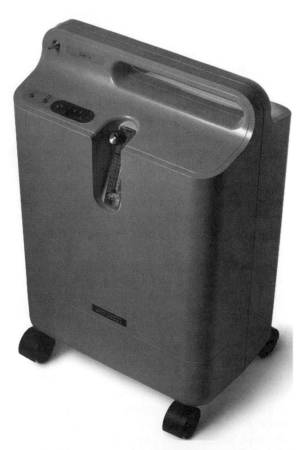

FIGURE 28-1 Oxygen concentrator: the EverFlo oxygen concentrator from Respironics (Murrysville, Pa.).

A recent technological development offers some new advantages to the patient. A specially designed O_2 concentrator now allows the patient to fill small compressed O_2 cylinders from the concentrator.[33] The patient can actually use the concentrator while the cylinder is filling. The filling process is slow to prevent heat buildup; although this is an important safety feature, patients needs to understand that it *is* slow and anticipate their needs for a full cylinder well ahead of time. Depending on the size of the cylinder, fill time can be up to 8 hours.

Another recent technological development is a *battery-powered* concentrator/O_2-conserving device. This is a very small unit with wheels and "luggage-carrier handle" that allows the user to roll the concentrator along with them. Battery life is limited, only certain patients can use the devices, and maximal liter flow limitations exist, but the battery-powered device does offer another viable option for ambulatory patients.

Liquid Oxygen Systems

The third method of providing continuous O_2 therapy in the home is the LOX. Oxygen is stored in its liquid state at $-273°$ F $(-182.9°$ C) in specially manufactured containers that are in essence sophisticated thermos bottles. These containers, called dewars, keep the O_2 in its liquid state and control the rate of evaporation through warming coils to provide sufficient gaseous O_2 for administration.

The primary advantage of the LOX is portability. Most stationary LOX dewars can be used to refill a smaller, lightweight version of the larger stationary unit. Figure 28-2 shows an example of a stationary LOX container with its smaller portable unit. Portable LOX containers, when filled with 1 to 2 lb (3.6 to 4.5 kg) of liquid O_2, weigh approximately 10 to 12 lb and can provide continuous O_2 for up to 8 hours at a flow rate of 2 lpm. A portable LOX unit can be refilled from its stationary tank any number of times as long as the stationary tank contains an ample quantity of liquid O_2, and the refilling procedure can be done by the patient.

Other favorable features associated with LOX systems include the availability of flow rates up to 15 lpm and the fact that they operate without the need for electricity. Although the stationary tank needs to be refilled by the provider, it will last approximately 1 week with continuous use at 2 lpm. The stationary LOX tank can be placed on a roller base and moved around the home easily.

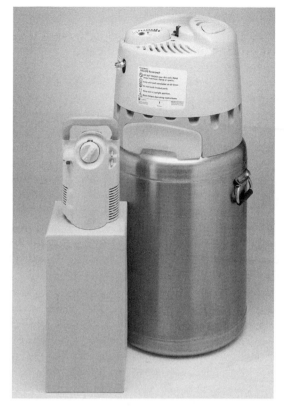

FIGURE 28-2 Liquid oxygen system.

The LOX system is also quiet, producing only a small hissing sound from evaporation. This evaporation, however, is the biggest disadvantage to using the LOX. Simply stated, dewars are not capable of maintaining O_2 in the liquid state for an extended period. Under normal conditions, the amount of evaporation is controlled, and the O_2 is immediately made available for administration. However, when the system is not being used, evaporation will occur. Warmer room temperatures and frequent transfilling of the portable tank cause the evaporative loss to be greater. An LOX not used for days may run dry solely through evaporative loss. The same applies to a portable LOX tank, so that if a patient fills the portable tank the previous night, the tank will have lost much of its contents by the next day.

Another disadvantage to the LOX is that O_2 in its liquid state is extremely cold and requires special handling. Gloves and protective eyewear must be worn by delivery personnel while filling the stationary tank to protect them from burns that occur when liquid O_2 comes in contact with skin. The tanks themselves are more costly for the HME provider to own and operate compared with the other O_2 delivery systems. Some patients find the portable tank transfilling procedure difficult and do not like the noise created by the fill procedure. Patients must also be prepared to handle problems that can occur while filling the portable, such as freezing at the coupling of the portable and stationary tanks or overfilling or underfilling of the small tank.

An advancement in LOX technology is the low-loss container. Its enhanced insulation reduces the evaporative loss common to stationary LOX tanks. The low-loss system is designed to be used primarily to fill a portable LOX tank. It has a content indicator like that on a traditional stationary tank but no flow control valve; a separate flow control valve can be added, however. Home O_2 providers frequently use the low-loss system in conjunction with an O_2 concentrator; patients use the concentrator as their stationary system and use the low-loss system to fill a portable LOX tank. This combination reduces the number of deliveries the company needs to make to refill the stationary LOX tank or provide full compressed gas cylinders and provides the patient with the ultimate in portability.

Portable and Ambulatory Oxygen Equipment

Contrary to what many patients think, they are not confined to their homes just because they use O_2. Options are available that will allow them to be away from their stationary source of O_2 for several hours at a time. Small compressed O_2 cylinders and the portable LOX tank are the options, but determining which is the better option is complex.

Usually referred to as a portable O_2 system, it is important to categorize this equipment appropriately.[34] *Portable* O_2 equipment is small enough in size and weight to allow the patient to move it about, usually in a wheeled cart. *Ambulatory* systems are even smaller and lighter and can be carried on the body, usually by a shoulder carrying strap or in a bag. Box 28-6 outlines suggested criteria for selecting the most appropriate O_2 system for the patient. It may take some time before it can be decided which equipment is most appropriate. The patient's activities dictate their equipment needs, but the patient's activities may be limited when O_2 is first ordered for them. The home care RT will be able to identify the patient's changing needs during subsequent visits.

BOX 28-6	Suggested Criteria for Selecting the Most Appropriate Oxygen System for the Patient

Stationary O_2 delivery system alone:
- Patient is bed bound or unable to ambulate beyond the limits of a 50-foot length of tubing
- Patient requires nocturnal O_2 only
- Patient requires an O_2 source for a ventilator, continuous positive airway pressure, etc.

Stationary and portable O_2 delivery system (e.g., concentrator with E tank or LOX):
- Continuous O_2 therapy is needed for a patient who only occasionally travels beyond the limits of a 50-foot length of tubing (e.g., occasional visits to the physician)

Stationary and ambulatory O_2 delivery system (e.g., concentrator with lightweight cylinders weighing less than 10 lb or an LOX):
- Continuous O_2 therapy is needed for a patient who frequently travels beyond the limits of a 50-foot length of tubing (e.g., frequent trips outside the home for medical care, activities of daily living, recreation)

LOX, *Liquid oxygen system;* O_2, *oxygen.*
Adapted from McInturff SL, O'Donohue WJ: Respiratory care in the home and alternate sites. In Burton GC, Hodgkin JE, Ward JJ, editors: Respiratory care: a guide to clinical practice, ed 4, Philadelphia, 1997, Lippincott.

Oxygen-Conserving Devices

O_2-conserving devices are popular and useful additions to home O_2 therapy. These devices, which use either a passive reservoir system or electronic or pneumatic technology, help extend the use time of a liquid or gaseous O_2 tank. They offer significant cost savings to the O_2 provider and a nice option for portability to the patient.[35]

O_2-conserving devices reduce the total amount of O_2 contents used in several ways. The reservoir system is a continuous flow device, but the O_2 flows into a reservoir, where it is stored during the patient's expiratory phase. The reservoir system is disposable and is replaced at regular intervals. This allows a bolus of O_2 to be made available to the patient at the beginning of their next inhalation (Figure 28-3). Although reservoir-type devices are continuous flow systems, they accomplish oxygenation goals at substantially lower flow rates than would otherwise be required using a conventional nasal cannula. For example, a reservoir device operating at 0.5 lpm can usually match the oxygenation levels attained with a conventional cannula at 2 lpm (assuming no increased demand exists for O_2 as during exertion).

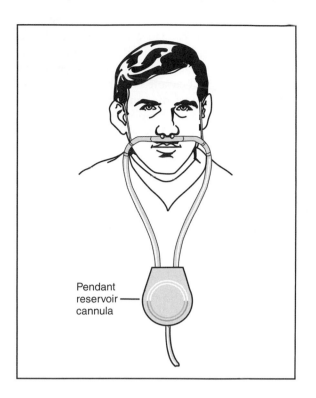

FIGURE 28-3 Reservoir cannula.

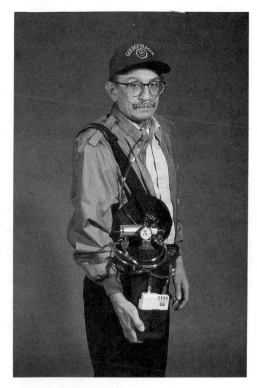

FIGURE 28-4 Oxygen-conserving device ambulatory system.

The major disadvantage to the mustache-type reservoir—nasal cannula is that it is rather unsightly to wear. Patients who dislike wearing a nasal cannula for cosmetic reasons would find this device even more unacceptable. For this reason and because other O_2-conserving options are available, reservoir cannulas are not frequently used. Pendant-type reservoir cannulas are less conspicuous and more commonly used.

Electronic and pneumatic O_2-conserving devices are widely used. These devices work by pulsing small volumes of O_2 to the nasal cannula only during the first part of inspiration. These devices have been reported to reduce the amount of O_2 used by 50% to 85%.[35] Pulsed-dose conserving devices can be used on stationary, portable, and ambulatory O_2 systems and are suitable for use on either liquid or compressed O_2 tanks.

A disadvantage of using a pulsed-O_2 conserving device is that because it is delivered on demand, the patient will not receive O_2 should periodic interruptions occur in breathing, such as during sleep. Another concern is whether the patient will be adequately oxygenated during exertion; the patients' O_2 saturation should be monitored at rest and during exertion when they first start using a pulsed-dose conserving device. Careful

patient and device selection is essential: it should meet the patient's physiologic and ambulatory needs during all their activities.[35,36]

O_2-conserving devices have found their greatest acceptance when used to prolong the duration of ambulatory O_2 systems. When paired with a small aluminum cylinder (e.g., B, M6, or ML6), the conserving device makes for a lightweight ambulatory system that can last 10 hours or more (Figure 28-4). Using such a system greatly enhances a patient's sense of freedom. The drawback to this, however, is that these units are costly and not covered by many insurance companies, Medicare in particular. HME providers see the value added to both the patient and themselves by using these devices. Traditionally, a patient who is very active uses more O_2 and requires more frequent O_2 deliveries. With a conserving device, the patient can remain active and use less O_2, thereby requiring less frequent deliveries, which is advantageous to the provider.

Transtracheal Oxygen Systems

The development of the transtracheal O_2 catheter in the 1980s occurred as a result of the desire to increase patient compliance when continuous O_2 therapy was ordered. Patients using traditional

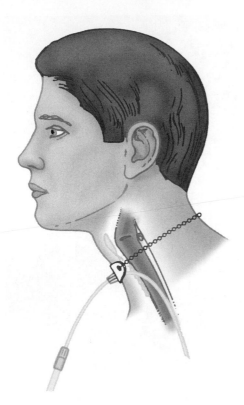

FIGURE 28-5 Transtracheal oxygen catheter.

nasal O_2 tend to remove the cannula because of discomfort around the nares or ears or because they feel restricted or inconvenienced by it. Some patients refuse to use O_2 when they are in public because they are embarrassed by it. It is also difficult to keep the nasal prongs in place during sleep, contributing to interrupted O_2 therapy and concomitant desaturation.

The transtracheal O_2 system is an invasive method of O_2 delivery. A small silastic catheter, approximately 20 cm long with a 9-French tract, is inserted into the trachea somewhere between the cricothyroid membrane and the notch of the manubrium (Figure 28-5). The transtracheal catheter bypasses a considerable volume of anatomic deadspace (e.g., the hypopharynx), thereby reducing the amount of O_2 flow necessary to achieve the desired oxygenation. These flow rates, even though they are continuous, have been reported to be up to 50% less than with a conventional nasal cannula.[35]

The O_2-conserving and aesthetic benefits of transtracheal O_2 therapy must be balanced with other aspects of a less desirable nature. Problems reported with its use include stoma site infection, stoma maintenance, inadvertent catheter displacement, kinking, and mucus plugs that adhere to the catheter. Other less prevalent complications include subcutaneous emphysema, mild hoarseness, and tract discomfort. Careful patient selection, training, and monitoring are essential, and if done so, these side effects can be significantly reduced.

Traveling with Oxygen

Many patients using O_2 admit that they feel tethered to their O_2 tank and that they cannot leave their home. This chapter has described several portable and ambulatory systems that allow a patient to do just that, but what about the patient who wishes to travel? It is certainly possible to do long-distance traveling with O_2. Car, train, bus, and commercial air travel can all be done by the patient with O_2. It takes planning, however, and several details must be considered before traveling to ensure a safe and positive experience (see Chapter 29).

Healthy persons maintain an arterial partial pressure of oxygen (Pa_{O_2}) between 50 and 60 mm Hg at elevations of about 8000 to 10,000 feet (2440 to 3050 m). Patients with COPD whose normal Pa_{O_2} is 60 mm Hg have been shown to maintain Pa_{O_2} levels in the 30—mm Hg range at these altitudes.[37] As a consequence, it is important to carefully assess the patient for general health and to identify contraindications before attempting air travel.[38] The normal response to hypoxemia is to increase ventilation, which may be difficult or impossible for a patient with severe pulmonary disease, making the patient unable to compensate for the resultant drop in blood O_2 level.

In-flight O_2 administration can assist the patient in managing this acute altitude stress. Most domestic airlines can supply O_2 at 2 to 4 lpm to patients requiring supplemental O_2. They will not, however, allow patients to carry their own compressed or liquid O_2 onboard, but they will allow the patient's empty O_2 cylinders to be checked as baggage. FAA regulations in August 2005 approved the use of specific portable concentrators in flight (e.g., the Inogen One and AirSep's LifeStyle model concentrators). The airlines will not supply O_2 for use in the airport terminal, so it is advisable to have someone with the patient who can take the patient's O_2 equipment home once the patient has boarded the plane. It is also advisable to fly direct and have O_2 waiting at the arriving airport and at the traveler's ultimate destination. Airlines require a medical certificate from the patient's physician along with up to 2 weeks' advance notice. They also charge fees for this service, for which the patient is responsible. The patient's O_2 provider can assist in making the necessary arrangements for onboard O_2 and for the delivery of O_2 equipment for use at the patient's travel destination.

Traveling by bus or train is also possible. The Greyhound bus line will allow a patient to bring a portable O_2 container on its buses, but the patient's stationary system cannot be checked as baggage. Prior arrangements need to be made to have O_2 available at the arriving bus terminal and the patient's final destination. Check ahead with private bus lines for their policies on traveling with O_2. Patients traveling on Amtrak can bring their stationary liquid tank or concentrator on board, but they must travel in the nonsmoking sections of the train. If traveling with liquid O_2, prior arrangements need to be made for having the tank refilled at the traveler's destination.

Travel by car is an easy way for a patient to make trips. Liquid O_2 tanks can be secured by a seat belt into the back seat of the car, but the patient will need assistance in placing it into the car, and great care must be taken when doing so. The stationary system must be removed from the car before filling the portable tank off of it, and both units must be kept upright at all times; allowing them to tip over will result in venting of the liquid O_2, posing a safety hazard. The patient's O_2 provider can identify other O_2 suppliers along the patient's itinerary who can fill the stationary tank. It is essential that these locations be contacted before traveling because different suppliers carry different brands of equipment and all liquid systems are not compatible. Patients must also have a copy of their prescription available for these suppliers because the suppliers cannot legally provide O_2 without it.

Resources for the O_2 patient who wishes to travel are abundant. One such resource is the Web site *Breathin' Easy Travel Guide*, a comprehensive guide for O_2 suppliers and patients alike, and can be accessed at www.breathineasy.com/. The American Association for Respiratory Care developed this Internet Web site specifically for O_2 patients who travel.

Aerosol Therapy Devices

Many patients with chronic lung disease require inhaled medication therapy as part of the plan of treatment when they are discharged home. Several options are available: metered dose inhalers, dry-powder inhalers (DPIs), compressor nebulizers, and bland aerosol delivery devices.

Metered Dose Inhalers

The metered dose inhaler (MDI) is a cost-effective, convenient, and routinely prescribed method of inhaled medication delivery. Its small size and ease of use make it the preferred method. It is ideal for the patient who attends school, works, or is otherwise away from home and needs to use inhaled medicine.

Technique is important when using an inhaler. It is necessary for the patient to inhale slowly and actuate the MDI at the beginning of this inspiration. This can be a difficult skill for some patients to master, particularly for the patient who is extremely short of breath. Difficulty in actuating the inhaler, and rapid, shallow inspiration are common. A valved holding chamber can make it easier for the patient to get a proper dose and is particularly recommended for older adults and younger children, and when inhaled corticosteroids are used.[39]

Dry-Powder Inhalers

DPIs are a more recent development and are becoming more widely used. Instead of a liquid medication with a liquid propellant, a DPI is breath-actuated, wherein the powder is broken into small particles by the patient's inhalation.[40] The primary difficulty in using a DPI is that the patient must have adequate lung function to actuate the dose. Also, if a patient uses both types of inhaler, he or she must remember the proper breathing maneuvers for each.[41]

Compressor Nebulizers

When a patient is unable to use an MDI, a compressor nebulizer is a relatively inexpensive and simple way for the patient to self-administer inhaled medications. A compressor nebulizer is a small, oil-free machine that puts out an approximately 10-lpm flow to power medication nebulizers. A compressor nebulizer is usually powered by electricity, but battery-operated ones are also available at a substantially higher cost. Battery-operated compressors can be plugged into a cigarette lighter receptacle or run on their own internal battery. It is essential to check with the patient's medical insurance company to determine whether a battery-operated compressor nebulizer is a covered benefit, because many will not cover this item.

Bland Aerosol Therapy

Bland aerosol therapy is most frequently used with home care patients who have tracheostomies or laryngectomies for secretion control. This type of setup is composed of a large-volume nebulizer that is driven by an electrically powered high-output compressor. The aerosol is delivered through large-bore, usually disposable, tubing to a tracheostomy mask. It can be heated or room temperature.

Whereas large-volume nebulizers are powered by O_2 with room air entrainment in the hospital, O_2 is bled into the circuit at the outlet of the nebulizer in the home care setting because the hospital can run the nebulizer on O_2 at 15 lpm; the equipment needed to provide O_2 at 15 lpm in the home is much more difficult to provide. Setup and maintenance of a high-output compressor with a nebulizer are not difficult for the patient or caregiver; however, a primary focus should be on cleaning the equipment and infection control.

Airway Clearance Devices

Adjuncts to therapy for patients needing secretion control include airway clearance devices. The most commonly prescribed device for this purpose is an *aspirator*. This device is used for oral and endotracheal suction. The aspirator can be either an electrically powered, heavy-duty type that is usually kept at the patient's bedside, or a smaller, battery-operated version. The battery-operated aspirator is used most frequently for patients who leave home for school, work, and recreational activities. It is also used as a backup to the heavy-duty type in the event of a power failure and when airway clearance is a critical issue.

Patients and caregivers are taught to perform the suctioning procedure, which for the most part is done as it is in the acute care setting. Clean technique and reuse of the suction catheters are the primary differences in the way this procedure is done in the home.[42]

Another common airway clearance device used in home care is the mechanical percussor. Similar to those used in the acute care setting, this is an electrically powered alternative to manual percussion and vibration. The patient and caregivers are taught proper positioning techniques for optimal mobilization of secretions. A more recent development in vibratory clearance is a "vest" that resembles a life jacket and vibrates as the person wears it. It is ideally suited for patients with bronchiectasis and cystic fibrosis.[43]

Manual cough assist devices such as the *flutter valve* and *mechanical exsufflator*, and *positive expiratory pressure therapy*, are being used with increasing frequency in home care. Many patients are taught to use these devices while in the acute care setting, and their use is part of the discharge plan. The home care RT can evaluate the patient's technique and compliance during home visits and retrain as necessary.

Ventilatory Assist Devices

Major advancements in the technology of HME give us the ability to treat patients with chronic respiratory insufficiency, ventilatory failure, and other breathing disorders. These devices are made to be "user friendly," allowing the home care RT to train the patient and other lay personnel to care for the ventilator-assisted individual.

Intermittent Positive-Pressure Breathing

Although not used frequently, intermittent positive-pressure breathing has its place in home care. It is used to improve lung expansion in patients with ventilatory muscle weakness and to assist in clearing secretions when other methods fail to prove effective.[44] The chief problem with using intermittent positive-pressure breathing at home is that these devices usually need a 50-psi air source to power them. A high-output compressor can be used, but is noisy and quite large.

Continuous Positive Airway Pressure and Bilevel Therapy

Second to home O_2 therapy, continuous positive airway pressure (CPAP) and bilevel positive airway pressure therapy may be the next most common HME being used. It is used to treat obstructive sleep apnea, a condition wherein the patient's airway closes during sleep, causing snoring, O_2 deprivation, and sleep fragmentation. Patients with obstructive sleep apnea experience extreme daytime hypersomnolence, hypertension, and cardiac arrhythmias. It is estimated that the incidence of sleep apnea in the general population is as much as 10%, and undiagnosed and untreated sleep disorders constitute a pandemic.

CPAP therapy works by delivering pressurized airflow from a small blower at the bedside to a mask that the patient wears over the nose (and, infrequently, via a full-face mask). Figure 28-6 illustrates commonly used CPAP facial appliances. The air has been pressurized somewhere in the range of 5 to 15 cm H_2O or higher and acts as a "pneumatic splint," preventing the airway from closing off during sleep. Bilevel pressure therapy works the same way but gives the patient one pressure during inhalation and a lower pressure during exhalation. Bilevel pressure is useful when a patient has difficulty tolerating CPAP because it is easier to exhale. CPAP and bilevel therapy is the single most effective way to treat obstructive sleep apnea; surgical remedies, weight loss, oral appliances, and other methods have met with limited success.

The most difficult issue to be faced when CPAP or bilevel therapy is started with a patient is compliance. It takes a few weeks to adjust to the treatment, and many patients have difficulty tolerating a mask that is strapped onto the face. Proper mask fitting and patience are essential to ensuring the patient's success. Studies have reported improved compliance through the use of heated humidification inline.[45]

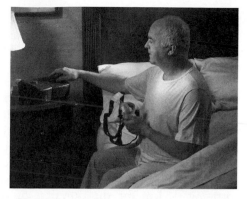

FIGURE 28-6 Continuous positive airway pressure machine and mask.

Home Mechanical Ventilation

The subject of home care would not be complete without a discussion of the management of patients using assisted ventilation. No longer are many of these patients kept in the hospital or long-term care facility. Although home ventilator care is complex, it is being done with increasing frequency. Proper patient selection, training, and follow-up care are essential to the success of a home ventilator program.[46,47] The reader is urged to refer to Chapter 22 of this book for comprehensive descriptions of mechanical ventilation performed in the United States and internationally.

Diagnostic and Monitoring Devices

Pulse Oximetry

Pulse oximeters are used routinely in the home care setting. They are used for oxygen saturation "spot checks," continuous monitoring in certain patients, and oxygen titration. Advances in technology have made them much easier to use, battery powered, and especially portable. Pulse oximetry must only be done by order of the patient's physician.[48]

As convenient as they are, pulse oximeters do have drawbacks. Readings can be inaccurate under certain conditions, and the RT and patient must be aware of those conditions. For example, poor perfusion at the probe site can cause lower than expected readings; this is encountered often with the elderly patient with cold hands or the patient with diabetes who has poor peripheral circulation. Warming the patient's hand or using an ear or forehead probe will result in more accurate readings

Excessive movement at the probe site can prevent the oximeter from working at all or can make the heart rate reading inaccurately high. Excessive ambient light interferes with the function of the sensor and so no reading will be taken; this is important to remember when trying to titrate a patient's ambulatory O_2 needs by taking them out for a walk on a sunny day. Low batteries can also give low readings.

One of the biggest drawbacks to home oximetry is the dependence the patient and family have on it. Patients may experience benign momentary changes in O_2 saturation that can throw patients and families into a panic. It is important that they understand that the oximetry readings are only a small part of the patient's medical picture and should be used in conjunction with other aspects of the patient's condition, such as heart rate, respiratory rate, and color. Another major drawback is that oximeters are seldom reimbursed by medical insurance payers.

Sleep-Recording Devices

It is now possible to perform a limited sleep study in the comfort of the patient's own bed. Portable sleep-recording devices are being used with increasing frequency to confirm a suspected diagnosis of obstructive sleep apnea. They present the patient with an alternative to the formal polysomnogram performed in a traditional sleep disorders center.

Portable sleep-recording devices usually measure airflow, snoring, O_2 saturation, heart rate, and body position. They do not record neurologic data and are not intended to diagnose other types of sleep disorders. Beyond that, automatically adjusting CPAP and bilevel devices are used to titrate pressure; some patients continue using autotitrating devices for the duration of their CPAP therapy.

REIMBURSEMENT ISSUES

This chapter has referred repeatedly to medical insurance and reimbursement issues and for good reason. A good home care program for a patient cannot be established without reimbursement for the equipment or services rendered. It is vital to establish which aspects of the patient's home care needs are reimbursable before initiation of these services. Patients and their families are seldom willing or able to accept the financial burden of HME and home care services. For example, on finding out that they do not qualify under Medicare's criteria for home O_2, many patients refuse the equipment if they have to pay for it themselves. Although a patient with severe obstructive sleep apnea needs a CPAP device, he or she may not want it if it turns out that medical equipment is not a benefit of his or her health insurance policy, even though his or her apnea is considered critical.

It is important for the referral source, the home care provider, and the patient to understand how reimbursement works. Managed care, Medicare, health maintenance organizations, preferred or participating providers—it can all be confusing, particularly to the beneficiaries, our patients.

Medicare

Medicare, a federally funded health insurance program, is probably the most commonly billed insurance company. Its beneficiaries include people aged 65 years and older and people who have been 100% medically disabled for 2 consecutive years. (This is why a 30-year-old quadriplegic patient undergoing mechanical ventilation can be covered by Medicare.) Medicare has two distinct parts: Part A, funded by payroll taxes, covers hospitalization, skilled nursing facility care, and home health and hospice care; Part B, a voluntary supplement to Part A paid in part by the beneficiary in monthly premiums, covers things such as doctors' services, outpatient clinical laboratory services, and HME.

Medicare has specific coverage guidelines for items such as O_2 equipment, hospital beds, and electric wheelchairs. It is important to understand that although the patient's physician orders a piece of equipment or a service for him or her, it does not mean that it is automatically covered by Medicare. Medicare does not cover some commonly used items, such as grab bars and other bathroom safety aids, at all.

Medicaid

Medicaid is a jointly funded federal and state medical assistance program for the economically disadvantaged. It serves low-income mothers and children for acute and ambulatory medical services; nonelderly disabled persons who use health insurance services and long-term care; and low-income elderly people who use it as a supplement to their Medicare benefits. As with Medicare, Medicaid has specific coverage guidelines, and it cannot be assumed that Medicaid will pay for something because the physician has ordered it.

Private Commercial Insurance

Private commercial health insurance is another source of reimbursement for home care services. Employers frequently provide it as part of their employee benefits package. Private insurance is also purchased individually by the consumer. In either case, the beneficiary pays premiums. Benefits and coverage vary widely among the different types of commercial insurance plans. Many follow Medicare's criteria for defining their coverage; however, policy coverage varies for each beneficiary, so it is essential to verify coverage before providing the service.

Managed Care

Managed care has drastically changed the way medical care is administered. Its primary objective is to control the cost of health care through rigorous management of the use of health care resources. Some managed care organizations provide services directly, whereas others enter into contracts with health care providers to obtain these services at greatly reduced rates.

Some require preauthorization, others require that the primary physician be the "gatekeeper" for all the services a patient needs. Managed care is, at the very least, complex, and the patient, the referral source, and the provider should contact the managed care organization to verify coverage issues.

Documentation of Medical Necessity

A prescription for equipment or services that are included as a benefit of a patient's health insurance plan does not automatically guarantee that it will be reimbursed. For example, a prescription stating "home O_2 at 2 lpm PRN shortness of breath" would not qualify for Medicare payment of home O_2 services although Medicare pays for home O_2. Third-party payers, especially Medicare, require justification that services are medically necessary and reasonable. Insurance carriers will only pay for the services the patient has been shown to medically need, not for what is convenient to the patient or family and not necessarily what the patient or physician may desire. Common requirements for documenting medical necessity are as follows:

- Diagnosis(es)
- Prognosis
- Length of need
- Height, weight
- Place of service
- Results of medical tests (e.g., sleep study, blood gas, or oximetry)
- Goals of treatment
- Other treatments tried that have been unsuccessful

The physician must be concise when writing a prescription or completing a certificate of medical necessity and should avoid ambiguous verbiage such as "PRN" or "for emergency use." Neither Medicare nor Medicaid will pay for medical equipment or services when prescribed in that manner. Instead, the specific use times, such as "during sleep" or "during exertion/exercise" should be indicated.

Obtaining reimbursement for home O_2 equipment is more complicated than for other types of home care equipment. Medicare has specific and rigid coverage criteria. They also require the patient's physician to complete a special certificate of medical necessity to document that the patient has met those criteria. Box 28-7 reviews Medicare's coverage criteria for home O_2.

BOX 28-7 | **Medicare Coverage Criteria for Home Oxygen**

A. Continuous long-term O_2 therapy when
   1. $Pao_2 \leq 55$ mm Hg or $Sao_2 \leq 88\%$, or
   2. Pao_2 56 to 59 mm Hg or Sao_2 89%, with
      a. Edema owing to congestive heart failure, or
      b. Evidence of pulmonary hypertension or cor pulmonale, or
      c. Elevated hematocrit, ≥ 56
   3. ABGs or Sao_2 by pulse oximetry obtained after optimal medical management
   4. ABGs or Sao_2 by pulse oximetry obtained either with the patient in a chronic stable state as an outpatient or within 2 days of discharge from an inpatient facility to home
   5. Repeat ABGs or pulse oximetry 3 months after initial certification when
      a. Initial $Pao_2 \geq 56$ mm Hg or Sao_2 89%, or
      b. The physician's initial estimated length of need was 1 to 3 months
   6. Certificate of medical necessity and prescription for O_2 therapy have been completed by the physician
   7. Revised certificate of medical necessity when the O_2 prescription changes (e.g., flow rate, hours of use, change in equipment)
B. O_2 with exercise when
   1. $Sao_2 \leq 88\%$ or $Pao_2 \leq 55$ mm Hg during exercise, while resting $Pao_2 \geq 56$ mm Hg or Sao_2 89% and
   2. Demonstration of improvement in hypoxemia that was evidenced when the patient exercised while breathing supplemental O_2
C. Nocturnal O_2 when
   1. $Sao_2 \leq 88\%$ or $Pao_2 \leq 56$ mm Hg evidenced during sleep, with $Sao_2 \geq 89\%$ or $Pao_2 \geq 56$ mm Hg during the day, or
   2. A decrease in $Pao_2 > 10$ mm Hg or desaturation of $>5\%$ associated with nocturnal restlessness, insomnia, or other physical or mental impairments attributable to nocturnal hypoxemia

ABGs, Arterial blood gases; O_2, oxygen; Pao_2, partial pressure of oxygen; Sao_2, arterial oxygen percent saturation.

Reimbursement for Respiratory Therapy Services

Much discussion has been given to the home care team and the professional services provided by the various professionals on the team. Medicare and most other insurers do provide nursing care as part of their covered benefits, as well as those of physical, occupational, and speech therapists. Social workers, home health aides, and other paid caregivers are reimbursed as well.

Unfortunately, however, services provided by RTs in the home are still not covered by Medicare or by many other insurance plans. Medicaid reimbursement for RTs varies by state, and services are often limited when they are covered. Managed care presents the greatest hope for the home care RT because medical equipment providers and home health agencies negotiate their services into contracts with individual managed care plans. Despite the lack of reimbursement for RTs, most HME providers have them on staff to work with and monitor their pulmonary patients.

CONCLUSION

The need for home care services in the immediate and long-term future is not expected to diminish. Rather, as previously stated, our aging population will actually spur home care services to even greater utilization levels than ever before. Moreover, it is inevitable that technological advances will add yet another impetus to home care, as procedures and techniques once thought to be the exclusive domain of the hospital are now considered commonplace for in-home application.

However, reimbursement issues will continue to be the primary challenge facing home care providers, those prescribing home care services, and ultimately those receiving home care services. In this regard, it will be essential that archaic and nonsensical coverage–payment guidelines be abandoned and replaced with reimbursement strategies that accurately reflect the complexity and related expense of appropriately prescribed and provided home care services. The irony is that "appropriately prescribed and provided home care services" represents a significant and proven cost-effective alternative to more costly institutional care. And, home care has repeatedly been identified by consumers as being preferable to institutional care.

Public and private health care policy makers can no longer ignore the tremendous benefits and value that high-quality home care can offer the nation's beleaguered health care system. Our aging population is staring them right in the face; they themselves are part of our aging population. The cost of caring for all of us as we age would be crippling without home care.

References

1. Hoyert D, Heron M, Murphy S et al: Deaths: final data for 2003, Hyattsville, Md, 2003, National Center for Health Statistics, Centers for Disease Control and Prevention, U.S. Department of Health and Human Services.
2. National Center for Health Statistics: Fast stats A to Z; chronic obstructive pulmonary disease, data for the year 2003, Hyattsville, Md, 2003, Centers for Disease Control and Prevention, U.S. Department of Health and Human Services. Available at www.cdc.gov/nchs/fastats/copd.htm. Retrieved October 2007.
3. U.S. Census Bureau News: Dramatic Changes in U.S. aging highlighted in new census: NIH report, Hyattsville, Md, 2006, Centers for Disease Control, U.S. Department of Health and Human Services.
4. Centers for Disease Control and Prevention: Health, United States, 2005, with chartbook on trends in the health of Americans, Hyattsville, Md, 2005, Centers for Disease Control and Prevention, U.S. Department of Health and Human Services.
5. Federal Interagency Forum on Aging-Related Statistics: Older Americans 2004: key indicators of well-being, Washington DC, 2004, U.S. Government Printing Office.
6. Garland A, Dawson N, Altmann I et al: Outcomes up to 5 years after severe, acute respiratory failure, Chest 126:1897-1904, 2004.
7. Leff B, Burton L, Mader S et al: Hospital at home: feasibility and outcomes of a program to provide hospital-level care at home for acutely ill older patients, Ann Intern Med 143:798-808, 2005.
8. Ram F, Wedzicha J, Wright J et al: Hospital at home for patients with acute exacerbations of chronic obstructive pulmonary disease: systematic review of evidence, BMJ 329:315, 2004.
9. Spratt G, Petty T: Partnering for optimal respiratory home care: physicians working with respiratory therapists to optimally meet respiratory home care needs, Respir Care 46:475-488, 2001.
10. Make B: Chronic obstructive pulmonary disease: developing comprehensive management, Respir Care 48:1225-1237, 2003.
11. National Center for Health Statistics: Home health care patients: data from the 2000 National Home Care and Hospice Survey, Hyattsville, Md, 2004, Centers for Disease Control and Prevention, U.S. Department of Health and Human Services.
12. Caples S, Gami A, Somers V: Obstructive sleep apnea, Ann Intern Med 142:187-197, 2005.
13. Respiratory Home Care Focus Group: AARC clinical practice guideline: discharge planning for the respiratory care patient, Respir Care 40:1308-1312, 1995.
14. Hoisington E, Miller D, Adams C et al: Impact of a program to provide patients with comparative information about providers of durable medical equipment for home respiratory care, Respir Care 49:1309-1315, 2004.
15. Malloy N: Home care 101: tips for ensuring properly trained HME delivery personnel, Adv Manage Respir Care November:26, 1998.
16. American Association for Respiratory Care: Position statement on home respiratory care services, Irving, Tex, 2000, American Association for Respiratory Care.
17. McInturff SL: Proceed with caution, Adv Manage Respir Care 1999; October:24.

18. Lenfant C, Khaltaev N et al: Global strategy for the diagnosis, management, and prevention of chronic obstructive pulmonary disease, executive summary, Bethesda, Md, 2005, National Heart, Lung, and Blood Institute and Geneva, Switzerland, World Health Organization.

19. Marlow S, Stoller J: Smoking cessation, Respir Care 48:1238-1254, 2003.

20. Harper SA, Fukuda K, Uyeki TM et al: Advisory Committee on Immunization Practices (ACIP), Centers for Disease Control and Prevention (CDC): Prevention and control of influenza: recommendations of the Advisory Committee on Immunization Practices (ACIP), MMWR Recomm Rep 54(RR-8):1-40, 2005.

21. Peters J: Nutritional assessment of patients with respiratory disease. In Wilkins R, Krider S, Sheldon R, editors: Clinical assessment in respiratory care, ed 4, St. Louis, 2000, Mosby.

22. Larsen PD, Hazen SE, Hoot Martin JL: Assessment and management of sensory loss in elderly patients, AORN J 65:432, 1997.

23. Salmen J: The do-able renewable home: making your home fit your needs, Washington DC, 1985, Consumer Affairs, Program Department, American Association of Retired Persons.

24. U.S. Consumer Product Safety Commission: Safety for older consumers home safety checklist (document 701), Washington DC, Office of Information and Public Affairs.

25. McInturff S: Assessment of the home care patient. In Wilkins R, Krider S, Sheldon R, editors: Clinical assessment in respiratory care, ed 4, St. Louis, 2000, Mosby.

26. Tangalos E, Bignotti D, Evans J et al: Geriatric patient reference guide, ed 7, American Board of Family Practice, MDchoice.com, 2006.

27. Lim J, Zebrack B: Caring for family members with chronic physical illness: a critical review of caregiver literature. Health Quality Life Outcomes 2:50, 2004.

28. Koens J: Respiratory report card: acuity scoring for home oxygen care scores one for patient assessment, Adv Manage Respir Care 5:63, 1999.

29. Dunne PJ, McInturff SL: The home visit. In Dunne PJ, McInturff SL, editors: Respiratory home care: the essentials, Philadelphia, 1998, FA, Davis.

30. Gourley D: Care planning, AARC Home Care Bull March/April:3, 1999.

31. Belda T: Computers in patient education and monitoring, Respir Care 49:480-487, 2004.

32. Criner G: Effects of long-term oxygen therapy on mortality and morbidity, Respir Care 45:105-118, 2000.

33. Cuvelier A, Nuir J, Chakroun N et al: Refillable oxygen cylinders may be an alternative for ambulatory oxygen therapy in COPD, Chest 122:451-456, 2002.

34. McInturff SL, O'Donohue WJ: Respiratory care in the home and alternate sites. In Burton GC, Hodgkin JE, Ward JJ, editors: Respiratory care: a guide to clinical practice, ed 4, Philadelphia, 1997, Lippincott.

35. McCoy R: Oxygen-conserving techniques and devices, Respir Care 45:95-103, 2000.

36. Sclafani J: Pulse oxygen delivery systems: which system is best for which patient? AARC Times October:12, 1998.

37. Gong H: Advising pulmonary patients about commercial air travel, J Respir Dis 2:484, 1990.

38. Stoller J: Patient information: supplemental oxygen on commercial air carriers. In Rose BD, editor: UpToDate [Internet], version 14.1, Wellesley, Mass, 2006, UpToDate. Available at www.uptodate.com. Retrieved October 2007.

39. National Asthma Education and Prevention Program: Expert Panel Report 3 (EPR-3): Guidelines for the Diagnosis and Management of Asthma-Summary Report 2007, J Allergy Clin Immunol 120:S94-S138, 2007.

40. Geller D: Comparing clinical features of the nebulizer, metered-does inhaler, and dry powder inhaler, Respir Care 50:1313-1321, 2005.

41. Hess D: Metered dose inhalers and dry powder inhalers in aerosol therapy, Respir Care 50:1376-1383, 2005.

42. Home Care Focus Group: AARC clinical practice guideline: suctioning of the patient in the home care setting, Respir Care 1:99, 1999.

43. Wagener J, Headley A: Cystic fibrosis: current trends in respiratory care, Respir Care 48:234-245, 2003.

44. Aerosol Therapy Guidelines Committee: Clinical practice guideline: intermittent positive pressure breathing—2003 revision and update, Respir Care 48:540-546, 2003.

45. Neill A, Wai H, Bannan S et al: Humidified nasal continuous positive airway pressure in obstructive sleep apnoea, Eur Respir J 22:258-262, 2003.

46. Make BJ, Hill NS, Goldberg Al et al: Mechanical ventilation beyond the intensive care unit, Chest 5:289s, 1998.

47. Home Care Focus Group: AARC clinical practice guideline: invasive mechanical ventilation in the home, Respir Care 40:1313, 1995.

48. Bartow S: Home care oximetry: a practice under scrutiny, AARC Times 24:51-55, 2000.

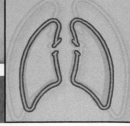

Chapter 29

Travel for the Patient with Respiratory Disease

BRUCE P. KRIEGER*

CHAPTER OUTLINE

Effects of Hypobaric Hypoxia
Physiology
**Acute Pulmonocardiac Responses
to Hypobaric Hypoxia**
Healthy Individuals
Patients with Pulmonary Disease
Effect of Hypobaric Hypoxia on Sleep
Air Travel
Aircraft Cabin Conditions
In-flight Medical Incidents
Medical Evaluation Before Flying

Planning Air Travel for Patients
with Pulmonary Disease
Medicolegal Aspects of Traveling
with Medical Equipment
**Travel at Sea Level for the Technology-
Dependent Patient with Pulmonary
Disease**
Cruise Ships
Travel by Private Auto
Travel by Bus and Rail
**Traveling with Advanced Medical
Technology**

PROFESSIONAL SKILLS

On completion of this chapter, the reader will be able to do
the following:

♦ Describe the cause of altitude-related hypoxemia
♦ Evaluate whether patients will require supplemental oxygen (O_2) when they fly
♦ Prepare a plan to help technology-dependent patients travel safely

Air and sea travel has expanded from a relatively exclusive few to more than 500 million domestic airline passengers and millions more enjoying luxury cruises throughout the world.[1] These passengers include individuals with chronic pulmonary disease, many of whom require special equipment such as medications, supplemental oxygen (O_2), and mechanical ventilators. As one O_2-dependent patient remarked, being tethered to a tank need not be the same as being chained to an anchor.[2] Advances in technology, such as lightweight O_2 systems and portable mechanical ventilators, have allowed patients more freedom to experience meaningful trips. O_2 concentrators and mechanical ventilators are now portable enough to fit in staterooms and hotel rooms.[3] Coupled with these advances in technology, pulmonary rehabilitation programs have emphasized the goal of maintaining as normal a life pattern as possible,[4] including traveling for leisure and business.

Travel for the technology-dependent patient with pulmonary disease can pose vexing problems. Airline travel requires exposure to a physiologically

*I greatly appreciate the financial support of the Bertha Abess
Pulmonary Research Fund.

hostile environment because of the occurrence of hypobaric hypoxia and other adverse environmental changes.[1] Therefore the travel industry has had to adapt to passenger needs within the restraint that their prime concern is to provide safe transportation for the public while maintaining a high standard of service that is economically feasible.[5] This chapter explores the physiologic effects of hypobaric hypoxia on healthy individuals and on those with cardiopulmonary disease. It emphasizes the pretravel evaluation of the traveler and provides recommendations on how to procure appropriate medical needs during travel.

EFFECTS OF HYPOBARIC HYPOXIA

Physiology

Travel by commercial aircraft poses complex problems for the patient with pulmonary or cardiopulmonary disease because of the occurrence of hypobaric hypoxia in flight. The etiology of hypobaric hypoxia is best understood by a review of the alveolar gas equation (Box 29-1).[6] Alveolar partial

pressure of oxygen (P_{AO_2}) is directly related to barometric pressure (P_B). P_{AO_2} determines arterial partial pressure of oxygen (P_{aO_2}) based on the alveolar minus arterial gradient $[P(A - a)O_2]$ for the patient. Subjects with pulmonary disease frequently have widened $P(A - a)O_2$ gradients, resulting in abnormal O_2 tension. At an altitude of 8000 feet, which is equivalent to Sun Valley, Idaho,[7] or the lowest P_B allowed in a commercial aircraft (564 mm Hg), the P_{aO_2} in healthy individuals is approximately 60 mm Hg, which corresponds to an arterial oxygen percent saturation (S_{aO_2}) of approximately 90% (Figure 29-1). However, in a patient with a $P(A - a)O_2$ gradient of 20 mm Hg, the P_{aO_2} is predicted to be approximately 50 mm Hg, with a corresponding S_{aO_2} of 85%. It is in this range of the oxyhemoglobin dissociation curve that small changes in P_{aO_2} can translate to significant decreases in S_{aO_2} and therefore oxygen delivery ($\dot{D}_{O_2}$) (Box 29-2).

The ceiling of air under which we reside at sea level is equal to 1 atm absolute, which is equivalent to 760 mm Hg or 14.70 psi. As altitude increases, P_B decreases, which results in lower partial pressure of inspired oxygen (P_{IO_2}). For each 1000 feet of elevation, P_{IO_2} decreases by approximately 5 mm Hg.[8] Table 29-1 displays the gas pressures under hypobaric conditions for altitudes that are encountered by the traveling public. For example, in-cabin altitude is usually maintained between 5000 and 8000 feet, whereas visitors to Santa Fe, New Mexico, are exposed to an altitude of 10,000 feet. Other commonly visited destinations that are at moderate or high

BOX 29-1	Alveolar Gas Equation

$$P_{AO_2} = (P_B - PH_2O)F_{IO_2} - (P_{aCO_2}/R)$$

F_{IO_2}, *Fraction (%) of inspired oxygen (O_2); P_{aCO_2}, arterial partial pressure of carbon dioxide (in millimeters of mercury); P_{AO_2}, alveolar partial pressure of oxygen (in millimeters of mercury); P_B, barometric pressure; PH_2O, water vapor tension (47 mm Hg); R, respiratory exchange coefficient (carbon dioxide production/oxygen consumption).*

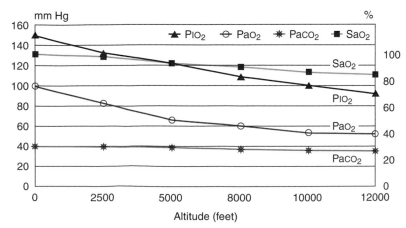

FIGURE 29-1 Arterial gas tensions at increasing altitude. Partial pressure of inspired oxygen (P_{IO_2}), arterial partial pressure of oxygen (P_{aO_2}), and arterial partial pressure of carbon dioxide (P_{aCO_2}) are measured in millimeters of mercury (vertical axis on the left). Arterial oxygen percent saturation (S_{aO_2}) is depicted as a percentage (vertical axis on the right).

BOX 29-2 $\dot{D}o_2$ Equation

$$\dot{D}o_2 = CO \times CaO_2$$

$\dot{D}o_2$, *Oxygen (O_2) delivery; CO, cardiac output (heart rate × stroke volume); CaO_2, arterial oxygen content (Hgb × 1.34 × SaO_2 + [0.0031][PaO_2]); Hgb, hemoglobin (in grams %); SaO_2, arterial oxygen percent saturation; PaO_2, arterial partial pressure of oxygen (in millimeters of mercury).*

---

altitudes are depicted in Figure 29-2. At the ultimate altitude obtainable by human beings while breathing ambient air (Mount Everest), the PIO_2 is only approximately one third that of sea level, resulting in a PIO_2 of 43 mm Hg and a PaO_2 of

---

TABLE 29-1   Gas Pressures Under Hypobaric Conditions

Altitude (ft)	ATA	psi	B_P	PIO_2
		AMBIENT PRESSURE		
0	1	14.70	760	150
5,000	0.83	12.19	630	122
6,000	0.80	11.76	608	118
8,000	0.74	10.91	564	109
10,000	0.69	10.12	523	100
12,000	0.64	9.34	483	92

ATA, *Atmosphere absolute;* B_P, *barometric pressure (in milliliters of mercury);* PIO_2, *partial pressure of inspired oxygen (in milliliters of mercury) corrected for water pressure (47 mm Hg); psi, pounds per square inch.*
Adapted from Hultgren H: High altitude medicine, Stanford, Calif, 1997, Hultgren Publications, Section 3, p 9; and de la Hoz RE, Krieger BP: Dysbarism. In Rom WN, editor: Environmental and occupational medicine, ed 3, Philadelphia, 1998, Lippincott-Raven, pp 1359-1375.

---

28 mm Hg, which corresponds to an SaO_2 of 70% despite extreme hypocarbia (end-tidal carbon dioxide (CO_2), 7.5 mm Hg).[9]

At moderate or high elevations, the inspired gas density is decreased, which is thought to be the reason for the improved midexpiratory flow rates that have been reported at altitude.[10] Associated with the decreased gas density, however, is the possibility of expansion of enclosed gases according to Boyle's law (P × V = K, where P = pressure, V = volume, and K = constant). At 5000 feet, an enclosed gas volume is estimated to be approximately 20% greater than at sea level, whereas at 8000 feet, an approximately 40% expansion occurs. A patient with a giant intrapulmonary bronchogenic cyst experienced a fatal air embolus on a commercial aircraft.[11] The authors hypothesized that the cyst enlarged and ruptured as predicted by Boyle's law, which allowed air to enter the systemic circulation. Although barotrauma in commercial aviation records is rare, other cases of air embolism and pneumothoraces have been reported.[12,13]

ACUTE PULMONOCARDIAC RESPONSES TO HYPOBARIC HYPOXIA

Healthy Individuals

Although "hypoxia" and "hypoxemia" are often used interchangeably, in physiologic terms they are distinctly different.[14,15] Understanding this distinction is integral to comprehending how individuals acutely adapt to hypobaric hypoxia. *Hypoxemia* is defined as a decrease in the oxygenation of blood as measured by PaO_2 or as SaO_2, whereas *hypoxia* is

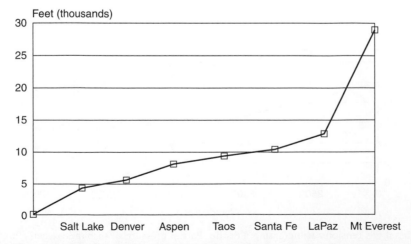

FIGURE 29-2 Altitudes of popular travel destinations. The in-cabin barometric pressure on commercial aircraft is the equivalent of that between Denver and Aspen's altitude (5000 to 8000 feet).

defined as a decrease in Do_2 to the tissues. Therefore hypoxemia can occur without hypoxia (such as at moderate to high altitude) if an appropriate cardiac response to desaturated blood occurs. As can be seen in the Do_2 equation (see Box 29-2), a decrease in Sao_2 will result in a decrease in arterial O_2 content. However, Do_2 can be maintained by a compensatory increase in cardiac output (CO).

As the Pao_2 decreases to less than 60 mm Hg, the peripheral hypoxemia-mediated chemoreceptors in the carotid bodies are stimulated, which results in hyperventilation.[16-18] The increase in minute ventilation is caused more by an increase in tidal volume than by changes in breathing frequency.[19] This results in hypocarbia and respiratory alkalosis, which may partially suppress the hypoxic drive,[10,16] but also results in an elevation in Pao_2 and therefore Pao_2. In addition, the $P(A - a)o_2$ gradient is narrowed, even in patients with chronic obstructive pulmonary disease (COPD).[19,20]

The acute ventilatory response to hypobaric hypoxia has been shown to be blunted by the ingestion of alcoholic beverages. Roeggla and colleagues[21] demonstrated that when healthy individuals ingested the equivalent of 1 L of beer, no significant changes in Pao_2 or $Paco_2$ occurred at an altitude of 5061 feet. However, when the same amount of alcohol was consumed at 9840 feet in these 10 volunteers, the median Pao_2 decreased from 69.0 to 64.0 mm Hg (P <.01) and the median $Paco_2$ increased from 32.5 to 34.0 mm Hg (P <.01). This blunted response to the acute effects of hypobaric hypoxia is similar to what has been reported when individuals ingested diazepam.[21] Although this may not be deleterious in healthy individuals, patients with diseases that lower their baseline oxygenation may be more severely affected.

When hyperventilation becomes inadequate in preventing further decrements in Sao_2 and arterial O_2 content, the cardiovascular system responds by increasing CO. The increase in CO offsets the decrease in arterial O_2 content, and $\dot{D}o_2$ is preserved. An early study[22] performed under isocarbic conditions ascribed the hypoxemia-induced increase in CO to reflexive tachycardia without an associated increase in stroke volume. However, a study done in our laboratory[23] under hypoxic, hypocarbic conditions, using noninvasive measurements of stroke volume, CO, tidal volume, and Sao_2, showed statistically significant increases in heart rate, stroke volume, and CO in 10 healthy men subjected to lower concentrations of inspired O_2.

Patients with Pulmonary Disease

A few investigators have studied how outpatients with COPD acutely adapt to altitude. Graham and Houston[19] exposed men with nonhypoxemic COPD who had a mean forced expiratory volume in 1 second (FEV_1)/forced vital capacity (FVC) ratio of 43% and a mean FEV_1 of 1.27 L to an altitude equivalent to 8000 feet at rest and during exercise and compared the changes with the same degree of activity at sea level (Figure 29-3). Subjectively, the patients complained of mild fatigue and insomnia. Although the minute ventilation at rest did not change between sea level and altitude, it was significantly increased during exercise at altitude (17% higher, P <.05). Pao_2 was significantly lower at altitude, but this reached statistical significance only with exercise. Interestingly, the $P(A - a)o_2$ gradient

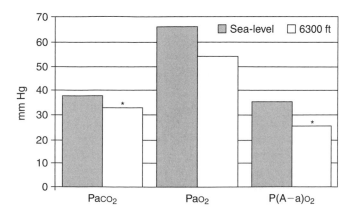

FIGURE 29-3 Arterial blood gas values at rest and at 6300 feet in eight patients with COPD. *P < .05 compared with measurements at sea level. $Paco_2$, arterial partial pressure of carbon dioxide; Pao_2, arterial partial pressure of oxygen; $P(A - a)o_2$, alveolar minus arterial oxygen gradient.

narrowed at altitude because of hypocarbia. Respiratory rate, pulse rate, and dead space ratio (dead space volume/tidal volume) did not change significantly at rest or with exercise at altitude. Dyspnea was not a major complaint even when patients with COPD had a PaO_2 as low as 40 mm Hg.[20,24] One explanation for this lack of dyspnea may be adaptation by these subjects to hypoxemia that they regularly experience at sea level, especially during sleep.

The cardiovascular responses to altitude noted by Graham and Houston[19] were similar to those in a study performed by Berg and colleagues.[25] They exposed 18 men with nonhypoxemic COPD (mean PaO_2, 72 mm Hg; mean FEV_1, 0.97 L) to the equivalent of 8000 feet, which resulted in a mean PaO_2 at altitude of 47 mm Hg. No significant changes between sea level and altitude were noted for arterial pressure, heart rate, cardiac ectopy, or pulsus paradox until supplemental O_2 was administered at altitude. After O_2 was begun, pulse pressure diminished, blood pressure declined, and pulsus paradox was reduced. It was hypothesized that the administration of O_2 resulted in decreased intrathoracic pressure swings because of a decrease in work of breathing. However, no measurements of oxygenation were recorded in the study to compare with the work of Graham and Houston. Other studies have also noted that patients report that it "is easier to breathe" at altitude, perhaps because of reduced gas density.[26]

Hypoxemia causes an acute increase in pulmonary arterial pressure mainly because of precapillary vasoconstriction,[27] although the compensatory increase in CO also contributes slightly. This response is not lost in patients with primary pulmonary hypertension.[28] Therefore in patients with significant pulmonary hypertension, ascent to even moderate altitudes may result in an increase in pulmonary vascular resistance resulting in acute right heart strain, which could be fatal. In addition, the rise in pulmonary arterial pressure may suddenly open a patent foramen ovale, resulting in worsening hypoxemia owing to an acute right-to-left shunt.[29,30]

Theoretically, hypobaric-induced hypoxemia and the associated hyperventilation and compensatory increase in CO could predispose susceptible persons to myocardial ischemia. However, a study of almost 100 visitors (mean age, 70 years) to Vail, Colorado (8200 feet), showed no electrocardiographic signs of myocardial ischemia.[31] Even so, travelers who have a predisposition to cardiac dysrhythmias may experience an increase in their arrhythmia when at moderate altitude.[32]

EFFECT OF HYPOBARIC HYPOXIA ON SLEEP

Cheyne-Stokes respirations were noted by climbers in the 19th century at altitudes less than 12,000 ft.[33] Cheyne-Stokes respiration consists of a progressive and repetitive crescendo-decrescendo pattern of breathing in which hyperpnea and tachypnea is followed by bradypnea, hypopnea, and usually short apneas. This cycle then repeats throughout the night.[34] During the hyperventilatory phase of Cheyne-Stokes respirations, pulse oximetry recordings show a decrease in O_2 saturation. This nocturnal desaturation is thought to be the underlying mechanism for acute mountain sickness, which is experienced by 25% of travelers to moderate altitudes.[35] Acetazolamide moderates the O_2 desaturation during periodic breathing by inducing a metabolic acidosis and compensatory hyperventilation.[36] Acetazolamide has been recommended to prevent acute mountain sickness when traveling to altitudes of 8000 feet or higher.[37,38] Alternative prophylactic agents include dexamethasone, long-acting theophylline, or ginkgo biloba.

AIR TRAVEL

Aircraft Cabin Conditions

A common misconception by the general public and health care personnel is that commercial aircraft cabins are pressurized to sea level.[16,18,20,39-41] In actuality, aircraft cabins are maintained at a pressure relative to the aircraft's altitude, which can range from 20,000 to 40,000 feet. Cabin pressure is regulated by a series of outlet valves that maintain the cabin pressure between 7.5 and 8.7 psi greater than the outside environment; the exact pressure differential differs for each type of aircraft. For example, the differential in an L-1011 aircraft between the ambient pressure and the cabin is approximately 8.4 psi.[8] At an altitude of 40,000 feet, the outside P_B is 2.72 psi (140 mm Hg).[39] Therefore the cabin pressure would be equivalent to 11.12 psi (8.4 + 2.72), which equals approximately 575 mm Hg or the equivalent altitude of Aspen, Colorado (see Figure 29-2). At this altitude, the PIO_2 is approximately 110 mm Hg (see Figure 29-1), which corresponds to a PaO_2 in healthy individuals of approximately 60 mm Hg.

In a comparison of 204 commercial aircraft, Cottrell[8] calculated the median cabin altitude to be 6214 feet, with a range up to 8915 feet. During the study, cruising altitude ranged from 10,000 to 60,000 feet, with higher altitudes (mean, 7004 feet) being obtained for older aircraft compared with newer planes (mean, 5280 feet). The largest cabin-atmospheric differential was obtained by the (retired) supersonic Concord (10.7 psi), which is necessary because of the craft's high cruising altitude (> 40,000 feet). According to Federal Aviation Administration (FAA) requirements, the cabin altitude pressure is required to be maintained at less than 8000 feet unless temporary diversions are required to avoid inclement weather.[18] As noted earlier in the section describing adaptations to hypobaric hypoxia, the resistance to airflow at altitude is slightly decreased, thus resulting in an increase in peak expiratory flow rate.[10] However, other conditions that are unique to airline cabins may worsen the status of patients with pulmonary disease.[15,42] Cabin humidity and temperature are usually low, which may result in the drying of secretions and the ineffective expectoration of sputum. In addition, if a flight allows cigarette smoking, carbon monoxide will be recirculated,[43] which may worsen O_2 desaturation in patients who are on the steep portion of the oxyhemoglobin dissociation curve.[17] Boyle's law[44] predicts that hyperinflation may worsen at altitude in patients with bullous lung disease if they have areas with extremely prolonged time constant (resistance × compliance). If a bulla overexpands, this could compromise lung function by encroaching on adjacent lung tissue[45] and by causing hyperinflation and worsening diaphragmatic function.[46]

Newer aircraft recirculate more in-cabin air as a means of saving fuel. Although not unique to the patient with pulmonary disease, this enclosed environment can promote exposure to aerosolized pathogens such as atypical bacteria, viruses, and granulomatous organisms. A case report of multidrug-resistant *Mycobacterium tuberculosis* being transmitted to passengers and crew during a long international flight has been well documented.[47]

Another factor to consider on airplane flights is the prolonged immobilization of the patient. This increases the risk for developing deep venous thrombosis and subsequently pulmonary thromboembolic disease.[48,49] Cases of pulmonary embolism have been reported both on disembarkation and a few days after long trips. This is especially important in the traveling patient with pulmonary disease, who may be predisposed to hypercoagulability because of older age and underlying chronic disease states. However, hypobaric hypoxia does not appear to be prothrombotic as demonstrated in healthy subjects who underwent simulated prolonged air travel in a hypobaric chamber.[50] A report of sudden death occurring during airline flights noted that 18% were caused by pulmonary thromboembolic disease.[48] Women who had a history of deep venous thrombosis and were older than 40 years were at higher risk.[48] Relative to the number of air travelers, the incidence of pulmonary embolism is low. The frequency of pulmonary embolism is relative to the distance traveled: 0.01 case per million flyers when the distance is less than 3100 miles; 1.5 cases per million when more than 3100 miles; and 4.8 cases per million when flying more than 6,200 miles.[51]

In-flight Medical Incidents

Because airlines are only required to report in-flight deaths, the reported numbers of in-flight medical emergencies probably represent an underestimation.[52] Statistics from the Seattle-Tacoma Airport indicate that the frequency of medical occurrences were 1 per 39,600 inbound passengers,[53] whereas foreign carriers reported an incident of 1 per 13,000 to 21,000 passengers.[54] However, for patients who have disabilities that were reported to the airlines preflight, the incidence of a medical occurrence during flight was 1 per 350 passengers.[54] Although the incidence seems low, it translates into at least two emergency calls per day from inbound flights to the Seattle-Tacoma Airport and an estimated incidence of 3000 in-flight medical emergencies annually on domestic airlines.[55]

The most common respiratory complaint encountered in flight is dyspnea. As expected, this is more frequent in passengers with known obstructive lung disease.[55] However, cardiovascular, neurologic, and gastrointestinal tract complaints are more common than respiratory complaints according to reported statistics.[18,54-57] The most frequent cause of death reported on commercial aircraft is cardiac, and frequently the afflicted passenger has no known pre-existing conditions. The estimated incidence of this is 1 per 3 million to 10 million passengers.[52,54]

Medical Evaluation Before Flying

Although respiratory complaints are only the fourth leading cause of medical incidents in flight, pulmonary diseases are the most common reason for preflight medical evaluations.[15] In one study of 233 passengers referred to a major domestic airline's private advisory service for pre-flight clearance during a 3-month period in 1991,[18] two thirds of the diagnoses were of a pulmonary nature, including COPD (39%), lung cancer (7%), pre—lung transplantation (2%), and other respiratory diagnoses (20%). Before mobilized jetways were used to board and disembark from commercial aircraft, the routine way of determining whether a patient was medically cleared to fly was whether he or she could walk up the set of stairs to the aircraft's entrance way.[40,58] Since then, multiple physiologic and clinical parameters have been evaluated to assess passengers' fitness to fly, including the presence of hypoxemia or hypercarbia, dyspnea on minimal exertion, abnormal pulmonary function tests, pulmonary hypertension, or unstable cardiac conditions.[5,24] With the recognition that hypobaric hypoxia is the major physiologic stress while flying, attention has focused on being able to predict in-flight oxygenation.[8,15,58] Therefore the most pragmatic recommendation concerning who should be evaluated before commercial airline flight is to screen patients who have a predicted PaO_2 of less than 50 mm Hg at altitude (5000 to 8000 feet).[18,24,59-61] For an ambulatory patient with COPD who is not hypercarbic, a PaO_2 greater than or equal to 72 mm Hg recorded at sea level should be adequate to safely fly in commercial aircraft.[59] However, complicating conditions such as cardiac disease, anemia, active bronchospasm, pulmonary hypertension, or bullous lung disease may compromise patients with COPD even if the PaO_2 is 72 mm Hg or higher.[15] In addition, patients with active sinusitis or otitis media may not be able to equilibrate their inner ear and be distressed because of this.[44] A more dangerous situation occurs in patients who have recently undergone abdominal surgery because of the possibility of wound dehiscence owing to expansion of gas within the gastrointestinal tract, as predicted by Boyle's law.[5,44] Similarly, patients who have had thoracic surgery or a pneumothorax within 3 weeks may be at risk when flying.[5]

Since the early 1980s, various studies have made efforts to predict in-flight oxygenation. One of the first studies to measure the PaO_2 during flight was undertaken by Schwartz, Bencowitz, and Moser.[20] In this study, 13 patients with COPD had arterial blood gases measured at rest at sea level and then again while flying in an unpressurized cabin at 5412 and 7380 ft. In addition, they were exposed to a 17.2% O_2 mixture at rest and with light exercise at sea level. All the patients had an FEV_1/FVC ratio less than or equal to 50% and no evidence of restrictive lung disease, ischemic heart disease, or cerebral vascular disease. They all had PaO_2 values greater than or equal to 55 mm Hg at rest while on room air at sea level. This study found that the patients' PaO_2 decreased from 68.0 ± 0.3 mm Hg (mean ± 1 SD) to 51.0 ± 9.1 mm Hg at 5412 ft and further declined to 44.7 ± 8.7 mm Hg at 7380 feet. There was only a weak correlation between the PaO_2 measured a few weeks before the flight at sea level and the in-flight PaO_2, whereas a PaO_2 measured within 2 hours of flight had a better predictive value for estimating the in-flight PaO_2. The part of the study in which the patients breathed a fraction of inspired oxygen (FIO_2) of 17.2% showed a strong correlation with in-flight PaO_2 at 5412 ft (52.5 ± 9.6 vs. 51.0 ± 9.1 mm Hg). In a subsequent letter to the editor,[62] the same authors recommended that breathing an FIO_2 of 15% O_2 at sea level would predict in-flight oxygenation at a cabin altitude of 8000 ft.

During the same year that Schwartz, Bencowitz, and Moser[20] published their data on unpressurized in-flight oxygenation, Gong[24] proposed the acronym "hypoxia—altitude simulation test" (HAST) to describe the use of hypoxic gas mixtures to predict oxygenation at altitude.[59] This acronym has subsequently been termed the "high-altitude simulation test" to better describe its purpose to patients and their families.[15] The HAST is relatively easy to perform and requires only a premixed hypoxic (O_2 plus nitrogen) gas mixture (or an O_2 blender), a pulse oximeter (or arterial blood gas analyzer), an electrocardiogram, and a mouthpiece with a noseclip (or a tight-fitting mask with the least amount of dead space possible). By using lower concentrations of O_2 (Table 29-2), hypobaric hypoxia is simulated. As originally described, steady state conditions were assumed to be attained within 15 minutes, at which time the

TABLE 29-2   **High-Altitude Simulation Test**

	SIMULATED ALTITUDE	
Feet	Meters	FIO_2 (%)
0	0	20.9
5,000	1524	17.1
8,000	2438	15.1
10,000	3048	13.9

FIO_2, *Fraction of inspired oxygen.*

patient was asked to walk in place to simulate having to ambulate around the cabin of an aircraft.[15,20,59] Confirmation of the accuracy of the HAST was provided by a group from Australia, who measured oxygenation in a hypobaric chamber and with the HAST.[63] They found that the HAST accurately predicted hypobaric hypoxemia at altitudes of 6000 and 8000 ft and that steady state conditions were met within 5 minutes both in healthy individuals and in patients with COPD. They also noted a significant reduction in Pa_{O_2} with light exercise, thus confirming the need for simulated walking during the HAST. However, the HAST does not reproduce the other in-cabin changes that occur at altitude such as the lower air density, lower P_B, and reduced humidity.[15]

Other investigators have developed regression equations to predict Pa_{O_2} at altitude by evaluating patients with COPD in hypobaric chambers.[40,64] Dillard, Rosenberg, and Berg[65] recommended that the FEV_1 be incorporated into these equations to improve the accuracy, although others have questioned whether the added expense and inconvenience are justified.[66] These equations are listed in Box 29-3. As mentioned previously, the patient with normoxic COPD who is in a stable state and has a recent Pa_{O_2} greater than or equal to 72 mm Hg does not necessarily need to be screened unless other concomitant conditions exist. Testing with the HAST has advantages over prediction equations,[15,58] including (1) allowing the patient to subjectively experience the sensation of hypoxemia; (2) allowing prediction of oxygenation during light exercise, such as walking around the cabin; and (3) allowing the evaluation of patients regardless of the cause of pulmonary disease or whether concomitant diseases (cardiac, hematologic, cerebrovascular, or psychological) are present to affect the patient's subjective and objective responses to a simulated cabin environment. The HAST also

permits adjustment of supplemental O_2 to meet the requirement of the patient under hypoxemic conditions.

A pragmatic article showed that the addition of supplemental O_2 at 2 L/minute in an enclosed environment with an Fi_{O_2} of 15% was adequate to return the pulse oximetry to values obtained while breathing ambient air at sea level (Fi_{O_2} = 21%).[67,68] Three groups of 10 patients each were studied, including healthy individuals, patients with restrictive lung disease, and patients with obstructive lung disease. However, only two patients had resting pulse oximetry at sea level of less than 92%, and both of these were inpatients with obstructive lung disease. Still, the study provides a guideline as to how much supplemental O_2 may be necessary for patients to maintain adequate in-flight oxygenation when arrangements must be made without the availability of an HAST.

Because hypoxia can adversely affect other medical conditions, screening of the traveler also needs to include a detailed history of possible cardiovascular problems and anemia (especially sickle cell disease and sickle cell β-thalassemia).[69] Patients with recent cerebral infarction may have worsening of their neurologic deficits because of cerebral hypoxia. Similarly, any of the following cardiac conditions should be considered a contraindication to air travel if they occurred within the preceding 2 weeks: myocardial infarction, angioplasty, intracoronary stent placement, angina, poorly compensated heart failure, uncontrolled cardiac dysrhythmias, or coronary artery bypass grafting (3-week limit).[70] Of interest for these patients is the finding that airport security devices have not been shown to have any deleterious effects on implantable pacemakers or cardiac defibrillators.[70] As mentioned earlier, recent thoracic surgery, pneumothorax, or giant bronchogenic cysts[11] are relative contraindications to fly because of the potential expansion of enclosed gas according to Boyle's law.[5]

Planning Air Travel for Patients with Pulmonary Disease

Planning for air travel with supplemental O_2 requires preparation by the patient well ahead of takeoff.[2,71] Although most major domestic and international airlines allow O_2 to be used in flights, many of the smaller airlines and regional carriers will not accept passengers with supplemental O_2.[2,15] Until an August 2005 ruling by the FAA,

---

BOX 29-3	**Regression Equations for Predicting Pa_{O_2} at Altitude**

Patients with chronic obstructive pulmonary disease:
  a. $22.8 - 2.74x + 0.68y$
  b. $0.453y + (0.386)(FEV_1\%$ predicted$) + 2.44$
Patients with restrictive lung disease:
  a. $25.0 - 3.12x + 0.62y$

Pa_{O_2}, *Arterial partial pressure of oxygen (O_2);* x, *altitude (in thousands of feet);* y, Pa_{O_2} *(in milliliters of mercury) at sea level;* $FEV_1\%$ predicted, *forced expiratory volume in 1 second (relative to predicted normal).*

no domestic carrier allowed passengers to use their own O_2 tanks. Most, but not all carriers, still require that the airline supplies the source of O_2. Liter flow is 2 to 8 L/minute via face mask or cannula.[2,58,71] Some carriers will contact the patient's personal physician directly, whereas others only require a letter. The fee for the supplemental O_2 varies and is based on the number of flight segments. In addition, the carriers will not supply O_2 while on the ground, so that if the patient requires supplemental O_2 at rest or when in an airport at altitude, these arrangements must be made separately. If transportation (such as a wheelchair) between flight segments or to ground transportation is necessary, then arrangements are required before takeoff. Various publications have listed the differences between air carriers, although these policies frequently change.[24,61,71-73] Therefore the traveler will always need to make arrangements at least 48 hours ahead of time for domestic airlines and as long as 1 week before traveling on an international carrier.

Other arrangements are required before embarkation. Seat selection should ideally be at the front of the aircraft or near a lavatory. Nonstop flights are preferable for convenience and to limit the extra cost of using O_2, which is based on a per-segment charge. Furthermore, it is advisable to travel during normal business hours in case any equipment fails or a need arises for changes that might occur because of flight plan alterations.[2,71]

Before even contacting the air carrier, however, patients should have a detailed evaluation by their treating physician. Recommendations can be based on previous experience or may require an HAST or other estimation of O_2 requirements. The physician should supply the patient with a brief summary of his or her medical history, medication requirements, O_2 requirements, stability to travel, and a list of physicians en route and at their final destinations who may be contacted in case of emergencies.[15,71] In addition, airports have emergency physicians available, and their names and numbers can be provided before travel by the travel agent. Some travel agencies specialize in arranging trips for patients with medical problems and can be helpful, especially for international trips.[2]

Any patient traveling with O_2 will need to have a companion who is able to help with their equipment and their medications. Some international carriers require that an extra seat be purchased in lieu of a charge for O_2. Most carriers will allow empty O_2 tanks to be checked as luggage. Because of in-flight O_2 generator—related disasters, these restrictions are becoming much more stringent. Patients should carry all their medications on board as well as packing duplicates in their luggage.[58,71] Moreover, they should bring tape, scissors, extra tubing, cannulas, and adapters, especially if they use an O_2-conserving device.[15] Along with their medications, the traveler should have a copy of all medical information and advanced directives, and these directives need to be understood by their traveling companion.

On the day of departure, the patient should be well rested and void before boarding the plane. Simple measures such as not overeating and avoiding sedatives, alcohol, caffeine (which may cause diuresis), and tight-fitting clothing should be taken. Also, on flights longer than 1 to 2 hours, patients should stand up and exercise their leg muscles periodically to avoid the risk of deep venous thrombosis. If the flight is longer than 6 to 8 hours, especially if the passenger has risk factors for venous thromboembolic disease, then below-the-knee graduated compression stocking or low molecular weight heparin is advised. There is no evidence that aspirin lowers the risk in this situation.[70]

Most of these arrangements need to be organized by the patient. Therefore the patient should have either experience with traveling with O_2 or a knowledgeable travel agent. Most travelers should obtain extra trip cancellation insurance and medical air transport insurance, especially if traveling outside their home country. Although seemingly arduous, these arrangements can be done relatively expediently by the experienced traveler.[2]

Medicolegal Aspects of Traveling with Medical Equipment

The prime concern of any carrier is to provide safe transportation for its passengers. Therefore it is considered reasonable for an air carrier to refuse passage to passengers who they think are not medically fit to travel by air.[5]

When a passenger is stricken in flight, it is common for airline personnel to ask for the assistance of any physician who may be on board in the role of a "good Samaritan."[54,61] A survey of 577 in-flight deaths noted that in 43% of cases, on-board physicians offered medical assistance.[52] However, one survey of 42 physicians who responded to in-flight emergencies found a certain degree of reservation about volunteering their services, mainly because the physicians thought that emergency care was outside their field of expertise.[74] Other concerns included medicolegal implications, which vary widely among countries.[54] For example, in the British and American legal systems, no legal obligation for a physician to provide aid to a stranger exists, whereas some European countries consider it a criminal offense if assistance is not rendered by a physician even if that physician is not "qualified" to provide the required medical services. Moreover, even qualified physicians may not be knowledgeable about the various physiologic changes that could affect diagnosis and treatment while at altitude.[54] Furthermore, no consensus exists as to whether a physician should be reimbursed for services rendered, as publicized by a legal battle that occurred in London.[75] Many physicians noted that their services were not acknowledged and that no effort was made to deal with their ambivalence, especially when a passenger dies while under their emergency care.[54,61,76] However, most physicians face difficult decisions on a daily basis and should be psychologically prepared to respond appropriately.[15]

Since 1986, domestic airline carriers have been required by the FAA to carry a medical kit that contains a sphygmomanometer, a stethoscope, an oropharyngeal airway, and various medications (epinephrine, diphenhydramine, 50% dextrose, and nitroglycerin tablets) along with an instruction book.[55] Although not an FAA requirement, many major domestic carriers are now equipped with cardiac defibrillators and have trained their personnel in the proper use of these defibrillators along with basic and advanced life support methods. These changes have been popularized by incidents in which journalists have written that passengers could have been saved if such equipment had been available. The exact impact of this equipment, both favorable and harmful, has yet to be determined.[54,55] This is especially pertinent given the extremely low incidence of fatal medical emergencies that occur in flight.[52,55]

TRAVEL AT SEA LEVEL FOR THE TECHNOLOGY-DEPENDENT PATIENT WITH PULMONARY DISEASE

Cruise Ships

Although the cruise industry does not have a uniform policy, most cruise lines allow patients to bring their own equipment on board, including O_2 concentrators, without charging a fee.[71] Some actually rent O_2 concentrators when cruising is done internationally. Usually more than 4 weeks' advance notice is required before departure. Although allowing patients to bring their own equipment eliminates one of the problems of traveling, frequently the patient needs to fly to the cruise ship and therefore will still need to deal with the airline industry.

If the patient requires continuous supplemental O_2 or portable O_2 when ambulating, adequate equipment needs to be prearranged for excursions away from their concentrator. Therefore the patient needs to contact his or her O_2 vendor along with the cruise line to be certain that tanks can be refilled and that the O_2 supplier will be open when the ship is docked.[2]

When booking a cruise, patients need to work closely with their travel agent. A detailed letter should be sent to the cruise line with an expected response confirming the date and destination of the cruise, the cabin number, the equipment that is going to be brought on board, the electrical requirements of such equipment, the portable equipment that will be used, the wheelchair that will be required, and the electrical supply for any electrical equipment that may be necessary (such as a nebulizer, a nasal continuous positive airway pressure machine, a percussor, or a suction device).[2] In addition, the astute cruiser may want to ask whether the cabin has been newly painted or carpeted before sailing because this may adversely affect the patient. The passenger should have a letter that contains the name and telephone number of the O_2 supplier at home so that further details can be worked out and to ask for confirmation that all arrangements have been made.

The problem of hypobaric hypoxia will not be encountered when cruising because travel is occurring at sea level. However, travel sickness may occur, which could adversely affect the overall medical status of the patient. Appropriate steps can be taken to prevent this. However, many medications used to prevent sea sickness have cardiovascular and drying side effects that need to be discussed with the patient's physician before departure. The patient should also request a cabin near an elevator and in a nonsmoking area of the ship. Most large cruise ships have medical personnel on board for assistance. However, most carriers are foreign and therefore the qualifications of health care personnel can vary, as can the quality and presence of advanced medical equipment.[77] More recently, cruise ship lines have begun to associate themselves with medical advisory teams that can be reached via satellite to help diagnose and treat patients. This is made easier if patients provide a summary of their medical history, medications, and advance directives.

The United States Coast Guard has a hazardous material branch (202-267-1577), as does the Department of Transportation under the regulation DOT-E 9856 (202-366-4535), for more specific questions about cruising with O_2.[71]

Travel by Private Auto

Patients who require supplemental O_2 and other medical technology frequently opt to travel by private car or recreational vehicle.[15] Large-volume tanks can be secured in the back seat or in an appropriately designed auto or recreational vehicle. In the latter, O_2 concentrators can also be used. It is advisable that a backup, portable system be available in case of vehicle breakdown or accidents. Patients need to make arrangements with O_2 suppliers so that refills can be obtained throughout the trip. Therefore travel should be done during usual business hours.[2] In addition, patients and their companions need to be warned against allowing tanks to overheat when left in the trunk or the back of a vehicle and to be certain that inflammable materials are not in close proximity to O_2 tanks. Not only are O_2 concentrators convenient for recreational vehicles, they can also be moved to most motel and hotel rooms. If travel is going to take the patient to higher altitudes, adjustments need to be made in the O_2 flow, and this needs to be discussed with their physician before departure.

Travel by Bus and Rail

Most long-distance bus carriers and commercial railroads allow passengers to travel with their own portable O_2 containers and frequently with O_2 concentrators for longer trips.[71] As with other forms of transportation, arrangements need to be made with the carrier before departure. In addition, a seat in a nonsmoking area of the bus or train should be sought in advance. Each carrier has limits as to how many O_2 containers can be stowed as baggage. It is advised that an extra supply of O_2 be available to the traveler and that he or she be familiar with how to have their equipment serviced (in case of an unexpected problem).

TRAVELING WITH ADVANCED MEDICAL TECHNOLOGY

Increasing numbers of patients now rely on portable mechanical ventilator support for use at home on either a continuous or a nocturnal basis. A growing number of patients rely on a noninvasive method of full or partial mechanical ventilator support.[3] Similar to the requirements for portable O_2, policies concerning the use of mechanical ventilators on aircraft and on ships vary with each carrier. Usually, a portable ventilator is allowed in flight but must be able to fit under the seat in front of the traveler and be powered by a dry- or gel-cell battery.[71,78] Some European carriers have electrical hookup; even so, it is best to have a battery backup, especially if the patient is dependent on assisted ventilation. Similarly, noninvasive mechanical ventilator support devices, such as bilevel positive airway pressure devices, may require electrical adapters or batteries. One study showed that the accuracy of the delivered tidal volume and flow rates of mechanical ventilators, including continuous positive airway pressure units, may be altered by the lower P_B encountered at altitude.[79] The lower density of gas at altitude alters the ability of the system to make the appropriate calculation of pressure. Therefore adjustments for this need to be considered before air flight. Similarly, because of Boyle's law, the cuffs of endotracheal or tracheostomy tubes will expand if filled with air in flight, which could be dangerous to the patient. An alternative is to use saline to inflate the cuff while at altitude.[80]

Reports have emerged describing the use of commercial aircraft to transport patients with advanced lung disease to medical centers for lung transplantation or pulmonary thromboendarterectomy.[80,81] These flights will require six to nine seats in the plane so that the patient's gurney can be placed above the seat and adequate room is available for the accompanying medical personnel, usually a critical care nurse and physician.[80] Because of the lower P_B in flight, intravenous solutions need to be regulated by battery-powered pumps to ensure proper delivery of medication if this is critical to the patient's hemodynamic status. In addition, the delivered F_{IO_2} will need to be adjusted either before or during flight with noninvasive monitors (pulse oximetry) or end-tidal CO_2 monitors. It should be noted, however, that some air carriers do not allow the use of suction equipment on board because it may interfere with the aircraft navigational system. Furthermore, detailed calculations will be necessary so that enough portable O_2 is available, especially on longer flights. Even though these medically complicated patients can be safely transported on commercial aircraft,[80,81] it is usually advisable that a qualified air ambulance service transport these patients when feasible.

References

1. Harding RM, Mills FJ: Medical aspects of airline operations. I. Health and hygiene, BMJ 286:2049-2051, 1983.
2. Petersen P: Good if not great travel with oxygen, Charlotte, NC, 1996, Raven.
3. Make J, Hill NS, Goldberg AI et al: Mechanical ventilation beyond the intensive care unit, Chest 113(suppl):289S-344S, 1998.
4. Rodrigues JC, Ilowite JS: Pulmonary rehabilitation in the elderly patient, Clin Chest Med 14:429-436, 1993.
5. Mills FJ, Harding RM: Fitness to travel by air. I. Physiological considerations, BMJ 286:1269-1271, 1983.
6. Weinberger SE: Principals of pulmonary medicine, Philadelphia, Pa, 1992, WB Saunders, p 16.
7. Hultgren H: High altitude medicine, Stanford, Calif, 1997, Hultgren Publications, Section 3, p 9.
8. Cottrell JJ: Altitude exposure during aircraft flight: flying higher, Chest 92:81-84, 1988.
9. West J, Hackett P, Maret K et al: Pulmonary gas exchange on the summit of Mt. Everest, J Appl Physiol 55:678-687, 1983.
10. Coates G, Gray G, Mansell A et al: Changes in lung volume, lung density, and distribution of ventilation during hypobaric decompression, J Appl Physiol 46:752-755, 1979.
11. Zaugg M, Kaplan V, Widmer U et al: Fatal air embolism in an airplane passenger with a giant intrapulmonary bronchogenic cyst, Am J Respir Crit Care Med 157:1686-1689, 1998.
12. Neidmart P, Suter PM: Pulmonary bulla and sudden death in a young aeroplane passenger, Intensive Care Med 11:45-47, 1985.
13. Gil HS, Stetz FK, Chong K et al: Nonresolving spontaneous pneumothorax in a 38-year-old woman, Chest 110:835-837, 1996.
14. Block ER: In: Fishman AP, ed. Update: pulmonary diseases and disorders, New York, 1982, McGraw-Hill, pp 349-365.
15. Krieger BP: Travel for the technology-dependent patient with lung disease, Clin Pulm Med 2:1-29, 1995.
16. Lenfant C, Sullivan K: Adaptation to high altitude, N Engl J Med 284:1298-1309, 1971.
17. Harding RM, Mills FJ: Problems of altitude. I. Hypoxia and hyperventilation, BMJ 286:1408-1410, 1983.
18. Gong H: Air travel and oxygen therapy in cardiopulmonary patients, Chest 101:1104-1113, 1992.
19. Graham WGB, Houston CS: Short-term adaptation to moderate altitude: patients with obstructive lung disease, JAMA 240:1491-1494, 1978.
20. Schwartz JS, Bencowitz H, Moser KM: Air travel hypoxemia with chronic obstructive pulmonary disease, Ann Intern Med 100:473-477, 1984.
21. Roeggla G, Roeggla H, Roeggla M et al: Effect of alcohol on acute ventilatory adaptation to mild hypoxia at moderate altitude, Ann Intern Med 122:925-927, 1995.
22. Phillips BA, McConnell JW, Smith MD: The effects of hypoxemia on cardiac output: a dose–response curve, Chest 93:471-475, 1988.
23. Sackner MA, Hoffman RA, Stroh D et al: Thoracocardiography. 1. Noninvasive measurement of changes in stroke volume comparison to thermodilution, Chest 99:613-622, 1991.
24. Gong H: Advising COPD patients about commercial air travel, J Respir Dis 5:28-39, 1984.
25. Berg BW, Dillard TA, Derderian SS et al: Hemodynamic effects of altitude exposure and oxygen administration in chronic obstructive pulmonary disease, Am J Med 94:407-412, 1993.
26. Christopherson JK, Hlasita MD: Pulmonary gas exchange during altered gas density breathing, J Appl Physiol 52:221-225, 1982.
27. Marshall C, Marshall B: Site and sensitivity of hypoxia pulmonary vasoconstriction, J Appl Physiol 55:711-716, 1983.
28. Hultgren H: High altitude medicine, Stanford, Calif, 1997, Hultgren Publications, p 475.
29. Wilmshurst PT, Byrne JC, Webb-Peploe MM: Relation between interstitial shunts and decompression sickness in divers, Lancet 2:1302-1306, 1989.
30. Moon RE, Camporesi EM, Kisslo JA: Patent foramen ovale and decompression sickness in divers, Lancet 1:513-514, 1989.
31. Yaron M, Alexander J, Hultgren H: Low risk of myocardial ischemia in the elderly at moderate altitude, J Wilderness Med 6:20-28, 1995.
32. Hultgren H: High altitude medicine, Stanford, Calif, 1997, Hultgren Publications, p 429.
33. Mosso A: Life of man on the high alps, London, 1989, Fisher Unwin, p 44.
34. West JB, Peters RM, Aksner G et al: Nocturnal periodic-breathing at altitudes of 6,300 and 8,050 m, J Appl Physiol 61:280-287, 1986.
35. Honigman B, Theis MK, Koziol-McLain J et al: Acute mountain sickness in a general tourist population at moderate altitudes, Ann Intern Med 118:587-592, 1993.
36. Larson EB, Roach RC, Schoene RB: Acute mountain sickness and acetazolamide: clinical efficiency and effect on ventilation, JAMA 248:328-332, 1982.
37. Cain SM, Dunn JE: Low doses of acetazolamide to aid accommodation of men to altitude, J Appl Physiol 21:1195-2000, 1966.
38. Birmingham Medical Research Expeditionary Society Mountain Sickness Group: Acetazolamide in the control of acute mountain sickness, Lancet 1:180-183, 1981.
39. Liebman J, Lucas R, Moss A et al: Airline travel for children with chronic pulmonary disease, Pediatrics 57:408-410, 1976.

40. Shillito FH, Tomashefski JF, Ashe WF: The exposure of ambulatory patients to moderate altitudes, Aerosp Med 34:850-857, 1963.

41. Gong H: Air travel and patients with chronic obstructive pulmonary disease [editorial], Ann Intern Med 100:595-597, 1984.

42. Latimer KM, O'Byrne PM, Morris MM et al: Bronchoconstriction stimulated by airway cooling, Ann Rev Respir Dis 128:440-443, 1983.

43. Mattson ME, Boyd G, Byar D et al: Passive smoking on commercial airline flights, JAMA 261:867-872, 1989.

44. de la, Hoz RE, Krieger BP: In Rom WN, editor: Dysbarism, ed 3, Philadelphia, 1998, Lippincott-Raven, pp 1359-1375.

45. Wade JF, Mortenson R, Irvin CG: Physiologic evaluation of bullous emphysema, Chest 100:1151-1154, 1991.

46. Travaline JM, Addonizio P, Criner GJ: Effect of bullectomy on diaphragm strength, Am J Respir Crit Care Med 152:1697-1701, 1995.

47. Kenyon TA, Valway SE, Ihle WW et al: Transmission of multidrug-resistant *Mycobacterium tuberculosis* during a long airplane flight, N Engl J Med 334:933-938, 1996.

48. Cruickshank J, Gorlin R, Jennett B: Air travel and thrombotic episodes: the economy class syndrome, Lancet 2:497-498, 1988.

49. Ferrari E, Chevallier T, Chapelier A et al: Travel as a risk factor for venous thromboembolic disease: a case–control study, Chest 115:440-444, 1999.

50. Toff WD, Jones CI, Ford I et al: Effect of hypobaric hypoxia, simulating conditions during long-haul air travel on coagulation, fibrinolysis, platelet function, and endothelial function, JAMA 295:2251-2261, 2006.

51. Lapostolle F, Surget V, Borrin SW et al: Severe pulmonary associated with air travel, N Engl J Med 345:779-783, 2001.

52. Cummins RO, Chapman PJC, Chamberlain DA et al: In-flight deaths during commercial air travel: how big is the problem? JAMA 259:1983-1988, 1988.

53. Cummins RO, Schubach JA: Frequency and types of medical emergencies among commercial air travelers, JAMA 261:1295-1299, 1989.

54. Mills FJ, Harding RM: Medical emergencies in the air. I. Incidence and legal aspects, BMJ 286:1131-1132, 1983.

55. Cottrell JJ, Callaghan JT, Kohn GM et al: Inflight emergencies: one year of experience with the enhanced medical kit, JAMA 262:1653-1656, 1989.

56. Speizer C, Rennie CJ III, Breton H: Prevalence of in-flight medical emergencies on commercial airlines, Ann Emerg Med 18:26-29, 1989.

57. Skjenna OW, Evans JF, Moore MS et al: Helping patients travel by air, CMAJ 144:287-293, 1991.

58. Krieger BP: Oxygen in the air, Emerg Med 29:77-82, 1997.

59. Gong H, Tashkin DP, Lee EY et al: Hypoxia—altitude simulation test, Am Rev Respir Dis 130:980-986, 1984.

60. Bjorkman BA, Selecky PA: High-altitude simulation at rest and exercise to determine oxygen therapy needs in hypoxemic patients during airplane travel: a community hospital experience [abstract], Chest 94(suppl):31S, 1988.

61. AMA Commission on Emergency Medical Service: Medical aspects of transportation aboard commercial aircraft, JAMA 247:1007-1011, 1982.

62. Schwartz J: Hypoxemia during air travel [letter], Ann Intern Med 112:147-148, 1990.

63. Naughton MT, Rochford PD, Pretto JJ et al: Is normobaric simulation of hypobaric hypoxia accurate in chronic airflow limitation? Am J Respir Crit Care Med 152:1956-1960, 1995.

64. Dillard TA, Berg BW, Rajagopal KR et al: Hypoxemia during air travel in patients with chronic obstructive pulmonary disease, Ann Intern Med 111:362-367, 1989.

65. Dillard TA, Rosenberg AP, Berg BW: Hypoxemia during altitude exposure: a meta-analysis of chronic obstructive pulmonary disease, Chest 103:422-425, 1993.

66. Apte NM, Karnad DR: Altitude hypoxemia and the arterial-to-alveolar oxygen ratio [letter], Ann Intern Med 112:547-548, 1990.

67. Cramer D, Ward S, Geddes P: Assessment of oxygen supplementation during air travel, Thorax 51:202-203, 1996.

68. Kelly PT, Swanney MP, Seccombe LM et al: Air travel hypoxemia vs the hypoxia inhalation test in passengers with COPD, Chest 133:920-926, 2008.

69. Green RL, Huntsman RG, Serjeant GR: Sickle-cell and altitude, BMJ 4:593-595, 1971.

70. Possick SE, Barry M: Evaluation and management of the cardiovascular patient embarking on air-travel, Ann Intern Med 141:148-154, 2004.

71. Stoller JK: Travel for the technology-dependent individual, Respir Care 39:347-362, 1994.

72. Gong H: Air travel and altitude in hypoxemic patients, Pulm Perspect 6:8-12, 1989.

73. American Association for Respiratory Care (AARC): Requirements for traveling with oxygen, Dallas, Tex, 1992, AARC.

74. Hays MB: Physicians and airline medical emergencies, Aviat Space Environ Med 48:468-470, 1977.

75. Goldsmith C: Is there a doctor on the plane? Yes, if he can bring his bill pad, Wall Street Journal, October 8, 1998:B1.

76. Wakeford R: Death in the clouds, BMJ 293:1642-1643, 1986.

77. Perrin W: Cruise ships and medical care, Condé Nast Traveler 1994;December:37-46.

78. Lifecare: Heading south this winter? Tips for traveling with a ventilator. In Alert: new ideas in respiratory care, Lafayette, Colo, November/December 1993, Lifecare.

79. Fromm R, Varon J, Lechin AE et al: CPAP machine performance and altitude, Chest 108:1577-1580, 1995.

80. Wachtel AS, Allen HN, Lewis HI: Aeromedical transport of the mechanically ventilated patients, J Intensive Care Med 12:310-315, 1997.

81. Kramer MR, Jakobson DJ, Springer C et al: The safety of air transportation of patient with advanced lung disease: experience with 21 patients requiring lung transplantation or pulmonary thromboendarterectomy, Chest 12:310-315, 1995.

Chapter 30

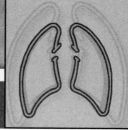

Management of and Reimbursement for Pulmonary Rehabilitation

GERILYNN L. CONNORS • THOMAS P. MALINOWSKI • LANA R. HILLING • JAMES P. LAMBERTI

CHAPTER OUTLINE

Management Overview
Scope of Program
Organization
Information and Data Management
Data Management
Operational Performance
Quality
Evaluating Organizational and Staff Performance
Evaluating Operational Performance
Time Standards and Productivity
Financial Performance
Customer Service
Improvement in Internal Operations
Quality and Performance Improvement
Foundations of Quality Improvement
Integrating Performance Improvement
    into Job Performance
Accreditation and Standards Agencies

The Joint Commission
American Association of
    Cardiovascular and Pulmonary
    Rehabilitation Program
    Certifications
Reimbursement
Historical Perspective
Sources of Health Care Financing
Federal and State Health Insurance
    Programs
Comprehensive Outpatient
    Rehabilitation Facility
Nongovernmental Health Insurance
    Programs
Documentation
Medicare Documentation
    Requirements
UB-04
Conclusion

PROFESSIONAL SKILLS

On completion of this chapter, the reader will be able to do the following:

* Discuss the management issues to be addressed when orchestrating a pulmonary rehabilitation program
* Describe the essential components of comprehensive pulmonary rehabilitation
* List the conditions appropriate for pulmonary rehabilitation beyond chronic obstructive pulmonary disease
* State the role outcomes, performance improvement, and benchmarking has in a pulmonary rehabilitation program
* Understand the sources of health care financing and their role in pulmonary rehabilitation reimbursement
* Know how to document the skilled level of intervention for pulmonary rehabilitation procedures to optimize outcomes and reimbursement

Program management starts with understanding the mission, vision, and values of the organization, the scope of the program and the customers (e.g., patients, families, physicians, other allied health departments) who will receive pulmonary rehabilitation (PR). Program management also includes information and data management, evaluating organization and staff performance, regulatory and accreditation agencies, and reimbursement. The reimbursement status, on which revenue projections are based, is essential but difficult to project because of the changing regulatory controls imposed by third-party payers and Medicare in the United States.

MANAGEMENT OVERVIEW

Scope of Program

The science- and evidence-based papers pertaining to PR have increased in response to the intensification in the prevalence of the patient populations treated by PR.[1-6] The efficacy and scientific foundation of PR have been firmly established from the first definition of PR in 1974 by the American College of Chest Physicians (ACCP) to the 2007 Joint ACCP/AACVPR (American Association of Cardiovascular and Pulmonary Rehabilitation) *Evidence-based Clinical Practice Guidelines* for PR. Box 30-1 presents a PR historical and scientific walk through time. Continued collaboration with national organizations and our colleagues across the world will bring PR into the 21st century as an integral part of the clinical management, health maintenance, and disease prevention of people with chronic pulmonary disease.

The essential components of a comprehensive PR program have emerged from the various published guidelines and consensus statements and include the following: assessment, patient education and training, therapeutic exercise, psychosocial intervention, and promotion of long-term adherence, with prevention strategies and outcome assessment incorporated into every component. Patient goals and objectives are established during each component, which reinforces the foundation of the program. PR is not just an exercise or education program. It is an individualized, multidisciplinary program that meets the special needs of each patient with pulmonary disease through assessment, patient education/training, exercise, psychosocial intervention, and long-term adherence.

Patients with chronic obstructive pulmonary disease (COPD) account for the majority of

BOX 30-1	Historical Perspective of the Scientific Evidence-based Medicine of Pulmonary Rehabilitation
1974	ACCP: Pulmonary rehabilitation defined
1981	ATS: Position statement on pulmonary rehabilitation
1990	AACVPR: Position paper on the scientific basis of PR
1993	AACVPR: First published guidelines for PR programs
1994	NIH Workshop summary: New PR definition
1997	ACCP/AACVPR Pulmonary Rehabilitation Guidelines Panel: evidence-based guidelines
1997	ERS Task Force position paper: selection criteria for pulmonary rehabilitation of patients with COPD
1998	AACVPR: Second edition of guidelines for PR programs
1999	ATS: Official statement on pulmonary rehabilitation
2000	AARC: Clinical practice guidelines: pulmonary rehabilitation
2001	GOLD, in collaboration with NHLBI, NIH, USA, and WHO
2001	British Thoracic Society Standards of Care Subcommittee on Pulmonary Rehabilitation
2002	AARC: Clinical practice guidelines: pulmonary rehabilitation
2004	AACVPR: Third edition of guidelines for pulmonary rehabilitation
2004	ATS/ERS: Standards for the diagnosis and management of patients with COPD
2005	GOLD Workshop Report: annual updates
2006	ATS/ERS: Statement on pulmonary rehabilitation
2007	Pulmonary rehabilitation: joint ACCP/AACVPR evidence-based clinical practice guidelines

AACVPR, *American Association of Cardiovascular and Pulmonary Rehabilitation;* AARC, *American Association for Respiratory Care;* ACCP, *American College of Chest Physicians;* ATS, *American Thoracic Society;* COPD, *chronic obstructive pulmonary disease;* ERS, *European Respiratory Society;* GOLD, *Global Initiative for Chronic Obstructive Lung Disease;* NHLBI, *National Heart, Lung, and Blood Institute;* NIH, *National Institutes of Health;* PR, *pulmonary rehabilitation.*

patients entering and participating in PR programs.[7] This is traditional, but program options should be expanded to other chronic lung conditions.[1,2,4,5,8] Tobacco smoking is the main cause of COPD, and encouragement and support from the PR program to terminate this addiction are critical. Promotion of awareness of risk factors and identification of at-risk populations are areas in which the rehabilitation program should become involved. In fact, although neuromuscular disorders and thoracic wall deformities are incurable, supportive treatment to improve the patient's quality of life is used. This supportive treatment should consider PR as a standard of care to meet the patient's needs.[9] Cystic fibrosis is a disease for which PR is appropriate. Box 30-2 lists various patient conditions appropriate for PR. These patients will challenge the PR specialist beyond the continuum of traditional care.

The components of a comprehensive PR program (assessment, patient training, exercise, psychosocial intervention, and long-term adherence) are the same for these patients, but individualizing the program components is vital to address the specific needs of the patients. It means redesigning the PR program for disease specification. The key to successful patient outcomes is individualization of the program to the patient's needs. Innovative strategies for each component of PR need to be developed and enhanced for the nontraditional diseases. The continuum of care for chronic pulmonary disease begins at birth and ends with death. PR must become integrated into this continuum of care for earlier detection and prevention of pulmonary disease[10-12] and for the chronic lung diseases beyond COPD.

Organization

Interdisciplinary Team

PR benefits from an interdisciplinary team of health care specialists. Members of each specialty use their expertise to assess, treat, and follow up the patient in the program as appropriate.[1] Box 30-3 provides an extensive list of the interdisciplinary team members of a PR program.

Not every member of the interdisciplinary team will assess the patient, but if a specific patient deficit is evaluated, then the appropriate specialist intervenes. The composition of the interdisciplinary team will depend on the facility resources and patients' needs. Each interdisciplinary team member must possess the knowledge and skills to assess,

---

BOX 30-2	Traditional and Nontraditional Conditions Appropriate for Pulmonary Rehabilitation

OBSTRUCTIVE DISORDERS
- Asthma
- Asthmatic bronchitis
- Chronic bronchitis
- Emphysema
- Chronic obstructive pulmonary disease
- Bronchiectasis
- Cystic fibrosis
- Bronchiolitis obliterans

RESTRICTIVE DISORDERS
- Interstitial fibrosis
- Rheumatoid lung disease
- Lung disorders secondary to collagen-vascular disease
- Occupational lung disease
- Environmental lung disease
- Sarcoidosis
- Kyphoscoliosis
- Spondylitis
- Parkinson's disease
- Postpolio syndrome
- Amyotrophic lateral sclerosis
- Diaphragm dysfunction
- Multiple sclerosis

OTHER DISORDERS
- Nicotine addiction
- Lung cancer
- Primary pulmonary hypertension
- Post-thoracic surgery
- Lung transplantation, pre/post
- Lung volume reduction surgery, pre/post
- Ventilator dependency
- Pediatric patients with pulmonary disease
- Morbid obesity
- Sleep apnea
- Primary tuberculosis

BOX 30-3	Interdisciplinary Team Members of a Pulmonary Rehabilitation Program*

- Patient
- Primary care physician
- Medical director
- Program coordinator/director/team leader
- Respiratory therapist or technician
- Registered or licensed vocational nurse
- Physical therapist
- Occupational therapist
- Exercise physiologist
- Dietitian
- Social worker
- Clinical psychologist
- Social worker
- Psychiatrist
- Chaplain or pastoral care associate
- Speech therapist
- Physiatrist
- Recreational therapist
- Pulmonary function technologist
- Patient graduate volunteers
- Home care personnel
- Business office representative
- Vocational rehabilitation counselor

Not every member of the interdisciplinary team may be involved with the patient. It depends on the individual patient assessment.

treat, train/educate, reevaluate, document, and determine home recommendations for the pulmonary patient. Program strength and success are based on the unique talents, traits, and dedication of the interdisciplinary team. PR is a "team effort," not a "one-person operation."

Administrative Director

A designated administrative director will manage the program. The individual should be a health care professional with clinical experience and expertise in the care of patients with pulmonary disease and PR. The administrative director must understand the philosophy and goals of PR and work under the guidance and supervision of the program medical director. The role of the administrative director may encompass program development, management, marketing, education, and research. The administrative director functions as a liaison with the team, facilitator of the patient's total treatment program, leader, educator, and communicator.

Medical Director

Guidelines for Pulmonary Rehabilitation Programs, published by the AACVPR,[1,13] provides a description of the role of the medical director in PR. These guidelines are recommendations and are not binding but serve as a framework for an effective and safe PR program. The medical director of a PR program should be a licensed physician who has special interest and expertise in the care of patients with chronic pulmonary diseases. Within the hospital setting, the medical director, as the agent of the medical staff, is responsible for ensuring that PR is in compliance with federal and state regulations and the requirements of The Joint Commission (TJC). The medical director participates in the development of appropriate comprehensive program elements regarding evaluation, patient education, and exercise.

The medical director provides medical expertise to the administrative director of the program. The medical director's pulmonary medicine background is important in all aspects of the establishment and ongoing functioning of a program. The medical director should review and approve the mission statement, policies, procedures, and protocols. Although referrals may come from various physicians in the community, the medical director is ultimately responsible for determining the appropriateness of the plan of care for the patient. The medical director should participate in the review of all referrals for an appropriate diagnosis and level of impairment. The medical director should understand the current coverage guidelines for PR used by various insurers and assist staff members in the interpretation of the guidelines. After a patient starts a comprehensive program, the medical director needs to be readily available to review changes in a participant's medical condition that would be an impediment to continued participation in the program.

As PR extends into non-COPD diagnoses (see Box 30-2), involvement by a medical director assumes increased importance. For example, patients with interstitial lung diseases may require high-flow oxygen (O_2) during exercise. Patients with cystic fibrosis may be colonized with organisms that require special attention to infectious precautions. As PR is used in new disease states, the medical director should work closely with the staff to establish medically appropriate policies and procedures. The medical director should actively participate to improve the quality of the program.

The medical director should be a resource in the education of PR patients and should be actively involved in the continuing education of staff members. Medical students, residents, and pulmonary fellows should be encouraged to undertake electives in PR under the direction of the medical director. The medical director should lead clinical research efforts within the department and should be an advocate for the importance of PR among members of the hospital medical staff and community. The medical director should work to progress the stature of PR with various governmental and private insurers.

INFORMATION AND DATA MANAGEMENT

Data Management

Data and documentation serve three main functions: medical record information, financial and billing elements, and provision of information about the operational characteristics of the program. All too often, the focus is solely on either the medical record or billing capture issues; the untapped operational management elements are often overlooked. Quality improvement (QI) strategies are often described as "data driven." This term refers to the requirement for supporting evidence or information. How do we know we are performing well, or performing poorly? QI decisions are based on knowledge, confirmed with facts and data, and driven by an understanding of variation and statistical thinking. Data are used to validate the presence or absence of a problem. For example, if a complaint is lodged from a physician regarding the amount of time required to enroll a patient in a PR program, data help determine the validity that such complaints actually occur. This allows managers the opportunity to focus on problems that can be validated, and that may occur more frequently than sporadic events. Data are also important for benchmarking performance before implementation of improvements, and for demonstrating improvement after process changes. Data drive issues. Data identify the presence or absence of quality and verify process improvement.

Patient's Medical Record

Health information technology is changing rapidly, but the ultimate goal is patient safety, and increasing the quality of the care delivered. Elimination of errors and efficiency has been reported with computerized medical records.

The patient's record in a PR program requires specific documentation that is significant, concise, to the point, and uses standardized terms. Handwritten notes or computer-generated notes facilitate the data entry of pertinent patient information. Each institution has general rules that govern medical record keeping.[14,15] The medical records department has the specifications. The patient record improves communication and continuity of care among the interdisciplinary team members. PR documentation is the only means the program has to prove that they are providing an appropriate skilled level of care and meeting established standards. No matter how frustrating charting may be, it must be done, and thus it should be as simple, straightforward, and specific as possible, easy to follow and read. The PR patient's medical record is an information-intensive document. The chart is a legal document that can be sent into court.

The PR progress note is the repository of medical facts and critical thinking pertaining to the patient with pulmonary disease. It must be concise: a vehicle of communication about the patient's condition to those who access the health record. The progress notes must be readable, easily understood, complete, accurate, and completed in black ink. The interdisciplinary team's documentation must be flexible enough to logically convey what happened during the therapy, the chain of events occurring during the treatment session, as well as guaranteeing full accountability for the documented material, and clearly documenting who recorded the information, and when it was recorded.

Computers in the health care setting are standard, and the interdisciplinary team should become familiar with the hospital's computer information systems, and how integration of the patient's record and test results can be achieved to make documentation more efficient. Computerized patient records support patient-focused care by points of documentation that give the interdisciplinary team greater time with the patient through reduced manual and clerical activities. The handwritten medical record can be used by only one person, at one location, at one time and is often poorly organized and illegible; data retrieval for outcome documentation is time-consuming. Moving from the handwritten pathway to the automated system is an important transition to a computerized interdisciplinary documentation system. The use of computers may allow the development, quantitative perspective, and realization of the virtual patient record; the documentation of all health-relevant data that accumulate during a person's lifetime at the touch of a finger, using the age of networked computers.

Three basic methods are used for patient record keeping: the traditional chart, the problem-oriented medical record (POMR), and computer documentation.[14]

Traditional Chart

The traditional chart (block chart or source-oriented record) is divided into specific areas of blocks. These blocks may include the admission sheet, physician order sheet, progress notes, history and physical examination, medication sheet, medical test reports, care plans, and discharge summaries. This format is easy to record but makes it more difficult to monitor a specific problem/event.

Problem-Oriented Medical Record

The POMR, known as the Weed system after its developer, is one format of documentation. It is used to systematically gather clinical data, formulate an assessment, and select an appropriate treatment plan and record changes made to the original treatment plan. The POMR consists of four basic components: the database, problem list, progress notes, and plan. The exact format each of these components takes varies between institutions. In the PR POMR chart the database includes past medical records, assessments done by the interdisciplinary team, and diagnostic test results. The database builds the baseline for the individualized program. The problem list will include the target areas/deficits found in the evaluation process that interfere with the pulmonary patient's physical/psychological health and ability to function. The problem list is dynamic, with the deletion and addition of problems as indicated. Goals and outcome data are developed from the problem list and supported by the progress notes. The progress notes of the medical record chart may be narrative or written in the SOAP format, which entails *s*ubjective, *o*bjective, *a*ssessment, and *p*lan documentation.

SOAPing systematically reviews one health problem. The subjective information is obtained from the patient receiving PR, a family member, or a significant other. The objective information is based on the interdisciplinary team's assessment of the patient, observations, and test results as measured, factually described, or collected. The assessment is the analysis of/critical thinking about the patient's problems as found during the subjective and objective gathering phase. The plan of action consists of the steps to be taken to address, treat, and resolve the problems. The implementation occurs under the plan and is the actual administration of the specific treatment. Evaluation occurs through the collection of measurable data concerning the patient's response to the intervention, and revision addresses any changes made to the original treatment plan on the basis of the evaluation.

Patient documentation requires critical thinking on the part of the interdisciplinary team members.[16] Critical thinking is defined as the process of purposeful, self-regulatory judgment. This process gives reasoned consideration to evidence-based medicine, contexts, conceptualizations, methods, and criteria in PR. The future of patient documentation may become a blueprint, a critical pathway alternative because good documentation is the cornerstone of quality data. Medical records are documents that can travel from the courtroom to the hospital to the team conference. Medical records are an indelible defense if the documentation is precise and meticulous.

Operational Performance
Policy and Procedures
The PR policy and procedure manual defines the rules of program operations and the PR interdisciplinary staff must be familiar with them. It provides a narrative description of the program services and protocols developed for patient care and is required by TJC for compliance. Box 30-4 shows a sample table of contents for a PR policy and procedure manual.

Location, Facility, Equipment, and Staffing Ratios
PR programs have typically been hospital based, in the respiratory therapy or rehabilitation department or as part of a cardiovascular and PR department. The latter allows for diversification and cross-training of staff, which impacts revenue sources and possibly reduces duplication of staff and equipment. In addition to hospital-based programs, physician clinics and comprehensive outpatient rehabilitation facilities are also considerations. The key factors in site selection are accessibility for patients, safe environmental conditions, and appropriate medical and emergency supervision. Box 30-5 lists location options for PR programs.

The facilities and equipment used in PR programs must meet state, federal, and TJC safety code standards. Box 30-6 provides a list of facility considerations for PR programs.[1] Regardless of the facility design and equipment, the most important aspect to any successful PR program is the interdisciplinary team, which projects confidence, enthusiasm, and a positive attitude in meeting the goals and objectives of PR.

Participants in a PR program are typically in small groups or on one-on-one staffing. The AACVPR staffing ratio minimal requirements are as follows: a medical director, a PR administrative director, and at least one PR specialist (may also be the PR administrative director). During the therapeutic exercise program a minimum of one PR specialist per four exercising patients is suggested, except for patients with severe pulmonary disease or significant comorbidity, for whom one-on-one staffing may be needed. For education/training a staffing ratio of one PR specialist per eight patients is suggested, except with patients needing one-on-one education/training. It is important that each facility determines whether there exists a state Medicare local coverage determination (LCD) with requirements for staffing that must be complied with for reimbursement.

Quality
Accrediting agencies, TJC, payers (e.g., Medicare, Blue Cross), and providers (integrated delivery systems) mandate documentation of outcomes. It is helpful for the program to use accepted,

BOX 30-4	Sample of Contents for the Pulmonary Rehabilitation Policy and Procedure Manual

ORGANIZATIONAL CHART
Pulmonary rehabilitation services
Facility organizational plan

SCOPE OF SERVICE
Scope of service and staffing plan

DEPARTMENT POLICIES, PROCEDURES, AND PROTOCOLS
Information management/medical records
Budget plan
Patient rights
Facility mission, vision, and values
Pulmonary rehabilitation mission statement and values
Americans with Disabilities Act
Interpreting services
Security
Epidemiology, overview, definition, and philosophy
Program description
Smoking policy
Program admission/physician referral
Patient selection and assessment criteria
Patient/program goals
Exercise protocols
Safety guidelines for exercise equipment
O_2 medication indications, titration, and reconciliation
Management of emergencies
Home exercise prescription
Documentation
Discharge criteria
Long-term adherence
Outcomes
Maintenance exercise program
Outpatient safety/emergency procedure
Staffing policy
Patient and family training/education
Staff and team member teaching skills
National definitions/guidelines
• ACCP/AACVPR evidence-based guidelines
• NIH definition
• ATS statements
• Medicare Bulletin
Cleaning of equipment
Space and facilities
Outside services

ORIENTATION PROGRAM
Staff orientation policy
Dress code
Exercise instructor orientation
Interdisciplinary team therapist orientation
Employee evaluation of orientation
Volunteer orientation policy and checklist

EDUCATION PROGRAM
Staff education policy
Staff education plan
Education record form
Staff competency/skills fair
Exercise specialist skills/assessment
Interdisciplinary team therapist skills/assessment

REGISTRY/AGENCY/CONTRACT/STUDENTS
Temporary/agency personnel policy
Temporary/agency personnel orientation policy
Contract employee policy
Contract employee orientation policy
Competency report for temporary/agency and contracted personnel
Respiratory student responsibilities and objectives of clinical rotation
Pulmonary fellow responsibilities and objectives of clinical rotation

PERFORMANCE IMPROVEMENT
CQI plan
Performance improvement

JOB DESCRIPTIONS
Administrative director
Pulmonary rehabilitation respiratory therapist II-IV
Exercise specialist
Medical director job responsibilities
Interdisciplinary team members job responsibilities
• Physical therapist
• Dietitian
• Pharmacist
• Social worker
Volunteers

STAFF MEETING MINUTES
In-service policy/staff meetings rehabilitation

AACVPR, American Association of Cardiovascular and Pulmonary Rehabilitation; ACCP, American College of Chest Physicians; ATS, American Thoracic Society; CQI, continuous quality improvement; NIH, National Institutes of Health; O_2, oxygen.

standardized tools for outcome evaluations. See Chapter 21 on outcomes for an extensive discussion on the domains and outcome measurements used in PR.

Benchmarking

Benchmarking is one form of documenting outcomes (Box 30-7). A significant component of effective program management is the tracking of clinical outcomes (TJC requirement) and partaking in benchmarking activities.[17] Benchmarking and QI go hand in hand. In the past, benchmarking relied on more subjective identification of "leaders in the field." Achievable benchmark of care is now determined by measuring and analyzing performance on process-of-care indicators.[18] Important characteristics for benchmarking are able to measure level of excellence; are demonstrable and attainable; and are

BOX 30-5	Location Options for Pulmonary Rehabilitation Programs

INPATIENT OPTIONS
Acute care during hospitalization
Transitional care unit
Rehabilitation hospital

OUTPATIENT OPTIONS
Outpatient hospital setting
Physician office
Clinic setting
Skilled nursing facility
Subacute care facility
Long-term care facility
Residential outpatient facility
Comprehensive outpatient rehabilitation facility
Shared facility with other rehabilitation programs (e.g., cardiac)

ALTERNATIVE SITES OPTIONS
Storefront
Home resident
Fitness center or spa
Wellness center
Senior citizen center
Local high school or community college
Adult education center
Places of worship
Club meeting halls

BOX 30-6	Facility Considerations for Pulmonary Rehabilitation Programs

PHYSICAL GROUND
Adequate and convenient parking, including handicapped accessibility
Elevator access, not only stairs
Safety hazards

PROGRAM LOCATION
Easy access to water/drinking source
Restrooms, including handicapped access, alarms
Education classroom: size, tone of environment, access, and ventilation
Exercise facility: space, ventilation, and safety
Clinical assessment locations
ADL facility: teaching kitchen, bed, and so on, to assess/train patients in specific ADL needs with adaptive equipment

ADMINISTRATIVE SERVICES LOCATION
Confidentiality of patient records
Patient privacy
Displayed copy of the Patient's Bill of Rights
Emergency supplies (e.g., O_2 source, delivery apparatus, resuscitation bag/mask, first-aid supplies, rescue bronchodilator medication, standard defibrillator or AED)
O_2 source, delivery apparatus, and monitoring device for O_2 saturation
Storage space for equipment
Hand-washing facilities: antibacterial and/or waterless soap

ENVIRONMENTAL ISSUES
Optimal light, temperature, and ventilation control
Avoidance of chemical odors, scented perfumes, and so on
Hazardous material requirements

ADL, *Activities of daily living;* AED, *automatic external defibrillator;* O_2, *oxygen.*
Adapted from American Association of Cardiovascular and Pulmonary Rehabilitation: Program management. In Guidelines for Pulmonary Rehabilitation Programs ed 3, Champaign, Ill, 2004, Human Kinetics.

derived from data in an objective, reproducible, and predetermined fashion; therefore providers with high performance are selected to define a level of excellence. Benchmarking in PR is the comparison of value indicators with those high-performing organizations. The goal of PR benchmarking is to identify outstanding performance regarding cost-effectiveness, quality of life, and best practices in relation to PR treatment interventions.

Medical Coding

To understand quality it is necessary to understand medical coding, which originated in the 1850s. The importance of accurate coding in PR starts with the referral diagnosis and ends with the billing for PR therapeutic treatments. Medical coding assigns a numeric value to medical diagnoses, procedures, surgery, signs and symptoms of disease and ill-defined conditions, poisoning and adverse effects of drugs, and complications of surgery and medical care. The *International Classification of Diseases* (ICD) is the standard diagnostic coding system for epidemiologic and many health management purposes, such as analysis of the general health of population groups and monitoring of the incidence and prevalence of diseases and other health problems. ICD coding

serves an important function for quality review, benchmarking outcome measurements, collection of medical statistical data, physician reimbursement, and payment for hospital and outpatient services. The American Hospital Association is the only official clearinghouse for information about the use of the clinical coding systems used in the United States.[19-22] The *International Classification of Diseases, 9th Revision, Clinical Modification* (ICD-9-CM) and the Healthcare Common Procedure Coding System (HCPCS) are used to report hospital outpatient procedures and physician services (level 1 CPT [*Current Procedural Terminology*] codes and level II national codes).

BOX 30-7 | Key Elements of Benchmarking

- Determine what processes are to be defined in the benchmarking initiative
- Understand the process in detail
- Determine the benchmarking project scope
- Choose relevant, common, and consistent measurements or data
- Study programs that reflect best practice as based on the data
- Judge whether the proposed work practices are appropriate to the program and should be adopted
- Plan and implement the new evidence-based practices
- Measure the effects of the new work practice to determine whether the change had an impact on performance

---

In future there will be a major change in the codes used. The ICD-9-CM has been used for the standard reporting of diagnosis and institutional procedures for almost two decades. Improving the health terminology systems in the United States with guidelines, criteria selection, and public policy implication is never-ending. The current ICD-9-CM classification groups patients in broad categories that do not allow for the development of refined guidelines or the comparison of patient outcomes or benchmarks. Because of an international treaty, the United States moved in 1999 to the updated 10th edition (ICD-10, copyrighted by the World Health Organization [WHO]) to code and classify mortality data from death certificates; the ICD-10 has been implemented for mortality throughout much of the world since the mid-1990s.

The clinical modification of the classification for morbidity purposes, the ICD-10-CM, replaces the older book for the reporting of diagnoses. This new edition has thousands of improved codes, and the Centers for Medicare and Medicaid Services (CMS) has funded the development of a procedure coding system (PCS) for the ICD-10 (ICD-10-PCS). The PCS codes body systems, operations, body parts, approaches, and devices. The new codes do not resemble the American Medical Association Current Procedural Terminology codes (AMA CPT codes) that the CMS now requires physicians and other disciplines to use in coding services. The new reporting system, based on the ICD-10-CM and ICD-10-PCS, will require extensive training of physicians and other providers with substantial changes in the health information technology systems. The benefits of the new coding system

are as follows: accurate payments for new procedures; fewer miscoded, rejected reimbursement claims; better understanding of the values of new procedures; improved disease management; and better understanding of health care outcomes. This new coding will affect the referral diagnosis and billing codes currently used in PR.

EVALUATING ORGANIZATIONAL AND STAFF PERFORMANCE

Evaluating Operational Performance

The PR manager is often faced with many complex decisions and actions. How does a manager or a department know when they are doing a good job? The answer lies in monitoring and measuring operational performance and improving levels of service. Healthy organizations make a balanced commitment to quality, service, cost and financial management, growth, and improvement in internal performance. This commitment results in their ability to stay at the forefront of the industry. Balancing efforts in multiple areas fosters an environment that empowers and encourages all employees to be innovative and resolve roadblocks that limit organizational performance. During the course of business it can become extremely difficult to keep a department focused and on course, headed in the right direction. Managers may be expected to track and monitor performance in multiple categories, but often gravitate to evaluating departmental performance by one or two key indices (e.g., productivity and operational costs). This type of "tunnel vision" approach, focusing all of the department's efforts on one performance area, can lead to imbalance, poor performance, and operational failure.

PR managers and hospital administrators are also susceptible to performance imbalance. Managers and administrators often drive departments down single-focus pathways. Relying exclusively on financial indicators ignores the status of other tools and resources that reflect the organizational health of the system: patient satisfaction and customer loyalty, skill levels of staff, best practice processes, centers of excellence, and so on. This imbalance often leads to suboptimal organizational performance. Consequently, departments and systems fail to meet strategic objectives and the organizational mission. This leads to discordance and frustration for employees and customers alike, driving costs up and system performance down.

The concept of a "balanced scorecard," first reported by Robert Kaplan and David Norton in 1990, was based on a study of 12 high-performance companies in the private sector.[23,24] The results implied that successful organizations do not rely on financial indicators alone to manage the business environment, but instead strive to improve product and services, exceed customer expectations, and increase share through innovation. This approach is particularly important for service-centered organizations that strive to be more customer-focused. The balanced scorecard approach complements financial indicators with customer satisfaction information, status updates on improvements in the internal operations, and the capacity of the organization to learn, lead, and be innovative.

The PR department can develop similar indicators that are tailored to the strategic initiatives of the hospital system. Linking departmental indicators to systems initiatives accomplishes multiple tasks. It aligns departmental performance with institution strategy. It provides visible indicators on departmental performance. It also links staff contributions to the institution strategic initiatives, enhancing ownership and responsibility.

Time Standards and Productivity

Time standards and productivity allow the PR administrative manager to determine staffing needs, ways to manage the cost of providing the rehabilitation services, set realistic fees for self-pay maintenance exercise programs, and also negotiate more profitable contracts with third-party payers when indicated.

The relative value unit (RVU), a cost accounting method, is a valuable practice management tool that allows common denominator analyses and per-unit comparisons for both clinical productivity and expense data. RVUs were originally developed as a physician payment mechanism and has expanded into all areas of health care. The PR administrative manager can use the analysis of RVUs for program strategic planning, resource allocation, budgeting, payer analysis, contract

---

TABLE 30-1   Example of Pulmonary Rehabilitation Procedure Counts, Times Standards, and Relative Value Units

Procedure	Quantity	Time Standard (TS) (min)	Minutes	RVUs (1 RVU = 6 min)	Total (%)
Assess transplant clinic	3	60	180	30.0	0.28
Assess inpatient	7	60	420	70.0	
Assess inpatient transplant	5	60	300	50.0	0.47
Assess outpatient	No new program patients this month	120	0	0	0
Extended therapy	**69**	**Actual minutes**	**2,612**	**435.3**	**4.17**
HAD/knowledge test	**19**	**25**	**475**	**79.2**	**0.75**
Inpatient exercise/ education training	51	60	3,060	510.0	4.83
Maintenance exercise	327	38	12,427	2,071.0	19.63
PR nonbillable time	**419**	**Actual minutes**	**33,467**	**5,577.8**	**52.87**
Patient education/ training group	51	10	510	85.0	0.81
SGRQ data	8	15	120	20.0	0.19
6MWT	26	80	2,080	346.7	3.29
Supervised exercise	85	90	7,650	1,275.0	12.08
Totals:	1,020	Time standard/ procedure	63,300	10,550	100
Billed procedures	555	TS	26,627	4,437.7	42
Insurance billed procedures (excluding maintenance exercise)	228	TS	14,200	1,091.7	10.35
Nonbilled procedures*	**515**	**TS**	**36,674**	**6,112.3**	**58**

*For examples of nonbilled procedures, see Box 30-8.
6MWT, 6-Minute Walk Test; HAD, Hospital Anxiety and Depression Scale; PR, pulmonary rehabilitation; SGRQ, St. George's Respiratory Questionnaire.
Courtesy Inova Fairfax Hospital Pulmonary Rehabilitation Department, Falls Church, Virginia.

review and maintenance, and per-rehabilitation procedure profitability analysis. Table 30-1 provides an example of PR procedure counts, times standards, and RVUs.

RVUs can be used to determine appropriate staffing, and to obtain data to make optimal decisions regarding resource allocation and cost containment to ensure PR program viability. RVUs are more comprehensive than just looking at rehabilitation procedures and charges in terms of measuring program productivity and resource consumption. RVUs also take into consideration the nonbillable time for patient activities that have no charges attached: patient activities without time standards, such as calling the referring physician for a new O_2 delivery device because a patient desaturated during the 6-Minute Walk Test (6MWT) and requires higher liter flow; patient care support procedures such as cleaning the gymnasium and ordering equipment; staff education and training; and QI. Box 30-8 lists PR nonbillable time examples.

RVUs are an objective measure and quantify a PR program's productivity and performance data versus traditional productivity measures such as the number of PR patients in a program or billed program charges. RVU cost analysis gives the PR program administrator the power and knowledge to analyze expenditures, control cost, and determine appropriate and safe staffing. RVU benchmarking in PR has yet to be established, but we should take notes from respiratory care RVU benchmarking. The American Association for Respiratory Care (AARC) has developed a *Uniform Reporting Manual for Acute Care Hospitals* that is a wonderful reference for the PR administrative manager.[25]

RVUs help determine the full-time equivalents required to deliver PR services, based on service demand. The PR administrator must look beyond the assigned PR therapist workload procedure count as the indicator of workload intensity. For example: One procedure count of supervised exercise lasts 60 minutes and one procedure count of PR assessment lasts 90 to 120 minutes excluding the 6MWT. This is not an accurate reflection of each therapist's workload because the therapist performing the PR assessment is treating the patient for an additional 30 to 60 minutes. Patient volume needs to be discussed in terms of RVUs and not just the indicators of procedures/activities completed, billed services, diagnosis codes, or patient days. This information is useful but cannot address the intensity of each procedure like RVUs can. The accounting for clinical and nonclinical support activities provided to patients receiving PR must be tracked, a task which RVUs can accomplish. RVUs can also be used to examine the efficiency of the PR staff to set up process improvements. Hospital/facility administrators review productivity in terms of target efficiency level. PR departments should know this number to understand top administration staffing expectation. The development of time standards for PR procedures and RVUs is needed for best management practice to move PR into the 21st century.

Financial Performance

Financial or productivity indicators are far and away the most commonly monitored and used performance indices.[28-34] Most departments track multiple financial parameters including direct expenses, cost per revenue/procedure, workload volume, and productive hours. These indices are frequently linked to strategic organizational indices such as achieving a system-wide target for operating income and operating margin, or implementing a profitability strategy that results in increased operating income. Most managers have developed specific target goals and monitoring methodologies to trend performance (e.g., program census, case mix load, inpatient and outpatient volume). Financial indicators are considered outcome indicators. Outcome indicators lag behind an action and measure performance that

---

BOX 30-8	**Examples of Pulmonary Rehabilitation Nonbillable Time**

- Gymnasium/classroom setup and cleaning
- Billing
- Follow-up with patients
- Follow-up with physicians
- Program administration
- Program inquiries
- New patient registration
- Team conferences
- Home recommendation write-up
- Preoperative lung transplantation program
- Support group
- Lung Games involvement
- Precepting/orientation
- In-service time
- Staff meetings
- QI
- Research
- Unlisted; see therapist's comment

QI, Quality improvement.

TABLE 30-2   Example of Pulmonary Rehabilitation Operation Financial Indicators

Objective Performance Plan	Outcome Indicator(s)	Strategic Initiative
Strict (±2% variance) adherence to operational budgets for 2008	K, LGA	
Implement copayment program for maintenance program members	LGA, K	Achieve system-wide operational budget
Transition from a fixed-cost center to variable productivity cost center	DPR, K	
Expand OP revenue by adding four additional programs in 2008	LGA	

DPR, *Daily productivity report;* K, *biweekly productivity report;* LGA, *general ledger;* OP, *operating.*

TABLE 30-3   Performance Objective Plan for Customer Service

Performance Objective Plan	Outcome Indicators	Strategic Initiative
Improve quality of service perception by physicians, parents/families, and support staff in ICUs and general floor care areas	QI survey reports; direct interview with unit manager and physician	Improved customer loyalty, improvement of overall satisfaction scores
Develop child-friendly exercise solutions within pulmonary rehabilitation	Presence of new signage, equipment	

ICUs, *Intensive care units;* QI, *quality improvement.*

occurred in the past (e.g., cost-per-case expenses decrease, productivity increases). Table 30-2 provides an example of PR operation financial indicators. As a consequence, financial performance is going to be the "effect" of an action. This describes the dependency of financial performance indicators on the other scorecard categories. Substandard customer satisfaction performance or poor system design of day-to-day operations will ultimately have a substantial impact on the financial bottom line via referral pattern, case volume, and so on.

It often becomes difficult for the PR manager to obtain real net revenue statistics from hospital information systems. Actual numbers often are provided only 4 to 6 months after services have been provided. Reimbursement often varies from payer to payer, and consequently it becomes extremely important for the manager to know their patient "market." Clearly, the majority of patients seen within PR programs have a Medicare component, but copayer mix becomes an important element for the manager to know.

Customer Service

The customer perspective is essentially how patients, families, and physicians see the PR department. The general term applied to this perspective is *customer satisfaction,* but this should be transitioned to specific strategic initiative goals. For example, strategic initiatives might include establishing a target of improved customer satisfaction for new program attendees, or demonstrate an increasing trend in maintenance exercise program loyalty within designated control limits. The department should develop a more focused perspective on specific target audiences (e.g., referring physicians) with detailed data on performance. Table 30-3 provides a performance objective plan for customer service.

Improvement in Internal Operations

The internal business perspective asks "How do we make our internal operations better?" The core to any organization is an understanding of the primary mission, or the reason for operations. PR departments should focus on excelling at the delivery of interventional services. Examples of improvement in internal business measurements include the continual evaluation of quality performance indicators, services, and initiatives that focus on reducing emergency department or hospital readmissions, quality of life, and duration of hospital stay. The key is to identify indicators that contribute to the strategic organization initiatives. Table 30-4 provides an objective performance plan for PR improvement in internal operations.

TABLE 30-4 Improvement in Internal Operations		
Objective Performance Plan	**Outcome Indicator(s)**	**Strategic Initiative**
Revise job descriptions, with establishment of clinical ladder	New job descriptions completed and online by end of year	Strengthen clinical ladder, responsibilities of staff, financial incentives
Review, refine assessment activity in charting	Availability of new activity within database	Strengthen clinical services and documentation
Expand inpatient coverage to address lung transplant patient coverage	Increase inpatient visits, activities	Strengthen clinical services, earlier involvement in clinical management
Review/revise pulmonary hypertension patient access	Corrections to existent pathway	

TABLE 30-5 Performance Improvement Plan for Innovation and Learning		
Objective Performance Plan	**Outcome Indicator(s)**	**Strategic Initiative**
Develop alternative O_2 delivery systems to allow exercise programs for pulmonary hypertensive patients	Clinical application, procedure	Strengthen clinical services
Review and refine pulmonary rehabilitation exercise protocols	Newly revised protocols in procedure manual	
Encourage exercise certification programs within clinical staff	Two additional certified staff in 2007	Enhanced community presence, recognition as world-class in rehabilitation
Continuation of research related to pulmonary rehabilitation and select groups	At least three abstracts, papers, studies presented during year	

O_2, *Oxygen.*

The differentiation between driving or leading indicator and outcome indicator is important. Think of it as a cause-and-effect relationship. An outcome indicator often lags behind an action, because it measures performance that occurred in the past (e.g., cost-per-case expense decrease, productivity increases). Financial indicators are always outcome indicators. Driving or leading indicators, on the other hand, are the direct cause for the outcome (e.g., by instructing staff to apply an O_2 titration protocol to 95% of cases, cost-per-case expenses were reduced). Table 30-5 provides a performance improvement (PI) plan for PR program innovation and learning.

Quality and Performance Improvement

Quality and performance improvement are a pivotal part of the charge and mission of any PR department. PR departments are continually challenged with finding ways of "doing things better, faster, less expensively" and incorporating these changes into their daily operations.

Quality

Quality is often referred to as a trait or characteristic referenced to a level of excellence or high performance.[28,35,36] These observed quality traits are measurable elements that are important to the consumer. Performance, cost, and delivery are each examples of aspects of quality. Performance and cost may predominate when describing quality aspects for products, and delivery often predominates in service industries such as health care.

Aspects of quality can be further refined to become performance indicators. Aspects of quality are equally important and definable in PR. What characteristics describe the "quality" of service? The time between referral and starting the program? The percentage of improvement in Borg Index or 6MWT distance while in maintenance exercise? Multiple aspects may be evaluated, but an expected level of performance has still been established, and defines the quality and performance level for the service. The take-home message is that we can define and measure quality, and we can know when it is and is not present.

Performance Improvement

Performance improvement (PI) is the process of continually evaluating and refining with the intent to improve the delivery of services.[37] PI is dependent on monitoring; monitoring provides the department with internal tracking and trending, and when used by external groups, provides accountability for department performance. Performance monitoring helps the department provide data-driven, statistically valid measurements that continuously feed information about departmental performance. This helps the department better understand, adjust, and benchmark operations, and optimize performance of the organization. A PR annual skills fair is a PI process. It provides an opportunity for the team to review, relearn, and explore new evidence-based treatment procedures in PR.[38] The ultimate goal is for staff development of strong critical thinking processes. Figure 30-1 gives an example of a PI annual skills fair checkoff sheet.

Foundations of Quality Improvement

Programs that make a commitment to quality and performance improvement develop a competitive edge. This advantage comes from embracing the foundations of quality and performance improvement and creating a generative culture that empowers and encourages all employees to be innovative. Innovative employees practice with confidence, generate solutions, and practice a higher level of care. They maintain this high performance by understanding and applying the foundations of quality and performance improvement. QI is customer driven, and requires alignment, collaboration, and statistical analysis of data.[28,39,40]

Determining Characteristics of Quality and Performance

A central point of PI is recognition of whose opinion counts. Ultimately it is the customer who determines what is important for any business

---

Pulmonary Rehabilitation Skills Fair

RCP name _____   Date _____

Clinical competency (to be completed the day of Skills Fair)

Initials = Competency achieved

a. Be able to state the different PH medications and what we need to key in on   _____

b. Know the documentation language needed to prove skilled level of intervention in
    Pulmonary Rehabilitation Treatment   _____

c. Understand the "other systems" involvement in sarcoidosis and how it will result in
    pulmonary rehabilitation exercise program modification   _____

d. Recognize the importance of the ACCP/AACVPR evidence based guidelines in
    pulmonary rehabilitation and how the pulmonary rehabilitation program follows the
    national standards   _____

e. Know the latest IPF medications and resources available   _____

Practical competency (to be completed the day of Skills Fair)

f. Demonstrate the Nustep and the Biodex correct arm and seat setting placements   _____

g. Use the Dinamap BP monitor with correct cuff placement   _____

h. Demonstrate walker height setting and where to document on the exercise chart   _____

i. Verbalize the pre-registration process/knowing the script and how to use the
    "cube" files   _____

FIGURE 30-1 Example of an annual skills fair performance improvement checkoff sheet.

to focus on. A *customer* is any individual or group of individuals who rely on our product or service. Examples of PR customers would include patients, families, and physicians. The *ultimate customer* is the patient. Physicians, peers, and other health care team members often are described as *intermediate customers*: customers who rely on our service to provide another component of care. Much of PR quality improvement focuses on providing quality services to intermediate customers.

Opportunities for improvement are identified by the customers. These often share the following characteristics: problems that are chronic in nature, and that significantly limit the ability of the department to maximize their impact; problems that have not been resolved in the past, despite attempts to do so; and problems that cross over multiple areas or departments.

Customers determine the quality aspects of services, either directly or indirectly as a service request through another health care provider. Using the Borg Index and 6MWT examples, patients are most concerned with aspects related to comfort, level of dyspnea, and quality of life. The referring physician, on the other hand, may be more concerned with the improvement in 6MWT distance. Insurance carriers would be extremely interested in the impact of the program on emergency department visits or hospital readmission rates. Monitoring both intermediate and ultimate customer needs maximizes the understanding of the desired aspects of quality.

Quality Improvement Team

All PR team members need to take a role in improving quality care for QI/PI to be truly effective. Leadership and managers are responsible for sharing the vision of the department, and providing guidance and support for process improvement. In addition, leaders frequently have access to the issues most important to customers. As a result, they can provide the PI team with guidance on processes that may need improvement. Leadership has the responsibility of helping people to become accustomed to the quality improvement process: defining quality, tools used in QI processes, and so on.

Any process that involves more than one individual will use a team. Processes that cross departmental boundaries are best approached with members from other departments. Team members must have ownership of the process. Because they are close to the process, they are the people most suited to describing process problems and improvements.

The team will be responsible for defining the problem, and for developing meeting guidelines, ground rules, and a process roadmap, also known as a Gantt chart. The process roadmap serves as a visual reminder of the steps and schedule projections that need to be accomplished for completion of the project.

Integrating Performance Improvement into Job Performance

Core to the tenet of continual QI is staff involvement. For QI/PI to be embraced by the staff, leaders must show a sustained and heartfelt commitment to QI/PI. Leadership buy-in is essential to success. The QI/PI process avoids blame but focuses on process improvement. This does not mean that individuals should not take ownership for QI/PI. On the contrary, the principles of QI/PI need to be understood and applied by all team members. One place to start defining the expectations of PI is in the job description. The job description provides a venue for addressing the various levels of QI/PI participation. Departments can tailor the expectations for PI to the individual's job description and performance level. For example, a new employee who is a recent graduate from a local respiratory therapy program may have little knowledge of QI and not understand its value and importance to the organization. Consequently, the expectations for QI/PI knowledge and performance will be different from those of a front-line supervisor. Over time the new graduate could be expected to become better acquainted with the reason and methodology of QI/PI. Box 30-9 describes how one could approach developing PI across the different job descriptions of the PR department.

Clinical Ladder: Job Descriptions

The opportunity for the PR administrative manager to recognize and reward excellence in PR clinical practice, leadership, professional growth, and contributions to the organization is through the development of a clinical ladder for PR staff.[41,42] The nursing and respiratory care community has used the clinical ladder for years. It is time to develop a process improvement to specifically recognize the PR staff. Staff retention and the hiring of competent PR team members are critical to the strength of a program. The clinical ladder can financially compensate and recognize superior staff for their PR clinical skills. The starting

---

BOX 30-9 | **Pulmonary Rehabilitation Services Job Description**

Pulmonary Rehabilitation Therapist 1 (entry level): Understands the basics of the QI/PI process, and can list the primary indicators being followed within the department

Pulmonary Rehabilitation Therapist 2 Understands the value of QI, the tools used in QI, and the performance indicators being tracked within the department

Pulmonary Rehabilitation Therapist 3: Understands the value of QI/PI, the tools used in QI, and the performance indicators. Actively participates in QI with the department as evidenced by team or project participation

Pulmonary Rehabilitation Therapist 4 (highest level): Is thoroughly knowledgeable in QI/PI. Actively participates or leads multiple QI projects with department or institution

---

PI, *Performance improvement*; QI, *quality improvement*.

---

point is the development of job descriptions that builds on greater clinical skills, has an expectation of greater responsibility, allows staff to set and achieve goals, and has accountability for performance. Box 30-10 provides an example of job descriptions for the PR respiratory therapy clinical ladder, from entrance level PR Respiratory Therapist—RCP II, Senior PR Respiratory Therapist—RCP III, to the PR Team Leader—RCP IV.

ACCREDITATION AND STANDARDS AGENCIES

Accreditation and standards groups provide key guidance information that health care institutions can use to continually improve their level of patient care. Virtually all of these standards are intended to establish baseline levels of care, or to prevent care issues from occurring. There are multiple national and international agencies or groups committed to patient safety and quality health care improvement, and it is beyond the scope of this chapter to address all. The following examples are of particular interest to the PR department.

The Joint Commission

The Joint Commission, or simply TJC, is arguably the most influential accrediting agency in the nation. TJC, formerly called the Joint Commission

of Accreditation of Hospitals, or JCAHO, was formed in 1951 by the American College of Surgeons, the American Hospital Association, and the American Medical Association. In 1999, TJC cosponsored a world symposium on improving health care worldwide through accreditation[41] summarizing greater emphasis on accountability in the United States and worldwide, which has triggered growth within the internal (organizational) quality management program and external (cross-organizational) benchmarking arena with comparative data, accreditation, and certification.

TJC is an independent, not-for-profit organization whose mission is to "continuously improve the safety and quality of health care provided to the public through the provision of health care accreditation and related services that support performance improvement in health care organizations." TJC sets the standards by which most health care delivery systems are measured in the United States. TJC evaluates the quality and safety of care for nearly 17,000 health care organizations. To maintain and earn accreditation, organizations must have an extensive on-site review by a team of TJC health care professionals, at least once every 3 years. The purpose of the review is to evaluate each organization's performance in areas that affect patient care. Accreditation may then be awarded on the basis of how well the organizations met TJC standards.[37]

Patient safety—related issues are of particular importance to TJC.[43] Key principal elements include sentinel events: patient safety—related incidents that have occurred at multiple health delivery sites. PR departments have historically used the TJC accreditation process to direct their performance improvement initiatives. Box 30-11 provides a list of the national patient safety goals applicable to PR.

The TJC survey process is continually evolving to better meet the needs of consumers and health care organizations. As part of this evolution, TJC is changing the way surveys will be performed. TJC has developed a list of core performance measures to better evaluate performance within facilities.[44,45] Surveys require a periodic performance review process, which places greater emphasis on health care organizations identifying indicators of performance. In addition, TJC requires focus and survey of significant areas of patient safety and the quality process. PR departments should strive to direct QI processes to be inclusive of the

BOX 30-10	Example of a Pulmonary Rehabilitation Respiratory Therapy Clinical Ladder

PULMONARY REHABILITATION RESPIRATORY THERAPIST—RCP II LEVEL

Overview

The position of Pulmonary Rehabilitation (PR) Therapist is an entry-level position in pulmonary rehabilitation for a Registered Respiratory Therapist. It is expected that mastery of the components of pulmonary rehabilitation from assessment, education, psychosocial intervention, and therapeutic exercise to long-term adherence will be achieved within 1 year of accepting the Pulmonary Rehabilitation Therapist position.

Job Specifications

	Description	Minimum Required	Preferred/Desired
Education	COARC-accredited respiratory therapy program	Graduate from an entry- or advanced-level education program with at least an associate degree	Bachelor's degree from an advanced-level education program
Experience	Postgraduate clinical respiratory care	2 to 3 yr of clinical respiratory therapy experience, including ICU	1 to 3 yr of pulmonary rehabilitation clinical experience
Training	Age-specific criteria: children, adolescents, adults, and geriatrics	Training in selected age populations	
Certification		RRT	ACSM credential as Health/Fitness Instructor, *or*
		BLS	Exercise Specialist,
		ACLS	Asthma Educator
Licensure	Valid/current license as a Respiratory Care Practitioner	Possession of license as a Respiratory Care Practitioner	
Special skills		Proficient in English	Area-specific experience and training, and bilingual
Requirements	Clinical ladder requirements	1 Initiative 0 QI projects 12 CEUs/CRCEs 0 In-services	

ACLS, *Advanced cardiac life support;* ACSM, *American College of Sports Medicine;* BLS, *basic life support;* CEU, *continuing education unit;* COARC, *Committee on Accreditation for Respiratory Care;* CRCE, *continuing respiratory care education;* ICU, *intensive care unit;* RRT, *Registered Respiratory Therapist;* QI, *quality improvement.*

SENIOR PULMONARY REHABILITATION THERAPIST—RCP III LEVEL

Overview

The Senior Pulmonary Rehabilitation Therapist is an advanced-level Pulmonary Rehabilitation Therapist with advanced assessment and pulmonary rehabilitation therapeutic skills in multiple patient populations, areas, and age groups. The Senior Pulmonary Rehabilitation Therapist is expected to have higher knowledge, skills, ability levels, and critical thinking than the Pulmonary Rehabilitation Therapist. The Senior Pulmonary Rehabilitation Therapist can handle virtually any circumstance that may arise pertaining to pulmonary rehabilitation without supervision; is able to coordinate projects, assist in PR program development, and continuous quality improvement (CQI); and is able to perform daily staff assignments and be responsible for coordinating, monitoring, and evaluating the shift-to-shift pulmonary rehabilitation services of the operational area. The Senior Pulmonary Rehabilitation Therapist ensures that staff performs pulmonary rehabilitation in a manner consistent with departmental standards and requirements; resolves problems and strives continuously to improve the quality of patient care; and is responsible for operational functions of pulmonary rehabilitation.

Continued

BOX 30-10	Example of a Pulmonary Rehabilitation Respiratory Therapy Clinical Ladder—cont'd		
	Job Specifications		
	Description	Minimum Required	Preferred/Desired
Education	COARC-accredited respiratory therapy program	Graduate from an entry- or advanced-level education program with at least an associate degree	Bachelor's degree from an advanced-level education program
Experience	Postgraduate clinical respiratory care	5 yr of clinical experience in respiratory care services, with ICU experience ≥3 yr of clinical experience working in pulmonary rehabilitation	>5 yr of clinical experience working in pulmonary rehabilitation
Training	Age-specific criteria: children, adolescents, adults, and geriatrics Hospital and departmental orientation	Training in selected age populations Completion of Inova system/hospital/ department leadership training	Previous supervisory training
Certification		RRT BLS ACLS ACSM credential as Health/ Fitness Instructor or Exercise Specialist	Certified as Tobacco Treatment Specialist or Asthma Educator
Licensure	Valid/current license as a Respiratory Care Practitioner	Possession of license as a Respiratory Care Practitioner	
Special skills	Critical thinking skills, preceptor skills, presentation/instructional techniques	Critical thinking skills, preceptor skills, proficient in English	Area-specific experience and training, and bilingual Pulmonary rehabilitation, clinical specialist problem solving, bilingual skills
Requirements	Clinical ladder requirements	2 Initiatives 1 QI project 16 CEUs/CRCEs >1 In-service, staff and/or community	

For definitions, see Job Specification for Pulmonary Rehabilitation Respiratory Therapist—RCP II level.

PULMONARY REHABILITATION TEAM LEAD—RCP IV LEVEL

Overview

The Pulmonary Rehabilitation Clinical Specialist is an advanced-level senior Pulmonary Rehabilitation Therapist with higher knowledge, skill, abilities, and critical thinking levels than the Senior Pulmonary Rehabilitation Therapist, and has advanced assessment and pulmonary rehabilitation therapeutic skills in multiple patient populations, areas, and age groups. The PR Clinical Specialist can handle virtually any circumstance that may arise pertaining to pulmonary rehabilitation without supervision. The PR Clinical Specialist is expected to routinely perform and interact as a professional with exemplary interpersonal skills. The PR Clinical Specialist takes a leadership role in managing research, CQI, and investigational and educational projects to advance the science of pulmonary rehabilitation. The PR Clinical Specialist is able to perform daily staff assignments and is responsible for coordinating, monitoring, and evaluating the shift-to-shift pulmonary rehabilitation services of the operational area. The PR Clinical Specialist ensures that staff performs pulmonary rehabilitation in a manner consistent with departmental standards and requirements. The PR Clinical Specialist resolves problems and strives to continuously improve the quality of patient care. The PR Clinical Specialist is expected to have advanced teaching skills and is proficient in developing educational tools, including lesson plans and course outlines.

BOX 30-10	Example of a Pulmonary Rehabilitation Respiratory Therapy Clinical Ladder—cont'd

Job Specifications

	Description	Minimum Required	Preferred/Desired
Education	COARC-accredited respiratory therapy program	Graduate from an entry- or advanced-level education program with at least an associate degree	Bachelor's degree from an advanced-level education program/master's degree
Experience	Postgraduate clinical respiratory care	8 yr of clinical experience in respiratory care services, with ICU experience ≥5 yr of clinical experience working in pulmonary rehabilitation	>10 yr of clinical experience working in pulmonary rehabilitation
Training	Age-specific criteria: children, adolescents, adults, and geriatrics	Training in selected age populations	Previous supervisory training
	Hospital and departmental orientation	Completion of Inova system/ hospital/department leadership training	
Certification		RRT BLS ACLS ACSM credential as Health/ Fitness Instructor or Exercise Specialist	Certified as a Tobacco Treatment Specialist or Asthma Educator
Licensure	Valid/current license as a Respiratory Care Practitioner	Possession of license as a Respiratory Care Practitioner	
Special skills	Critical thinking, preceptorship/mentoring, presentation skills/ instructional technologies	Proficient in English	Area-specific experience and training, and bilingual
		Relief team leader	Submit and publish case study/abstract/review article in medical journal
Requirements	Clinical ladder requirements	6 Initiatives 2 QI projects 16 CEUs/CRCEs 3 In-services, staff and/or community	

For definitions, see Job Specification for Pulmonary Rehabilitation Respiratory Therapist—RCP II level.
Courtesy Inova Fairfax Hospital, Pulmonary Rehabilitation Department, Falls Church, Virginia.

new performance indicators within their health care organization.

TJC has developed disease-specific care certifications programs that sets standards, outlines clinical practice guidelines applicable to the disease-specific care, and measures performance outcomes. The TJC certification programs that pertain to PR are as follows: chronic obstructive pulmonary disease,[46] lung volume reduction surgery,[47] and transplant center[48] (specifically lung transplantation). Each certification program has specific standards with requirements that may require PR involvement and outcome data (Box 30-12).

American Association of Cardiovascular and Pulmonary Rehabilitation Program Certifications

The impetus to develop a national PR program certification process came from the membership of the American Association of Cardiovascular and Pulmonary Rehabilitation (AACVPR).[1] It was thought that a standard should be developed with

| BOX 30-11 | The Joint Commission National Patient Safety Goals Applicable to Pulmonary Rehabilitation: 2003-2008 |

2003 NATIONAL PATIENT SAFETY GOALS

Goal 1   Improve the accuracy of patient identification.

Goal 1A   Use at least two patient identifiers (neither to be the patient's room number) whenever taking blood samples or administering medications or blood products.

Goal 2   Improve the effectiveness of communication among caregivers.

Goal 2A   Implement a process for taking verbal or telephone orders that requires a verification "read-back" of the complete order by the person receiving the order.

Goal 2B   Standardize the abbreviations, acronyms, and symbols used throughout the organization, including a list of abbreviations, acronyms, and symbols not to use.

Goal 6   Improve the effectiveness of clinical alarm systems.

Goal 6A   Implement regular preventive maintenance and testing of alarm systems.

Goal 6B   Ensure that alarms are activated with appropriate settings and are sufficiently audible with respect to distances and competing noise within the unit.

2004 NATIONAL PATIENT SAFETY GOALS

Goal 7   Reduce the risk of health care–acquired infections

Goal 7A   Comply with current CDC hand hygiene guidelines.

2005 NATIONAL PATIENT SAFETY GOALS

Goal 2C   Measure, assess and, if appropriate, take action to improve the timeliness of reporting, and the timeliness of receipt by the responsible licensed caregiver, of critical test results and values.

Goal 8A   During 2005, for full implementation by January 2006, develop a process for obtaining and documenting a complete list of the patient's current medications upon the patient's admission to the organization and with the involvement of the patient. This process includes a comparison of the medications the organization provides with those on the list.

Goal 8B   A complete list of the patient's medications is communicated to the next provider of service when it refers or transfers a patient to another setting, service, practitioner, or level of care within or outside the organization.

Goal 9A   Reduce the risk of patient harm resulting from falls. Assess and periodically reassess each patient's risk for falling, including the potential risk associated with the patient's medication regimen, and take action to address any identified risks.

2006 NATIONAL PATIENT SAFETY GOALS

Goal 8B   The complete list of medications is also provided to the patient on discharge from the facility.

Goal 13   Encourage patients' active involvement in their own care as a patient safety strategy.

Goal 13A   Define and communicate the means for patients and their families to report concerns about safety and encourage them to do so.

Goal 15   The organization identifies safety risks inherent in its patient population.

2007 NATIONAL PATIENT SAFETY GOALS

Goal 8B   A complete list of the patient's medications is communicated to the next provider of service when a patient is referred or transferred to another setting, service, practitioner, or level of care within or outside the organization. The complete list of medications is also provided to the patient on discharge from the facility. [Ambulatory, Assisted Living, Behavioral Health Care, Critical Access Hospital, Disease-Specific Care, Home Care, Hospital, Long-Term Care, Office-Based Surgery]

Goal 13A   Define and communicate the means for patients and their families to report concerns about safety and encourage them to do so. [Ambulatory, Assisted Living, Behavioral Health Care, Critical Access Hospital, Disease-Specific Care, Home Care, Hospital, Lab, Long-Term Care, Office-Based Surgery]

Goal 15   The organization identifies safety risks inherent in its patient population.

Goal 15B   The organization identifies risks associated with long-term O_2 therapy such as home fires. [Home Care] Although this pertains to Home Care, the Pulmonary Rehabilitation program should reinforce O_2 safety in the home.

2008 NATIONAL PATIENT SAFETY GOALS

Goal 7A   Comply with current WHO Hand Hygiene Guidelines or CDC hand hygiene guidelines. [Ambulatory, Assisted Living, Behavioral Health Care, Critical Access Hospital, Disease-Specific Care, Home Care, Hospital, Lab, Long-Term Care, Office-Based Surgery]

Goal 16   Improve recognition and response to changes in a patient's condition.

Goal 16A   The organization selects a suitable method that enables health care staff members to directly request additional assistance from a specially trained individual(s) when the patient's condition appears to be worsening. [Critical Access Hospital, Hospital]

CDC, *Centers for Disease Control and Prevention;* O_2, *oxygen;* WHO, *World Health Organization.*

BOX 30-12	The Joint Commission Disease Certification Program Requirements with Pulmonary Rehabilitation Involvement

LVRS REQUIREMENTS

- Delivering or facilitating clinical care: How is PR involved
- Performance measurement: PR outcomes
- Supporting self-management: PR patient training/ education
- Program management: Role
- Clinical information management

COPD REQUIREMENTS

- Staff education requirements
- The use of spirometry
- Smoking cessation
- Risk factor reduction
- Patient education on self-management of COPD
- Coordination of care

TRANSPLANT CENTER REQUIREMENTS

- Organization leadership
- Selection of patients and living donors, as well as managing care and respecting patient and donor rights
- Coordination of care, including pre- and postsurgical processes
- Qualifications of caregivers
- Staff competency and training
- Information management
- Standardized performance measurement and data submission
- Performance assessment and improvement

COPD, *Chronic obstructive pulmonary disease;* LVRS, *lung volume reduction surgery.*

---

which PR programs in the United States could compare/benchmark themselves. The national certification is based on the following documents:

- AACVPR *Guidelines for Pulmonary Rehabilitation Programs*, third edition[1]
- AACVPR clinical competency guidelines for pulmonary rehabilitation professionals[42]
- AACVPR Outcomes Committee: Outcome measurement in cardiac and pulmonary rehabilitation[49]

The first program certification process began in the fall of 1998. A total of 291 applications were submitted for review, which included both pulmonary and cardiac rehabilitation programs. The recommendations of the National Program Oversight Committee with the approval of the AACVPR Board of Directors granted 254 programs certification in 1999. In 2007, a total of 91 applications were approved for certification and 275 were approved for recertification. In 2008, 125 programs applied for certification and

480 applied for recertification. Program certification is annual and recertification is every 3 years.

The feedback from the membership of the AACVPR and other professionals in the field of PR continues to be positive regarding certification. The future of program certification is strong and programs have improved by committing to the national standards as outlined by the AACVPR.

REIMBURSEMENT

PR program directors need to be as familiar with all aspects of reimbursement for PR as they are with evidence-based medicine. They need to become experts in understanding reimbursement terminology, know what a billable service is and whether it is necessary to obtain preauthorization from an insurance company, and how to proceed with the request. Learning the mechanics of all types of insurances is a basic skill that should be mastered. It is also important to know who the Medicare administrative contractor (MAC) is and whether the MAC has a local coverage determination (LCD) for PR. If the MAC does not have an LCD, what is their policy for reimbursing the PR services?[50]

The health care organization's contract coordinator or the contracting department should be aware of the provided PR services so that they will keep the program in mind while negotiating contracts. The business office should communicate changes or billing problems related to reimbursement.

PR staff members should belong to state and national pulmonary organizations to help stay current with the ever-changing reimbursement arena. *Recently, on July 15, 2008, history was made with the passage of the law designating pulmonary rehabilitation as a Medicare benefit.* The impact of this law will benefit patients with chronic lung disease who need pulmonary rehabilitation.

Historical Perspective

Historically, the demand for health insurance originated in the breakdown of a household economy, as families depended on the employment of the primary wage earner for income and on the services of physicians and hospitals for medical treatment. Illness caused an interruption in the flow of income to a household, causing economic hardship. The need for health insurance in the United States was more than a private problem. The strain of the rising cost of health care imposed on society as a whole generated great debate in the politics of health insurance in the early 1900s and continues to do so today as we move into the 21st century.

Before the enactment of the Medicare and Medicaid programs, health care was financed through private commercial insurance or was paid for privately. As early as 1900, a few states became involved with workmen's compensation laws, and by 1920 these laws were accepted by 42 states. Cash payments for a worker's time lost from the job because of injury or illness was the first benefit, later followed by coverage for health care and rehabilitation services.

The Medicare and Medicaid programs evolved during a 53-year period, starting with Theodore Roosevelt's Bull Moose Party platform, which first promoted the ideas of having national health insurance. In 1935 the Social Security Act was passed and in 1949 a bill was introduced calling for comprehensive and universal health care coverage. Intense debate occurred over some form of national health insurance from 1949 to 1965, when at last the Medicare and Medicaid laws were finally passed under the guidance of the Kennedy and Johnson administrations. The great complexity between governmental process and social policy is evident in the health insurance arena.

Sources of Health Care Financing

In the United States, the financing of health care services originates from three basic sources: (1) federal and state governmental health insurance programs,[51-53] (2) nongovernmental health insurance programs, and (3) private pay. A further explanation of the different sources for reimbursement is shown in Box 30-13. Payment of health care services is made by third-party payers or by the patient. A third-party payer is an organization (e.g., a commercial insurance company) that pays or insures medical/health expenses on behalf of its beneficiaries, members, or clients. Therefore the patient receiving the medical service is considered the first party, the provider of the medical service is considered the second party, and the organization paying for the medical service is the third party (Figure 30-2).

Federal and State Health Insurance Programs
Medicare
Medicare, established by Congress in 1965, is the federal health insurance program for people age 65 years and older, people younger than 65 years with disabilities, people with end-stage renal disease, and certain otherwise noncovered aged persons who choose to buy into Medicare. The Medicare Act is known as Title XVIII of the Social Security Act. When Medicare was implemented in 1966, the

---

BOX 30-13	Sources of Health Care Financing

NONGOVERNMENTAL HEALTH INSURANCE PROGRAMS
- Private/commercial health insurance plans
- Managed care organizations
- Medicare Supplement/Medigap plans

FEDERAL AND STATE HEALTH INSURANCE PROGRAMS
- Medicare
- Medicaid
- Hill-Burton Program
- Comprehensive Outpatient Rehabilitation Facility
- Veterans Health Administration Program
- Civilian Health and Medical Program of the Uniformed Services/TRICARE
- Federal Employees Health Benefit (FEHB) program

CASUALTY INSURANCE PROGRAM
- Workers' compensation, related to accidents on the job

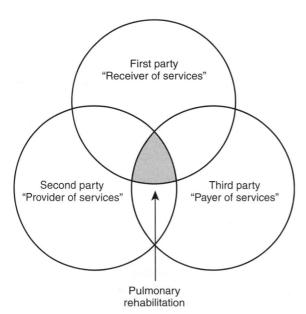

FIGURE 30-2 The correlation of insurance terminology to pulmonary rehabilitation is necessary for effective communication with the insurance industry and for program reimbursement. Pulmonary rehabilitation involves first-, second-, and third-party involvement, with each party having a specific function as it relates to pulmonary rehabilitation.
Understanding the party function is essential to ensure reimbursement for the program.

program covered persons age 65 years and older. In 1972, the program was expanded to cover persons who are entitled to Social Security or Railroad Retirement disability benefits for at least 24 months, persons with end-stage renal disease, and certain otherwise noncovered aged persons. The intent of Medicare's architects was to provide the elderly and the disabled with a program that would help to decrease their out-of-pocket costs for medically necessary health service. Medicare, however, is neither a comprehensive health care system nor cost free; many health care services are not covered, and Medicare beneficiaries are required to share the costs of such coverage.

Medicare Coverage

Medicare coverage consists of: Part A (Hospital), Part B (Medical), Part C (Medicare Advantage Plans, such as health maintenance organizations and preferred provider organizations),[54] and Part D (Medicare prescription drug coverage).

Medicare Part A (Hospital Insurance) helps cover inpatient care in hospitals, and skilled nursing facilities (not custodial or long-term care). It also helps cover hospice care and some home health care. Certain conditions must be met to obtain these benefits. A Medicare national coverage policy on pulmonary rehabilitation will be written as a result of the July 2008 law making pulmonary rehabilitation a Medicare benefit.

Medicare Part B (Medical Insurance) helps cover doctors' services and outpatient care. It also covers some other medical services that Part A does not cover, such as some of the services of physical and occupational therapists, and some home health care.

Medicare Claims Processing

The processing of Medicare claims is handled by nongovernment, private organizations or agencies (e.g., a commercial insurance company) that contract to serve as the fiscal agent between health care providers (e.g., hospitals and physicians) and the federal government. These private contractors process claims locally for Medicare Part A and Part B and have been known as *intermediaries* and *carriers*. Until recently, the fiscal intermediaries were processing Part A claims for institutional services including inpatient hospital services, skilled nursing facilities, home health agencies, hospice services, and hospital outpatient claims for Medicare Part B, which includes PR. Medicare carriers processed Part B claims for services by physicians and medical

suppliers, including durable medical equipment and ambulance services. In 2003, the Medicare Modernization Act required "Medicare contracting reform," which will integrate Parts A and B for the fee-for-service benefit to new entities called Medicare administrative contractors (MACs).[55] The purpose of the integration is to centralize information that was once held separately, creating a platform for advances in the delivery of comprehensive care to Medicare beneficiaries. There is open competition for all claims administration contracts. This should lead to more efficiency and greater accountability, as well as promote the ability of the CMS to negotiate incentives to reward Medicare contractors that perform well. When the MACs are in place there will be a single point of contact for providers and they are required to be responsive to the providers. Some of the MACs are already in place and the CMS is hoping to transfer all work to MACs by October 2011.

Comprehensive Outpatient Rehabilitation Facility

A comprehensive outpatient rehabilitation facility (CORF) is a Medicare-certified health care facility that is defined as:

> A nonresidential facility that is established and operated exclusively for the purpose of providing diagnostic, therapeutic, and restorative services to outpatients for the rehabilitation of injured, disabled, or sick persons, at a single fixed location, by and under the supervision of a physician (Code of Federal Regulations 42: Section 485.51).[56]

CORFs are required to provide at least physical therapy and social services and to either contract with or employ a medical director. Additional CORF services are occupational therapy, speech–language pathology, respiratory therapy, psychological services, orthotic and prosthetic device services, nursing care services, drugs and biologicals, and durable medical equipment. In the federal regulations, respiratory therapy services are defined as "services for the assessment, diagnostic evaluation, treatment, management, and monitoring of patients with deficiencies or abnormalities of cardiopulmonary function" (Section 410.100 [3e]).

Nongovernmental Health Insurance Programs
Private Health Insurance Programs

Private health insurance programs are a method of redistributing the financial risk associated with major illnesses from individuals to collectives mediated by commercial insurance companies.

TABLE 30-6 National Managed Care Enrollment in the United States: 2008	
Health Plan	**Number Enrolled**
HMO	88.8 million
PPO	60.1 million
Total	148.9 million

Adapted from Managed Care On-Line Web site. Available at http://www.mcol.com. Retrieved April 3, 2008.

Private insurers underwrite the coverage without becoming involved in the delivery system. Insurance was developed to protect people from economic hardships. A high percentage of private coverage is obtained through a current or former employer or union.

Managed Care

The concept of managed care[57-60] in the United States as it is known today is an outgrowth of the private sector and dates back to the late 1920s. Between 1930 and 1960 numerous other major prepaid group practice plans emerged and experienced significant success in attracting enrollees. In early 1970, the term *health maintenance organization* (HMO) was given to prepaid group practice plans to emphasize the focus on health promotion and prevention, thus making HMOs more attractive. The growth of managed care increased significantly when Congress enacted the HMO Act of 1973 (PL 93-222). The legislation provided grants and loans to develop new HMOs. To qualify for funding, an HMO had to offer specific basic services and charge premiums based on "community"-wide health care costs.

The term *managed care* is used in many ways, so it is essential to recognize that not all managed care plans are the same. Risk-based managed care describes care from organizations that provide or contract to provide health care in broad specified areas for a defined population for a predetermined prepaid fee. In addition, managed care organizations (MCOs) take on the financial risk to deliver the services for the predetermined fee. MCOs use various cost-controlling techniques.

MCOs are typically classified into two dominant forms: (1) HMOs and (2) preferred provider organizations (PPOs). An HMO is a prepaid health plan delivering comprehensive care to members through designated providers. HMOs combine insurer and providers into one entity. Enrollees choose a primary care physician (i.e., a gatekeeper) to coordinate their care. PPOs are entities through which employer health benefit plans and health insurance carriers contract to purchase health care for beneficiaries. Typically, PPOs offer the flexibility for beneficiaries to use non-PPO providers. In exchange for this freedom of choice, usually substantial deductibles and/or copayments apply to care from non-PPO providers. A third form of managed care is the exclusive provider organization, a variation of the PPO with characteristics of an HMO. Beneficiaries are limited to using specific providers and hospitals, and exclusive provider organizations may use gatekeeper approaches similar to HMOs for authorizing specialty services. Table 30-6 shows the National Managed Care Enrollment in the United States for 2008.

DOCUMENTATION

PR reimbursement is a dynamic arena in which regulatory changes occur rapidly. To optimize the revenue for PR, the administrative manager must be familiar with the facility's business office and contracting department, where decisions are made regarding the negotiation of contracts and reimbursement.[61] A business office representative and the facility contracting specialist should be invited to be on the PR team. The liaison developed with these departments will expand the PR program's understanding and exposure to the constantly changing reimbursement field from managed care to Medicare. Uniformity in handling and reimbursing PR claims is not consistent in the United States. What is known are the do's and don'ts of Medicare. Because other third-party payers will often follow the rules set by Medicare, it is helpful to clearly understand Medicare's rules.

Human error can cause reimbursement nightmares as it pertains to a patient's billing claim, medical record, and rehabilitation program documentation. A claim denial by a third-party payer may be due to technical errors as it relates to program documentation, the billing office electronic bill submission, or the medical records department chart completeness. The golden rule for documentation does not exist, but specific guidelines apply. Some third-party payers have developed policy statements for reimbursement of PR services. Administrative directors must determine whether such a document exists in their state or with their MAC. Where no policy is available, collaboration with other local program administrative directors should be to offer PR expertise and assistance to the third-party payer to develop such a document, to help set standards. Understanding the current third-party payer guidelines for reimbursement of the interdisciplinary team home departments, such as respiratory therapy, physical therapy, and occupational therapy services, may also be helpful in understanding the current trends for reimbursement and how changes or directives seen in those disciplines may also impact the PR program.

Medicare Documentation Requirements

Medicare requires that documentation reflect an individualized, skilled needs evaluation within the interdisciplinary team's scope of practice, license, and expertise. Initial patient evaluations must identify the problems, develop specific plans of treatment in accordance with evidence-based practice, and set concrete goals. All documentation must demonstrate the clinical rationale for the skilled intervention, reflect medical necessity, and track outcomes. Patient documentation that leads to outcome analysis entails critical thinking on the part of the interdisciplinary team. The cognitive skills the interdisciplinary team uses in critical thinking include interpretation, analysis, evaluation, inference, explanation, and self-regulation. It is interesting to note that the scientific method uses these skills as well. Self-regulation refers to the ability of PR team members to competently, efficiently, and promptly adapt to changes in PR clinical practice. The PR team must continually assess quality improvement outcomes and evidence-based outcomes to modify the PR treatment to the patient's needs. Box 30-14 lists PR treatment documentation requirements.

The program documentation must match the itemized bill (UB-04) for date of service and duration of treatment. The documentation must refer to patient outcomes. The documentation must cover the following areas: treatments must be ordered by a physician; qualify as a covered service or policy benefit; be reasonable and necessary for the diagnosis and/or treatment of the pulmonary illness; be consistent with the nature and severity of the individual's symptoms and diagnosis; be reasonable in terms of procedure/modality, amount, frequency, and duration of treatment; be accepted by the professional community as being safe and effective treatment for the purpose used; be of a level of complexity such that the services can

---

BOX 30-14 **Pulmonary Rehabilitation Treatment Documentation Requirements**

- Physician order for therapy is required
- Documentation must be individualized and show medical necessity
- Interdisciplinary teams work in their scope of practice in accordance with state and federal regulations
- Initial assessment must identify the problems
- Plan of treatment must be specific and show need for skilled level of intervention
- Goals must be specific to promote recovery and restore function, and be measurable
- Treatment must be reasonable, necessary, and clinically based for the diagnosis and procedure
- Treatment is accepted by the professional community as safe and effective for the diagnosis and evidence based

---

be rendered only by a skilled clinician; and be delivered by qualified health professionals in accordance with state and federal regulations; also, the PR services must not exceed the patient's particular PR needs, must promote recovery, must restore function, and must ensure safety affected by the illness or injury, have an expectation that there will be measurable improvement of the patient's condition in a reasonable and generally predictable period of time, and demonstrate practical improvement. To optimize program reimbursement under Medicare guidelines, a clear understanding of what is *not* covered is also important. These noncovered services should never show up as a billed procedure on the patient's UB-04 or in documentation. Box 30-15 lists the Medicare noncovered services.

Reasons for Medicare denial may include the following: the patient is being provided known noncovered services; the patient is expected to spontaneously return to his or her previous level of function without skilled therapeutic intervention; the treatment is for maintenance of a chronic baseline condition; the treatment is merely to maintain a functional level; the patient has an acute and or unstable disease; the patient is incapable of participating in PR because of mental or physical limitations; the patient is smoking; documentation does not support measurable benefit; and the patient is unable or unwilling to benefit from the treatment.

The physical medicine community has used documentation language accepted by Medicare, called functional assessment measures (FAMs), functional independent measures (FIMs),[62] and the World Health Organization International

---

BOX 30-15 | **Medicare Noncovered Services**

- Nonindividualized treatment, education, and training
- Routine psychological screening and/or routine psychological therapy
- Duplication of services between occupational, physical, and respiratory therapy and nursing
- Treatment that exceeds the patient's needs for the identified condition
- Routine, nonskilled, and/or maintenance care
- Repetitive services for chronic baseline conditions
- Plateau in patient's progress toward goals
- Inability to sustain gains
- No overall improvement
- Generalized exercise
- Poor rehabilitation potential exists with the patient
- Treatment that is not reasonable and necessary because of lack of significant objective findings in preliminary pulmonary diagnostic testing
- Routine follow-up visits
- Viewing of films or videotapes, listening to audiotapes, completing interactive computer programs
- Any supervised or independent technology-based instruction
- Exercise equipment or supplies
- Biofeedback services for relaxation
- Nutritional counseling
- Social services
- Team and/or family conferences
- Documentation time
- Discharge summaries
- Educational materials such as books

Classification of Functioning (ICF), that allows for precise documentation of the skilled treatment intervention. The specific content areas to document include level of physical assistance and cueing. Physical assistance is categorized as independent, modified dependence, or complete dependence:

The *independent patient* (I) is independent and safe with mobility without an adaptive device—no wall, railings, walkers, canes, etc.

The *modified independent* (Mod I or MI) patient is independent with mobility with an adaptive device—use of a walker, cane, etc. The patients in this category who are inpatients *would not* be expected to be cotreated with physical therapy and PR simultaneously.

The next level is *modified dependence*. There are a number of criteria in this level:

Standby assist or set-up (SBA or s/u) describes a patient who can complete an exercise or task with someone present to provide needed tools.

Supervision (S) describes a patient who requires direct supervision for safety, but completes 100% of a task if the patient is cued.

Contact Guard Assist (CGA) describes a patient who requires close, hands-on contact for safety.

Hand-held Assist (HHA) describes a patient who requires minimal support of hands for balance and safety.

Minimal Assist (Min A) describes a patient who completes 75% to 99% of a task, referring to the effort the patient exhibits. This would mean the therapist's effort represents about 25%.

Moderate Assist (Mod A) describes a patient who completes 50% to 74% of a task. This would mean the therapist's effort represents about 50%. In this situation *cotreatment* with physical therapy and PR simultaneously is expected for an inpatient. An example would be a post-lung transplantation patient being treated in the intensive care unit immediately after the operation.

The last level is *complete dependence*:

Maximum Assist (Max A) describes a patient who completes 25% to 49% of a task. This would mean the therapist's effort is about 75%. This is another situation in which simultaneous cotreatment of an inpatient with physical therapy and PR is possible.

Dependent (Dep or D) describes a patient who completes less than 25% of a task. The patient is not able to do transfers at this time, and is not able to stand and support weight. The therapist actually moves the patient, such as by in-bed rotation. This level of care is often seen in the intubated patient. The dependent patient is not able to do PR exercise, but the PR therapist may work with the patient on breathing techniques, panic control, etc.

Assistance of two (A of 2) describes a patient who requires two people to physically assist for safety with mobility.

The other documentation used by physical medicine concerns cueing. Cueing is divided into verbal cues and tactile cues. *Verbal cues* (VC) include the following: *Minimal verbal cueing* (Min VC) describes when the patient completes a task with verbal cues given less than 25% of the time. An example of this would be a patient who, after numerous supervised exercise sessions, is able to perform warm-up exercises with Min VC. *Moderate verbal cueing* (Mod VC) describes when the patient requires verbal cues for 25% to 49% of the task. *Maximal verbal cueing* (Max VC) describes when the patient requires verbal cues for more than 50% of the task. A new patient in PR exercise would be expected to have Max VC for the first few sessions or as indicated. *Tactile cues* describe when physical touch is needed to complete a certain task or attend to a certain body part. Other abbreviations used in physical medicine documentation are as follows: adaptive device (AD), which is the general term for a mobility aid such as a walker, cane, rolling walker (RW), straight point cane (SPC), and quad cane (QC).

Medicare understands this language to document the need for skilled level of therapist intervention and the PR community must begin to use this language to document the cueing needed in education and level of physical assistance needed during the therapeutic supervised exercise.

UB-04

Billing for PR charges must follow Medicare guidelines: charges are itemized to reflect the date of service, revenue code, and current procedural terminology codes and units, and each treatment procedure or modality billed must match the documentation in the daily therapy notes by date and units. The patient's bill is submitted electronically on an itemized UB-04.[63]

CONCLUSION

The intent of this chapter is to provide a framework to build on in the process of program management and in learning and understanding the financing of health care and ultimately the reimbursement of PR. The 21st century brings this nation the challenges of an increase in the morbidity and mortality of chronic lung disease. It is up to the PR administrative director and medical director to establish the standards of excellence in patient care and program outcomes. The key elements needed to achieve long-term success are critical.

PR specialists are constantly striving for excellence to bring the evidence-based practice of PR to the patient populations we serve. PR must expand beyond the traditional COPD program admission to include "other" chronic lung conditions. To have a personal and economic global impact, prevention must be incorporated into each component of a comprehensive PR program. These essential components include assessment, patient training/education, exercise, psychosocial intervention, and long-term follow-up. Collaboration with colleagues around the world will bring a new energy and optimism to PR.

The cost of chronic lung disease, both economic and personal, is staggering. To lessen this burden, PR must become the "standard of care" for the treatment and prevention of chronic lung disease, not just an "alternative of care." The evolution of health insurance in the United States has been dynamic and noncomplacent. The rising cost of health care has impacted society, creating great political debates. The sources of health care financing have had changing faces over the centuries.

The need for accurate documentation for outcomes, benchmarking, and reimbursement cannot be overemphasized. The e-commerce highway will drive the PR program documentation to the next level. The realization of the virtual patient record through networked computers is in the future. There must be collaboration with colleagues throughout the world to improve the standard of care for pulmonary patients and forge differences into strengths. The evidence-based medicine of PR must become a standard in the pulmonary health care network. Through collaboration with colleagues, the focus of PR programs must shift from treatment to prevention, ultimately impacting the patients' quality of life and the country's economy.

References

1. American Association of Cardiovascular and Pulmonary Rehabilitation: Guidelines for pulmonary rehabilitation programs, ed 3, Champaign, Ill, 2004, Human Kinetics.
2. Ries AL, Bauldoff GS, Carlin BW et al: Pulmonary rehabilitation: Joint ACCP/AACVPR evidence-based clinical practice guidelines, Chest 131:4-42, 2007.
3. American Association for Respiratory Care: AARC clinical practice guidelines: pulmonary rehabilitation, Respir Care 47:617-625, 2002.
4. Fishman AP, editor: Lung biology in health and disease, Vol 91: Pulmonary rehabilitation, New York, 1996, Marcel Dekker.
5. Nici L, Donner C, Wouters E et al: American Thoracic Society/European Respiratory Society statement on pulmonary rehabilitation, Am J Respir Crit Care Med 173:1390-1413, 2006.
6. Troosters T, Casaburi R, Gosselink R et al: Pulmonary rehabilitation in chronic obstructive pulmonary disease, Am J Respir Crit Care Med 172:19-38, 2005.
7. Donner CF, Muir JF; Rehabilitation and Chronic Care Scientific Group of the European Respiratory Society: Selection criteria and programmes for pulmonary rehabilitation in COPD patients, Eur Respir J 10:744-757, 1997.
8. Donner CF, Ambrosino N, Goldstein RS, editors: Part 4: Delivering pulmonary rehabilitation: specific

problems. In Pulmonary rehabilitation, New York, 2005, Oxford University Press, pp 247-352.

9. Hodson ME, Gyi KM, Elkin SL: Rehabilitation of patients with cystic fibrosis. In Donner CF, Ambrosino N, Goldstein RS, editors: Pulmonary rehabilitation, New York, 2005, Oxford University Press, pp 288-296.

10. National Lung Health Education Program Executive Committee: Strategies in preserving lung health and preventing COPD and associated diseases: the National Lung Health Education Program (NLHEP), Chest 113(suppl):123S-155S, 1998.

11. Connors GL, Hilling L: Prevention, not just treatment, Respir Care Clin N Am 4:1-12, 1998.

12. Morris JF, Temple W: Spirometric "lung age" estimates for motivating smoking cessation, Prev Med 14:655-662, 1985.

13. American Association of Cardiovascular and Pulmonary Rehabilitation: AACVPR Pulmonary Rehabilitation Medical Directors Newsletter, Summer 2007, Chicago, Ill, 2007, AACVPR. Available at www.aacvpr.org. Retrieved July 2007.

14. Wilkins RL: Patient safety, communication, and recordkeeping. In Wilkins RL, Stoller JK, Kacmarek, editors: Egan's fundamental of respiratory care, ed 9, St. Louis, Mo, 2009, Mosby-Elsevier, pp 35-52.

15. Mussa CC, Langsam Y: Management and processing of respiratory care information in respiratory care departments, Respir Care 52:730-739, 2007.

16. Des Jardins T, Burton GG: Recording skills: the basis for data collection, organization, assessment skills (critical thinking), and treatment plans. In Clinical manifestations and assessment of respiratory disease, ed 3, St. Louis Mosby, pp 141-151.

17. Goodfellow LT: Using and developing clinical practice guidelines, respiratory care protocols. And critical pathways. In: Mishoe SC, Welch MA, editors: Critical thinking in respiratory care: a problem-based learning approach, New York, 2002, McGraw-Hill, pp 159-180.

18. Weissman NW, Allison JJ, Kiefe CL et al: Achievable benchmarks of care: the ABCs of benchmarking, J Eval Clin Pract 5:269-281, 1999.

19. AHA Central Office: American Hospital Association coding. Available at http://www.ahacentraloffice.org/ahacentraloffice/html/hcpcs.html. Retrieved March 2008.

20. National Association for Medical Direction of Respiratory Care (NAMDRC): Coding and reimbursement. Available at http://www.namdrc.org/coding.html. Retrieved March 2008.

21. American Hospital Association: Health information technology. Available at http://www.aha.org/aha_app/issues/HIT/news-hit.jsp. Retrieved March 2008.

22. American Hospital Association: Coding. Available at http://www.ahacentraloffice.org/ahacentraloffice/html/hcpcs.html. Retrieved March 2008.

23. Kaplan RS, Norton DP: The balanced scorecard: measures that drive performance, Harvard Business Review, 1992, January-February, pp 71-79.

24. Kaplan RS, Norton DP: The balanced scorecard, Boston, Mass, 1996, Harvard Business School Press.

25. American Association for Respiratory Care: Uniform reporting manual for acute care hospitals, Irving, Tex, 2004, American Association for Respiratory Care. Available at http://www.aarc.org/media_center/press_releases/urm_04.asp. Retrieved March 2008.

26. Glass KP, Anderson JR: Relative value units and cost analysis, part 3 of 4, J Med Pract Manage 18(2):66-70, 2002.

27. Wright J: Time and resource management. In Mishoe SC, Welch MA, editors: Critical thinking in respiratory care: a problem-based learning approach, New York, 2002, McGraw-Hill, pp 281-312.

28. James B: Quality management in health care delivery, Chicago, Ill, 1989, Hospital Research and Education Trust.

29. Griffits TL, Bourbeau J: The economics of pulmonary rehabilitation and self-management education for patients with chronic obstructive pulmonary disease. In: Donner CF, Ambrosino N, Goldstein RS, editors: Pulmonary rehabilitation, New York, 2005, Oxford University Press, pp 164-172.

30. Ries AL: Effects of pulmonary rehabilitation on dyspnea, quality of life, and healthcare costs in California, J Cardiopulm Rehab 24:52-62, 2004.

31. Goldstein RS, Gort EH, Guyatt GH et al: Economic analysis of respiratory rehabilitation, Chest 112:370-379, 1997.

32. Reina-Rosenbaum R, Bach JR, Penek J: The costs/benefits of outpatient-based pulmonary rehabilitation, Arch Phys Med Rehabil 78:240-244, 1997.

33. Griffiths TL, Phillips CJ, Davies S et al: Cost effectiveness of an outpatient multidisciplinary pulmonary rehabilitation programme, Thorax 56:779-784, 2001.

34. Monninkhof E, Valk PVD, Schermer T et al: Economic evaluation of a comprehensive self-management programme in patients with COPD, Chron Respir Dis 1:7-16, 2004.

35. Webster's II New Riverside University Dictionary, ed 3, Boston, 1994, Houghton Mifflin.

36. Malinowski TP: Quality and performance improvement in respiratory care, Respir Care Clin N Am 10:235-251, 2004.

37. Executive Learning: Continual improvement principles: an introduction to concepts and tools for healthcare leaders, Brentwood, Tenn, 1993, Executive Learning, p 7-7.

38. Hess DR: What is evidence-based medicine and why should I care? Respir Care 49:730-741, 2004.

39. Schunemann HJ, ZuWallack R: Evaluation of impairment and disability and outcome measures for rehabilitation. In: Donner CF, Ambrosino N, Goldstein RS, eds. Pulmonary Rehabilitation, Oxford University Press Inc., New York, NY, 2005;150-163.

40. Goldstein RS, ZuWallack R: Long-term compliance after chronic obstructive pulmonary disease rehabilitation. In: Donner CF, Ambrosino N, Goldstein RS, editors: Pulmonary rehabilitation, New York, 2005, Oxford University Press, pp 369-376.

41. Frymyer T, Trevino M, Weinstein G: The clinical ladder: a key element in recruitment, professional development, retention and work force planning, Abstr Respir Care 48:1060, 2003.

42. Nici L, Limberg T, Hilling L et al: Clinical competency guidelines for pulmonary rehabilitation professionals: AACVPR position statement, J Cardiopulm Rehabil 27:355-358, 2007.

43. The Joint Commission: 2008 national patient safety goals. Available at http://www.jcaho.org/Patient Safety/NationalPatientSafetyGoals/. Retrieved March 2008.

44. The Joint Commission on Accreditation of Healthcare Organizations: Information on final specifications for national implementation of hospital core measures. http://www.jcaho.org/pms/core+measures/information+on+final+specifications.htm. Retrieved August 25, 2003.

45. The Joint Commission on Accreditation of Healthcare Organizations: Core measure set for public comment. http://www.jcaho.org/pms/core+-measures/core+measure+sets.htm. Retrieved August 25, 2003.

46. The Joint Commission: Chronic obstructive pulmonary disease certification. Available at www.jcaho.org/CertificationPrograms/COPD. Retrieved March 2008.

47. The Joint Commission: Lung volume reduction surgery certification program. Available at http://www.jcaho.org/CertificationPrograms/LungVolume ReductionSurgery/. Retrieved March 2008.

48. The Joint Commission: Transplant Center Certification Program. Available at http://www.jcaho.org/CertificationPrograms/TransplantCenter Certification. Retrieved March 2008.

49. AACVPR Outcomes Committee: Outcome measurement in cardiac and pulmonary rehabilitation, J Cardiopulm Rehabil 15:394-405, 1995.

50. Centers for Medicare and Medicaid Services: Available at http://www.cms.hhs.gov/. Retrieved March 2008.

51. U.S. Department of Veterans Affairs: Health care—Veterans Health Administration home. Available at http://www1.va.gov/health/index.asp. Retrieved March 2008.

52. TRICARE Management Activity, Military Health System: TRICARE information: the history of CHAMPUS and its evolving role in TRICARE. Available at http://www.tricare.osd.mil. Retrieved March 2008.

53. TRICARE Management Activity, Military Health System: What is TRICARE? Available at http://www.tricare.mil/mybenefit/ProfileFilter.do;jsessio-nid=LvXY9wLnQwbRHjTppQFTJzqGkFqh74XQ3-B14bdyw01nJgJwQSkWR!-1344581246?puri=%2Fhome%2Foverview%2FWhatIsTRICARE. Retrieved March 2008.

54. Centers for Medicare & Medicaid Services, U.S. Department of Health and Human Services: Medicare Managed Care Manual. Available at http://www.cms.hhs.gov/Transmittals/Downloads/R4MCM.pdf. Retrieved March 2008.

55. Centers for Medicare & Medicaid Services, U.S. Department of Health and Human Services: Medicare Contracting Reform: Part A/Part B Medicare administrative contractor. Available at http://www.cms.hhs.gov/MedicareContractingReform/07_PartAandPartBMedicareAdministrativeContractor.asp. Retrieved March 2008.

56. Centers for Medicare & Medicaid Services, U.S. Department of Health and Human Services: Comprehensive outpatient rehabilitation facility: rules and regulations, Fed Regist 47:56282, 1982. Available at http://www.cms.hhs.gov/CertificationandComplianc/17_CORFs.asp. Retrieved March 2008.

57. Iglehart J: The American health care system: Medicare, N Engl J Med 340:327-332, 1999.

58. Ellis RP, McGurie TG: Insurance principles and the design of prospective payment systems, J Health Econ 7:215, 1988.

59. U.S. Department of Veterans Affairs: Veterans Health Administration home. Available at http://www1.va.gov/health/index.asp. Retrieved March 2008; TRICARE Management Activity, Military Health System: TRICARE information. Available at http://www.tricare.mil. Retrieved March 2008.

60. Henry J. Kaiser Family Foundation, Kaiser Commission on Medicaid Basics: Medicaid: a primer, an introduction and overview, Washington DC, 1999, Kaiser Commission.

61. Limberg T: How does pulmonary rehabilitation survive in a managed care market? Respir Care Clin N Am 4:1, 1998.

62. World Health Organization: International Classification of Functioning and Disability and Health. ICF. Geneva: WHO; 2001.

63. Medicare Learning Network: Uniform billing (UB-04) implementation—UB-92 Replacement. Available at http://www.cms.hhs.gov/MLNMattersArticles/downloads/MM5072.pdf. Retrieved March 2008.

Chapter 31

Pulmonary Rehabilitation for Patients with Disorders Other Than Chronic Obstructive Pulmonary Disease

CAROLYN L. ROCHESTER

CHAPTER OUTLINE

Rationale for Providing Pulmonary Rehabilitation to Patients with Diagnoses Other Than Chronic Obstructive Pulmonary Disease
General Considerations and Challenges
Conditions of Airflow Obstruction Other Than Chronic Obstructive Pulmonary Disease
Asthma
Cystic fibrosis
Non—Cystic Fibrosis Bronchiectasis

Respiratory Disorders Associated with Restrictive Ventilatory Impairment
Interstitial Lung Disease/Pulmonary Fibrosis
Restrictive Chest Wall Disease
Respiratory Disorders Associated with Obesity
Pulmonary Hypertension
Lung Cancer
Neuromuscular Disease
Conclusion

PROFESSIONAL SKILLS

On completion of this chapter, the reader will be able to do the following:
- Gain insight about the rationale for providing pulmonary rehabilitation to patients with diagnoses other than chronic obstructive pulmonary disease (COPD)
- Understand the physiologic rationale to expect benefits in patients with respiratory compromise other than COPD
- Review the existing evidence that supports the use of pulmonary rehabilitation in those diseases
- Better comprehend the rationale behind some of the possible forms of treatment for specific physiologic conditions and the challenges faced by this new area of pulmonary rehabilitation

Pulmonary rehabilitation (PR) is "an evidence-based, multidisciplinary, and comprehensive intervention for patients with chronic respiratory diseases who are symptomatic and often have decreased daily activities. Integrated into the individualized treatment of the patient, pulmonary rehabilitation is designed to reduce symptoms, optimize functional status, increase participation and reduce health care costs through stabilizing or reversing systemic manifestations of the disease."[1] Together with smoking cessation, optimized pharmacotherapy and disease prevention through immunizations, comprehensive PR, including exercise training, education, breathing retraining, and psychosocial support, improves exercise tolerance, reduces dyspnea and fatigue, improves quality of life (QOL), and can reduce health care costs of patients with chronic obstructive pulmonary disease (COPD).[1-3] Indeed, PR is a crucial component of the comprehensive care of patients with COPD.[4]

The success of PR for patients with COPD has fostered interest in whether PR is also beneficial for patients with respiratory disorders other than COPD. To date, the evidence base demonstrating the scientific rationale, as well as beneficial outcomes, of PR for such patients is far less comprehensive than that available for COPD. As such, health care providers, third-party payers, and patients with non-COPD diagnoses themselves often regard referral to PR with skepticism, and many patients who may benefit from PR are not referred at all. However, in more recent years, several studies have been conducted that do support the use of PR for patients with non-COPD diagnoses, and no study has convincingly shown a lack of benefit. Thus on the basis of existing data and the recognized success of PR for patients with COPD, patients with a wide variety of respiratory disorders who remain symptomatic despite routine medical therapy are being referred increasingly to PR programs worldwide. In turn, PR programs with a long-standing history of having provided care almost exclusively to patients with COPD are facing new challenges as to how to incorporate patients with non-COPD diagnoses. This chapter reviews current knowledge regarding the rationale for and benefits of PR, as well as special considerations in providing PR to patients with respiratory disorders other than COPD.

RATIONALE FOR PROVIDING PULMONARY REHABILITATION TO PATIENTS WITH DIAGNOSES OTHER THAN CHRONIC OBSTRUCTIVE PULMONARY DISEASE

Early skepticism regarding the benefits of PR for patients with COPD was based on the findings that PR did not result in improved lung function per se, and on concerns that patients with advanced stages of disease would not be able to exercise at an intensity high enough to lead to gains in exercise tolerance or aerobic fitness. These concerns proved to be unfounded, when it was demonstrated clearly that patients of all ages with COPD, including those with severely impaired pulmonary function, could benefit from PR incorporating low-intensity, high-intensity, and/or interval-type exercise training.[1-3,5,6] Extensive investigation has illuminated the scientific basis by which PR benefits patients with COPD in spite of negligible effects on lung function. In addition to the structural and functional changes in the airways and lung parenchyma, patients with COPD are commonly affected by systemic inflammation,[7] and skeletal muscle dysfunction,[8] as well as skeletal and cardiac manifestations of the disease[9] that have a major impact on patients' exercise tolerance, symptoms, ability to participate in activities of daily living (ADLs), and quality of life.[1,2,8,10,11] Improvements demonstrated subsequent to PR among patients with COPD thus stem largely from improvement or stabilization of these systemic manifestations of the disease[1,2,8] after exercise training or nutritional intervention and psychosocial support. Comprehensive pulmonary education, breathing retraining, training with pacing, energy conservation techniques, assistance managing oxygen (O_2) therapy, and use of self-management disease intervention strategies[12] also help to stabilize and minimize the ventilatory limitation associated with the disease.[3]

As such, it stands to reason that patients with respiratory diseases other than COPD, including persons with asthma, cystic fibrosis (CF), non-CF bronchiectasis, interstitial lung disease (ILD) (including survivors of adult respiratory distress syndrome), restrictive chest wall disease, respiratory disorders associated with obesity, pulmonary vascular disease, lung cancer, and selected patients with neuromuscular disease might also benefit from PR

BOX 31-1	Respiratory Disorders for Which to Consider Pulmonary Rehabilitation as a Therapeutic Option

CONDITIONS OF AIRFLOW OBSTRUCTION OTHER THAN COPD
Asthma
Cystic fibrosis
Diffuse bronchiectasis of other causes

RESPIRATORY DISORDERS ASSOCIATED WITH RESTRICTIVE VENTILATORY IMPAIRMENT
Interstitial lung disease/pulmonary fibrosis
  • Idiopathic (e.g., UIP and NSIP)
  • Sarcoidosis
  • Collagen vascular disease
  • Chronic hypersensitivity pneumonitis
  • Asbestosis (or other occupational exposures)
  • Survivors of ARDS
  • Other
Restrictive chest wall disease
  • Post-thoracoplasty
  • Kyphosis or kyphoscoliosis
Obesity-related respiratory disease
Neuromuscular disease with respiratory manifestations

PULMONARY VASCULAR DISEASE
Idiopathic pulmonary hypertension
Secondary causes of pulmonary hypertension

LUNG CANCER
Preoperative short intervention
Post-therapeutic intervention (surgery, chemotherapy, radiation therapy)

ARDS, *Adult respiratory distress syndrome;* COPD, *chronic obstructive pulmonary disease;* NSIP, *nonspecific interstitial pneumonia;* UIP, *usual interstitial pneumonia.*

(Box 31-1). Indeed, as is true for COPD, the symptoms of dyspnea, fatigue, exercise intolerance, and functional disability with difficulty performing activities of daily living, often with associated anxiety and depression, social isolation, and inability to participate in recreational or occupational activities, are protean manifestations of these disorders as well. Importantly, although the mechanisms of exercise limitation are multifactorial and vary widely across these conditions, it is likely that skeletal muscle dysfunction is an important contributing factor to exercise limitation in many patients with non-COPD respiratory disease. Indeed, deconditioning, systemic inflammation, nutritional impairments, aging, anemia, and hypoxemia—important components of skeletal muscle dysfunction found in COPD (which is responsive to PR intervention), as well as other systemic manifestations of disease similar to those found in COPD—are commonly present among patients with non-COPD respiratory

disease as well. Moreover, medical therapy such as corticosteroids (e.g., used commonly for patients with asthma, CF, and ILD) may cause myopathy and worsen skeletal muscle dysfunction and weakness. Thus the scientific rationale for providing PR to patients with COPD also exists for patients with non-COPD respiratory disease. In addition, promotion of compliance with complex medication regimens, O_2 therapy, or noninvasive assisted ventilation, chest physiotherapy techniques; training in the use of adaptive/assistive equipment (such as walking aids, sock reachers, toilet/tub equipment); and preparation of patients for lung transplantation require more intensive training and education, time for patient questions, behavior modification, and partnering between patients and their health care providers than can usually be accomplished in the routine outpatient clinical setting. PR programs wherein patients have steady contact with multidisciplinary health care providers over an extended period of time are an ideal setting in which to address such issues.

Importantly, studies conducted to date, wherein patients with a wide variety of disorders other than COPD have been included in a PR program administered also to patients with COPD, have shown that patients with non-COPD diagnoses achieved benefits in exercise tolerance[13-16] and quality of life[14,16] comparable to those made by the patients with COPD. For example, the study by Foster and Thomas[13] included patients with interstitial lung disease, fibrothorax, bronchiectasis, restrictive chest wall disease, and neuromuscular disease. More recently, Ferreira, Feuerman, and Spiegler[14] evaluated the outcomes of an 8-week, multidisciplinary outpatient, hospital-based PR program among 309 patients with COPD and 113 patients with diagnoses other than COPD. Non-COPD diagnoses included asthma (n = 27), pulmonary fibrosis or other ILD (n = 44), chest wall restriction (n = 14), bronchiectasis (n = 12), pulmonary arterial hypertension (n = 5), diaphragm paralysis (n = 5), patients requiring lung resection surgery (n = 4), and tracheomalacia (n = 2). Both patients with COPD and those with non-COPD respiratory disease had significant improvements in exercise tolerance (assessed by the 6-Minute Walk Test [6MWT])[17] and health-related QOL (assessed by the Chronic Respiratory Disease Questionnaire [CRQ]).[18] Moreover, as was true in the study by Foster and Thomas,[13] there was no significant difference in the magnitude of gains between the COPD and non-COPD patient groups. Although the total "n" for some of the diagnoses was small, subgroup analysis performed on the non-COPD group failed to demonstrate any disease category that derived greater versus lesser benefit from PR. Indeed, the joint American Thoracic Society/European Respiratory Society statement on pulmonary rehabilitation[1] and American College of Chest Physicians/American Association of Cardiovascular and Pulmonary Rehabilitation evidence-based guidelines for pulmonary rehabilitation[3] both suggest that, on the basis of existing knowledge, consideration should be given to referral of patients with diseases other than COPD to PR programs. Collectively, therefore, a strong rationale exists for providing PR to patients with respiratory disorders other than COPD. Studies supporting this rationale, and demonstrating benefits of PR among patients with individual types of non-COPD disorders, are discussed in the following sections.

BOX 31-2	Educational Topics for Selected Patients with Non-COPD Diagnoses

- Peak flow monitoring
- Bronchial hygiene/chest physiotherapy techniques
- Use of adaptive/assistive equipment
- Noninvasive ventilation (e.g., CPAP, BiPAP)
- Tracheostomy care
- Home mechanical ventilation
- Advance directives/end of life care
- Community resources, support groups, long-term care facilities
- Immunosuppressive (or other specialized) medications
- Vasodilator/antiproliferative therapy
- Lung transplantation
- Recovery from thoracic surgery and prevention of postoperative complications (e.g., importance of early mobilization, incentive spirometry, assisted cough)

BiPAP, *Bilevel positive airway pressure;* CPAP, *continuous positive airway pressure.*

GENERAL CONSIDERATIONS AND CHALLENGES

Although there exist no formal guidelines for providing PR to patients with non-COPD respiratory disease and currently the core components of PR are the same as those for patients with COPD, several important issues merit consideration. To provide safe and effective PR to patients with various types of respiratory disease, it is necessary for PR care providers to be familiar with the anatomic, physiologic, and clinical features of these diverse disorders, as well as treatment interventions used for them. This poses the challenge of providing educational sessions and reading materials to staff members whose clinical experience may have been limited to caring for patients with COPD. A multidisciplinary PR team, including a physiotherapist or exercise physiologist, nurse, respiratory therapist, occupational therapist, nutritional therapist, pharmacologist, psychologist, and dedicated medical director, is desirable, although resources may be limited at some programs. Close partnering between PR staff and referring health care providers is crucial. Consideration must be given to how best to incorporate patients with non-COPD diagnoses (often a single patient or a few patients) into a group of patients with COPD undergoing PR. As discussed in the following sections, this issue encompasses staffing needs, logistics, time and patient safety considerations, as well as the need to broaden the scope of didactic educational

sessions and written educational materials. Topics that may be beneficial to include in addition to those covered routinely in PR (depending on the patient population) are shown in Box 31-2. It is clearly essential that patients with diverse diagnoses in a given program not be confused regarding their condition by educational or exercise training information that does not pertain to them.

Also, the optimal strategies for exercise training for patients with non-COPD diagnoses are as yet unknown. Individualized, realistic goal setting is crucial, and circumstances may arise wherein nontraditional goals may be considered to enable patients to maintain functional independence. Moreover, specialized equipment may be needed. Finally, it cannot be assumed that the tests and tools used routinely to assess exercise tolerance, symptoms, and health status to formulate the exercise prescription and measure outcomes among patients with COPD[1,2] have comparable validity and/or sensitivity to change after PR among patients with other forms of respiratory disease. Information about this topic relevant to individual diagnoses, where available, is also considered in the following sections. Age- and disease-appropriate tools should be used in PR programs whenever possible. In summary, an individualized, disease-appropriate approach to providing PR, designed to meet realistic goals, is required.

CONDITIONS OF AIRFLOW OBSTRUCTION OTHER THAN CHRONIC OBSTRUCTIVE PULMONARY DISEASE

PR for the pediatric patient is considered in detail elsewhere in this book (see Chapter 33), and most of the available clinical data regarding PR/exercise training for asthma and CF have been gathered in studies conducted in the pediatric population. Nevertheless, because patients with asthma and CF may also be referred to adult PR programs, these conditions also merit consideration here.

Asthma

Patients with well-controlled asthma whose lung function remains normal or only mildly impaired between disease exacerbations, who are otherwise healthy and do not have significant deconditioning, disturbing symptoms despite medical therapy or steroid-induced myopathy typically do not require PR. PR should, however, be considered for those patients whose asthma is more severe, who remain symptomatic with dyspnea and exercise impairment despite optimal medical therapy, who experience exacerbations leading to a decline in functional ability, and who could benefit from comprehensive pulmonary education to assist in self-management of disease.[19] Exercise impairment in patients with asthma may result from increased airway resistance and dynamic hyperinflation (especially if there is a fixed, permanent component of airflow obstruction), deconditioning, anxiety, or steroid-induced muscle weakness.[20-22] Some patients have reduced perceived self-efficacy to perform exercise as compared with persons without asthma.[23] Exercise-induced bronchospasm (EIB) is a key consideration of particular importance in patients with asthma.[22] Use of cardiopulmonary exercise testing (CPET), when available, is useful before initiation of PR to identify factors contributing to exercise intolerance for individual patients, and to formulate an exercise prescription targeted to the specific existing problems. When CPET is not available, consideration should be given to measurement of flow rates before and after a field test of exercise tolerance (e.g., the 6MWT or the Incremental Shuttle Walk Test [ISWT][24]) in an effort to detect EIB, before initiation of exercise training. Although such measurement has not been shown to alter outcomes of exercise training, it is conducive to provision of optimal bronchodilator therapy before initiation of exercise.

The optimal tools for measurement of health status/health-related QOL and other outcomes of PR among patients with asthma have not been rigorously investigated. Instruments used to date in studies of other therapeutic interventions in asthma include the Medical Outcomes Study Short-Form 36 (SF-36),[25,26] the Juniper Asthma Quality of Life Scale,[25] the CRQ,[27] the Pediatric Asthma Quality of Life Questionnaire,[28] and the St. George's Respiratory Questionnaire (SGRQ).[26] One study in elderly persons from the general population found that adult persons with a diagnosis of "asthma" reported impaired health-related QOL as indicated by worse mean scores on the SF-36 and SGRQ health status instruments.[26] The optimal QOL tools best suited to detecting change after PR in patients with asthma remain unknown, and may differ in adult and pediatric patient groups.

Physical rehabilitation programs for patients with asthma have been undertaken in a wide variety of settings, and have incorporated several types of exercise, including cycling,[29] walking or running,[30] swimming,[30,31] yoga,[32] and basketball,[28] at variable exercise intensities, frequency of exercise sessions, and program duration. Although large randomized controlled trials are lacking, studies in both children[28,29,31,33,34] and adults[20,27,30,35-37] with asthma conducted to date have consistently demonstrated gains in exercise endurance and/or aerobic fitness (with improved maximal oxygen consumpion [$\dot{V}o_2max$] and/or delay in anaerobic threshold[27-29,31,33-36]) as well as reduced ventilation for a given exercise workload[35] after physical training, conducted either alone or in the context of a PR program. The existing randomized controlled trials have demonstrated significant differences in exercise tolerance among the training, as compared with control groups.[28,29] For example, a randomized controlled trial of 6 weeks' cycle ergometer training among 16 adolescents with mild to moderate asthma demonstrated an 18% increase in $\dot{V}o_2max$ among patients in the training group as compared with a 9% increase in control subjects who did not undergo exercise training ($P < .05$), and a 32% increase in maximal aerobic power in the training group versus a 12% increase in control subjects ($P < .05$).[29] Likewise, in the trial by Cochrane and Clark,[35] young adults with asthma who were randomized to receive multimodality exercise training had a 5 ml/kg/min improvement in $\dot{V}o_2max$ ($P < .001$) whereas control subjects had no change. Two studies have suggested that patients with asthma with the greatest baseline degree of impairment in fitness may derive the greatest benefit from physical training.[30,33] Physical training for patients with asthma also reduces symptoms (e.g., breathlessness measured by the Borg Dyspnea Scale)[27,30,35,36,38] and improves QOL,[27] and preliminary data suggest it may also reduce the requirement for acute asthma care.[30,38] Significant changes in pulmonary function or reductions in EIB after exercise training have not been demonstrated consistently. The optimal exercise training regimen, and impact/role of PR components other than exercise training, and optimal methods for measuring health status outcomes after PR among patients with asthma, are as yet unknown.

Special considerations for patients with asthma enrolled in PR include the importance of an adequate warm-up period before exercise and measurement of and monitoring for EIB. To this end, the temperature and humidity of the rehabilitation environment may be important. Outcomes of relevance to patients with asthma, in addition to those measured routinely in PR, include the impact of PR on measures of health care costs, school and/or work absenteeism, adherence to medication use, and the question of reduction of EIB after training.[39]

Cystic Fibrosis

As is true for patients with asthma, patients with CF experience various degrees of respiratory symptoms, exercise intolerance, and impairment in QOL. They too have varying frequency and severity of acute disease exacerbations, which may lead not only to worsening of symptoms and increased sputum production, but also to decline in functional status (particularly if the patient requires hospitalization). As compared with healthy age- and gender-matched control subjects, patients with CF tend to have reduced maximal exercise capacity,[40,41] impaired muscle strength,[42] greater resting energy expenditure, lower peak anaerobic power,[43] and, among those with severe pulmonary impairment, reduced arm work capacity.[44] Exercise impairment in CF can result from increased airway resistance, dynamic hyperinflation (with resultant respiratory muscle mechanical disadvantage and increased elastic load to breathing), or cardiocirculatory limitation (including pulmonary hypertension),[41,45,46] osteopenia, and hypertrophic osteopathy (that may impair joint flexibility),[46] in addition to the skeletal muscle impairments already noted. EIB, reported to

occur in 22% to 55% of patients with CF, may also impair exercise tolerance for some persons.[46] Interestingly, impaired nutritional status correlates with exercise intolerance independently of impairments in pulmonary function.[41]

Although exercise capacity tends to worsen with worsening pulmonary function impairment, resting pulmonary function does not reliably predict the response of patients to exercise. Thus given the multiple possible causes of exercise impairment, as well as the inability to predict exercise performance from resting parameters, CPET is the ideal way to assess exercise tolerance and formulate the PR exercise prescription for patients with CF.[46] Identification of exercise impairment is important not only for identifying patients who may benefit from PR and designing an appropriate training regimen, but is also important in predicting patient outcomes, because low exercise capacity in CF is associated with work and school impairment[47] and with lower long-term survival.[41,45,48] A faster rate of decline in $\dot{V}o_2max$ over time was predictive of greater 8-year mortality in one study.[49] When CPET is unavailable or the patient is unable to tolerate CPET, the 6MWT[50] or the modified Shuttle Walk Test[51,52] may be used to measure exercise tolerance before and at the end of PR. Given that endurance for walking may remain normal and baseline maximal exercise capacity tends to be impaired, it may be optimal to use the modified SWT—a test that uses incremental exercise loads—although it is not clear which of these tests is more sensitive to changes after exercise training/PR for patients with CF.

CF can also be associated with impaired health-related QOL.[53] Outcome tools geared toward the activities and concerns of children and adolescents, such as instruments that address issues pertaining to school, friendships, self-worth, physical appearance, and romance, as well as athletics and daily activity performance, should be considered for use among patients with CF in these younger age groups.[54] The Quality of Well-being Scale, CRQ, Cystic Fibrosis Questionnaire, and other[55-58] instruments have been used to measure health status/QOL, and the Borg Dyspnea Scale score[59] has been used to measure dyspnea among adult patients with CF.

Short-term, nonrandomized uncontrolled trials, as well as randomized controlled trials, have shown that aerobic exercise training conducted in a wide variety of settings involving training modalities such as running, swimming, hiking/climbing, and cycling improves the exercise tolerance of children and adolescents with CF.[43,54,56,60-62] Training effects have been demonstrated not only among persons with mild to moderate severity of disease, but also among persons with severe impairment in pulmonary function.[63] Although some studies suggest that the best results have occurred among patients who trained in supervised settings,[55,64] the randomized controlled trial by Moorcroft and colleagues[65] demonstrated that adult patients with CF who undertook unsupervised, home-based upper and lower body exercise (according to individual preference) over a 1-year period had reduced blood lactate concentrations and heart rate for an identical constant work rate (suggestive of a training effect), as compared with a control group that did not undergo training. Importantly, this benefit resulted from an unsupervised home-based intervention, which may be more feasible for the patients and have greater impact on long-term outcomes than shorter term (e.g., several weeks) or facility-based interventions.

The optimal methods of exercise training in CF are as yet unknown. In keeping with the COPD patient population, strength/resistance training in patients with CF improves muscle size, strength,[43,55,66] and mass.[43] One randomized controlled trial comparing 12 months of home-based aerobic stair-stepping exercise training with upper body strength training among 67 children and teenagers with CF demonstrated that both interventions improved upper body strength and overall physical work capacity (watts).[55] Clinical trials comparing outcomes of aerobic versus strength training versus the combination of both among patients with CF are lacking. Inspiratory muscle training (IMT) can improve inspiratory muscle strength and endurance[67-69] but may[68] or may not[67] lead to generalized improvement in overall exercise capacity. Interestingly, some studies, particularly those that have included exercise training over a long period (e.g., 1 to 3 years) have demonstrated that exercise training is associated with better maintenance of lung function over time.[64,65,70-72] The mechanisms for this are not yet clear. The use of supplemental O_2 for patients who desaturate during exercise may optimize the benefits of exercise training.[45]

Exercise training among patients with CF can also lead to a reduction in symptoms[70] and improved sense of well-being (measured by the Quality of Well-being Scale)[43,60,73] that have been associated with change in aerobic capacity.[43] Rehabilitation programs that provide structured calorie supplementation can also impact nutrition.

Notably, most trials of exercise training for patients with CF have been conducted either at home or in a supervised setting but not as part of a comprehensive PR program such as those used routinely for patients with COPD. Thus it is not currently possible to draw conclusions about the outcomes of PR per se, as opposed to exercise training as a sole intervention, among patients with CF. Also, because few of the existing studies have systematically measured dyspnea, QOL, health care use, or survival, the impact of exercise training or PR on these outcomes is as yet unknown.

Special considerations in provision of PR to patients with CF include the need to assess and monitor patients for EIB and to maintain rigorous hygiene and adequate spacing of exercise equipment to avoid cross-patient contamination/colonization with virulent organisms such as *Burkholderia cepacia*,[60] which carries risk of added patient morbidity. Because patients with CF may lose exaggerated amounts of sodium and chloride, especially in hot exercise environments, and may not sense their degree of fluid loss or thirst, rigorous efforts should be made to encourage patients to maintain fluid intake, for example, of electrolyte-rich fluids.[41,46,54,56] The importance of maintaining adequate caloric intake should also be emphasized during exercise training.[54,74] Training of patients regarding strategies to maintain optimal bronchial hygiene/secretion clearance is also essential.

Non–Cystic Fibrosis Bronchiectasis

A randomized controlled trial assessed outcomes of a comprehensive, 8-week, outpatient hospital-based PR program among 32 adult patients with non-CF diffuse bronchiectasis.[75] Patients were randomized to receive PR plus sham IMT or PR plus targeted threshold IMT at 30% of maximal inspiratory pressure versus no training.[75] The exercise training in the PR group consisted of 45 minutes of multimodality aerobic exercise at 80% peak heart rate, three times weekly for 8 weeks. PR also included comprehensive pulmonary education. PR led to significant gains in exercise endurance (measured by treadmill endurance time at 85% peak baseline $\dot{V}O_2$; 17% increase in PR–sham IMT group and 20.6% increase in

PR–IMT group) and overall exercise capacity (measured by ISWT; up to a 124.5-m increase over baseline for the PR–IMT group).[75] The addition of the IMT component of training led to improvement in maximal inspiratory pressure and better maintenance of exercise capacity 3 months after training as compared with sham IMT. Patients who underwent PR also had significant gains in QOL (measured by SGRQ score) as compared with control subjects. No significant change in sputum volume was noted after PR. Another study has also since demonstrated beneficial effects of PR on exercise tolerance among patients with bronchiectasis.[76] Although additional studies are needed to corroborate these findings, referral of selected adults with non-CF diffuse bronchiectasis to PR seems reasonable and appropriate.

RESPIRATORY DISORDERS ASSOCIATED WITH RESTRICTIVE VENTILATORY IMPAIRMENT

Interstitial Lung Disease/ Pulmonary Fibrosis

Interstitial lung disease (ILD) is a clinically and pathologically heterogeneous group of disorders characterized by varying degrees of inflammation and fibrosis of the lung parenchyma. Pulmonary fibrosis with severe derangements in pulmonary function is the end result of many forms of ILD. Because the response to medical therapy is often limited, many patients ultimately require consideration for lung transplantation. Severe exertional dyspnea, cough, and exercise intolerance are characteristic and disabling features of ILD.[77,78] Exercise intolerance in patients with ILD results from several processes, including altered lung mechanics with low lung compliance,[79,80] alterations in respiratory drive,[80] and gas exchange disturbances (with diffusion impairment, inceased dead space, and ventilation–perfusion mismatch). Exercise-induced hypoxemia tends to be particularly severe among patients with ILD, especially those persons with moderate to severe disease.[80-83] A subset of patients with ILD also develop expiratory flow limitation during exercise.[79] Persons with moderate–severe disease with capillary destruction may also have resting and/or exertion-induced pulmonary hypertension, with resultant cardiocirculatory limitation to exercise,[81] and some also have low resting left ventricular ejection fraction.[84]

Collectively, these disturbances lead to ventilatory[80,82] limitation, low breathing reserve, low peak $\dot{V}o_2$, and reduced maximal work capacity.[77,80] As is true for patients with COPD, resting pulmonary function does not predict exercise tolerance of patients with ILD.[80,82] Moreover, $\dot{V}o_2$max can be impaired among patients without severe impairment in lung function. Deconditioning and nutritional impairments are also common among patients with ILD, and for some patients exercise is limited by leg fatigue, either alone or in combination with dyspnea.[78,79]

One study demonstrated that many patients with idiopathic pulmonary fibrosis (IPF) have significant quadriceps weakness, and that quadriceps force is an independent predictor of exercise capacity among these persons.[85] Moreover, patients with ILD commonly still experience exercise limitation and impaired functional capacity after lung transplantation, despite improvement in (or normalization of) lung function.[86] Collectively, these findings suggest that patients with IPF may have skeletal muscle dysfunction. Whether disturbances of skeletal muscle function among patients with ILD are similar to those found among patients with COPD is as yet unknown. Muscle function can be compromised as well by steroid-induced myopathy. Importantly, walking endurance is an important predictor of survival post-transplantation,[87] as well as of outcomes after transplantation. Moreover, patients with ILD/pulmonary fibrosis have significant impairments in QOL[88-91] and the benefits of pharmacologic/medical therapy are often limited. Finally, the American Thoracic Society/European Respiratory Society international consensus statement on the diagnosis and treatment of IPF suggests that patients with IPF "should be encouraged to enroll in a physical rehabilitation program."[92] All of these issues provide a strong rationale for the use of PR as a treatment intervention for patients with ILD.

Because of the complex multifactorial basis of exercise limitation in ILD, CPET is desirable, when feasible, to assess the basis of patients' exercise limitation and to guide formulation of the PR exercise prescription.[93] The 6MWT and ISWT are also effective as measures of exercise tolerance among patients with ILD.[93-96] These field tests of exercise capacity can be used to measure baseline exercise tolerance, assist in formulating the exercise prescription, and assess gains in exercise tolerance after PR.

The validity of several health status/QOL questionnaires (both generic and disease specific, designed initially for use among patients with COPD) has been assessed among patients with ILD. Chang and colleagues[89] showed that scores from the SF-36, Quality of Well-being Scale, CRQ, and SGRQ all correlated with exercise limitation and dyspnea among a group of 50 patients with various forms of ILD. The SF-36 and SGRQ scores correlated best with the degree of physical impairment in that study,[89] and other studies have confirmed that these tools are useful to measure QOL among patients with ILD.[90,91,97] The World Health Organization QOL scale is another generic 100-question health status instrument useful to measure QOL among patients with ILD.[87,98] The health status instruments most sensitive to detect change in QOL after PR among patients with ILD are unknown. The Borg Dyspnea Scale, Baseline Dyspnea Index/Transitional Dyspnea Index, and Medical Research Council and Visual Analog Dyspnea Scales have been used to measure dyspnea,[91,97,99] but their responsiveness to change resulting from PR needs to be further validated among patients with ILD.

Although large randomized, controlled trials are lacking, 10 of the 32 patients with non-COPD diagnoses in the study by Foster and Thomas[13] (which demonstrated comparable gains in exercise tolerance among both COPD and non-COPD patient groups) had either pulmonary fibrosis or fibrothorax. Several more recent small studies have confirmed that PR is indeed beneficial for patients with ILD. In the study by Ferreira, Feuerman, and Spiegler,[14] patients with pulmonary fibrosis, sarcoidosis, asbestosis, cryptogenic organizing pneumonia, eosinophilic granuloma, Churg-Strauss syndrome, hypersensitivity pneumonitis, lymphangioleiomyoma, and ILD due to adult respiratory distress syndrome comprised 44 of the 113 patients with non-COPD respiratory disease shown to achieve significant gains in 6MWT distance and QOL (based on CRQ scores) after an 8-week outpatient PR program. In the study by Jastrzebski and colleagues,[99] 31 patients with various forms of ILD had reduced severity of dyspnea (Borg Dyspnea Scale) and improved QOL (including gains in the activity, impact, and total scores of the SGRQ and the role physical subscore of the SF-36) after PR. Likewise, Naji and colleagues[95] demonstrated that 8 weeks of outpatient PR led to significant gains in treadmill endurance time (mean gain, 10.2 ± 7.4 min) and distance walked in the ISWT

(mean gain, 27.2 ± 75.9 m), as well as significant improvements in dyspnea, QOL, and depression (measured by the CRQ, SGRQ, and Hospital Anxiety and Depression Scale, respectively) among 46 patients with restrictive lung disease (35 with ILD and 11 with restrictive chest wall disease). Intriguingly, gains in treadmill endurance time persisted at 1-year follow-up, and a significant reduction in number of hospital admission days was noted for the group of patients in the year after (10.4 ± 9.7 days) as compared with the year before (13.5 ± 13.1 days) rehabilitation. However, one third of the patients enrolled failed to complete the PR program. The basis for this high dropout rate is unclear.

Further work is needed to clarify the optimal exercise training regimen and PR program content for patients with ILD. Close attention should be paid to maintenance of adequate oxygenation during exercise, because O_2 supplementation improves exercise performance among hypoxemic patients with ILD,[83,100] although to date there is no clear evidence that this impacts outcomes of PR. Some patients may require high inspired O_2 concentration, even 100% O_2 via nonrebreather mask, to maintain O_2 saturation at greater than 88% during exercise.

Educational topics of particular importance to patients with ILD include symptom management (including training with pursed lips and a relaxed coordinated breathing pattern to minimize dyspnea, discussion of strategies to control cough, and performance of chest wall stretching exercise to minimize reductions in chest wall compliance), training with energy conservation and pacing techniques to assist in performance of ADLs, body positioning to decrease the work of breathing, importance and expected benefits of supplemental O_2, coping and relaxation techniques, and introduction of recreational therapies such as yoga or tai chi. Additional important educational topics include the risks versus benefits of pharmacologic therapies, the importance of proper nutrition, and preparation for as well as recovery from lung transplantation. Program staff must be aware of any orthopedic or other systemic medical problems associated with the patient's ILD that might impact patient safety during exercise (e.g., joint involvement among persons with rheumatoid arthritis, or cardiac or neurologic involvement in patients with sarcoidosis). Because outcomes of patients with pulmonary fibrosis who develop respiratory failure requiring mechanical ventilation are so dismal,[101] issues pertaining to advance directives, mechanical ventilation, and end of life care also merit discussion during PR.

Restrictive Chest Wall Disease

Patients with restrictive chest wall disease such as scoliosis, kyphoscoliosis, or changes in the chest wall after thoracoplasty typically have restrictive physiology on pulmonary function testing (resulting from thoracic deformity), progressive dyspnea, and exercise impairment. Indeed, respiratory failure can develop over time as the mechanics of breathing become progressively impaired. Randomized controlled trials evaluating benefits of PR among patients with restrictive chest wall disease are lacking. However, a few small studies, some published to date only in abstract form, suggest benefits of rehabilitation for such patients. For example, a 4-month program of exercise training led to improvements in pulmonary function (forced vital capacity, forced expiratory volume in 1 second [FEV_1], inspiratory capacity, and expiratory reserve volume) and exercise endurance (measured by the 6MWT) among 34 adolescents with idiopathic scoliosis.[102] Significant gains in 6MWT (42 m; P <.01), daily activity score, and dyspnea (measured by the Medical Research Council Dyspnea Scale and Transitional Dyspnea Index) were made after 9 weeks of outpatient PR among 32 patients with restrictive chest wall disease due to post-tuberculosis thoracoplasty, of comparable magnitude to the gains made by 32 age- and FEV_1-matched patients with COPD.[94] Patients with restrictive chest wall disease were also among the groups of patients with non-COPD diagnoses who improved after PR in the studies by Foster and Thomas[13] and by Ferreira, Feuerman, and Spiegler.[14] Importantly, patients with restrictive chest wall disease often have nocturnal alveolar hypoventilation with nocturnal O_2 desaturations and/or disrupted sleep, and may also develop O_2 desaturation during exercise. In one study, a 1-week course of nocturnal noninvasive positive pressure ventilation (NIPPV) not only reduced nocturnal O_2 desaturations but also led to improved daytime exercise endurance as measured by the 6MWT.[103] The role of NIPPV used either at night or during exercise training sessions in PR for patients with restrictive chest wall disease is as yet undefined. Nevertheless, it seems prudent to include education about and acclimatization to NIPPV as a component of PR for such patients, given that many persons do require it at some point during the course of their disease.

RESPIRATORY DISORDERS ASSOCIATED WITH OBESITY

Obesity is a major cause of morbidity and mortality worldwide. Patients with morbid obesity, including those who are eucapnic (i.e., with "simple obesity," who maintain normal partial pressure of carbon dioxide and have normal respiratory drive) and those with obesity hypoventilation syndrome, commonly have restrictive defects on pulmonary function testing and disturbances in gas exchange[104,105] or obstructive sleep apnea. Dyspnea, impaired exercise tolerance, and impaired quality of life[106,107] are experienced commonly by obese persons, even in the absence of other comorbid respiratory conditions. Exercise intolerance in obese persons has a multifactorial basis, including the noted derangements in pulmonary function, as well as reduced respiratory system compliance, hypoxemia, increased O_2 cost of breathing, an exaggerated cardiorespiratory response to exercise, and reductions in respiratory muscle strength.[104,105] Pulmonary hypertension and other cardiocirculatory disturbances (such as systemic hypertension, diastolic dysfunction, myocardial ischemia, claudication, or microvascular disease) and musculoskeletal disturbances also commonly contribute to exercise impairment. Impaired exercise capacity in obese persons often leads to decreased participation in social, recreational, or work activities and may ultimately result in decreased ability to perform activities of daily living, with associated deconditioning, anxiety, and depression. Weight loss can lead to improvements in lung function, exercise tolerance, and sleep-disordered breathing.[108-110] Exercise training together with nutritional interventions can facilitate weight loss and improve exercise tolerance. Moreover, promotion of patient compliance with continuous positive airway pressure or bilevel positive airway pressure therapy requires training, education, and troubleshooting to ensure patient comfort and acclimatization. As such, comprehensive PR programs that encompass exercise training, pulmonary education (including training with NIPPV), nutritional intervention (weight loss strategies), and psychosocial support (to assist in the management of anxiety and/or depression and to facilitate behavioral change) are ideal settings in which such patients may improve.

To date, two small studies, published in abstract form only, have demonstrated benefits of PR for patients with severe obesity-related respiratory disease. The first demonstrated that comprehensive inpatient PR (mean length of stay, 33 days) led to improvements in motor skills, locomotion, mobility, and self-care (assessed by Functional Independence Measurement scores[111]) among 12 patients with severe obesity (mean body mass index, 54 kg/m^2) who had experienced a recent episode of respiratory failure.[112] In the other study, 8 weeks of PR led to significant weight loss as well as improvements in treadmill walking endurance, health status (assessed by the SF-36), and sleep quality (measured by the Functional Outcomes of Sleep Questionnaire[113]) among 46 obese patients with obstructive sleep apnea.[114] Although small and uncontrolled, the results of these studies do suggest benefits of PR for persons with obesity-related respiratory disease. The potential benefits of PR in reducing symptoms of dyspnea or fatigue among morbidly obese persons have not been tested, and the validity of health status questionnaires designed and used for other forms of chronic respiratory disease also needs to be tested among patients with obesity-related respiratory disease. Additional outcomes of potential interest to be measured in PR for such patients include assessment of disease stability over time (especially among patients with pulmonary hypertension [PH] and repeated episodes of decompensated cor pulmonale and/or respiratory failure), hospitalizations, compliance with NIPPV, weight loss and adherence with nutritional interventions, cognitive or neuropsychiatric function, and survival. No knowledge exists in these areas to date. Outcomes of PR for patients with obesity-related respiratory disturbances and concurrent other lung disease (such as COPD or ILD) are also unknown.

The safety of exercise training merits special consideration when considering PR for patients with obesity-related respiratory disease, particularly those with severe morbid obesity and severely impaired mobility. Whereas patients with less severe obesity are usually able to undergo CPET or perform field tests such as the 6MWT or ISWT, persons with the most severe obesity and impaired mobility may be unable to perform exercise assessment tests used routinely in PR for patients with other conditions. To ensure safety, a cardiac evaluation (including pharmacologic stress testing and echocardiography) is useful before initiation of exercise training, to avoid unanticipated cardiac ischemia, arrhythmias, or syncope (such as may occur with obesity hypoventilation syndrome–related

PH). A physiatry or physical therapy evaluation may be useful to ensure that exercise training will not pose excess risk of musculoskeletal injury. Close attention must be paid to weight limits of the exercise equipment and furniture available in the PR program, and specialized bariatric equipment (including lifts, beds, wheelchairs, commodes, or walkers) may be needed by some patients. Consideration must be given as to whether adequate staffing is available to provide rehabilitation safely to morbidly obese persons with severely impaired functional status, to avoid patient falls and staff injuries. Inpatient PR programs, wherein a multidisciplinary PR team and specialized equipment are more likely available, are ideally suited to meet the needs of severely impaired persons with morbid obesity, particularly those with multiple comorbid medical conditions and/or the need for specialized nursing care.

PULMONARY HYPERTENSION

For many years pulmonary hypertension (PH) was considered to be a contraindication to performing PR because of concerns about the risk of inducing cardiocirculatory collapse or worsening PH due to shear stress associated with higher blood flow during exercise.[115,116] However, the advent of newer medical therapies that improve exercise tolerance[117-120] and survival[117] of patients with severe PH, as well as the general recommendation that patients with PH undergo PR while preparing for lung transplantation, has led to reconsideration of this issue. As is true for patients with COPD, patients with PH (due to primary or secondary causes) experience exercise intolerance[77,93,121] and symptoms of dyspnea,[93] and report impaired health-related QOL.[122] The exercise intolerance of patients with PH has a complex and multifactorial basis, which depends in part on whether the patient has idiopathic primary PH versus secondary PH; for those with secondary PH, it also depends on the underlying cause (e.g., obesity hypoventilation syndrome vs. advanced ILD or end-stage COPD). Apart from any disturbances of mechanics or gas exchange caused by parenchymal lung disease, exercise impairment in PH results from high pulmonary vascular resistance, which limits or prevents the normal increase in cardiac output necessary to meet increased metabolic demand during exercise. Exercise testing among patients with pulmonary vascular disease typically demonstrates reduced peak O_2 consumption, increased O_2 cost of work, reduced peak O_2 pulse, high ventilatory equivalent for carbon dioxide (the ratio of minute ventilation to carbon dioxide production: $\dot{V}_E/\dot{V}_{CO_2}$) with a high ratio of dead space volume to tidal volume, and increased alveolar–arterial O_2 gradient or exercise-induced O_2 desaturation[123] as well as O_2 transport abnormalities, higher minute ventilation relative to low work rates with rapid shallow breathing pattern, and at times, lactic acidosis at low work rates.[77,93] These disturbances are typically associated with exertional dyspnea, atypical chest pain, and among patients with more severe disease, may include dizziness, presyncope, or overt syncope due to circulatory failure[124] or cardiac arrhythmia. Patients with these disturbances also tend to exercise less, and in turn may become deconditioned. Importantly, low exercise tolerance has been associated with reduced survival among patients with primary pulmonary hypertension.[121]

The best means of assessing exercise capacity among patients with PH is debated. Resting pulmonary artery pressure often does not predict exercise capacity. Because of the multifactorial basis of exercise limitation, CPET may be considered as a means of identifying the cause(s) of each individual's impairment and of formulating an appropriate exercise prescription to be used in PR, provided that the PH is optimally treated and controlled with pharmacologic therapy. Incremental CPET should be avoided among persons with exercise-induced syncope, presyncope, or ventricular arrhythmia. When CPET is considered unsafe or is unavailable, the 6MWT can be used as an alternative method to test the exercise tolerance of patients with PH.[93,121] The 6MWT distance correlates with the severity of the New York Heart Association (NYHA) functional class, as well as peak $\dot{V}_{O_2}$ O_2 pluse, and $\dot{V}_E/\dot{V}_{CO_2}$ slope of PH patients as determined by CPET.[121] The 6MWT is also sensitive to detect changes in exercise capacity that result from vasodilator pharmacologic therapy, and correlates with survival of patients with primary pulmonary hypertension.[121] In the study by Miyamoto and colleagues,[121] patients with baseline 6MWT distance less than 332 m had lower survival than those able to walk greater distances. Exercise O_2 desaturation during the 6MWT is also a predictor of poor prognosis among such patients.[125,126]

Several studies have shown that QOL is also impaired among patients with PH,[127-129] especially those with worse NYHA functional class[130,131] and those who experience side effects from medical therapy.[132] As is true for exercise tolerance, QOL improves after pharmacologic treatment for PH.[128,132-135] Health status measurement tools shown to be useful among patients with PH include the SF-36, SGRQ, and Minnesota Living with Heart Failure Questionnaire.[127,129,131] Cognitive defects, as well as anxiety and depression, are also common among patients with PH.[127,136] Importantly, QOL scores do not correlate with resting hemodynamic parameters,[129,131] hence QOL must be measured as an independent outcome of therapeutic interventions for the disease. QOL scores do correlate better with exercise capacity assessed by the 6MWT and functional class (WHO or NYHA).[129,131]

To date, only one small, prospective randomized controlled trial has evaluated the benefits of PR among patients with PH.[137] Thirty patients with moderate PH of various causes (mean pulmonary artery pressure, 50 ± 15 mm Hg) with impaired functional status and a mean 6MWT distance of 420 to 430 m despite optimized medical therapy were randomized to receive PR versus ongoing medical therapy plus massage and counseling over a 15-week study period.[137] The PR in this study consisted of low workload (WL) and interval-type cycle ergometry (low WL for 0.5 minute alternating with high WL for 1 minute at a level adjusted to 60% to 80% of the heart rate reached at peak $\dot{V}_{O_2}$ during a baseline CPET) for 10 to 25 min/day, as well as low-intensity free weight training three times per week and respiratory training five times per week. The intensity of training was increased over time as tolerated, but treatment was limited to avoid a peak heart rate exceeding 120 beats/minute. Supplemental O_2 was given to maintain arterial oxygen saturation at greater than 88%. This training was followed by 12 weeks of outpatient treatment wherein the PR patients received individual training manuals and were given cycle ergometers for home use. Patients were asked to exercise 15 to 30 minutes/day, 5 days/week, and to walk two times per week as well as continue weight and respiratory training for 15 to 30 minutes at least every other day. Patients received telephone contact from PR staff every 2 weeks. Patients who underwent PR achieved significant gains in 6MWT distance, peak $\dot{V}_{O_2}$, $\dot{V}_{O_2}$ at anaerobic threshold, WHO functional class, and improved QOL measured by the SF-36 questionnaire.[137] No significant change was noted in Borg Dyspnea Scale scores. Importantly, this exercise regimen was well tolerated, and there were no adverse events other than two episodes of patients experiencing dizziness after cycling. Overall compliance with the home-based component of the exercise program was excellent. Patients randomized initially to the control group were subsequently offered PR, and they too achieved gains comparable to those made by the primary training group. This important study demonstrates that it is feasible to provide PR to selected patients with moderate PH under carefully controlled conditions, and that PR can lead to significant gains in exercise tolerance and QOL for such persons. The optimal program content and means of exercise training, and health status measurement tools most sensitive to change after PR are as yet unknown, and it is unclear whether these results can be generalized to a larger group of patients or persons with more severe PH awaiting transplantation. Further clinical trials are awaited.

There are several special considerations for maintaining safety for patients with PH during PR. No guidelines exist regarding the safest methods of exercise training. Apart from the study discussed previously, wherein interval-type cycle ergometry training was used as part of the exercise program (at intensities up to a peak heart rate of 120 beats/minute), experts have suggested that high-intensity aerobic exercise and any exercise (such as high-intensity resistive exercise or exercise involving sit-ups or rising from the floor) that may lead to Valsalva-like maneuvers that may increase intrathoracic pressure should be avoided, to minimize risk of preload reduction and circulatory collapse,[138] particularly among persons with severe PH awaiting transplantation. Activities such as walking on level ground or low-intensity treadmill walking or cycling, stretching, and active range of motion exercises have been advocated. The potential role of training strategies such as neuromuscular electrical stimulation has not been investigated. Extreme caution must be taken to avoid falls among patients who are anticoagulated, and patients receiving continuous intravenous vasodilator therapy must not have therapy interrupted inadvertently during the course of exercise. Whenever possible, arterial oxygen saturation should be maintained at greater than 90% to avoid hypoxic vasoconstriction that may worsen pulmonary vascular resistance during exercise. Telemetry monitoring during exercise is considered advisable for patients with a history of cardiac arrhythmias.

Patients must also be monitored for exercise-induced systemic hypertension or hypotension, and exercise should be stopped immediately if the patient develops dizziness, chest pain, or presyncope. Educational topics of particular importance to patients with PH include benefits and risks of vasodilator/antiproliferative therapy as well as anticoagulation therapy, and issues pertaining to preparation for and recovery from lung transplantation.

LUNG CANCER

Patients preparing for, or recovering from, various treatments for lung cancer are another group of individuals who may benefit from PR. Some patients with lung cancer, including those with or without COPD, who are candidates for surgical resection may be deconditioned. Because preoperative exercise tolerance is one factor that predicts outcomes of thoracic surgery,[139] preoperative PR may improve outcomes for some patients with lung cancer. PR also offers an opportunity to educate patients regarding aspects of postoperative symptoms and care strategies such as incentive spirometer use, bronchial clearance techniques, controlled coughing, and other strategies that may reduce risk of postoperative complications. In considering PR for patients with lung cancer awaiting resection, care providers clearly must weigh both the potential benefits of the PR intervention and the duration of the intervention so as not to place the patient at risk by postponing the resection. Although the minimal duration and optimal components of PR that may be effective for patients with lung cancer awaiting resection are unknown, and no randomized controlled trials have yet studied comprehensive outcomes of PR in this situation, Wall[140] demonstrated greater postoperative improvements in sense of hope and power among patients with non–small cell lung cancer who had undergone a preoperative exercise training program as compared with patients who received no exercise. Exercise capacity, dyspnea, and other aspects of QOL were not measured in this study. Sekine and colleagues[141] conducted an analysis of 22 patients with lung cancer and COPD who underwent PR that included an intensive exercise program for 2 weeks preoperatively, and compared outcomes with a group of historical control subjects who had not received preoperative PR. Despite lower baseline FEV_1 and forced vital capacity, patients in the group that underwent PR had shorter hospital length of stay, and better actual (compared with predicted) postoperative FEV_1 as compared with the historical control group. Traditional outcomes of PR such as gains in postoperative exercise tolerance, symptom reduction, and QOL were also not tested. This small study nevertheless suggests that short-duration preoperative PR may help maintain postoperative pulmonary function and reduce postoperative complications, but its findings need to be confirmed in a randomized controlled study. However, such studies are difficult to conduct, given the well-placed concerns of patients and health care providers about avoiding any delays in performing potentially curable lung cancer resection. At present, the potential benefits of conducting preoperative PR relative to the risks of cancer spread posed by delaying surgery by 2 to 3 weeks to enable patients to undergo PR are not defined.

Of note, exercise tolerance is also often impaired after treatment for lung cancer.[142] Exercise training has led to improved exercise tolerance and sense of well-being among patients with other forms of cancer,[143] and as such, interest has arisen in PR as a therapeutic intervention for patients with lung cancer as well. Although minimal data exist in this area, Spruit and colleagues conducted a small pilot trial wherein 10 patients with severely impaired lung function and impaired exercise tolerance after treatment for lung cancer (surgery, chemotherapy, and/or radiation therapy) underwent 8 weeks of inpatient, multidisciplinary PR.[144] The exercise program included daily walking, gymnastics, and cycling exercise, with exercise intensity increased over time as tolerated. This PR program led to significant improvements in exercise endurance (145 m, 43.2% increase; $P = .002$) and peak exercise capacity (26 W, 34.4% increase; $P = .0078$) as compared with baseline. Larger, randomized controlled trials are also needed to confirm these findings, and to assess the impact of PR on other outcomes such as symptoms, well-being, QOL, ability to perform ADLs, health care use, and survival among these patients.

In providing exercise training to patients with lung cancer, caution must be taken to ensure that patients do not have metastatic disease (such as brain or bone metastases) that might render exercise training unsafe (e.g., due to risk of falls, seizures, or bone fractures). Indeed, some patients with lung cancer may not be able to participate in conventional exercise training. Interestingly, one case report has demonstrated that a 4-week program of neuromuscular electrical stimulation of the lower extremities, (an alternative method of training muscle without the requirement for conventional exercise) resulted in a significant (183 m, 44% increase) improvement in 6MWT and improvement in QOL (measured by the SF-36 questionnaire) for a patient with advanced lung cancer with brain and bone metastases. Thus, novel alternative strategies for maintaining functional ability should also be considered for use within PR for patients with lung cancer.[145] Finally, PR programs (particularly inpatient programs) have the potential to enable severely disabled, even long-term ventilator-dependent patients with lung cancer who may otherwise require institution-based living, to return to live at home with their loved ones, and in turn to improve patient QOL. In this situation, goals of PR may not include conventional exercise training but may include training of the patient and their family members with the use of adaptive/assistive equipment to optimize independence with and ability to perform ADLs and maintain mobility, as well as training of the patient in the areas of symptom control, stress, anxiety or depression management and training for tracheostomy or home mechanical ventilation equipment. Thus an expanded view of the scope of PR may be needed to enable provision of PR to the most severely disabled patients.

NEUROMUSCULAR DISEASE

Patients with a wide variety of neuromuscular disorders, including stroke, Parkinson's disease, postpolio syndrome, muscular dystrophy, multiple sclerosis, survivors of critical illness-related neuropathy and myopathy; patients with Guillain-Barré syndrome and other myopathies, Charcot-Marie-Tooth disease, amyotrophic lateral sclerosis, spinal cord injury, disorders of the neuromuscular junction, and diaphragm paralysis can have several disturbances of respiratory function, particularly if there is associated weakness of the respiratory and/or bulbar muscles or reduced chest wall compliance.[146-148] In addition to disturbances in pulmonary function (typically a restrictive ventilatory defect), patients with neuromuscular disease commonly experience swallowing dysfunction or episodes of aspiration, difficulty clearing respiratory secretions, sleep-disordered breathing (alveolar hypoventilation or obstructive sleep apnea), gas exchange disturbances, and disturbances of respiratory control.[148,149] The specific respiratory manifestations of various forms of neuromuscular disease have been reviewed elsewhere.[146,147] Depending on the nature and severity of the disease, these disturbances, together with abnormalities of the peripheral muscles, can lead to significant exercise impairment and disability during daily life activities, daytime fatigue, and impairment in QOL.[150] Patients with disability due to neuromuscular disease may become sedentary and have secondary deconditioning.[151]

To date, published discussions of "pulmonary rehabilitation" in neuromuscular disease have focused primarily on breathing strategies, noninvasive ventilation, and secretion clearance techniques.[152] Comprehensive PR programs have the potential to improve the functional status of selected patients with neuromuscular disease in several ways.[153] Patients may benefit from exercise training of the extremity or respiratory muscles to counteract reductions in strength or endurance resulting from deconditioning. Indeed, some patients with neuromuscular disease were among those who improved in PR in the trials conducted by Foster and Thomas[13] and by Ferreira, Feuerman, and Spiegler,[14] and modest benefits of PR on 6MWT, dyspnea, and pulmonary function were noted in a small, uncontrolled study among patients with Parkinson's disease.[154] There is, as well, a sizeable body of literature examining the use of physical activity and various strategies of exercise training to maintain maximal function and QOL of patients with neuromuscular diseases, wherein disturbances of respiratory function were not specifically considered.[153,155-157] Multiple small trials have confirmed benefits of aerobic or strength training conducted in various rehabilitation settings for patients with multiple sclerosis,[158-161] Parkinson's disease,[162-164] stroke,[165] postpolio syndrome,[166] myopathies,[167-171] and amyotrophic lateral sclerosis.[172-174] Inspiratory muscle training can also lead to at least short-term improvements in pulmonary function, cough, and dyspnea among patients with neuromuscular disease.[175-180] In addition to exercise training, PR may benefit patients with neuromuscular disease (particularly those with greater disability, who may not be able to undertake conventional exercise training) by training them in the use of adaptive/assistive equipment to enable them to maintain functional independence and live in their own home. Importantly also, as mentioned earlier, PR programs, particularly inpatient ones, are an ideal setting in which patients can be acclimatized to and trained in the use of NIPPV and to learn assisted coughing techniques, and to use devices such as the insufflator–exsufflator[181,182] or intermittent positive-pressure breathing equipment. The use of NIPPV by patients with pulmonary impairment due to neuromuscular disease leads to improved functional independence[183] and may prolong survival.[184] Inpatient PR can also be conducted while patients are gradually weaned from mechanical ventilation after an episode of respiratory failure. Thus, collectively, it is likely that selected patients with respiratory impairment due to neuromuscular disease would benefit from comprehensive PR. To date, however, no randomized controlled clinical trials have yet investigated the benefits of conventional comprehensive PR (including exercise training, pulmonary education and self-management training, and psychosocial support) on the outcomes of exercise tolerance, symptoms, QOL, health care use, or survival specifically for patients with neuromuscular disease.

The safety of conducting exercise training in PR for patients with neuromuscular disease is controversial, but in general depends on the nature and severity of the condition and the precise functional impairments present. No formal exercise training guidelines exist for such patients. A reasonable goal is to maintain and/or improve muscle conditioning to optimize the ability of patients to perform ADLs while avoiding excess muscle fatigue, inflammation, or injury that may worsen muscle function. High-intensity strength training may indeed cause muscle injury in some situations.[185] Further work is needed to determine how much and what type of exercise is beneficial and not harmful in patients with different neuromuscular disorders at various stages of disease. Additional study is needed to identify optimal tools for assessing health status and activity participation after PR for patients with neuromuscular disease.

CONCLUSION

PR is an effective therapeutic intervention that leads to significant gains in exercise tolerance, reduction in symptoms, and improved quality of life for patients with several forms of chronic respiratory disease. Existing evidence suggests that not only are the scientific basis and rationale for providing PR to patients with non-COPD diagnoses similar to those for patients with COPD, but also, where studied, outcomes of PR are similar. Although the core components of PR for patients with respiratory disorders other than COPD are the same as those for COPD, a disease-appropriate approach, based on careful consideration of the physiology and clinical manifestations of the individual disease states, patient safety, and goal setting to meet patient needs, is required. Additional research is needed to identify optimal exercise training strategies, symptom and health status assessment tools, and other important outcomes of PR for patients with disorders other than COPD. PR is an important component of a multidisciplinary, integrated treatment approach for patients with chronic respiratory disease.

References

1. Nici L, Donner C, Wouters E et al: American Thoracic Society/European Respiratory Society statement on pulmonary rehabilitation, Am J Respir Crit Care Med 173:1390-1413, 2006.
2. Troosters T, Casaburi R, Gosselink R et al: Pulmonary rehabilitation in chronic obstructive pulmonary disease: state of the art, Am J Respir Crit Care Med 172:19-38, 2005.
3. Ries A Bauldoff GS, Carlin BW et al: Pulmonary rehabilitation: joint ACCP/AACVPR evidence-based clinical practice guidelines, Chest 131(suppl):4S-42S, 2007.
4. Rabe KF, Hurd S, Anzueto A et al: Global strategy for the diagnosis, management, and prevention of chronic obstructive pulmonary disease: GOLD executive summary, Am J Respir Crit Care Med 176:532-535, 2007.
5. Bourjeily G, Rochester CL: Exercise training in chronic obstructive pulmonary disease, Clin Chest Med 21:763-781, 2000.
6. Puhan MA, Busching G, Schunemann HJ et al: Interval versus continuous high-intensity exercise in chronic obstructive pulmonary disease, Ann Intern Med 145:816-825, 2006.
7. Remels AH, Gosker HR, van der Velden J et al: Systemic inflammation and skeletal muscle dysfunction in chronic obstructive pulmonary disease: state of the art and novel insights in regulation of muscle plasticity, Clin Chest Med 28:537-552, 2007.
8. American Thoracic Society/European Respiratory Society: Skeletal muscle dysfunction in chronic obstructive pulmonary disease, Am J Respir Crit Care Med 159:S1-S40, 1999.
9. Stone AC, Nici L: Other systemic manifestations of chronic obstructive pulmonary disease, Clin Chest Med 28:553-557, 2007.
10. Gosselink R, Troosters T, Decramer M: Peripheral muscle weakness contributes to exercise limitation in COPD, Am J Respir Crit Care Med 153:976-980, 1996.
11. Hamilton AL, Killian KJ, Summers E et al: Muscle strength, symptom intensity, and exercise capacity in patients with cardiorespiratory disorders, Am J Respir Crit Care Med 152:2021-2031, 1995.
12. Bourbeau J, Julien M, Maltais F et al: Reduction of hospital utilization in patients with chronic obstructive pulmonary disease: a disease-specific self-management intervention, Arch Intern Med 163:585-591, 2003.
13. Foster S, Thomas HM: Pulmonary rehabilitation in lung disease other than chronic obstructive pulmonary disease, Am Rev Respir Dis 141:601-604, 1990.
14. Ferreira G, Feuerman M, Spiegler P: Results of an 8-week, outpatient pulmonary rehabilitation program on patients with and without chronic obstructive pulmonary disease, J Cardiopulm Rehabil 26:54-60, 2006.
15. Smidt N, de Vet HCW, Bouter LM et al: Effectiveness of exercise therapy: a best-evidence summary of systematic reviews, Austr J Physiother 51:71-85, 2005.
16. Congleton J, Bott J, Hindell A et al: Comparison of outcome of pulmonary rehabilitation in obstructive lung disease, interstitial lung disease and chest wall disease, Thorax 52(6S)Supplement6:p11A, 1997.
17. American Thoracic Society: ATS statement: guidelines for the Six-Minute Walk Test, Am J Respir Crit Care Med 166:111-117, 2002.
18. Guyatt GH, Berman LB, Townsend M et al: A measure of quality of life for clinical trials in chronic lung disease, Thorax 42:773-778, 1987.
19. Chung KF: Unmet needs in adult asthma, Clin Exp Allergy 30(suppl 1):66-69, 2000.
20. Clark CJ: The role of physical training in asthma. In Casaburi R, Petty T, editors: Principles and practice of pulmonary rehabilitation, Philadelphia, 1993, WB Saunders, pp 424-437.
21. Folgering H, van Herwaarden C: Pulmonary rehabilitation in asthma and COPD: physiological basics, Respir Med 87(suppl B):41-44, 1993.
22. Satta A: Exercise training in asthma, J Sports Med Phys Fitness 40:277-283, 2000.
23. Kitsantas A, Zimmerman BJ: Self-efficacy, activity participation, and physical fitness of asthmatic and nonasthmatic adolescent girls, J Asthma 37:163-174, 2000.
24. Singh SJ, Morgan MD, Hardman AE et al: Development of a shuttle walking test of disability in patients with chronic airways obstruction, Thorax 47:1019-1024, 1992.
25. Carlin BW: Outcome measurement in pulmonary rehabilitation, Respir Care Clin N Am 4:113-127, 1998.
26. Dyer CAE, Hill SL, Stockley et al: Quality of life in elderly subjects with a diagnostic label of asthma from general practice registers, Eur Respir J 14:39-45, 1999.
27. Cambach W, Wagenaar RC, Koelman TW et al: The long-term effects of pulmonary rehabilitation in patients with asthma and chronic obstructive pulmonary disease: a research synthesis, Arch Phys Med Rehabil 80:103-111, 1999.

28. Basaran S, Guler-Uysal F, Ergen N et al: Effects of physical exercise on quality of life, exercise capacity and pulmonary function in children with asthma, J Rehabil Med 38:130-135, 2006.

29. Counil FP, Varray A, Matecki S et al: Training of aerobic and anaerobic fitness in children with asthma, J Pediatr 142:179-184, 2003.

30. Emtner M, Herala M, Stalenheim G: High-intensity physical training in adults with asthma: A 10 week rehabilitation program, Chest 109:323-330, 1996.

31. Matsumoto I, Araki H, Odajima H et al: Effects of swimming training on aerobic capacity and exercise induced bronchoconstriction in children with bronchial asthma, Thorax 54:196-201, 1999.

32. Ernst E: Breathing techniques: adjunctive treatment modalities for asthma? A systematic review, Eur Respir J 15:969-972, 2000.

33. Neder JA, Nery LE, Silva AC et al: Short term effects of aerobic training in the clinical management of moderate to severe asthma in children, Thorax 54:202-206, 1999.

34. Ram FS, Robinson SM, Black PN: Effects of physical training in asthma: a systematic review, Br J Sports Med 34:162-167, 2000.

35. Cochrane LM, Clark CJ: Benefits and problems of a physical training programme for asthmatic patients, Thorax 45:345-351, 1990.

36. Emtner M, Finne M, Stalenheim G: High-intensity physical training in adults with asthma: a comparison between training on land and in water, Scand J Rehab Med 30:201-209, 1998.

37. Hallstrand TS, Bates PW, Schoene RB: Aerobic conditioning in mild asthma decreases the hyperpnea of exercise and improves exercise and ventilatory capacity, Chest 118:1460-1469, 2000.

38. Emtner M, Finne M, Stalenheim G: A 3-year follow up of asthmatic patients participating in a 10-week rehabilitation training program with emphasis on physical training, Arch Phys Med Rehabil 79:539-544, 1998.

39. Carroll N, Sly P: Exercise training as an adjunct to asthma management? Thorax 54:190-191, 1999.

40. Freeman W, Stableforth DE, Cayton RM et al: Endurance exercise capacity in adults with cystic fibrosis, Respir Med 87:541-549, 1993.

41. Orenstein DM, Noyes BE: Cystic fibrosis. In: Casaburi R, Petty TL, editors: Principles and practice of pulmonary rehabilitation, Philadelphia, 1993, WB Saunders, pp 439-458.

42. Sahlberg ME, Svantesson U, Magnusson Thomas EML et al: Muscular strength and function in patients with cystic fibrosis, Chest 127:1587-1592, 2005.

43. Selvadurai HC, Blimkie CJ, Meyers N et al: Randomized controlled study of in-hospital exercise training programs in children with cystic fibrosis, Pediatr Pulmonol 33:194-200, 2002.

44. Alison JA, Regnis JA, Donnelly PM et al: Evaluation of supported upper limb exercise capacity in patients with cystic fibrosis, Am J Respir Crit Care Med 156:1541-1548, 1997.

45. McKone EF, Barry SC, FitzGerald MX et al: The role of supplemental oxygen during submaximal exercise in patients with cystic fibrosis, Eur Respir J 20:134-142, 2002.

46. Boas SR: Exercise recommendations for individuals with cystic fibrosis, Sports Med 24:17-37, 1997.

47. Frangiolas DD, Holloway CL, Vedal S et al: Role of exercise and lung function in predicting work status in cystic fibrosis, Am J Respir Crit Care Med 167:150-157, 2003.

48. Nixon PA, Orenstein DM, Kelsey SF et al: The prognostic value of exercise testing in patients with cystic fibrosis, New Engl J Med 327:1785-1788, 1992.

49. Pianosi P, LeBlanc J, Almudevar A: Peak oxygen uptake and mortality in children with cystic fibrosis, Thorax 60:50-54, 2005.

50. Chetta A, Pisi G, Zanini A et al: Six-minute walking test in cystic fibrosis adults with mild to moderate lung disease: a comparison to healthy subjects, Respir Med 95:986-991, 2001.

51. Bradley J, Howard J, Wallace E et al: Reliability, repeatability, and sensitivity of the modified shuttle test in adult cystic fibrosis, Chest 117:1666-1671, 2000.

52. Bradley J, Howard J, Wallace E et al: Validity of a modified shuttle test in adult cystic fibrosis, Thorax 54:437-439, 1999.

53. De Jong W, Kaptein AA, van der Schans CP et al: Quality of life in patients with cystic fibrosis, Pediatr Pulmonol 23:95-100, 1997.

54. Gulmans VA, de Meer K, Brackel HJ et al: Outpatient exercise training in children with cystic fibrosis: physiological effects, perceived competence, and acceptability, Pediatr Pulmonol 28:39-46, 1999.

55. Orenstein DM, Hovell MF, Mulvihill M et al: Strength vs. aerobic training in children with cystic fibrosis: a randomized controlled trial, Chest 126:1204-1214, 2004.

56. Nixon PA: Role of exercise in the evaluation and management of pulmonary disease in children and youth, Med Sci Sports Exerc 28:414-420, 1996.

57. Rickert KA, Bartlett SJ, Boyle MP et al: The association between depression, lung function and health-related quality of life among adults with cystic fibrosis, Chest 132:231-237, 2007.

58. Hogg M, Braithwaite M, Barley M et al: Work disability in adults with cystic fibrosis and its relationship to quality of life, J Cyst Fibros 6:223-227, 2007.

59. Moorcroft AJ, Dodd ME, Webb AK: Exercise limitations and training for patients with cystic fibrosis, Disabil Rehabil 20:247-253, 1998.

60. Blau H, Mussaffi-Georgi H, Fink G et al: Effects of an intensive 4-week summer camp on cystic fibrosis: pulmonary function, exercise tolerance and nutrition, Chest 121:1117-1122, 2002.

61. O'Neill PA, Dodd ME, Abbott JV et al: The benefits of exercise and reduction of breathlessness in cystic fibrosis, Br J Dis Chest 81:62-69, 1987.

62. Bradley J, Moran F: Physical training for cystic fibrosis, Cochrane Database Syst Rev 2:CD002768, 2002.

63. De Jong W, Grevink RG, Roorda RJ et al: Effect of a home exercise training program in patients with cystic fibrosis, Chest 105:463-468, 1994.

64. Orenstein DM, Higgins LW: Update on the role of exercise in cystic fibrosis, Curr Opin Pulm Med 11:519-523, 2005.

65. Moorcroft AJ, Dodd ME, Morris J et al: Individualised unsupervised exercise training in adults with cystic fibrosis: a 1 year randomized controlled trial, Thorax 59:1074-1080, 2004.

66. Strauss GD, Osher A, Wang C-I et al: Variable weight training in cystic fibrosis, Chest 92:273-276, 1987.

67. De Jong, W, van Aalderen WM, Kraan J et al: Inspiratory muscle training in patients with cystic fibrosis, Respir Med 95:31-36, 2001.

68. Sawyer EH, Clanton TL: Improved pulmonary function and exercise tolerance with inspiratory muscle conditioning in children with cystic fibrosis, Chest 104:1490-1497, 1993.

69. Enright S, Chatham K, Ionescu AA et al: Inspiratory muscle training improves lung function and exercise capacity in adults with cystic fibrosis, Chest 126:405-411, 2004.

70. Schneiderman-Walker J, Pollock SL, Corey M et al: A randomized controlled trial of a 3-year home exercise program in cystic fibrosis, J Pediatr 136:304-310, 2000.

71. Stanghelle JK, Skyberg D, Haanaes OC: Eight year follow-up of pulmonary function and oxygen uptake during exercise in 16-year old males with cystic fibrosis, Acta Pediatr 81:527-531, 1992.

72. Nikolaizik WH, Simon H-U, Iseli P et al: Effect of 3 weeks' rehabilitation on neutrophil surface antigens and lung function in cystic fibrosis, Eur Respir J 15:942-948, 2000.

73. Klijn PHC, Oudshoorn A, van der Ent CK et al: Effects of anaerobic training in children with cystic fibrosis, Chest 125:1299-1305, 2004.

74. Heijerman HGM: Chronic obstructive lung disease and respiratory muscle function: the role of nutrition and exercise training in cystic fibrosis, Respir Med 87(suppl B):49-51, 1993.

75. Newall C, Stockley RA, Hill SL: Exercise training and inspiratory muscle training in patients with bronchiectasis, Thorax 60:943-948, 2005.

76. Bradley J, Moran F: Pulmonary rehabilitation improves exercise tolerance in patients with bronchiectasis, Austr J Physiother 52:65, 2006.

77. Wasserman K, Hansen JE, Sue DY et al: Pathophysiology of disorders limiting exercise. In Principles of exercise testing and interpretation, ed 3, Philadelphia, 1999, Lippincott Williams & Wilkins, pp 95-114.

78. O'Donnell DE, Chau LKL, Webb KA: Qualitative aspects of exertional dyspnea in patients with interstitial lung disease, J Appl Physiol 84:2000-2009, 1998.

79. Marciniuk DD, Sridhar G, Clemens RE et al: Lung volumes and expiratory flow limitation during exercise in interstitial lung disease, J Appl Physiol 77:963-973, 1994.

80. Markovitz GH, Cooper CB: Exercise and interstitial lung disease, Curr Opin Pulm Med 4:272-280, 1998.

81. Hsia CC: Cardiopulmonary limitations to exercise in restrictive lung disease, Med Sci Sports Exerc 31(1 suppl):S28-S32, 1999.

82. Hansen JE, Wasserman K: Pathophysiology of activity limitation in patients with interstitial lung disease, Chest 109:1566-1576, 1996.

83. Harris-Eze AO, Sridhar G, Clemens RE et al: Oxygen improves maximal exercise performance in interstitial lung disease, Am J Respir Crit Care Med 150:1616-1622, 1994.

84. Kaltreider NL, McCann WS: Respiratory response during exercise in pulmonary fibrosis and emphysema, J Clin Invest 16:23-40, 1937.

85. Nishiyama O, Taniguchi H, Kondoh Y et al: Quadriceps weakness is related to exercise capacity in idiopathic pulmonary fibrosis, Chest 127:2028-2033, 2005.

86. Reinsma GD, ten Hacken NH, Grevink RG et al: Limiting factors of exercise performance 1 year after lung transplantation, J Heart Lung Transplant 25:1310-1316, 2006.

87. Kadikar A, Maurer J, Kesten S: The Six-Minute Walk Test: a guide to assessment for lung transplantation, J Heart Lung Transplant 16:313-319, 1997.

88. DeVries J, Kessels BLJ, Drent M: Quality of life of idiopathic pulmonary fibrosis patients, Eur Respir J 17:954-961, 2001.

89. Chang JA, Curtis JR, Patrick DL et al: Assessment of health-related quality of life in patients with interstitial lung disease, Chest 116:1175-1182, 1999.

90. Martinez TY, Pereira CA, dos Santos ML et al: Evaluation of the short form 36 item questionnaire to measure health-related quality of life in patients with idiopathic pulmonary fibrosis, Chest 117:1627-1632, 2000.

91. Khanna D, Clements PJ, Furst DE et al: Correlation of the degree of dyspnea with health-related quality of life, functional abilities, and diffusing capacity for carbon monoxide in patients with systemic sclerosis and active alveolitis, Arthritis Rheum 52:592-600, 2005.

92. American Thoracic Society: Idiopathic pulmonary fibrosis: diagnosis and treatment. International consensus statement. American Thoracic Society (ATS), and the European Respiratory Society (ERS), Am J Respir Crit Care Med 161:646-664, 2000.

93. Palange P, Ward SA, Carlsen K-H et al: ERS Task Force recommendations on the use of exercise testing in clinical practice, Eur Respir J 29:185-209, 2007.

94. Ando M, Mori A, Esaki H et al: The effect of pulmonary rehabilitation in patients with post-tuberculosis lung disorder, Chest 123:1988-1995, 2003.

95. Naji NA, Connor MC, Donnelly SC et al: Effectiveness of pulmonary rehabilitation in restrictive lung disease, J Cardiopulm Rehabil 26:237-243, 2006.

96. Moloney ED, Clayton N, Mukherjee DK et al: The shuttle walk test in idiopathic pulmonary fibrosis, Respir Med 97:682-687, 2003.

97. Beretta L, Santaniello A, Lemos A et al: Validity of the Saint George's Respiratory Questionnaire in the evaluation of health-related quality of life in patients with interstitial lung disease secondary to systemic sclerosis, Rheumatology 46:296-301, 2007.

98. De Vries J, Seebregts A, Drent M: Assessing health status and quality of life in idiopathic pulmonary fibrosis: which measure should be used? Respir Med 94:273-278, 2000.

99. Jastrzebski D, Gumola A, Gawlik R et al: Dyspnea and quality of life in patients with pulmonary fibrosis after six weeks of respiratory rehabilitation, J Physiol Pharmacol 57(suppl 4):139-148, 2006.

100. Anderson SD, Bye PT: Exercise testing in the evaluation of diffuse interstitial lung disease, Aust N Z J Med 14(5 suppl 3):762-768, 1984.

101. Fumeaux T, Rothmeier C, Jolliet P: Outcome of mechanical ventilation for acute respiratory failure in patients with pulmonary fibrosis, Intensive Care Med 27:1868-1874, 2001.

102. Dos Santos Alves VL, Stirbulov R, Avanzi O: Impact of a physical rehabilitation program on the respiratory function of adolescents with idiopathic scoliosis, Chest 130:500-505, 2006.

103. Fuschillo S, De Felice A, Gaudiosi C et al: Nocturnal mechanical ventilation improves exercise capacity in kyphoscoliotic patients with respiratory impairment, Monaldi Arch Chest Dis 59:281-286, 2003.

104. Mohsenin V, Gee JBL: Effect of obesity on the respiratory system and pathophysiology of sleep apnea, Curr Pulmonol 14:179-197, 1993.

105. Rochester DF: Obesity and pulmonary function. In Alpert MA, Alexander JK, editors: The heart and lung in obesity, New York, 1998, Futura Publishing, pp 109-131.

106. Teixeira CA, Dos Santos JE, Silva GA et al: Prevalence of and the potential pathophysiological mechanisms involved in dyspnea in individuals with class II or III obesity, J Bras Pneumol 33:28-35, 2007.

107. Hopman WM, Berger C, Joseph L et al: The association between body mass index and health-related quality of life: data from CaMos, a stratified population study, Qual Life Res 16(10):1595-1603, 2007.

108. Sugerman HJ, Fairman RP, Baron PL et al: Gastric surgery for respiratory insufficiency of obesity, Chest 90:81-86, 1986.

109. Hakala K, Mustajoki P, Aittomaki J et al: Improved gas exchange during exercise after weight loss in morbid obesity, Clin Physiol 16:229-238, 1996.

110. Olsen EJ, Moore WR, Morgenthaler TI et al: Obstructive sleep apnea hypopnea syndrome, Mayo Clin Proc 78:1545-1552, 2003.

111. Granger CV, Hamilton BB, Linacre JM et al: Performance profiles of the functional independence measure, Am J Phys Med Rehabil 72:84-89, 1993.

112. Whittaker LA, Rochester CL: Functional outcome of inpatient pulmonary rehabilitation for patients with severe obesity [abstract], Am J Respir Crit Care Med 161:A495, 2000.

113. Devine EB, Hakim Z, Green J: A systematic review of patient-reported outcome instruments measuring sleep dysfunction in adults, Pharmacoeconomics 23:889-912, 2005.

114. Knipper J, Nielsen K, Lane-Gipson N et al: Outcomes of pulmonary rehabilitation in obstructive sleep apnea [abstract], Am J Respir Crit Care Med 161:A496, 2000.

115. Badesch DB, Abman SH, Ahearn GS et al: Medical therapy for pulmonary arterial hypertension: ACCP evidence-based clinical practice guidelines, Chest 126:35S-62S, 2004.

116. Gaine SP, Rubin LJ: Primary pulmonary hypertension, Lancet 352:719-725, 1998.

117. Badesch DB, Abman SH, Simonneau G et al: Medical therapy for pulmonary arterial hypertension: updated ACCP evidence-based clinical practice guidelines, Chest 131:1917-1928, 2007.

118. Palevsky HI: Therapeutic options for severe pulmonary hypertension, Clin Chest Med 18:595-609, 1997.

119. Nagaya N, Shimizu Y, Satoh T et al: Oral beraprost sodium improves exercise capacity and ventilatory efficiency in patients with primary or thromboembolic pulmonary hypertension, Heart 87:340-345, 2002.

120. Riley MS, Pórszász J, Engelen MP et al: Responses to constant work rate bicycle ergometry exercise in primary pulmonary hypertension: the effect of inhaled nitric oxide, J Am Coll Cardiol 36:547-556, 2000.

121. Miyamoto S, Nagaya N, Satoh T et al: Clinical correlates and prognostic significance of Six-Minute Walk Test in patients with primary pulmonary hypertension: comparison with cardiopulmonary exercise testing, Am J Respir Crit Care Med 161:487-492, 2000.

122. Archibald CJ, Augger WR, Fedullo PF et al: Long-term outcome after pulmonary thromboendarterectomy, Am J Respir Crit Care Med 160:523-528, 1999.

123. Markowitz DH, Systrom DM: Diagnosis of pulmonary vascular limit to exercise by cardiopulmonary exercise testing, J Heart Lung Transplant 23:88-95, 2004.

124. Matthay RA, Matthay MA: Pulmonary thromboembolism and other pulmonary vascular diseases. In George RB, Light RW, Matthay MA et al, editors: Chest medicine: essentials of pulmonary and critical care medicine, ed 2, Baltimore, 1990, Williams & Wilkins, pp 249-276.

125. Wensel R, Opitz CF, Anker SD et al: Assessment of survival in patients with primary pulmonary hypertension: importance of cardiopulmonary exercise testing, Circulation 106:319-324, 2002.

126. Paciocco G, Martinez FJ, Bossone E et al: Oxygen desaturation on the Six-Minute Walk Test and mortality in untreated primary pulmonary hypertension, Eur Respir J 17:647-652, 2001.

127. White J, Hopkins RO, Glissmeyer EW et al: Cognitive, emotional, and quality of life outcomes in patients with pulmonary arterial hypertension, Respir Res 7:55-64, 2006.

128. Shafazand S, Goldstein MK, Doyle RL et al: Health-related quality of life in patients with pulmonary arterial hypertension, Chest 126:1452-1459, 2004.

129. Taichman DB, Shin J, Hud L et al: Health-related quality of life in patients with pulmonary arterial hypertension, Respir Res 6:92-101, 2005.

130. Frank H, Miczoch J, Huber K et al: The effect of anticoagulant therapy in primary and anorectic

drug-induced pulmonary hypertension, Chest 112:714-721, 1997.

131. Chua R, Keogh AM, Byth K et al: Comparison and validation of three measures of quality of life in patients with pulmonary hypertension, Int Med J 36:705-710, 2006.

132. Anderson RB, Hollenberg NK, Williams GS: Physical symptoms distress index, Arch Intern Med 159:693-700, 1999.

133. Mikhail G, Prasad SK, Li W et al: Clinical and haemodynamic effects of sildenafil in pulmonary hypertension: acute and mid-term effects, Eur Heart J 25:431-436, 2004.

134. Olschewski J, Simonneau G, Galie N et al: Inhaled iloprost for severe pulmonary hypertension, N Engl J Med 347:322-329, 2002.

135. Testa MA, Turner RR, Simonson DC et al: Quality of life and calcium channel blockers with nifedipine GITS versus amlodipine in hypertensisive patients in Spain, J Hypertension 16:1839-1847, 1998.

136. Lowe B, Grafe K, Ufer C et al: Anxiety and depression in patients with pulmonary hypertension, Psychosom Med 66:831-836, 2004.

137. Mereles D, Ehlken N, Kreuscher S et al: Exercise and respiratory training improve exercise capacity and quality of life in patients with severe chronic pulmonary hypertension, Circulation 114:1482-1489, 2006.

138. Crouch R, MacIntyre NR: Pulmonary rehabilitation of the patient with nonobstructive lung disease, Respir Care Clin N Am 4:59-70, 1998.

139. Schuurmans MM, Diacon AH, Bolliger CT: Functional evaluation before lung resection, Clin Chest Med 23:159-172, 2002.

140. Wall LM: Changes in hope and power in lung cancer patients who exercise, Nurs Sci Q 13:234-242, 2000.

141. Sekine Y, Chiyo M, Iwata T et al: Perioperative rehabilitation and physiotherapy for lung cancer patients with chronic obstructive pulmonary disease, Jpn J Thorac Cardiovasc Surg 53:237-243, 2005.

142. Bobbio A, Chetta A, Carbognani P et al: Changes in pulmonary function test and cardiopulmonary exercise capacity in COPD patients after lobar pulmonary resection, Eur J Cardiothorac Surg 28:754-758, 2005.

143. Horowitz MB, Littenberg B, Mahler DA: Dyspnea ratings for prescribing exercise intensity in patients with COPD, Chest 109:1169-1175, 1996.

144. Spruit MA, Janssen PP, Willemsen SCP et al: Exercise capacity before and after an 8-week multidisciplinary inpatient pulmonary rehabilitation program in lung cancer patients: a pilot study, Lung Cancer 52:257-260, 2006.

145. Crevenna R, Marosi C, Schmidinger M et al: Neuromuscular electrical stimulation for a patient with metastatic lung cancer—a case report, Supportive Care Cancer 14:970-973, 2006.

146. Hill NS, Lynch JP: Pulmonary complications of neuromuscular diseases, Semin Respir Crit Care Med 23:189-314, 2002.

147. Respiratory dysfunction in neuromuscular disease, Clin Chest Med 15:607-795, 1994.

148. Aboussouan LS: Respiratory disorders in neurologic diseases, Cleve Clin J Med 72:511-520, 2005.

149. Piper A: Sleep abnormalities associated with neuromuscular disease: pathophysiology and evaluation, Semin Respir Crit Care Med 23:211-219, 2002.

150. Sabate M, Rodriguez M, Mendez E et al: Obstructive and restrictive pulmonary dysfunction increases disability in Parkinson disease, Arch Phys Med Rehabil 77:29-34, 1996.

151. Stanghelle JK, Festvag L, Aksnes AK: Pulmonary function and symptom-limited exercise stress testing in subjects with late sequelae of poliomyelitis, Scand J Rehabil Med 25:125-129, 1993.

152. Kang S-C: Pulmonary rehabilitation in patients with neuromuscular disease, Yonsei Med J 47:307-314, 2006.

153. Shneerson JM: Rehabilitation in neuromuscular disorders and thoracic wall deformities, Monaldi Arch Chest Dis 53:415-418, 1998.

154. Koseoglu F, Inan L, Ozel S et al: The effects of a pulmonary rehabilitation program on pulmonary function tests and exercise tolerance in patients with Parkinson's disease, Funct Neurol 12:319-325, 1997.

155. Fowler WM: Consensus conference summary: role of physical activity and exercise training in neuromuscular diseases, Am J Phys Med Rehabil 81(suppl):S187-S195, 2002.

156. Kilmer DD: Response to resistive strengthening exercise training in humans with neuromuscular disease, Am J Phys Med Rehabil 81(suppl):S121-S126, 2002.

157. Eldar R, Marineek C: Physical activity for elderly persons with neurological impairment: a review, Scand J Rehabil Med 32:99-103, 2000.

158. Reitberg MB, Brooks D, Uitdehaag BM et al: Exercise therapy for multiple sclerosis, Cochrane Database Syst Rev 1:CD003980, 2005.

159. White LJ, Dressemdorfer RH: Exercise and multiple sclerosis, Sports Med 34:1077-1100, 2004.

160. Surakka J, Romberg A, Ruutiainen J et al: Effects of aerobic and strength exercise on motor fatigue in men and women with multiple sclerosis: a randomized controlled trial, Clin Rehabil 18:637-646, 2004.

161. Romberg A, Virtanen A, Ruutiainen J et al: Effects of a 6-month exercise program on patients with multiple sclerosis, a randomized study, Neurology 63:2034-2038, 2004.

162. de Goede CJT, Keus SHJ, Kwakkel G et al: The effects of physical therapy in Parkinson's disease: a research synthesis, Arch Phys Med Rehabil 82:509-515, 2001.

163. Bergen JL, Toole T, Elliott RG et al: Aerobic exercise intervention improves aerobic capacity and movement initiation in Parkinson's disease patients, Neurorehabilitation 17:161-168, 2002.

164. Baatile J, Langbein WE, Weaver F et al: Effect of exercise on perceived quality of life in individuals with Parkinson's disease, J Rehabil Res Dev 37:529-534, 2000.

165. Ouellette MM, LeBrasseur NK, Bean JF et al: High-intensity resistance training improves

muscle strength, self-reported function, and disability in long-term stroke survivors, Stroke 35:1404-1409, 2004.

166. Chan KM, Amirjani N, Sumrain M et al: Randomized controlled trial of strength training in post-polio patients, Muscle Nerve 27:332-338, 2003.

167. Alexanderson H, Lundberg IE: The role of exercise in the rehabilitation of idiopathic inflammatory myopathies, Curr Opin Rheumatol 17:164-171, 2005.

168. Alexanderson H, Dastmalchi M, Esbjornsson-Liljedahl M et al: Benefits of intensive resistance training in patients with chronic polymyositis or dermatomyositis, Arthritis Rheum 57:768-777, 2007.

169. Jeppesen TD, Schwartz M, Olsen DB et al: Aerobic training is safe and improves exercise capacity in patients with mitochondrial myopathy, Brain 129:3402-3412, 2006.

170. Phillips BA, Mastaglia FL: Exercise therapy in patients with myopathy, Curr Opin Neurol 13:547-552, 2000.

171. Orngreen MC, Olsen DB, Vissing J: Aerobic training in patients with myotonic dystrophy type I. Ann Neurol 57:754-757, 2005.

172. Drory VE, Goltsman E, Goldman Reznik J et al: The value of muscle exercise in patients with amyotrophic lateral sclerosis, J Neurol Sci 191:133-137, 2001.

173. Bello-Haas VD, Kloos FJM, Scheirbecker J et al: A randomized controlled trial of resistance exercise in individuals with ALS, Neurology 68:2003-2007, 2007.

174. Morris ME, Perry A, Bilney B et al: Outcomes of physical therapy, speech pathology, and occupational therapy for people with motor neuron disease: a systematic review, Neurorehabil Neurol Repair 20:424-434, 2006.

175. Inzelberg R, Peleg N, Nisipeanu P et al: Inspiratory muscle training and the perception of dyspnea in Parkinson's disease, Can J Neurol Sci 32:213-217, 2005.

176. McCool FD, Tzelepis GE: Inspiratory muscle training in the patient with neuromuscular disease, Phys Ther 75:1006-1014, 1995.

177. Gosselink R, Kovacs l, Ketelaer P et al: Respiratory muscle weakness and respiratory muscle training in severely disabled multiple sclerosis patients, Arch Phys Med Rehabil 81:747-751, 2000.

178. Gross D, Meiner Z: The effect of ventilatory muscle training on respiratory function and capacity in ambulatory and bed-ridden patients with neuromuscular disease, Monaldi Arch Chest Dis 48:322-326, 1993.

179. Koessler W, Wanke T, Winkler G et al: 2 years' experience with inspiratory muscle training in patients with neuromuscular disorders, Chest 120:765-769, 2001.

180. Wanke T, Toifl Kate, Merkle M et al: Inspiratory muscle training in patients with Duchenne muscular dystrophy, Chest 105:475-482, 1994.

181. Chatwin M, Ross E, Hart N et al: Cough augmentation with mechanical insufflation/exsufflation in patients with neuromuscular weakness, Eur Respir J 21:502-508, 2003.

182. Winck JC, Goncalves MR, Lourenco C et al: Effects of mechanical insufflation–exsufflation on respiratory parameters for patients with chronic airway secretion encumbrance, Chest 126:774-780, 2004.

183. Baydur A, Layne E, Aral H et al: Long term noninvasive ventilation in the community for patients with musculoskeletal disorders: 46 year experience and review, Thorax 55:4-11, 2000.

184. Nugent A-M, Smith IE, Shneerson JM: Domiciliary-assisted ventilation in patients with myotonic dystrophy, Chest 121:459-464, 2002.

185. Kilmer DD, Aitkens SG, Wright NC et al: Response to high-intensity eccentric muscle contractions in persons with myopathic disease, Muscle Nerve 24:1181-1187, 2001.

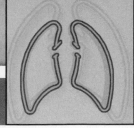

Chapter 32

Exercise and Pulmonary Hypertension

SHELLEY SHAPIRO • GLENNA L. TRAIGER

CHAPTER OUTLINE

Background
Role and Types of Exercise Testing
    Six-Minute Walk Test
    Cardiopulmonary Exercise Testing:
        CPET Gas Exchange
    Treadmill Testing
Pulmonary Function Tests

Purpose of Exercise in Patients with
    Pulmonary Hypertension
Risk of Exercise
Benefits of Exercise and Pulmonary
    Rehabilitation
Conclusion

PROFESSIONAL SKILLS

On completion of this chapter, the reader will be able to do
the following:
* Differentiate between pulmonary hypertension (PH) and pulmonary arterial hypertension (PAH).
* Discuss the classification, etiology, prevalence, and treatment of pulmonary arterial hypertension.
* Perform or assist with testing for the PAH patient including the 6-minute walk test, cardiopulmonary exercise testing, treadmill testing and pulmonary function test.
* Provide an exercise prescription and counsel the PAH patient on the risks and benefits of exercise.
* Recognize the role of pulmonary rehabilitation in the patient with pulmonary hypertension.

BACKGROUND

Pulmonary arterial hypertension (PAH) is defined as mean pulmonary arterial pressures greater than 25 mm Hg, caused by abnormalities of the pulmonary vascular bed and associated with normal left filling pressures. It is a result of smooth muscle cell and intimal vascular proliferation and ongoing changes in the cellular components of the small arteries. It is a degenerative, incurable disease process, the progression of which can be slowed with treatment. Over time, progressive lumen obliteration and microvascular thrombosis cause loss of the vascular bed. The reduced vascular bed and increased vascular resistance increase the load on the right ventricle,

ultimately resulting in right heart failure and falling cardiac output. Figure 32-1 illustrates this gradual process and the hypothesized hemodynamic changes associated with it. At first the vascular changes are associated with reduced function only at high levels of activity, but ultimately they impact functional status as the disease progresses.

Pulmonary arterial hypertension needs to be distinguished from elevated pulmonary pressures due to left heart disease, for example, left heart failure or left valvular heart disease. Left diseases result in elevated left atrial pressure and backward heart failure with compensatory changes (vasoconstriction of the pulmonary arteries). Reduction of

PAH: Hemodynamics over time

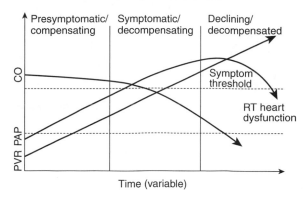

FIGURE 32-1 Schematic representation of histologic changes in the pulmonary arterial wall juxtaposed to the hypothesized hemodynamic changes that occur over time. CO, cardiac output; PAH, pulmonary arterial hypertension; PAP, pulmonary artery pressure; PVR, pulmonary vascular resistance, RT, right.

BOX 32-1	World Health Organization (WHO) Classification of Pulmonary Hypertension

GROUP I: PULMONARY ARTERIAL HYPERTENSION (PAH)
Idiopathic PAH
Familial PAH
PAH associated with
- Collagen vascular disease
- Congenital systemic-to-pulmonary shunts (large, small, repaired, or unrepaired)
- Portal hypertension
- HIV infection
- Drugs and toxins
- Other (glycogen storage disease, Gaucher disease, hereditary hemorrhagic telangiectasia, hemoglobinopathies, myeloproliferative disorders, splenectomy)

PAH associated with significant venous or capillary involvement:
- Pulmonary veno-occlusive disease
- Pulmonary capillary hemangiomatosis

GROUP II: PULMONARY VENOUS HYPERTENSION
Left atrial or ventricular heart disease
Left valvular heart disease

GROUP III: PULMONARY HYPERTENSION ASSOCIATED WITH LUNG DISEASES AND/OR HYPOXEMIA
Chronic obstructive pulmonary disease
Interstitial lung disease
Sleep-disordered breathing
Alveolar hypoventilation disorders
Chronic exposure to high elevation

GROUP IV: PULMONARY HYPERTENSION DUE TO CHRONIC THROMBOTIC AND/OR EMBOLIC DISEASE
Thromboembolic obstruction of proximal pulmonary arteries
Thromboembolic obstruction of distal pulmonary arteries
Nonthrombotic pulmonary embolism (tumor, parasites, foreign material)

GROUP V: MISCELLANEOUS
Sarcoidosis, histiocytosis X, lymphangiomatosis, compression of pulmonary vessels (adenopathy, tumor, fibrosing mediastinitis)

---

the left atrial pressure resolves the pulmonary hypertension significantly and with that the dyspnea and decreased exercise tolerance. Thus pulmonary hypertension from left heart disease is managed and treated differently from a pulmonary arteriopathy and vascular process occurring in the pulmonary bed. It responds to treatments for left heart failure and the exercise programs and issues for patients with pulmonary hypertension due to left heart disease are not discussed here.

Box 32-1 lists the World Health Organization (WHO) classification of pulmonary hypertension (PH), which classifies PH according to etiology.[1] WHO group I includes pulmonary arterial hypertension (PAH) caused by pulmonary arteriopathies, and represents the group of diseases treated with PAH medications. The incidence of idiopathic pulmonary arterial hypertension has been estimated at 1 or 2 per million persons.[2] Idiopathic pulmonary arterial hypertension can occur sporadically or as an inherited predisposition (familial). PAH that occurs in the setting of a variety of other systemic diseases is termed associated pulmonary arterial hypertension. These include connective tissue diseases such as scleroderma, lupus, mixed connective tissue disease, and rheumatoid arthritis.

The UNCOVER study estimated the prevalence of PAH by echocardiography in 791 patients with scleroderma or mixed connective tissue disease at 26.7%.[3] Liver disease can result in "portopulmonary hypertension," which is the pulmonary arteriopathy associated with liver disease. Between 5% and 10% of patients who are seen for liver transplantation evaluation have PAH.[4] Approximately 1 in 200 patients infected with human immunodeficiency virus have pulmonary hypertension and it is not clear whether it is the virus or associated viruses that are the cause.[5] Drugs and toxins can also cause pulmonary hypertension, in particular, anorexigens and amphetamines. Patients with congenital heart disease (intracardiac shunts causing systemic to

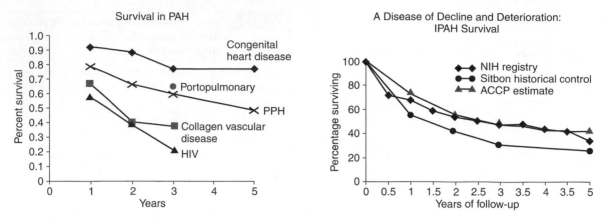

FIGURE 32-2 Survival over time for patients with untreated idiopathic pulmonary hypertension and pulmonary hypertension due to other World Health Organization group 1 disease processes. IPAH, idiopathic pulmonary arterial hypertension; PAH, pulmonary arterial hypertension.

pulmonary flow) may have pulmonary hypertension. Data from the National Institutes of Health (NIH) Registry of patients with idiopathic pulmonary arterial hypertension (previously called primary pulmonary hypertension), from 1985 and before treatment was available, showed dismal survival, particularly once right heart failure developed.[6] In the NIH Registry[6] the 6-month survival for patients with pulmonary hypertension and right heart failure (New York Heart Association class IV) was about 50%. The incidence in and survival of patients with pulmonary hypertension is changing as greater awareness of the clinical signs and symptoms, as well as improved therapy, develops.[7]

Figure 32-2 illustrates the survival of patients with untreated idiopathic pulmonary arterial hypertension and those with various other WHO group I disease processes. The outcome is variable, with some patients rapidly deteriorating and failing to respond to therapy whereas others may have extended life expectancy if they have vasoreactivity or respond to medication. This is often due in large part to the systemic nature of their disease process and is not necessarily due to the PAH. Patients with connective tissue disease, in particular scleroderma and pulmonary arterial hypertension, have the worst prognosis, with rapid deterioration after its development.

Patients with pulmonary hypertension who fall into WHO group I, pulmonary arterial hypertension, are treated similarly. Evidence for treating patients in WHO groups III through V is not established. Patients with recurrent pulmonary emboli (chronic thromboembolic pulmonary hypertension) can have a pulmonary arteriopathy and

appear to respond to PAH, therapy. The cumulative incidence of PAH after acute pulmonary embolism without prior venous thromboembolism is 3.8% at 2 years.[8] There remains controversy and active research on whether and how to treat pulmonary hypertension in patients with disorders such as sarcoidosis, interstitial lung disease, chronic obstructive pulmonary disease (COPD), and obesity hypoventilation. Our approach to patients with sarcoidosis, interstitial lung disease, sickle cell disease, and other blood dyscrasias has been to treat patients in these categories who have pulmonary hypertension that results in right heart failure and decreasing cardiac function. There is a theoretical rationale for this, particularly in light of data[9] that there is considerable vasoreactivity in patients with sarcoidosis. The treatment of pulmonary hypertension is used in many cases as a bridge to transplantation, particularly in patients with interstitial lung disease, for whom there are currently no effective therapies. The development of PH, in addition to interstitial lung disease, marks rapid clinical deterioration and death.

Before 1994 there were essentially no medications available to treat PAH except for a small number of patients who had pulmonary vasoreactivity and responded to calcium channel blockers.[10] In 1994 epoprostenol (Flolan) was studied and found to be effective in prolonging life and improving exercise capacity and survival.[11] In 2001 the first oral medication, an endothelin receptor blocker, bosentan (Tracleer), was approved.[12] Treprostinil (Remodulin) was first approved for subcutaneous and later for intravenous use.[13] Sildenafil (Revatio) was approved for use in 2005.[14] Iloprost (Ventavis), an inhaled prostacyclin, was approved in 2006.[15]

Most recently a selective endothelin receptor blocker, ambrisentan (Letairis), was approved for use.[16] Several medications are being studied clinically, including tadalafil (Cialis), and experimental oral and inhaled treprostinil. Imitanib (Gleevec) blocks platelet-derived growth factor and is being studied as a new approach to treating pulmonary hypertension.[17] Finally, multidrug therapy, which is occurring clinically, is being studied through ongoing blinded and open label clinical trials to determine the efficacy of combination therapy. Thus an ever-increasing armamentarium of medications is becoming available to treat patients. Treatment of PAH has resulted in prolongation of life and increased functional capacity. The average decrease in mean pulmonary artery pressure for most of the clinical drug trials was about 5 mm Hg after 12 to 16 weeks of treatment. The primary end point and basis of U.S. Food and Drug Administration approval for medications was the 6-Minute Walk Test (6MWT) distance. For most of the drugs evaluated in 12-week placebo-controlled trials, the 6MWT distance increased between 20 and 60 m when compared with control subjects. Although this appears to be a rather modest change, in terms of both hemodynamics and walk distance, it translates into a significant improvement for patients. Long-term data on survival and maintenance of functional status indicate that patients are living longer as a result of therapy, particularly when compared with historical NIH data. With patients living longer and the downward spiral associated with right heart failure and decreased cardiac output delayed or averted, attention needs to be turned to other factors that can improve quality of life and functional status.

ROLE AND TYPES OF EXERCISE TESTING

Exercise testing in pulmonary hypertension is performed to help make the diagnosis and to assess prognosis and response to therapy. Patients with pulmonary hypertension are initially asymptomatic at rest and manifest symptoms only with physical activity. Because the physical findings of pulmonary hypertension and the initial symptoms are subtle the diagnosis is often missed. Diagnostic tests are used to clarify the etiology of the symptoms. Subsequently, repeated exercise testing is used clinically as a noninvasive approach to monitor functional status, to assess response to therapy, and to assess the need for increased therapy.

As with other chronic conditions, pulmonary hypertension results in deconditioning as patients voluntarily and unconsciously restrict their activity to avoid symptoms. The patients are often unaware of their voluntary restriction and underestimate their limitations. Family members who live with the patient may provide a more accurate description of a patient's usual activity level. Exercise testing provides quantitation and can validate these observations.

In addition to formal exercise testing we ask patients to set exercise goals for themselves (e.g., walking up a flight of stairs or walking a particular circuit in their neighborhood) and to use that as a marker of performance. By regularly performing these tasks the patient can monitor how easy or difficult they have become. Their observations can be used to further clinical assessment. As an aside, this approach also encourages the patients to continue to perform somewhat more strenuous activity than they otherwise might and therefore has benefit by requiring that they perform some exercise or activity routinely.

Functional classification is another method used to assess patients' functional status according to symptoms at progressive levels of activity. The New York Heart Association Functional Classification was modified by the World Health Organization for patients with PAH (Table 32-1). Functional class

TABLE 32-1	Functional Classification* of Pulmonary Arterial Hypertension: Predictor of Prognosis
Class I	No limitation of physical activity Ordinary physical activity does not cause undue dyspnea or fatigue, chest pain, or near syncope
Class II	Slight limitation of physical activity Ordinary physical activity causes undue dyspnea or fatigue, chest pain, or near syncope
Class III	Marked limitation of physical activity Less than ordinary physical activity causes undue dyspnea or fatigue, chest pain, or near syncope
Class IV	Inability to perform any physical activity without symptoms Signs of right heart failure Dyspnea or fatigue may be present at rest, and discomfort is increased by any physical activity

*New York Heart Association/World Health Organization modification.
Adapted from Rich S, editor: Executive summary from the World Congress on Primary Pulmonary Hypertension, 1998. Available at http://www.who.int/ncd/cvd/pph.html.

I describes asymptomatic patients, whereas functional class IV describes patients with symptoms at rest. Functional class has been shown to correlate with outcome and is also used as a marker for response to therapy (clinically and in research drug trials). We estimate the patient's functional class at each clinic visit to assess changes in status and response to therapy.

It should also be noted that research on the effects, prescription, and safety of exercise in patients with pulmonary hypertension is limited.[18] Therefore the approaches below reflect our experience in treating patients with pulmonary hypertension over many years. Further research is needed on the efficacy and safety of various rehabilitation programs for patients with PH. In the past, before drug therapy was available, patients were advised not to exercise because of the concerns about syncope and sudden death. As therapy has improved, patients are doing better and want to be physically active. To maintain function they will need to be physically active. We will need to be able to provide safe and efficacious ways to achieve this.

Six-Minute Walk Test

The 6-Minute Walk Test (6MWT)[19] is a submaximal, patient-limited exercise test. It is safe to perform in patients with cardiopulmonary limitations, for example, heart failure or pulmonary hypertension, and it is a valid outcome measure. It may be a surrogate predictor for mortality. The 6MWT has provided the foundation for approval of medications for PAH. It is extremely easy to perform; requiring only a stop watch and a flat, straight, 30- to 35-m measured walkway with enough room to turn at each end. For reliable, reproducible results, the 6MWT must be performed in a consistent manner with attention to the following details (see also Chapter 12):

- Patients should be instructed on the procedure each time, using a standard script.
- The test should be uncoached because various forms of encouragement or discouragement can result in markedly different results.
- The test should be performed in the same location, with markers indicating where the patient needs to turn. Even the quality of the walking surface can alter the results.
- During the performance of the test, the patient is advised of the time remaining at 2-minute intervals. The patient is advised to cover as much distance as he or she can.

- It is important for the patient to be rested before the test, particularly if the walk area is a distance from the clinic or waiting area.
- At the conclusion, the total distance covered is measured and the degree of dyspnea is estimated on the basis of a 0- to 10-point Borg Scale. Vital signs (heart rate, blood pressure, and oxygen [O_2] saturation) may be measured before and at the end of the test to assess heart rate and blood pressure response to activity and to screen for desaturation with activity.

There are a number of factors that can confound the performance of the test, including patient cooperation and understanding; type of shoes used; and walking surface, which can change the ease of walking. Patients with musculoskeletal problems may be limited more by joint or back pain than PH symptoms.

Patients using O_2 tanks need to have someone else push or carry the tank to avoid the additional work impacting on the outcome of the test. However, arguments can be made for having patients perform the test while pushing or carrying their O_2 supply. Having someone else do it does not provide an accurate estimate of their functional status in their regular environment. Providing advice regarding exercise should take this workload into account.

In pulmonary function laboratories, walking tests are frequently terminated when the O_2 saturation drops below 88%. In the 6MWT, patients are symptom limited; thus patients are permitted to stop if short of breath, dizzy, or tired and O_2 saturation is not used as a predetermined end point. In particular, patients with PH may have a patent foramen ovale that can open during exertion and allow right-to-left shunting at the atrial level. Some patients have other forms of congenital heart disease that also permit intracardiac right-to-left shunting. The associated drop in O_2 saturation does not have the same implication as the desaturation associated with hypoxemia from underlying lung disease and an inability of the lungs to transfer O_2. Patients performing daily activities do not routinely measure their O_2 saturation and stop activities because of low saturation. They stop activity because of shortness of breath or dizziness. It is therefore reasonable to let symptoms rather than a specific saturation determine the end point of exercise for patients with PAH during a 6MWT. O_2 desaturation measured during the test may trigger a formal desaturation study to quantify the amount of O_2 required to maintain an acceptable saturation. Although this may vary from patient to patient, American College of Chest Physicians guidelines for PAH recommend maintaining saturation at more than 90% at all times.[20]

Essentially none of the studies of pulmonary arterial hypertension have shown an improvement in 6MWT distance for untreated patients, and therefore it becomes a reasonable test for evaluating response to therapy or other nondrug interventions.[21] Studies of patients with "primary" pulmonary hypertension (now called *idiopathic pulmonary arterial hypertension*) have shown that a 6MWT distance less than 332 m is associated with reduced survival. It is also correlated with results of maximal oxygen uptake ($\dot{V}o_2$max) in cardiopulmonary exercise testing (CPET) and functional status.[21]

In our clinic, for example, a 6MWT is performed by the trained clinic nurse at almost every visit. The walk test is integrated into the nursing intake along with the taking of vital signs and medication history. The results of the walk are evaluated and discussed as part of the clinic visit. The results are graphed and monitored over time as therapy is adjusted. Although mild changes in 6MWT results may not be acted on immediately, over time evidence of decreasing 6MWT distance indicates a need for adjustment in therapy and discussion of potential reversible causes. It is also a red flag that necessitates additional testing, for example, an echocardiogram or right heart catheterization to reassess the disease.

Cardiopulmonary Exercise Testing: CPET Gas Exchange

Cardiopulmonary exercise testing (CPET) is a quantified exercise test based on graded exercise. Unlike routine exercise testing for coronary artery disease, which looks at heart rate, blood pressure, and electrocardiogram as physiologic parameters, CPET also measures ventilatory markers, consumption of O_2, and production of carbon dioxide (CO_2). In some centers lactate production and continuous monitoring of blood gases, using an arterial line, also allows measurement of pH. However, useful information can be obtained without this, using peripheral O_2 saturation rather than blood gases, yielding a safer and easier, noninvasive test. It can be performed on either a bicycle ergometer or a treadmill. Various exercise protocols can be used, based on the patient's level of functioning. A standard bicycle

test for a patient with pulmonary hypertension would be a continuous ramp increase of 10 to 15 watts/minute. The ideal test lasts about 10 minutes, long enough to allow physiological response to exercise and determination of maximal O_2 consumption and the anaerobic threshold but short enough to avoid muscle fatigue. The advantage of exercise gas exchange is the ability to quantify the effort and compare it with that of healthy subjects matched for age, sex, height, and weight. The test also allows determination of the ventilatory as well as cardiovascular impact on exercise by measuring the ratio of minute ventilation to carbon dioxide uptake ($\dot{V}_E/\dot{V}co_2$), heart rate, and blood pressure responses to exercise, as well as some of the ventilatory parameters. The test requires sophisticated equipment, which measures inhaled and exhaled gases, blood pressure, heart rate and electrocardiogram, and workload second by second. The CPET can be performed on a bicycle ergometer or treadmill. The bike is preferred because it allows for issues related to patient's leg length and weight. The output from these collections of data appears continuously as plots of the various measured and derived parameters and is summarized in a "nine-panel plot" as well as a table of measurements at rest, anaerobic threshold, and peak exercise. Figure 32-3 demonstrates the results of a CPET in a patient with functional class III pulmonary arterial hypertension due to an uncorrected atrial septal defect. Her $\dot{V}o_2$max is only 31% of predicted for her age and size, consistent with her symptoms. Her $\dot{V}_E/\dot{V}co_2$ is elevated above a predicted normal of approximately 25. That, in conjunction with her relatively normal spirometry (data not shown), made the diagnosis of pulmonary vascular disease likely.

In laboratories where equipment is routinely standardized and calibrated and there are well-trained personnel, there is excellent reproducibility of results and valuable information about the etiology and severity of a patient's limitations. However, there have been problems with interlaboratory variability and quality of reports that indicate that testing is very much center dependent. Exercise gas exchange parameters were used as end points in multicenter trials of new therapies for pulmonary arterial hypertension. Two studies provided a stark comparison. In one study of beraprost, CPET was carefully controlled. Technique in each laboratory was validated. Each patient test was repeated within 1 week. A central

Nine Panel Plot
Cardiopulmonary Exercise Test

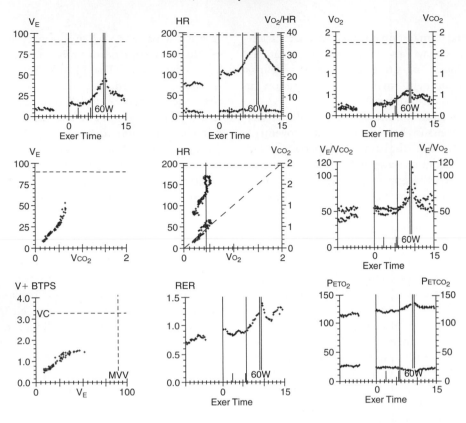

CPET in Patient with Pulmonary Hypertension

	Rest	AT	Peak Exe	Peak Vo₂	Pred Max	Max/Pred
Work						
Total time	9:19	15:15	18:45	16:45		
Exercise time		5:53	9:23	7:23		
Watts		27	60	40	141	28.3%
Oxygen consumption						
Vo₂/kg	5.4	8.9	9.7	10.9	34.6	31.5%
Vo₂	272	446	486	543	1726	31.5%
Vco₂	234	410	634	571		
RER	0.86	0.92	1.31	1.05		
METs	1.6	2.6	2.8	3.1	9.9	31.5%
Ventilation						
V_E BTPS	13.3	22.2	47.2	34.4	88.9	38.6%
Vt BTPS	653	983	1473	1352		
RR	20	23	32	25		
Br reserve	85.1	75.0	46.9	61.4		
V_E/Vo₂	49	50	97	63		
V_E/Vco₂	57	54	74	60		
Cardiac						
HR	97	126	169	153	195	78.2%
Vo₂/HR	3	4	3	4	9	40.2%
HR reserve	100.0	69.7	26.3	43.3		
Systolic BP	100				166	
Diastolic BP	66					
RPP	97				324	

FIGURE 32-3 Nine-panel plot (*top*) and selected measured values (*bottom*) obtained during cardiopulmonary exercise testing in a patient with pulmonary arterial hypertension before treatment. The patient was exercised on an upright bicycle ergometer. BP, blood pressure; HR, heart rate; METs, metabolic equivalents; Pᴇᴛᴄᴏ₂, end-tidal (partial) carbon dioxide pressure; RER, respiratory exchange ratio; RPP, rate pressure product; RR, respiratory rate; V̇co₂, carbon dioxide uptake; V̇_E, minute ventilation; V̇o₂, oxygen uptake.

laboratory was used for monitoring and calculation of results.[21] Although the drug itself was not clinically approved for therapy, the data from the study demonstrated the reproducibility and value of CPET for evaluation of patients. In contrast, in studies of sitaxsentan, another drug tested for pulmonary arterial hypertension, the degree of variability between centers resulted in the approach being abandoned and the 6MWT being used as the primary end point.

CPET has been shown to be safe even in patients with significant PAH[23-25] There is strong literature to support both the prognostic and diagnostic value of CPET both in heart failure and in pulmonary hypertension. In heart failure, $\dot{V}o_2$max, or maximal O_2 consumption, has been used to determine the need for heart transplantation. It correlates better than right heart catheterization data in predicting survival.[23] In contrast, for lung transplant, O_2 desaturation and 6MWT distance have been more commonly used. In comparing heart failure and pulmonary arterial hypertension findings on CPET, it appears that patients with PAH have more dyspnea at comparable workloads and greater reductions in the efficiency of respirations as measured by the $\dot{V}_E/\dot{V}co_2$.[25] $\dot{V}o_2$max generated during CPET provides valuable survival information about patients with PAH.[24] Patients with pulmonary arterial hypertension have significantly reduced maximal O_2 consumption, and achieve lower workloads and anaerobic thresholds with elevated $\dot{V}_E/\dot{V}co_2$. Treatment with effective agents can result in improvement in these parameters.

Treadmill Testing

Some pulmonary hypertension centers have advocated using a modified treadmill regimen to examine duration of exercise as a measure of response to therapy. One advantage may be a greater ability to provide a measured stress than the 6MWT. However, it requires availability of equipment and more highly trained personnel than the 6MWT. Use of a treadmill makes it somewhat more difficult for patients to terminate exercise when short of breath. In the clinic setting it may be more difficult to coordinate treadmill testing with routine visits.

PULMONARY FUNCTION TESTS

Patients with pulmonary hypertension due to pulmonary arteriopathy (PAH) may have normal underlying lung tissue and airways, as in idiopathic pulmonary arterial hypertension. These patients often have abnormal pulmonary function test results that point toward the diagnosis.[25] These include mild reductions in forced vital capacity and forced expiratory volume in 1 second, and lung volumes consistent with a restrictive picture.[26] The diffusing capacity of the lung for carbon monoxide ($DLco$) is often moderately reduced and to a greater extent than the forced vital capacity, usually below 80% of predicted. However, patients with pulmonary hypertension due to connective tissue disease or other underlying lung diseases may demonstrate abnormal pulmonary function test results based on airway or lung tissue abnormalities rather than a pulmonary arteriopathy, complicating interpretation. In patients with combined lung disease a disproportionately reduced $DLco$ may suggest pulmonary vascular disease out of proportion to the parenchymal disease.

PURPOSE OF EXERCISE IN PATIENTS WITH PULMONARY HYPERTENSION

Patients with pulmonary hypertension initially have normal respiratory function at rest and have symptoms only with increased demand. Over time, as cardiac output becomes more limited due to decreased right ventricular function and increased right ventricular afterload, dyspnea occurs at lower levels of activity and becomes limiting as right heart failure develops. This is associated with reduced exercise and deconditioning, similar to the loss of muscle mass seen in patients with chronic heart failure and lung disease. Worsening deconditioning and muscle wasting further limit activity, and patients become unable to perform the activities of daily living. It becomes a vicious cycle: reduced activity results in deconditioning, which leads to further decreased activity and worsening dyspnea at lower workloads. Pulmonary rehabilitation that includes exercise training therefore presents a way of maintaining physical conditioning. Patients with PAH are not usually limited in a ventilatory sense, nor do they have airway disease for which certain types of breathing medications and treatments would be useful as for patients with obstructive lung disease (e.g., COPD, asthma, and emphysema). Breathing retraining is useful for dyspnea and anxiety control in patients with obstructive lung disease and may also be useful in patients with pulmonary hypertension.

RISK OF EXERCISE

In recommending exercise, providing an exercise prescription, and ultimately supervising performance of exercise by patients with pulmonary hypertension, certain provisos should be remembered. Most importantly as pulmonary hypertension worsens, the ability of patients to generate increased cardiac output or to increase their O_2 consumption becomes limited. Thus pushing patients beyond their ability to increase cardiac output results in syncope and collapse. An exercise prescription can be developed on the basis of the results of cardiopulmonary exercising testing. The patient with PAH often demonstrates low maximal O_2 consumption that occurs early in exercise and an early and low anaerobic threshold. This is an indication in the patient with PAH that sufficient O_2 is not being provided to the muscles to meet the metabolic needs generated with exercise. In developing the exercise prescription, the metabolic equivalents (METs) performed at the anaerobic threshold, heart rate, and blood pressure response during the CPET should be used. This approach makes it possible to set a reasonable estimate of the amount and intensity of activity that can be performed before exceeding the patient's capacity. These are only estimates and guidelines. Physical conditions and the patient's physical state at the time of exercise may be different from when the assessment was performed. For example, patients may have worsening right heart failure with fluid overload, and if this was not present at the time of exercise testing, the exercise capacity noted during the test would be higher than what the patient is able to achieve in his or her worsening physiologic state.

For independent, unsupervised exercise patients must be able to terminate activity immediately in a safe location. Thus, swimming alone, hiking alone, or rock climbing can be dangerous, especially if it is not possible to stop easily or obtain help. A particularly telling example occurred when one of our patients went to the Grand Canyon and decided to walk down. While hiking out of the canyon the patient's workload was significantly increased; the patient was unable to climb out and became near syncopal. The people with him were unaware of his limitations or of how to handle them, and kept encouraging him to push on. Help was finally obtained but the potential for a disastrous outcome was clear. Participating in contact sports or sports that do not allow one to rest poses a potential risk with the patient unable to adjust to developing symptoms. Competitive activities that require abrupt high-intensity bursts of activity, for example, racquetball or water polo, also pose a potential risk with the patient not being able to adjust the workload or warm up. Patients with pulmonary hypertension do not tolerate heat when trying to perform activity. The added vasodilatation and increased cardiac output add to the workload but are not translated into more power. The added output is wasted in perfusing the skin and losing heat. The drop in blood pressure can result in significant dizziness. Thus patients need to be advised to reduce workload and expectations when exercising at higher temperatures. High altitude is also limiting. Although patients with pulmonary hypertension often have normal resting O_2 saturations, higher altitudes with lower O_2 concentrations result in hypoxemia. This is not well tolerated with activity and patients need to be aware of their reduced capacity at higher elevations. It is not infrequent that patients become symptomatic and often syncopal when trying to exercise at higher elevations. For a patient needing to remain at higher elevation for extended periods of time we often recommend an HAST (high-altitude simulation test) with exercise to determine whether the patient will require supplemental O_2 to function at higher elevations. Then supplemental O_2 can be given, improving the patient's functional status at altitude.

BENEFITS OF EXERCISE AND PULMONARY REHABILITATION

As in patients with chronic heart failure, progressive loss of muscle function and mass provides an obstacle to exercise but also to the performance of many activities of daily living. It also results in deteriorating quality of life and loss of functional independence. In addition to developing overall weakness, deconditioned patients with PAH also develop respiratory muscle dysfunction,[27] which increases the work of breathing and creates a sensation of breathlessness. Poor overall muscle function also results in inefficient use of energy and thus increases the work associated with a given activity. Preservation of muscle function and mass as well as exercise training can improve exercise capacity and quality of life. This has been demonstrated in heart failure[28] and in a careful study of patients with chronic severe pulmonary hypertension.[18] Using a cross-over design, the effect of a formal exercise program and respiratory training was tested. Patients were hospitalized and participated in 3 weeks of vigorous training and counseling with a 12-week follow-up monitored home program. WHO functional class, QOL scores, and O_2 consumption improved with training. There was a significant change (111 m) in the 6MWT distance, which is comparable (and perhaps better) than those achieved with medical therapy in other studies. The exercise protocols were adjusted as patients improved, but in general aimed for 60% to 80% of the heart rates obtained during CPET. The study demonstrated both safety and efficacy of exercise in patients with pulmonary hypertension. Although this is the first study demonstrating the benefit of exercise training and pulmonary rehabilitation in PH, there are comparable models in pulmonary disease, COPD, and heart failure that support the concept.

Thus we encourage patients to maintain ongoing physical training with a walking program, treadmill, or stationary bicycle. Light weights are used for upper body conditioning. Monitored exercise in a pulmonary rehabilitation program is optimal, particularly if a patient is already compromised and needs consistent monitoring and rehabilitation. The availability of pulmonary rehabilitation programs and insurance reimbursement varies from place to place in the United States. Therefore obtaining supervised exercise is often not achievable because of access and cost. Many nonmedical programs are reluctant to take patients using O_2. Thus patients may need to improvise. The CPET results can provide a basis for an exercise prescription with regard to heart rate and workload. However, even a walking program can result in functional improvement for patients with PH if performed consistently. The addition of stairs to a walking program provides a modest amount of resistance training not achieved with level walking.

CONCLUSION

Patients with pulmonary arterial hypertension have significant limitations regarding exercise. Treatments are now available that improve functional capacity and survival. Exercise testing can be used to help diagnose pulmonary hypertension and measure the degree of limitation. Exercise testing can also be used to monitor response to therapy. Finally, exercise training as a component of comprehensive pulmonary rehabilitation is necessary to reverse and prevent the muscle wasting and deterioration associated with this chronic disease. Exercise with certain provisos is both safe and beneficial. Pulmonary rehabilitation programs are beneficial for patients with PAH and provide both structure and monitoring but may not be easily accessible.

References

1. Galiè N, Rubin LJ: Proceedings of the 3rd World Symposium on Pulmonary Arterial Hypertension. Venice, Italy, June 23-25, 2003, J Am Coll Cardiol 43(12 suppl 1):1S-90S, 2004.
2. Rich S, Chomka E, Hasara L et al: The prevalence of pulmonary hypertension in the United States: adult population estimates obtained from measurements of chest roentgenograms from the NHANES II survey, Chest 96:236-241, 1989.
3. Wigley FM, Lima JA, Mayes M et al: The prevalence of undiagnosed pulmonary arterial hypertension in subjects with connective tissue disease at the secondary health care level of community-based rheumatologists (the UNCOVER Study), Arthritis Rheum 52:2125-2132, 2005.
4. Kuo PC, Plotkin JS, Gaine S, et al: Portopulmonary hypertension and the liver transplant candidate, Transplantation 67:1087-1093, 1999.
5. Mesa RA, Edell ES, Dunn WF et al: Human immunodeficiency virus infection and pulmonary hypertension: two new cases and a review of 86 reported cases. Mayo Clin Proc 73:37-45, 1998.
6. D'Alonzo GE, Barst RJ, Ayres SM et al: Survival in patients with primary pulmonary hypertension: results of a national prospective registry, Ann Intern Med 115:343-349, 1991.
7. McLaughlin VV, Presberg KW, Doyle RL et al: Prognosis of pulmonary arterial hypertension: ACCP evidence-based clinical practice guidelines, Chest 126(1 suppl):78S-92S, 2004.
8. Pengo V, Lensing AW, Prins MH et al: Incidence of chronic thromboembolic pulmonary hypertension after pulmonary embolism, N Engl J Med 350:2257-2264, 2004.
9. Barst RJ, Ratner SJ: Sarcoidosis and reactive pulmonary hypertension, Arch Intern Med 145:2112-2114, 1985.
10. Rich S, Brundage BH: High-dose calcium channel-blocking therapy for primary pulmonary hypertension: evidence for long-term reduction in pulmonary arterial pressure and regression of right ventricular hypertrophy, Circulation 76:135-141, 1987.
11. Rubin LJ: Treatment of primary pulmonary hypertension with continuous intravenous prostacyclin (epoprostenol), Ann Intern Med 112:485-491, 1990.
12. Rubin LJ, Badesch DB, Barst RJ et al: Bosentan therapy for pulmonary arterial hypertension, N Engl J Med 346:896-903, 2002.
13. Simonneau G, Barst RJ, Galiè N et al: Continuous subcutaneous infusion of treprostinil a prostacyclin analogue, in patients with pulmonary arterial hypertension, Am J Respir Crit Care Med 165:800-804, 2002.

14. Galiè N, Ghofrani HA, Torbicki A et al: Sildenafil citrate therapy for pulmonary arterial hypertension, N Engl J Med 353:2148-2157, 2005.

15. Olschewski H, Simonneau G, Galiè N et al: Inhaled iloprost for severe pulmonary hypertension, N Engl J Med 347:322-329, 2002.

16. Galiè N, Badesch D, Oudiz R et al: Ambrisentan therapy for pulmonary arterial hypertension, J Am Coll Cardiol 46:529-535, 2005.

17. Ghofrani HA, Seeger W, Grimminger F: Imatinib for the treatment of pulmonary arterial hypertension, N Engl J Med 353:1412-1413, 2005.

18. Mereles D, Ehlken N, Kreuscher S et al: Exercise and respiratory training improve exercise capacity and quality of life in patients with severe chronic pulmonary hypertension, Circulation 114:1482-1489, 2006.

19. Meyer FJ, Lossnitzer D, Kristen AV et al: Respiratory muscle dysfunction in idiopathic pulmonary arterial hypertension, Eur Respir J 25:125-130, 2005.

20. Badesch DB, Abman SH, Ahearn GS et al: Medical therapy for PAH, Chest 126:35s-62s, 2004.

21. Helman DL Jr, Brown AW, Jackson JL et al: Analyzing the short-term effect of placebo therapy in pulmonary arterial hypertension: potential implications for the design of future clinical trials, Chest 132:764-772, 2007.

22. Miyamoto S, Nagaya N, Satoh T et al: Clinical correlates and prognostic significance of Six-Minute Walk Test in patients with primary pulmonary hypertension: comparison with cardiopulmonary exercise testing, Am J Respir Crit Care Med 161:487-492, 2000.

23. Barst RJ, McGoon M, McLaughlin V et al: Beraprost therapy for pulmonary arterial hypertension, J Am Coll Cardiol 41:2119-2125, 2003.

24. Myers J, Gullestad L, Vagelos R et al: Clinical, hemodynamic, and cardiopulmonary exercise test determinants of survival in patients referred for evaluation of heart failure, Ann Intern Med 129:286-293, 1998.

25. Deboeck G, Niset G, Lamotte M et al: Exercise testing in pulmonary arterial hypertension and in chronic heart failure, Eur Respir J 23:747-751, 2004.

26. Sun XG, Hansen JE, Oudiz RJ et al: Pulmonary function in primary pulmonary hypertension, J Am Coll Cardiol 41:1028-1035, 2003.

27. Wensel R, Opitz CF, Anker SD et al: Assessment of survival in patients with primary pulmonary hypertension: importance of cardiopulmonary exercise testing, Circulation 106:319-324, 2002.

28. Jonsdottir S, Andersen KK, Sigurosson AF et al: The effect of physical training in chronic heart failure, Eur J Heart Fail 8:97-101, 2006.

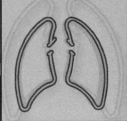

Chapter 33

Rehabilitation for the Pediatric Patient with Pulmonary Disease

CHRISTOPHER L. CARROLL

CHAPTER OUTLINE

The Pediatric Patient
Asthma
 Medical
 Rehabilitation Program
 Exercise Program
Cystic Fibrosis
 Medical
 Airway Clearance Techniques
 Exercise Program
 Precautions
Obesity
 Medical
 Exercise Program

Bronchopulmonary Dysplasia
 Medical
 Physical Rehabilitation
 Exercise Program
Neuromuscular Disease
 Medical
 Duchenne Muscular Dystrophy
 Exercise Program
Scoliosis
Conclusion

PROFESSIONAL SKILLS

On completion of this chapter, the reader will be able to do
the following:
* Provide an overview of pathophysiology of each disease and the impact on rehabilitation
* Apply theories and definitions of rehabilitation to the individual with a pediatric pulmonary disease
* Discuss barriers to growth and development of the individual and name at least one strategy to overcome these barriers
* Discuss precautions to establishing an exercise prescription in this patient population

THE PEDIATRIC PATIENT

There are few guidelines for the rehabilitation of pediatric patients with pulmonary disease. In part, this is due to the diverse population that is served by pediatric pulmonary rehabilitation. With advances in pediatric pulmonary and critical care medicine, there are a growing number of children in need of rehabilitation who may not have previously survived. The goals for rehabilitation of these children are not well established and there are few evidence-based treatment strategies. In adult patients, pulmonary rehabilitation aims to reduce symptoms, optimize functional status, and increase participation through a multidisciplinary, patient-centered approach involving patient assessment, exercise training, education, nutritional intervention, and psychosocial support. This chapter presents an adaptation of these principles of pulmonary rehabilitation,

BOX 33-1 | **Suggested Goals of Pediatric Pulmonary Rehabilitation**[2-6]

PSYCHOSOCIAL

- Improve self-esteem
- Enable the patient or family/caregiver to independently perform medical care
- Minimize the impact of the disease on the daily activity and lifestyle of the patient/family/caregiver
- Decrease complaints of shortness of breath
- Teach the individual self-monitoring skills for safe play and exercise
- Decrease fear of the individual and family/caregiver to allow participation in play and exercise
- Teach independent pursed-lips breathing
- Allow the child to participate in a play activity with peers

MEDICAL

- Improve secretion clearance techniques
- Improve ventilation and perfusion matching
- Develop effective coughing techniques and breath control
- Improve and help normalize growth and development when possible
- Teach independent and safe/effective home suctioning techniques
- Decrease episodes of exacerbations, bronchospasm, and hospitalizations
- Teach independence in airway clearance technique

KNOWLEDGE

- Increase knowledge of disease
- Identify signs and symptoms of exacerbation and plan for appropriate medical care
- Instruct in proper use and administration of medications
- Promote adherence with plan of care
- Teach family/caregiver safe and effective home manual ventilation techniques
- Increase knowledge/application of techniques to improve airflow
- Teach individual/family/caregiver to be independent with effective cough or assisted cough
- Increase knowledge and practice of relaxation techniques

EXERCISE

- Increase endurance and activity level
- Improve trunk range of motion and efficiency
- Decrease complaints of shortness of breath with a specific activity
- Improve distance walked on the 6-Minute Walk Test
- Improve heart rate response, respiratory rate, rating of perceived exertion, and level of dyspnea for a given activity or exercise

and supportive environment during rehabilitation. However, children also have a strong desire to join in with play, sports, and other activities. This can be a powerful motivator for pediatric patients. Rehabilitation is more successful in children when creative efforts are used that are designed to be both fun and beneficial.

Rehabilitation of the pediatric patient can also be rewarding. In general, children have more rehabilitation potential than adults. Because lung development continues into young adulthood, some chronic pulmonary diseases can improve with age. However, even in diseases with progressive decline in pulmonary function over time, there can be a greater capacity for healing. The pediatric patient can be incredibly resilient, both physically and emotionally. Successful rehabilitation of the pediatric patient can lead to a lifetime of health and well-being.

This chapter includes a discussion of asthma, cystic fibrosis (CF), bronchopulmonary dysplasia (BPD), and neuromuscular diseases. Obesity is also discussed because of its profound effect on pediatric pulmonary disease. The objectives of the chapter are to describe a clinical overview of each disease, to discuss the pathophysiology of the disease, and to define rehabilitation theories and practice in the pediatric pulmonary population. In pediatric pulmonary rehabilitation, the child is rehabilitated to his or her highest potential of medical, mental, emotional, social, developmental, and vocational level (Box 33-1).[2-6] Considerations of disease severity, oxygenation, limitations in ventilation owing to secretions and musculoskeletal pump deficits, responses to exercises, and exercise testing and prescriptions are also discussed.

ASTHMA

Asthma has become the most common chronic disease of childhood.[7,8] In the United States, the annual prevalence of self-reported asthma in children is between 4% and 8% and asthma accounts for 6% to 10% of all pediatric office visits.[9] Hospitalization for asthma is also increasing in the United States and worldwide.[7,8] Asthma is now the leading cause of absence from work and school, the most frequent admission diagnosis at many children's hospitals, and the most frequent cause of admission to a pediatric intensive care unit.

Medical

Asthma is characterized by diffuse lower airway obstruction.[7] This obstruction is caused by

which have been modified and applied to the pediatric pulmonary population.[1-6]

Rehabilitation of the pediatric patient can be challenging. The child's age and developmental level can interfere with traditional adult rehabilitation practices. Children require an encouraging inflammation of the airways, bronchial smooth muscle hypertrophy, and mucous plugging.[7] The inflammation is present even during asymptomatic periods. The consequences of this chronic process include episodic or persistent symptoms, bronchial hyperreactivity, and the development of irreversible airflow obstruction.[7] Patients may have symptoms of wheezing, shortness of breath, chest tightness, and cough that may progress to attacks of bronchoconstriction that may require emergency care or hospitalization. These symptoms may lead to significant impairment in a patient's quality of life, even in children with "mild" disease.

The role of chronic airway inflammation, rather than smooth muscle contraction alone, has been recognized as playing the key role in the pathogenesis of asthma.[7-14] This inflammatory process causes the already hyper-responsive airway to be even more sensitive to stimuli such as inhaled allergens, environmental factors, and viral infections. To treat this underlying inflammation, anti-inflammatory medications, such as inhaled corticosteroids and leukotriene receptor antagonists, have become the mainstay of treatment in the outpatient management of patients with persistent asthma.[7-14]

Asthma is a wide-spectrum disease with distinct subtypes or phenotypes. Response to therapy differs from individual to individual and as a result, maintenance therapies and rehabilitation programs need to be individualized. In 2007, the National Asthma Education and Prevention Program updated the guidelines for the diagnosis and management of asthma.[15] Clinical symptoms and pulmonary function are used to classify a patient's asthma severity and asthma control, and a treatment plan is determined from these classifications. These guidelines encourage the development of individualized action plans that tailor asthma management during periods of sickness and wellness.[15]

Rehabilitation Program

The goals of a rehabilitation program for children with asthma are to allow the child to have as normal a life as possible, with the fewest symptoms, the fewest disruptions to the normal routine, and the fewest side effects from the therapies received. Exercise programs and physical activity should not be restricted as a result of the child's disease. Rather, medical therapy should be adjusted to allow the child to participate fully in school and play.

BOX 33-2	Asthma Rehabilitation: Objectives of Education[2,15]

ESTABLISH A PARTNERSHIP

TEACH ASTHMA SELF-MANAGEMENT

Teach Basic Facts about Asthma
- The contrast between asthmatic and normal airways
- What happens to the airways in an asthma attack

Roles of Medications
- How medications work (long-term control and quick relief)
- The importance of long-term control medications and why quick relief should not be expected with their use

Skills
- Inhaler use
- Spacer/holding chamber use
- Symptom monitoring, peak flow monitoring, and recognition of early signs of deterioration

Environmental Control Measures
- Identifying and avoiding environmental precipitants or exposures

When and How to Take Rescue Actions
- Responding to changes in asthma severity

JOINTLY DEVELOP TREATMENT GOALS
- Developing a written asthma action plan to help patient manage exacerbations

---

Asthma rehabilitation programs aim to promote self-management and to improve quality of life. Patient or caregiver education is one tool in achieving self-management. Suggested objectives of education are described in Box 33-2.[2,15] The child should be taught to assess his or her respiratory status. The measurement of peak flow can help to assess respiratory status during acute exacerbations; however, the routine use of peak flow for asymptomatic children is not useful.[16,17] The most critical aspect of self-management is the most difficult to control: motivation and adherence with the plan of care. The establishment of individualized and mutually agreed on goals encourages compliance. However, the episodic nature of asthma, with relatively long periods of stability, discourages adherence with a plan of care.

When poorly controlled, asthma interferes with the daily life of the individual and the family. Days are missed from school and work and the family dynamic is changed. Patients and families can experience fear, frustration, and anger. Children with asthma may think that they cannot compete with other children in athletic activities or may accommodate their illness by avoiding strenuous exercise.

BOX 33-3	Exercise Prescription for the Child with Asthma[19]

GENERAL
- As per the American Academy of Pediatrics guidelines for sports participation in children*: "With proper medication and education, only athletes with the most severe asthma will need to modify their participation."

PRE-EXERCISE
- Warm-up
  - Keep at low to moderate intensity, heart rate less than 75% predicted maximum for a few minutes
  - Do not use intermittent sprinting
- Premedication
  - For example, 200 µg of albuterol or equivalent via large-volume spacer at least 10 minutes before starting warm-up
  - Long-acting bronchodilator medication may be useful for children when exercise is unplanned

PREFERRED ACTIVITIES
- Swimming (but note possible chlorine sensitivity)
- Cycling
- Walking
- Other aerobic activities (e.g., running and playing games)
Competitive sports (e.g., soccer and basketball)

MONITORING
- Children should be encouraged to "listen to their bodies" and learn how to take their heart rate and monitor signs of both exertional breathlessness and asthma
- Further "rescue" medication should be available
- Children should be encouraged to take appropriate rests during high-intensity competitive sports (e.g., basketball)

CONTRAINDICATIONS
- As for normal recommendations (e.g., fever and headache, but especially respiratory infections)

*American Academy of Pediatrics Committee on Sports Medicine and Fitness: Medical conditions affecting sports participation, Pediatrics 94:757-760, 1994.

asthma can safely participate in exercise.[19,20] Medical therapy can and should be adjusted to control exercise-induced symptoms. In addition, there is growing evidence that physical conditioning can improve pulmonary function and asthma symptoms in some children with asthma, thereby reducing the number of hospitalizations and missed days of school.[20] Exercise training is particularly beneficial in obese children with moderate to severe asthma, who tend to be more sedentary. As a result, regular physical exercise is recommended for children with asthma.[20,21]

However, care should be taken when starting an exercise program in a child with asthma. Exercise is known to provoke symptoms of bronchospasm in 70% to 90% of patients with asthma.[2,20] These symptoms can include coughing, wheezing, dyspnea, chest tightness, and a reduction in exercise capacity. Pretreatment with bronchodilators, such as the short-acting albuterol or the long-acting formoterol, can prevent the development of most symptoms.[19,21,22] In children with persistent exercise-induced symptoms, a maintenance anti-inflammatory drug can also be added.[22]

The type of exercise can be tailored to the child's interest in consideration of the child's asthma triggers (Box 33-3).[19] The development of exercise-induced symptoms is related to the type, duration, and intensity of the exercise and to the environment in which the exercise takes place. Exercising in cold, dry air tends to cause more problems than exercising in warm, humid air.[15,23,24] There is considerable evidence that the indoor swimming pool environment, with its moist, warm inspired air, is less likely to trigger exacerbations. However, there are numerous examples of successful professional athletes with asthma in sports as diverse as ice hockey and track. With proper education and medical management, an exercise plan can be initiated in almost all children with asthma.

CYSTIC FIBROSIS

Medical

CF is the most common genetic disease in the white population, affecting 1 in 2500 live births, with upward of 1000 new cases being diagnosed each year.[25-28] CF results from defects in the gene encoding the CF transmembrane conductance receptor, which in turn lead to impairment of chloride ion transport in epithelial cells. This causes changes in multiple organ systems; however, overall prognosis is most related to a patient's pulmonary and

This may result in reduced self-esteem and a pattern of inactivity and deconditioning.

Exercise Program

Children with asthma tend to be less active than their peers.[18] In part, this is due to a misconception that children with asthma are unable to participate in athletics or in exercise programs. Well-meaning parents may discourage their child from physical activity because of concern regarding increased symptoms. Children may also avoid exercise for this reason. However, multiple studies have shown that children with mild to moderate nutritional status.[26-28] Children with CF have abnormally thick and tenacious mucous secretion in the airways, leading to airway obstruction and mucous plugging. The airway is predisposed to infection and inflammation, which in turn leads to more mucous secretion. Other important medical complications of CF include the development of osteoporosis, malnutrition/poor growth, and diabetes mellitus.

Nutritional support and pulmonary rehabilitation are the cornerstones of maintenance therapy for CF. Although there is a steady decline in pulmonary function over time, successful rehabilitation programs have been shown to improve outcomes including survival in patients with CF.[29] Anti-inflammatory medications, antibiotics, pancreatic replacement enzymes, airway clearance techniques, exercise, and nutritional supplements are key elements of medical treatment.[28] Treatment methods that improve mucous clearance are also considered essential in optimizing respiratory status and reducing the progression of lung disease. A variety of methods are aimed at reducing airway inflammation, thinning secretions, and treating infections. These include airway clearance techniques, inhaled antibiotics, and human deoxyribonuclease.[28-35]

Airway Clearance Techniques

Airway clearance is a crucial component of a successful rehabilitation program for children with CF.[3-4,26,36-38] Techniques to improve airway clearance can improve secretion mobilization, gas exchange, and measures of pulmonary function such as total lung capacity and functional residual volume.[29-35] Examples include postural drainage, percussion, vibration, and shaking of the chest wall. Taken together, these techniques are termed *chest physiotherapy* and are the "gold standard" for airway clearance in patients with CF.[37,38] Examples of specific airway clearance techniques are described in Box 33-4.[29-35]

Choosing the best airway clearance technique for a patient is important to the success of this facet of the overall care program. Developing an individualized airway clearance program incorporates multiple factors including medical history, clinical presentation, severity of illness, cost and efficacy of devices, availability of assistance, needs of the patient and the family, cognitive level, age, and time constraints.[37] Patients may benefit from a combination treatment as determined in partnership with a multidisciplinary CF team. Airway

---

BOX 33-4   Airway Clearance Techniques[29-35]

ASSISTED TECHNIQUES

Manually Assisted Cough[31-32]
- Assistant applies pressure with both hands to upper abdomen after an inspiratory effort and forced glottic closure
- Often not well tolerated and ineffective in patients with stiff chest walls

UNASSISTED TECHNIQUES

Forced Expiratory Technique (Also Known as "Huffing")[33]
- One or two forced exhalations without closure of the glottis, starting from mid- to low lung volumes, followed by relaxed breathing
- Provides better clearance than coughing alone

Autogenic Drainage[34]
- Mobilizes secretions in peripheral airways and moves them centrally
- First breath at low tidal volumes to "unstick" the mucus
- Second breath at low to mid-volume to "collect" the mucus in the intermediate-sized airways
- Third breath at mid- to high volume to "evacuate" the mucus from the central airways; the mucus can then be coughed up

DEVICES

Positive Expiratory Pressure Physiotherapy
- Administration of positive pressure (5 to 20 cm H_2O) via mask

Oscillatory Devices
- FlutterCreates oscillations in the airway by exhaling through the device
- Intrapulmonary percussive ventilationUses small, frequent (200 to 300/minutes) bursts of aerosol delivered via mouthpiece
- High-frequency chest wall oscillation: High-frequency oscillation applied to the external chest wall via a vest

Mechanical Insufflation–Exsufflation
Applies negative pressure for 1 to 3 seconds during airway opening

---

clearance techniques must be performed at least once per day and should be increased in frequency during an exacerbation.[28]

Exercise Program

Exercise training has been shown to be beneficial in patients with CF, improving aerobic fitness, slowing the decline in pulmonary function, improving quality of life, and possibly extending longevity.[39] An ideal rehabilitation program includes components of airway clearance, endurance activities, flexibility training, postural exercises, and weight training.[4,28] Exercise is beneficial as an adjunct to airway clearance and as a way to

BOX 33-5	Suggested Components of an Exercise Prescription for Children with Cystic Fibrosis

MODE
- Tricycle, bicycle, swimming, tennis, crab soccer, basketball, wheelchair basketball, aerobic dancing, jogging, running, walking, climbing, wheelbarrow racing, cross-country skiing, skating, weight lifting, elastic bands, step aerobics, snowshoeing, and so on

FREQUENCY
- Four or five times per week; in some cases the individual is able to perform only short bouts of exercise (<5 to 10 continuous minutes; progress first to two or three times per day and then increase duration)

DURATION
- Progress to 20 to 30 continuous minutes of "aerobic" activity (may take 6 to 8 weeks to progress to that level if untrained)

INTENSITY
- Heart rate range, 70% to 85% of peak heart rate determined in exercise tolerance test
- Eleven to 15 (on a scale of 6 to 20) or 3 to 5 (on a scale of 0 to 10) on the Borg Rating of Perceived Exertion Scale
- Zero to 1 on Dyspnea Levels Scale (number of breaths to count to 15 in an 8-second period, score 0 to 4)

PRECAUTIONS
- Undergo a thorough medical examination before starting any exercise program (include O_2 saturation at rest, with activity, and recovery)
- Supplemental O_2 should be used as per physician order (should be determined from results of exercise tolerance test)
- No exercise/play should cause any level of pain
- Evaluate sudden rib pain/soreness (even with a cough)
- Allow extra fluids for hydration and extra calories for nutritional support
- Check blood glucose levels if diabetic
- Avoid heat and extreme temperatures and high-pollution times of day
- Watch for decline in activity/play level
- Use metered dose inhalers before exercise if indicated by previous symptoms
- Airway clearance regimen should be incorporated into program
- Practice good hand washing (2 min) and cleaning of equipment
- Watch for complaints of increased dyspnea or shortness of breath

O_2, Oxygen.

improve self-esteem, endurance, and flexibility; to build or maintain muscle mass; and to slow progression of osteoporosis.[3-5,40] A standard exercise prescription (Box 33-5) consists of mode (device or type of exercise to be performed [e.g., walking, cycling, or basketball]), duration (length of time for exercise), frequency (number of times per day or week), and intensity (the level at which the exercise is performed, usually measured in heart rate or oxygen (O_2) consumption).[26-28,41,42]

A thorough evaluation of the individual should be performed before initiating an exercise program.[3,5,26,28] O_2 saturation should be evaluated at rest and during exercise in all patients with CF to evaluate hypoxemia.[26] A musculoskeletal screen to evaluate posture, flexibility, and strength is important to isolate specific needs of the individual.[3] A functional test such as a 6-Minute Walk Test, which is standardized and easily repeatable, is a good clinical tool to evaluate O_2 saturation and hemodynamic response to a normal activity.[26] Suggestions then can be made regarding the use of supplemental O_2 for a home exercise program. Monitoring heart rate, respiratory rate, and blood pressure and rating of perceived exertion during the timed walk test help the clinician to formulate an exercise prescription for the patient. Rating of perceived exertion is a subjective measure of work.[5,41] Scales ranging from 6 to 20 (perceived exertion) and from 0 to 10 (breathlessness) are used to estimate a level of work as a measure of intensity. A child or adolescent may not be able to find a pulse to check for a target heart rate. The use of a simple scale that correlates with a measure of exercise intensity, such as heart rate, may be easier for the child to understand. Measuring the number of coughs and secretions expectorated during the walk test helps to assess efficacy of the present airway clearance program and how the patient handles secretions with exercise. All of this information will help establish the level of intensity for the home exercise program. Bronchodilators may be useful before initiation of exercise to improve airflow in those patients with reactive airways.[26]

Precautions

There are several medical concerns that may affect a successful rehabilitation program in children with CF. Concern regarding increased symptoms is frequently expressed. However, pretreatment with bronchodilators and incorporation of airway clearance techniques into the exercise program can alleviate many of these symptoms. Concern regarding weight loss is another natural fear and common excuse for not exercising, given the importance placed on weight gain in children with CF. Proper nutrition, caloric intake, and supplementation should therefore be part of the foundation to an exercise program for an individual with CF and enzymes and nutritional supplementation may need to be increased.[28] In children with CF who have diabetes, careful monitoring of blood glucose is important when initiating an exercise program. However, diabetes does not preclude exercise in patients with CF. Osteopenia, which is thought to develop in part from the malnutrition associated with CF, is another important concern when initiating an exercise program. As a result, fractures are an important consideration. However, exercise has been shown to improve osteopenia. In general, the potential benefits of exercise in children with CF outweigh these concerns in the majority of instances.

OBESITY

Obesity is as growing problem in the United States. According to data from the National Health and Nutrition Examination Survey (1999-2002), 31% of the children in the United States are at risk for becoming overweight (>85% for body mass index [BMI]), and 16% are overweight (>95% for BMI).[43] The prevalence of childhood obesity has also increased steadily.[43-46] Childhood obesity can have significant pulmonary consequences, impairing pulmonary function and increasing the symptoms of chronic pulmonary diseases. In addition, given the strong correlation between childhood and adult obesity, there is significant risk of lifelong morbidity and early mortality in these children.

Medical

Obesity has been shown to adversely affect the health of children with a variety of respiratory diseases. Compared with nonobese children, obese children have decreased static lung volumes, functional residual capacities, and chest wall compliance. Baseline work of breathing tends to be increased in obese children. Ventilatory function, however, appears to be normal, and the adverse effects to lung function are potentially reversible after weight loss.[47]

Obstructive sleep apnea is a common sequela of obesity. In obstructive sleep apnea, partial or complete obstruction to breathing occurs during sleep, which in turn leads to hypoxia, arousal, and sleep disturbances. The child's interrupted sleep pattern can be associated with symptoms of daytime sleepiness, fatigue, morning headaches, behavioral issues, and poor school performance. If untreated, obstructive sleep apnea can cause serious life-threatening cardiopulmonary problems such as pulmonary hypertension and cor pulmonale.[47] Children should be referred to a pediatric pulmonologist for a sleep study when obstructive sleep apnea is suggested by symptoms of heavy snoring, witnessed obstruction or apnea during sleep, morning headaches, morning nausea/vomiting, or excessive daytime sleepiness. The ideal treatment is weight loss. However, given the poor success rates of weight loss programs, tonsillectomy, adenoidectomy, or both may also be appropriate therapies. Continuous positive airway pressure while sleeping is also used to prevent obstruction and improve symptoms.

Obesity hypoventilation syndrome is characterized by a combination of obesity and hypercapnia in the absence of other causes of hypo-ventilation. This syndrome is well described in adults, and with the growing prevalence of childhood obesity there are isolated case reports of this disease in children. These patients may be seen with symptoms similar to those of patients with obstructive sleep apnea, including excessive daytime sleepiness and fatigue. On blood gas analysis, a metabolic alkalosis is present, reflecting compensation for chronic hypercapnia associated with the hypoventilation. The hormone leptin may play a role in the development of this syndrome; however, this association is not proven. Treatment includes weight loss and continuous positive airway pressure while sleeping.

Along with obesity, the prevalence of childhood asthma has also been increasing. Because these increases have been concomitant, some have suggested a casual relationship. However, the link between asthma and obesity is controversial.[48-56] Although some clinicians think that obesity may contribute to the development of asthma, associations with objective asthma-related indices are less consistent. The hormone leptin, a protein produced by fat cells, has been linked to hypoventilation associated with obesity and to asthma in children.[55,56] Several large studies have been performed, some independently linking asthma and obesity[48,49] and some finding no association.[50,51] Although obesity has been associated with increased subjective symptoms of asthma and wheezing,[54] increased medication use,[54] and increased hospital admission and duration of hospitalization for asthma, obesity itself has not been linked to the development of airway hyper-responsiveness, the hallmark of asthma.[53]

Exercise Program

Regular exercise and lifestyle modification are the foundation of effective weight loss in children. Several investigators have demonstrated that unstructured exercise programs (e.g., encouraging "free play") are not effective for weight loss.[57,58] Heavier children tend to choose indoor or sedentary activity to avoid negative situations. Structured exercise is more effective for weight loss, but simply prescribing vigorous, aerobic exercise may result in injury or noncompliance. Gradual increases in exercise within a structured multidisciplinary program are more effective at encouraging compliance and avoiding injury.

However, few centers have reported success in treating moderate to severe conditions of pediatric obesity.[58,59] Epstein and colleagues[59] found that lifestyle modification combined with exercise was more effective at maintaining weight loss than diet or exercise alone. In this study of obese girls, although there was no difference in short-term weight loss, children who underwent a program targeted at lifestyle modification in addition to exercise were significantly more likely to maintain their weight loss. Nemet and colleagues[58] also found that a structured multidisciplinary program that included combined dietary, behavioral, and physical activity interventions was effective at producing short-term and long-term weight loss in children.

Calorie restriction is controversial in weight reduction programs for children. Although successful initially, some clinicians think that calorie restriction may result in poor long-term compliance. If caloric restriction is used, it should be accompanied by gradual increases in exercise and daily physical activity, together with consistent behavior modification that includes nutrition and fitness education.

Picking the types of physical activity for obese children can seem daunting to the practitioner and to the patient. Several authors have suggested strategies that tailor type of exercise on the basis of degree of obesity. The protocol recommended by Sothern is a good example.[57] In this structured exercise protocol, severely obese children (>200%

of ideal boy weight; >97% for BMI) have weekly supervision with a trained exercise professional. Non—weight-bearing aerobic activities are recommended including swimming, recline bicycling, arm-specific ergometrics, seated (chair) aerobics, or seated/lying circuit training. Obese children (150% to 200% of ideal boy weight; >95% to 97% for BMI) are recommended to perform primarily non—weight-bearing aerobic activities such as swimming, cycling, strength or aerobic circuit training, arm-specific ergometrics, recline bicycling, and interval walking (gradually working up to longer walks with fewer stops). Overweight children (100% to 150% of ideal boy weight; >85% to 95% for BMI) may perform weight-bearing aerobic activities such as brisk walking, exercising on a treadmill or stair climber, jumping rope, dancing, hiking, or roller blading. Participation in sports is also encouraged and provides an excellent structured exercise opportunity for overweight children.

BRONCHOPULMONARY DYSPLASIA

Bronchopulmonary dysplasia (BPD) is a chronic lung disease associated with premature birth. This condition was first described in 1966 by Northway in a group of newborn infants with secondary pulmonary injury.[60] A combination of factors, including pulmonary immaturity, high O_2 concentrations, and positive-pressure ventilation with high airway pressure, is thought to contribute to the development of BPD. With advances in obstetrics and neonatology and with the discovery of surfactant, the incidence of BPD has fallen markedly. However, BPD remains a significant source of morbidity and mortality in children born prematurely.

Medical

Clinically, BPD is characterized by tachypnea, retractions, crackles, wheezing, hypoxemia, and hypercarbia. Anatomically, the alveolar structure is abnormal with fibrosis of the alveolar septa, interstitial edema, and thickening of the alveolar basement membrane.[61] Mucosal hyperplasia further reduces the lumen of small airways and excessive production of mucus compromises mucociliary transport. Frequently, the large airways are involved, manifested as tracheomalacia or bronchomalacia. Pulmonary artery hypertension is commonly present, and cor pulmonale may occur in severely affected children.

These anatomic abnormalities have significant physiologic impacts.[61] Chronic respiratory disease results from damage to the lung parenchyma and airways. Lung compliance is decreased from pulmonary fibrosis and interstitial edema. Resistance to airflow is increased from narrowing of the airway lumen and the presence of excess mucus. Impaired growth and development result from this combination of factors.

The severity of BPD varies from thriving infants with minimal O_2 requirements to infants with chronic respiratory failure, dependent on mechanical ventilation via tracheostomy. Supplemental O_2 therapy is used to avoid the long-term consequences of chronic hypoxia, such as pulmonary hypertension and cor pulmonale. Oxygenation may need to be monitored by pulse oximetry, particularly during sleep and feeding, when the child is more prone to hypoxemia. Diuretics, bronchodilators, and anti-inflammatory medications are used to reduce airway resistance and work of breathing.[60] In children with large airway involvement or significant pulmonary impairment, positive end-expiratory pressure is used to prevent airway collapse, particularly during exhalation.

In children severely affected by BPD, who require chronic mechanical ventilation via tracheostomy, long-term outcomes depend on pulmonary rehabilitation, avoidance of infections, and nutritional support. Regular chest physiotherapy and techniques to improve mucociliary clearance are important to maintain airway patency. These techniques are similar to those used in children with CF (see Box 33-4). Viral respiratory infections, particularly influenza and respiratory syncytial virus in the fall and winter months, can be devastating and immunization is important. Adequate nutrition is important for growth, improvement in muscle strength, and the ability to wean from ventilation. The baseline calorie requirements for these children are high, estimated to be 25% to 50% higher than for a healthy child because of increased work of breathing.[6] Inadequate nutrition can result from these increased requirements and can be exacerbated by the underlying feeding disorders and oral aversion associated with endotracheal intubation and the fluid restrictions used to treat the child's chronic lung disease. Enteral feeding via a gastrostomy tube may be required to supplement oral intake and to provide adequate calories.

Physical Rehabilitation

Infants with BPD have a diverse set of clinical needs that are best handled by a multidisciplinary team emphasizing growth and development. These interdisciplinary goals require teamwork at the bedside. The speech pathologist and respiratory therapist work together to help the child learn to vocalize via the tracheostomy. Speech and occupational therapists work together to develop feeding plans to help overcome a child's oral aversion that results from prolonged endotracheal intubation. The child life specialist and physical therapist develop a list of play activities to address motor deficits. The respiratory therapist works with physical therapy to make the child as mobile as possible and monitors the patient during activities. Treatment is directed toward two goals: preventing further harm, either neurologic or pulmonary, and promoting growth, both physical and developmental.

Long-term outcomes of patients with BPD are difficult to predict. Pulmonary function results are abnormal for many years in children recovering from BPD.[61] Reactive airway disease, a common comorbidity, can also significantly affect the quality of life for children with BPD, resulting in frequent symptoms and exacerbations. However, many children with BPD are generally able to participate in normal childhood activities. Even the most severely affected children have the potential for recovery. A study by Buschbacher[62] found that 70% to 80% of ventilator-dependent patients with BPD can be weaned from a ventilator. Even when weaning and decannulation are not possible, ventilator support can often be reduced and these children can learn to speak, to feed orally, and to interact with their environment in meaningful ways.

When reducing ventilatory support, the child must be carefully observed. Failure to tolerate weaning can be demonstrated in a variety of subtle ways: a decrease in oral feeding, slowed weight gain or weight loss, or change in social interaction. The needs of the child and family can determine the goals of weaning. Even a short period of freedom from mechanical ventilation can make a tremendous impact on the life of a family.

The ideal goal for these children is a safe discharge home. For some children this means discharge home on ventilatory support. For other children, discharge home is not an option, and long-term care facilities need to be considered.

Wherever the location, each child deserves to be in a program or environment that will allow them to fulfill their potential.

Exercise Program

Rehabilitation programs for children with BPD can promote growth and development, reduce the time required for weaning from mechanical ventilation, and shorten the discharge process.[63] Therapies may be prescribed to address specific motor impairments or for areas of developmental delay. However, for infants and children, play is exercise therapy. Therapeutic play sessions, including interdisciplinary sessions with occupational, physical, and speech therapies, are an important part of rehabilitation. These children need every opportunity to explore and interact with their environment and other people. Rather than prescribe specific activities, efforts should be directed toward removing barriers to physical activity. The child should be as mobile as possible by simplifying the equipment required for care. Portable ventilators are used, if tolerated, to facilitate these activities and to provide more effective play therapy.

Children receiving ventilatory support need to be carefully monitored when active or stressed. Acceptable ranges for carbon dioxide (CO_2), O_2 saturation, respiratory rate, and heart rate should be set on the basis of individual status. Because some children have elevated respiratory and heart rate at rest, ranges given as activity guidelines in textbooks may not apply to these patients. The tracheostomy tube must be protected during physical activity and the child monitored for signs of hypoxemia and respiratory distress. Measurements of O_2 saturation must be combined with clinical assessments. End-tidal CO_2 levels may need to be measured before and after exercise in some children. If necessary, ventilatory support can be increased during periods of increased activity. Even patients who no longer require supplemental O_2 should be monitored for hypoxemia during exercise.

NEUROMUSCULAR DISEASE

Medical

Neuromuscular disorders, degenerative muscle diseases, and paralytic syndromes involving the chest wall can reduce pulmonary function through limitation of spontaneous respiration and tidal volumes, and through impairment of the coordination of muscle movement during inspiration and expiration.[4,64-66] This limitation may be slow and progressive, as in Duchenne muscular dystrophy, or abrupt, as in a traumatic accident. Cerebral palsy, muscular dystrophy, and Down syndrome are examples of diseases in which the musculoskeletal deficits have profound implications for the pulmonary system.[36] Muscle weakness, muscle imbalance, or alterations in muscle tone (either high tone in the case of cerebral palsy or low tone in the case of Down syndrome) may result in scoliotic changes in the rib cage, further restricting air movement.[36,65] A pulmonary rehabilitation program for these patients should focus on enhancing movement and coordination of the thorax and shoulder girdle musculature.[25] Ensuring and augmenting an effective cough, either through manual techniques or devices that mobilize and clear secretions, are also crucial for maintaining airway patency and for prevention of pulmonary complications in these patients.[36]

Duchenne Muscular Dystrophy

Duchenne muscular dystrophy (DMD) is an inherited disease in boys that leads to a progressive loss of muscle control, tone, and function.[64,65,67] The ability to cough and clear secretions effectively becomes impaired.[5,26,64,68] Prevention of infection and secretion retention are key to avoid further impairment of pulmonary function leading to respiratory distress and eventual failure, the leading cause of death in patients with DMD.[65,69,70] Educating parents, caregivers, and patients to recognize signs and symptoms of decline in the respiratory system is also important to delay pulmonary compromise.[5] Any change in sleep pattern, vivid nightmares or dreams, morning headaches, confusion, or increasing level of fatigue may be signs of CO_2 retention and the need for medical intervention. Myocardial damage occurs in more than 90% of patients with DMD.[65] Precautions should include evaluation of both the cardiac and pulmonary systems before initiating an exercise program in this patient population.

Exercise Program

Exercises to improve and maintain respiratory muscle function are the major components of an exercise program for patients with neuromuscular disease.[5,25] These exercises start with simple diaphragmatic breathing exercises and stacking of breaths with or without manual assistance. Inspiratory muscle training can also play a role in improving the force and endurance of the respiratory muscles.[71] However, the efficacy of inspiratory muscle training is limited by disease progression and type of training regimen used. Wanke and colleagues[72] found that inspiratory muscle training was most effective in the early stages of the disease. Standard chest physiotherapy, breathing exercises, and intermittent positive-pressure breathing have also been shown to improve pulmonary function and diaphragmatic breathing patterns in patients with DMD.

An individual treatment plan and ongoing reassessment of the plan are important to meet a patient's needs. The individual's level of disease severity and progression will limit progress with the exercise program. Functional activities such as walking may initially be part of the rehabilitation program, but as the child progresses to a wheelchair the goals of the program will shift more toward maintaining posture, flexibility, and enhancement of cough.[67] The use of abdominal binders is recommended as strength decreases.[25] A decline in activity level, increased shortness of breath, or complaints of tiredness are signals from the patient about fatigue. In a degenerative type of disorder, this is not a desired outcome. Alert the family, caregiver, and patient to these signals to slow down or even stop the pulmonary rehabilitation program and contact the team for assistance.

SCOLIOSIS

Scoliosis is usually idiopathic but can also be due to spinal deformities that develop from muscle weakness, imbalance in muscle tone, and denervation.[5,25,64] Treatment for scoliosis ranges from conservative observation to surgical intervention depending on the age of the patient, the severity of the curve, the progressive nature of the deformity, and the underlying etiology.[64] The role of exercise in the treatment of scoliosis is controversial. Deconditioning and associated progressive muscle weakness are thought to contribute to the impaired pulmonary function in patients with scoliosis. Some studies have shown no benefit from exercise, but others have shown improvements in pulmonary function without further progression of the disease.[73,74]

Pulmonary function and risk for pulmonary complications should be considered when planning a program for an individual with scoliosis.[5,64] Providing effective cough, airflow, and volume of air movement are key components to any program for a patient with a restrictive lung disorder.[5] Teaching positions to improve ventilation and chest expansion and instructing ways to strengthen and enhance respiratory muscle endurance will help with secretion mobilization, cough, and prevention of atelectasis.[25] The ability to stack breaths to enhance air volume for cough and development of an exercise plan to enhance chest wall movement and conditioning should not be overlooked. The patient's breathing pattern may be shallow and rapid at rest and during exercise, owing to the length–tension relationship of the respiratory muscles from the change in the angle of the thorax. The heart rate may also be elevated at rest, owing to these abnormalities in the pulmonary system. Teaching signs and symptoms of fatigue and decline in activity should also be included in the overall plan.

CONCLUSION

There is a growing need for the rehabilitation of pediatric patients with pulmonary disease. However, guidelines for the care of these children are not well established and there are few evidence-based treatment strategies. Children requiring pulmonary rehabilitation have medical problems and issues that differ from those of the adult patient and are unique to their disease and to their physical and psychological development. Adaptation of pulmonary rehabilitation goals and techniques that are used in adult patients may provide useful methods of rehabilitation in this population. Importantly, successful rehabilitation of the pediatric patient can lead to a lifetime of health and well-being.

References

1. American Association of Cardiovascular and Pulmonary Rehabilitation: Guidelines for pulmonary rehabilitation programs, ed 3, Champaign, Ill, 2004, Human Kinetics.
2. Magee C: Asthma. In Campbell SK, Vander Linden DW, Palisano RJ, editors: Physical therapy for children, Philadelphia, 1995, WB Saunders.
3. Tecklin JS: Physical therapy for children with chronic lung disease. Phys Ther 61:1774-1782, 1981.
4. Watchie J: Cardiopulmonary physical therapy: a clinical manual, Philadelphia, 1995, WB Saunders.
5. Dean E, Frownfelter D: Chronic primary cardiopulmonary dysfunction. In Frownfelter DL, Dean E,

editors: Principles and practice of cardiopulmonary physical therapy, ed 3, Chicago, 1996, Mosby-Year Book.

6. Kelly M: Children with ventilator dependence. In Campbell SK, Vander Linden DW, Palisano RJ, editors: Physical therapy for children, Philadelphia, 1995, WB Saunders.

7. Werner HA: Status asthmaticus in children, Chest 119:1913-1929, 2001.

8. DeNicola LK, Monem GF, Gayle MO et al: Treatment of critical status asthmaticus in children, Pediatr Clin North Am 41:1293-1324, 1994.

9. Mannino DM, Homa DM, Akinbami LJ et al: Surveillance for asthma—United States, 1980-1999, MMWR Surveill Summ 51:1-13, 2002.

10. Suissa S, Ernst P: Inhaled corticosteroids: impact on asthma morbidity and mortality, J Allergy Clin Immunol 107:937-944, 2001.

11. Suissa S, Ernst P, Kezouh A: Regular use of inhaled corticosteroids and the long term prevention of hospitalization for asthma, Thorax 57:880-884, 2002.

12. Eisner MD, Lieu TA, Chi F et al: Beta aAgonists, inhaled steroids, and the risk of intensive care unit admission for asthma, Eur Respir J 17:233-240, 2001.

13. Sin DD, Man J, Sharpe H et al: Pharmacological management to reduce exacerbations in adults with asthma: a systematic review and meta-analysis, JAMA 292:367-376, 2004.

14. Boushey HA: Effects of inhaled corticosteroids on the consequences of asthma, J Allergy Clin Immunol 102:S5-S16, 1998.

15. National Asthma Education and Prevention Program. Expert Panel Report 3 (EPR-3): guidelines for the diagnosis and management of asthma-summary report 2007, J Allergy Clin Immunol 120:S94-S138, 2007.

16. Reddel HK, Vincent SD, Civitico J: The need for standardization of peak flow charts, Thorax 60:164-167, 2005.

17. Kamps AW, Roorda RJ, Brand PL: Peak flow diaries in childhood asthma are unreliable, Thorax 56:180-182, 2001.

18. Lang DM, Butz AM, Duggan AK et al: Physical activity in urban school-aged children with asthma, Pediatrics 113:e341-e346, 2004.

19. Welsh L, Kemp JG, Roberts RGD: Effects of physical conditioning on children and adolescents with asthma, Sports Med 35:127-141, 2005.

20. Carroll N, Sly P: Exercise training as an adjunct to asthma management? Thorax 54:190-191, 1999.

21. Ram FS, Robinson SM, Black PN: Effects of physical training in asthma: a systematic review, Br J Sports Med 34:162-167, 2000.

22. National Heart, Lung and Blood Institute: Practical guide for the diagnosis and management of asthma (NIH publication No. 97-4053), Bethesda, 1997, National Heart, Lung and Blood Institute.

23. Fitch KD, Morton AR: Specificity of exercise in exercise induced asthma, BMJ 4:577-581, 1971.

24. Inbar O, Dotan R, Dlin RA et al: Breathing dry or humid air and exercise-induced asthma during swimming, Eur J Appl Physiol 44:43-50, 1980.

25. DeCesare JA, Graybill-Tucker CA, Gould AL: Physical therapy for the child with respiratory dysfunction. In Irwin S, Tecklin J, editors: Cardiopulmonary physical therapy, ed 3, St. Louis, 1995, Mosby-Year Book.

26. Nixon PA: Cystic fibrosis. In ACSM's exercise management for persons with chronic diseases and disabilities, Champaign, Ill, 1997, Human Kinetics.

27. Orenstein DM, Nixon PA: Patients with cystic fibrosis. In Franklin BA, Gordon S, Timmis GC, editors: Exercise in modern medicine, Baltimore, 1989, Williams & Wilkins.

28. Orenstein DM, Noyes BE: Cystic fibrosis. In Casaburi R, Petty TL, editors: Principles and practice of pulmonary rehabilitation, Philadelphia, 1993, WB Saunders.

29. McCool FD, Rosen MJ: Nonpharmacologic airway clearance therapies: ACCP evidence-based clinical guidelines, Chest 129:250S-259S, 2006.

30. Suri R: The use of human deoxyribonuclease (rhDNase) in the management of cystic fibrosis, Biodrugs 19:135-144, 2005.

31. Braun SR, Giovannoni R, O'Connor M: Improving the cough in patients with spinal cord injury, Am J Phys Med 63:1-10, 1982.

32. Bach JR, Smith WH, Michaels J et al: Airway secretion clearance by mechanical exsufflation for post-poliomyelitis ventilator-assisted individuals, Arch Phys Med Rehabil 74:170-177, 1993.

33. Sutton PP, Parker RA, Webber BA et al: Assessment of the forced expiration technique, postural drainage and directed coughing in chest physiotherapy, Eur J Respir Dis 64:62-68, 1983.

34. Miller S, Hall DO, Clayton CB et al: Chest physiotherapy in cystic fibrosis: a comparative study of autogenic drainage and the active cycle of breathing techniques with postural drainage, Thorax 50:165-169, 1995.

35. Elkins MR, Jones A, van der Schans C: Positive expiratory pressure physiotherapy for airway clearance in people with cystic fibrosis, Cochrane Database Syst Rev 1:CD003147, 2004.

36. Moerchen VA, Crane LD: The neonatal and pediatric patient. In Frownfelter DL, Dean E, editors: Principles and practice of cardiopulmonary physical therapy, ed 3, Chicago, 1996, Mosby-Year Book.

37. Hardy KA: A review of airway clearance: new techniques, indications, and recommendations, Respir Care 39:440-452, 1994.

38. Downs AM: Physiological basis for airway clearance techniques. In Frownfelter DL, Dean E, editors: Principles and practice of cardiopulmonary physical therapy, ed 3, Chicago, 1996, Mosby-Year Book.

39. Orenstein DM, Higgins LW: Update on the role of exercise in cystic fibrosis, Curr Opin Pulm Med 11:519-523, 2005.

40. Bachrach LK: Osteopenia in cystic fibrosis: symposium session, Pediatr Pulm Suppl 14: 200-201, 1997.

41. Downs AM: Clinical application of airway clearance techniques. In Frownfelter DL, Dean E, editors: Principles and practice of cardiopulmonary physical therapy. ed 3, Chicago, 1996, Mosby-Year Book.

42. Temes WC: Cardiac rehabilitation. In Hillegass EA, Sadowsky HS, editors: Essentials of cardiopulmonary physical therapy, Philadelphia, 1994, WB Saunders.

43. Hedley AA, Ogden CL, Johnson CL et al: Prevalence of overweight and obesity among US children, adolescents, and adults, 1999-2002, JAMA 291: 2847-2850, 2004.

44. Flegal KM, Ogden CL, Wei R et al: Prevalence of overweight in US children: comparison of US growth charts from the Centers for Disease Control and Prevention with other reference values for body mass index, Am J Clin Nutr 73:1086-1093, 2001.

45. Troiano RP, Flegal KM, Kuczmarski RJ et al: Overweight prevalence and trends for children and adolescents: the National Health and Nutrition Examination Surveys, 1963 to 1991, Arch Pediatr Adolesc Med 149:1085-1091, 1995.

46. Strauss RS, Pollack HA: Epidemic increase in childhood overweight, 1986-1998, JAMA 286: 2845-2848, 2001.

47. Deane S, Thomson A: Obesity and the pulmonologist, Arch Dis Child 91:188-191, 2006.

48. von Mutius E, Schwartz J, Neas LM et al: Relation of body mass index and atopy in children: the National Health and Nutrition Examination III, Thorax 56:835-838, 2001.

49. Shaheen SO, Sterne JAC, Montgomery SM et al: Birth weight, body mass index and asthma in young adults, Thorax 54:396-402, 1999.

50. To T, Vydykhan TN, Dell S et al: Is obesity associated with asthma in young children? J Pediatr 144:162-168, 2004.

51. Tantisira KG, Litonjua AA, Weiss ST et al: Association of body mass with pulmonary function in the childhood asthma management program, Thorax 58:1036-1041, 2003.

52. Conway B, Rene A: Obesity as a disease: no lightweight matter, Obes Rev 5:145-151, 2004.

53. Schacter LM, Salome CM, Peat JK et al: Obesity is a risk factor for asthma but not for airway hyperresponsiveness, Thorax 56:4-8, 2001.

54. Belamarich PF, Luder E, Kattan M et al: Do obese inner-city children with asthma have more symptoms than nonobese children with asthma? Pediatrics 106:1436-1441, 2001.

55. Phipps PR, Starritt E, Caterson I et al: Association of serum leptin with hypoventilation in human obesity, Thorax 57:75-76, 2002.

56. Guler N, Kirerleri E, Ones U et al: Leptin: does it have any role in childhood asthma? J Allergy Clin Immunol 114:254-259, 2004.

57. Sothern MS: Exercise as a modality in the treatment of childhood obesity, Pediatr Clin North Am 48:995-1015, 2001.

58. Nemet D, Barkan S, Epstein Y et al: Short- and long-term beneficial effects of a combined dietary–behavioral–physical activity intervention for the treatment of childhood obesity, Pediatrics 115:e443-e449, 2005.

59. Epstein LH, Wing RR, Penner BC et al: Effect of diet and controlled exercise on weight-loss in obese children, J Pediatr 7:358-361, 1985.

60. Barrington KJ, Finer N: Treatment of bronchopulmonary dysplasia: a review. Clin Perinatol 25: 177-197, 1998.

61. Boyle K, Baker V, Cassaday C: Neonatal pulmonary disorders. In Barhart S, Czervinske M, editors: Perinatal and pediatric respiratory care, Philadelphia, 1995, WB Saunders.

62. Buschbacher R: Outcomes and problems in pediatric pulmonary rehabilitation, Am J Phys Med Rehabil 74:287-293, 1995.

63. Buschbacher R, Tsangaris M, Shay T: Rehab and bronchopulmonary dysplasias, J Respir Care Pract 9:75-77, 1996.

64. Clough P: Restrictive lung dysfunction. In Hillegass EA, Sadowsky HS, editors: Essentials of cardiopulmonary physical therapy, Philadelphia, 1994, WB Saunders.

65. Bach JR: Neuromuscular and skeletal disorders leading to global alveolar hypoventilation. In Bach JR, editor: Pulmonary rehabilitation: the obstructive and paralytic conditions, Philadelphia, 1996, Hanley & Belfus.

66. Adkins HV: Improvement of breathing ability in children with respiratory muscle paralysis, Phys Ther 48:577-581, 1968.

67. Bach JR: Pulmonary rehabilitation in musculoskeletal disorders. In Fishman AP, editor: Pulmonary rehabilitation, New York, 1996, Marcel Dekker.

68. Bach JR: Conventional approaches to managing neuromuscular ventilatory failure. In Bach JR, editor: Pulmonary rehabilitation: the obstructive and paralytic conditions, Philadelphia, 1996, Hanley & Belfus.

69. Bach JR, Ishikawa Y, Kim H: Prevention of pulmonary morbidity for patients with Duchenne muscular dystrophy, Chest 112:1024-1028, 1997.

70. De Troyer A, Estenne M: Neuromuscular disorders. In Fishman AP, ed: Pulmonary rehabilitation, New York, 1996, Marcel Dekker.

71. McCool FD, Tzelepis GE: Inspiratory muscle training in the patient with neuromuscular disease, Phys Ther 75:1006-1014, 1995.

72. Wanke T, Toifl K, Merkle M et al: Inspiratory muscle training in patients with Duchenne muscular dystrophy, Chest 105:475-482, 1994.

73. Weiss HR, Lohschmidt K, el-Obeidi N et al: Preliminary results and worst-case analysis of inpatient scoliosis rehabilitation, Pediatr Rehabil 1:35-40, 1997.

74. dos Santos Alves VL, Stirbulov R, Avanzi O: Impact of a physical rehabilitation program on the respiratory function of adolescents with idiopathic scoliosis, Chest 130:500-505, 2006.

Chapter 34

Benefits and the Future of Pulmonary Rehabilitation

JOHN E. HODGKIN

CHAPTER OUTLINE

**Overall Benefits of Pulmonary
   Rehabilitation**
**Benefits of Individual Components
   of Care**
   General Care
   Medications
   Respiratory Therapy Techniques

Occupational Therapy
Psychosocial Rehabilitation
Vocational Rehabilitation
Lung Surgery
**Future Challenges of Pulmonary
   Rehabilitation**
Conclusion

PROFESSIONAL SKILLS

On completion of this chapter, the reader will be able to do
the following:
* Describe the reported benefits to those patients who participate in a pulmonary rehabilitation
  program
* Discuss the benefits of the individual components of care used for those with chronic lung disease
* List issues of concern in pulmonary rehabilitation that still need to be resolved or clarified

As emphasized in the preceding chapters, pulmonary rehabilitation requires the use of many individually tailored treatment modalities and a management system that can be used to help the patient achieve and maintain the highest functional capacity possible. Box 34-1 outlines the components of a pulmonary rehabilitation program. Many benefits, which allow those with

chronic lung disease to appreciate a more enjoyable life, have been reported by pulmonary rehabilitation programs using these components of care.[1-6] Reported benefits span the last 50 years. In this chapter, early studies along with more recent studies are referenced. The advantage of many of the studies reported in the last 15 years is that participants were randomized between a

BOX 34-1	Components of Pulmonary Rehabilitation

GENERAL
- Patient and family education
- Proper nutrition, including weight control
- Avoidance of smoking and other inhaled irritants
- Avoidance of infection (e.g., immunization)
- Proper environment
- Adequate hydration

MEDICATIONS
- Bronchodilators
- Expectorants
- Antimicrobials
- Corticosteroids
- Cromolyn sodium/nedocromil sodium
- Leukotriene antagonists/inhibitors
- Diuretics
- Psychopharmacologic agents

RESPIRATORY THERAPY TECHNIQUES
- Aerosol therapy
- O_2 therapy
- Home use of ventilators

PHYSICAL THERAPY MODALITIES
- Relaxation training
- Breathing retraining
- Chest percussion and postural drainage
- Deliberate coughing and expectoration
- Exercise conditioning

OCCUPATIONAL THERAPY
- Evaluate activities of daily living
- Outline energy-conserving maneuvers
- Psychosocial rehabilitation

VOCATIONAL REHABILITATION

O_2, *Oxygen.*

pulmonary rehabilitation group and a control group. The overall benefits reported for pulmonary rehabilitation programs, the demonstrated benefits for each individual component of care, and the future of pulmonary rehabilitation are discussed in this chapter.

OVERALL BENEFITS OF PULMONARY REHABILITATION

A list of benefits of pulmonary rehabilitation has been reported by the Global Initiative on Chronic Obstructive Lung Disease (GOLD) report.[1] See Table 34-1 for a description of levels of evidence used in the GOLD document and Box 34-2 for the benefits of pulmonary rehabilitation in chronic obstructive pulmonary disease (COPD). Early observational studies reported such things as reduction in respiratory symptoms, reversal of anxiety and

depression, and improvement in their sense of control over their status.[7-9] Essentially all of the studies have reported an enhanced ability to carry out activities of daily living,[10-18] improved exercise ability,[19-57] better quality of life,[10-18,31,34,35,46,49-58] and decreased dyspnea.[31,33,45-47,51,59-61] Some patients were able to return to or continue gainful employment.[10,13,32,33,35,52,62-65] Unfortunately, patients are commonly referred to pulmonary rehabilitation programs only after they are severely impaired and no longer able to consider working at a regular job.

There have been many scientific advances both in our understanding of the systemic effects of chronic respiratory disease as well as of the changes induced by the process of pulmonary rehabilitation.[2] A meta-analysis in 2006 reviewed the published reports of 31 randomized, controlled pulmonary rehabilitation programs.[66] These crucial randomized, controlled studies, reported since the early 1990s, have demonstrated unequivocally that pulmonary rehabilitation is valuable. The science in support of pulmonary rehabilitation has come a long way since the first official position statement supporting pulmonary rehabilitation by the American Thoracic Society in 1981.[67]

Early studies reported a reduction in the need for hospitalization following pulmonary rehabilitation programs, suggesting that there could be a reduction in the cost of care as a result of such programs.[8,15,17,63,64,68-77] More recent reports have concluded that pulmonary rehabilitation programs are cost-effective.[6,78,79]

Although the decrement in forced expiratory volume in 1 second (FEV_1) for a normal population is estimated to be 20 to 30 ml/year,[80,81] the reported decrement for patients with COPD ranges from 40 to 80 ml/year.[76,82-88] Studies reporting on the results of pulmonary rehabilitation have not documented a significant alteration in the mean rate of decrease in the FEV_1 of patients with COPD who have significant respiratory impairment. A reduction in dynamic hyperinflation through components of pulmonary rehabilitation (including the use of medications, exercise training, and supplemental oxygen [O_2] use) has been reported.[3,89]

It has been commonly stated that no evidence exists that pulmonary rehabilitation for patients with COPD improves survival. Although it is clear that O_2 therapy significantly improves survival among patients with COPD who are seriously hypoxemic,[90,91] many think that the other aspects of care commonly used in these persons do not significantly prolong life. However, some reports

TABLE 34-1	Description of Levels of Evidence	
Evidence Category	Sources of Evidence	Definition
A	Randomized controlled trials (RCTs): rich body of data	Evidence is from end points of well-designed RCTs that provide a consistent pattern of findings in the population for which the recommendation is made; category A requires substantial numbers of studies involving substantial numbers of participants
B	Randomized controlled trials (RCTs): limited body of data	Evidence is from end points of intervention studies that include only a limited number of patients, post hoc or subgroup analysis of RCTs, or meta-analysis of RCTs; in general, category B pertains when few randomized trials exist, they are small in size, they were undertaken in a population that differs from the target population of the recommendation, or the results are somewhat inconsistent
C	Nonrandomized trials: observational studies	Evidence is from outcomes of uncontrolled or nonrandomized trials or from observational studies
D	Panel consensus judgment	This category is used only when the provision of some guidance was deemed valuable but the clinical literature addressing the subject was deemed insufficient to justify placement in one of the other categories; the panel consensus is based on clinical experience or knowledge that does not meet the criteria for the other categories

suggest that pulmonary rehabilitation can lead to improved survival.[13,74,76,92-98]

One of the early randomized, controlled trials compared the effect of a pulmonary rehabilitation program with a group education program in 119 patients with COPD.[31] Survival at 6 years was slightly better in the group participating in the pulmonary rehabilitation program—that is, 67% compared with 56% for the education-only group. This difference, however, was not statistically significant, possibly because of the lack of power, that is, not enough individuals were enrolled in the study to detect a significant survival advantage.

A review article on pulmonary rehabilitation states that, to conclusively establish whether pulmonary rehabilitation impacts the progression of disease and survival, a large-scale multicenter randomized trial with up to 750 to 1000 patients in both the treatment and control groups, with at least 3 years of follow-up, would be required.[3] Because pulmonary rehabilitation is now considered to be a standard of care for patients with COPD, it is doubtful this study will ever be done. Of note is the fact that the GOLD report[1] stated that pulmonary rehabilitation for patients with COPD improves survival (see Box 34-2); however, the 2007 pulmonary rehabilitation evidence-based clinical practice guidelines, produced by the American College of Chest Physicians and the American Association of Cardiovascular and Pulmonary Rehabilitation,[6] concluded that there is insufficient evidence to determine whether

---

Box 34-2   Benefits of Pulmonary Rehabilitation in Chronic Obstructive Pulmonary Disease

- Improves exercise capacity (Evidence A)
- Reduces the perceived intensity of breathlessness (Evidence A)
- Improves health-related quality of life (Evidence A)
- Reduces the number of hospitalizations and days in the hospital (Evidence A)
- Reduces anxiety and depression associated with chronic obstructive pulmonary disease (Evidence A)
- Strength and endurance training of the upper limbs improves arm function (Evidence B)
- Benefits extend well beyond the immediate period of training (Evidence B)
- Improves survival (Evidence B)
- Respiratory muscle training is beneficial, especially when combined with general exercise training (Evidence C)
- Psychological intervention is helpful (Evidence C)

pulmonary rehabilitation improves survival among patients with COPD.

The factors that affect survival of patients with COPD have been reviewed.[99] COPD is associated with clinical manifestations not closely related to the FEV_1, such as worsened dyspnea, reduction in exercise capacity, peripheral muscle weakness, and malnutrition. All of these factors have proven to be more important predictors of mortality than the FEV_1.[100] It seems logical that if a significant prolongation of life is to be achieved, the principles of pulmonary rehabilitation discussed in this book must be applied earlier in the course of the disease rather than waiting until severe, irreversible impairment of function is present.

A joint committee of the American College of Chest Physicians and the American Association of Cardiovascular and Pulmonary Rehabilitation developed the first evidence-based guidelines on pulmonary rehabilitation.[5] This report reviewed the scientific basis for pulmonary rehabilitation in patients with COPD, with whom most of the research in this area has been conducted. These two organizations have produced an updated report.[6]

BENEFITS OF INDIVIDUAL COMPONENTS OF CARE

General Care

Most of the professional association position statements regarding the benefits of pulmonary rehabilitation relate to patients with COPD, because it is this population of patients that makes up the majority of people referred to pulmonary programs.[2,3,5,6] However, there are a growing number of reports that patients with other reasons for pulmonary dysfunction also benefit from pulmonary rehabilitation programs.[101-104]

Although it is difficult to measure the direct contribution of education to the overall outcomes of pulmonary rehabilitation,[1,4] teaching patients about their disease process and its treatment is an integral part of pulmonary rehabilitation.[105-107] A pulmonary rehabilitation knowledge test has been developed and validated.[108] Self-management education is replacing didactic lectures in teaching behavior modification.[2] It is most effective when it is interactive and conducted in small workshops designed to improve both knowledge and skills.[109] Education is particularly

important in helping people stop smoking,[1] and has been reported to improve a patient's response to exacerbations.[110]

A careful evaluation of nutritional factors and diet patterns is performed as part of the initial assessment of most pulmonary rehabilitation programs. There is an association between underweight status and increased mortality among patients with COPD.[111-113] A high-protein diet, along with multiple small feedings, has long been recommended for underweight patients with chronic respiratory disease.[114]

Nutritional enhancement has been reported to improve exercise performance in patients with COPD[115] and, combined with exercise training, increased body weight and fat-free mass in underweight patients.[116,117] It has been stated that nutritional interventions, in general, are not effective in outpatients with COPD [118]; however, when undernourished patients with COPD gain weight, survival is improved.[112,119] Nutritional supplements may lead to a greater exercise training effect in terms of functional status[115,117] and health-related quality of life.[117] In obese patients with pulmonary impairment, nutritional education and restricted calories can lead to weight loss and improved functional status and quality of life.[2,120,121] Proper nutrition has been reported to help patients resist respiratory infections[122] and may help restore the ventilatory response to hypoxemia[123] and hypercapnia[124] in severely malnourished individuals. Studies suggest that further research regarding the role of nutrition support is warranted.[112,125,126]

Cessation of smoking is fundamental to achieving subjective and objective improvement. Stopping smoking generally results in an improved appetite, decreased dyspnea, a reduction in cough and sputum, and improved pulmonary function.[127,128] The Lung Health Study[129] demonstrated that patients with mild degrees of airway obstruction had improvements in their FEV_1 and a slower rate of decline compared with patients who continued to smoke. Smoking has been shown to increase the risk of getting an influenza infection.[130] Stopping smoking was reported, in 1989, to improve survival among patients with COPD[95] and this has been confirmed through long-term follow-up of subjects enrolled in the Lung Health Study.[131]

The GOLD report[1] states that smoking cessation is the single most effective and cost-effective intervention by which most people may reduce the risk of having COPD and stop its progression.

There is no evidence that smokers will benefit less than nonsmokers from pulmonary rehabilitation.[1,4] Some data indicate that continuing smokers are less likely to complete pulmonary rehabilitation programs.[132] Obviously, any smoker enrolled in a pulmonary rehabilitation program should be provided with the support needed to help the individual stop smoking.

Influenza vaccinations, yearly, are recommended for individuals with chronic lung disease.[1] The GOLD report stated that the pneumococcal polysaccharide vaccine is recommended for those patients with COPD who are 65 years of age and older, and for patients with COPD who are younger than age 65 with an FEV_1 less than 40% of predicted.[1] It has been stated that the pneumococcal vaccination should be repeated in individuals older than 65 years if it has been more than 5 years since their initial vaccination.[133]

Medications

Almost all patients benefit from a consistent program of medications. On the other hand, all these agents have significant side effects and, when not used appropriately, can lead to a worsening of the patient's condition. Bronchodilators not only help relieve bronchospasm but also can enhance mucociliary clearance, reduce dyspnea, and improve exercise tolerance.[134-137] Antimicrobial agents limit the airway irritation and inflammation that result from bacterial respiratory infections. Corticosteroids lessen airway inflammation and the adverse effects of allergy; in addition, they facilitate bronchodilator action. Two nonsteroidal anti-inflammatory medications, cromolyn sodium and nedocromil sodium, available for inhalation, and leukotriene antagonists, available in oral form, can reduce the need for corticosteroids in patients with bronchial asthma. Diuretics are beneficial for the fluid retention of left ventricular decompensation and cor pulmonale. Proper use of psychopharmacologic agents can significantly improve the ability of some patients with COPD to function effectively. Anabolic steroids in patients with COPD have been found to increase muscle strength[138] but not to improve exercise endurance.[3,139,140] A landmark study reported that the combination of inhaled salmeterol and fluticasone (compared with placebo or the use of salmeterol or fluticasone alone) in patients with COPD resulted in improved health status and spirometric values and a borderline improvement in survival.[141,142]

Respiratory Therapy Techniques

Aerosol Therapy

Various devices have been used to aerosolize bronchodilators, corticosteroids, nonsteroidal anti-inflammatory agents, mucolytic agents, bland mist, and antimicrobials. Although little support exists for aerosolization of the latter three agents, clearly inhalation of bronchodilators and the anti-inflammatory medications are of tremendous benefit. Inhalation of a sympathomimetic medication accomplishes faster bronchodilation, with fewer systemic side effects, than oral ingestion or parenteral administration of the same agent. The addition of inhaled tiotropium to pulmonary rehabilitation enhanced the benefits reported from pulmonary rehabilitation alone.[137] Inhalation of corticosteroids accomplishes much of the anti-inflammatory effect while significantly reducing the risk of systemic side effects.

Oxygen Therapy

Supplemental O_2 has clearly been shown to lessen the adverse effects of significant hypoxemia, such as pulmonary hypertension, polycythemia, and neuropsychological dysfunction, in patients with COPD. Specifically, patients with an arterial partial pressure of O_2 of 55 mm Hg or less (O_2 saturation, $\leq$88%) on room air or less than 60 mm Hg (O_2 saturation, <90%) and evidence of polycythemia or right-sided heart dysfunction, when stable, have achieved a significant prolongation of life with continuous O_2 compared with nocturnal O_2 only.[90,91] Patients who have significant hypoxemia during exercise testing can improve their exercise tolerance by using supplemental O_2 during exercise training.[19,143-147] Supplemental O_2 has also been reported to improve the level of maximal exercise that can be achieved, even among patients who do not become hypoxemic during exercise.[148-152] Despite the consistent improvements found in exercise tolerance, most studies seeking to determine whether providing supplemental O_2 during exercise training improved the gains in exercise tolerance elicited by rehabilitative training have failed to show an additional benefit.[3,153-155] Obviously, O_2 during exercise training is warranted for those who meet the criteria for the use of O_2 because of significant hypoxemia when resting.[90,91]

The GOLD report has stated that there is no benefit from using short bursts of O_2 for symptomatic relief before or after exercise.[1] The importance of supplemental O_2 for those patients with COPD who become hypoxemic only while asleep is yet to be determined. Obviously, those with obstructive

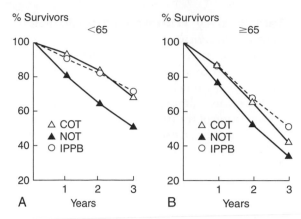

FIGURE 34-1 Comparison of survival in the National Institutes of Health Intermittent Positive-Pressure Breathing (IPPB) trial and the Nocturnal Oxygen Therapy Trial (NOTT). All patients had a baseline FEV_1 of less than 30% of predicted. **A**, Data from patients younger than 65 years at the beginning of the studies. **B**, Patients 65 years of age and older. *Circles*, patients in the IPPB trial; *open triangles*, patients with hypoxemia receiving continuous oxygen therapy (COT); *solid triangles*, patients with hypoxemia receiving 12 hours of nocturnal oxygen therapy (NOT).

sleep apnea may need supplemental O_2 in addition to continuous positive airway pressure. Supplemental O_2 administered to patients with severe hypoxemia can result in a survival similar to that of patients with similar levels of impairment (i.e., FEV_1) but without severe hypoxemia (Figure 34-1).[97]

Assistance with Mechanical Ventilation

Although intermittent positive-pressure breathing (IPPB) therapy was used for many years in patients with pulmonary disorders, no evidence suggests that in outpatients with chronic disease such therapy has any advantage over less expensive and simpler methods of aerosol therapy, such as cartridge inhalers or compressor nebulizers. The National Heart, Lung, and Blood Institute–sponsored study comparing IPPB devices with compressor nebulizers in outpatients with COPD showed no difference in morbidity or mortality between patients in the two groups.[156] This evaluation of 985 patients did not demonstrate any role for periodic IPPB treatments in outpatients with COPD.

The addition of noninvasive positive pressure ventilation (NPPV) at night in combination with pulmonary rehabilitation in patients with severe COPD improved exercise tolerance and quality of life.[157] Studies in progress are assessing the possible benefit of NPPV during exercise training, through unloading the respiratory muscles; however, it is labor intensive and cannot be currently recommended.[3]

Physical Therapy Modalities

Relaxation training; breathing retraining; deliberate cough, chest percussion, and postural drainage; and exercise conditioning are considered physical therapy modalities. However, it is recognized that these services are often carried out by other experts besides physical therapists (e.g., respiratory care practitioners and nurses).

Relaxation Training

Relaxation techniques, such as biofeedback or listening to soothing music, can help anxious patients reduce fear and tension and may be useful for persons with the high-fear, high-anxiety personality type[158,159]; however, long-term benefits from these brief interventions have not been demonstrated.[160] Some relaxation exercises, such as contracting and then relaxing skeletal muscle groups, can help reduce dyspnea and anxiety in patients with COPD.[161] Other demonstrated benefits include a slowing of the respiratory rate and heart rate, as well as lowering O_2 consumption.[162,163]

Breathing Retraining

Training patients with COPD to slow their respiratory rate with a prolonged exhalation (with or without the use of pursed lips) helps control dyspnea and results in improved ventilation, increased tidal volume, decreased respiratory rate, and a reduced alveolar–arterial O_2 difference.[164-169] A study of the value of pursed lips breathing in patients with COPD reported a reduction in respiratory rate, dyspnea, and arterial partial pressure of carbon dioxide, while improving tidal volume and O_2 saturation under resting conditions.[170] Such a breathing pattern not only helps relieve dyspnea but can improve the ability to exercise and carry out activities of daily living.[170-173] The benefits of pursed lips breathing are often discovered by patients before instruction from health care providers. An early study reported benefit from diaphragmatic breathing[174]; however, more recent studies do not support the use of this technique in patients with COPD.[175-177]

An improvement in respiratory muscle strength and endurance has been reported through voluntary normocapnic hyperpnea,[178-182] and inspiratory resistive loading.[183] Inspiratory muscle training in patients with poor initial inspiratory muscle strength has been shown in some studies to improve exercise capacity in patients with COPD.[181-186] Its effect on symptoms and functional limitation has not been firmly established.[4,186] Inspiratory muscle training is inferior to general exercise training in COPD, as far as improving quality of life or function.[3] The routine addition of inspiratory muscle training to whole body exercise training cannot be justified on the basis of studies to date.[6]

Deliberate Cough, Chest Percussion, and Postural Drainage

Teaching patients how to cough properly can result in more effective expectoration. The forced expiration technique for coughing has been recommended for expectorating sputum.[187,188] Postural drainage, when accompanied by chest percussion or vibration, has also been recommended to help clear secretions from obstructed airways. Positive expiratory pressure therapy has been advocated as an adjunct for individuals who have difficulty expectorating airway secretions.[189,190] The combination of postural drainage, percussion, and forced expiration has been reported to improve airway clearance, but not pulmonary function in patients with COPD and bronchiectasis[191]; its routine use in stable patients is not warranted.[2]

Exercise Conditioning

Exercise training should be an essential component of any pulmonary rehabilitation program. Many studies have reported an enhanced exercise level following such general conditioning exercises as walking, bicycle riding, and swimming.[19-48] A combination of improved mechanical efficiency, improved muscle force[40] and oxidative capacity,[39,192] and adaptations in the breathing pattern[193,194] and consequently reduced dynamic hyperinflation[195] is likely to contribute to the improved exercise tolerance that is consistently reported.[2] Favorable outcomes from exercise training among patients with COPD include increases in maximal exercise tolerance, peak O_2 uptake, endurance time during submaximal testing, functional walking distance, and peripheral and respiratory muscle strength.[4]

One of the greatest benefits of exercise conditioning is that it allows patients to do more work for any given O_2 consumption. In effect, patients become more efficient, and increased muscular strength and endurance enable them to accomplish more. As a result, the patients can better tolerate daily activities. Although exercise training has little effect on pulmonary function, it has been shown to improve sleep, appetite, and tolerance of dyspnea.[193] Studies demonstrate that patients with COPD can exercise at a considerably higher percentage of their maximal exercise capacity than had originally been recommended.[28,42,196,197] Exercise training above the anaerobic threshold has been reported to achieve more benefit than training at a lower intensity level in patients with COPD who can exercise to a high enough intensity to reach an anaerobic threshold.[36,37,42,48,198-200] Adding upper extremity exercise training to traditional lower extremity training is recommended for patients with COPD.[1-5,44,201-205]

Adding strength (resistance) training to endurance training provides additional benefit in treating peripheral muscle dysfunction[200,206,207]; however, this has not been shown to translate into superior benefits in terms of health-related quality of life or symptomology.[3] For those patients with severe respiratory impairment, interval training (alternating brief periods of high-intensity exercise with periods of low-intensity exercise or rest) allows patients who cannot exercise continuously at a high intensity for 20 to 30 minutes to achieve the significant benefits associated with exercise training.[208-211]

The optimal length of pulmonary rehabilitation programs and exercise training is unknown. However, longer duration programs yield greater benefits.[1-3,35,57,66,212-214] Programs with 28 or more rehabilitation sessions had more effect than programs with fewer sessions.[3,66] It has been stated that a minimum of about 8 weeks seems necessary.[3]

Although the benefits of pulmonary rehabilitation extend well beyond the immediate period of training, they do begin to decline after a year or so.[31] Outpatient rehabilitation three times a week for up to 15 months after completion of the program maintained benefits better than simply advising patients to exercise at home.[215]

Occupational Therapy

An occupational therapy evaluation will help identify reasonable short- and long-term goals for the patient, will disclose tasks important for the patient that are precluded by functional limitations, and will reveal patterns of daily activities in which energy can be conserved for other productive and worthwhile activities.[35,216] A home visit will often disclose unexpected architectural barriers and often leads to significant improvement in the patient's ability to function in his or her real world.

Psychosocial Rehabilitation

Patients disabled from COPD commonly exhibit emotional reactions, such as depression, fear, anxiety, hostility, and denial, all of which impair functional capacity. Dealing with anxiety and depression can make a significant difference in the patient's quality of life.[217] Pulmonary rehabilitation programs including psychological interventions improve anxiety and depression more than those consisting of exercise training only.[218] Psychotherapy, sometimes requiring a psychologist or psychiatrist and the appropriate use of psychopharmacologic agents, can help such patients better cope with their disease process. Patients with chronic respiratory disease who have positive social support have less depression and anxiety than those who do not.[219]

Sexual dysfunction is often a crucial obstacle to overall rehabilitation and should be addressed positively. The attitudes transmitted by the entire rehabilitation team and the interactions among the patients themselves contribute significantly to the psychological rehabilitation of the patients.

Vocational Rehabilitation

Although some individuals will be able to continue working in their current occupations, many others will either need to quit their jobs or alter the type of work performed. A proper evaluation and categorization of the patient's capacities are important for successful rehabilitation. The goals of vocational and functional rehabilitation may vary after careful evaluation of the patient. Possible goals include the following:

- Returning the patient to the job he or she is holding
- Returning the patient to the same occupational field or plant but in a different job or location
- Changing the occupational field to a totally different one in which the patient can use previous training or existing skills
- Job retraining and reemployment
- Entering the patient in a sheltered workshop program

- Retraining the individual in daily self-care with an eye to conservation of effort and efficiency of motion[220]

When a patient is employed in an unhealthy environment or if further progression of disease is anticipated and continued employment is therefore unlikely, it may be desirable to train the patient for a sedentary occupation in anticipation of the future course of the disease. One reason that vocational rehabilitation is not considered more often is that by the time patients with chronic respiratory disease are referred for pulmonary rehabilitation they often have severe impairment.

Lung Surgery

Lung volume reduction surgery after rehabilitation in patients with severe emphysema improved survival, exercise capacity, and quality of life more effectively than pulmonary rehabilitation alone in a select group of patients (i.e., those with predominantly upper lobe emphysema and low exercise capacity).[221] There was no survival advantage with surgery in those with predominantly upper lobe emphysema and a high exercise capacity, but they did achieve better exercise and quality of life. Those with emphysema throughout the lungs and a low exercise capacity, who underwent surgery, showed only a mild improvement in quality of life. Those who had emphysema throughout the lungs and a high exercise capacity actually experienced higher mortality after surgery than those receiving only pulmonary rehabilitation. Lung volume reduction surgery also had a prohibitively high postsurgical mortality if they had preoperative FEV_1 or diffusing capacity values less than 20% of predicted.[222] The cost of lung volume reduction surgery is high.[223]

Lung transplantation in patients with serious lung impairment from diseases including COPD, cystic fibrosis, and pulmonary fibrosis should be considered,[2,224] as a way of improving quality of life, decreasing the need for O_2, and prolonging life. Also, pulmonary rehabilitation should be used routinely, preoperatively and postoperatively in patients with respiratory disease before they undergo lung volume reduction surgery or lung transplantation.[222,225]

FUTURE CHALLENGES OF PULMONARY REHABILITATION

- Although no slowing of the rate of pulmonary function deterioration has been shown, reports of improvement in survival through pulmonary rehabilitation were reviewed earlier in this chapter. Clearly, instituting a comprehensive respiratory care program earlier in the course of a patient's disease will provide more potential for favorably altering the course of the disease.

- Unfortunately, only 20% to 35% of participants in most smoking cessation programs quit permanently. An enhanced effort needs to be directed toward the prevention of respiratory diseases rather than waiting until significant respiratory impairment has occurred to begin instituting therapy.

- The evidence that patients with pulmonary disease reap psychological, psychosocial, or behavior benefits from pulmonary rehabilitation is weak. Well-controlled studies using validated measures of psychological and behavior functioning are needed. A standardized and accepted tool for assessing quality of life changes in patients with respiratory disease would be beneficial.

- Each member of the pulmonary rehabilitation team needs to be aware of the factors that can lead to failure of rehabilitation so that the potential for success can be optimized. Reasons for failure include lack of competent and dedicated medical supervision, inclusion of inappropriate patients, lack of individualization so that the very sick and the nearly well receive the same treatment, poor communication with referring physicians, lack of objective documentation, excessive commercialization, poor organization of the program, lack of personal access between the patients and the program on an ongoing basis, failure to establish realistic goals, and lack of flexibility in the therapeutic offerings.

- One of the major limitations continues to be the failure of many primary care physicians and even pulmonologists to refer their pulmonary patients for rehabilitation. Teams must redouble their efforts to familiarize these physicians with the benefits of rehabilitation.

- The problem of inadequate reimbursement for pulmonary rehabilitation in some areas needs to be resolved. Third-party payers must be educated about the cost savings (e.g., reduction in hospital days) that can be achieved through pulmonary rehabilitation. Further studies proving the cost-effectiveness of pulmonary rehabilitation are needed.

- Steps should be taken to ensure that the special needs and problems of respiratory patients are incorporated into the curricula of allied health schools, including nursing, respiratory therapy, physical therapy, occupational therapy, and dietetics. Psychologists, psychiatrists, chaplains, social workers, and others involved in counseling patients and their families need to be knowledgeable about the special needs of respiratory patients to fully meet their needs.

- The routine use of spirometry in the office can assist in identifying respiratory disease before clinical signs and symptoms appear. Decreasing the number of persons who smoke remains the key to a major reduction in disability from respiratory disease.

- The optimal duration of a pulmonary rehabilitation program has not yet been determined. Further studies are needed to determine how best to maintain the benefits achieved from pulmonary rehabilitation programs for a longer period of time.

- The value of pulmonary rehabilitation in patients with chronic respiratory impairment due to diseases other than COPD and asthma has been reported, but more data would help clarify the specific components of pulmonary rehabilitation that are needed to treat these individuals.

- Further studies are needed on the potential value of neuromuscular electrical stimulation of peripheral muscles to elicit beneficial training effects for those with severe peripheral muscle dysfunction.[226,227]

- More thorough evaluation of the role, if any, for the use of anabolic steroids combined with pulmonary rehabilitation is needed.

- The number of pulmonary rehabilitation programs needs to be increased so it can be available to all patients with chronic lung disease who need rehabilitation.

- More studies to clarify the value of the non-exercise components of pulmonary rehabilitation would be helpful.

- Studies are needed to clarify whether O_2 supplementation in patients during exercise training sessions is useful when they do not use O_2 during the remainder of the day.

- More data are needed to assess the potential value of O_2 supplementation in patients who are hypoxemic only while asleep.

- Further evaluation of the role of NPPV during exercise training and at night in patients with severe COPD and hypercapnia is needed.

- Whether or not nutritional support can more effectively improve function and outcome in malnourished and underweight patients with COPD needs further research.

- The potential that erythropoietin therapy could help patients with COPD who have chronic anemia, as it has those with chronic renal disease, deserves to be assessed.

CONCLUSION

This chapter has reviewed the current thinking regarding the benefits of pulmonary rehabilitation and has mentioned some of the future challenges. It is satisfying to have seen pulmonary rehabilitation evolve from an underutilized resource with many critics, in the 1970s, to its current status as the standard of care for patients with chronic lung disease in the 21st century.

References

1. Pauwels RA, Buist AS, Calverly PM et al. GOLD Scientific Committee: Global strategy for the diagnosis, management, and prevention of chronic obstructive pulmonary disease. NHLBI/WHO Global Initiative for Chronic Obstructive Lung Disease (GOLD) workshop summary, Am J Respir Crit Care Med 163:1256-1276, 2001. Available at http://www.goldcopd.com (last major revision, November 2006). Retrieved June 5, 2008.
2. American Thoracic Society/European Respiratory Society: Statement on pulmonary rehabilitation, Am J Respir Crit Care Med 173:1390-1413, 2006. Available at http://www.thoracic.org/sections/publications/statements/index.html. Retrieved June 5, 2008.
3. Troosters T, Casaburi R, Gosselink R et al: Pulmonary rehabilitation in chronic obstructive pulmonary disease [state of the art]. Am J Respir Crit Care Med 172:19-38, 2005.
4. American Thoracic Society/European Respiratory Society Task Force: Standards for the diagnosis and management of patients with COPD [Internet], version 1.2. New York, American Thoracic Society, 2004. Available at http://www.thoracic.org/go/copd (last updated September 8, 2005). Retrieved June 5, 2008.
5. ACCP-AACVPR Pulmonary Rehabilitation Guidelines Panel: Pulmonary rehabilitation: joint ACCP/AACVPR evidence-based guidelines, J Cardiopulm Rehabil 17:371-405, 1997.
6. Ries AL, Bauldoff GS, Carlin BW et al: Pulmonary rehabilitation: joint ACCP/AACVPR evidence-based clinical practice guidelines, Chest 131(5 suppl):4S-42S, 2007.
7. Fishman DB, Petty TL: Physical, symptomatic, and psychological improvement in patients receiving comprehensive care for chronic airway obstruction, J Chronic Dis 24:775-785, 1971.
8. Agle DP, Baum GL, Chester EH et al: Multidiscipline treatment of chronic pulmonary insufficiency. 1. Psychologic aspects of rehabilitation, Psychosom Med 35:41-49, 1973.
9. Dudley DL, Glaser EM, Jorgenson BN et al: Psychosocial concomitants to rehabilitation in chronic obstructive pulmonary disease, Chest 77:413-420, 544-551, 677-684, 1980.
10. Kass I, Dyksterhuis JE: The Nebraska COPD Rehabilitation Project: a program to identify the factors involved in the rehabilitation of patients with chronic obstructive pulmonary disease: a multidisciplinary study of 140 patients. Omaha, Neb. 1971, University of Nebraska. Final Report, Social and Rehabilitation Service, DHEW Project RD-2517-m.
11. Daughton DM, Fix AJ, Kass I et al: Physiological—intellectual components of rehabilitation success in patients with chronic obstructive pulmonary disease (COPD), J Chronic Dis 32:405-409, 1979.
12. Miller WF, Taylor HF, Pierce AK: Rehabilitation of the disabled patient with chronic bronchitis and pulmonary emphysema, Am J Public Health 53:18-24, 1963.
13. Haas A, Cardon H: Rehabilitation in chronic obstructive pulmonary disease: a five-year study of 252 male patients, Med Clin North Am 53:593-606, 1969.
14. Cherniack RM, Handford RG, Svanhill E: Home care of chronic respiratory disease, JAMA 208:821-824, 1969.
15. Petty TL, Nett LM, Finigan MM et al: A comprehensive care program for chronic airway obstruction: methods and preliminary evaluation of symptomatic and functional improvement, Ann Intern Med 70:1109-1120, 1969.
16. Kimbel P, Kaplan AS, Alkalay I et al: An in-hospital program for rehabilitation of patients with chronic obstructive pulmonary disease, Chest 60(suppl):6S-10S, 1971.
17. Moser RM: Rehabilitation of the COPD patient: lesson 40. in Weekly update: pulmonary medicine, Princeton, NJ, 1979, Biomedia.
18. Balchum OJ: Rehabilitation in chronic obstructive pulmonary disease, Arch Environ Health 16:614, 1968.
19. Pierce AK, Paez PN, Miller WF: Exercise therapy with the aid of a portable oxygen supply in patients with emphysema, Am Rev Respir Dis 91:653-659, 1965.
20. Miller WF: Rehabilitation of patients with chronic obstructive lung disease, Med Clin North Am 51:349-361, 1967.
21. Woolf CR, Suero JT: Alterations in lung mechanics and gas exchange following training in chronic obstructive lung disease, Dis Chest 55:37-44, 1969.
22. Bass H, Whitcomb JF, Forman R: Exercise training: therapy for patients with chronic obstructive pulmonary disease, Chest 57:116-121, 1970.
23. Rusk HA: Pulmonary problems. In Rehabilitation medicine, ed 3, St. Louis, 1971, CV Mosby.
24. McGavin CR, Gupta SP, Lloyd EL et al: Physical rehabilitation of chronic bronchitis: results of a controlled trial of exercises in the home, Thorax 32:307-311, 1977.
25. Chester EH, Belman MJ, Bahler RC et al: Mutlidisciplinary treatment of chronic pulmonary insufficiency. 3. The effect of physical training on cardiopulmonary performance in patients with

chronic obstructive pulmonary disease, Chest 72:695-702, 1977.

26. Cockcroft AE, Saunders MT, Berry G: Randomized controlled trial of rehabilitation in chronic respiratory disability, Thorax 36:200, 1981.

27. Holle RH, Williams DV, Vandree JC et al: Increased muscle efficiency and sustained benefits in an outpatient community hospital-based pulmonary rehabilitation program, Chest 94:1161-1168, 1988.

28. Carter R, Nicotra B, Clark L et al: Exercise conditioning in the rehabilitation of patients with chronic obstructive pulmonary disease, Arch Phys Med Rehabil 69:118-122, 1988.

29. Mall RW, Medeiros M: Objective evaluation of results of a pulmonary rehabilitation program in a community hospital, Chest 94:1156-1160, 1988.

30. Strijbos JH, Koeter GH, Meinesz AF: Home care rehabilitation and perception of dyspnea in chronic obstructive pulmonary disease (COPD) patients, Chest 97:109s-110s, 1990.

31. Ries AL, Kaplan RM, Limberg TM et al: Effects of pulmonary rehabilitation on physiologic and psychosocial outcomes in patients with chronic obstructive pulmonary disease, Ann Intern Med 122:823-832, 1995.

32. Wijkstra PJ, Van der Mark TW, Kraan J et al: Effects of home rehabilitation on physical performance in patients with chronic obstructive pulmonary disease (COPD), Eur Respir J 9:104-110, 1996.

33. Strijbos JH, Postma DS, Van Altena R et al: A comparison between an outpatient hospital-based pulmonary rehabilitation program and a home-care pulmonary rehabilitation program in patients with COPD, Chest 109:366-372, 1996.

34. Goldstein RS, Gort EH, Stubbing D et al: Randomised controlled trial of respiratory rehabilitation, Lancet 344:1394-1397, 1994.

35. Bendstrup KE, Ingemann Jensen J, Holm S et al: Out-patient rehabilitation improves activities of daily living, quality of life and exercise tolerance in chronic obstructive pulmonary disease, Eur Respir J 10:2801-2806, 1997.

36. Casaburi R, Patessio A, Ioli F et al: Reductions in exercise lactic acidosis and ventilation as a result of exercise training in patients with obstructive lung disease, Am Rev Respir Dis 143:9-18, 1991.

37. Casaburi R, Wasserman K, Patessio A et al: A new perspective in pulmonary rehabilitation: an-aerobic threshold as a discriminant in training, Eur Respir J 2(suppl 7):618s-623s, 1989.

38. Maltais F, Leblanc P, Simard C et al: Skeletal muscle adaptation to endurance training in patients with chronic obstructive pulmonary disease, Am J Respir Crit Care Med 154:442-447, 1996.

39. Maltais F, Leblanc P, Jobin J et al: Intensity of training and physiologic adaptation in patients with chronic obstructive pulmonary disease, Am J Respir Crit Care Med 155:555-561, 1997.

40. Casaburi R, Porszasz J, Burns MR et al: Physiologic benefits of exercise training in rehabilitation of patients with severe chronic obstructive pulmonary disease, Am J Respir Crit Care Med 155:1541-1551, 1997.

41. Horowitz MB, Littenberg B, Mahler DA: Dyspnea ratings for prescribing exercise intensity in patients with COPD, Chest 109:1169-1175, 1996.

42. Punzal PA, Ries AL, Kaplan RM et al: Maximum intensity exercise training in patients with chronic obstructive pulmonary disease, Chest 100:618-623, 1991.

43. Celli BR: Pulmonary rehabilitation in patients with COPD, Am J Respir Crit Care Med 152:861-864, 1995.

44. Lake FR, Henderson K, Briffa T et al: Upper-limb and lower-limb exercise training in patients with chronic airflow obstruction, Chest 97:1077-1082, 1990.

45. Reardon J, Awad E, Normandin E et al: The effect of comprehensive outpatient pulmonary rehabilitation on dyspnea, Chest 105:1046-1052, 1994.

46. Grosbois J-M, Lamblin C, Lemaire B et al: Long-term benefits of exercise maintenance after out-patient rehabilitation program in patients with chronic obstructive pulmonary disease, J Cardiopulm Rehabil 19:216-225, 1999.

47. O'Donnell DE, McGuire M, Samis L et al: The impact of exercise reconditioning on breathlessness in severe chronic airflow limitation, Am J Respir Crit Care Med 152:2005-2013, 1995.

48. Casaburi R: Mechanisms of the reduced ventilatory requirement as a result of exercise training, Eur Respir Rev 5:42-46, 1995.

49. Atkins CJ, Kaplan RM, Timms RM et al: Behavioral exercise programs in the management of chronic obstructive pulmonary disease, J Consult Clin Psychol 52:591-603, 1984.

50. Guyatt GH, Berman LB, Townsend M: Long-term outcome after respiratory rehabilitation, Can Med Assoc J 137:1089-1095, 1987.

51. Wijkstra PJ, Van Altena R, Krann J et al: Quality of life in patients with chronic obstructive pulmonary disease improves after rehabilitation at home, Eur Respir J 7:269-273, 1994.

52. Wedzicha JA, Bestall JC, Garrod R et al: Randomized controlled trial of pulmonary rehabilitation in severe chronic obstructive pulmonary disease patients, stratified with the MRC Dyspnoea Scale, Eur Respir J 12:363-369, 1998.

53. Wijkstra PJ: Pulmonary rehabilitation at home [editorial], Thorax 51:117-118, 1996.

54. Vale F, Reardon JZ, ZuWallack RL: The long-term benefits of outpatient pulmonary rehabilitation on exercise endurance and quality of life, Chest 103:42-45, 1993.

55. Griffiths TL, Burr ML, Campbell IA et al: Results at 1 year of outpatient multidisciplinary pulmonary rehabilitation: a randomized clinical trial, Lancet 355:362-368, 2000.

56. Finnerty JP, Keeping I, Bullough I et al: The effectiveness of outpatient pulmonary rehabilitation in chronic lung disease: a randomized controlled trial, Chest 119:1705-1710, 2001.

57. Troosters T, Gosselink R, Decramer M: Short- and long-term effects of outpatient rehabilitation in patients with chronic obstructive pulmonary disease: a randomised trial, Am J Med 109:207-212, 2000.

58. Reardon J, Patel K, ZuWallack RL: Improvement in quality of life is unrelated to improvement in exercise

endurance after outpatient pulmonary rehabilitation, J Cardiopulm Rehabil 13:51-54, 1993.

59. Strijbos JH, Sluiter HJ, Postma DS et al: Objective and subjective performance indicators in COPD, Eur Respir J 2:666-669, 1989.

60. Reardon J, Awad E, Normandin E et al: The effect of comprehensive outpatient pulmonary rehabilitation on dyspnea, Chest 105:1046-1052, 1994.

61. American Thoracic Society: Dyspnea: mechanisms, assessment, and management: a consensus statement, Am J Respir Crit Care Med 159:321-340, 1999.

62. Petty TL, MacIlroy ER, Swigert MA et al: Chronic airway obstruction, respiratory insufficiency, and gainful employment, Arch Environ Health 21:71-78, 1970.

63. Lustig FM, Haas A, Castillo R: Clinical and rehabilitation regime in patients with chronic obstructive pulmonary disease, Arch Phys Med Rehabil 53:315-322, 1972.

64. Kass I, Dyksterhuis JE, Rubin H et al: Correlation of psychophysiological variables with vocational rehabilitation outcome in patients with chronic obstructive pulmonary disease, Chest 67:433-440, 1975.

65. Fix AJ, Daughton D, Kass I et al: Personality traits affecting vocational rehabilitation success in patients with chronic obstructive pulmonary disease, Psychol Rep 43:939-944, 1978.

66. Lacasse Y, Goldstein R, Lasserson TJ et al: Pulmonary rehabilitation for chronic obstructive pulmonary disease, Cochrane Database Syst Rev 4:CD003793, 2006.

67. American Thoracic Society: Pulmonary rehabilitation, Am Rev Respir Dis 124:663-666, 1981.

68. Burton GG, Gee G, Hodgkin JE et al: Respiratory care warrants studies for cost-effectiveness, Hospitals 49:61-71, 1975.

69. Hudson LD, Tyler ML, Petty TL: Hospitalization needs during an outpatient rehabilitation program for severe chronic airway obstruction, Chest 70:606-610, 1976.

70. Lertzman MM, Cherniack RM: Rehabilitation of patients with chronic obstructive pulmonary disease, Am Rev Respir Dis 114:1145-1165, 1976.

71. Jensen PS: Risk, protective factors, and supportive interventions in chronic airway obstruction, Arch Gen Psychiatry 40:1203-1207, 1983.

72. Johnson HR, Tanzi F, Balcham OJ et al: Inpatient comprehensive pulmonary rehabilitation in severe COPD, Respir Ther May/June: 15-19, 1980.

73. Nichol J, Hodgkin JE, Connors G et al: Strategies for developing a cost-effective pulmonary rehabilitation program, Respir Care 28:1451-1455, 1983.

74. Sneider R, O'Malley JA, Kahn M: Trends in pulmonary rehabilitation at Eisenhower Medical Center: an 11-years' experience (1976-1987), J Cardiopulm Rehabil 8:453-461, 1988.

75. Lewis D, Bell SK: Pulmonary rehabilitation, psychosocial adjustment and use of healthcare services, Rehabil Nurs 20:102, 1995.

76. Sahn SA, Nett LM, Petty TL: Ten-year follow-up of a comprehensive rehabilitation program for severe COPD, Chest 77:311-314, 1980.

77. Wright RW, Larsen DF, Monie RG et al: Benefits of a community-hospital pulmonary rehabilitation program, Respir Care 28:1474-1479, 1983.

78. Griffiths TL, Phillips CJ, Davies S et al: Cost-effectiveness of an outpatient multidisciplinary pulmonary rehabilitation programme, Thorax 56:779-784, 2001.

79. Goldstein RS, Gort EH, Guyatt GH et al: Economic analysis of respiratory rehabilitation, Chest 112:370-379, 1997.

80. Ferris BG Jr, Anderson DO, Zickmantel R: Prediction values for screening tests of pulmonary function, Am Rev Respir Dis 91:252, 1965.

81. Kory RC, Callahan R, Boren HG et al: Veterans Administration—Army cooperative study of pulmonary function. 1. Clinical spirometry in normal men, Am J Med 30:243, 1961.

82. Burrows B, Earle RH: Course and prognosis of chronic obstructive lung disease, N Engl J Med 280:397, 1969.

83. Boushy SF, Thompson HK, North LB et al: Prognosis in chronic obstructive pulmonary disease, Am Rev Respir Dis 108:1373-1382, 1973.

84. Diener CF, Burrows B: Further observations on the course and prognosis of chronic obstructive lung disease, Am Rev Respir Dis 111:719, 1975.

85. Emergil C, Sobol BJ: Long-term course of chronic obstructive pulmonary disease: a new view of the mode of functional deterioration, Am J Med 51:504, 1971.

86. Postma DS, Burema J, Gimeno F et al: Prognosis in severe chronic obstructive pulmonary disease, Am Rev Respir Dis 119:357, 1979.

87. Rezetti AD Jr, McClement JH, Litt BD: The Veterans Administration Cooperative Study of Pulmonary Function. III. Mortality in relation to respiratory function in chronic obstructive pulmonary disease, Am J Med 41:115, 1966.

88. Davis AL, McClement JH: The course and prognosis of chronic obstructive pulmonary disease. In Current research in chronic respiratory disease: Proceedings of the 11th Aspen Emphysema Conference, Arlington, Va, 1968, Department of Health, Education, and Welfare, p 219.

89. Porszasz J, Emtner M, Whipp BJ et al: Endurance training decreases exercise-induced dynamic hyperinflation in patients with COPD, Eur Respir J 22:205s, 2003.

90. Medical Research Council Working Party: Long-term domiciliary oxygen therapy in chronic hypoxic cor pulmonale complicating chronic bronchitis and emphysema, Lancet 1:681-686, 1981.

91. Nocturnal Oxygen Therapy Trial Group: Continuous or nocturnal oxygen therapy in hypoxemic chronic obstructive pulmonary disease: a clinical trial, Ann Intern Med 93:391-398, 1980.

92. Petty TL: Pulmonary rehabilitation, Am Rev Respir Dis 122(suppl):159-161, 1980.

93. Bebout DE, Hodgkin JE, Zorn EG et al: Clinical and physiological outcomes of a university-hospital pulmonary rehabilitation program, Respir Care 28:1468-1473, 1983.

94. Hodgkin JE, Branscomb BV, Anholm JD et al: Benefits, limitations and the future of pulmonary

rehabilitation. In Hodgkin JE, Zorn EG, Connors GL, editors: Pulmonary rehabilitation: guidelines to success, Boston, 1984, Butterworth.

95. Postma DS, Sluiter HJ: Prognosis of chronic obstructive pulmonary disease: the Dutch experience, Am Rev Respir Dis 140(suppl):S100, 1989.

96. Burns MR, Sherman B, Madison R et al: Pulmonary rehabilitation outcome, J Respir Care Pract 2:25-30, 1989.

97. Anthonisen NR, Wright EC, Hodgkin JE et al: Prognosis in chronic obstructive pulmonary disease, Am Rev Respir Dis 133:14-20, 1986.

98. Cote CG, Celli BR: Pulmonary rehabilitation and the BODE Index in COPD, Eur Respir J 26:630-636, 2005.

99. Martinez FJ, Foster G, Curtis JL et al: Predictors of mortality in patients with emphysema and severe airflow obstruction, Am J Respir Crit Care Med 173:1326-1334, 2006.

100. Celli BR: Predicting mortality in chronic obstructive pulmonary disease: chasing the "Holy Grail", Am J Respir Crit Care Med 173:1298-1299, 2006.

101. Foster S, Thomas HM: Pulmonary rehabilitation in lung disease other than chronic obstructive pulmonary disease, Am Rev Respir Dis 141:601-604, 1990.

102. Crouch R, MacIntyre NR: Pulmonary rehabilitation of the patient with nonobstructive lung disease, Respir Care Clin North Am 4:59-70, 1998.

103. Ando M, Mori A, Esaki H et al: The effect of pulmonary rehabilitation in patients with post-tuberculosis lung disorder, Chest 123:1988-1995, 2003.

104. Ferreira G, Feuerman M, Spiegler P: Results of an 8-week, outpatient pulmonary rehabilitation program on patients with and without chronic obstructive pulmonary disease, J Cardiopulm Rehabil 26:54-60, 2006.

105. Gilmartin ME: Patient and family education, Clin Chest Med 7:619-627, 1986.

106. Neish CM, Hopp JW: The role of education in pulmonary rehabilitation. In Hodgkin JE, editor: Pulmonary Rehabilitation Symposium, J Cardiopulm Rehabil 11:439-441, 1988.

107. Ashikaga T, Vacek PM, Lewis SO: Evaluation of a community-based education program for individuals with chronic obstructive pulmonary disease, J Rehabil Res Dev 46:23-27, 1980.

108. Hopp JW, Lee JW, Hills R: Development and validation of a pulmonary rehabilitation knowledge test, J Cardiopulm Rehabil 7:273-280, 1989.

109. Toshima MT, Kaplan RM, Ries AL: Experimental evaluation of rehabilitation in chronic obstructive pulmonary disease: short-term effects on exercise endurance and health status, Health Psychol 9:237-252, 1990.

110. Bourbeau J, Julien M, Maltais F et al: Reduction of hospital utilization in patients with chronic obstructive pulmonary disease: a disease-specific self-management intervention, Arch Intern Med 163:585-591, 2003.

111. Wilson DO, Rogers RM, Wright EC et al: Body weight in chronic obstructive pulmonary disease: the National Institutes of Health Intermittent Positive Pressure Breathing Trial, Am Rev Respir Dis 139:1435-1438, 1989.

112. Schols AMWJ, Slangen J, Volovics L et al: Weight loss is a reversible factor in the prognosis of chronic obstructive pulmonary disease, Am J Respir Crit Care Med 157:1791-1797, 1998.

113. Gray-Donald K, Gibbons L, Shapiro SH et al: Nutritional status and mortality in chronic obstructive pulmonary disease, Am J Respir Crit Care Med 153:961-966, 1996.

114. Arora NS, Rochester DF: Respiratory muscle strength and maximal voluntary ventilation in undernourished patients, Am Rev Respir Dis 126:5-8, 1982.

115. Steiner MC, Barton RL, Singh SJ et al: Nutritional enhancement of exercise performance in chronic obstructive pulmonary disease: a randomised controlled trial, Thorax 58:745-751, 2003.

116. Schols AM, Soeters PB, Mostert R et al: Physiologic effects of nutritional support and anabolic steroids in patients with chronic obstructive pulmonary disease: a placebo-controlled randomized trial, Am J Respir Crit Care Med 152:1268-1274, 1995.

117. Creutzberg EC, Wouters EF, Mostert R et al: Efficacy of nutritional supplementation therapy in depleted patients with chronic obstructive pulmonary disease, Nutrition 19:120-127, 2003.

118. Ferreira IM, Brooks D, Lacasse Y et al: Nutritional supplementation in stable chronic obstructive pulmonary disease, Cochrane Database Syst Rev 3:CD000998, 2000.

119. Prescott E, Almdal T, Mikkelsen KL et al: Prognostic value of weight change in chronic obstructive pulmonary disease: results from the Copenhagen City Heart Study, Eur Respir J 20:539-544, 2002.

120. Whittaker LA, Brodeur LE, Rochester CL: functional outcome of inpatient pulmonary rehabilitation for patients with morbid obesity [abstract]. Am J Respir Crit Care Med 161:A495, 2000.

121. Guerneli J, Wainapel SF, Pack S et al: Morbidly obese patients with pulmonary disease: a retrospective study of four cases, Am J Phys Med Rehabil 78:60-65, 1999.

122. Wilson DO, Rogers RM, Sanders MH et al: Nutritional intervention in malnourished patients with emphysema. Am Rev Respir Dis 134:672-677, 1986.

123. Doekel RC, Zwillich CW, Scoggin CH et al: Clinical semistarvation: depression of hypoxic ventilatory response, N Engl J Med 295:358-361, 1976.

124. Askanazi J, Weissman C, La Sala PA et al: Effect of protein intake on ventilatory drive, Anesthesiology 60:106, 1984.

125. Rogers RM, Donahoe M, Costantino J: Physiologic effects of oral supplemental feeding in malnourished patients with chronic obstructive pulmonary disease, Am Rev Respir Dis 146:1511-1517, 1992.

126. Efthimiou J, Fleming J, Gomez C et al: The effect of supplementary oral nutrition in poorly nourished patients with chronic obstructive pulmonary disease, Am Rev Respir Dis 137:1075-1082, 1988.

127. Buist AS, Nagy JM, Sexton GJ: Effect of smoking cessation on pulmonary function: a 30-month follow-up to two smoking cessation clinics, Am Rev Respir Dis 120:953, 1979.

128. Camilli AE, Burrows B, Knudson RJ et al: Longitudinal changes in forced expiratory volume in one second in adults, Am Rev Respir Dis 135:794, 1987.

129. Anthonisen NR, Connett JE, Murray RP et al: Smoking and lung function of Lung Health Study participants after 11 years, Am J Respir Crit Care Med 166:675-679, 2002.

130. Kark JD, Lebiush M, Rannon L: Cigarette smoking as a risk factor for epidemic A(H1N1) influenza in young men, N Engl J Med 307:1042-1046, 1982.

131. Anthonisen NR, Skeans MA, Wise RA et al: The effects of a smoking cessation intervention on 14.5-year mortality, Ann Intern Med 142:233-239, 2005.

132. Young P, Dewse M, Fergusson W et al: Improvements in outcomes for chronic obstructive pulmonary disease (COPD) attributable to a hospital-based respiratory rehabilitation programme, Aust N Z J Med 29:59-65, 1999.

133. Butler JC, Shapiro ED, Carlone GM: Pneumococcal vaccines: history, current status, and future directions, Am J Med 107:69S, 1999.

134. Belman MJ, Botnick WC, Shin JW: Inhaled bronchodilators reduce dynamic hyperinflation during exercise in patients with chronic obstructive pulmonary disease, Am J Respir Crit Care Med 153:967-975, 1996.

135. O'Donnell DE, Lam M, Webb KA: Spirometric correlates of improvement in exercise performance after anticholinergic therapy in chronic obstructive pulmonary disease, Am J Respir Crit Care Med 160:542-549, 1999.

136. O'Donnell DE, Voduc N, Fitzpatrick M et al: Effect of salmeterol on the ventilatory response to exercise in COPD, Eur Respir J 24:86-94, 2004.

137. Casaburi R, Kukafka D, Cooper CB et al: Improvement in exercise tolerance with the combination of tiotropium and pulmonary rehabilitation in patients with COPD, Chest 127:809-817, 2005.

138. Casaburi R: Rationale for anabolic therapy to facilitation rehabilitation in chronic obstructive pulmonary disease, Baillieres Clin Endocrinol Metab 12:407-418, 1998.

139. Hartgens F, Kuipers H: Effects of androgenic—anabolic steroids in athletes, Sports Med 34:513-554, 2004.

140. Casaburi R, Storer T, Bhasin D: Testosterone effects on body composition and muscle performance. In Bhasin D, Gabelnick H, Spieler J et al, editors: Biology, pharmacology and clinical applications of androgens, New York, 1996, Wiley Liss, pp 283-288.

141. Calverley PMA, Anderson JA, Celli B et al: Salmeterol and fluticasone propionate and survival in chronic obstructive pulmonary disease, N Engl J Med 356:775-789, 2007.

142. Rabe KF: Treating COPD: the TORCH trial, P values, and the dodo, N Engl J Med 356: 851-854, 2007.

143. Barach AL: Ambulatory oxygen therapy: oxygen inhalation at home and out of doors, Dis Chest 35:229-241, 1959.

144. Bradley BL, Garner AE, Billiu D et al: Oxygen-assisted exercise in chronic obstructive lung disease: the effect on exercise capacity and arterial blood gas tensions, Am Rev Respir Dis 118:239-243, 1978.

145. Cotes JE, Gilson JC: Effect of oxygen on exercise ability in chronic respiratory insufficiency, Lancet 1:872, 1956.

146. Leggett RJE, Flenley DC: Portable oxygen and exercise tolerance in patients with chronic hypoxic cor pulmonale, BMJ 2:84, 1977.

147. Stein DA, Bradley BL, Miller WC: Mechanisms of oxygen effects on exercise in patients with chronic obstructive pulmonary disease, Chest 81:6-10, 1982.

148. O'Donnell DE, D'Arsigny C, Webb KA: Effects of hyperoxia on ventilatory limitation in advanced COPD, Am J Respir Crit Care Med 163: 892-898, 2001.

149. Emtner M, Porszasz J, Burns M et al: Benefits of supplemental oxygen in exercise training in nonhypoxemic chronic obstructive pulmonary disease patients, Am J Respir Crit Care Med 168:1034-1042, 2003.

150. Somfay A, Porszasz J, Lee SM et al: Dose—response effect of oxygen on hyperinflation and exercise endurance in nonhypoxaemic COPD patients, Eur Respir J 18:77-84, 2001.

151. Fujimoto K, Matsuzawa Y, Yamaguchi S et al: Benefits of oxygen on exercise performance and pulmonary hemodynamics in patients with COPD with mild hypoxemia, Chest 122:457-463, 2002.

152. Brusasco V, Pellegrino R: Oxygen in the rehabilitation of patients with chronic obstructive pulmonary disease: an old tool revisited, Am J Respir Crit Care Med 168:1021-1022, 2003.

153. Garrod R, Paul EA, Wedzicha JA: Supplemental oxygen during pulmonary rehabilitation in patients with COPD with exercise hypoxaemia, Thorax 55:539-543, 2000.

154. Rooyackers JM, Dekhuijzen PN, van Herwaarden CL et al: Training with supplemental oxygen in patients with COPD and hypoxaemia at peak exercise, Eur Respir J 10:1278-1284, 1997.

155. Wadell K, Henriksson-Larsen K, Lundgren R: Physical training with and without oxygen in patients with chronic obstructive pulmonary disease and exercise-induced hypoxaemia, J Rehabil Med 33:200-205, 2001.

156. Intermittent Positive-Pressure Breathing Trial Group: Intermittent positive-pressure breathing therapy of chronic obstructive disease, Ann Intern Med 99:612-620, 1983.

157. Garrod R, Mikelsons C, Paul EA et al: Randomized controlled trial of domiciliary noninvasive positive pressure ventilation and physical training in severe chronic obstructive pulmonary disease, Am J Respir Crit Care Med 162: 1335-1341, 2000.

158. Sexton DL: Relaxation techniques and biofeedback. In Hodgkin JE, Petty TL, editors: Chronic obstructive pulmonary disease: current concepts, Philadelphia, 1987, WB Saunders, pp 99-112.

159. Gift AG, Moore T, Soeken K: Relaxation to reduce dyspnea and anxiety in COPD patients, Nurs Res 41:242, 1992.

160. American Thoracic Society: Pulmonary rehabilitation—1999, Am J Respir Crit Care Med 159:1666-1682, 1999.

161. Renfroe KL: Effect of progressive relaxation on dyspnea and anxiety in patients with chronic obstructive pulmonary disease, Heart Lung 17:408-413, 1988.

162. Benson H: The relaxation response, New York, 1975, Morrow.

163. Benson H, Kotch JB, Crassweller KD: The relaxation response: a bridge between psychiatry and medicine, Med Clin North Am 61:929-938, 1977.

164. Mueller RE, Petty TL, Filley GF: Ventilation and arterial blood gas changes induced by pursed lip breathing, J Appl Physiol 28:784-789, 1970.

165. Motley HL: The effects of slow deep breathing on the blood gas exchange in emphysema, Am Rev Respir Dis 88:484-492, 1963.

166. Paul G, Eldridge F, Mitchell J et al: Some effects of slowing respiration rate in chronic emphysema and bronchitis, J Appl Physiol 21:877, 1966.

167. Sergysels R, Willeput R, Lenders D et al: Low frequency breathing at rest and during exercise in severe chronic obstructive bronchitis, Thorax 34:536-539, 1979.

168. Thoman RL, Stoker GL, Ross JC: The efficacy of pursed-lips breathing in patients with chronic obstructive pulmonary disease, Am Rev Respir Dis 93:100-106, 1966.

169. Tiep BL, Burns M, Kao D et al: Pursed lips breathing training using ear oximetry, Chest 90:218-221, 1986.

170. Bianchi R, Gigliotti F, Romagnoli I et al: Chest wall kinematics and breathlessness during pursed-lip breathing in patients with COPD, Chest 125:459-465, 2004.

171. Breslin EH: The pattern of respiratory muscle recruitment during pursed-lip breathing, Chest 101:75-78, 1992.

172. Jones AY, Dean E, Chow CC: Comparison of the oxygen cost of breathing exercises and spontaneous breathing in patients with stable chronic obstructive pulmonary disease, Phys Ther 83:424-431, 2003.

173. Sharp JT, Drutz WS, Moisan T et al: Postural relief of dysnpea in severe chronic obstructive pulmonary disease, Am Rev Respir Dis 122:201-211, 1980.

174. Miller WF: A physiologic evaluation of the effects of diaphragmatic breathing training in patients with chronic pulmonary emphysema, Am J Med 17:471-477, 1954.

175. Willeput R, Vachaudez JP, Lenders D et al: Thoracoabdominal motion during chest physiotherapy in patients affected by chronic obstructive lung disease, Respiration 44:204-214, 1983.

176. Vitacca M, Clini E, Bianchi L et al: Acute effects of deep diaphragmatic breathing in COPD patients with chronic respiratory insufficiency, Eur Respir J 11:408-415, 1998.

177. Gosselink RA, Wagenaar RC, Rijswijk H et al: Diaphragmatic breathing reduces efficiency of breathing in patients with chronic obstructive pulmonary disease, Am J Respir Crit Care Med 151:1136-1142, 1995.

178. Leith DE, Bradley ME: Ventilatory muscle strength and endurance training, J Appl Physiol 41:508-510, 1976.

179. Peress L, McClean P, Woolf C et al: Respiratory muscle training in severe chronic obstructive pulmonary disease, Am Rev Respir Dis 119:157, 1979.

180. Celli BR: Respiratory muscle function, Clin Chest Med 7:567-584, 1986.

181. Pardy RL, Reid WD, Belman MJ: Respiratory muscle training, Clin Chest Med 9:287-296, 1988.

182. Belman MJ, Mittman D, Weir R: Ventilatory muscle training improves exercise capacity in chronic obstructive pulmonary disease patients, Am Rev Respir Dis 121:273-280, 1980.

183. Pardy RL, Rivington RN, Despas PJ et al: Inspiratory muscle training compared with physiotherapy in patients with chronic airflow limitation, Am Rev Respir Dis 123:421-425, 1981.

184. Larson JL, Kim MJ, Sharp JT et al: Inspiratory muscle training with a pressure threshold breathing device in patients with chronic obstructive pulmonary disease, Am Rev Respir Dis 138:689-696, 1988.

185. Lisboa C, Villafranca C, Leiva A et al: Inspiratory muscle training in chronic airflow limitation: effect on exercise performance, Eur Respir J 10:537-542, 1997.

186. Lotters F, Van Tol B, Kwakkel G et al: Effects of controlled inspiratory muscle training in patients with COPD: a meta-analysis, Eur Respir J 20:570-576, 2002.

187. Pryor JA, Webber BA, Hodson ME et al: Evaluation of the forced expiration technique as an adjunct to postural drainage in treatment of cystic fibrosis, BMJ 2:417-418, 1979.

188. Sutton PP, Parker RA, Webber BA et al: Assessment of the forced expiration technique, postural drainage and directed coughing in chest physiotherapy, Eur J Respir Dis 64:62-68, 1983.

189. Mahlmeister MJ, Fink JB, Hoffman GL et al: Positive-expiratory-pressure mask therapy: theoretical and practical considerations and a review of the literature, Respir Care 36:1218-1230, 1991.

190. AARC Clinical practice guideline: use of positive airway pressure adjuncts to bronchial hygiene therapy. American Association for Respiratory Care, Respir Care 38:516-521, 1993.

191. Jones AP, Rowe BH: Bronchopulmonary hygiene physical therapy for chronic obstructive pulmonary disease and bronchiectasis, Cochrane Database Syst Rev 2:CD000045, 2000.

192. Schols AM, Soeters PB, Dingemans AM et al: Prevalence and characteristics of nutritional depletion in patients with stable COPD eligible for pulmonary rehabilitation, Am Rev Respir Dis 147:1151-1156, 1993.

193. American Thoracic Society/European Respiratory Society: Skeletal muscle dysfunction in chronic obstructive pulmonary disease: a statement of the American Thoracic Society and European Respiratory Society, Am J Respir Crit Care Med 159:S1-S40, 1999.

194. Bernard S, Le Blanc P, Whittom F et al: Peripheral muscle weakness in patients with chronic obstructive pulmonary disease, Am J Respir Crit Care Med 158:629-634, 1998.

195. Gosselink R, Troosters T, Decramer M: Peripheral muscle weakness contributes to exercise limitation in COPD, Am J Respir Crit Care Med 153:976-980, 1996.

196. Ries AL, Archibald CJ: Endurance exercise training at maximal targets in patients with chronic obstructive pulmonary disease, J Cardiopulm Rehabil 7:594-601, 1987.

197. Wasserman K, Sue DY, Casaburi R et al: Selection criteria for exercise training in pulmonary rehabilitation, Eur Respir J 2(suppl 7): 604s-610s, 1989.

198. Puente-Maestu L, Sanz ML, Sanz P et al: Effects of two types of training on pulmonary and cardiac responses to moderate exercise in patients with COPD, Eur Respir J 15:1026-1032, 2000.

199. Sala E, Roca J, Marrades RM et al: Effects of endurance training on skeletal muscle bioenergetics in chronic obstructive pulmonary disease, Am J Respir Crit Care Med 159:1726-1734, 1999.

200. Bernard S, Whittom F, LeBlanc P et al: Aerobic and strength training in patients with chronic obstructive pulmonary disease, Am J Respir Crit Care Med 159:896-900, 1999.

201. Celli BR, Rassulo J, Make BJ: Dyssynchonous breathing during arm but not leg exercise in patients with chronic airflow obstruction, N Engl J Med 314:1485-1490, 1986.

202. Ries AL, Ellis B, Hawkins RW: Upper extremity exercise training in chronic obstructive pulmonary disease, Chest 93:688-692, 1988.

203. Ellis B, Ries AL: Upper extremity exercise training in pulmonary rehabilitation, J Cardiopulm Rehabil 11:227-231, 1991.

204. Martinez FJ, Vogel PD, Dupont DN et al: Supported arm exercise vs unsupported arm exercise in the rehabilitation of patients with severe chronic airflow obstruction, Chest 103:1397-1402, 1993.

205. Couser JI Jr, Martinez FJ, Celli BR: Pulmonary rehabilitation that includes arm exercise reduces metabolic and ventilatory requirements for simple arm elevation, Chest 103:37-41, 1993.

206. Spruit MA, Gosselink R, Troosters T et al: Resistance versus endurance training in patients with COPD and skeletal muscle weakness, Eur Respir J 19:1072-1078, 2002.

207. Ortega F, Toral J, Cejudo P et al: Comparison of effects of strength and endurance training in patients with chronic obstructive pulmonary disease, Am J Respir Crit Care Med 166:669-674, 2002.

208. Vogiatzis I, Nanas S, Roussos C: Interval training as an alternative modality to continuous exercise in patients with COPD, Eur Respir J 20:12-19, 2002.

209. Vogiatzis I, Nanas S, Kastanakis E et al: Dynamic hyperinflation and tolerance to interval exercise in patients with advanced COPD, Eur Respir J 24:385-390, 2004.

210. Sabapathy S, Kingsley RA, Schneider DA et al: Continuous and intermittent exercise responses in individuals with chronic obstructive pulmonary disease, Thorax 59:1026-1031, 2004.

211. Puhan MA, Büsching PT, Schünemann HJ et al: Interval versus continuous high-intensity exercise in chronic obstructive pulmonary disease: a randomized trial, Ann Intern Med 145: 816-825, 2006.

212. Green RH, Singh SJ, Williams J et al: A randomised controlled trial of four weeks versus seven weeks of pulmonary rehabilitation in chronic obsructive pulmonary disease, Thorax 56:143-145, 2001.

213. Guell R, Casan P, Belda J et al: Long-term effects of outpatient rehabilitation of COPD: a randomized trial, Chest 117:976-983, 2000.

214. Rossi G, Florini F, Romagnoli M et al: Length and clinical effectiveness of pulmonary rehabilitation in outpatients with chronic airway obstruction, Chest 127:105-109, 2005.

215. Berry MJ, Rejeski WJ, Adair NE et al: A randomized controlled trial comparing long-term and short-term exercise in patients with chronic obstructive pulmonary disease, J Cardiopulm Rehabil 23:60-68, 2003.

216. Lorenzi CM, Cilione C, Rizzardi R et al: Occupational therapy and pulmonary rehabilitation of disabled COPD patients, Respiration (Herrlisheim) 71:246-251, 2004.

217. Kim HF, Kunik ME, Molinari VA et al: Functional impairment in COPD patients: the impact of anxiety and depression, Psychosomatics 41: 456-471, 2000.

218. de Godoy DV, de Godoy RF: A randomized controlled trial of the effect of psychotherapy on anxiety and depression in chronic obstructive pulmonary disease, Arch Phys Med Rehabil 84:1154-1157, 2003.

219. McCathie HC, Spence SH, Tate RL: Adjustment to chronic obstructive pulmonary disease: the importance of psychological factors, Eur Respir J 19:47-53, 2002.

220. Matzen RV: Vocational rehabilitation: the culmination of physical reconditioning, Chest 60(suppl):21S, 1971.

221. Weinmann GC, Hyatt R: Evaluation and research in lung volume reduction surgery, Am J Respir Crit Care Med 154:1913-1918, 1996.

222. National Emphysema Treatment Trial Research Group: A randomized trial comparing lung-volume-reduction surgery with medical therapy for severe emphysema, N Engl J Med 348:2059-2073, 2003.

223. National Emphysema Treatment Trial Research Group: Cost-effectiveness of lung-volume-reduction surgery for patients with severe emphysema, N Engl J Med 348:2092-2102, 2003.

224. Trulock EP, Egan TM, Kouchoukos NT et al: Single lung transplantation for severe chronic obstructive pulmonary disease, Chest 96:738-742, 1989.

225. Goldstein RS, Hall MJ: Pulmonary rehabilitation before and after lung transplantation. In Fishman AP, editor: Pulmonary rehabilitation, New York, 1996, Marcel Dekker, p 739.

226. Neder JA, Sword D, Ward SA et al: Home based neuromuscular electrical stimulation as a new rehabilitative strategy for severely disabled patients with chronic obstructive pulmonary disease (COPD), Thorax 57:333-337, 2002.

227. Zanotti E, Felicetti G, Maini M et al: Peripheral muscle strength in bed-bound patients with COPD receiving mechanical ventilation: effect of electrical stimulation, Chest 124:292-296, 2003.

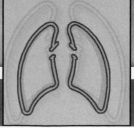

Credits

Chapter 1

Figure 1-1: Modified from National Heart, Lung, and Blood Institute, National Institutes of Health, Public Health Service, U.S. Department of Health and Human Services: Morbidity & mortality: 2007 chart book on cardiovascular, lung, and blood diseases. Available at http://www.nhlbi.nih.gov/resources/docs/07-chtbk.pdf. Retrieved July 21, 2008.

Chapter 4

Figure 4-1: Modified from Agustí AG: COPD, a multi-component disease: implications for management, Respir Med 99:670-682, 2005.

Chapter 5

Figure 5-3: Modified from American Thoracic Society: Dyspnea: mechanisms, assessment, and management [consensus statement], Am J Respir Crit Care Med 159:321-340, 1999.

Chapter 8

Figure 8-1: Modified from Raimondi AC, Schottlender J, Lombardi D et al: Treatment of acute severe asthma with inhaled albuterol delivered via jet nebulizer, metered dose inhaler with spacer, or dry powder, Chest 97:24-28, 1997.

Figure 8-2: From Hess D, MacIntyre N, Mishoe S et al. Respiratory care: principles & practice, Philadelphia, 2002, WB Saunders.

Figure 8-3: Modified from Hess D, Fisher D, Williams P et al: Medication nebulizer performance: effects of diluent volume, nebulizer flow and nebulizer brand, Chest 110:498-505, 1996.

Figure 8-4: From Rau JL Jr: Practical problems with aerosol therapy in COPD, Respir Care 57:158-172, 2006.

Figure 8-5: From Gardenhire DS: Rau's respiratory care pharmacology, ed 7, St. Louis, 2008, Mosby.

Figure 8-6: Modified from Wilkes W, Fink J, Dhand R: Selecting an accessory device with a metered-dose inhaler: variable influence of accessory devices on fine particle dose, throat deposition, and drug delivery with asynchronous actuation from a metered-dose inhaler, J Aerosol Med 14:351-360. 2001; as cited in Hess D, MacIntyre N, Mishoe S et al: Respiratory care: principles and practice, Philadelphia, 2002, WB Saunders.

Figure 8-7: Modified from materials courtesy 3M Corp. (St. Paul, Minn); as cited in Hess D, MacIntyre N, Mishoe S et al: Respiratory care: principles and practice, Philadelphia, 2002, WB Saunders.

Figure 8-8: Modified from Dhand R, Fink J: Respir Care 44:940, 1999; as cited in Hess D, MacIntyre N,

Mishoe S et al: Respiratory care: principles and practice, Philadelphia, 2002, WB Saunders.

Figure 8-9: Modified from Dhand R, Fink J: Respir Care 44:940, 1999; as cited in Hess D, MacIntyre N, Mishoe S et al: Respiratory care: principles and practice, Philadelphia, 2002, WB Saunders.

Chapter 12

Figure 12-1: Courtesy of the Pulmonary Rehabilitation Program, Inova Fairfax Hospital (Falls Church, Va).

Figure 12-2: Courtesy of the Pulmonary Rehabilitation Program, Duke University Medical Center (Durham, NC).

Figure 12-3: Courtesy of the Pulmonary Rehabilitation Program, Inova Fairfax Hospital (Falls Church, Va).

Figure 12-4: From Wilkins RL: Bedside assessment of the patient. In Wilkins RL, Stoller JK, Kacmarek RM: Egan's fundamentals of respiratory care, ed 9, St. Louis, 2009, Mosby.

Figure 12-6: Courtesy of the Pulmonary Rehabilitation Program, Inova Fairfax Hospital (Falls Church, Va).

Figure 12-7: Courtesy of the Pulmonary Rehabilitation Program, Duke University Medical Center (Durham, NC).

Chapter 13

Figure 13-1: Data from International Classification of Functioning, Disability and Health (ICF). Available at http://www.who.int/classifications/icf/en/. Retrieved January 2008.

Figure 13-3: From Byers-Cannon S, Lohman HL, Padilla RL: Occupational therapy with elders: strategies for the COTA, ed 2, St. Louis, 2004, Mosby.

Figure 13-4: From Byers-Cannon S, Lohman HL, Padilla RL: Occupational therapy with elders: strategies for the COTA, ed 2, St. Louis, 2004, Mosby.

Chapter 20

Figure 20-1: From Ries AL, Kaplan RM, Limberg TM et al: Effects of pulmonary rehabilitation on physiologic and psychosocial outcomes in patients with chronic obstructive pulmonary disease, Ann Intern Med 122:823-832, 1995.

Figure 20-2: From Eakin EG, Kaplan RM, Ries AL: Measurement of dyspnoea in chronic obstructive pulmonary disease, Qual Life Res 2:181-191, 1993.

Figure 20-3: From Heppner PS, Morgan C, Kaplan RM et al: Regular walking and long-term maintenance of outcomes after pulmonary rehabilitation, J Cardiopulm Rehabil 26:44-53, 2006.

Figure 20-4: Modified from Atkins CJ, Kaplan RM, Timms RM et al: Behavioral exercise programs in the management of chronic obstructive pulmonary disease, J Consult Clin Psychol 52:591-603, 1984.

Chapter 21

Figure 21-1: Modified from Casaburi R, Patessio A, Loli F et al: Reductions in exercise lactic acidosis and ventilation as a result of exercise training in patients with obstructive lung disease, Am Rev Respir Dis 143:9-18, 1991.

Figure 21-2: Modified from Ries AL, Kaplan RM, Limberg TM et al: Effects of pulmonary rehabilitation on physiologic and psychosocial outcomes in patients with chronic obstructive pulmonary disease, Ann Intern Med 122:823-832, 1995.

Figure 21-3: From Lacasse Y, Wong E, Guyatt GH et al: Meta-analysis of respiratory rehabilitation in chronic obstructive pulmonary disease, Lancet 348:1115-1119, 1996.

Figure 21-4: Data from Reardon J, Awad E, Normandin E et al: The effect of comprehensive outpatient pulmonary rehabilitation on dyspnea, Chest 105:1046-1052, 1994.

Figure 21-5: Data from Goldstein RS, Gort EH, Stubbing D et al: Randomized controlled trial of respiratory rehabilitation, Lancet 344:1394-1397, 1994.

Figure 21-6: From Shoup R, Dalsky G, Warner S et al: Body mass and quality of life in obstructive airway disease, Eur Respir J 10:1576-1580, 1997.

Figure 21-7: From Jones PW, Bosh TK: Quality of life changes in COPD treated with salmeterol, Am J Respir Crit Care Med 155:1283-1289, 1997.

Figure 21-8: From Leidy NK: Using functional status to assess treatment outcomes, Chest 106:1645-1646, 1994.

Figure 21-9: From Votto J, Bowen J, Scalise P et al: Short-stay comprehensive inpatient pulmonary rehabilitation for advanced chronic obstructive pulmonary disease, Arch Phys Med Rehabil 77:1115-1118, 1996.

Figure 21-10: Modified from Shoup R, Dalsky G, Warner S et al: Body composition and health-related quality of life in patients with obstructive airways disease, Eur Respir J 10:1576-1580, 1997.

Figure 21-11: From Cote CG, Celli BR: Pulmonary rehabilitation and the BODE Index in COPD, Eur Respir J 26:630-636, 2005.

Figure 21-12: From Ries AL, Kaplan RM, Limberg TM et al: Effects of pulmonary rehabilitation on physiologic and psychosocial outcomes in patients with chronic obstructive pulmonary disease, Ann Intern Med 122:823-832, 1995.

Figure 21-13: Courtesy Lorraine ZuWallack.

Chapter 23

Figure 23-1: From Nathan SD: Lung transplantation: disease-specific approach, Chest 127:1006-1016, 2005.

Chapter 24

Figure 24-1: Redrawn from Ries A, Make B, Lee S et al; for the National Emphysema Treatment Trial Research

Group: The effects of pulmonary rehabilitation in the National Emphysema Treatment Trial, Chest 128:3799-3809, 2005.

Chapter 28

Figure 28-1: Courtesy Respironics, Inc.

Figure 28-2: From Czervinske MP, Barnhart SL: Perinatal and pediatric respiratory care, Philadelphia, 2003, WB Saunders.

Figure 28-3: From Cairo JM, Pilbeam SP: Mosby's respiratory care equipment, ed 7, St. Louis, 2004, Mosby.

Figure 28-4: From Noble J: Textbook of primary care medicine, ed 3, St. Louis, 2001, Mosby.

Figure 28-5: From Wilkins RL, Stoller JK, Kacmarek RM: Egan's fundamentals of respiratory care, ed 9, St. Louis, 2009, Mosby.

Figure 28-6: Courtesy Respironics, Inc.

Chapter 29

Figure 29-1: Adapted from Krieger BP: Travel for the technology-dependent patient with lung disease, Clin Pulm Med 2:1-29, 1995; and Hecht H: A sea-level view of altitude problems, Am J Med 50:703-708, 1971.

Figure 29-2: Adapted from Hultgren H: High altitude medicine, Stanford, Calif, 1997, Hultgren Publications, Section 3, p 9.

Figure 29-3: Data from Graham WGB, Houston CS: Short-term adaptation to moderate altitude: patients with obstructive lung disease, JAMA 240:1491-1494, 1978.

Chapter 30

Figure 30-1: Courtesy Inova Fairfax Hospital (Falls Church, Va).

Chapter 32

Figure 32-2: Data from McLaughlin VV, Presberg KW, Doyle RL et al: Prognosis of pulmonary arterial hypertension: ACCP evidence-based clinical practice guidelines, Chest 126(1 suppl):78S-92S, 2004; adapted from Sitbon O, Humbert M, Nunes H et al: Long-term intravenous epoprostenol infusion in primary pulmonary hypertension: prognostic factors and survival, J Am Coll Cardiol 40:780-788, 2002; and D'Alonzo GE, Barst RJ, Ayres SM et al: Survival in patients with primary pulmonary hypertension: results of a national prospective registry, Ann Intern Med 115:343-349, 1991.

Chapter 34

Figure 34-1: From Anthonisen NR, Wright EC, Hodgkin JE et al: Prognosis in chronic obstructive pulmonary disease, Am Rev Respir Dis 133:14-20, 1986.

Index

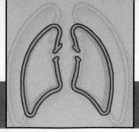

A

AACVPR. *See* American Association of Cardiovascular and Pulmonary Rehabilitation 472

AARP. *See* American Association of Retired Persons 288

Abdominal breathing, 51

ABG. *See* Arterial blood gas 117

Abnormal breathing patterns, occupational therapist observation, 192

Abnormal gas exchange, 130

Accessory muscles
  activity, loss, 425
  function, 25

Accessory respiratory muscles, activity (loss), 421

ACE, 108**f**

Acetylcysteine, usage. *See* Topical acetylcysteine 102
  limitation, induced bronchoconstriction (impact), 102

Acid-base balance, acute changes (ABG detection), 118

Acid-base status, state, 23

Acidosis, suspicion, 121

Active nicotine nasal spray, transdermal nicotine (combination), 250-251

Activities of daily living (ADLs), 275
  assessment, 13
  division, 343
  dyspnea
    association, 339
    relationship, 149
  exercise training, factor, 277
  initiation, 168
  participation, ability, 498
  performing, 343
  performing ability, 510
    improvement, 167

Activity
  dimensions, 190
  endurance, improvement, 168
  grading, 198
    therapeutic strategy, 198-199
  limitations, chronic conditions (impact), 3**t**
  loss, tracking, 45-46
  modification, 50, 202. *See also* Specific activities 203-204**t**
  performance, occupational therapist observation, 195**f**
  physical response monitoring, vital signs, 192**t**
  WHO International Classification, 182**f**

Activity-specific recommendations, 202

Acuity scoring, 440
  example, 440**t**

Acupressure, 58
  studies, 58
  therapy, 229
  treatment, single-blind crossover design, 58
  usage. *See* Dyspnea 58

Acupuncture, 58
  relationship. *See* Cancer-related breathlessness 58
  studies, 58
  usage. *See* Dyspnea 58

Acupuncture points, 58

Acute care settings, pulmonary therapy (PT provision), 155

Acute exacerbations (outcome), weight loss predictor, 210

Acute respiratory failure
  mechanical ventilation, 85
  prediction ability, limitation, 394

Adaptive device (AD), 492-493

Adenosine triphosphate (ATP), creation, 227-228

Adipocyte-derived hormone, representation, 213

Adipose tissue, loss, 130

ADLs. *See* Activities of daily living 13

Adult education, 75
  cooperative self-management, 75
  facilitation, examples. *See* Family education 76; Patient education 76
  importance. *See* Health 75
  teaching/teaching styles, 76

Adult learning, principles, 76**b**

Adult teaching-learning interactions, 75

Advance care planning
  barriers, 395
    existence, 396
  communication barriers, 395
  component, 399
  curricula, effectiveness. *See* Pulmonary rehabilitation 397
  definition, expansion, 399
  discussions, promotion, 396
  end-of-life discussions, physician reluctance, 396
  goals, 400
  information, pulmonary rehabilitation (value), 397
  initiation, pulmonary rehabilitation (role), 396
  occurrence, observational studies, 396
  patient education, formal curricula (absence), 398
  psychological impact, 397-398
  rationale, 394

Advance directives, 400
  end-of-life care promotion, 399
  sources, preferences, 397**t**
  success. *See* Written advance directives 399

Advanced lung disease, 393
  care, ethical dilemmas, 394
  end-of-life decisions, opportunity, 395
  end-of-life issues, patient attitudes, 397
  patients, transport. *See* Commercial aircraft 464-465

Advanced medical technology, usage. *See* Travel 464

AeroChamber, 108**f**

Aerolizer, 106**f**

Aerosolized drugs, usage, 101-102

Aerosolized recombinant human DNase I, mucolytic role, 102

Aerosols. *See* Bland aerosols 101; Combination aerosols 101**t**
  administration, DPI popularity, 102
  delivery, modes, 102

Aerosol therapy, 547
  devices, 447

Afferent stimuli (decrease), peripheral receptors (impact), 54

Agency for Health Care Policy and Research (AHCPR), smoking cessation guidelines, 326

Agency for Healthcare Research and Quality (AHRQ), 264

Aging, physical changes (expectation), 288

Aging female, sexual relations, 288

Aging process, relationship. *See* Sexuality 287

AHRQ. *See* Agency for Healthcare Research and Quality 264

AIDS pharmacotherapy, 258-259

Air carrier, travel contact, 462

Aircraft cabin altitude, calculation. *See* Median aircraft cabin altitude 458-459

Aircraft cabin conditions, 458

Airflow limitation, 21
  progression, 24**f**

Airflow obstruction, 130. *See also* Body mass index, airflow Obstruction, Dyspnea level, and Exercise capacity 84-85
  change, absence, 133
  conditions, 499**b**, 501
  pharmacologic therapy, 86
  physiological evidence, 22
  significance, 423

Air hunger, 40

Air travel
  departure day, preparations, 462
  expansion, 454
  planning. *See* Pulmonary disease 461
  supplemental O_2, planning, 461-462

Airway anastomosis, dehiscence, 375-376

Airway clearance
  devices, 448
  techniques, 533
    list, 533**b**
    selection, 533

Airway complications. *See* Lung transplantation 375

Airway disease, distribution (unevenness), 22-23

Airway hyperresponsiveness, 99

Airway inflammation (decrease), inhaled corticosteroids (usage), 100

Airway mucosal edema, impact, 95-96

Airway secretions
  impact, 95-96
  vacuuming, 354-355

Airway tethering, loss, 95-96

Alae nasi dilator muscles, muscular activity, 420-421

Albuterol, 98**t**
  combination, availability. *See* Ipratropium/albuterol 97

Alcohol consumption, smoking predictor, 319

Alimentary tissue hypoxia, manifestation, 117

All-cause death prediction, BODE Index (usage), 34

Allergic rhinitis, boswellia (usage), 224

Allograft, denervation, 372

α_2-adrenergic agonists, 247, 237-240**t**

$\alpha_4\beta_2$ nicotinic acetylcholine receptor, binding, 240

α_1-antitrypsin, 89
  deficiency, impact, 3
  usage. *See* Chronic obstructive pulmonary disease 89

$\alpha_4\beta_2$ nicotinic acetylcholine receptor, Varenicline (relationship), 306

$\alpha_4\beta_2$ nicotinic receptor
  binding, 248**f**
  partial agonists, 240, 237-240**t**

α-linolenic acid, end products, 228

α-tocopherol, supplementation (study), 226

Altered breathing patterns, 51

Page numbers followed by *f* indicate figures; *t*, tables; *b*, boxes.

Altitude, cardiovascular responses, 458
Alveolar-capillary membrane,
    O_2 diffusion, 116
Alveolar gas equation, 455**b**
Alveolar minus arterial gradient [P(A-a)O_2], 455
Alveolar partial pressure of oxygen (P$_{AO2}$)
    barometric pressure, relationship, 455
    prediction, 459–460
        regression equations, development, 461
        regression equations, list, 461**b**
Ambulation
    ability, evaluation, 170–171
    performing, 371
    progression, 168
    training mode, 173
Ambulatory oxygen equipment, 444
Ambulatory oxygen systems, types, 441
American Association for Respiratory Care
    (AARC). See Uniform Reporting Manual for
    Acute Care Hospitals 477
American Association of Cardiovascular and
    Pulmonary Rehabilitation (AACVPR)
    clinical competency guidelines, 487
    Outcomes Committee: cardiac/pulmonary
        rehabilitation outcome
        measurement, 487
    program certifications, 485
    PR program certification process, impetus,
        485–487
    staffing ratio minimal requirements, 472
American Association of Retired Persons
    (AARP), sexuality survey, 288
American College of Chest Physicians
    (ACCP)
American College of Chest Physicians Tobacco
    Cessation Tool Kit, 264
    educational information, providing, 265
American College of Radiology and
    Physiotherapy, founding, 155
American Thoracic Society (ATS)
    European Respiratory Society, joint
        statement, 5
    guidelines, 30
    6-Minute Walk Test performance
        guidelines, 335
    obstruction degree, study, 364
    position statement. See Pulmonary
        rehabilitation 2
    principles, importance, 4
    pulmonary rehabilitation, statement
        (1999), 5
    Statement on Pulmonary Rehabilitation,
        goals, 331
American Urological Association guidelines,
    287–288
Aminoglycosides, aerosolization, 102
AMPS. See Assessment of Motor and Process
    Skills 194
Amyotrophic lateral sclerosis, 510–511
Andragogy
    definition, 75
    Knowle's principles, 75
Andropause, 287–288
Ankle edema, signs, 428
Annual mammography, 258–259
Anthropometry, usage, 345
Antibiotics, 89, 102
    therapy, impact, 367–368
    usage. See Chronic obstructive pulmonary
        disease 89
Anticholinergics, 87
    agents, usage. See Inhalation 97**t**
    therapy, 96
    usage. See Chronic obstructive pulmonary
        disease 87
Antidepressant therapy. See Dyspnea
Anti-inflammatory drugs, 88
    usage. See Chronic obstructive pulmonary
        disease 88

Antioxidant enzymes, body synthesis, 117–118
Antioxidant nutrients, NHANES III
    examination, 226
Antioxidant supplementation, 226
    consumption, 224
Anxiety, 270
    presence, 78
Anxiolytics, 256
    ineffectiveness, 256
Apnea-arousal mechanism, phenomena,
    427–428
Appetite, stimulation, 214
Arformoterol, impact, 99
Arformoterol tartrate, 99**t**
Arm ergometry training, comparison.
    See Unsupported arm training 138
Arm exercise. See Unsupported arm exercise
    136–137
    controlled studies. See Chronic obstructive
        pulmonary disease 139**t**
    training, training method. See Supported
        arm exercise training 140**b**
Arm training
    effect, 137
    studies, 137–138
    training method. See Unsupported arm
        training 140**b**
Arterial blood gas (ABG)
    measurement, 117
    noninvasive alternative, 117
    values, 457**f**
Arterial gas tensions (increase), altitude
    (increase), 455**f**
Arterial hypoxemia, TNF-α circulating levels
    (relationship), 32
Arterial oxygenation, measurement, 117
Arterial oxygen percent saturation (Sa$_{O2}$), 455,
    455–456
Arterial oxygen saturation, determination, 116
Arterial partial pressure of carbon dioxide
    (Pa$_{CO2}$), change, 420
Arterial partial pressure of oxygen (Pa$_{O2}$),
    change, 420
Ask advise assess assist arrange (5 As).
    See Smoking cessation 306
Assertiveness training, 201
Assessment of Motor and Process Skills
    (AMPS), 194
Assistance of two (A of 2), description, 492
Assistive devices, usage, 201
Asthma, 236, 425, 501, 530
    children, exercise prescription, 532**b**
    chronic airway inflammation, role, 531
    chronic childhood disease, 530
    control, 501
        worsening, 99
    education programs, positive effects, 55
    exercise programs, 532
    existence, debate. See Nocturnal asthma
        425–426
    inflammation, presence, 530–531
    lower airway obstruction, 522
    medical characteristics, 530
    QOL, improvement, 523
    rehabilitation program, 531
        goals, 531
        self-management promotion, 531
    symptoms, prevalence (reduction), 225
    wide-spectrum disease, 523
Asthma, bronchodilator use (monitoring), 225
Astragalus root, 224
    Cochrane Database, 224
Atelectasis, 372
ATP. See Adenosine triphosphate 227–228
Atrial arrhythmias, 117
Atropa belladonna. See Nightshade plant 96–97
Atropine, anticholinergic bronchodilator,
    96–97
Attentional coping strategies, usage, 56

Attention strategies, 56
    contrast. See Distraction strategies 56
    examples, 56
    usage. See Dyspnea 56
Autofluorescence bronchoscopy, 311–312
Autogenic drainage, 533**b**
Aventyl. See Nortriptyline HCl 247
Azathioprine (AZA), 373
    allopurinol, coadministration
        (contraindication), 374
    immunosuppressive medication, 374**t**
    lymphocyte replication/function, inhibition,
        373–374
    side effects, 374

B

Backpacking regimen, impact, 135–136
Bacterial pneumonias, 376–377
BAI. See Beck Anxiety Inventory 272
Balanced scorecard, concept, 476
Barach, Alvan L., 1–2, 155
Barometric pressure (P$_B$), P$_{AO2}$
    relationship, 455
Barrel chest, 163
Basal metabolic rate, total energy expenditure
    component, 212
Baseline Dyspnea Index (BDI), 12–13
    interviewer-administered
        questionnaires, 338
    outcome measure, 338
    usage, 149
Baseline/Transition Dyspnea Index
    (BDI/TDI), 44
Battery-powered concentrator/O_2-conserving
    device, 443
BBC. See Better Breathers Club 407
BCSS. See Breathlessness, Cough and Sputum
    Scale 46
BDI. See Baseline Dyspnea Index 12–13;
    Beck Depression Inventory 272
BDI/TDI. See Baseline/Transition Dyspnea
    Index 44
Beck Anxiety Inventory (BAI), 272
Beck Depression Inventory (BDI), 272
Beclomethasone dipropionate, 100**t**
Beddoes, Thomas, 115
Behavioral contracts, usage, 321
Behavioral functioning, 275
Behavioral intervention, 256
Behavior (performing), physical capacity, 78
Benchmarking, 473
    elements, 475**b**
    usage. See Outcome documentation
        473–474
Best breathing times, 293–294
    chores, 51
β-agonists, 86
β_2-agonists, 98. See also Long-acting β_2-agonists
    98**t**; Short-acting β_2-agonists 98**t**
    bronchodilators, potential, 98
    peak effect, comparison, 97
    rescue therapy limitation, 97
Beta carotene, usage, 226
β-lactam antibiotics, aerosolization, 102
Better Breathers Club (BBC)
    BOD offices, 409
    development, absence, 408
    establishment, 407
    first meeting, importance, 407–408
    funding, 409
    meetings
        frequency, 407
        location, 407
        planning, 407
    operations (oversight), BOD (usage),
        408–409
    organization name, 409
    respiratory rally, 413–414
    telephoning, 408

Bicycle ergometrer, incremental exercise testing, 332

Bicycle ergometry, advantages/disadvantages. *See* Graded exercise testing 156**t**

Bilateral lung transplantation, indications, 362**b**

Bilateral LVRS, result, 385–386

Bilevel positive airway pressure, 53

Bilevel therapy, 448

Bioelectrical impedance analysis, 211
  usage, 345

Biofeedback. *See* Dyspnea 57; Heart rate variability biofeedback 57
  treatments, receiving, 230

Biofeedback-assisted relaxation/breathing exercises, 228

Biomass fuel, exposure (decrease), 86

Bitolterol mesylate, 98**t**

Bland aerosols, 101
  therapy, 448
    usage, frequency, 448
  usage. *See* Chronic obstructive pulmonary disease 101–102

Block chart, division, 471

Blood-brain barrier, nicotine (entry), 235–236

Blood diseases, economic cost, 5**t**

Blood gases
  abnormalities, severity, 394
  changes. *See* Sleep 420

Blood pressure, occupational therapist monitoring, 190–191

Blood volume, increase, 130

BMI. *See* Body mass index 210

BNP. *See* Brain natriuretic peptide 48

Board of directors. *See* Patient board of directors 408

BODE. *See* Body mass index, airflow Obstruction, Dyspnea level, and Exercise capacity 346**f**

Bodily symptoms, misinterpretations (psychological treatments), 273

Body composition, 210
  change, 130
  evaluation, 345

Body functions, sexual affirmation, 288

Body functions/structures
  dimension, 194
  evaluation, efficiency/comprehensiveness, 194–195
  ICF functional dimension, 196
  observation, 194–195
  top-down approach, 194–195

Body mass index, airflow Obstruction, Dyspnea level, and Exercise capacity (BODE)
  Index, 20, 34
    mortality predictor, 21
    usage. *See* All-cause death prediction 34
  score, 364
    pulmonary rehabilitation (impact), 346**f**

Body mass index (BMI), 210
  airflow obstruction, dyspnea, and exercise capacity (BODE), 84–85

Body position, variations. *See* Lovemaking 294

Body systems, monitoring (technological advances), 57

Body ventilators, 353–354

Body weight/composition, relationship, 345**f**

Borg Scale, 12–13
  exertional dyspnea measurement, 337
  measurement, 57
  modification, 58
  usage, 192

Borg visual analog scale, usage, 132

BOS. *See* Bronchiolitis obliterans syndrome 376

Bostrom, A.G., 253

Boswellia, 224
  herbs, usefulness, 225

Botanicals, 222

Boundary violations, 297

BPD. *See* Bronchopulmonary dysplasia 522

Bradycardia-tachycardia pattern, emergence, 427–428

Brain energy metabolism, abnormality, 34

Brain function, imaging function, 41

Brain natriuretic peptide (BNP), measurement, 48

Brain tissue hypoxia, 117

Breath, shortness. *See* Shortness of breath 42
  impact, 50–51
  position, impact, 52
  self-management strategies, 55–56

Breath-actuated Maxair Autohaler, schematic illustration, 109**f**

Breath-actuated MDIs, 108

Breath-actuated pMDI, 106**f**

Breath hold, necessity, 109–110

Breathin' Easy Travel Guide, oxygen resource, 447

Breathing
  component integration, schematic model, 27**f**
  depth, 40
  discomfort, categories, 40
  drive, decrease, 50
  exercises, 155, 228
  frequency, 40
    increase, 22
  patterns. *See* Altered breathing patterns 51
    assessment, 163
    study, 136–137
    therapist observation, 163
  reserve, measurement usefulness, 49–50
  stations, 50–51
  strategies, 51
    modeling, 59–60
  training process, 199**b**
  work, 140**t**
    increase, 24**f**

Breathing techniques, 199
  achievement, 169
  improvement, 168
  process, 199**b**
  review, 168
  teaching, 199

Breathlessness. *See* Exertional breathlessness 337
  cause, 156
  comparison, 133
  language, 46
  severity, 156
  studies, 149
  treatment, oral/parenteral opioids (usage), 54

Breathlessness, Cough and Sputum Scale (BCSS)
  clinical change, threshold, 47
  usage, 46

Breathlessness, Modified Borg Scale
  dyspnea descriptors, inclusion, 44**f**
  ten-point category ratio (CR-10) scale, 43–44
  usage, 43

Breath sounds, intensity (decrease), 48

Brief Symptom Inventory (BSI), 272

British Medical Research Council, COPD study, 307

Bronchi, lymphocytes (presence), 19

Bronchial asthma, diagnosis estimates, 2–3

Bronchiolitis obliterans syndrome (BOS), physiologic entity, 376

Bronchoalveolar lavage cytology studies, 311

Bronchoconstrictiion, impact, 95–96

Bronchodilators, 53, 96
  dose, manipulation, 53
  effects, tolerance, 97
  usage, 86

Bronchogenic carcinoma, 236

Bronchopulmonary dysplasia (BPD), 530, 536
  anatomic abnormalities, 537
  chronic lung disease, 536
  chronic mechanical ventilation, requirement, 550
  exercise program, 538
  goals, 537–538
  impact. *See* Childhood BPD 537
  infants, clinical needs, 537
  medical characteristics, 536
  patients, long-term outcomes, 537
  physical rehabilitation, 537
  severity, variation, 537
  ventilatory support, reduction, 537

Bronchospasm, 117

BSI. *See* Brief Symptom Inventory 272

Budesonide, 100**t**

Budesonide/formoterol, combination, 101**t**

Bupropion
  association. *See* Smoking cessation 306**t**
  controller medications, first line, 252
  dose, reduction (guidelines), 246
  double-blind treatment, 242–243
  effectiveness, 242**t**
  maintenance study, 242–243
  metabolite concentration, 253
  usage, 86

Bupropion hydrochloride
  receiving, 306–307
  sustained-release formulation, 244–246

Bupropion hydrochloride immediate acting (Wellbutrin), 244–246

Bupropion hydrochloride sustained release (Wellbutrin SR), 244–246

Bupropion immediate acting, 246

Bupropion sustained release (Bupropion SR) (Zyban)
  action, mechanism, 244
  clinical trials, 244
  comparison, 241**f**
  controller medications, first line, 253
  effectiveness, 245–246**t**
  initiation, 244
    timing, 244
  pharmacokinetics, 244
  tobacco dependence clinical trials, 253
  usage, 246, 246, 246
    safety, 251

Burkholderia cepacia
  impact, 503
  infection, 368

Bus travel, 464

C

Cachexia, 210–211

California Thoracic Society Position Paper: Medical Management for Tobacco Dependence, 264

CAM. *See* Complementary alternative medicine 221

Canadian Occupational Performance Measure (COPM), 188

Cancer-related breathlessness, acupuncture (relationship), 58

Carbohydrate metabolism, data. *See* Chronic obstructive pulmonary disease 213

Carbon dioxide (CO_2)
  breathing, impact, 41
  concentration, 23
  concept, Lavoisier discussion, 1
  production, 523
  ranges, 538
  release, 220–221

Carbon monoxide (CO), diffusing capacity, 11

Cardiac β_1-receptor effects, dose dependence, 98

Cardiac diseases, respiratory diseases (coexistence), 156

Cardiac output, decline, 518

Cardiac performance, alterations, 130
Cardiac safety
  concepts/principles, 254
  controller/rescue nicotine medications, 253
Cardiopulmonary conditioning, progression, 168
Cardiopulmonary disease, acute/chronic
  progressive dyspnea (experience), 39–40
Cardiopulmonary exercise test, 49
  inclusion. *See* Patient assessment 13
Cardiopulmonary exercise testing
  safety, 525
Cardiopulmonary exercise testing (CPET)
  baseline, 508–509
  CPET gas exchange, 523
  graded exercise basis, 523
  maximal oxygen uptake, 523
  nine-panel plot, 524**f**
  performing, 523
  usage, 501
Cardiovascular conditioning,
  improvement, 331
Cardiovascular disease
  economic burden, 3
  economic cost, 5**t**
Cardiovascular effects, 33
Cardiovascular measurements,
  components, 156
Caregiver-patient relationship
  disruption, gender conflicts, 298
  sexual bias, 298
Caregiver-patient sexual attraction, 297
Caregivers
  analysis/interpretation. *See* Patients 297–298
  boundary blurring, 297**b**
  professional-patient boundaries,
    self-reflection, 298**b**
  seductive behavior, 297
Carriers, role, 489
Casualty insurance program, 488**b**
Catapres. *See* Clonidine 247
CCQ. *See* Chronic obstructive pulmonary
  disease Coping Questionnaire 272
CDC. *See* Centers for Disease Control and
  Prevention 264
CellCept, 374
Cellular function (impairment), chronic
  hypoxia (impact), 116
Cellular hypoxia, muscle exercise, 120
Center for Epidemiological Studies-
  Depression Inventory (CES-D), 272
Centers for Disease Control and Prevention
  (CDC), 264
Central drive
  decrease, 53
  noninvasive measurement, 24–25
Central nervous system (CNS)
  genetic systems (activation), nicotine
    (impact), 235
  neuronal changes, induction, 236
  nicotine medication delivery speed, 247
Central perception, alteration, 55
CES-D. *See* Center for Epidemiological
  Studies-Depression Inventory 272
CF. *See* Cystic fibrosis 367
CGA. *See* Contact Guard Assist 492
Chantix. *See* Varenicline 240
Charcot-Marie-Tooth disease, 510–511
Chemoreceptors, impact, 41
Chest
  auscultation, usage, 163–165
  iodinated contrast, spiral CT scanning
    (usage), 49
  mobility, therapist observation, 163
  pain, assessment, 167
  percussion, 549
  physical therapy techniques, 155
  physiotherapy, 533
  radiographs, usage, 48–49
  tightness, 40

Chest wall
  changes, 506
  diseases, 351
  receptors, impact, 40
  stimulation, 39
Cheyne-Stokes breathing, 428–429
Cheyne-Stokes respirations, 458
Childhood asthma, prevalence (increase),
  535–536
Childhood BPD, impact, 537
Childhood CF, exercise prescription, 534**b**
Children, sexual abuse, 299
Chiropractic spinal manipulation, beneficial
  outcomes, 230
Cholecalciferol. *See* Vitamin D$_3$ 227
Chronic airway inflammation, role, 531
Chronic asthma, chiropractic spinal
  stimulation, 230
Chronic bronchitis
  clinical definition, 18–19
  diagnosis estimates, 2–3
Chronic dyspnea
  exercise tolerance, 59–60
  fans, impact, 55
Chronic illness, relationship. *See* Sexuality 289
Chronic lung disease
  cigarette smoking, impact, 304
  complications, reduction, 305
  detection efforts, 304
  development
    factors, 312
    genetics, role, 312
    risk factor, 304
  health measures, 310–311
  prevention
    opportunities, 303
    potential, 304
    strategies, 304**b**
  preventive measures, 311
  primary prevention, 304
  psychosocial composite, 289**b**
  secondary prevention, 304
  spirometry
    performance, difficulties, 305
    usage, 304–305
  symptomatic disease, prevention, 304
  tertiary prevention, 305
Chronic obstructive pulmonary disease
  (COPD), 2, 84, 236
  adherence, 317
  airflow obstruction, 83–84
    development, reason, 22
    retained tracheobronchial mucus,
      impact, 101
  α$_1$-antitrypsin, usage, 84
  American Thoracic Society definition,
    usage, 96
  antibiotics, usage, 89, 102
  anticholinergics, usage, 87
  anti-inflammatory drugs, usage, 88
  association, 84–85. *See also* Weight loss 209
  bland aerosols, usage, 101–102
  burden, 86
  CAM
    therapies, usage, 222–223**t**
    treatments, research, 224
    usage, 221–222
  carbohydrate/fat metabolism, data
    limitation, 213
  characterization, 19–20, 30–31
  combination therapy, usage, 88
  comprehensive care programs, 2
  comprehensive management, algorithm, 85**f**
  coronary heart disease, coexistence, 293
  corticosteroids, usage, 88
  cure, 339–340
  death ranking, 18
  death rates, 3
  definition, 18

Chronic obstructive pulmonary disease
  (COPD) *(Continued)*
  depression, prevalence, 270
  diagnosis/care, update, 5
  diagnosis data, 434
  discharge criteria, 89
  disease-free interval, 303
  drug regimens, modification, 90
  end-of-life care, communication
    components, 395**b**
  evidence-based studies, 222
  exacerbations, 89
    development, viral infections
      (association), 308–309
    emergency department evaluation, 89**t**
    impact, 307–308
    oral agents, meta-analysis, 101
    patient approach, algorithm (usage), 90**f**
    prevention, 310
    rate reduction, pharmacologic
      interventions, 310
  exercise
    limitation, 228–229
    monitoring. *See* Symptomatic COPD 43
    tolerance, limitation, 228–229
  exercise training
    evidence benefits, 140**t**
    impact, 134–135
    supervision, 332
  FEV$_1$
    level, 131
    presence, evaluation, 21
  FFM depletion, 210–211
  first-listed discharge diagnosis, 3
  functional impairments, disease severity
    (impact), 276
  high-intensity exercise training, 334**f**
  high-risk patients, identification, 90
  hospitalization, 89
    indications, 91**b**
  inclusion, 303
  inflammatory mediators, increase, 215
  intervention studies, 274
  kidneys, chronic hypercapnia
    (compensation), 118
  lifestyle, 275
  long-term exercise maintenance, factors, 322
  low-intensity exercise training, 334**f**
  management issues, complexity, 91
  medical regimen, 279–280
  medication compliance, increase, 280
  morbidity/mortality predictor, 20
  mortality
    factors, literature, 20
    study, 224
  mucolytics, usage, 102
  multicomponent disease, 35**f**, 84
  multidimensional classification, 34
  multidimensional staging, 346
  nutritional abnormalities, 32
  outcomes, pharmacologic agents
    combination, impact, 87**t**
    impact, 86**t**
  pathogenesis, chronic/acute infection
    (role), 102
  pathophysiology, 19
  patients
    arm exercise, controlled studies, 139**t**
    electronic nebulizers, usage, 105
    evaluation, 274
    exercise, usage (rehabilitation studies),
      130**f**
    PR success, 498
  patient-specific objective clinical/laboratory
    features, 90
  pharmacologic therapy, requirement, 86
  phosphodiesterase inhibitors, usage, 87
  plasma amino acid pattern, abnormality,
    214–215

Chronic obstructive pulmonary disease (COPD) *(Continued)*
polysomnogram, schematic representation, 424**f**
presence. *See* Treadmill 56–57
prevention/treatment, docosahexaenoic acid (role), 228
PR patients, 468–469
psychological consequence, 270–271
pulmonary rehabilitation
benefits, 545
referrals, 10
respiratory rate, increase, 24**f**
respiratory system, integrative approach, 26
self-efficacy, increase, 55, 273
self-infliction, 236
sleep, presence, 423
SMD
clinical consequences, 33
mechanisms, 33**b**, 33
pathogenesis, systemic inflammation (role), 33
presence, 32
systemic inflammation, impact, 32–33
staging system, variables (inclusion), 21**b**
structure/function relationship, knowledge (uncertainty), 20
surgical options, algorithm (suggestion), 366**f**
symptom, 20–21
systemic effects, 30
list, 31**b**
systemic inflammation
nonpharmacologic therapy, impact, 34–35
origin, uncertainty, 32
presence, 31
therapeutic options, 34
treatable disease, 85
treatment
goals, 84
nutritional intervention, 224
underweight characteristic, 14
vaccination, usage, 89
ventilatory challenges, 425
Chronic obstructive pulmonary disease Coping Questionnaire (CCQ), 272
Chronic obstructive pulmonary disease Self-Efficacy Scale (CSES), 272
Chronic pulmonary disease
impact, 2–3
trajectory, 46–47
Chronic respiratory disease
overweight characteristic, 52
physical activity, decrease, 129
severity, 343
symptoms/functional limitations, clinical appearance, 11
Chronic Respiratory Disease Questionnaire (CRDQ), 276–277, 340
changes, 332
dyspnea domain, outcome measure, 338
Chronic Respiratory Disease Questionnaire (CRQ), 44
clinical change, threshold, 47
HRQL measurement, 339
interviewer administration, 340–341
usage, 149
Chronic respiratory failure, home mechanical ventilation (treatment), 351
Chronic Respiratory Questionnaire, inclusion, 386–387
Cigarette deprivation, 265–266
Cigarette smoking
addiction, association, 306
craving, 265–266
habit/lifestyle choice, examination, 236
inflammatory process, induction, 19
lifestyle choice, 258

Cigarette smoking *(Continued)*
medical management, 267
pathogen, predominance, 236
restlessness, 265–266
social habit, 258
Cilomilast, antiinflammatory/bronchodilator effects, 87
Circulating leptin, correlation, 213
Circulating neutrophils, alterations, 31
Citric synthase (CS), 136
Clinical ladder
example. *See* Pulmonary rehabilitation 483–485**b**
job descriptions, 481
Clinical relevance. *See* Chronic obstructive pulmonary disease 34
Clonidine (Catapres // Catapres-TTS), 247
controller medication, second line, 254
tablets, side effects, 254
Clotting cascade, nicotine nonactivation, 254
CMV. *See* Cytomegalovirus 376–377
Cochrane Database of Systematic Reviews, echinacea studies, 222–224
Coenzyme Q10 (ubiquinone // ubidecarenone), 227
immune function improvement, 228
usage, 225
Cognitive-behavioral group format, 272–273
Cognitive-behavior modification, 324–325
Cognitive defects, 508
Cognitive demands, responses, 193
Cognitive distortions, interactive cycle (model), 273**f**
Cognitive functioning, 273
assessment, 274
treatment, 274
Cognitive performance, self-perceptions (evaluation), 274
Cognitive techniques, usage, 325
Cold turkey
concentration difficulty, 266
irritability/anger, increase, 266–267
usage, 248**f**
Colistin, aerosolization, 102
Combination aerosols, 101**t**
Combination medications, 249
clinical trial, 251
concepts/principles, 251
published studies, 250
recommendations, 252
Combination therapy, 88
usage. *See* Chronic obstructive pulmonary disease 88
Comfort, Alex, 287
Commercial aircraft, advanced lung disease patient transport, 464–465
Communication barriers, 395. *See also* Advance care planning 395
Complementary alternative medicine (CAM), 221
evidence-based studies, 222
physician knowledge, 221–222
systematic review, 228
therapies
diet/lifestyle recommendations, involvement, 231**b**
usage. *See* Chronic obstructive pulmonary disease 222–223**t**
treatments, review, 221
Complete dependence, 492
Compliance/adherence, 279
education, 280
treatment, 280
Compliance quartile, exercise endurance (dose-response relationship), 324**f**
Comprehensive outpatient rehabilitation facility (CORF), 489
Medicare-certified health care facility definition, 489

Comprehensive pulmonary rehabilitation, long-term benefits (demonstration failure), 325
Compressed gas O_2, storage, 122–123
Compressor nebulizers, 447
Computerized axial tomography (CAT)
CAT-based morphology, 364
techniques, improvement, 364
usage. *See* Lungs 364
Concentrators. *See* Oxygen concentrators 122–123
low-pressure systems, 442
Congestive heart failure, 117
Constructive emotional state, expression, 78
Consumer Guide: You Can Quit Smoking, 264
Contact Guard Assist (CGA), description, 492
Continuous positive airway pressure (CPAP), 53, 448
difficulties, 449
machine/mask, 449**f**
therapy, 449
Controller medications, 237–240**t**
combinations, 251
usage, 251
first line, 240, 252
second line, 247
safety, 254
Controller nicotine medications, 254
concepts/principles, 254
Cooperative intention, sharing, 75
Cooperative self-management. *See* Adult education 75
COPD. *See* Chronic obstructive pulmonary disease 2
Coping skills
interventions. *See* Supportive coping skills interventions 273
usage, 271
Coping styles, attention (increase), 271
COPM. *See* Canadian Occupational Performance Measure 188
CORF. *See* Comprehensive outpatient rehabilitation facility 489
Coronary heart disease, death rate, 3
Cor pulmonale, 364, 535
Corticosteroid-dependent bronchial asthma, 227–228
Corticosteroids, 88, 100, 374
appetite, impact, 52
immunosuppressive mechanisms, 374–375
therapy
manipulation, 53
recommendations, 100
toxicities, 375
usage. *See* Chronic obstructive pulmonary disease 88; Inhaled corticosteroids 100
Cost-per-case expenses, decrease, 477–478
Cough
assessment, 167
augmentation, 354**b**
deliberateness, 549
history, 163–165
techniques
achievement, 169
improvement, 168
review. *See* Directed cough techniques 168
CoughAssist (Respironics), 354–355
Coupling, 23–24
CPAP. *See* Continuous positive airway pressure 53
CPET. *See* Cardiopulmonary exercise testing 501
Crackles, 536,
auscultation, 165–166
indications, 163–165
CRDQ. *See* Chronic Respiratory Disease Questionnaire 276–277
C-reactive protein, involvement, 212

Critical illness-related neuropathy, survivors, 510–511
Critical thinking, definition, 472
CRP levels, increase, 33
CRQ. See Chronic Respiratory Disease Questionnaire 44
Crude death rates, 4f
Cruise ships, travel, 463
CS. See Citric synthase 136
CSES. See Chronic obstructive pulmonary disease Self-Efficacy Scale 272
Cuff weights, usage, 171
Cushing's syndrome, steroid use (impact), 163
Customer service, 478
    performance objective plan, 478t
Cycle ergometer
    usage, 49–50
    work, comparison, 133
Cyclic adenosine monophosphate-dependent, decrease, 98
Cyclosporine A (CSA), 373
    hepatotoxicity, occurrence, 373
    immunosuppressive medication, 374t
    nephrotoxicity, 373
    side effects, 373
    Tacrolimus, relationship, 373
    usage. See Lung transplantation 373
Cystic fibrosis (CF), 367, 502, 530, 532
    airway clearance techniques, 533
    children, exercise prescription, 534b
    evaluation, 534
    exercise program, 533
    exercise training
        impacts, 503
        methods, 503
        trials, 503
    genetic disease, commonness, 532–533
    medical characteristics, 532
    nutritional support, 533
    precautions, 534
    short-term nonrandomized uncontrolled trials, 502–503
Cystic Fibrosis Foundation National Patient Registry, 368
Cytomegalovirus (CMV)
    commonness, 377
    survival, 376–377

D

Daily living groups, problematic aspects (focus), 202–204
Data management, 470. See also Pulmonary rehabilitation programs 470
Davy, Humphry, 115
Daytime O_2 setting, prescription. See Sleep 119
Dead space-to-tidal volume (V_D/V_T) ratio, increase, 118
Dead volume, presence. See Small-volume nebulizers 104
Death rates. See Crude death rates 4f
Deep venous thrombosis, history, 459
Deltasone, 374
Denison, Charles L., 1
Dependent (Dep // D), description, 492
Depression, 270
    prevalence. See Chronic obstructive pulmonary disease 270
Desaturations, association. See REM sleep 119
Detraining effect, 130, 132
    impact, 132
Device-appropriate education, problem, 110
Dewar flask, usage, 122–123
Diagnostic tests, 12
Dial, Lanyard, 287
Diamon, Jared, 286
Diaphragm
    electric stimulation, 354
    innervation, 25
    paralysis, 510–511

Diaphragmatic breathing
    breathing techniques/training process, 199b
    recommendation, 199
    research, 199–200
Diaphragmatic flattening, 163
Diaphragmatic pressure excursion, increase, 137
Dietary factors. See Pulmonary rehabilitation 278
    treatment, 278
Dietary intake, 213
Diet-induced thermogenesis, 212
Diet study, 226
Diffusing capacity of the lung for carbon monoxide (DLCO), 525
Digital clubbing, 166f
    hyponychial angle, increase, 166f
    severity, 166f
Digoxin, usage, 224
Directed cough techniques, review, 168
Disease management/self-care, information (sharing), 76
Disease severity, impact. See Chronic obstructive pulmonary disease 276
Diskhaler (Rotadisk), 106f
Diskus, 106f
Distance walked, field measures, Printing it would be ten cents per page. p0510
Distraction strategies, 56
    attention strategies, contrast, 56
    usage. See Dyspnea 56
Distress, experience (measurement), 46–47
DLCO. See Diffusing capacity of the lung for carbon monoxide 525
DMD. See Duchenne muscular dystrophy 538
Ḋo2. See Oxygen delivery 455
Docosahexaenoic acid
    α-linolenic acid end product, 228
    role. See Chronic obstructive pulmonary disease 228
Dopamine reuptake, occurrence, 248f
Dopaminergic neurons, schematic. See Mesolimbic dopaminergic pathway 248f
Dopaminergic-noradrenergic reuptake inhibitors, 244, 237–240t
    concepts/principles, 246
    dosage, 244
    double-blind placebo-controlled studies, 244
    relapse prevention trial, 244
Dose-response relationship. See Compliance quartile 324f
Double-lung transplantation, 168
Doubly labeled water, usage, 212
DPIs. See Dry powder inhalers 102
Drive/inspiratory pressure, relation, 23–24
Driving gas, decrease, 104
Drug aerosolization, DPI usage, 109f
Drug delivery, factors, 109
    inclusion, 109
Drug delivery maximization, MDI usage, 106
Drug-induced thermogenesis, 212
Dry mouth. See Xerostomia 253
Dry-powder inhalers, 447
Dry powder inhalers (DPIs)
    advantages, 110
        comparison, 111t
        explanation, 110
    chlorofluorocarbons, absence, 110
    disadvantages, 110
        comparison, 111t
        explanation, 110
    drug, availability, 103
    environmental humidity, impact, 109
    particle deposition, electrostatic charge (impact), 109
    technique differences. See Metered dose inhaler 111b

Dry powder inhalers (DPIs) (Continued)
    usage, 102. See also Drug aerosolization 109f
        technique, 109
        technique, list, 110b
Dual-energy X-ray absorptiometry, usage, 345
Duchenne muscular dystrophy (DMD), 538
    inheritance, 538
Dumbbells, usage, 171
Durham Veterans Administration Medical Center
    residential programs, establishment, 257
    residential treatment programs, 257
Dynamic hyperinflation
    conditions, 212
    reduction, 51–52
Dyspnea, 25
    acupressure/acupuncture, usage, 58
    affective dimension, 41
    affective responses, measurement, 46
    antidepressant therapy, 54
    anxiety, source, 271
    assessment, 167, 337
    attention strategies, usage, 56
    BDI, relationship, 342f
    biofeedback, 57
    cause/extent, laboratory evaluation (usage), 48
    causes
        uncertainty, 156
        understanding, 40
    central perception, alteration, 40
    changes, understanding, 174
    clinical assessment, 47–48
    clinical measurements, 42
        performing, 42
    clinical states, presence, 47
    clinical term, 40
    cognitive-behavioral strategies, 55
    daily outline, 51
    database, inclusion, 48–49
    decrease
        exercise training, impact, 59
        physiologic mechanisms, 334–335
        self-care strategies. See Eating 52b
        strategies. See Sexual activity 51
    description, 40
    descriptors, usage, 46
    development, 130
    diagnostic approach, 47
    diseases, presence, 47
    distraction strategies, usage, 56
    distress, 41
    education, 55
    evaluation instructions. See Perceived dyspnea 193t
    factors, awareness (absence), 42
    fans, usage. See Chronic dyspnea 55
    fatigue, relationship, 50
    fibromyalgia, impact, 54
    guided imagery, usage, 58
    HRQL, relationship, 342f
    impact. See Exercise 25–26
    improvement, exercise training (impact), 60
    increase, 45–46
    inhaled opiate therapy, usage, 54
    intensity, inverse relationship, 149
    intensity measurement, clinical instruments (usage), 45t
    laboratory evaluation, 48
    level. See Body mass index, airflow obstruction, dyspnea, and exercise capacity 84–85
    determination, 42
    limiting symptom, 138
    longitudinal placebo-controlled outpatient studies, 54
    lung disease symptom, 289
    malnutrition, impact, 52
    management

Dyspnea (Continued)
plan, availability. See Palliative care patients 54
self-efficacy, increase, 55
measurement, 42. See also Real-time dyspnea 42
questionnaires, example, 339t
reasons, 42
mechanisms, 40
laboratory studies, 41
medical regimens/action plans, manipulation, 53
medications, 54
multidimensional instruments, usage, 44. See also Recalled dyspnea 42
music, usage, 57
nebulized opiates, usage, 54
nonspecific effects, 56
obesity, impact, 52
opiates, usage, 54
patient history, 47
patient isolation, preference, 59
perception, 41
factors, 41
physical examination, usage, 48
physiologic causes, modification. See Pulmonary rehabilitation 41
physiologic mechanisms, 40
placebo effect, 56
position, impact, 52
progressive development, respiratory disease (association), 130f
psychometric testing, 46
pulmonary rehabilitation treatment, effectiveness. See Exertional dyspnea 337-338
questions, tailoring, 340
randomization, study, 132-133
reductions, IMT (impact), 53
referral usage, 12-13
relationship. See Activities of daily living 149
relaxation techniques, 56
relief, providing, 58
resting respiratory drive, impact, 26
sedatives, usage, 54
self-management strategies, 55-56
sensitization, reduction, 168
SGRQ, relationship, 342f
short-term goals, development, 59-60
social support, usage, 58-59
stimulus, uncertainty. See Exercise 43
subjective experience, 48
symptomatic treatment, 50b
usage, 50
symptom management, self-efficacy/control (increase), 59
symptoms, 20-21
monitoring, 46
target, 42
timing/measurement, relationship, 42
treatments, clinical studies, 41
unidimensional instruments, usage, 43. See also Recalled dyspnea 42
vibration, impact, 54
visceral sensation, 40

E

EADL. See Extended ADL 344
Eating, dyspnea decrease (self-care strategies), 52b
Echinacea, products (availability), 222-224
Echinacea purpurea, aerial parts, 222-224
Edema, assessment, 167
Education, direct contribution (measurement), 546
Educational assessment, 14
Educational program, curriculum (basis), 14-15

Effector cells, muscarinic receptors (impact), 96
Effort, sense (reduction), 50
Effort-dependent outcome measures, impact, 331
EIB. See Exercise-induced bronchospasm 501
Eicosapentaenoic acid, α-linolenic end product, 228
Eisenmenger syndrome, 369
Electrocardiogram, usage, 48-49
Electronic medical documentation (EMD), commonness, 157
Electronic medication monitors, value, 319
Electronic nebulizers, 105
Electronic oxygen-conserving devices, usage, 445
Ellipse, 108f
EMD. See Electronic medical documentation 157
Emergency department (ED)
evaluation. See Chronic obstructive pulmonary disease 89t
therapy, short-term response, 90
Emotional support, 58-59
Emotions, interactive cycle (model), 273f
Emphysema
categorization. See Advanced emphysema 394
diagnosis estimates, 2-3
heterogeneity, definition, 388
significance, 423
End-expiratory lung volume, decrease, 51
Endocrine dysregulation, 33
End-of-life care
communication components, 395b
patient selection, approach, 398
providing, physician skills, 401b
End-of-life decisions
dialogue, 400
mandates, 394-395
patient assistance, 399
End-of-life discussions
initiation, success, 396
physician reluctance. See Advance care planning 396
End-of-life issues, discussions, 398
End-of-life needs, support, 400
End-stage COPD, 507-508
Endurance
exercise testing, 334
usefulness, 334, 334-335
increase, 130, 145
training, 172
treadmill, usage, 42
Endurance Shuttle Walk Test, endurance test, 336-337
Energy balance (maintenance/improvement), nutritional intervention (usage), 213
Energy conservation, 50, 200
principles, 201b, 202-204
strategies, 201b
teaching, 200
Energy expenditure, division. See Total energy expenditure 212
Energy metabolism, 212
Energy-saving devices, advertisements, 201-202
Enteric gram-negative bacteria, isolate, 102
Environmental modification, 202
Environment safety, 77
Environment targets, assessment, 189
Eon, usage. See Lung transplantation 373
Epinephrine, 98t
Erectile dysfunction, 294
PDE5 inhibitor treatment, 295
treatment, 295
Erections
improvement, sildenafil (impact), 295
physiologic process, 294

Ergocalciferol. See Vitamin D_2 227
European Respiratory Society
guidelines (2006), 30
joint statement. See American Thoracic Society 5
Statement on Pulmonary Rehabiltation, goals, 331
EverFlo oxygen concentrator (Respironics), 442f
Exercise, 228
adherence, 322
studies, 323
alternative types, 60
assessment, 13
benefits, 171
capacity, predictor, 276
cessation, dyspnea (impact), 25-26
cognitive techniques, usage, 325
dyspnea (amelioration), oxygen (impact), 121
endurance
time, improvement, 134f
work, 140t
functional analysis, performing, 325
goals, setting, 521
importance, argument, 322-323
instruction/practice, treatment, 323
intensity, maintenance, 371-372
limitation, cause, 156
load
increase, 131
intensity/frequency/duration, 131
oxygen
therapeutic modality, 121
usage, 120
performance. See Inspiratory muscle training 149
tests, 332
PH, background, 518
physiologic adaptation, 334f
prescription, necessity, 156
program, design, 171
promotion, suggestions, 325
realistic goals, setting, 325
risk, 525
sessions, number (consideration), 131-132
supplemental oxygen, usage, 120
test, dyspnea stimulus (uncertainty), 43
testing, 42, 156. See also Incremental exercise testing 332
hypoxemia results, 11
role/types, 521
tolerance, impairment, 510
treatment, 279
Exercise capacity. See Body mass index, airflow Obstruction, Dyspnea level, and Exercise capacity 84-85
assessment, 508
decrease, 502
increase, absence, 121
measurement, 13
measures, 49-50
Exercise conditioning, 549
factor, importance, 130
knowledge, 129-130
short-term/long-term effects. See Systematic exercise conditioning 130
Exercise-induced bronchoconstriction, impact, 99
Exercise-induced bronchospasm (EIB)
assessment/monitoring, 503
consideration, 501
Exercise-induced oxygen desaturation, evaluation, 156
Exercise-induced symptoms, development, 532
Exercise training
components, 171
evidence benefits. See Chronic obstructive pulmonary disease 140t

Exercise training (Continued)
 high/low levels, comparison, 334f
 impact. See Dyspnea 59
 importance. See Pretransplantation
  rehabilitation 371
 IMT studies, combination, 150
 physiologic adaptation, 130
 program
  design, 171
   physiologic principles, consideration, 171
  usage, 120
 pulmonary rehabilitation, combination, 59
 randomized trials, 148t, 332
 safety, 507
 strategies, 500
Exercising muscle, cellular hypoxia
  protection, 120
Exertion, evaluation instructions. See Perceived
  exertion 193t
Exertional breathlessness, 337
Exertional dyspnea
 changes, 338f
  absence, 337-338
  example, 338
  pulmonary rehabilitation treatment,
   effectiveness, 337-338
Experimenting smoker, nicotine
  activation, 235
Expert Committee on Complementary
  Medicines in the Health System,
  221-222
Expiratory time, lengthening, 51
Extended ADL (EADL) Scale, 344
 discrimination ability, 344
 performance rating, 344
External stimuli, responses, 419-420
Extrapulmonary disorders, 425
Extrathoracic anchoring points, 136
Extremity exercise. See Lower extremity
  exercise 132; Upper extremity exercise 136

F

Facilitator-learner relationship,
  development, 75
Fagerström Test for Nicotine Dependence
  (FTND), 236
 measurement, 255-256
Family education, adult education
  (facilitation examples), 76
Fans, usage, 55
Fat-free mass (FFM)
 adjustment. See Metabolically active
  FFM 212
 depletion. See Chronic obstructive
  pulmonary disease 210-211
 estimation, 345
 improvements, 214
 muscle mass measure, 210
Fatigue
 assessment, 167
 referral usage, 12-13
 relationship. See Dyspnea 50
Fat mass, regulation, 213
Fat metabolism, data limitation. See Chronic
  obstructive pulmonary disease 213
Federal Aviation Administration (FAA)
 cabin pressure requirements, 458-459
 medical kit requirements, 463
Federal health insurance programs,
  488b, 488
Female sexual response, aging (impact), 287b
FEV$_1$. See Forced expiratory volume in 1
  second 10-11
FFM. See Fat-free mass 210
Fibrosis, Velcro-like lung sounds, 163-165
FIM. See Functional Independence
  Measure 194
Financial indicators, monitoring, 477-478
Financial performance, 477

Fish consumption, epidemiologic
  evidence, 225
5 As. See Smoking cessation 306
5 Rs. See Smoking cessation 306
FK506, 373
Flexibility/stretching, 172
Flow-sensitive loading, impact, 145
Flow-volume loop, 21
 difference, 21-22
 illustration, 22f
Flunisolide, 100t
Fluticasone, combination (impact).
  See Salmeterol-fluticasone
  combination 88
Fluticasone, effects, 34
Fluticasone-alone study, 100-101
Fluticasone propionate, 100t
Fluticasone/salmeterol, combination, 101t
fMRI. See Functional magnetic resonance
  imaging 41
Focused pressure, control (direction), 229
Forced expiratory technique, 533b
Forced expiratory volume in 1 second (FEV$_1$),
  10-11, 49
 absolute changes, 103f
 changes, 84
  increment, 86
 decrement, estimation, 544
 equivalent, 368t
 exacerbation rate, 88
 increase, 331
 objective abnormality, 11
 percent predicted, 346
 prediction, 44
 rate decline, 306
 reduction, 364
 usage, 83-84
Forced vital capacity (FVC)
 improvement, 367
 screening test, 49
Formal smoking cessation programs,
  availability, 307
Formoterol
 combination. See Budesonide/formoterol
  101t
 impact, 99
 usage, 88
Formoterol fumarate, 99t
FRC. See Functional residual capacity 144
Free play, encouragement, 536
Fruits, consumption, 224
 epidemiologic evidence, 225
 longitudinal data, 225
FTND. See Fagerström Test for Nicotine
  Dependence 236
Full facemask, usage, 353f
Full-time ventilation, accomplishment, 352
Function
 ICF definition, 182-183
 improvement, occupational therapy
  (impact), 182
 occupational therapy, relationship, 182
Functional activities, inpatient pulmonary
  rehabilitation (effect), 344f
Functional analysis, performance, 325
Functional assessment
 activity configuration, 188
 approach, advantages, 186, 187
 initiation interview questions, 188
 performance-based assessments,
  reliance, 190
 phase one, 187-188
 phase three, 194
 phase two, 190
Functional assessment, initiation, 166
Functional capacity utilization, 343
Functional disability, quantification, 49-50
Functional dyspnea levels, discriminative
  measure, 44

Functional Independence Measure (FIM), 194,
  491-492. See also WeeFIM 194
Functional magnetic resonance imaging
  (fMRI), usage, 41
Functional performance, 343
 physical components, 343
Functional reserve, 343
Functional residual capacity (FRC), 144
Functional status. See Questionnaire-measured
  functional status 343
 components, 343f
 factors, 276
 noninterchangeability, 343
 reference, 343
Functional Status Questionnaire, 188
FVC. See Forced vital capacity 49

G

Gas exchange
 alteration, 22
 derangement, severity, 20
 determination, 156-157
 occurrence, 23
Gas pressures, hypobaric conditions, 456t
Gastric acidity, alterations, 117
Gastric motility, impairment, 117
Gastrocnemius muscles, ROM limitation, 172
Gastroesophageal reflux, presence, 310
Gastrointestinal irritation, reduction, 87
Gender conflicts, impact. See Caregivers 298
Gengraf, usage. See Lung transplantation 373
Geriatric patients, survival likelihood
  (estimations), 395
Gingko, herbs (usage), 225
Ginseng, 224
Glandular hypertrophy, impact, 95-96
Global Initiative for Chronic Obstructive Lung
  Disease (GOLD)
 benefits report, 544
 guidelines meta-analysis, 236, 265
Global Initiative for Chronic Obstructive
  Pulmonary Disease guidelines (2006), 30
Global Strategy for Diagnosis, Management, and
  Prevention of COPD, 265
Glycopyrrolate, 97t
Goal development, 15
GOLD. See Global Initiative for Chronic
  Obstructive Lung Disease 236
GOLD Teaching Slide Set, 265
Good Samaritan, role, 462-463
Graded exercise testing
 bicycle ergometry, advantages/
  disadvantages, 156t
 treadmill, advantages/disadvantages, 156t
Gravity resistance, impact, 137-138
Greeley, Andrew, 288
Gross manual muscle test. See Lower extremity
  166; Upper extremity 166
Guided imagery, 58
 usage. See Dyspnea 58
Guidelines for Pulmonary Rehabilitation Programs
  (AACVPR), 470, 487
Guillain-Barré syndrome, 510-511

H

HADH. See 3-hydroxyacyl-CoA
  dehydrogenase 136
Haemophilus influenzae, 102
 impact, 89
Hamstring, ROM limitation, 172
Hand-held Assist (HHA), description, 492
HandiHaler, 106f
Hardy, James, 362
HAST. See Hypoxia-altitude simulation test
  460-461
Health
 adult education, importance, 75
 belief/promotion, models, 78
 information technology, change, 471

Health *(Continued)*
 insurance, demand, 487–488
 literacy, 78–79
 status. *See* Inspiratory muscle training 149
Health, Aging, and Body Composition Study,
  data analysis, 33
Health care
 financing, sources, 488
  list, 488**b**
 setting, computers (usage), 471
 use, 347
  uncontrolled studies. *See* Pulmonary
   rehabilitation 347
Health maintenance organization (HMO)
 MCO classification, 490
 term, usage, 490
Health-related quality of life (HRQL), 182, 339
 assessment, 340
 functional status component, 343
 gauges, 196
 impairment, 507–508
 instruments, usage, 343–344
 long-acting bronchodilator therapy,
  effect, 342**f**
 measure, SF-36 (comparison), 342–343
 measurement, 339–340
 multidimensional concept, 341
 noninterchangeability, 343
 pulmonary rehabilitation, impact, 340**f**
 questionnaire
  measurement, 331
  usage, 340
 relationship. *See* Dyspnea 342**f**
Health status/health-related QOL,
  measurement tools, 501
Health status/QOL questionnaires,
  validity, 505
Healthy behaviors, adherence
  (enhancement), 15
Heart burn, assessment, 167
Heart-lung transplantation
 evolution, 369
 indications, 362**b**
Heart rate, occupational therapist monitoring,
  190–191
Heart rate variability biofeedback, 57
Heart transplantation, 258–259
Heliox, decrease, 104
Hemoglobin, chemical attraction, 116
Hemoptysis, assessment, 167
Hepatojugular reflex, 48
Herbal preparations, 222
Heterogeneous spirometric response. *See* Lung
  volume reduction surgery, 386
HHA. *See* Hand-held Assist 492
High-altitude simulation test, 460**t**
High-flow oxygen
 administration, 101–102
 requirement, 171
High-intensity training program,
  initiation, 132**f**
High-pressure cylinders, 441. *See also* Small
  high-pressure cylinders 441
High-pressure stationary O₂ system,
  advantages, 441–442
High-resolution computed tomography
  (HRCT)
 fibrosis score, 365–366
 morphologic characteristics, 366–367
 scans, classification, 387–388
High-risk patients, identification.
  See Chronic obstructive pulmonary
  disease 90
Histologic UIP, 366–367
HME. *See* Home medical equipment
  432–433
HMG-CoA reductase inhibitors, 228
HMO. *See* Health maintenance
  organization 490

Holding chambers, 106**f**
 usage, 108
  concerns, 108
Home-based cycle ergometry, 150
Home care. *See* Respiratory home care 433
Home health agencies, medical specialists
  (employment list), 439**b**
Home mechanical ventilation, 351, 449
 costs, 356
 equipment, necessity, 439
 evidence, 357
 financial disincentive, 357
 in-hospital care, cost comparison, 356
 methods, 352
 patients
  personality characteristics, 355
  selection, 355
 techniques, 352**b**
 treatment. *See* Chronic respiratory
  failure 351
Home medical equipment (HME). *See*
  Respiratory home medical equipment 441
 ancillary services, necessity, 439
 companies, 432–433
 financial issues, 439
 necessity, 438
 ordering information, requirement, 435**t**
 provider, 435
  equipment maintenance,
   responsibilities, 436
  patient responsibilities, 436
  selection, factors, 435
 types, 439**t**
Home oxygen
 Medicare coverage criteria, 451**b**
 sources, 122–123
 therapy, ABG/Sao₂ indications, 121**b**
Home ventilation, demographics, 351
Hospice services, patient qualification
  (identification), 401**b**
HRCT. *See* High-resolution computed
  tomography 365–366
HRQL. *See* Health-related quality of life 182
Huffing, 533**b**
Human Interaction Research Institute,
  study, 2
Human leukocyte antigen (HLA) protein.
  See Non-HLA protein 376
 inclusion, 376
Human sexual response, changes (focus),
  287–288
Humidification, 124
 usage, 124
Hyperarousal/hypoarousal, impact, 271
Hyperbaric oxygen, usage, 115–116
Hypercapnia
 aggravation, 424
 suspicion, 121
Hypercarbia, 536
Hyperglycemia, occurrence, 98
Hyperinflation, 22
 decrease. *See* Dynamic hyperinflation 51–52
 dose-dependent reduction, 121
Hyperlipidemia pharmacotherapy, 258–259
Hypermetabolism, 213
Hyperpnea. *See* Sustained hyperpnea 145
Hypertension pharmacotherapy, 258–259
Hypertension screening, 258–259
Hypertriflyceridemia, Sirolimus (impact), 374
Hypobaric conditions. *See* Gas pressures 456**t**
Hypobaric hypoxia
 acute pulmonocardiac responses, 456
 effects, 455
 healthy individuals, reaction, 456
 impact. *See* Sleep 458
 physiology, 455
 problem, absence, 463–464
 pulmonary disease patients, response, 457
Hypobaric-induced hypoxemia, 458

Hypogonadism, 229
Hypokalemia, occurrence, 98
Hypoxemia, 536
 aggravation, 424
 impact. *See* Pulmonary arterial pressure 458
 sleep disorders, association, 273–274
Hypoxemic patients, recovery, 121
Hypoxia. *See* Brain tissue hypoxia 117;
  Hypobaric hypoxia 455
 clinical signs, 117
 impact, 461
Hypoxia-altitude simulation test (HAST),
  460–461
 availability, absence, 461

I

ICD-9-CM. *See* International Classification
  of Diseases, 9th Revision, Clinical
  Modification 474
ICD-10-CM. *See* International Classification
  of Diseases, 10th Revision, Clinical
  Modification 475
ICF. *See* International Classification of
  Functioning, Disability, and Health 182
Idiopathic pulmonary arterial hypertension
  (IPAH), 368
 medical management, advances, 368
 patients, listing (decision), 368–369
 survival, 520
  illustration, 520**f**
Idiopathic pulmonary fibrosis (IPF), 365
 diagnosis, referral, 365
 prognosis, 365–366
Idiopathic pulmonary hypertension, 523
IGF-I. *See* Insulin-like growth factor 214–215
ILD. *See* Interstitial lung disease 236
Illness-related impairment, reductions, 279
Iloprost (Ventavis), usage, 520–521
Immunosuppressive medications, 374**t**
Impaired ventilatory control, 351
Impairments, WHO International
  Classification, 182**f**
Impotence
 impact, 294
 nature, 294–295
IMT. *See* Inspiratory muscle training 144–145;
  Inspiratory muscle training 52
Imuran, 373
Incisional pain, reduction, 169
Incremental exercise testing, 332
 examples, 333**t**
Incremental Shuttle Walk Test, therapy
  response, 336
Independent patient, 492
Individualized home exercise program, usage,
  174–176
Individualized pulmonary rehabilitation
  program, planning, 170
Induced bronchoconstriction, impact.
  See Acetylcysteine 102
Induced sputum, inflammatory markers, 32
Inflammation (prevention), levalbuterol
  (advantages), 99–100
In-flight deaths, survey, 462–463
In-flight medical incidents, 459
In-flight oxygen administration, assistance,
  446–447
In-flight oxygenation, prediction, 459–460
Influenza
 administration, 310
 infection, impact, 309
 vaccination, recommendation, 309
 vaccines, usage, 85
Informational support, 58–59
Information seeking strategy, usage, 56
Inhalation
 anticholinergic agents, usage, 97**t**
 therapists, term (discontinuance), 155
 therapy techniques, 155

Inhaled albuterol, FEV₁ (absolute changes), 103**f**

Inhaled β-agonists, usage, 212

Inhaled corticosteroid/long-acting β-agonist combination, TORCH Study support, 88–89

Inhaled corticosteroids
airway effect, dose-response curve, 100
list, 100**t**
systemic manifestations, 100
usage, 100

Inhaled medications, long-term adherence, 319

Inhaled opiate therapy, usage. *See* Dyspnea 54

Inhaler-delivered β-agonists, systemic doses, 99

Inhaler devices, examples, 106**f**

Inhomogeneous upper lobe emphysema, 83–84

Innovation, performance improvement, 479**t**

Inpatient hospital training, 135–136

Inpatient pulmonary rehabilitation, effect. *See* Functional activities 344**f**

INR. *See* International normalized ratio 228

Inspiration, MDI actuation (coordination), 108

Inspiratory capacity, increase, 97

Inspiratory capacity to total lung capacity, ratio, 84

Inspiratory efforts, assistance, 166**f**

Inspiratory flow, rapidity, 109–110

Inspiratory flow/pressure, proportion, 21**f**

Inspiratory muscles
importance, 25
strength, increase, 145
weakness, diagnosis, 144

Inspiratory muscle training (IMT), 52
candidate selection, 150
device, usage, 145
exercise performance, 149
exercise prescription guidelines, 150
health status, 149
impact, 53, 503
outcomes, 146
measurement, decision, 151
programs, training characteristics, 146
published studies, review, 145
randomized controlled trials, 146
list, 147–148**t**
randomized trials, list, 148**t**
rationale, 144
receiving, 503–504
results, interpretation, 144
studies, combination. *See* Exercise training 150
types, 145

Inspiratory resistance breathing, 145

Inspirease, 108**f**

InspirEase (Schering-Plough), 108

Inspiring, MDI usage, 106

Institutional living environments, occupational therapist work, 189

Insulin-like growth factor (IGF)-I
anabolic pathway mediator, 214–215
IGF-I-mediated signaling pathways, 214–215
mRNA (stimulation), high-intensity exercise (usage), 214–215

Insurance terminology, PR correlation, 488**f**

Intensive therapy, 294. *See also* Permission, Limited Information, Specific Suggestion, Intensive Therapy 291
usage. *See* Sexual problems 294**b**

Interleukin-6 (IL-6) levels, increase, 33

Intermediaries, role, 489

Intermediate-acting β₂-agonists, 98

Intermittent flow devices (pulsed flow devices), 123
usage. *See* Oxygen 123

Intermittent Positive Pressure Breathing (IPPB), 448
Study, 319
therapy, usage, 548
Trial, data, 273–274

Internal operations, improvement, 478, 479**t**

Internal stimuli, responses, 419–420

International Classification of Diseases, 9th Revision, Clinical Modification (ICD-9-CM), 474
usage, 475

International Classification of Diseases, 10th Revision, Clinical Modification (ICD-10-CM), diagnoses replacement, 475

International Classification of Functioning, Disability, and Health (ICF), 182
occupation, relationship, 183, 184**t**
occupational therapy outcomes, 197**t**

International normalized ratio (INR), monitoring, 228

International Society for Heart and Lung Transplantation (ISHLT), 363
guidelines, 369
Official Adult Lung and Heart-Lung Transplantation Report, 377–378
recommendations, 367, 369–370

Interpersonal Support Evaluation List-Short Form (ISEL-SF), 275

Interstitial lung disease (ILD), 236, 504
advancement, 507–508
disorder, pathological heterogeneity, 504
education topics, importance, 505–506
exercise limitation, multifactorial basis, 504
randomized controlled trials, 505

Interstitial pneumonitis, 49

Intervention
documentation, 205
evidence-based principles. *See* Pulmonary disorders 196

Intestinal motility, impairment, 117

Intraocular pressure, elevation, 96–97

Intubation, life support intervention, 397**t**

Invasive positive-pressure ventilation (IPPV), 352

Invasive TPPV, receiving, 355

Investigator-associated pneumonia, 88

IPAH. *See* Idiopathic pulmonary arterial hypertension 368

IPF. *See* Idiopathic pulmonary fibrosis 365

IPPB. *See* Intermittent Positive Pressure Breathing 273–274

IPPV. *See* Invasive positive-pressure ventilation 352

Ipratropium/albuterol, combination, 101**t**
availability, 97

Ipratropium bromide, 97**t**
aerosol anticholinergic, 97

ISEL-SF. *See* Interpersonal Support Evaluation List-Short Form 275

ISHLT. *See* International Society for Heart and Lung Transplantation 363

Isoetharine mesylate, 98**t**

Isoproterenol hydrochloride, 98**t**

J

Jerry L. Pettis Memorial Veterans Administration Medical Center
pilot behavioral/pharmacotherapeutic approach, 257
residential programs, establishment, 257
residential treatment programs, 257

Job descriptions. *See* Clinical ladder 481

Job performance, performance improvement (integration), 481

Joint ROM, maintenance, 168

Jugular venous distention, 48

Juniper Asthma Quality of Life Scale, 501

K

Kaplan, Robert, 476

Kidneys, chronic hypercapnic compensation, 118

Kyphoscoliosis, 351, 506

Kyphotic postures, association. *See* Restrictive lung disease 166

L

Laboratory evaluation, usage. *See* Dyspnea 48

Lactate buildup, 116

Lactic acidosis, 116

Lactic acidosis, decrease, 134

Language usage, occupational therapist modeling, 200

Large-volume nebulizers, power, 448

Late-stage T-cell activation, MMF inhibition, 374

L-carnitine, usage, 225

Learners
characteristics. *See* Pulmonary rehabilitation 77
compliance, 78
cultural attributes, 79
decision makers, respect, 77
deficits/disabilities, 79
developmental stage, 77
language/perspective, sensitivity/response, 76
literacy, 78
motivation, 78
participation, encouragement, 76
relationship. *See* Teacher
socioeconomics, 79
understanding, 77

Learning
advanced planning skills, usage, 51
environment, creation, 76
interaction, 77
performance improvement, 479**t**

Learning interaction, facilitation (variables), 76

Leg exercise, training method, 136**b**

Leg fatigue, 26

Leg training
effect, 137
studies, 137–138

Length-tension hypothesis, suggestion, 40

Levalbuterol, bronchodilatory effects, 99–100

Levalbuterol hydrochloride, 98**t**

Licorice, 224

Life, health-related quality, 14
occupational therapy, relationship, 182

Lifestyle change, facilitation, 174

Life support interventions. *See* Intubation 397**t**; Mechanical ventilation 397**t**

Life-supportive care, forgoing, 400

Life-sustaining medical care, refusal, 394

Limb-strengthening exercises, 135–136

Limited information, 292. *See also* Permission, Limited Information, Specific Suggestion, Intensive Therapy 291

Linear VAS, usage, 337–338

Linton, Winifred, 154

Liquid gas O₂, creation, 122–123

Liquid oxygen (LOX) systems, 441, 443. *See also* Small LOX systems 441
advantage, 443, 443
disadvantage, 443, 443–444
flow rates, availability, 443
portability, 443
technology, advancement, 444

Literacy, impact, 78–79

Long-acting β₂-agonists, 98, 98**t**
list, 99**t**

Long-acting bronchodilator therapy, effect. *See* Health-related quality of life 342**f**

Long-term exercise maintenance. *See* Chronic obstructive pulmonary disease 322

Long-term goals, description, 205

Long-term mechanical ventilation, patient candidates, 355
Long-term oxygen therapy (LTOT), 83–84
  clinical efficacy, proof, 116
  hypoxemia, presence, 85
  patients
    evaluation, 121
    initial evaluation, 121–122
  prescribing, 124
    ATS/ERS flow diagram, 122f
    physiologic criteria, 121
  prescription, indications, 309b
  receiving, 117–118
  scientific basis, 116
Long-term survival, pulmonary rehabilitation (impact), 346
Loop diuretics, usage, 224
Lovemaking
  avoidance, 294
  body position, variations, 294
  couples advice, 296
  rehabilitation team advice, 293–294
  suggestions, 293b
Lower extremity, gross manual muscle test, 166
Lower extremity exercise, 132
  benefits, 136
  evidence, 134
  patient benefit, consideration, 134
  training, results, 136f
Lower respiratory tract infection, signs/symptoms (awareness), 310
Lower rib cage, movement (focus), 51
Low-intensity aerobic exercise, 131
LOX. See Liquid oxygen 441
LTOT. See Long-term oxygen therapy 83–84
Lung cancer, 509
  death rates, 3
  detection, sputum/bronchoalveolar lavage cytology studies, usage, 311
  diagnosis, American Cancer Society estimation, 311
  identification, 311
  preparation, 509–510
  prevention, 312
  recovery, 509–510
  respiratory disorder, 499b
Lung disease
  anxiety, experience, 201
  coping, 78
  economic cost, 5t
  incidence, continuation, 304
Lung function
  comparison, 226
  decline, study, 226
  impairment, 209
  improvement, breathing exercises, 228
  prevalence, reduction, 225
  screening, 221
Lung Health Study, 306, 319
Lungs
  age
    equations, development, 305
    estimation, equations, 305b
  allocation score, 362
  function abnormalities, early detection, 305
  hyperinflation, decrease, 97
  inflation, increase, 87
  morphology (determination), CAT techniques (usage), 364
  surgery, 550
  volume
    decrease, 87
    variation. See Pᴇmax 144
  volume-pressure relationship, 23f
Lung transplantation
  absolute contraindications, 362
  active malignancy, impact, 363

Lung transplantation (Continued)
  acute exacerbations, hospital admissions, 364
  acute rejection, 376
    absence, 376
    presentation, 376
  airway complications, 375
  candidate selection, 363
  cardiovascular/technical complications, 377
  chronic rejection, 376
  complications, 375
  conditions, consideration, 362b
  contraindications, 362
  Cyclosporine A, usage, 373
  diagnoses, 370–371
  discharge, patient expectations, 372–373
  drug/alcohol abuse problems, 363
  Eon, usage, 373
  functional outcomes, 378
  Gengraf, usage, 373
  graft failure, 377
  inclusion criteria, 362
  indications. See Bilateral lung transplantation 362b; Heart-lung transplantation 362b; Single lung transplantation 362b
  infection, 376
    complications, prevention (measures), 377
  initiation, 362
  medications, 373
  mortality, correlation, 364
  myopathy, development, 375
  Neoral, usage, 373
  non-CMV infections, 377
  outcomes, 377
  patients, pulmonary disease. See Pre-lung transplantation patients 371
  PGD, impact, 375
  postoperative rehabilitation, 372
    inclusion, 372
  post-transplantation rehabilitation, 372
    goal, 372
  pretransplantation rehabilitation, 370
  psychiatric disorders/psychosocial problems, impact, 363
  referral, timing, 363
  rehabilitation, 370
  rejection-related graft failure, impact, 362
  relative contraindications, 363
  Sandimmune, usage, 373
  smoking, impact, 362
  success, increase, 376
  systemic disease, impact, 363
  techniques, familiarity, 168
Lung volume reduction surgery (LVRS), 83–84.
  See also Upper lobe emphysema 85
  candidate, 364–365
  clinical evaluation, 387
  clinical features, 387
  comparisons, 366f
  controlled trials, onset, 389
  data, availability, 386
  functional changes, 385
  health status, 386
  heterogeneous spirometric response, 386
  imaging, 387
  improvement, 386–387
  incisions, types, 168
  lung transplantation candidates, 364–365
  patient selection, 387
  performing, 385
  physiologic features, 387
  physiologic/morphologic inclusion/exclusion criteria, 365b
  population, rehabilitation needs/results, 388
  preoperative exercise capacity, 387
  pulmonary function/exercise, 385
  pulmonary rehabilitation

Lung volume reduction surgery (LVRS) (Continued)
    approach, 390t
    case series, 388t
    role, 389
    role, recommendations, 389–390
    randomized trials, 388t
    result. See Bilateral LVRS 385–386
    surgical procedures, familiarity, 168
    thoracic imaging, importance, 387–388
    thorascopic procedure, 168
  LVRS. See Lung volume reduction surgery 83–84
  Lymphocytes, alterations, 31

M

MACs. See Medicare administrative contractors 489
Magnesium, 227
  involvement, 227
  maintenance, 227
Maintenance bronchodilating treatment, 212
Male sexual response, aging (impact), 287b
Malnutrition, impact, 130. See also Dyspnea 52
Mammalian target of Rapamycin (mTOR), 374
Managed care, 490
  advent, 433
  concept, 490
  impact. See Respiratory home care 450
  term, usage, 490
Managed care organizations (MCOs), 490
  classification, 490
Manually assisted cough, 533b
  method, 354
Manual therapies, 228, 229
  Cochrane Database, 229–230
  studies, 230
Marital functioning, 274
  assessment, 275
  treatment, 275
Mask-type noninvasive ventilation, 353
Maximal inspiratory pressure (Pɪmax), 49, 52–53
  improvement, 146–149
  volitional tests, 144
Maximal oxygen uptake, increase, 130
Maximal transdiaphragmatic pressure, work, 140t
Maximal verbal cueing (Max VC), 492–493
Maximum Assist (Max A), description, 492
Mayo Clinic
  behavioral treatment model, 257
  residential treatment programs, 257
MCID. See Minimal clinically important difference 47
MCOs. See Managed care organizations 490
MDI. See Metered dose inhaler 97
MDIhs. See Metered dose inhaler with a spacer/holding chamber 102
Mechanical insufflation-exsufflation, 533b
Mechanical insufflator-exsufflator
  availability, 354–355
  usage, 355f
Mechanical ventilation. See Noninvasive mechanical ventilation 353
  assistance, 548
  life support intervention, 397t
  usage, 352b
Median aircraft cabin altitude, calculation, 458–459
Median sternotomy, 168
Medicaid
  impact. See Respiratory home care 450
  programs, evolution, 488
Medi-Cal, 258–259
Medical advice
  adherence/nonadherence, traditional view, 319–320
  noncompliant behavior, viewpoints, 320–321

Medical advice *(Continued)*
　overadherence, 320
　rational nonadherence, 320
Medical advice, adherence problem
　extent, 317
　physician awareness, 317
　prediction, variables, 319
　studies, summary, 318t
Medical director, 470
　role. *See* Pulmonary rehabilitation 470
Medical evaluation. *See* Pre-flight medical
　　evaluation 459
Medical facilities, working (advantage), 202
Medical history, 12
Medical Outcomes Study, 275
Medical Outcomes Study Short-Form 36
　(SF-36), 501
Medical regimen, oxygen (role), 118
Medical Research Council (MRC)
　Breathlessness Scale, 44
　　ranking, 44f
　Dyspnea Scale, 20–21, 506
　　outcome measure, 338
　　usage, 134–135
　dyspnea scores, 386
　Scale, modification, 84–85
　study, 116
　study, NOTT study (results combination),
　　116f
Medical treatment, optimum (establishment),
　13
Medicare, 488
　claims processing, 489
　components, 489
　coverage, 489
　　criteria. *See* Home oxygen 451b
　denial, reasons, 491
　documentation requirements, 491
　establishment, 488–489
　impact. *See* Respiratory home care 450
　noncovered services, 492b
　Part A, 489
　Part B, 489
　programs, evolution, 488
　reimbursement, changes, 433
Medicare administrative contractors (MACs),
　489
Medicare Modernization Act (2003), 489
Medications, 547. *See also* Immunosuppressive
　medications 374t
　adherence, suggestions, 321
　aerosolization, 95
　usage, 185
　　optimization, 168
Medicine-taking adherence, increase, 321–322
MediSpacer, 108f
Mesolimbic dopaminergic pathway,
　dopaminergic neurons (schematic), 248f
Metabolically active FFM, adjustment, 212
Metabolic equivalent (MET) values.
　See Occupational performance 191t
　usefulness, 190
Metaproterenol, 98t
Metered dose inhaler (MDI), 105, 447.
　See also Breath-actuated MDIs 108
　actuation, coordination. *See* Inspiration 108
　actuations, delivery, 107
　advantages, 108
　　comparison, 111t
　components, 107f
　construction/operation, 105–106
　coordination, disadvantage, 108
　disadvantages, 108
　　comparison, 111t
　　explanation, 108, 108
　DPIs, technique differences, 111b
　drug
　　availability, 103
　　remainder, determination problem, 106–107

Metered dose inhaler (MDI) *(Continued)*
　issues, 106–107
　pharyngeal drug deposition, disadvantage,
　　108
　technique, importance, 447
　usage, 97, 102. *See also* Drug delivery
　　maximization 106; Inspiring 106
　　inability, 447–448
　　technique, 107b
Metered dose inhaler with a spacer/holding
　chamber (MDIhs)
　advantages/disadvantages, comparison, 111t
　drug delivery, 103
　usage, 102
Metering valve, function, 107f
Methylprednisolone sodium succinate,
　usage, 376
MET level, calculation, 161b
Midcial Research Council Dyspnea Scale,
　12–13
Middle-aged adults, changes, 77–78
Middle-aged nonathletes, exercise
　(requirement), 131
Miller, William F., 2
Mind-body relaxation, 228
Minimal Assist (Min A), description, 492
Minimal clinically important difference
　(MCID), 47. *See also* Transition Dyspnea
　Index 53
Minimal verbal cueing (Min VC), 492–493
Minnesota Living with Heart Failure
　Questionnaire, 508
Minute ventilation to carbon dioxide uptake,
　ratio, 507–508
MMF. *See* Mycophenolate Mofetil 374
MMRC. *See* Modified Medical Research
　Council 338
Mobility, increase, 169
Moderate Assist (Mod A), description, 492
Moderate verbal cueing (Mod VC), 492–493
Modified Borg Scale
　sensitivity, 43–44
　usage. *See* Breathlessness 43
Modified independence, 492
Modified independent patient, 492
Modified Medical Research Council (MMRC)
　Dyspnea Scale, 338, 346
Modified piezoelectric SVN, 106f
Modified proprioceptive neuromuscular
　facilitation, 137–138
Mometasone furoate, 100t
Monoamine oxidase inhibitors, benefits, 224
Monocytes, alterations, 31
Moraxella catarrhalis, 102
　impact, 89
Motivational interviewing, 278
　development, 278
　impact. *See* Smoking cessation 278
Mouth occlusion pressure, 24f
　measurement, 24–25
Mouthpiece ventilation (MPV)
　device, usage, 353f
　motorized wheelchair setup, 354f
　setup, schematic, 354f
MRC scale. *See* Medical Research Council
　84–85
MSPSS. *See* Multidimensional Scale of
　Perceived Social Support 275
mTOR. *See* Mammalian target of
　Rapamycin 374
Mucociliary transport, increase, 98
Mucoid sputum, production, 101
Mucokinetic agents, 101
Mucokinetic drugs, usage. *See* Sputum 89
Mucokinetic therapy, trials, 101
Mucolytics, 102
　usage. *See* Chronic obstructive pulmonary
　　disease 102
Multicomponent pulmonary rehabilitation, 59

Multidimensional functional assessment, 185
　conducting, preparation, 185
　outcomes, 196
Multidimensional instruments, usage, 44
Multidimensional Scale of Perceived Social
　Support (MSPSS), 275
Multidisciplinary pulmonary rehabilitation
　program, 137–138
Muscarinic receptors, impact. *See* Effector
　cells 96
Muscles
　atrophy, 214
　biopsy sample oxidative enzyme,
　　analysis, 134
　capacity, 143–144
　coordination, improvement, 130
　fibers
　　enlargement, 130
　　shift, 212–213
　force-generating capacity, reduction, 33
　mass, increase, 130
　metabolism, 215
　mitochondria, enzymatic content, 136
　oxidative capacity, decrease, 212–213
　strength, increase, 130–131
　stretching, 172
　tone (decrease), sleep (impact), 420–421
　training. *See* Inspiratory muscle training 52
　wasting, 211
　　significance, 229
　weakness, 229
　　diagnosis. *See* Inspiratory muscles 144
Muscular dystrophy, 351, 510–511
Muscular strength, increase, 130
Musculoskeletal assessment, initiation, 166
Musculoskeletal impairments/function,
　reduction, 167
Music, 57
　usage. *See* Dyspnea 57
Mustache-type reservoir-nasal cannula,
　disadvantage, 445
Mycobacterium tuberculosis, multidrug
　resistance, 459
Mycophenolate Mofetil (MMF), 374
　immunosuppressive medication, 374t
　inhibition. *See* Late-stage T-cell
　　activation 374
Myocardial infarction, 254
Myopathy, 510–511
　development. *See* Lung transplantation 375
Myst Assist, 108f

N

N-acetyl-L-cysteine, usage. *See* Topical
　acetylcysteine 102
Nasal cannula, 444
　disadvantage. *See* Mustache-type reservoir-
　　nasal cannula 445
Nasal mask, usage, 353f
Nasal spray, safety, 254
National Cancer Institute (NCI), 264
National Emphysema Therapy Trial, outcome
　variable, 335
National Emphysema Treatment Trial
　(NETT), 364–365
　results, 385
National Health and Nutrition Examination
　Survey, 535
National Health and Nutrition Examination
　Survey (NHANES II), 225
National Health and Nutrition Examination
　Survey (NHANES III), 226
National Heart, Lung, and Blood Institute,
　consensus conference on pulmonary
　rehabilitation (results), 5
National Hospice Organization, patient
　selection guidelines (revision), 401
National Institute for Health and Clinical
　Excellence (NICE) guidelines, 280–281

National Institutes of Health (NIH)
  IPPB trial, survival comparison, 548**f**
  Registry, idiopathic PAH data, 519–520
National managed care enrollment, 490**t**
National Patient Safety Goals (TJC), 486**b**
NCI. *See* National Cancer Institute 264
Nebulized-delivered β-agonists, systemic
  doses, 99
Nebulized hypertonic saline, airway irritant,
  101–102
Nebulized solution, temperature/humidity
  (impact), 104–105
Nebulized therapy, SGRQ compliance, 319
Nebulizers. *See* Electronic nebulizers 105
  usage, 86
Needs assessment, 77
Neoral, usage. *See* Lung transplantation 373
Net revenue statistics, obtaining
  (difficulty), 478
NETT. *See* National Emphysema Treatment
  Trial 364–365
Neuromuscular disease, 510, 538
  exercise program, 538
  medical characteristics, 538
  NPPV usage, preference, 357
  PR discussions, 511
Neuromuscular junction, disorders,
  510–511
Neuroventilatory disassociation, 40
Neutrophils, alterations. *See* Circulating
  neutrophils 31
New York Heart Association (NYHA)
  class III/IV symptoms, 368–369
    intravenous epoprostenol/treprostinil,
      usage, 369
  functional class, 521–522
  severity, 508
NICE. *See* National Institute for Health and
  Clinical Excellence 280–281
Nicotine, 246, 247
  addiction, 235
    management, 258
  concepts/principles, 253
  controller medications, first line, 252
  delivery systems
    arterial nicotine concentration, 249
    arterial-venous nicotine difference, 249
  dependence, severity (variation). *See* Physical
    nicotine dependence 236
  medication combinations, 251
  nasal spray, 247
  oral inhaler, 247
    arterial-venous nicotine gradient,
      absence, 249
  polacrilex lozenge, availability, 249
  replacement options, 327**t**
  rescue medications, 243, 250
    toleration, 254
Nicotine patch
  controller, 247
  controller medications, first line, 253
  impact, 249
  safety, 254
  toleration, 253–254
  usage, 247
Nicotine withdrawal, 234
  elimination, pharmacotherapy usage, 257
  occurrence, 236
  physical impact, 236
  symptoms. *See* Physiologically induced
    nicotine withdrawal symptoms 235**t**
  extent/severity, 257–258
Nicotinic receptor agonists, 246, 247, 237–240**t**
  concepts/principles, 247
Nicotinic receptor partial agonists, 237–240**t**
Nifedipine, usage, 224
Nightshade plant (*Atropa belladonna*), 96–97
NIPPV. *See* Noninvasive positive airway
  pressure 506

Nitric oxide synthase, encoding, 32–33
Nocturnal asthma, existence (debate), 425–426
Nocturnal breathing problems,
  assessment, 167
Nocturnal myoclonus, 426
Nocturnal noninvasive positive pressure
  ventilation, 506
Nocturnal-only desaturating patients,
  mortality rates, 119
Nocturnal-only desaturators, 119
Nocturnal Oxygen Therapy Trial (NOTT), 116
  data, 273–274
  performing, 116–117
  results combination. *See* Medical Research
    Council 116**f**
  study, 307
Nocturnal restless leg syndrome, 426–427
Noncompliance, viewpoints, 320–321
Non-COPD diagnoses, PR (extension), 470
Non-COPD patient diagnoses, educational
  topics, 500**b**
Non-cystic fibrosis bronchiectasis, 503
Nongovernmental health insurance programs,
  488**b**, 489
Non-HLA protein, inclusion, 376
Noninvasive mechanical ventilation, 353
Noninvasive positive airway pressure, 53
Noninvasive positive pressure ventilation
  (NIPPV), 506. *See also* Nocturnal
    noninvasive positive pressure
    ventilation 506
  usage, 506
Noninvasive positive pressure ventilation
  (NPPV), 351–352
  addition, 548
  candidate selection, criteria, 356**t**
  criteria, American College of Chest Physicians
    definition (consensus statement), 356
  interfaces, 353**f**
  selection factors, 355, 356
Noninvasive ventilation, usage (extensiveness),
  357–358
Noninvasive ventilatory support, impact, 53
Non-O$_2$-dependent subjects, exercise
  capacity, 276
Non-REM sleep
  frequency variability, reduction, 420
  stages, combination, 419**f**
Nonspecific bronchial hyperreactivity,
  improvement, 230
Nonspecific interstitial pneumonia (NSIP),
  366–367, 367
  conditions, heterogeneous group
    (conjunction), 367
  pathologic pattern, 367
  prognosis, 367
Non-upper lobe-predominant emphysema,
  387–388
Noradrenergic-serotonergic reuptake
  inhibitors, 247, 237–240**t**
Norton, David, 476
Nortriptyline, 247
  abstinence rate, 306–307
  controller medication, second line, 254
  side effects, 254
Nortriptyline HCl (Aventyl // Pamelor), 247
NOTT. *See* Nocturnal Oxygen Therapy
  Trial 116
Noxious agents inhalation, cellular/biologic
  response (schematic representation), 19**f**
NPPV. *See* Noninvasive positive pressure
  ventilation 351–352
NSIP. *See* Nonspecific interstitial pneumonia
  366–367
Nuclear factor (NF)-KB, activation. *See* Skeletal
  muscle 215
Nutritional abnormalities, 31**b**
  causes, 32
  weight loss, relationship, 32

Nutritional assessment, 14, 210
  screening, 14
Nutritional enhancement, impact, 546
Nutritional intervention, 506
  effectiveness, clinical trials, 213
  usage. *See* Energy balance 213
Nutritional repletion, positive outcome,
  213–214
Nutritional screening/therapy, flowchart, 211**f**
Nutritional status, 345
  abnormalities, 345
Nutritional supplementation, studies, 214
Nutritional support
  implementation, 215
  interest, renewal, 209
  rationale, 210
NYHA. *See* New York Heart Association
  368–369

O

Obese children, physical activity
  (selection), 550
Obesity, 535
  association. *See* Respiratory disorders 506
  calorie restriction, 536
  exercise program, 536
  impact. *See* Dyspnea 52; Sleep 424
  medical characteristics, 535
Obesity hypoventilation syndrome, 429, 535
Obesity-related respiratory disease, 506–507
Obstructive airway disease, prevalence
  data, 3**t**
Obstructive lung disease, 305
  early detection, 304
Obstructive sleep apnea (OSA)
  characterization, 427
  obesity, relationship, 535
  signs, absence, 119
  sleep failure manifestations, experience, 428
  syndrome, 427
    schematic representation, 427**f**
Occupation, 181
  action, 183
  core construct, 180–181
  importance, 181
  relationship. *See* International Classification
    of Functioning, Disability, and
    Health 183
Occupational performance
  areas, MET values, 191**t**
  assessment, 185
  documentation, 194
  therapeutic procedures/techniques,
    incorporation, 198
Occupational plan, devising, 200
Occupational project groups, 202–204
  organization, 204–205
Occupational projects, therapeutic
  characteristic, 198
Occupational therapists
  activity checklists, usage, 188–189
  evaluation, patient assumption, 187
  hook interventions, 189
  involvement, 181
  patient confusion, 201
  treatment regimen, imposition
    (avoidance), 187
  work. *See* Institutional living environments
    189; Private homes 189; Schools 189
  impact. *See* Pulmonary rehabilitation
    181–182
Occupational therapy, 549
  activities, direct matching, 198
  assessment form, sample, 186**f**
  dimension, 200
  multidimensional functional assessment
    ICF organization, 187**t**
    initiation, 185
  principles, incorporation, 198

Occupational Therapy Practice Framework: Domain and Process (AOTA publication), 185
Occupational therapy therapeutic process, 180–181, 185
Omega-3 fatty acids, 228
  Agency for Healthcare Research and Quality evidence report/technology assessment, 228
Operational performance. *See* Pulmonary rehabilitation 472
  evaluation, 475
Opiate receptors, usage, 54–55
Opioids, usage. *See* Breathlessness 54
OPOs. *See* Organ procurement organizations 370
OptiChamber, 108**f**
OptiHaler (Respironics), 108
  illustration, 108**f**
Oral steroids, usage, 88
Organ donors, 370
  pulmonary/surgical decisions, 370
Organizational performance, evaluation, 475
Organ procurement organizations (OPOs), 370
Organ rejection detection, 169
Orthopnea, 48
OSA. *See* Obstructive sleep apnea 119
Oscillatory devices, 533**b**
Oseltamivir, administration, 309
Osteoporosis
  development potential, 312
  progression, 533–534
Outcome assessment. *See* Pulmonary rehabilitation 80
  perspective, 331
  rationale, 330–331. *See also* Pulmonary rehabilitation 331**b**
Outcome documentation, 472–473
  benchmarking, usage, 473–474
Out-of-pocket costs, decrease, 488–489
Outpatient hospital training, 135–136
Outpatient pulmonary rehabilitation, controlled study, 347
Overadherence, 320
Overlap syndrome, 119
Over the door pulley system, usage, 172
Overweight smokers, demographics, 119
Oxidative phosphorylation, impairment, 212, 212–213
Oxygenation, state, 23
Oxygen-conserving devices, 444
  acceptance, 445
  ambulatory system, 445**f**
Oxygen Cost Diagram, 12–13
Oxygen delivery ($\dot{D}O_2$), 455
  device selection, 309**f**
  equation, 456**b**
  methods, 123
Oxygen-nitrogen mixtures, usage combination. *See* Small-volume nebulizers 104
Oxygen (O_2)
  adjustment/titration, 169
  administration. *See* High-flow oxygen 101–102
    immediate effects, 120
  bus travel, 447
  car travel, 447
  concept, Lavoisier discussion, 1
  exercise training, 124
  flow, titration, 118
  history, 115
  intake. *See* Sleep 119
  intermittent flow devices, usage, 123
  patient education, 124
  prescription, 121
    management, 54
    providing, 170

Oxygen (O_2) *(Continued)*
  pulsed flow devices, usage, 123
  pursed lips breathing, combination, 124
  reservoir cannulas, usage, 123
  saturation
    measurement, 49, 58
    rate, occupational therapist monitoring, 190–191
  storage, 441
  systems, 122
    selection criteria, 444**b**
    stationary/portable components, 123
  tanks, usage, 522
  therapeutic use, 1–2
  transport, 116
    blood/hemoglobin, usage, 423
  transtracheal catheters, usage, 124
  transtracheal delivery, challenges, 124
  travel, 446
  tubing, safety, 54
  uptake, 220–221
    increase. *See* Maximal oxygen uptake 130
  usage. *See* Exercise 120; Supplemental O_2 51
Oxygen (O_2) concentrators, 122–123, 441, 442.
  advantages, 442
  device, 442
  example, 442**f**
  usage, 464
  disadvantages, 442
Oxygen (O_2) therapy, 547
  adherence, 317–319
  concern, 118
  consideration, 124–126
  contribution, 34–35
  devices, 441
  equipment, design, 118
  hazards/pitfalls/cautions, 117
  indications, 170
  summary. *See* Pulmonary rehabilitation 125**f**
Oxygen uptake ($\dot{V}O_2$), 137
  impact, 138**f**
  rise, decrease, 138

P

P(A-a)O_2. *See* Alveolar minus arterial gradient 455
Paced breathing, exercise (inclusion), 173
PaCO_2. *See* Arterial partial pressure of carbon dioxide 420
PAH. *See* Pulmonary arterial hypertension 518
Pain assessment, 13
Palliative care patients, dyspnea management plan (availability), 54
Pamelor. *See* Nortriptyline HCl 247
Panax ginseng, 224
  immunostimulant effects, 224
Panic symptoms, 252
PaO_2. *See* Alveolar partial pressure of oxygen 455
PaO_2. *See* Arterial partial pressure of oxygen 420; Partial pressure of oxygen in the arteries 116
Parasympathetic innervation, presence, 96
Parenchymal destruction, 22
Parkinson's disease, 510–511
Partial nicotinic receptor agonist, 246–247
Partial pressure of oxygen in the arteries (PaO_2)
  determination, 116
  measurement, American Thoracic Society/European Respiratory Society guidelines, 121
Participation
  dimension, 187
  physical contexts, assessment, 189
  social contexts, assessment, 189
  WHO International Classification, 182**f**
Part-time ventilation, accomplishment, 352

Pathophysiological theories, 56
Patient assessment, 12
  cardiopulmonary exercise test, inclusion, 13
  psychosocial evaluation, inclusion, 15
Patient board of directors (BOD), 408
  boats, usage, 412
  buses, usage, 411
  events, guidelines, 410
  group trips, 411
  holidays, 410
  hospital policy, 411
  meetings, 409
  offices, 409
    inclusion, 409
  oxygen needs, 411
  picnics, 410
  rally/special event/timetable, 414
  refund policy, 411
  ships, usage, 412
  social activities, 410
  transportation, usage, 411
  usage. *See* Better Breathers Club 408–409
Patient education, 14
  adult development, importance, 75
  adult education, facilitation (examples), 76
  importance, 110
  knowledge/skills, translation, 80
  learning, readiness (importance), 75
Patient-physician dialogue, importance, 395
Patients
  activity, subjective experience (occupational therapist determination), 192
  adherence, evidence, 320
  behavior, caregiver analysis/interpretation, 297–298
  boundary blurring, 297**b**
  caregiver, sexual attraction, 296
  documentation, critical thinking (requirement), 472
  encounters, caregiver preparation (importance), 298–299
  environment elements, environmental explanations, 320
  history. *See* Dyspnea 47
  hospitalization, decision, 90
  involvement
    encouragement, 412
    increase, 322
  medical record, 471
  motivation, consideration, 11
  nonadherence, 320
    reason, 321
  occupational needs, performance-based assessment tools (overlap), 194
  overadherence, evidence, 320
  personal space, 296
  perspective, ascertainment, 186
  physical environment, occupational therapist assessment, 189
  relationship
    establishment/maintenance. *See* Provider-patient relationship 297
    uniqueness, 296
  seductiveness, responses, 298**b**
  self-esteem, preservation, 298
  training, 173
  vaccination, 309
Patient selection. *See* Pulmonary rehabilitation 10
  exclusions, 11
  program logistics, 12
Patient support group
  audiocassette recorder/videotape camera, usage, 408
  boats, usage, 412
  buses, usage, 411
  establishment, 407
  events
    guidelines, 410

Patient support group (Continued)
  timetables, 414
  first meeting, importance, 407
  funding, 409
  holidays, 410
    transportation, 411
  hospital policy, 411
  location, 407
  meetings, timing, 407
  organization name, 409
  oxygen needs, 411
  physical activity, encouragement, 413
  picnics, 410
  rally, 414
  refunds, 411
  respiratory rally, 413
  ships, usage, 412
  social activities, 410
  special events, 414
  telephone committee, 408
  trips, 411
Patient-ventilator dyssynchrony, impact,
    353-354
PDE5. See Phosphodiesterase-5 295
Peak carbon dioxide update ($\dot{V}CO_2$), 137
  rise, decrease, 138
Peak expiratory flow rate, addition.
    See Shortness of breath 46
Peak oxygen consumption, correlation.
    See Shuttle walking distance 336
Pedal edema, 48
Pediatric asthma, treatment, 531
Pediatric Asthma Quality of Life
    Questionnaire, 501
Pediatric patient, 529
  rehabilitation
    challenge, 530
    guidelines, 529-530
    rewards, 530
Pediatric pulmonary rehabilitation, goals, 530b
PEmax
  lung volume, variation, 144
  volitional tests, 144
PEP Pioneers, respiratory rally, 413-414
Perceived dyspnea, evaluation
    instructions, 193t
Perceived exertion, evaluation
    instructions, 193t
Percutaneous endoscopic gastrostomy tube,
    usage, 213-214
Performance
  characteristics, determination, 480
  imbalance, susceptibility. See Pulmonary
    rehabilitation 475
Performance-based assessments.
    See Standardized performance-based
    assessments 194
Performance improvement (PI), 480
  checkoff sheet, example, 480f
  embracing, 481
  integration. See Job performance 481
  process, 480
  relationship. See Quality 479
Periodic limb movements, 426
Peripheral muscle
  conditioning, improvement, 331
  dysfunction, 130
Peripheral muscle function, 26
Peripheral skeletal muscle function,
    improvements, 213
Permission, Limited Information, Specific
    Suggestion, Intensive Therapy
    (PLISSIT) model, 291. See also Sexual
    counseling 291b
Permission-giving questions, 291
Personal experiences, sharing, 75
Personality, impact, 271
Personality measures, adherence predictors
    (problem), 319

Petasites hybridus, usage, 226
PFlex (Respironics HealthScan), 145
PFSDQ. See Pulmonary Functional Status and
    Dyspnea Questionnaire 46
PFSDQ-M. See Pulmonary Functional Status
    and Dyspnea Questionnaire, modified
    version 46
PFSS, 344
  self-administered questionnaire, 344
PGD. See Primary graft dysfunction 375
PH. See Pulmonary hypertension 364
Pharmacologic interventions, adherence, 317
  studies, summary, 318t
Pharmacotherapy, usage. See Nicotine
    withdrawal 257
Phosphodiesterase E4 inhibitors,
    antiinflammatory/bronchodilator
    effects, 87
Phosphodiesterase inhibitors, 87
  therapeutic serum levels, 87
  usage. See Chronic obstructive pulmonary
    disease 87
Phosphodiesterase-5 (PDE5), 295
  inhibitors, availability, 295
Physical abilities, changes
    (understanding), 174
Physical activity, direct measurements, 345
Physical activity-induced thermogenesis,
    variation, 212
Physical changes, negative influence, 77-78
Physical contexts, assessment. See
    Participation 189
Physical demands, responses, 190
Physical disability, levels (increase), 56
Physical examination, 12
  usage. See Dyspnea 48
Physically caused nicotine withdrawal
    symptoms, reduction, 247
Physical medicine, documentation language
    (establishment), 491-492
Physical nicotine dependence, severity
    (variation), 236
Physical reconditioning, 130
  principles, 130
  training, physiologic adaptation, 130
Physical rehabilitation programs, 501-502
Physical symptoms, interactive cycle
    (model), 273f
Physical therapist (PT)
  chest physical therapy technique
    instruction, 155
  history, 154
  pulmonary therapy, providing. See Acute
    care settings 155
Physical therapy evaluation, 157
  form, example. See Pulmonary rehabilitation
    162-163f
  initiation, 157-161
Physical therapy modalities, 548
Physical well-being, self-efficacy (role), 272
Physiologically induced nicotine withdrawal
    symptoms, 235t
PI. See Performance improvement 480
PImax. See Maximal inspiratory pressure 49
Pirbuterol acetate, 98t
Pirbuterol inhalation, 109f
Plasma, inflammatory markers, 32
Platypnea, 48
PLB. See Pursed lips breathing 51
PLISSIT. See Permission, Limited Information,
    Specific Suggestion, Intensive
    Therapy 291
pMDIs. See Pressurized MDIs 106f
Pneumatic oxygen-conserving devices,
    usage, 445
Pneumobelt, usage, 136-137
Pneumococcal vaccination
  administration, 310
  recommendation, 310

Pneumococcal vaccine, recommendation, 310
Pneumococcal vaccine, usage, 85
Pneumocystis carinii, impact, 49
Pneumonia, diagnosis data, 434
Polacrilex gum/lozenge
  safety, 254
  usage, 243, 247
Polysomnography, recommendation (absence),
    119-120
POMR. See Problem-oriented medical
    record 471
POMS-SF. See Profile of Mood States-Short
    Form 272
Portable mechanical ventilator
  dry-cell/gel-cell battery power, 464
  reliance, 464
Portable oxygen equipment, 444
Portable oxygen systems, types, 441
Positive end-expiratory pressure, usage, 537
Positive expiratory pressure
  physiotherapy, 533b
Positron emission tomography, usage, 41
Postbronchodilator FEV_1, 20
Postmyocardial infarction thrombolytic
    therapy, 258-259
Postnasal drainage, assessment, 167
Postoperative complications, risk (reductions),
    509-510
Postpolio syndrome, 510-511
Post-transplantation rehabilitation, 372.
    See also Lung transplantation 372
Postural drainage, 549
Posture, problems (development), 166
POWERbreathe (Gaiam), 145
  device, diagram, 146f
PPOs. See Preferred provider organizations 490
PR. See Pulmonary rehabilitation 406
Praxis, action, 77
Precapillary vasoconstriction, impact, 458
Prednisolone, 374
Prednisone, 374
  immunosuppressive medication, 374t
Preferred provider organizations (PPOs), MCO
    classification, 490
Pre-flight arrangements, 462
Pre-flight medical evaluation, 459
Pregnancy, tobacco dependence medication
    (usage), 254
Pre-lung transplantation patients, pulmonary
    disease, 371
Prerandomization pulmonary rehabilitation
    program, changes, 389f
Pressure generation, pattern, 137
Pressurized MDIs (pMDIs), 106f
Presynaptic nerve terminals, acetylcholine
    (release), 96
Pretransplantation rehabilitation (PR), 370.
    See also Lung transplantation 370
  exercise capacity, maintenance/increase, 370
  exercise training, importance, 371
  program, 370
Primary graft dysfunction (PGD), 375
  impact. See Lung transplantation 375
  incidence, 375
    UNOS database, usage, 375
Primary pulmonary disease, 351
Primary pulmonary hypertension, 368, 523
Prime, loss, 106-107
PR-IMT. See Pulmonary rehabilitation-
    inspiratory muscle training 503-504
Private auto travel, 464
Private commercial insurance, usage.
    See Respiratory home care 450
Private health insurance programs, 489
  financial risk redistribution, 489-490
Private homes, occupational therapist
    work, 189
Probiotics, supplementation (research), 225

Problem-oriented medical record (POMR), 471
Productivity indicators, monitoring, 477-478
Professional-patient boundaries, self-reflection. *See* Caregivers 298**b**
Profile of Mood States-Short Form (POMS-SF), 272
Prograf, 373
Proinflammatory cytokines, concentrations (augmentation), 30-31
Proprioceptive neuromuscular facilitation. *See* Modified proprioceptive neuromuscular facilitation 137-138
Protein nitrotyrosination, cause, 32-33
Provider-patient relationship, establishment/ maintenance, 297
Proximal muscle weaknesses, 195
Pseudomonas species, isolate, 102
Psychiatric symptoms, 270
Psychological demands, responses, 192
Psychological distress, treatment, 273
Psychological functioning, 270
    treatments, behavioral research, 278
Psychological well-being, observation, 270
Psychometric testing. *See* Dyspnea 46
Psychomotor function, faltering, 117
Psychosocial assessment, 15
Psychosocial evaluation, inclusion. *See* Patient assessment 15
Psychosocial problems, patient referral, 15
Psychosocial rehabilitation, 550
Psychosocial support, 506
    providing, 168
Psychotherapy-related methods, usage, 228
Psychotic reactions, 252
Psychotropic medications, impact, 273
PT. *See* Physical therapist 154
Public Health Service Clinical Practice Guideline: Treating Tobacco Use and Dependence, 264
Pulmonary arterial hypertension (PAH)
    definition, 518
    distinction, 518-519
    occurrence, 519
    prognosis predictor, functional classification, 521**t**
    treatment, 520-521
    WHO group I, treatment, 520
Pulmonary arterial pressure (increase), hypoxemia (impact), 458
Pulmonary arterial wall, histologic changes (schematic representation), 519**f**
Pulmonary assessment, 163
Pulmonary complications, risk, 539
Pulmonary disease
    development, 166
    dyspnea, description, 171
    functional element, 166-167
    medical attention, reasons, 156
    medical encounters, advice/ recommendations, 316-317
    patients
        air travel, planning, 461
        health/psychological well-being, social support, 275
        involvement, encouragement, 412
        response. *See* Hypobaric hypoxia 457
    physical activity, encouragement, 413
    presence. *See* Sea-level travel 463
    sleep-related disorders, impact, 426
    supplemental O$_2$, usage, 280
    technology-dependent patient travel, 454-455
    therapeutic considerations, 429
Pulmonary disorders
    cognitive deficits, 193-194
    intervention, 196
        determination, 196
        evidence-based principles, 196
Pulmonary exercise protocol, cycle ergometer/ treadmill (usage), 156
Pulmonary fibrosis, 504

Pulmonary fibrosis *(Continued)*
    randomized controlled trials, 505
Pulmonary function
    impact, 276
    improvements, 373
    laboratories, walking tests (termination), 522
    NHANES III study, 226
    testing, usefulness, 387
    tests, 525
Pulmonary Functional Status and Dyspnea Questionnaire, modified version (PFSDQ-M), 46
    activity limitation, measures, 344-345
    development, 344
    measurement, 57
Pulmonary Functional Status and Dyspnea Questionnaire (PFSDQ), 46, 344
    activity limitation measures, 344-345
    self-administered questionnaire, 344
Pulmonary function testing, 155
    abnormal results, importance, 10-11
Pulmonary function tests, importance, 49
Pulmonary hygiene therapy, 168
Pulmonary hypertension (PH), 364, 507. *See also* Primary pulmonary hypertension 368
    consideration, 507-508
    deconditioning, 521
    exercise
        activity, termination, 526
        purpose, 525
        testing, 521
    pulmonary arteriopathy, impact, 525
    randomized control trial, 508-509
    respiratory function, 525
    safety, maintenance, 509
    signs, 428
    studies, 523
    suggestion, 48
    treadmill testing, 525
    treatment, 520-521
    UNCOVER study, 519-520
    WHO classification, 519
        list, 519**b**
Pulmonary mechanics, alterations, 130
Pulmonary patient
    limitations, 195
    treatment, cognitive-behavioral group format, 272-273
Pulmonary physiologic abnormalities, 331
Pulmonary Rehabilitation: Guidelines to Success, publication (1984), 2
Pulmonary Rehabilitation Health Knowledge Test, 14-15
Pulmonary rehabilitation-inspiratory muscle training (PR-IMT) group, 503-504
Pulmonary Rehabilitation Policy and Procedure Manual, contents (sample), 473**b**
Pulmonary rehabilitation (PR). *See* Multicomponent pulmonary rehabilitation 59
    accreditation/standards agencies, 482
    achievement, facilitation, 174
    active smoker enrollment, controversy, 11
    adherence, 279
    advance care planning curricula, effectiveness, 397
    American College of Chest Physicians definition, 3
    American Thoracic Society/European Respiratory Society statement, 74-75
    basis, 285
    behavioral medicine research, 269-270
    benefits, 544
    candidates, 5-6
    care
        components, benefits, 546
        standard, 406

Pulmonary rehabilitation (PR) *(Continued)*
    challenges, 550
    change, demonstration, 332
    clinical practice, impact, 269-270
    combination. *See* Exercise 59
    compliance, 78, 279
    components, 544**b**
    comprehensiveness, 307
    conditions, 11**b**
    consideration, 10
    cultural attributes, 79
    deficits/disabilities, 79
    definition, 3-5
    developmental stage, 77
    diagnosis, correctness (importance), 47
    disorders, considerations/challenges, 500
    documentation, 490
    educational component, 55
    educational topics, 173**b**
    education control groups, differences, 323
    educators, support, 400
    environmental considerations, 174
    evidence, levels (description), 545
    evidence-based support, 10
    exercise
        impact, 279
        training, 171
    general care, 546
    goals, 345
        setting, 174
    health care use, uncontrolled studies, 347
    home exercise program forms, examples, 176-177**f**
    hospital administrators, performance imbalance (susceptibility), 475
    importance, 388-389
    incisions, 168
    infection control, 169
    initial component, 10
    inpatient postoperative goals, 168
    interdisciplinary approach, 154
    intervention, 498
    involvement, TJC Disease Certification Program requirements, 487**b**
    learners, characteristics, 77
    lifestyle change, facilitation, 174
    literacy, 78
    management, overview, 468
    managers, performance imbalance (susceptibility), 475
    medical director, role, 470
    medications, effects, 375
    motivation, 78
    multidimensional staging, 346
    nonbillable time, examples, 477**b**
    noncompliance, treatment, 280
    nontraditional conditions, 469**b**
    nutritional services, impact, 170
    nutritional status, impact, 10
    occupational therapists, impact, 181-182
    occupational therapy, 180-181
    operational performance, 472
    operation financial indicators, example, 478**t**
    organization, 469
    outcome assessment, 80
        examples, 332**b**
        incremental exercise testing, examples, 333**t**
        rationale, 331**b**
    outcome measures, impact potential, 347**f**
    outcomes, scientific studies, 331
    outpatient postoperative goals, 169
    oxygen therapy, summary, 125**f**
    participant, psychosocial status/motivation (assessment), 161-163
    peripheral muscle weakness, impact, 10
    physical therapy evaluation form, example, 162-163**f**

Pulmonary rehabilitation (PR) (Continued)
  policy/procedure, 472
    manual, impact, 472
  postoperative outpatient objectives, 169
  potential, 15
  preoperative goals, 167–168
  procedure counts, example, 476t
  productivity, 476
  progress note, usage, 471
  providing, rationale, 498
  randomized controlled studies, examples,
      339t, 341t
  reimbursement, 487
    changes, 490
  respiratory therapy clinical ladder, example,
      483–485b
  RVUs, example, 476t
  schedule, example, 175f
  scientific evidence-based medicine, historical
      perspective, 468b
  services, 170, 170
    job description, 482b
  setting
    dyspnea, assessment, 42
    dyspnea, physiologic causes
      (modification), 41
  socioeconomics, 79
  specialists, impact, 75
  studies, BDI/TDI usage, 338–339
  support, ATS position statement, 2
  symptom assessment, impact, 12
  team approach, 170
  term, recognition, 3–4
  therapeutic intervention
    assessment/treatment, 272
    dietary factors, 278
    exercise, impact, 274
    social support, perception, 274–275
  therapeutic option, 499b
  times standards, example, 476t
  time standards, 476
  timing, 10
  traditional conditions, 469b
Pulmonary rehabilitation (PR) patients
  behavioral medicine evaluation,
      symptoms, 270t
  bronchodilators, prescribing, 124
  education, importance, 74
  evaluation, 155
  involvement, encouragement, 412
  medical director, education resource, 470
  selection, 10
  training, 173
Pulmonary rehabilitation (PR) programs.
    See Multidisciplinary pulmonary
      rehabilitation program 137–138
  acceptance/increase, 2
  appearance, 3–4
  benchmarking, 473
  changes. See Prerandomization pulmonary
      rehabilitation program 389f
  components, 468
    comparison, 469
    importance, 322
  customer service, 478
  data management, 470
  documentation, UB-04 matching, 491
  entry, 49–50
  equipment, 472
  facility, 472
    considerations, 474b
  financial performance, 477
  graduation, 176
  group size, consideration, 174
  information, 470
  interdisciplinary team, 469
    members, 469b
  internal operations, improvements, 478
  location, 472

Pulmonary rehabilitation (PR) programs
    (Continued)
    options, 474b
  management, administrative director, 470
  nutritional supplements, impact, 214
  organizational/staff performance,
      evaluation, 475
  participants, group size, 472
  participation sequence, 4
  patient record, 471
  patient self-reports, reliance, 14
  planning. See Individualized pulmonary
      rehabilitation program, planning 170
  preventive measures, inclusion, 313b
  provider, variation, 4
  quality, 472
  reimbursement, 487
  scope, 468
  staffing ratios, 472
  teamwork, usage, 194–195
  testing, completion, 136
  usefulness, 58–59
Pulmonary rehabilitation (PR) respiratory
    therapist, RCP II level, 483–485b
Pulmonary rehabilitation (PR) team lead, RCP
    IV level, 483–485b
Pulmonary rehabilitation (PR) treatment
  compliance, 280
  documentation requirements, 491b
  modalities, 543–544
  plan, retention/adherence, 173–174
Pulmonary thromboembolic disease, 459
Pulmonary vagal receptors, impact, 41
Pulmonary vascular disease, respiratory
    disorder, 499b
Pulmonary vasoconstriction, 117
Pulmonic sound, increase, 48
Pulsed flow devices. See Intermittent flow
    devices 123
Pulsed-oxygen conserving device, usage
    (disadvantage), 445
Pulse oximetry, 449
  feedback, combination. See Walking 57
  usage, 117
Pursed lips breathing (PLB), 51
  breathing techniques/training process, 199b
  combination. See Oxygen 124
  recommendation, 199

Q

Quad cane (QC), 492–493
Quadriceps strength, association, 31
Quality, 479
  aspects, refinement, 479
  characteristics, determination, 480
  definition, 479
  performance improvement, relationship, 479
Quality improvement (QI)
  embracing, 481
  foundations, 480
  strategies, 470–471
  team, 481
Quality of life (QOL). See Health-related
    quality of life 182
  concept, nebulousness, 339
  impairment, 502, 504
    studies, 508
  improvement, 498, 510
Quality of Well-Being (QWB) Scale, 324
  changes, 324f
  improvements, 324–325
  mean change, 325f
  measurement, 503
Questionnaire-measured functional status,
    343

R

Radiographs, usage. See Chest 48–49
Railroad travel, 464

Randomized controlled trials (RCTs), 53
  usage, 58
Range of motion (ROM)
  limitations, 196
  loss, 166
  performing, 155
Rapamune, 374
Rapamycin, 374
Rapid eye movement (REM) sleep, 418
  desaturations, association, 119
Rational nonadherence, 320
RCOPE. See Religious/Spiritual Coping Long
    Form 271
RCTs. See Randomized controlled trials 53
Real-time dyspnea, measurement, 42
Recalled dyspnea, unidimensional/
    multidimensional instruments (usage), 42
Recurrent hemoptysis, 367–368
REE. See Resting energy expenditure 212
Refractory/recurrent pneumothoraces,
    367–368
Rehabilitation
  basis. See Pulmonary rehabilitation 285
  exercise component, 322
  potential, 15
Rehabilitation, American Medical Association
    Council on Rehabilitation definition, 1
Reimbursement, 479
  historical perspective, 487
  human errors, impact, 490–491
Rejection-related graft failure, impact. See
    Lung transplantation 362
Relative value unit (RVU), 476–477
  example. See Pulmonary rehabilitation 476t
  objective measure, 477
  usage, 477
  usefulness, 477
Relaxation techniques. See Dyspnea 56
Relaxation training, 201, 548
Relevance risks rewards roadblocks repetition
    (5 Rs). See Smoking cessation 306
Religiosity/religious coping, 271
Religious/Spiritual Coping Long Form
    (RCOPE), 271
REM. See Rapid eye movement 418
Renal transplantation, 258–259
Replacement therapy, inference, 115
Rescue medications, 237–240t
  combination medications, 249
  concepts/principles, 249
  first line, 247
Rescue nicotine medications, 254
  concepts/principles, 254
Rescue therapy, limitation. See β_2-agonists 97
Reservoir cannulas, 123
  representation, 445f
  usage. See Oxygen 123
Resistance training, addition, 549
Respirable mass, SVN delivery, 104f
Respiration muscles, 166f
Respiratory allergies/infections, problems, 225
Respiratory center, location, 23
Respiratory defense mechanisms, vitamin C
    (role), 225–226
Respiratory disease
  coexistence. See Cardiac diseases 156
  dyspnea, association, 130f
  examination, physician participation, 4
  identification, diagnostic tests (usage), 12
  omega-3 supplementation, role, 228
  presence, 498–499
  sleep, presence, 423
  treatment, CAM therapies
      (recommendations), 231b
Respiratory disorders, 499b
  obesity, association, 506
    studies, 506–507
  PR program inclusion, studies, 499–500
Respiratory drive

Respiratory drive *(Continued)*
  decrease, 53
  suppression, occurrence, 118
Respiratory effort, increase, 40
Respiratory failure, eventuality, 117
Respiratory home care, 433
  ancillary services, necessity, 439
  assistance, necessity, 438–439
  benefits, 433
    list, 434**b**
  candidates, 434
    list, 434**b**
  caregiver involvement, 438
  diagnostic/monitoring devices, 449
  equipment, necessity, 439
  financial issues, 439
  follow-up care, 440
  home visit, 437
  managed care, usage, 450
  Medicaid, impact, 450
  medical necessity, documentation, 451
  Medicare, impact, 450
  patient evaluation, 437
  physical assessment, 437
  physical environment, assessment, 437
  plan, 440
  private commercial insurance, usage, 450
  psychosocial issues, 438
    evaluation, 438**b**
  pulse oximetry, 449
  reimbursement issues, 450
  respiratory therapist (RT)
    education/training, providing, 436
    role, 436
  services
    delivery, 434
    patient discharge, 441
  sleep-recording devices, 449
  team, 434
Respiratory home medical equipment
  (respiratory HME), 441
Respiratory muscles, 25
  dysfunction, 130
  endurance training, 229
  failure, 117
  function, 146
    improvement, 50, 50, 213
  rest, 53
  role, 40
  strength/endurance, improvement,
    548–549
  strength training program, initiation, 151
Respiratory muscle strength, 214
Respiratory physiologic abnormalities, 337
Respiratory rally, 413
Respiratory rate (RR)
  occupational therapist monitoring, 190–191
Respiratory rate (RR), decrease, 51, 51
Respiratory secretions, hydration, 101–102
Respiratory sensations, occurrence, 40
Respiratory system, function
  (representation), 26
Respiratory system, uniqueness, 220–221
Respiratory therapist (RT)
  history, 154
  responsibility, 436, 436–437
  role. *See* Respiratory home care 436
Respiratory therapy
  evaluation, 157
    initiation, 157–161
  services, reimbursement, 451
  techniques, 547
Resting energy expenditure (REE), 212
  increase, 33, 214
Resting hypoxemia, objective abnormality, 11
Restless leg syndrome, 427
Restrictive chest wall disease, 506
Restrictive lung disease, 144
  kyphotic postures, association, 166

Restrictive lung disease *(Continued)*
  scoliosis, association, 166
Restrictive neuromuscular diseases, 351
Restrictive pulmonary disorders, 425
Restrictive tissue, change, 24–25
Restrictive ventilatory defects, 425
Retractions, 536
Rib cage enlargement, 163
Rib cage stretching, 172
Right heart failure, 117
  signs, 428
Right ventricular heave, 48
Risk factor reduction, 221
Rocky Mountain Health Resorts (Denison), 1
Roflumilast, antiinflammatory/
  bronchodilator effects, 87
Rolling walker (RW), 492–493
ROM. *See* Range of motion 155
RR. *See* Respiratory rate 51
RT. *See* Respiratory therapist 154
RVU. *See* Relative value unit 476–477

S

Salbutamol sulfate, 98**t**
Salmeterol
  combination. *See* Fluticasone/salmeterol 101**t**
    effectiveness. *See* Theophylline/
      salmeterol 88
  effects, 34
  impact, 99
Salmeterol-fluticasone combination,
  impact, 88
Salmeterol xinafoate, 99**t**
Sandimmune, usage. *See* Lung
  transplantation 373
SaO₂. *See* Arterial oxygen percent
  saturation 455
Sarcoidosis, 369
  commonness, 369
  spontaneous reversal, possibility, 369
Sarcopenia, 210–211
School Function Assessment, 188
Schools, occupational therapist work, 189
Scoliosis, 506, 539
  association. *See* Restrictive lung disease 166
  exercise program, 539
  medical program, 539
Sea-level travel, technology-dependent patient
  (pulmonary disease, presence), 463
Sea travel, expansion, 454
Seattle-Tacoma Airport, medical occurrences
  (frequency), 459
Second Princeton Consensus Conference,
  erectile dysfunction treatment
  guidelines, 295
Secretion management, 354
  effectiveness, 354–355
  issue, importance, 354
  methods, 354**b**
Secretion mobilization, 354**b**
Sedimentation rate, elevation, 48
Seductive behavior, 297
Selective serotonin reuptake inhibitors
  (SSRIs), 256
  ineffectiveness, 256
Self-care activities, attention, 185
Self-care initiation, 168
Self-care strategies. *See* Eating 52**b**
Self-directedness, 75
Self-efficacy
  role. *See* Physical well-being 272
  usage, 271
Self-management principles, 56
Semistarvation, 210–211
Senior pulmonary rehabilitation therapist,
  RCP III Level, 483–485**b**
Set-up (s/u), 492
Sex

Sex *(Continued)*
  health care provider discussion, older adults
    suggestions, 290**b**
Sex, sexuality (contrast), 286
  list, 286**t**
Sex positive attitude, 290
Sexual abuse, 299
  occurrence, perception, 299
Sexual activity
  barriers, 289
  cardiac risk, 293
  dyspnea decrease, strategies, 51
Sexual bias, 298
Sexual concerns, education solution, 292
Sexual counseling, 290
  PLISSIT model, 291**b**
Sexual dysfunction, 294**b**
  medications, impact, 293
Sexual function
  hysterectomy, impact, 288
  stability, 287
Sexual functioning
  lung disease, impact, 289
  medications, impact, 293**t**
Sexual health
  care, 286
    ethical issues, 297
  WHO definition, 286
Sexual interactions, 299
Sexuality
  aging process, relationship, 287
  caregiver-patient relationship, 296
  chronic illness, relationship, 289
  continuation, 287
  intensive therapy, 294
  limited information, providing, 292**b**
  patient education, Internet resources, 292**b**
  periodic survey, 288
  permission, giving, 291**b**, 291
  rehabilitation program, introduction, 290
  specific suggestions, 293
  term, complexity, 286
  WHO definition, 286**b**
Sexual-organ changes, 287–288
Sexual partner
  availability, 287, 289
  privacy, absence, 289
Sexual problems
  intensive therapy, usage, 294**b**
  nonorganic causes, 295**b**
Sexual response, aging (impact), 287**b**
Sexual rights, WHO definition, 286**b**
Sexual well-being, correlation, 288
SF-36. *See* 36-item self-complete questionnaire
  342; Medical Outcomes Study Short-
  Form 36 501
SGRQ. *See* St. George's Respiratory
  Questionnaire 46
Short-acting β₂-agonists, 98, 98**t**
  impact, 53
Short Form Health Survey (SF-36), 275
Shortness of breath
  measurement reasons, 42
  rating, peak expiratory flow rate
    (addition), 46
  symptom, 192
Short-term bronchodilator response,
  absence, 99
Short-term goals, description, 205
Short-term weight loss, 536
Shoulder stretching, 172
Shuttle walk, usage, 49
Shuttle walking distance, peak oxygen
  consumption correlation, 336
Shuttle walking test, 49–50, 335
Sickness Impact Profile (SIP), 275
  measurement, 279
  short form, 276–277
Sildenafil

Sildenafil (*Continued*)
  availability, 295
  impact. *See* Erections
  usage, caution, 295
Simple Object Access Protocol (SOAP)
  action, 472
  format, 471–472
Single lung transplantation, indications, 362**b**
SIP. *See* Sickness Impact Profile 275
Sirolimus, 374
  immunosuppressive medication, 374**t**
  impact. *See* Hypertriglyceridemia 374
Six-minute walk speed, average (calculation), 161**b**
Six-minute walk test (6MWT), 13, 33, 522
  cessation, reasons, 157–159**b**
  changes, 332
  comparison, 133
  contraindications, 157–159**b**
  desaturation, 366–367
  distance, 346
    coverage, 44
    improvement, 55
    medications, usage, 520–521
  documentation
    flowsheet, sample, 160**f**
  documentation form, 157–159**b**
  equipment, requirement, 157–159**b**
  exercise gold standard, 157
  functional levels, calculation formulas, 161**b**
  impact, 135
  measurement, 57
  occupational therapist engagement, 196
  patient desaturation, 477
  physician assessment, 167
  policy/procedure, 157–159**b**
  pulmonary rehabilitation assessment, 164–165**f**
  purpose, 157–159**b**
  safety issues, 157–159**b**
  submaximal patient-limited exercise test, 522
  symptom assessment, 167
  usage, 42, 157
Skeletal muscle
  contraction, 420–421
  maximal strength, 144
  NF-KB activation, 215
  training, 145
Skeletal muscle dysfunction (SMD), 32
  list, 31**b**
  mechanisms. *See* Chronic obstructive pulmonary disease 33**b**
  presence. *See* Chronic obstructive pulmonary disease 32
Skin damage, complications, 88
Sleep, 418
  abnormality, 422
  active, energy-dependent process, 418
  apnea. *See* Obstructive sleep apnea 427
    types, 428
  architecture, variation, 418
  blood gases, change, 420
  continuity, impairment, 424
  daytime O_2 setting, prescription, 119
  duration
    impairment, 424
    sufficiency, 422
  facts, 418
  failure, 422
  function, uncertainty, 418
  hypobaric hypoxia, impact, 458
  mechanisms, 418
  obesity, impact, 424
  obstructive sleep apnea syndrome
    schematic representation, 427**f**
  oxygen intake, 119
  physiologic consequences, 419

Sleep (*Continued*)
  physiologic state, 418
  presence. *See* Chronic obstructive pulmonary disease 423; Respiratory disease 423
  problems, 422–423
  recording devices, 449
  respiratory consequences, 420
    schematic representation, 422**f**
  schematic representation, 419**f**
  ventilation, decrease, 420
  ventilatory challenges, 425
Sleep disorders, 417–418
  association. *See* Hypoxemia 273–274
  diagnostic approach, 429
Sleepiness, chronic consequences, 422
Sleep-related disorders, impact. *See* Pulmonary disease 426
Sleep-related respiratory failure, mechanism, 425
Small high-pressure cylinders, 441
Small LOX systems, 441
Small-volume nebulizers (SVNs), 103
  advantages, 105
    comparison, 111**t**
    explanation, 105
  dead volume, presence, 104
  delivery. *See* Respirable mass 104**f**
  disadvantages, 105
    comparison, 111**t**
    explanation, 105
  drug, delivery, 102–103
  oxygen-nitrogen mixtures, usage combination, 104
  particle removal, 103–104
  photograph, 106**f**
  schematic, 103**f**
  usage, 102
    technique, 105**b**
Smokers
  precontemplation phase, 326
  primary care provider visit, 305–306
  support, 277
Smoking
  behavior, COPD risk factor, 277
  behavioral medicine treatment, 277
  continuation, 254
  COPD, association, 325
  history, collection, 161
  interventions, suggestions, 326
  status, assessment, 161
  telephone counseling, 326
Smoking cessation, 86, 277, 546
  ask advise assess assist arrange (5 As), 306
  benefits, 325–326
  clinical practice guidelines recommendations, 308**t**
  effect, 251
  efficacy, increase, 278
  encouragement, importance, 304
  ICD-9 diagnosis code, absence, 258
  motivational interviewing, impact, 278
  motivation promotion, 5 Rs (usage), 306
  paradigms, 259
  programs
    adherence, 325
    availability. *See* Formal smoking cessation programs 307
  rates, Varenicline/Bupropion (association), 306**t**
  treatment, 277
    package, benefits, 278
  Varenicline, usage (approval), 306
Smoking Cessation Clinical Practice Guideline, application, 326–327
Smoking cessation rates, 256
  improvement, 247
    Varenicline, usage, 243–244

SOAP. *See* Simple Object Access Protocol 471–472
SOBQ. *See* University of California, San Diego Shortness of Breath Questionnaire and Pulmonary Functional Status and Dyspnea Questionnaire 45
Social cognitive learning theory, 56
Social contexts, assessment.
  See Participation 189
Social functioning, 274
  assessment, 275
  treatment, 275
Social resources, impact, 276
Social support, 56, 58
  perception, 276
  usage. *See* Dyspnea 58–59
Social support systems, variety, 78
Sore throats, boswellia (usage), 224
Source-oriented chart, division, 471
Spacer, usage, 86, 108
  concerns, 108
Spacer-specific instructions, usage, 108
SPC. *See* Straight point cane 492–493
Specific activities, modification, 203–204**t**
Specific suggestions, 293. *See also* Permission, Limited Information, Specific Suggestion, Intensive Therapy 291
Spinal cord injury, 351, 510–511
Spiral CT scanning. *See* Chest 49
Spirometry
  difficulties. *See* Chronic lung disease 305
  usage, 48–49. *See also* Chronic lung disease 304–305
Sputum
  assessment, 167
  studies, 311
  viscosity (decrease), mucokinetic drugs (usage), 89
SSRIs. *See* Selective serotonin reuptake inhibitors 256
St. George's Respiratory Questionnaire (SGRQ), 46, 341
  changes, 332
  clinical change, threshold, 47
  compliance. *See* Nebulized therapy 319
  components, 345**f**
  domain/total score, decrease, 341–342
  illness-specific measures of quality of life, 276–277
  inclusion, 386–387
  measurement, 210
  respiratory-specific self-administered questionnaire, 341
  studies, 501
  total scores, 505
St. Helena Center for Health
  residential tobacco dependency program, establishment, 257
  residential treatment programs, 257
Staffing ratios. *See* Pulmonary rehabilitation programs 472
Staff performance, evaluation, 475
STAI. *See* State-Trait Anxiety Inventory 272
Stair climbing, evaluation, 135
Stamina, improvement, 169
Standardized performance-based assessments, 194
Standby assist (SBA), 492
Staphylococcus aureus infection, 368
State anxiety
  decrease, 56–57
  measurement, 58
State health insurance programs, 488**b**, 488
State-Trait Anxiety Inventory (STAI), 272
Stationary bicycle
  endurance testing, 334
  ergometry, 371
Stationary O_2 systems, types, 441
Steady-state CNS levels, adequacy, 243

Steroid use, impact. *See* Cushing's syndrome 163
Straight point cane (SPC), 492–493
Strength
  increase, 169
  measure, 195–196
  program, initiation, 171–172
  training, 154
    addition, 549
Streptococcus pneumoniae, 102
  impact, 89
Stretching, equipment (usage), 172
Stroke (neuromuscular disease), 510–511
Structural support, 275
Study to Understand Prognoses and Preferences for Outcomes and Risks of Treatments (SUPPORT), 396
  dyspnea, experience, 400
Substrate metabolism, 212
Supervision (S), description, 492
Supplemental O₂
  administration, 307
  forms, administration, 307
  requirement, 463, 464
  therapy, 53
  usage, 51. *See also* Exercise 120
SUPPORT. *See* Study to Understand Prognoses and Preferences for Outcomes and Risks of Treatments 396
Supported arm exercise training, training method, 140**b**
Supportive coping skills interventions, 273
Surgical pulmonary rehabilitation
  challenges, 167
  education, 168
  evaluation parameters, 167
  exercise limitations, 168
  function, maximization, 167
  incisions, 168
  inpatient postoperative goals, 168
  preoperative goals, 167
Survival, 346
  changes, improvement, 130
  covariate influence, 368**t**
  promotion, life-supportive care (usage), 393
  pulmonary rehabilitation, impact. *See* Long-term survival 346
Sustained activity, ability (increase), 168
Sustained hyperpnea, 145
  IMT method, 145
SVNs. *See* Small-volume nebulizers 102
Swallowing problems, assessment, 167
Symptom assessment, 12
  impact. *See* Pulmonary rehabilitation 12
Symptomatic COPD, exercise monitoring, 43
Symptomatic stable COPD, therapy, 84**t**
Symptom monitoring strategy, usage, 56
Systematic exercise conditioning, short-term/long-term effects, 130
Systemic effects, 34
Systemic inflammation, 30
  impact. *See* Chronic obstructive pulmonary disease 32–33
  list, 31**b**
  therapeutic alternatives, role, 33

T

Tachycardia, 117
Tachypnea, 536
Tacrolimus, 373
  immunosuppressive medication, 374**t**
  relationship. *See* Cyclosporine A 373
Tactile cues, 492–493
Tadalafil, availability, 295
Talk Test, usage, 190–191
T cell-mediated immunity, 213
TDE. *See* Total daily expenditure 212
TDI. *See* Transition Dyspnea Index 44

Teachable moment, recognition, 75
Teacher, learner (relationship), 77
Teaching style, reference, 76
Technology-dependent patient. *See* Sea-level travel 463
Terbutaline, 98**t**
Tertiary ammonium alkaloid, 96–97
Testosterone replacement therapy, 287–288
The Joint Commission (TJC), 482
  Disease Certification Program Requirements, 487**b**
  formation, 482
  influence, 482
  mission, 482
  National Patient Safety Goals, 486**b**
  patient safety-related issues, importance, 482
  requirements, PR compliance, 470
  survey process, change, 482
Theophylline/salmeterol, combination (effectiveness), 88
Thera-Bands, usage, 171
Therapeutic groups, 202
  construction, issues, 202
  creation, 202
  membership, issues, 202
  types, 202–204
  uniqueness, 204
Thermogenesis. *See* Diet-induced thermogenesis 212; Drug-induced thermogenesis 212
  variation. *See* Physical activity-induced thermogenesis 212
Thermoregulation, 212
36-item self-complete questionnaire (SF-36), 342
Thoracic anchoring points, 136
Thoracic deformity, 506
Thoracic fulcrum, usage, 136
Thoracic imaging, importance. *See* Lung volume reduction surgery 387–388
Thorax, muscles/bony structures (assembly), 143
3-hydroxyacyl-CoA dehydrogenase (HADH), 136
Threshold IMT (Respironics HealthScan), 145
  device, diagram, 146**f**
Threshold loading, impact, 145
Thrombogenesis, facilitation, 254
Tidal volume (V_T)
  increase, 51
  restriction, 51–52
Timed walk test, 335
  bias, 335
  exclusion criteria, 336**b**
  incremental shuttle walking test, comparison, 337**t**
  popularity, 335
  protocol, recommendation, 336**b**
  pulmonary rehabilitation intervention responsiveness, 335
Tiotropium
  availability, 97
  prescribing, 124
  trial. *See* Understanding the Potential Long-term Impacts on Function with Tiotropium 87
Tiotropium bromide, 97**t**
Tissue depletion, pathogenesis, 212
Tissue hypoxia, signs (difference), 117
TJC. *See* The Joint Commission 470
TNF. *See* Tumor necrosis factor 212
TNF-α concentration, circulating levels, 32
TNF-α concentration, increase, 31
TNF-α receptors, plasma concentrations (increase), 32–33
Tobacco dependence, 235
  behavioral intervention, 256
  case examples, 265–267

Tobacco dependence (*Continued*)
  chronic/relapse characteristics, 236
  clinical cases, 265–266, 266, 266–267, 267
  controller medications, 252
    first line, 253
  cost-effectiveness, 259
    concepts/principles, 258
  counseling, 256
  CPT, usage, 258
  diagnosis coding, 258
  drug interactions, 251
  funding sources/financial disclosures, 259
  HMO-covered medical screening tests/interventions, 258–259
  ICD-9, usage, 258
  independent processes, occurrence, 235
  lifestyle problem, 235
  medical record, 258
  medication
    changes, 267
    clinical trials, 255
    concepts/principles, 255
    FDA reclassification, 254–255
    initiation, 268
    manufacturer recommendations, 255
  medication, usage. *See* Pregnancy 254
    concepts/principles, 255, 256
    duration, 255
    recommendations, 256
  patient resources, 264–265
  pharmacologic categories, 237
  pharmacotherapy, 256
  physician counseling, 256
  physician resources, 264
  physician treatment, 235
  practice concepts/principles, 236
  relapse
    anticipation, 236
    prevention, 243**t**
  residential study, 257
  residential treatment programs, 257
    data, limitation, 257
  resources, 264–265
  short-term medical treatment, 236
  side effects, 252
    concepts/principles, 253
  Social History, 258
  treat-to-effect, 259
Tobacco dependence treatment
  Bupropion SR, effectiveness, 245–246**t**
  combination, FDA approval, 250
  cost-effectiveness, 258**t**
  effectiveness, 259
    improvement, 250**t**
  medications, 237–240**t**
    ineffectiveness, 256
    ineffectiveness, concepts/principles, 256
    usage, 237
  Varenicline, impact, 243
  Varenicline/Bupropion, effectiveness, 242**t**
  work-related stress, 267
Tobacco-dependent patients
  nicotine, impact, 235–236
  physician-directed treatment, optimal cessation rates, 252
Tobacco smoke, substances (impact), 33
Tobacco usage, pulmonary consequences, 236
Tobacco use/exposure history, 258
Topical acetylcysteine (*N*-acetyl-L-cysteine), usage, 102
Total daily expenditure (TDE), 212
Total energy expenditure, division, 212
Toward Healthy Aging (Ebersole/Hess), 291
Towards a Revolution in COPD Health (TORCH), 85
  Study, 97
    mortality indications, 96
    usage, 34, 88–89

Tracheotomy Invasive positive-pressure
    ventilation (TPPV), 352
  complications, 352–353
  receiving. See Invasive TPPV 355
  requirement, 353
  selection factors, 355, 356
  usage, 351–352
    extensiveness, 357–358
    initiation, 353
  ventilators, usage, 353
Traditional chart, 471
  division, 471
Training. See Exercise training 130
  benefits, 130–131
  physiologic adaptation, 130
  program. See High-intensity training
    program 132f
  rationale. See Inspiratory muscle
    training 144
  specificity, 130
  stimulus, selection, 145
Transdermal nicotine, risk, 252
Transforming growth factor-B$_1$,
    alteration, 33
Transition Dyspnea Index (TDI), 44.
    See also Baseline/Transition Dyspnea
    Index 44
  changes, 332
  clinical change, threshold, 47
  dyspnea scores, 386
  interviewer-administered questionnaires, 338
  MCID, 53
  measurement, 53
  outcome measure, 338
  usage, 149
Transtracheal catheters, 124
  usage. See Oxygen 124
Transtracheal delivery, challenges.
    See Oxygen 124
Transtracheal oxygen catheters,
    representation, 446f
Transtracheal oxygen systems, 445
  oxygen delivery, invasiveness, 446
Travel
  advanced medical technology,
    usage, 464
  destinations, altitudes, 456f
  expansion. See Air travel 454;
    Sea travel 454
  medical equipment usage, medicolegal
    aspects, 462
Treadmill
  advantages/disadvantages. See Graded
    exercise testing 156t
  endurance exercise tests, 323f
  endurance testing, 334
  exercise
    COPD, presence, 56–57
    endurance time, comprehensive pulmonary
      rehabilitation (effect), 334f
  incremental exercise testing, 332
  testing, 525
  usage, 49–50
Trepopnea, 48
Triamcinolone acetonide, 100t
Trunk support, providing, 195–196
Tuberculosis, acid-fast smears (usage),
    101–102
Tumor necrosis factor (TNF), markers, 212
Turbuhaler (AstraZeneca), 106f
  components/airflow, 110f
12-minute walking distance, 135
Twisthaler, 106f
Tylophora asthmatica, usage, 226

U

UB-04, 491
Ubidecarenone. See Coenzyme Q10 227–228
Ubiquinone. See Coenzyme Q10 227–228

Ubiquitin-proteasome system, protein
    degradation (facilitation), 32–33
UCSD. See University of California,
    San Diego 45
UIP. See Usual interstitial pneumonitis 365
Understanding the Potential Long-term
    Impacts on Function with Tiotropium
    (UPLIFT) trial, 87, 97
Unidimensional instruments
  testing, 43
  usage, 43
Uniform Reporting Manual for Acute Care
    Hospitals (AARC), development, 477
United Network for Organ Sharing
    (UNOS), 362
  database, usage. See Primary graft
    dysfunction 375
  defined groups, 366f
United States Coast Guard, hazardous
    material branch, 464
University of California, San Diego (UCSD)
  Dyspnea Questionnaire, outcome
    measure, 338
  Shortness of Breath Questionnaire, 12–13
    development, 339
    psychosocial measures, 324
  Shortness of Breath Questionnaire
    and Pulmonary Functional Status
    and Dyspnea Questionnaire
    (SOBQ), 45
    clinical change, threshold, 47
UNOS. See United Network for Organ
    Sharing 362
Unsatisfied inspiration, 40
Unsupported arm exercise, 136–137
  usage, ventilatory response, 137
Unsupported arm training
  arm ergometry training, comparison, 138
  training method, 140b
UPLIFT. See Understanding the Potential
    Long-term Impacts on Function with
    Tiotropium 87
Upper body training, 171
Upper body weaknesses, 195
Upper extremity
  endurance training, 172
  gross manual muscle test, 166
  practical training, 138
  work, 171
  work, ventilatory demand
    (accompaniment), 371
Upper extremity exercise, 136
  training, evidence (indication), 138
Upper lobe emphysema, lung volume
    reduction surgery, 85
Usual interstitial pneumonitis
    (UIP), 365. See also Histologic UIP 366–367

V

Vaccination, 89
  usage. See Chronic obstructive pulmonary
    disease 89
Valsalva-like maneuvers, 509
Vardenafil, availability, 295
Varenicline (Chantix), 240
  action, mechanism, 240
  association. See Smoking cessation 306t
  Bupropion
    comparison, 252
    effectiveness, 243–244
  clinical trials, 240
  comparison, head-to-head trials, 241f
  concepts/principles, 243
  controller medication, first line, 252
  dosage, 243
  drug-drug interactions, absence, 252
  effectiveness, 242t
  impact, 86
  nicotine blockage, 251

Varenicline (Continued)
  partial agonist, 248f
  partial nicotinic receptor agonist, 246–247
  peak plasma concentration, 240
  pharmacokinetics, 240
  point-prevalence nonsmoking data, usage,
    241–242
  tobacco dependence treatment,
    effectiveness, 243t
  toleration, 253
  usage, 243–244
    approval. See Smoking cessation 306
Varenicline tartrate, release, 240
VAS. See Visual Analog Scale 12–13
Vascular safety
  concepts/principles, 254
  controller/rescue nicotine medications, 254
VATS. See Video-assisted thoracic surgery
    385–386
VC. See Verbal cues 492–493
$\dot{V}_{CO_2}$. See Peak carbon dioxide update 137
V_D/V_T. See Dead space-to-tidal volume 118
Vegetables, consumption, 224
  epidemiologic evidence, 225
Venous thromboembolism, 520
Ventilation
  control, 23
  demographics. See Home ventilation 351
  distribution, unevenness, 22–23
  feedback, combination (usage), 57
  frequency, 351–352
  treatment. See Chronic respiratory
    failure 351
  usage. See Mechanical ventilation 352b
Ventilation-perfusion matching, 116
Ventilation-to-perfusion ratio ($\dot{V}/\dot{Q}$), 22–23
Ventilatory assist devices, 448
Ventilatory impedance, increase, 40
Ventilatory muscle endurance,
    examination, 132
Ventilatory track oxidation/inflammation
    vulnerability, 117–118
Ventilatory variables, analysis, 24
Ventral tegmental area (VTA), dopaminergic
    neurons (schematic), 248f
Ventricular arrhythmias, 117
Verbal cues (VC), inclusion, 492–493
Vibration, impact. See Dyspnea 54
Video-assisted thoracic surgery (VATS) LVRS,
    385–386
Viral infections, 376–377
Visual Analog Scale (VAS), 12–13
  decrease, 58
  usage, 43. See also Linear VAS 337–338
Vital capacity (VC), 21f
  increase, 51
Vitamin C, 225
  increase, 226
  National Health and Nutrition Examination
    Survey (NHANES II), 225
  role. See Respiratory defence mechanisms
    225–226
Vitamin D$_3$ (cholecalciferol), 227
Vitamin D$_2$ (ergocalciferol), 227
Vitamin D (sunshine vitamin), 227
  cholesterol synthesis, 227
  immune system importance, 227
Vitamin E intake, 224–225
$\dot{V}_{O_2}$. See Oxygen uptake 137
Vocational rehabilitation, 550
Volitional control, sleep-related
    disappearance, 420
Volume-pressure relationship. See Lungs 23f
VTA. See Ventral tegmental area 248f

W

WAIS-III. See Wechsler Adult Intelligence
    Scale-III 274
Walking

Walking (Continued)
   ability, functional element, 166–167
   cumulative time, 324–325
   distance, pulmonary rehabilitation
      effect, 337**f**
   pulse oximetry feedback, combination, 57
   tests. *See* Shuttle walking test 335; Timed
      walk test 335
   termination, 522
Walk tests, 335
Warfarin, usage, 224
Water, evaporation (impact). *See* Nebulizers
   104–105
Wechsler Adult Intelligence Scale-III
   (WAIS-III), 274
WeeFIM, 194
Weight gain, fear, 253
Weight gain, suppression
   Bupropion, impact, 242
   Varenicline, usage, 243–244
Weight indices, 210

Weight limitations, 210
Weight-losing subjects, energy balance
   (impairment), 215–216
Weight loss, 31**b**, 210
   causes, 211
   COPD, association, 209
   predictor. *See* Acute exacerbations 210
   relationship. *See* Nutritional abnormalities 32
Weight machines, usage, 171
Weight management, behavioral approaches, 279
Wheezes
   assessment, 167
   auscultation, 165–166
   indications, 163–165
Wheezing, 536
Why Is Sex Fun? The Evolution of Human
   Sexuality (Diamond), 286
Work/effort, 40
Work rate, improvement, 134**f**
Work-related stress, impact. *See* Tobacco
   dependence treatment 267

World Health Organization (WHO).
   See Participation 182**f**
   classification. *See* Pulmonary
      hypertension 519**b**
Written advance directives, success, 399

X

Xerostomia (dry mouth), 253

Y

Yoga, 229
   exercises, evaluation, 229

Z

Zanamavir, administration, 309
Zinc, 226
   role, 226
   supplementation, 226
Zyban sustained release. *See* Bupropion
   SR 241**f**